D0472038

AACN Essentials of Critical Care Nursing

Marianne Chulay, RN, DNSc, FAAN
Consultant, Critical Care Nursing and Clinical Research
Chapel Hill, North Carolina

Suzanne M. Burns, RN, MSN, RRT, ACNP, CCRN, FAAN, FCCM
Professor of Nursing, Acute and Specialty Care
School of Nursing
Advanced Practice Nurse Level 2, Medicine/Medical Intensive Care Unit
University of Virginia Health System
Charlottesville, Virginia

McGraw-Hill
Medical Publishing Division

New York Chicago San Francisco Lisbon London Madrid Mexico City Milan
New Delhi San Juan Seoul Singapore Sydney Toronto

AACN Essentials of Critical Care Nursing

Copyright © 2006 by The McGraw-Hill Companies, Inc. All rights reserved. Printed in the United States of America. Except as permitted under the United States Copyright Act of 1976, no part of this publication may be reproduced or distributed in any form or by any means, or stored in a data base or retrieval system, without the prior written permission of the publisher.

1 2 3 4 5 6 7 8 9 0   QPD/QPD   0 9 8 7 6 5

ISBN 0-07-144771-7

NOTICE

Medicine is an ever-changing science. As new research and clinical experience broaden our knowledge, changes in treatment and drug therapy are required. The authors and the publisher of this work have checked with sources believed to be reliable in their efforts to provide information that is complete and generally in accord with the standards accepted at the time of publication. However, in view of the possibility of human error or changes in medical sciences, neither the authors nor the publisher nor any other party who has been involved in the preparation or publication of this work warrants that the information contained herein is in every respect accurate or complete, and they disclaim all responsibility for any errors or omissions or for the results obtained from use of the information contained in this work. Readers are encouraged to confirm the information contained herein with other sources. For example and in particular, readers are advised to check the product information sheet included in the package of each drug they plan to administer to be certain that the information contained in this work is accurate and that changes have not been made in the recommended dose or in the contraindications for administration. This recommendation is of particular importance in connection with new or infrequently used drugs.

This book was set in Times Roman by Mid-Atlantic Books and Journals, Inc.
The editor was Michael Brown.
The production supervisor was Sherri Souffrance.
Project management was provided by Jennsin Services.
Quebecor World Dubuque was printer and binder.

This book is printed on acid-free paper.

Please tell the author and publisher what you think of this book by sending your comments to nursing@mcgraw-hill.com. Please put the author and title of the book in the subject line.

Library of Congress Cataloging-in-Publication Data

AACN essentials of critical care / [edited by] Marianne Chulay, Suzanne M. Burns. — 1st ed.
    p. ; cm.
  Includes bibliographical references and index.
  ISBN 0-07-144771-7 (softcover)
  1. Intensive care nursing—Outlines, syllabi, etc. I. Title: American Association of Critical-Care Nurses essentials of critical care nursing. II. Title: Essentials of critical care nursing. III. Chulay, Marianne. IV. Burns, Suzanne M. V. American Association of Critical-Care Nurses.
  [DNLM: 1. Critical Care. 2. Critical Illness—nursing. 3. Nursing Care. WY 154 A111 2005]
RT120.I5A165 2005
610.73'6—dc22
                                                                                                    2005041551

*To our critical care nursing colleagues around the world
whose wonderful work and efforts ensure the safe passage of patients
through the critical care environment.*

Contents

Contributors xv

Reviewers xvii

Preface...xix

Section I. The Essentials 1

1. Assessment of Critically Ill Patients and Families...3
    Mary Fran Tracy

2. Planning Care for Critically Ill Patients and Families...17
    Mary Fran Tracy

3. Interpretation and Management of Basic Cardiac Rhythms 37
    Carol Jacobson

4. Hemodynamic Monitoring 65
    Leanna R. Miller

5. Airway and Ventilatory Management 111
    Robert E. St. John

6. Pain, Sedation, and Neuromuscular Blockade Management 145
    Joan Michiko Ching and Suzanne M. Burns

7. Pharmacology...165
    Earnest Alexander

8. Ethical and Legal Considerations..199
    Juanita Reigle

Section II. Pathologic Conditions 213

9. Cardiovascular System...215
    Barbara Leeper

10. Respiratory System 247
    Marianne Chulay

11. Multisystem Problems...267
    Ruth M. Kleinpell

12. Neurologic System 279
    Dea Mahanes

13. Hematology and Immunology Systems 305
    Diane K. Dressler

14. Gastrointestinal System...317
    Joanne Krumberger, Carol Reese Parrish, and Joe Krenitsky

15. Renal System...341
    Carol Hinkle

16. Endocrine System...357
    Joanne Krumberger

17. Trauma 371
    Carol A. Rauen and Jamie B. Sinks

SECTION III: Advanced Concepts in Caring for the Critically Ill Patient 389

18. Advanced ECG Concepts...391
    Carol Jacobson

19. Advanced Cardiovascular Concepts..431
    Barbara Leeper

20. Advanced Respiratory Concepts 463
    Suzanne M. Burns

21. Advanced Neurologic Concepts..477
    Dea Mahanes

SECTION IV: Key Reference Information 501

22. Normal Values Table 503
    Marianne Chulay

23. Pharmacology Tables 505
    Earnest Alexander

24. Advanced Cardiac Life Support Algorithms...519
    Marianne Chulay

25. Guidelines for the Transfer of Critically Ill Patients.....................................529
    Marianne Chulay

26. Hemodynamic Monitoring Troubleshooting Guide...533
    Leanna R. Miller

27. Ventilatory Troubleshooting Guide 539
    Robert E. St. John and Suzanne M. Burns

28. Cardiac Rhythms, ECG Characteristics, and Treatment Guide 551
    Carol Jacobson

Index...561

Contents in Detail

Contributors...*xv*

Reviewers...*xvii*

Preface...*xix*

Section I. The Essentials..1

1. Assessment of Critically Ill Patients and Families...3
   Mary Fran Tracy
   Assessment Framework   3
      Prearrival Assessment 4 / Admission Quick Check 4 / Comprehensive Admission Assessment 4 /
      Ongoing Assessment 4
   Prearrival Assessment: Before the Action Begins   4
   Admission Quick Check Assessment: The First Few Minutes   5
      Airway and Breathing 6 / Circulation and Cerebral Perfusion 6 / Chief Complaint 6 /
      Drugs and Diagnostic Tests 6 / Equipment 7
   Comprehensive Admission Assessment   7
      Past Medical History 8 / Social History 8 / Physical Assessment by Body System 9 /
      Psychosocial Assessment   12
   Ongoing Assessment   14

2. Planning Care for Critically Ill Patients and Families...17
   Mary Fran Tracy
   Multidisciplinary Plan of Care and Critical Pathways   17
   Prevention of Common Complications   18
      Physiologic Instability 18 / Deep Venous Thrombosis 18 / Hospital-Acquired Infections 23 /
      Skin Breakdown 24 / Sleep Pattern Disturbances 24 / Psychosocial Impact 25
   Patient and Family Education   26
      Assessment of Learning Readiness 26 / Strategies to Address Patient and Family Education 27 /
      Outcome Measurement 27
   Family-Focused Care   28
   Transporting the Critically Ill Patient   29
      Assessment of Risk for Complications 29 / Level of Care Required During Transport 30 /
      Preparation 31 / Transport 31 / Interfacility Transfers 32
   Transitioning to the Next Stage of Care   32
   Supporting Patients and Families During the Dying Process   33

3. Interpretation and Management of Basic Cardiac Rhythms...37
   Carol Jacobson
   Basic Electrophysiology   37

ECG Waveforms, Complexes, and Intervals   38
   P Wave 38 / QRS Complex 38 / T and U Waves 38 / ST Segment 38 / PR Interval 38 /
   QT Interval 39
Cardiac Monitoring   39
Determination of the Heart Rate   42
Determination of the Cardiac Rhythm   42
Common Arrhythmias   43
Rhythms Originating in the Sinus Node   43
   Sinus Bradycardia 44 / Sinus Tachycardia 44 / Sinus Arrhythmia 45 / Sinus Arrest 45
Arrhythmias Originating in the Atria   45
   Premature Atrial Complexes 46 / Wandering Atrial Pacemaker 46 / Atrial Tachycardia 47 /
   Atrial Flutter 47 / Atrial Fibrillation 48
Arrhythmias Originating in the Atrioventricular Junction   49
   Premature Junctional Complexes 50 / Junctional Rhythm, Accelerated Junctional Rhythm,
   and Junctional Tachycardia 50
Arrhythmias Originating in the Ventricles   50
   Premature Ventricular Complexes 51 / Ventricular Rhythm and Accelerated Ventricular Rhythm 51 /
   Ventricular Tachycardia 52 / Ventricular Fibrillation 53 / Ventricular Asystole 53
Atrioventricular Blocks   54
   First-Degree Atrioventricular Block 54 / Second-Degree Atrioventricular Block 54 / High-Grade
   Atrioventricular Block 56 / Third-Degree Atrioventricular Block (Complete Block) 56
Temporary Pacing   57
   Indications 57 / Transvenous Pacing 57 / Epicardial Pacing 57 / Components of a Pacing System 57 /
   Basics of Pacemaker Operation 58 / ECG Characteristics of Paced Rhythms 60 / Initiating
   Transvenous Ventricular Pacing 60 / Initiating Epicardial Pacing 60 / External (Transcutaneous)
   Pacemakers 60
Defibrillation and Cardioversion 60
   Defibrillation 60 / Automatic External Defibrillators 61 / Cardioversion 62

4. Hemodynamic Monitoring 65
   Leanna R. Miller
Hemodynamic Parameters   65
   Cardiac Output 65 / Components of Cardiac Output/Cardiac Index 67 / Stroke Volume and Stroke
   Volume Index 68 / Factors Affecting Stroke Volume/Stroke Volume Index 68
Basic Components of Hemodynamic Monitoring Systems   72
   Pulmonary Artery Catheter 72 / Arterial Catheter 72 / Pressure Tubing 72 / Pressure Transducer 73 /
   Pressure Amplifier 74 / Pressure Bag and Flush Device 74 / Alarms 74
Obtaining Accurate Hemodynamic Values   74
   Zeroing the Transducer 74 / Leveling the Transducer to the Catheter Tip 75 / Calibration of the
   Transducer/Amplifier System 77 / Ensuring Accurate Waveform Transmission 77
Insertion and Removal of Catheters   77
   Pulmonary Artery Catheters 77 / Arterial Catheters 80
Obtaining and Interpreting Hemodynamic Waveforms   84
   Patient Positioning 84 / Interpretation 84 / Artifacts in Hemodynamic Waveforms: Respiratory
   Influence 91 / Cardiac Output 92
Continuous Mixed Venous Oxygen Monitoring   97
   Svo_2 Monitoring Principles 97 / Selected Examples of Clinical Applications 98
Right Ventricular Ejection Fraction Catheters   99
   Monitoring Principles 99 / Troubleshooting 99
Minimally Invasive Hemodynamic Monitoring   100
   Thoracic Bioimpedance 100 / Esophageal Doppler Cardiac Output 100 / Carbon Dioxide
   Rebreathing 100 / Gastric Tonometry 100 / Sublingual Capnometry 101
Application of Hemodynamic Parameters   102
   Low Cardiac Output States 102 / High Cardiac Output States 106

5. Airway and Ventilatory Management 111
Robert E. St. John
Respiratory Assessment Techniques, Diagnostic Tests, and Monitoring Systems   111
Arterial Blood Gas Monitoring 111 / Analysis 112 / Venous Blood Gas Monitoring 116 / Pulse
Oximetry 116 / Assessing Pulmonary Function 118
Airway Management   118
Oropharyngeal Airway 118 / Nasopharyngeal Airway 120 / Artificial Airways 120
Oxygen Therapy   125
Complications 125 / Oxygen Delivery 127
Basic Ventilatory Management   129
Indications 129 / General Principles 129 / Modes 132 / Complications 135 / Weaning From
Short-Term Mechanical Ventilation 136 / Troubleshooting Ventilators 138 / Communication 139 /
Principles of Management 141

6. Pain, Sedation, and Neuromuscular Blockade Management 145
Joan Michiko Ching and Suzanne M. Burns
Physiologic Mechanisms of Pain   145
Peripheral Mechanisms 145 / Spinal Cord Integration 147 / Central Processing 147
Responses to Pain   147
Pain Assessment   148
A Multilevel Approach to Pain Management   148
Nonsteroidal Anti-Inflammatory Drugs   149
Side Effects   150
Opioids   150
Side Effects 150 / Intravenous Opioids 151 / Patient-Controlled Analgesia 151 / Switching From IV
to Oral Opioid Analgesia 152
Epidural Analgesia   153
Epidural Opioids 153 / Epidural Local Anesthetics 154
Cutaneous Stimulation   155
Distraction   155
Imagery   155
Relaxation and Sedation Techniques   155
Deep Breathing and Progressive Relaxation 156 / Presence 156
Special Considerations for Pain Management in the Elderly   156
Assessment 157 / Interventions 157
Sedation   157
Reasons for Sedation 157 / Drugs for Sedation 158 / Goals of Sedation, Monitoring, and
Management 159 / Sedation Scales: Goals and Monitoring 159 / Sedation Management 159
Neuromuscular Blockade   159
Neuromuscular Blocking Agents 160 / Monitoring and Management 161

7. Pharmacology 165
Earnest Alexander
Medication Administration Methods   165
Intravenous 165 / Intramuscular or Subcutaneous 165 / Sublingual 166 / Intranasal 166 /
Transdermal 166
Central Nervous System Pharmacology   167
Sedatives 167 / Analgesics 170 / Neuromuscular Blocking Agents 171 / Anticonvulsants 173
Cardiovascular System Pharmacology   176
Miscellaneous Agents 176 / Parenteral Vasodilators 177 / Antiarrhythmics 180 / Thrombolytic
Agents 182 / Vasoconstricting Agents 183 / Inotropic Agents 184 / Activated Protein C 185
Anti-Infective Pharmacology   185
Aminoglycosides 185 / Vancomycin 186 / Other Antibiotics 186

Pulmonary Pharmacology   187
Theophylline 187 / Albuterol 187
Gastrointestinal Pharmacology   188
Stress Ulcer Prophylaxis 188 / Acute Peptic Ulcer Bleeding 189 / Variceal Hemorrhage 189
Renal Pharmacology   190
Diuretics 190
Hematologic Pharmacology   191
Anticoagulants 191 / Direct Thrombin Inhibitors 193 / Glycoprotein IIb/IIa Inhibitor 193
Immunosuppressive Agents   193
Cyclosporine 193 / Tacrolimus (FK506) 194 / Sirolimus (Rapamycin) 194
Special Dosing Considerations   195
Continuous Renal Replacement Therapy 195 / Drug Disposition in the Elderly 195 / Therapeutic
Drug Monitoring 195

8. Ethical and Legal Considerations..199
Juanita Reigle
The Foundation for Ethical Decision Making   199
Professional Codes and Standards 199 / Position Statement and Guidelines 200 / Institutional
Policies 200 / Legal Standards 200 / Principles of Ethics 201 / Care 203 / Patient Advocacy 204
The Process of Ethical Analysis   204
Assessment 204 / Plan 204 / Implementation 205 / Evaluation 205
Contemporary Ethical Issues   205
Informed Consent 205 / Determining Capacity 205 / Advance Directives 206 / End-of-Life
Issues 207 / Resuscitation Decisions 209
Building an Ethical Environment   209
Values Clarification 209 / Provide Information and Clarify Issues 209 / Recognize Moral
Distress 210 / Engage in Collaborative Decision Making 210

Section II. Pathologic Conditions 213

9. Cardiovascular System..215
Barbara Leeper
Special Assessment Techniques, Diagnostic Tests, and Monitoring Systems   215
Assessment of Chest Pain 215 / Coronary Angiography 215 / Percutaneous Coronary
Interventions 216 / Other Percutaneous Coronary Interventions 217
Pathologic Conditions   218
Acute Ischemic Heart Disease 218 / Congestive Heart Failure 230 / Shock 238 / Hypertension 243

10. Respiratory System 247
Marianne Chulay
Special Assessment Techniques, Diagnostic Tests, and Monitoring Systems   247
Chest X-Rays 247 / Computed Tomography and Magnetic Resonance Imaging 251 /
Chest Tubes 252
Pathologic Conditions   252
Acute Respiratory Failure 252 / Acute Respiratory Distress Syndrome 256 / Acute Respiratory
Failure in the Patient With Chronic Obstructive Pulmonary Disease 258 / Pneumonia 260 /
Pulmonary Embolism 263

11. Multisystem Problems...267
Ruth M. Kleinpell
Pathologic Conditions   267
Sepsis and Multiple Organ Dysfunction Syndrome 267
Overdoses   274
Etiology, Risk Factors, and Pathophysiology 274

12. Neurologic System 279

Dea Mahanes

Assessment Techniques   279
Level of Consciousness 279 / Glasgow Coma Scale 280 / Mental Status 281 / Motor Assessment
283 / Sensation 283 / Cranial Nerve Assessment and Assessment of Brainstem Function 285 / Vital
Sign Alterations in Neurologic Dysfunction 286 / Death by Neurologic Criteria 287

Diagnostic Testing   287
Lumbar Puncture 287 / Computed Tomography 288 / Magnetic Resonance Imaging 288 / Cerebral
Angiography 289 / Transcranial Doppler Ultrasound 290 / Electroencephalography 290 /
Electromyography 290

Intracranial Pressure: Concepts and Monitoring   290
Cerebral Blood Flow 291 / Causes of Increased Intracranial Pressure 291

Acute Ischemic Stroke   296
Etiology, Risk Factors, and Pathophysiology 296 / Diagnostic Tests 297

Hemorrhagic Stroke   299
Etiology, Risk Factors, and Pathophysiology 299 / Clinical Presentation 300 / Diagnostic Tests 300 /
Principles of Management of Intracerebral Hemorrhage 300

Seizures   300
Etiology, Risk Factors, and Pathophysiology 300 / Clinical Presentation 300 / Principles of
Management of Seizures 301

Infections of the Central Nervous System   302
Meningitis 302 / Encephalitis 302 / Intracranial Abscess 302

Neuromuscular Diseases   303
Myasthenia Gravis 303 / Guillain-Barré Syndrome 303

13. Hematology and Immunology Systems 305

Diane K. Dressler

Special Assessment Techniques, Diagnostic Tests, and Monitoring Systems   305
Complete Blood Count 305 / Red Blood Cell Count 305 / Hemoglobin 306 / Hematocrit 306 /
Red Blood Cell Indices 306 / Total White Blood Cell Count 306 / White Blood Cell
Differential 306 / Platelet Count 307 / Erythrocyte Sedimentation Rate 307 / Coagulation
Studies 307 / Additional Tests and Procedures 308

Pathologic Conditions   308
Anemia 308 / Immunocompromise 310 / Coagulopathies 312

14. Gastrointestinal System..317

Joanne Krumberger, Carol Reese Parrish, and Joe Krenitsky

Pathologic Conditions   317
Acute Upper Gastrointestinal Bleeding 317 / Liver Failure 325 / Acute Pancreatitis 330 /
Bowel Infarction/Obstruction 331

Nutritional Support for Critically Ill Patients   332
Nutrition Needs 332 / Residual Volume 333 / Aspiration 334 / Bowel Sounds 335 / Nausea and
Vomiting 336 / Osmolality or Hypertonicity of Formula 336 / Diarrhea 337 / Flow Rates and Hours
of Infusion 337 / Formula Selection 337

15. Renal System...341

Carol Hinkle

Special Assessment Techniques, Diagnostic Tests, and Monitoring Systems   341

Pathologic Conditions   341
Acute Renal Failure 341 / Life-Threatening Electrolyte Imbalances 346

Renal Replacement Therapy   350
Access 351 / Dialyzer/Hemofilters/Dialysate 352 / Procedures 352 / Indications for and Efficacy of
Renal Replacement Therapy Modes 352 / General Renal Replacement Therapy Interventions 355

16. Endocrine System...357
    Joanne Krumberger
    Special Assessment Techniques, Diagnostic Tests, and Monitoring Systems   357
        Blood Glucose Monitoring 357
    Pathologic Conditions   359
        Hyperglycemic Emergencies 359 / Acute Hypoglycemia 364 / Syndrome of Inappropriate
        Antidiuretic Hormone Secretion 365 / Diabetes Insipidus 367

17. Trauma 371
    Carol A. Rauen and Jamie B. Sinks
    Specialized Assessment Techniques, Diagnostic Tests, and Monitoring Systems   371
        Primary and Secondary Trauma Survey Assessment 371 / Diagnostic Studies 374 / Mechanism of
        Injury 376 / Physiologic Consequences of Trauma 377
    Common Injuries in the Critically Ill Trauma Patient   378
        Thoracic Trauma 378 / Abdominal Trauma 380 / Musculoskeletal Trauma 381
    Complications of Traumatic Injury in Severe Multisystem Trauma   382
        Acute Respiratory Distress Syndrome 384 / Infection/Sepsis 385 / Systemic Inflammatory
        Response Syndrome 385
    Psychological Consequences of Trauma   385

Section III. Advanced Concepts in Caring for the Critically Ill Patient 389

18. Advanced ECG Concepts..391
    Carol Jacobson
    The 12-Lead Electrocardiogram   391
        Axis Determination 396 / Bundle Branch Block 399 / Myocardial Ischemia, Injury,
        and Infarction 401 / Preexcitation Syndromes 407
    Advanced Arrhythmia Interpretation   411
        Supraventricular Tachycardias 412 / Differentiating Wide QRS Beats and Rhythms 415
    ST-Segment Monitoring   419
        Measuring the ST Segment 420 / Choosing the Best Leads for ST-Segment Monitoring 421
    Cardiac Pacemakers   418
        Evaluating Pacemaker Function 423 / VVI Pacemaker Evaluation 423 / DDD Pacemaker
        Evaluation 427

19. Advanced Cardiovascular Concepts...431
    Barbara Leeper
    Pathologic Conditions   431
        Cardiomyopathy 431 / Valvular Disease 436 / Pericarditis 441 / Aortic Aneurysm 443 / Cardiac
        Transplantation 446 / Intra-Aortic Balloon Pump Therapy 452 / Ventricular Assist Devices 455

20. Advanced Respiratory Concepts 463
    Suzanne M. Burns
    Advanced Modes of Mechanical Ventilation   463
        New Concepts: Mechanical Ventilation 463 / Volume Versus Pressure Ventilator 464 / Alternative
        Ventilator Options 469
    Weaning Patients From Long-Term Mechanical Ventilation   470
        Wean Assessment 470 / Wean Planning 471 / Weaning Trials, Modes, and Methods 471 /
        Respiratory Fatigue, Rest, and Conditioning 471 / Wean Trial Protocols 472 / Other Protocols for
        Use 473 / Critical Pathways 473 / Systematic Institutional Initiatives for the Management of the
        LTMV Patient Population 473

21. Advanced Neurologic Concepts...477
    Dea Mahanes
    Subarachnoid Hemorrhage   477
        Etiology, Risk Factors, and Pathophysiology 477 / Clinical Presentation 477 / Diagnostic Tests 479

Traumatic Brain Injury   481
    Etiology, Risk Factors, and Pathophysiology 481 / Clinical Presentation 485 / Diagnostic Tests 485
Traumatic Spinal Cord Injury   487
    Etiology, Risk Factors, and Pathophysiology 487 / Clinical Presentation 489 / Diagnostic Tests 490 /
    Future Spinal Cord Injury Treatment 490
Brain Tumors   494
    Etiology, Risk Factors, and Pathophysiology 494 / Diagnostic Tests 495 / Advanced Technology:
    Brain Tissue Oxygen Monitoring 497

Section IV. Key Reference Information 501

22. Normal Values Table 503
    Marianne Chulay

23. Pharmacology Tables 505
    Earnest Alexander

24. Advanced Cardiac Life Support Algorithms..519
    Marianne Chulay

25. Guidelines for the Transfer of Critically Ill Patients...529
    Marianne Chulay
    Transfers Within the Hospital   529
        Transport Personnel 529 / Transport Equipment Requirements 529 / Monitoring During
        Transfer 529 / Pretransfer Coordination and Communication 529
    Transfers Between Hospitals   530
        Transport Personnel 530 / Transport Medication Requirements 530 / Transfer Equipment 530 /
        Monitoring During Transfer 531 / Transfer Algorithm 532

26. Hemodynamic Monitoring Troubleshooting Guide 533
    Leanna R. Miller

27. Ventilatory Troubleshooting Guide 539
    Robert E. St. John and Suzanne M. Burns

28. Cardiac Rhythms, ECG Characteristics, and Treatment Guide 551
    Carol Jacobson

Index..561

Acknowledgments

Special thanks to those who made contributions to the predecessor of this book, *AACN Handbook of Critical Care Nursing*. To Cathie Guzzetta, RN, PhD, FAAN and Barbie Dossey, RN, MS, FAAN for their editorial contributions and mentoring. And to the following authors for their contributions to chapter content:

Tom Ahrens, RN, DNS, CS, FAAN (*Chapters 4, 26*)
Deb Byram, RN, MS (*Chapter 1*)
Anita Sherer, RN, MSN (*Chapter 2*)
Sue Simmons-Alling, RN, MSN (*Chapter 2*)
Marlene Yates, RN, MSN (*Chapter 2*)
Susan Woods, PhD, RN (*Chapters 3, 18*)
Maria Connolly, RN, DNSc (*Chapters 5, 10*)
Lorie Wild, RN, PhD (*Chapter 6*)
Greg Susla, PharmD, FCCM (*Chapters 7, 23*)
Bradi Granger, RN, PhD (*Chapter 9*)
Debbie Tribett, RN, MS, CS, LNP (*Chapter 13*)
Karen Carlson, RN, MN (*Chapter 15*)
Dorie Fontaine, RN, DNSc, FAAN (*Chapter 17*)
Anne Marie Gregoire, RN, MSN, CRNP (*Chapter 19*)
Debra Lynn-McHale, RN, PhD, CS (*Chapter 19*)

Contributors

Earnest Alexander, PharmD
Critical Care Pharmacotherapy Specialist
Tampa General Hospital
Clinical Assistant Professor
University of Florida and Florida A&M University
Tampa, Florida
Chapter 7: Pharmacology
Chapter 23: Pharmacology Tables

Suzanne M. Burns, RN, MSN, RRT, ACNP, CCRN, FAAN, FCCM
Professor of Nursing, Acute and Specialty Care
Advanced Practice Nurse Level 2, Medicine/Medical
   Intensive Care Unit
School of Nursing
University of Virginia Health System
Charlottesville, Virginia
Chapter 6: Pain, Sedation, and Neuromuscular Blockade
   Management
Chapter 20: Advanced Respiratory Concepts
Chapter 27: Ventilatory Troubleshooting Guide

Joan Michiko Ching, RN, MN
Clinical Faculty
University of Washington
Pain Management Clinical Nurse Specialist
University of Washington Medical Center
Seattle, Washington
Chapter 6: Pain, Sedation, and Neuromuscular Blockade
   Management

Marianne Chulay, RN, DNSc, FAAN
Consultant, Critical Care Nursing and Clinical Research
Chapel Hill, North Carolina
Chapter 10: Respiratory System
Chapter 22: Normal Values Table
Chapter 24: Advanced Cardiac Life Support Algorithms
Chapter 25: Guidelines for the Transfer of Critically Ill
   Patients

Diane K. Dressler, RN, MSN, CCRN
Clinical Assistant Professor
Marquette University College of Nursing
Milwaukee, Wisconsin
Chapter 13: Hematology and Immunology Systems

Carol Hinkle, RN, MSN, CCRN
Education Consultant—Critical Care
Education Department
Brookwood Medical Center
Birmingham, Alabama
Chapter 15: Renal System

Carol Jacobson, RN, MN, FACCN III
Director, Quality Education Services
Per diem Clinical Nurse Specialist, Swedish Medical Center
Per diem Clinical Nurse Specialist, Children's Medical
   Center
Seattle, Washington
Chapter 3: Interpretation and Management of Basic
   Cardiac Rhythms
Chapter 18: Advanced ECG Concepts
Chapter 28: Cardiac Rhythms, ECG Characteristics, and
   Treatment Guide

Ruth M. Kleinpell, PhD, RN-CS, FAAN, ACNP, CCRN
Associate Professor
Rush University College of Nursing
Chicago, Illinois
Chapter 11: Multisystem Problems

Joe Krenitsky, MS, RD
Nutrition Support Specialist
Digestive Health Center of Excellence and Department of
   Nutrition Services
University of Virginia Health System
Charlottesville, Virginia
Chapter 14: Gastrointestinal System

Joanne Krumberger, RN, MSN, CHE, FAAN
Manager, Performance Improvement
Milwaukee VA Medical Center
Milwaukee, Wisconsin
Chapter 14: Gastrointestinal System
Chapter 16: Endocrine System

Barbara Leeper, MN, RN, CCRN
Clinical Nurse Specialist, Cardiovascular Services
Baylor University Medical Center
Dallas, Texas
Chapter 9: Cardiovascular System
Chapter 19: Advanced Cardiovascular Concepts

Dea Mahanes, RN, MSN, CCRN, CNRN, CCNS
Advanced Practice Nurse Level 1, Nerancy Neuro-
    Intensive Care Unit
University of Virginia Health System
Charlottesville, Virginia
Chapter 12: Neurologic System
Chapter 21: Advanced Neurologic Concepts

Leanna R. Miller, RN, MN, CCRN, CEN, NP
Educator for Trauma, Burn, Neurocare, Flight
Vanderbilt University Medical Center
Nashville, Tennessee
Chapter 4: Hemodynamic Monitoring
*Chapter 26: Hemodynamic Monitoring Troubleshooting
    Guide*

Carol Reese Parrish, MS, RD
Nutrition Support Specialist
Digestive Health Center of Excellence and
Department of Nutrition Services
University of Virginia Health System
Charlottesville, Virginia
Chapter 14: Gastrointestinal System

Carol A. Rauen, RN, MS, CCNS, CCRN
Assistant Professor
School of Nursing & Health Studies
Georgetown University
Washington, DC
Lecturer
Barbara Clark Mims Associates
Dallas, Texas
Chapter 17: Trauma

Juanita Reigle, RN, MSN, ACNP
Associate Professor of Nursing, Acute and Specialty Care
Advanced Practice Nurse Level 2, Heart Center
School of Nursing
University of Virginia Health System
Charlottesville, Virginia
Chapter 8: Ethical and Legal Considerations

Jamie B. Sinks, RN, MS
Trauma Resuscitation Nurse
MedSTAR
Washington Hospital Center
Washington, DC
Chapter 17: Trauma

Robert E. St. John, MSN, RN, RRT
Director Post-Market Clinical Research
Nellcor/Tyco Healthcare
Pleasanton, California
Chapter 5: Airway and Ventilatory Management
Chapter 27: Ventilatory Troubleshooting Guide

Mary Fran Tracy, PhD, RN, CCRN, CCNS, FAAN
Critical Care Clinical Nurse Specialist
Fairview-University Medical Center
Minneapolis, Minnesota
Chapter 1: Assessment of Critically Ill Patients and Families
*Chapter 2: Planning Care for Critically Ill Patients and
    Families*

Reviewers

Tom Ahrens, DNS, RN, CS
Research Scientist
Barnes-Jewish Medical Center
St. Louis, Missouri

Mary Kay Bader, RN, MSN, CCRN, CNRN
Neuro/Critical Care Clinical Nurse Specialist
Mission Hospital
Mission Viejo, California

Toni Balistrieri, RN, MSN, CCRN
Clinical Nurse Specialist, Critical Care
Milwaukee VA Medical Center
Milwaukee, Wisconsin

Connie Barden, RN, MSN, CCRN, CCNS
Cardiovascular Clinical Nurse Specialist
Mercy Hospital
Miami, Florida

Debbie Barnes, RN, MSN
Clinical Practice Specialist
American Association of Critical Care Nurses
Aliso Viejo, California

Linda Bell, RN, MSN
Clinical Practice Specialist
American Association of Critical Care Nurses
Aliso Viejo, California

Liz Browne, RN
Clinician 3, Medical Intensive Care Unit
University of Virginia Health System
Charlottesville, Virginia

Sarah Delgado, RN, MSN, ACNP
Clinical Instructor
School of Nursing
University of Virginia
Charlottesville, Virginia

Charles Fisher, RN, MSN, CCRN, ACNP
Advanced Practice Nurse Level 1 Outcomes Manager,
   Long-term Ventilated Patients
University of Virginia Health System
Charlottesville, Virginia

Lisa W. Forsyth, RN, MSN
Clinician 4, Clinical Educator
University of Virginia Health System
Charlottesville, Virginia

Ann B. Hamric, PhD, RN, FAAN
Associate Professor
School of Nursing
University of Virginia
Charlottesville, Virginia

Dave Hanson, MSN, RN, CCRN
Clinical Nurse Specialist
JPS Health System
Ft. Worth, Texas

Rebecca H. Hockman, Pharm DBCPS
Clinical Pharmacy Specialist, Medical Intensive Care Unit
University of Virginia Health System
Charlottesville, Virginia

Kimmith M. Jones, RN, MS
Advanced Practice Nurse/Clinical Nurse Specialist
Critical Care/Emergency Center
Sinai Hospital of Baltimore
Baltimore, Maryland

Kerry Kosmoski-Goepfert, PhD, RN
Clinical Assistant Professor/Acute Care Nurse Practitioner
   Option Coordinator
Marquette University
College of Nursing
Milwaukee, Wisconsin

Mary Beth Flynn Makic, RN, MS, CNS, CCRN
Clinical Nurse Specialist/Educator and Senior Instructor
University of Colorado Hospital and University of
  Colorado
Health Sciences Center, School of Nursing
Denver, Colorado

Mary Marshall, RN, MSN
Clinical Research Coordinator
University of Virginia Health System
Charlottesville, Virginia

Laura H. Mcilvoy, PhD, RN, CNRN, CCRN
Assistant Professor
University of Louisville School of Nursing
Louisville, Kentucky

Paul Merrel, RN, MSN, CCRN
Advanced Practice Nurse Level 1, Outcomes Manager,
  Long-term Ventilated
  Patients
University of Virginia Health System
Charlottesville, Virginia

Sue Sendelback, PhD, RN, FAHA
Clinical Nurse Specialist
Abbott-Northwestern Hospital
St. Paul, Minnesota

Christine Shaw, PhD, APRN-BC
Clinical Associate Professor
Marquette University College of Nursing
College of Nursing
Milwaukee, Wisconsin

Cheri Smith, RN, BSN
Clinician 4, Medical Intensive Care Unit
University of Virginia Health System
Charlottesville, Virginia

Greg Susla, PharmD, FCCM
Pharmacy Manager
VHA Consulting Services
Frederick, Maryland

Sherrie Walker, RD
Nutrition Support Specialist
University of Virginia Health System
Charlottesville, Virginia

Teresa A. Wavra, RN, MSN, CCRN, CCNS
Clinical Practice Specialist
American Association of Critical Care Nurses
Aliso Viejo, California

Lorie Wild, PhD, RN
Director, Patient Care Services
University of Washington Medical Center
Seattle, Washington

Susan L. Woods, PhD, RN, FAAN, FAHA
Professor and Associate Dean
University of Washington
School of Nursing
Seattle, Washington

Susan Yeager, MS, RN, CCRN, ACNP
Neuroscience Nurse Practitioner
Grant Riverside Methodist Hospital
Hillard, Ohio

Preface

Critical care nursing is a complex, challenging area of nursing practice, where clinical expertise is developed over time by integrating critical care knowledge, clinical skills, and caring practices. Finding a textbook that comprehensively yet succinctly presents essential information about how best to safely and competently care for critically ill patients and their families is a challenge for those charged with the education of new critical care practitioners. Most current textbooks deal with critical care content by combining essential and advanced concepts, rather than by providing the essential concepts first and introducing more advanced concepts later. In-depth discussion of these advanced concepts, although meaningful and important for advanced practitioners, often overwhelms the novice practitioner.

Current texts also include too much information for entry-level courses in critical care nursing or for use as a review tool for the critical care certification (CCRN) examination. Orientation programs in most hospitals are extremely short (2 to 6 weeks), and undergraduate programs that provide critical care content often do so in short elective courses, or integrate the content into an advanced medical-surgical nursing course. Instructors are reluctant to suggest or require students to buy expensive books that include more information than they need at that time or that repeat material that appears in other student-owned textbooks (anatomy and physiology, nursing diagnosis, non–critical care assessment, medical diagnostic reasoning). Although clinicians may purchase these books to prepare for certification examinations, many would benefit from a more concise textbook and clinical reference.

The *AACN Essentials of Critical Care Nursing* provides essential information on the care of adult critically ill patients and families. The book recognizes the learner's need to assimilate foundational knowledge before attempting to master more complex critical care nursing concepts. Written by nationally acknowledged clinical experts in critical care nursing, this handbook sets a new standard for critical care nursing education.

The *AACN Essentials of Critical Care Nursing* represents a departure from the way in which most critical care books are written because it

- Succinctly presents essential information for the safe and competent care of critically ill adult patients and their families, building on the clinician's significant medical-surgical nursing knowledge base, avoiding repetition of previously acquired information.
- Stages the introduction of advanced concepts in critical care nursing after essential concepts have been mastered.
- Presents practical approaches to patient and family teaching when time is short and acuity is high.
- Provides clinicians with clinically relevant tools and guides to use as they care for critically ill patients and families.

The *AACN Essentials of Critical Care Nursing* is divided into four sections:

- *Section I: The Essentials* presents essential information that new clinicians must understand to provide safe, competent nursing care to all critically ill patients, regardless of their underlying medical diagnoses. This section includes content on essential concepts of assessment, diagnosis, planning, and interventions common to critically ill patients and families; interpretation and management of cardiac rhythms; hemodynamic monitoring; airway and ventilatory management; pharmacology; and pain management. Chapters in Section I present content in enough depth to ensure that essential information is available for the new critical care clinician to develop competence, while deferring more advanced content to a later section of the handbook (Section III).
- *Section II: Advanced Concepts* covers pathologic conditions and management strategies commonly encountered in medical and surgical critical care units,

closely paralleling the blueprint for the CCRN examination. Chapters in this section are organized by body system (cardiovascular, respiratory, neurologic, hematology and immunology, gastrointestinal, renal, and endocrine) and include chapters on trauma and multisystem problems. Case studies assist clinicians in understanding the magnitude of the pathologic problems and their impact on patients and families. Brief descriptions of the pathophysiology, etiology, clinical manifestations, diagnostic testing, and complications associated with conditions presented in the case studies are provided. The focus of each pathologic presentation is the multidisciplinary management of key patient needs and problems.

- *Section III: Advanced Concepts in Caring for the Critically Ill Patient* presents advanced critical care concepts or pathologic conditions that are less common or more specialized than expected in general medical-surgical critical care units. The format of this section is identical to Section II.
- *Section IV: Key Reference Information* contains reference information that clinicians will find helpful in the clinical area (normal laboratory and diagnostic values;

algorithms for advanced cardiac life support; troubleshooting guides for hemodynamic monitoring and ventilator management; and summary tables of critical care drugs and cardiac rhythms). Content is presented primarily in table format for quick reference.

Each chapter begins with Knowledge Competencies that can be used to guide informal or formal teaching and to gauge the learner's progress. Case studies are presented in many of the chapters and can be read before proceeding with the chapter to obtain an overall picture of the clinical problem, or in context with the chapter content to reinforce concepts. A "Critical Thinking" case study concludes many of the chapters to challenge the clinician to apply chapter information to a realistic clinical scenario.

We believe that there is no greater way to protect our patients than to ensure that an educated clinician cares for them. Safe passage in critical care is ensured by competent, skilled, knowledgeable, and caring clinicians. We sincerely believe that this textbook will help you make it so!

Marianne Chulay
Suzi Burns

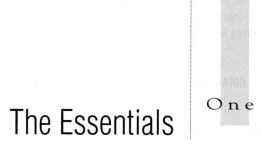

The Essentials

Assessment of Critically Ill Patients and Families

One 1

Mary Fran Tracy

▶ Knowledge Competencies

1. Discuss the importance of a consistent and systematic approach to assessment of critically ill patients and their families.
2. Identify the assessment priorities for different stages of a critical illness:
   • Prearrival assessment
   • Admission quick check

   • Comprehensive admission assessment
   • Ongoing assessment
3. Describe how the assessment is altered based on the patient's clinical status.

The assessment of critically ill patients and their families is an essential competency for critical care practitioners. Information obtained from an assessment identifies the immediate and future needs of the patient and family so a plan of care can be initiated to address or resolve these needs.

Traditional approaches to patient assessment include a complete evaluation of the patient's history and a comprehensive physical examination of all body systems. This approach, although ideal, rarely is possible in critical care as clinicians struggle with life-threatening problems during admission and must balance the need to gather data while simultaneously prioritizing and providing care. Traditional approaches and techniques for assessment must be modified in critical care to balance the need for information, while considering the critical nature of the patient and family's situation.

This chapter outlines an assessment approach that recognizes the emergent and dynamic nature of a critical illness. This approach emphasizes the collection of assessment data in a phased, or staged, manner consistent with patient care priorities. The components of the assessment can be used as a generic template for assessing most critically ill patients and families. The assessment can then be individualized by adding more specific assessment requirements depending on the specific patient diagnosis. These specific components of the assessment are identified in subsequent chapters.

Crucial to developing competence in assessing critically ill patients and their families is a consistent and systematic approach to assessments. Without this approach, it would be easy to miss subtle signs or details that may identify an actual or potential problem and also indicate a patient's changing status. Assessments should focus first on the patient, then on the technology. The patient needs to be the focal point of the critical care practitioner's attention, with technology augmenting the information obtained from the direct assessment.

There are two standard approaches to assessing patients, the head-to-toe approach and the body systems approach. Most critical care nurses use a combination, a systems approach applied in a "top-to-bottom" manner. The admission and ongoing assessment sections of this chapter are presented with this combined approach in mind.

ASSESSMENT FRAMEWORK

Assessing the critically ill patient and family begins from the moment the nurse is made aware of the pending admission of the patient and continues until transitioning to the next phase of care. The assessment process can be viewed as four distinct stages: prearrival, admission quick check ("just the basics"), comprehensive admission, and ongoing assessment.

Prearrival Assessment

A prearrival assessment begins the moment information is received about the upcoming admission of the patient. This notification comes from the initial health care team contact. The contact may be paramedics in the field reporting to the emergency department (ED), a transfer from another facility, or a transfer from other areas within the hospital such as the emergency room (ER), operating room (OR), or medical/surgical nursing unit. The prearrival assessment paints the initial picture of the patient and allows the critical care nurse to begin anticipating the patient's physiologic and psychological needs. This prearrival assessment also allows the critical care nurse to determine the appropriate resources that are needed to care for the patient. The information received in the prearrival phase is crucial because it allows the critical care nurse to adequately prepare the environment to meet the specialized needs of the patient and family.

Admission Quick Check

An admission quick check assessment is obtained immediately upon arrival and is based on assessing the parameters represented by the ABCDE acronym (Table 1–1). The admission quick check assessment is a quick overview of the adequacy of ventilation and perfusion to ensure early intervention for any life-threatening situations. Energy is also focused on exploring the chief complaint and obtaining essential diagnostic tests to supplement physical assessment findings. The admission quick check is a high-level view of the patient, but is essential because it validates that basic cardiac and respiratory function is sufficient.

Comprehensive Admission Assessment

A comprehensive admission assessment is performed as soon as possible, with the timing dictated by the degree of physiologic stability and emergent treatment needs of the patient. The comprehensive assessment is an in-depth assessment of the past medical and social history and a complete physical examination of each body system. The comprehensive assessment is vital to successful outcomes because it provides the nurse invaluable insight into proactive interventions that may be needed.

TABLE 1–1. ABCDE ACRONYM

*A*irway
*B*reathing
*C*irculation, *C*erebral perfusion, and *C*hief complaint
*D*rugs and *D*iagnostic tests
*E*quipment

Ongoing Assessment

After the baseline comprehensive assessment is completed, ongoing assessments, an abbreviated version of the comprehensive admission assessment, are performed at varying intervals. The assessment parameters outlined in this section are usually completed for all patients, in addition to other ongoing assessment requirements related to the patient's specific condition, treatments, and response to therapy.

PREARRIVAL ASSESSMENT: BEFORE THE ACTION BEGINS

A prearrival assessment begins when information is received about the pending arrival of the patient. The prearrival report, although abbreviated, provides key information about the chief complaint, diagnosis, or reason for admission, pertinent history details, and physiologic stability of the patient (Table 1–2). It also contains the gender and age of the patient and information on the presence of invasive tubes and lines, medications being administered, other ongoing treatments, and pending or completed laboratory or diagnostic tests. It

TABLE 1–2. SUMMARY OF PREARRIVAL AND ADMISSION QUICK CHECK ASSESSMENTS

Prearrival Assessment
- Abbreviated report on patient (age, sex, chief complaint, diagnosis, pertinent history, physiologic status, invasive devices, equipment and status of laboratory/diagnostic tests)
- Room setup complete, including verification of proper equipment functioning

Admission Quick Check Assessment
- General appearance (consciousness)
- *A*irway:
  Patency
  Position of artificial airway (if present)
- *B*reathing:
  Quantity and quality of respirations (rate, depth, pattern, symmetry, effort, use of accessory muscles)
  Breath sounds
  Presence of spontaneous breathing
- *C*irculation and *C*erebral Perfusion:
  ECG (rate, rhythm, and presence of ectopy)
  Blood pressure
  Peripheral pulses and capillary refill
  Skin, color, temperature, moisture
  Presence of bleeding
  Level of consciousness, responsiveness
- Chief Complaint:
  Primary body system
  Associated symptoms
- *D*rugs and *D*iagnostic Tests:
  Drugs prior to admission (prescribed, over-the-counter, illegal)
  Current medications
  Review diagnostic test results
- *E*quipment:
  Patency of vascular and drainage systems
  Appropriate functioning and labeling of all equipment connected to patient
- Allergies

is also important to consider the potential isolation requirements for the patient (e.g., neutropenic precautions or special respiratory isolation). Being prepared for isolation needs prevents potentially serious exposures to the patient or the health care providers. This information assists the clinician in anticipating the patient's physiologic and emotional needs prior to admission and in ensuring that the bedside environment is set up to provide all monitoring, supply, and equipment needs prior to the patient's arrival.

Many critical care units have a standard room setup, guided by the major diagnosis-related groups of patients each unit receives. The standard monitoring and equipment list for each unit varies; however, there are certain common requirements (Table 1–3). The standard room setup is modified for each admission to accommodate patient-specific needs (e.g., additional equipment, intravenous [IV] fluids, medications). Proper functioning of all bedside equipment should be verified prior to the patient's arrival.

It is also important to prepare the medical records forms, which usually consist of a manual flow sheet or computerized data entry system to record vital signs, intake and output, medication administration, patient care activities, and patient assessment. The prearrival report may suggest pending procedures, necessitating the organization of appropriate supplies at the bedside. Having the room prepared and all equipment available facilitates a rapid, smooth, and safe admission of the patient.

ADMISSION QUICK CHECK ASSESSMENT: THE FIRST FEW MINUTES

From the moment the patient arrives in the intensive care unit (ICU) setting, his or her general appearance is immediately observed and assessment of ABCDEs is quickly performed

---

AT THE BEDSIDE
► *Prearrival Assessment*

The charge nurse notifies Sue that she will be receiving a 26-year-old man from the ER who was involved in a serious car accident. The ED nurse caring for the patient has called to give Sue a report. The patient suffered a closed head injury and chest trauma with collapsed left lung. The patient was intubated and placed on a mechanical ventilator. IV access had been obtained, and a left chest tube had been inserted. After obtaining a computed tomographic (CT) scan of the head, the patient will be transferred to the ICU. Sue asks additional questions of the ED nurse including whether the patient has been agitated, had a Foley catheter placed, and whether family had been notified of the accident.

Sue goes to check the patient's room prior to admission and begins to do a mental check of what will be needed. "The patient is intubated so I'll connect the ambu bag to the oxygen source, check for suction catheters, and make sure the suction systems are working. The pulse oximetry and the ventilator are ready to go. I have an extra suction gauge to connect to the chest tube system. I'll also turn on the ECG monitor and have the ECG electrodes ready to apply. The arterial line flush system and transducer are also ready to be connected. The IV infusion devices are set up. This patient has an altered LOC, which means frequent neuro checks and potential insertion of an ICP catheter for monitoring. I have my pen light handy, but I better check to see if we have all the equipment to insert the ICP catheter in case the physician wants to perform the procedure here after the CT scan. I think I'm ready."

TABLE 1–3. EQUIPMENT FOR STANDARD ROOM SETUP

- Bedside ECG and invasive pressure monitor with appropriate cables
- ECG electrodes
- Blood pressure cuff
- Pulse oximetry
- Suction gauges and canister setup
- Suction catheters
- Bag-valve mask device
- Oxygen flow meter, appropriate tubing, and appropriate oxygen delivery device
- IV poles and infusion pumps
- Bedside supply cart that contains such things as alcohol swabs, nonsterile gloves, syringes, chux, and dressing supplies
- Admission kit that usually contains bath basin and general hygiene supplies
- Admission and critical care documentation forms

(see Table 1–1). The seriousness of the problem(s) is determined so that life-threatening emergent needs can be addressed first. The patient is connected to the appropriate monitoring and support equipment, critical medications are administered, and essential laboratory and diagnostic tests are ordered. Simultaneous with the ABCDE assessment, the nurse must validate that the patient is appropriately identified through a hospital wristband, personal identification, or family identification. In addition, the patient's allergy status is determined, including the type of reaction that occurs and what, if any, treatment is used to alleviate the allergic response.

There may be other health care professionals present to receive the patient and assist with admission tasks. The critical care nurse, however, is the leader of the receiving team. While assuming the primary responsibility for assessing the ABCDEs, the critical care nurse directs the team in completing delegated tasks, such as changing over to the ICU equipment or attaching monitoring cables. Without a leader of the receiving team, care can be fragmented and vital assessment clues overlooked.

The critical care nurse rapidly assesses the ABCDEs in the sequence outlined in this section. If any aspect of this preliminary assessment deviates from normal, interventions are immediately initiated to address the problem before continuing with the admission quick check assessment. Additionally, regardless of whether the patient appears to be conscious or not, it is important to talk to him or her throughout this admission process regarding what is occurring with each interaction and intervention.

Airway and Breathing

Patency of the patient's airway is verified by having the patient speak, watching the patient's chest rise and fall, or both. If the airway is compromised, verify that the head has been positioned properly to prevent the tongue from occluding the airway. Inspect the upper airway for the presence of blood, vomitus, and foreign objects before inserting an oral airway if one is needed. If the patient already has an artificial airway, such as a cricothyrotomy, endotracheal (ET) tube, or tracheostomy, ensure that the airway is secured properly. Note the position of the ET tube and size marking on the ET tube that is closest to the teeth, lips, or nares to assist future comparisons for proper placement. Suctioning of the upper airway, either through the oral cavity or artificial airway, may be required to ensure that the airway is free from secretions. Note the amount, color, and consistency of secretions removed.

Note the rate, depth, pattern, and symmetry of breathing; the effort it is taking to breathe; the use of accessory muscles; and, if mechanically ventilated, whether breathing is in synchrony with the ventilator. Observe for nonverbal signs of respiratory distress such as restlessness, anxiety, or change in mental status. Auscultate the chest for presence of bilateral breath sounds, quality of breath sounds, and bilateral chest expansion. Optimally, both anterior and posterior breath sounds are auscultated, but during this admission quick check assessment, time generally dictates that just the anterior chest is assessed. If noninvasive oxygen saturation monitoring is available, observe and quickly analyze the values. If the patient is receiving assistive breaths from a bag-valve mask or mechanical ventilator, note the presence of spontaneous breaths and evaluate whether ventilation requires excessive pressure.

If chest tubes are present, note whether they are pleural or mediastinal chest tubes. Ensure that they are connected to suction, if appropriate, and are not clamped or kinked.

Circulation and Cerebral Perfusion

Assess circulation by quickly palpating a pulse and viewing the electrocardiogram (ECG) monitor for the heart rate, rhythm, and presence of ectopy. Obtain blood pressure and temperature. Assess peripheral perfusion by evaluating the color, temperature, and moisture of the skin along with capillary refill. Based on the prearrival report and reason for ad-

mission, there may be a need to inspect the body for any signs of blood loss and determine if active bleeding is occurring.

Evaluating cerebral perfusion in the admission quick check assessment is focused on determining the functional integrity of the brain as a whole, which is done by rapidly evaluating the gross level of consciousness (LOC). Evaluate whether the patient is alert and aware of his or her surroundings, whether it takes a verbal or painful stimulus to obtain a response, or whether the patient is unresponsive. Observing the response of the patient during movement from the stretcher to the ICU bed can supply additional information about the LOC. Note whether the patient's eyes are open and watching the events around him or her. For example, does the patient follow simple commands such as "Place your hands on your chest" or "Slide your hips over"? If the patient is unable to talk because of trauma or the presence of an artificial airway, note whether the patient's head nods appropriately to questions.

Chief Complaint

Optimally, the description of the chief complaint is obtained from the patient, but this may not be realistic. The patient may be unable to respond or may not speak English. Data may need to be gathered from family, friends, or bystanders. In the absence of a history source, practitioners must depend exclusively on the physical findings (e.g., presence of medication patches, permanent pacemaker, or old surgery scars) and knowledge of pathophysiology to identify the potential causes of the admission.

Assessment of the chief complaint focuses on determining the body systems involved and the extent of associated symptoms. Additional questions explore the time of onset, precipitating factors, and severity. Although the admission quick check phase is focused on obtaining a quick overview of the key life-sustaining systems, a more in-depth assessment of a particular system may need to be done at this time. For example, in the prearrival case study scenario presented, completion of the ABCDEs is followed quickly by more extensive assessment of both the nervous and respiratory systems.

Drugs and Diagnostic Tests

Information about drugs and diagnostic tests is integrated into the priority of the admission quick check. If IV access is not already present, it should be immediately obtained and intake and output records started. If IV medications are presently being infused, check the drug(s) and verify the correct infusion of the desired dosage and rate.

Obtain critical diagnostic tests. Augment basic screening tests (Table 1–4) by additional tests appropriate to the underlying diagnosis and chief complaint. Review any available laboratory or diagnostic data for abnormalities or indications of potential problems requiring immediate intervention. The abnormal laboratory and diagnostic data for

TABLE 1–4. COMMON DIAGNOSTIC TESTS OBTAINED DURING ADMISSION QUICK CHECK ASSESSMENT

Serum electrolytes
Glucose
Complete blood count with platelets
Coagulation studies
Arterial blood gases
Chest x-ray
ECG

TABLE 1–5. EVIDENCE-BASED PRACTICE: FAMILY NEEDS ASSESSMENT

Quick Assessment
- Offer realistic hope[a,b]
- Give honest answers and information[a,b]
- Give reassurance[a]

Comprehensive Assessment
- Use open-ended communication and assess their communication style[a]
- Assess family members' level of anxiety[a,c]
- Assess perceptions of the situation (knowledge, comprehension, expectations of staff, expected outcome)[a]
- Assess family roles and dynamics (cultural and religious practices, values, spokesperson)[a]
- Assess coping mechanisms and resources (what do they use, social network and support)[a,b,d,e]

Sources: Compiled from [a]Leske (1997), [b]Leske (1992), [c]Raleigh, Lepczyk, and Rowley (1990), [d]Roman and co-workers (1995), and [e]Sabo and associates (1989).

specific pathologic conditions will be covered in subsequent chapters.

Equipment

Quickly evaluate all vascular and drainage tubes for location and patency, and connect them to appropriate monitoring or suction devices. Note the amount, color, consistency, and odor of drainage secretions. Verify the appropriate functioning of all equipment attached to the patient and label as required.

The admission quick check assessment is accomplished in a matter of a few minutes. After completion of the ABCDEs assessment, the comprehensive admission assessment begins. If at any phase during the admission quick check a component of the ABCDEs has not been stabilized and controlled, energy is focused first on resolving the abnormality before proceeding to the comprehensive admission assessment.

After the admission quick check assessment is complete, and the if the patient requires no urgent intervention, there may now be time for a more thorough report from the health care providers transferring the patient to the ICU. This is an opportunity for you to confirm your observations such as dosage of infusing medications, abnormalities found on the quick check assessment, and any potential inconsistencies noted between your assessment and the prearrival report. It is easier to clarify questions while the transporters are still present if possible.

This may also be an opportunity for introductory interactions with family members or friends, if present. Introduce yourself, offer reassurance, and confirm the intention to give the patient the best care possible (Table 1–5). If feasible, allow them to briefly see the patient. If this is not feasible, give them an approximate time frame when they can expect to receive an update from you on the patient's condition. Have another member of the health care team escort them to the appropriate waiting area.

COMPREHENSIVE ADMISSION ASSESSMENT

Comprehensive admission assessments determine the physiologic and psychosocial baseline so that future changes can be compared to determine whether the status is improving or deteriorating. The comprehensive admission assessment also defines the patient's pre-event health status, determining problems or limitations that may impact patient status during this admission as well as potential issues for future transitioning of care. The content presented in this section is a template to screen for abnormalities and determine the extent of injury to the patient. Any abnormal findings or changes from baseline warrant a more in-depth evaluation of the pertinent system.

The comprehensive admission assessment includes the patient's medical and brief social history, and physical examination of each body system. The comprehensive admission assessment of the critically ill patient is similar to admission assessments for non-critically ill patients. This section describes only those aspects of the assessment that are unique to critically ill patients or require more extensive information than is obtained from a non-critical care patient. The entire assessment process is summarized in Tables 1–6 and 1–7.

Changing demographics of critical care units indicate that an increasing proportion of patients are elderly, requiring assessments to incorporate the effects of aging. Although assessment of the aging adult does not differ significantly from the younger adult, understanding how aging alters the physiologic and psychological status of the patient is important. Key physiologic changes pertinent to the critically ill elderly adult are summarized in Table 1–8. Additional emphasis must also be placed on the past medical history because the aging adult frequently has multiple coexisting illnesses and is taking several prescriptive and over-the-counter medications. Social history must address issues related to home environment, support systems, and self-care abilities. The interpretation of clinical findings in the elderly must also take into consideration the fact that the coexistence of several disease processes and the diminished reserves of most body systems often result in more rapid physiologic deterioration than in younger adults.

TABLE 1–6. SUMMARY OF COMPREHENSIVE ADMISSION ASSESSMENT REQUIREMENTS

Past Medical History
Medical conditions, surgical procedures
Psychiatric/emotional problems
Hospitalizations
Previous medications (prescription, over-the-counter, illicit drugs) and
  time of last medication dose
Allergies
Review of body systems (see Table 1–7)

Social History
Age, gender
Ethnic origin
Height, weight
Highest educational level completed
Occupation
Marital status
Primary family members/significant others
Religious affiliation
Advanced Directive or Durable Power of Attorney for Health Care
Substance use (alcohol, drugs, caffeine, tobacco)
Domestic Abuse or Vulnerable Adult Screen

Psychosocial Assessment
General communication
Coping styles
Anxiety and stress
Expectations of critical care unit
Current stresses
Family needs

Spirituality
Faith/spiritual preference
Healing practices

Physical Assessment
Nervous system
Cardiovascular system
Respiratory system
Renal system
Gastrointestinal system
Endocrine, hematologic, and immune systems
Integumentary system

Past Medical History

Besides the primary event that brought the patient to the hospital, it is important to determine prior medical and surgical conditions, hospitalization, medications, and symptoms (see Table 1–7). In reviewing medication use, ensure assessment of over-the-counter medication use as well as any herbal or alternative supplements. For every positive symptom response, additional questions should be asked to explore the characteristics of that symptom (Table 1–9).

Social History

Inquire about the use and abuse of caffeine, alcohol, tobacco, and other substances. Because the use of these agents can have major implications for the critically ill patient, questions are aimed at determining the frequency, amount, and duration of use. Honest information regarding alcohol and

TABLE 1–7. SUGGESTED QUESTIONS FOR REVIEW OF PAST HISTORY CATEGORIZED BY BODY SYSTEM

Body System	History Questions
Nervous	• Have you ever had a seizure? • Have you ever fainted, blacked out, or had delirium tremens (DTs)? • Do you ever have numbness, tingling, or weakness in any part of your body? • Do you have any difficulty with your hearing, vision, or speech? • Has your daily activity level changed due to your present condition? • Do you require any assistive devices such as canes?
Cardiovascular	• Have you experienced any heart problems or disease such as heart attacks? • Do you have any problems with extreme fatigue? • Do you have an irregular heart rhythm? • Do you have high blood pressure? • Do you have a pacemaker or an implanted defibrillator?
Respiratory	• Do you ever experience shortness of breath? • Do you have any pain associated with breathing? • Do you have a persistent cough? Is it productive? • Have you had any exposure to environmental agents that might affect the lungs? • Do you have sleep apnea?
Renal	• Have you had any change in frequency of urination? • Do you have any burning, pain, discharge, or difficulty when you urinate? • Have you had blood in your urine?
Gastrointestinal	• Has there been any recent weight loss or gain? • Have you had any change in appetite? • Do you have any problems with nausea or vomiting? • How often do you have a bowel movement and has there been a change in the normal pattern? Do you have blood in your stools? • Do you have dentures? • Do you have any food allergies?
Integumentary Endocrine and Hematologic Immunologic Psychosocial	• Do you have any problems with your skin? • Do you have any problems with bleeding? • Do you have problems with chronic infections? • Have you recently been exposed to a contagious illness? • Do you have any physical conditions which make communication difficult (hearing loss, visual disturbances, language barriers, etc.)? • How do you best learn? Do you need information repeated several times and/or require information in advance of teaching sessions? • What are the ways you cope with stress, crises, or pain? • Who are the important people in your "family" or network? Who do you want to make decisions with you, or for you? • Have you had any previous experiences with critical illness? • Have you ever been abused? • Have you ever experienced trouble with anxiety, irritability, being confused, mood swings, or suicide attempts? • What are the cultural practices, religious influences, and values that are important to the family? • What are family members' perceptions and expectations of the critical care staff and the setting?
Spiritual	• What is your faith or spiritual preference? • What practices help you heal or deal with stress? • Would you like to see a chaplain, priest, or other type of healer?

TABLE 1–8. PHYSIOLOGIC EFFECTS OF AGING

Body System	Effects
Nervous	Diminished hearing and vision, short-term memory loss, altered motor coordination, decreased muscle tone and strength, slower response to verbal and motor stimuli, decreased ability to synthesize new information, increased sensitivity to altered temperature states, increased sensitivity to sedation (confusion or agitation), decreased alertness levels.
Cardiovascular	Increased effects of atherosclerosis of vessels and heart valves, decreased stroke volume with resulting decreased cardiac output, decreased myocardial compliance, increased workload of heart, diminished peripheral pulses.
Respiratory	Decreased compliance and elasticity, decreased vital capacity, increased residual volume, less effective cough, decreased response to hypercapnia.
Renal	Decreased glomerular filtration rate, increased risk of fluid and electrolyte imbalances.
Gastrointestinal	Increased presence of dentition problems, decreased intestinal mobility, decreased hepatic metabolism, increased risk of altered nutritional states.
Endocrine, hematologic, and immunologic	Increased incidence of diabetes, thyroid disorders, and anemia; decreased antibody response and cellular immunity.
Integumentary	Decreased skin turgor, increased capillary fragility and bruising, decreased elasticity.
Miscellaneous	Altered pharmacokinetics and pharmacodynamics, decreased range of motion of joints and extremities.
Psychosocial	Difficulty falling asleep and fragmented sleep patterns, increased incidence of depression and anxiety, cognitive impairment disorders, difficulty with change.

substance abuse, however, may not be always forthcoming. Family or friends might provide additional information that might assist in assessing these parameters. The information revealed during the social history can often be verified during the physical assessment through the presence of signs such as presence of needle track marks, nicotine stains on teeth and fingers, or the smell of alcohol on the breath.

Physical Assessment by Body System

The physical assessment section is presented in the sequence in which the combined system, head-to-toe approach is followed. Although content is presented as separate components, generally the history questions are integrated into the physical assessment. The physical assessment section uses the techniques of inspection, auscultation, and palpation. Although percussion is a common technique in physical examinations, it is infrequently used in critically ill patients.

TABLE 1–9. IDENTIFICATION OF SYMPTOM CHARACTERISTICS

Characteristic	Sample Question
Onset	How and under what circumstances did it begin? Was the onset sudden or gradual? Did it progress?
Location	Where is it? Does it stay in the same place or does it radiate or move around?
Frequency	How often does it occur?
Quality	Is it dull, sharp, burning, throbbing, etc.?
Intensity	Rank pain on a scale (numeric, word description, FACES, FLACC)
Quantity	How long does it last?
Setting	What are you doing when it happened?
Associated findings	Are there other signs and symptoms that occur when this happens?
Aggravating and alleviating factors	What things make it worse? What things make it better?

Pain assessment is generally linked to each body system rather than considered as a separate system category. For example, if the patient has chest pain, assessment and documentation of that pain is incorporated into the cardiovascular assessment. Rather than have general pain assessment questions repeated under each system assessment, they are presented here.

Pain and discomfort are clues that alert both the patient and the critical care nurse that something is wrong and needs prompt attention. Pain assessment includes differentiating acute from chronic pain, determining related physiologic symptoms, and investigating the patient's perceptions and emotional reactions to the pain. Explore the qualities and characteristics of the pain by using the questions listed in Table 1–9. Pain is a very subjective assessment and critical care practitioners sometime struggle with applying their own values when attempting to evaluate the patient's pain. To resolve this dilemma, use the patient's own words and descriptions of the pain whenever possible and use a patient-preferred pain scale (see Chapter 6, Pain, Sedation, and Neuromuscular Blockade Management) to objectively and consistently evaluate pain levels.

Nervous System

The nervous system is the "master computer" of all systems and is divided into the central and peripheral nervous systems. With the exception of the peripheral nervous system's cranial nerves, almost all attention in the critically ill patient is focused on evaluating the central nervous system (CNS). The physiologic and psychological impact of critical illness, in addition to pharmacologic interventions, frequently alters CNS functioning. The single most important indicator of cerebral functioning is the LOC. The LOC is assessed in the critically ill patient using the Glasgow Coma Scale (see Chapter 12, Neurological System).

Assess pupils for size, shape, symmetry, and reactivity to direct light. When interpreting the implication of altered pupil size, remember that certain medications such as atropine or morphine may affect pupil size. Baseline pupil assessment is important even in patients without a neurologic diagnosis because some individuals have unequal or unreactive pupils normally. If pupils are not checked as a baseline, a later check of pupils during an acute event could inappropriately attribute pupil abnormalities to a pathophysiologic event.

LOC and pupil assessments are followed by motor function assessment of the upper and lower extremities for symmetry and quality of strength. Traditional motor strength exercises include having the patient squeeze the nurse's hands and plantar flexing and dorsiflexing of the patient's feet. If the patient cannot follow commands, an estimate of strength and quality of movements can be inferred by observing activities such as pulling against restraints or thrashing around. If the patient has no voluntary movement or is unresponsive, check the gag and Babinski reflexes.

If head trauma is involved or suspected, check for signs of fluid leakage around the nose or ears, differentiating between cerebral spinal fluid and blood (see Chapter 12, Neurological System). Complete cranial nerve assessment is rarely warranted, with specific cranial nerve evaluation based on the injury or diagnosis. For example, extraocular movements are routinely assessed in patients with facial trauma. Sensory testing is a baseline standard for spinal cord injuries, extremity trauma, and epidural analgesia.

Now is a good time to assess mental status if the patient is responsive. Assess orientation to person, place, and time. Ask the patient to state their understanding of what is happening. As you ask the questions, observe for eye contact, pressured or muted speech, and rate of speech. Rate of speech is usually consistent with the patient's psychomotor status. Underlying cognitive impairments such as dementia and developmental delays are typically exacerbated during critical illness due to physiologic changes, medications, and environmental changes. It may be necessary to ascertain baseline level of functioning from the family.

Laboratory data pertinent to the nervous system include serum and urine electrolytes and osmolarity and urinary specific gravity. Drug toxicology and alcohol levels may be evaluated to rule out potential sources of altered LOC. If the patient has an intracranial pressure (ICP) monitoring device in place, note the type of device (e.g., ventriculostomy, epidural, subdural) and analyze the baseline pressure and waveform. Check all diagnostic values and monitoring system data to determine if immediate intervention is warranted.

Cardiovascular System

Cardiovascular system assessment factors are directed at evaluating central and peripheral perfusion. Revalidate your admission quick check assessment of the blood pressure,

heart rate, and rhythm. Assess the ECG for T-wave abnormalities and ST segment changes and determine the PR, QRS, and QT intervals and the QT_c measurements. Note any abnormalities or indications of myocardial damage, electrical conduction problems, and electrolyte imbalances. Note the pulse pressure. If treatment decisions will be based on the cuff pressure, blood pressure is taken in both arms. If an arterial pressure line is in place, compare the arterial line pressure to the cuff pressure. In either case, if a 10- to 15-mm Hg difference exists, a decision must be made as to which pressure is the most accurate and will be followed for future treatment decisions. If a different method is used inconsistently, changes in blood pressure might be inappropriately attributed to physiologic changes rather than anatomic differences.

Note the color and temperature of the skin, with particular emphasis on lips, mucous membranes, and distal extremities. Also evaluate nail color and capillary refill. Inspect for the presence of edema, particularly in the dependent parts of the body such as feet, ankles, and sacrum. If edema is present, rate the quality of edema by using a 0 to +4 scale (Table 1–10).

Auscultate heart sounds for S_1 and S_2 quality, intensity, and pitch, and for the presence of extra heart sounds, murmurs, clicks, or rubs. Listen to one sound at a time, consistently progressing through the key anatomic landmarks of the heart each time. Note whether there are any changes with respiration or patient position.

Palpate the peripheral pulses for amplitude and quality, using the 0 to +4 scale (Table 1–11). Check all pulses simultaneously, except the carotid, comparing each pulse to its partner. If the pulse is difficult to palpate, an ultrasound (Doppler) device should be used. To facilitate finding a weak pulse for subsequent assessments, mark the location of the pulse with an indelible pen. It is also helpful to compare quality of the pulses to the ECG to evaluate the perfusion of heart beats.

Electrolyte levels, complete blood counts (CBCs), coagulation studies, and lipid profiles are common laboratory tests evaluated for abnormalities of the cardiovascular system. Cardiac enzyme levels (creatine kinase-MB, troponin, B natriuretic peptide) are obtained for any complaint of chest pain or suspected chest trauma. Drug levels of commonly used cardiovascular medications, such as digoxin, may be warranted for certain types of dysrhythmias. A

TABLE 1–10. EDEMA RATING SCALE

Following the application and removal of firm digital pressure against the tissue, the edema is evaluated for one of the following responses:
- 0   No depression in tissue
- +1 Small depression in tissue, disappearing in <1 second
- +2 Depression in tissue disappears in less than 1–2 seconds
- +3 Depression in tissue disappears in less than 2–3 seconds
- +4 Depression in tissue disappears in ≥4 seconds

TABLE 1-11. PERIPHERAL PULSE RATING SCALE

- 0 Absent pulse
- +1 Palpable but thready; easily obliterated with light pressure
- +2 Normal; cannot obliterate with light pressure
- +3 Full
- +4 Full and bounding

12-lead ECG is typically evaluated on all patients, either due to their chief reason for admission (e.g., with complaints of chest pain, irregular rhythms, or suspected myocardial bruising from trauma) or as a baseline for future comparison if needed.

Note the type, size, and location of IV catheters, and verify their patency. If continuous infusions of medications such as vasopressors or antidysrhythmics are being administered, ensure that they are being infused into an appropriately sized vessel and are compatible with any piggybacked IV solution.

Verify all monitoring system alarm parameters as active with appropriate limits set. Note the size and location of invasive monitoring lines such as arterial, central venous, and pulmonary artery (PA) catheters. Confirm the appropriate flush solution is hanging and that the correct amount of pressure is applied to the flush solution bag. Level the invasive line to the appropriate anatomic landmark and zero the monitor as needed. For PA catheters, note the size of the introducer and the size (in centimeters) marking where the catheter exits the introducer. Interpret hemodynamic pressure readings against normals and with respect to the patient's underlying pathophysiology. Assess waveforms to determine the quality of the waveform (e.g., dampened or hyperresonant) and whether the waveform appropriately matches the expected characteristics for the anatomic placement of the invasive catheter (see Chapter 4, Hemodynamic Monitoring). For example, a right ventricular waveform for a central venous pressure line indicates a problem with the position of the central venous line that needs to be corrected. If the PA catheter has continuous mixed venous saturation (SvO_2) capabilities or continuous cardiac output data, these numbers are also evaluated in conjunction with vital sign data and any concurrent pharmacologic and/or volume infusions.

Respiratory System

Oxygenation and ventilation are the focal basis of respiratory assessment parameters. Reassess the rate and rhythm of respirations and the symmetry of chest wall movement. If the patient has a productive cough or secretions are suctioned from an artificial airway, note the color, consistency, and amount of secretions. Evaluate whether the trachea is midline or shifted. Inspect the thoracic cavity for shape, anterior–posterior diameter, and structural deformities (e.g., kyphosis or scoliosis). Palpate for equal chest excursion,

presence of crepitus, and any areas of tenderness or fractures. If the patient is receiving supplemental oxygen, verify the mode of delivery and percentage of oxygen against physician orders.

Auscultate all lobes anteriorly and posteriorly for bilateral breath sounds to determine the presence of air movement and the presence of adventitious sounds such as crackles or wheezes. Note the quality and depth of respirations, and the length and pitch of the inspiratory and expiratory phases.

Arterial blood gases (ABGs) are frequently used diagnostic tests to assess for both interpretation of oxygenation, ventilatory status, and acid–base balance. Hemoglobin and hematocrit values are interpreted for impact on oxygenation and fluid balance. If the patient's condition warrants, the oxygen saturation values may be continuously monitored via connection to a noninvasive oxygen saturation monitor or SvO_2 PA catheter monitoring device.

If the patient is intubated, note the size of the tube and record the centimeter marking at the teeth or nares to assist future comparisons for proper placement. If the patient is connected to a mechanical ventilator, verify the ventilatory mode, tidal volume, respiratory rate, positive end expiratory pressure, and percentage of oxygen against prescribed settings. Observe whether the patient has spontaneous breaths, noting both the rate and average tidal volume of each breath. Note the amount of pressure required to ventilate the patient for later comparisons to determine changes in pulmonary compliance. If available, continuous end-tidal CO_2 is integrated into the respiratory picture and compared to the ABGs.

If chest tubes are present, assess the area around the insertion site for crepitus. Note the amount and color of drainage and whether an air leak is present. Verify whether the chest tube drainage system is under water seal or connected to suction.

Renal System

Urinary characteristics and electrolyte status are the major parameters used to evaluate the function of the kidneys. In conjunction with the cardiovascular system, the renal system's impact on fluid volume status is also assessed.

Most critically ill patients have a Foley catheter in place to evaluate urinary output every 1 to 2 hours. Note the amount and color of the urine and, if warranted, obtain a sample to assess for the abnormal presence of glucose, protein, and blood. Inspect the genitalia for inflammation, swelling, ulcers, and drainage. If suprapubic tubes or a ureterostomy are present, note the position as well as the amount and characteristics of the drainage. Observe whether any drainage is leaking around the drainage tube.

In addition to the urinalysis, serum electrolyte levels, blood urea nitrogen, creatinine, and urinary and serum osmolarity are common diagnostic tests used to evaluate kidney function.

Gastrointestinal System

The key factors when reviewing the gastrointestinal system are the nutritional and fluid status. Inspect the abdomen for overall symmetry, noting whether the contour is flat, round, protuberant, or distended. Note the presence of discoloration or striae. Nutritional status is evaluated by looking at the patient's weight and muscle tone, the condition of the oral mucosa, and laboratory values such as serum albumin and transferrin.

Auscultation of bowel sounds should be done in all four quadrants in a clockwise order, noting the frequency and presence or absence of sounds. Bowel sounds are usually rated as absent, hypoactive, normal, or hyperactive. Before noting absent bowel sounds, a quadrant should be listened to for at least 60 to 90 seconds. Characteristics and frequency of the sounds are noted. After listening for the presence of normal sounds, determine if any adventitious bowel sounds such as friction rubs, bruits, or hums are present.

Light palpation of the abdomen helps to determine areas of tenderness, pain, and guarding or rebound tenderness. Remember to auscultate before palpating because palpation may change the frequency and character of the patient's peristaltic sounds.

Assess any drainage tube for location and function, and for the characteristics of any drainage. Validate the proper placement of the nasogastric tube and assess nasogastric secretions for pH and occult blood. Check emesis and stool for occult blood as appropriate. Evaluate ostomies for location, color of the stoma, and the type of drainage.

Endocrine, Hematologic, and Immune Systems

The endocrine, hematologic, and immune systems often are overlooked when assessing critically ill patients. The assessment parameters used to evaluate these systems are included under other system assessments, but it is important to consciously consider these systems when reviewing these parameters. Assessing the endocrine, hematologic, and immune systems is based on a thorough understanding of the primary function of each of the hormones, blood cells, or immune components of each of the respective systems.

Assessing the specific functions of the endocrine system's hormones is challenging because much of the symptomatology related to the hyposecretion or hypersecretion of the hormones can be found with other systems' problems. The patient's history may help to differentiate the source, but any abnormal assessment findings detected with regard to fluid balance, metabolic rate, altered LOC, color and temperature of the skin, electrolytes, glucose, and acid–base balance require the critical care nurse to consider the potential involvement of the endocrine system. For example, are the signs and symptoms of hypervolemia related to cardiac insufficiency or excessive amounts of antidiuretic hormone? Serum blood tests for specific hormone levels may be required to rule out involvement of the endocrine system.

Assessment parameters specific to the hematologic system include laboratory evaluation of the red blood cells (RBCs) and coagulation studies. Diminished RBCs may affect the oxygen-carrying capacity of the blood as evidenced by pallor, cyanosis, light headedness, tachypnea, and tachycardia. Insufficient clotting factors are evidenced by bruising, oozing of blood from puncture sites or mucous membranes, or overt bleeding.

The immune system's primary function of fighting infection is assessed by evaluating the white cell and differential counts from the CBC, and assessing puncture sites and mucous membranes for oozing drainage and inflamed, reddened areas. Spiking or persistent low-grade temperatures often are indicative of underlying infections. It is important to keep in mind, however, that many critically ill patients have impaired immune systems and the normal response to infection, such as white pus around an insertion site, may not be evident.

Integumentary System

The skin is the first line of defense against infection so assessment parameters are focused on evaluating the intactness of the skin. Assessing the skin can be undertaken while performing other system assessments. For example, while listening to breath sounds or bowel sounds, the condition of the thoracic cavity or abdominal skin can be observed, respectively.

Inspect the skin for overall integrity, color, temperature, and turgor. Note the presence of rashes, striae, discoloration, scars, or lesions. For any abrasions, lesions, pressure ulcers, or wounds, note the size, depth, and presence or absence of drainage. Consider use of a skin integrity risk assessment tool to determine immediate interventions that may be needed to prevent further skin integrity breakdown.

Psychosocial Assessment

The rapid physiologic and psychological changes associated with critical illnesses, coupled with pharmacologic and biological treatments, can profoundly affect behavior. Patients are suffering illnesses that have psychological responses that are predictable, and, if untreated, may threaten recovery or life. To avoid making assumptions about how a patient feels about his or her care, there is no substitute for asking the patient directly or asking a collateral informant, such as the family or significant other.

General Communication

Factors that affect communication include culture, developmental stage, physical condition, stress, perception, neurocognitive deficits, emotional state, and language skills. The nature of a critical illness, coupled with pharmacologic and airway technologies, interferes with the patients' usual methods of communication. It is essential to determine pre-illness communication methods and styles to ensure optimal communication with the critically ill patient and family. The inability of many critically ill patients to communicate verbally necessitates that critical care practitioners become expert at assessing nonverbal clues to determine important information from, and needs of, patients. Important assessment data are gained by observation of body gestures, facial expressions, eye movements, involuntary movements, and changes in physiologic parameters, particularly heart rate, blood pressure, and respiratory rate. Often, these nonverbal behaviors may be more reflective of the patients' actual feelings, particularly if they are denying symptoms and attempting to be the "good patient" by not complaining.

Anxiety and Stress

Anxiety is both psychologically and physiologically exhausting. Being in a prolonged state of arousal is hard work and uses adaptive reserves needed for recovery. The critical care environment is full of constant auditory and tactile stimuli, very stressful, and may contribute to a patient's anxiety level. The critical care setting may force isolation from social supports, dependency, loss of control, trust in unknown care providers, helplessness, and an inability to problem solve or attend. Restlessness, distractibility, hyperventilation, and unrealistic demands for attention are warning signs of escalating anxiety.

Medications such as interferon, corticosteroids, angiotensin-converting enzyme inhibitors, and vasopressors can induce anxiety. Abrupt withdrawal from benzodiazepines, caffeine, nicotine, and narcotics, as well as akathisia from phenothiazines, may mimic anxiety. Additional etiologic variables associated with anxiety include pain, sleep loss, delirium, hypoxia, ventilator synchronization or weaning, fear of death, loss of control, high-technology equipment, and a dehumanizing setting. Admission to or repeated transfers to the critical care unit may also induce anxiety.

Coping Styles

Individuals cope with a critical illness in different ways and their pre-illness coping style, personality traits, or temperament will assist you in anticipating coping styles in the critical care setting. Include the patient's family when assessing previous resources, coping skills, or defense mechanisms that strengthen adaptation or problem-solving resolution. For instance, some patients want to be informed of everything that is happening with them in the ICU. Providing information reduces their anxiety and gives them a sense of control. Other patients prefer to have others receive information about them and make decisions for them. Giving them detailed information only exacerbates their level of anxiety and diminishes their ability to cope. It is most important to understand the meaning assigned to the event by the patient and family, and the purpose the coping defense serves. Does the coping resource fit with the event and meet the patient's and family's need?

This may also be the time to conduct a brief assessment of the spiritual beliefs and needs of the patient and how those assist them in their coping. Minimally, patients should be asked if they have a faith or spiritual preference and wish to see a chaplain or priest. However, patients should also be asked about spiritual and cultural healing practices that are important to them to determine whether those can possibly be maintained during their ICU stay.

Patients express their coping styles in a variety of ways. Persons who are stoic by personality or culture usually present as the "good" patient. Assess for behaviors of not wanting to "bother" the busy staff or not admitting pain because family or others are nearby. Some patients express their anxiety and stress through "manipulative" behavior. Critical care nurses must understand that patients' and families' impulsivity, deception, low tolerance for frustration, unreliability, superficial charm, splitting among the provider team, and general avoidance of rules or limits are modes of interacting and coping and attempts to feel safe. Still other patients may withdraw and actually request use of sedatives and sleeping medications to blunt the stimuli and stress of the environment.

Fear has an identifiable source and has an important role in the ability of the patient to cope. Treatments, procedures, pain, and separation are common objects of fear. The dying process elicits specific fears, such as fear of the unknown, loneliness, loss of body, loss of self-control, suffering, pain, loss of identity, and loss of everyone loved by the patient. The family, as well as the patient, experiences the grieving process, which includes the phases of denial, shock, anger, bargaining, depression, and acceptance.

Family Needs

The concept of family is not simple today and extends beyond the nuclear family to any loving, supportive person regardless of social and legal boundaries. Ideally the patient should be asked who they identify as family, who should receive information about patient status, and who should make decisions for the patient if he or she becomes unable to make decisions for self. This may also be an opportune time to ask if they have an advanced directive or if they have discussed their wishes with any family members or friends. Critical care practitioners need to be flexible around traditional legal boundaries of "next of kin" so that communication is extended to, and sought from, surrogate decision makers and whomever the patient designates.

Families can have a positive impact on the patient's ability to cope with and recover from a critical illness. Each family system is unique and varies by culture, values, religion, previous experience with crisis, socioeconomic status, psychological integrity, role expectations, communication patterns, health beliefs, and ages. It is important to assess the family's needs and resources to develop interventions that will optimize the impact of the family on the patient and their interactions with the health care team. Areas for family needs assessments are outlined in Table 1–5.

Unit Orientation

The critical care nurse must take the time to educate the patient (if alert) and family about the specialized ICU environment. This orientation should include a simple explanation of the equipment being used in the care of the patient, visitation policies, the routines of the unit, and how the patient can communicate needs to the unit staff. Additionally, the family should be given the unit telephone number and the names of the nurse manager as well as the nurse caring for the patient in case problems or concerns arise during the ICU stay.

Referrals

After completing the comprehensive admission assessment, analyze the information gathered for the need to make referrals to other health care providers and resources (Table 1–12). With length of stay and appropriate resource management a continual challenge, it is important to start referrals as soon as possible to maintain continuity of care and avoid worsening decline of status.

ONGOING ASSESSMENT

After the admission quick check and the comprehensive admission assessments are completed, all subsequent assessments are used to determine trends, evaluate response to therapy, and identify new potential problems or changes from the comprehensive baseline assessment. Ongoing assessments become more focused and the frequency is driven by the stability of the patient; however, routine periodic assessments are the norm. For example, ongoing assessments can occur every few minutes for extremely unstable patients to every 2 to 4 hours for very stable patients. Additional assessments should be made when any of the following situations occur:

- When caregivers change;
- Before and after any major procedural intervention, such as intubation or chest tube insertion;

TABLE 1–12. EXAMPLES OF POTENTIAL REFERRALS NEEDED FOR CRITICALLY ILL PATIENTS

Referral	Resources Needed
Social work	• Financial needs/resources for patient and/or family • Coping resources for patient and/or family
Nutrition	• Nutritional status at risk and in need of in-depth nutritional assessment • Altered nutritional status on admission
Therapies	• Physical therapy for maintaining or improving physical flexibility and strength • Occupational therapy for assistive devices • Speech therapy for assessment of ability to swallow or communication needs
Chaplaincy	• Spiritual guidance for patient and/or family • Coping resources for patient and/or family
Enterostomal nursing	• Stoma assessment and needs • In-depth skin integrity needs
Ethics committee	• Decisions involving significant ethical complexity • Decisions involving disagreements over care between care providers or between care providers and patient/family • Decisions involving withholding or withdrawing life-sustaining treatment not adequately addressed in policy

TABLE 1–13. ONGOING ASSESSMENT TEMPLATE

Body System	Assessment Parameters
Nervous	• LOC • Pupils • Motor strength of extremities
Cardiovascular	• Blood pressure • Heart rate and rhythm • Heart sounds • Capillary refill • Peripheral pulses • Patency of IVs • Verification of IV solutions and medications • Hemodynamic pressures and waveforms • Cardiac output data
Respiratory	• Respiratory rate and rhythm • Breath sounds • Color and amount of secretions • Noninvasive technology information (e.g., pulse oximetry, end-tidal CO_2) • Mechanical ventilatory parameters • Arterial and venous blood gases
Renal	• Intake and output • Color amount of urinary output • BUN/creatinine values
Gastrointestinal	• Bowel sounds • Contour of abdomen • Position of drainage tubes • Color and amount of secretions • Bilirubin and albumin values
Endocrine, hematologic, and immunologic	• Fluid balance • Electrolyte and glucose values • CBC and coagulation values • Temperature • WBC with differential count
Integumentary	• Color and temperature skin • Intactness of skin • Areas of redness
Pain/discomfort	• Assessed in each system • Response to interventions
Psychosocial	• Mental status and behavioral responses • Reaction to critical illness experience (e.g., stress, anxiety, coping, mood) • Presence of cognitive impairments (dementia, delirium), depression, or demoralization • Family functioning and needs • Ability to communicate needs and participate in care • Sleep patterns

- Before and after transport out of the critical care unit for diagnostic procedures or other events;
- Deterioration in physiologic or mental status; and
- Initiation of any new therapy.

As with the admission quick check, the ongoing assessment section is offered as a generic template that can be used as a basis for all patients (Table 1–13). More in-depth and system-specific assessment parameters are added based on the patient's diagnosis and pathophysiologic problems.

SELECTED BIBLIOGRAPHY

Critical Care Assessment

Barry PD: *Psychosocial Nursing: Care of Physically Ill Patients and Their Families,* 3rd ed. Philadelphia: Lippincott; 1996.

Bickley LS, Szilagyi PG: *Bates' Guide to Physical Examination and History Taking,* 8th ed. Philadelphia: Lippincott Williams & Wilkins; 2003.

Chulay M, Guzetta C, Dossey B: *AACN Pocket Handbook of Critical Care Nursing.* Stamford, CT: Appleton & Lange; 1997.

Ely W, Margolin R, Francis J et al. Evaluation of delirium in critically ill patients: Validation of the Confusion Assessment Method for the Intensive Care Unit (CAM-ICU). *Crit Care Med* 2001;29:1370–1379.

Kinney M, Dunbar S, Brunn J, Molter N, Vittello-Cicciu J: *Clinical Reference for Critical Care Nursing,* 4th ed. St. Louis: Mosby; 1998.

Evidence-Based Practice

Leske JS: Family needs and interventions in the acute care environment. In Chulay M, Molter NC (eds): *AACN's Protocols for Practice: Creating a Healing Environment Series.* Aliso Viejo, CA: American Association of Critical-Care Nurses; 1997.

Leske JS: Needs of family members after critical illness: Prescriptions for interventions. *Crit Care Nurs Clin N Am* 1992;4:587–596.

Raleigh E, Lepczyk M, Rowley C. Significant others benefit from preoperative information. *J Adv Nurs* 1990;15:941–945.

Roman L, Lindsay J, Boger R, et al. Parent-to-parent support initiated in the neonatal intensive care unit. *Res Nurs Health* 1995;18:385–394.

Sabo KA, Kraay C, Rudy E, et al. ICU family support group sessions: Family members' perceived benefits. *Appl Nurs Res* 1989, 2:82–89.

Planning Care for Critically Ill Patients and Families

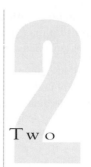

Two

Mary Fran Tracy

▶ Knowledge Competencies

1. Discuss the importance of a multidisciplinary plan of care for optimizing clinical outcomes.
2. Describe interventions for prevention of common complications in critically ill patients:
   • Deep venous thrombosis
   • Infection
   • Sleep pattern disturbances
   • Skin breakdown
3. Discuss interventions to maintain psychosocial integrity and minimize anxiety for the critically ill patient and family members.
4. Describe interventions to promote family-focused care and patient and family education.
5. Identify necessary equipment and personnel required to safely transport the critically ill patient within the hospital
6. Describe transfer-related complications and preventive measures to be taken before and during patient transport.

The achievement of optimal clinical outcomes in the critically ill patient requires a coordinated approach to care delivery by multidisciplinary team members. Experts in nutrition, respiratory therapy, critical care nursing and medicine, psychiatry, and social work, as well as other disciplines, must work collaboratively to effectively, and efficiently, provide optimal care.

The use of multidisciplinary plan of care is a useful approach to facilitate the coordination of a patient's care by the multidisciplinary team and optimize clinical outcomes. These multidisciplinary plans of care are increasingly being used to replace individual, discipline-specific plans of care. Each clinical condition presented in this text discusses the management of patient needs or problems with an integrated, multidisciplinary approach.

The following section provides an overview of multidisciplinary plans of care and their benefits. In addition, this chapter discusses common patient management approaches to needs or problems during critical illnesses that are not diagnosis specific, but common to a majority of critically ill patients, such as sleep deprivation, skin breakdown, and patient and family education. Additional discussion of these needs or problems is also presented in other chapters if management is specific to disease management.

MULTIDISCIPLINARY PLAN OF CARE AND CRITICAL PATHWAYS

A *multidisciplinary plan of care* is a set of expectations for the major components of care a patient should receive during the hospitalization to manage a specific medical or surgical problem. Other names for these types of plans include *clinical pathways, interdisciplinary care plans,* and *care maps.* The multidisciplinary plan of care expands the concept of a medical or nursing care plan and provides an interdisciplinary, comprehensive blueprint for patient care. The result is a diagnosis-specific plan of care that focuses the entire care team on expected patient outcomes.

The multidisciplinary plan of care outlines what tests, medications, care, and treatments are needed to discharge the patient in a timely manner with all patient outcomes met (Figure 2–1). Multidisciplinary plans of care have a variety of benefits to both patients and the hospital system:

- Improved patient outcomes
- Increased quality and continuity of care
- Improved communication and collaboration
- Identification of hospital system problems
- Coordination of necessary services and reduced duplication
- Prioritization of activities
- Reduced length of stay (LOS) and health care costs

Multidisciplinary plans of care are developed by a team of individuals who closely interact with a specific patient population. It is this process of multiple disciplines communicating and collaborating around the needs of the patient that creates benefits for the patients. Representatives of disciplines commonly involved in pathway development include physicians, nurses, respiratory therapists, physical therapists, social workers, and dieticians. The format for the multidisciplinary plans of care typically includes the following categories:

- Discharge outcomes
- Patient goals (e.g., pain control, activity level, absence of complications)
- Assessment and evaluation
- Consultations
- Tests
- Medications
- Nutrition
- Activity
- Education
- Discharge planning

The suggested activities within each of these categories are divided into daily activities or grouped into phases of the hospitalization (e.g., preoperative, intraoperative, and postoperative phases). All staff members who use the path require education as to the specifics of the pathway. This team approach in development and utilization optimizes communication, collaboration, coordination, and commitment to the pathway process.

Multidisciplinary plans of care are used by a wide range of disciplines. As individuals assess and implement various aspects of the multidisciplinary plan of care, documentation occurs directly on the pathway. Each item on the pathway is evaluated and documented as met, unmet, or not applicable. Items on the plan of care that are not completed typically are termed *variances,* which are deviations from the expected activities or goals outlined. Events outlined on the plans of care that occur early are termed *positive variances. Negative variances* are those planned events which are not accomplished on time. Negative variances typically include items not completed due to the patient's condition, hospital system problems, or lack of orders. Assessing patient progression on the pathway helps caregivers to have an overall picture of patient recovery as compared to the goals and can be helpful in early recognition and resolution of problems.

PREVENTION OF COMMON COMPLICATIONS

The development of a critical illness, regardless of its cause, predisposes the patient to a number of physiologic and psychological complications. A major focus when providing care to critically ill patients is the prevention of complications associated with critical illness. The following content overviews some of the most common complications.

Physiologic Instability

Ongoing assessments and monitoring of critically ill patients (see Table 1–13) are key to early identification of physiologic changes and to ensuring that the patient is progressing to the identified transition goals. It is important for the nurse to use critical thinking skills throughout the provision of care to accurately analyze patient changes.

After each assessment, the data obtained should be looked at in totality as they relate to the status of the patient. When an assessment changes in one body system, rarely does it remain an isolated issue, but rather it frequently either impacts or is a result of changes in other systems. Only by analyzing the entire patient assessment can the nurse see what is truly happening with the patient and anticipate interventions and responses.

When you assume care of the patient, define what goals the patient should achieve by the end of the shift, either as identified by the pathway or by your assessment. This provides opportunities to evaluate care over a period of time. It prevents a narrow focus on the completion of individual tasks and interventions rather than the overall progression of the patient toward various goals. In addition, it is key to anticipate the potential patient responses to interventions. For instance, have you noticed that you need to increase the insulin infusion in response to higher glucose levels every morning around 10 A.M.? When looking at the whole picture, you may realize that the patient is receiving several medications in the early morning that are being given in a dextrose diluent. Recognition of this pattern helps you to stabilize swings in blood glucose.

Deep Venous Thrombosis

Critically ill patients are at increased risk of deep venous thrombosis (DVT) due to their underlying condition and immobility. Routine interventions can prevent this potentially devastating complication from occurring. Increased mobility should be emphasized as soon as the patient is stable. Even transferring the patient from the bed to the chair can change positioning of extremities and improve circulation. Additionally, use of sequential compression devices and/or TED hose can assist in circulation of the lower extremities. Avoid

Short-term – Interdisciplinary Plan of Care for: PCI

Admitting DX _____   **Allergies**

Anticipated date of D/C _____

Date/Surgery/Procedure _____

_____

_____

_____

Needs: ☐ visual impairment ☐ contacts ☐ hearing impairment ☐ communication impairment
☐ glasses ☐ dentures ☐ hearing aid ☐ interpreter - lang. _____

Patient's Story/Significant Events this admission: _____

Inactive Problems

Initials	Signature/Title	Initials	Signature/Title	Initials	Signature/Title

PATIENT LABEL

SHORT-TERM
INTERDISCIPLINARY
PLAN OF CARE
PCI

**ABBOTT
NORTHWESTERN
HOSPITAL**
Allina Hospitals & Clinics

Page 1 of 6
form#
REV. 04/2003

Figure 2–1. Interdisciplinary plan of care for percutaneous coronary intervention (PCI). (*Source: Used with permission, Abbott-Northwestern Hospital, Minneapolis, MN.*)

Short-term – Interdisciplinary Plan of Care for: PCI

Disciplines Involved	Problem and Date Initiated	Outcome/Goal *When outcome/goals not met revise plan and outcomes.	INTERVENTIONS		
			Pre-procedure	0–12 hours Post-PCI	12–24 hours Post-PCI
	Discharge Planning	Patient discharges to a safe destination	Complete admission profile and assess need for SS consult

Assess family resources and involvement | Start referral, if needed

Determine if patient able to return to current living situation | Evaluate need for OPCR
☐ Referral done
☐ Not appropriate
☐ Patient declined |
| | | | Activities
Done: Initials
D ☐   _____
E ☐   _____
N ☐   _____ | Activities
Done: Initials
D ☐   _____
E ☐   _____
N ☐   _____ | Activities
Done: Initials
D ☐   _____
E ☐   _____
N ☐   _____ |
| | Knowledge Deficit | Patient/family able to verbalize understanding of medical diagnosis, treatment,plan of care,and discharge instructions | Appraise patients current level of knowledge related to specific disease process taking into account cultural and spiritual influences and age-related factors

Patient to view CV procedure video

Give handouts related to patients procedure and CV folder

Assess need for dietary and tobacco cessation consult | Educate patient on sheath pull

Establish mutual goals to enable a timely discharge | Educate patient/family on:
• Cardiac risk factors
• Activity limitations and home walking program
• Groin site precautions
• NTG SL use
• Medications
• S/S of infection
• When to call MD/911
• Cardiac diet |
| | | | Activities
Done: Initials
D ☐   _____
E ☐   _____
N ☐   _____ | Activities
Done: Initials
D ☐   _____
E ☐   _____
N ☐   _____ | Activities
Done: Initials
D ☐   _____
E ☐   _____
N ☐   _____ |
| | Activity Intolerance | Patient tolerates activity progression and limitations | Minimize over exertion | Educate patient on bedrest and activity restrictions post procedure | Patient tolerates first ambulation after bedrest then up ad lib |
| | | | Activities
Done: Initials
D ☐   _____
E ☐   _____
N ☐   _____ | Activities
Done: Initials
D ☐   _____
E ☐   _____
N ☐   _____ | Activities
Done: Initials
D ☐   _____
E ☐   _____
N ☐   _____ |

SHORT-TERM
INTERDISCIPLINARY
PLAN OF CARE
PCI

**ABBOTT
NORTHWESTERN
HOSPITAL**
Allina Hospitals & Clinics

Page 2 of 6
form#
REV. 04/2003

PATIENT LABEL

Figure 2–1. (Continued)

Short-term – Interdisciplinary Plan of Care for: PCI

Time of Discharge	INTERVENTIONS		Outcome/Goal Evaluation
	Day 2 Post-PCI (if needed)	Day 3 Post-PCI (if needed)	
Referral completed,if needed Appropriate facilities aware of transfer, if appropriate Patient has filled prescriptions or plans to fill independently Patient has a safe ride home			☐ Met Date_____ Initials _____ ☐ Not Met Date_____ Initials _____ **Plan at D/C:**
Activities Done: Initials D ☐ _____ E ☐ _____ N ☐ _____	Activities Done: Initials D ☐ _____ E ☐ _____ N ☐ _____	Activities Done: Initials D ☐ _____ E ☐ _____ N ☐ _____	
Review Discharge folder and instructions			☐ Met Date_____ Initials _____ ☐ Not Met Date_____ Initials _____ **Plan at D/C:**
Activities Done: Initials D ☐ _____ E ☐ _____ N ☐ _____	Activities Done: Initials D ☐ _____ E ☐ _____ N ☐ _____	Activities Done: Initials D ☐ _____ E ☐ _____ N ☐ _____	
Patient tolerates walking 5 min/ 5X day. Patient will climb stairs,if applicable			☐ Met Date_____ Initials _____ ☐ Not Met Date_____ Initials _____ **Plan at D/C:**
Activities Done: Initials D ☐ _____ E ☐ _____ N ☐ _____	Activities Done: Initials D ☐ _____ E ☐ _____ N ☐ _____	Activities Done: Initials D ☐ _____ E ☐ _____ N ☐ _____	

SHORT-TERM INTERDISCIPLINARY PLAN OF CARE PCI

ABBOTT NORTHWESTERN HOSPITAL
Allina Hospitals & Clinics

Page 3 of 6
form#
REV. 04/2003

PATIENT LABEL

Figure 2–1. (Continued)

Interdisciplinary Education Record

☐ See patient profile for education needs   ☐ See SCD for education record

READINESS TO LEARN	PARTICIPANTS	METHOD/MATERIALS	EVIDENCE OF LEARNING
W = willing to learn N = needs encouragement R = refusal	D = disoriented A = anxious L = LOC inadequate	P = patient O = other* F = family I = interpreter* * identify in comments	AV = audio/visual P = phone call C = class V = verbal D = demonstration W = written	N = needs additional teaching P = performs routinely V = verbalizes understanding R = returns accurate demonstration * = see interdisciplinary notes

Date	Initials/ Discipline	Readiness To Learn	Par- ticipants	Method/ Materials	Educational Needs	Evidence of Learning/ Date/ Initials	Evidence of Learning/ Date/ Initials	Evidence of Learning/ Date/ Initials
					Pre-op Teaching			
					Illness/Condition			
					Medication			
					Diet			
					Food-Drug Interactions			
					Equipment			
					Pain Management			
					Self-Care Skills			
					Mobility			

SHORT-TERM
INTERDISCIPLINARY
PLAN OF CARE
PCI

ABBOTT
NORTHWESTERN
HOSPITAL
Allina Hospitals & Clinics

Page 6 of 6
form#
REV. 04/2003

PATIENT LABEL

Figure 2–1. (Continued)

placing intravenous (IV) access in the groin site or lower limbs as this impedes mobility and potentially blood flow, and can thus increase risk of DVT. Ensure adequate hydration. Many patients may also be placed on low-dose heparin or enoxaparin protocols as a preventative measure.

Hospital-Acquired Infections

Critically ill patients are especially vulnerable to infection during their stay in the critical care unit. It is estimated that 20% to 60% of critically ill patients acquire some type of infection. In general, intensive care units (ICUs) have the highest incidence of hospital-acquired, or nosocomial, infections due to the high use of multiple invasive devices and the frequent presence of debilitating underlying diseases. Hospital-acquired infections increase the patient's LOS and hospitalization costs, and can markedly increase mortality rates depending on the type and severity of the infection and the underlying disease. Although urinary tract infections are the most common hospital-acquired infections in the critical care setting, hospital-acquired pneumonias are the second most common infection and the most common cause of mortality from infections. Details of specific risk factors and control measures for the prevention of hospital acquired pneumonias are presented in Chapter 10, Respiratory System. Other frequent infections include urinary tract, bloodstream, and surgical site infections. It is imperative for critical care practitioners to understand the processes that contribute to these potentially lethal infections and their role in preventing these untoward events.

Prevention

Standard precautions, sometimes referred to as "universal precautions" or "body substance isolation," refer to the basic precautions that are to be used on all patients, regardless of their diagnosis. The general premise of standard precautions is that all body fluids have the potential to transmit any number of infectious diseases, both bacterial and viral. Certain basic principles must be followed to prevent direct and indirect transmission of these organisms. Nonsterile examination gloves should be worn when performing venipuncture, touching nonintact skin or mucous membranes of the patient or for touching any moist body fluid. This includes urine, stool, saliva, emesis, sputum, blood, and any type of drainage. Other personal protective equipment, such as face shields and protective gowns, should be worn whenever there is a risk of splashing body fluids into the face or onto clothing. This protects not only the health care worker, but also prevents any contamination that may be transmitted between patients via the caregiver. Specific control measures are aimed at specific routes of transmission. See Table 2–1 for examples of isolation precaution categories and the types of infections for which they are instituted.

Other interventions to prevent nosocomial infections are similar regardless of the site. Maintaining glycemic con-

TABLE 2–1. ISOLATION CATEGORIES AND RELATED INFECTION EXAMPLES

Isolation Categories	Infection Examples When Used
Standard precautions	Used with care of all patients
Airborne precautions	Tuberculosis, measles (rubeola), varicella
Contact precautions	*Nisseria meningitidis, Haemophilus influenza,* pertussis, mumps
Droplet precautions	Vancomycin-resistant enterococcus (VRE), Methicillin-resistant *Staphylococcus aureus* (MRSA), *Clostridium difficile,* scabies, impetigo, respiratory syncitial virus (RSV)

trol in both diabetic and nondiabetic patients may help to decrease the patient's risk for developing an infection. Invasive lines or tubes should never remain in place longer than absolutely necessary and never simply for staff convenience. Avoid breaks as much as possible in systems such as urinary drainage systems, IV lines, and ventilatory tubing. Use of aseptic technique is essential if breaks into these systems are necessary. Hand washing before and after any manipulation of invasive lines is essential.

The current recommendation from the Centers for Disease Control and Prevention (CDC) is that peripheral IV lines remain in place no longer than 72 to 96 hours. There is no standard recommendation for routine removal of central venous catheters when required for prolonged periods. If the patient begins to show signs of sepsis that could be catheter related, these catheters should be removed. More important than the length of time the catheter is in place is how carefully the catheter was inserted and cared for while in place. All catheters that have been placed in an emergency situation should be replaced as soon as possible or within 48 hours. Dressings should be kept dry and intact and changed at the first signs of becoming damp, soiled, or loosened. IV tubing should be changed no more frequently than every 72 hours, with the exception of tubing for blood, blood products, or lipid-based products, which are changed every 24 hours.

Strategies to prevent hospital-acquired pneumonia in critically ill patients include the following for patients at high risk of aspiration, which is the primary risk factor: maintain the head of the bed at $\geq 30°$; use of a special endotracheal tube (ET), which removes secretions from above the ET cuff; assess residual volumes during enteral feeding and adjust feeding rates accordingly; and wash hands before and after contact with patient secretions or respiratory equipment.

One of the most important defenses to preventing infection, though, is hand washing. *Hand washing* is defined by the CDC as vigorous rubbing together of lathered hands for 15 seconds followed by a thorough rinsing under a stream of running water. Particular attention should be paid around rings and under fingernails. It is best to keep natural fingernails well trimmed and unpolished. Cracked nail polish is a good place for microorganisms to hide. Artificial fingernails should not be worn in any health care setting because they are virtually impossible to clean without a nail brush and vigorous scrubbing. Hand washing should be performed prior to donning exam gloves to carry out patient care activities and after removing exam gloves. Washing should occur any time bare hands become contaminated with any wet body fluid and should be done before the body fluid dries. Once it dries, microorganisms begin to colonize the skin, making it more difficult to remove them. Use of alcohol-based waterless cleansers are convenient and effective when no visible soiling or contamination has occurred.

Dry, cracked skin, a long-standing problem associated with hand washing, has new significance with the emergence of blood-borne pathogens. Frequent hand washing, especially with antimicrobial soap, can lead to extremely dry skin. The frequent use of latex exam gloves has been associated with increased sensitivities and allergies, causing even more skin breakdown. All of this skin breakdown can put the health care provider at risk for blood-borne pathogen transmission, as well as for colonization or infection with bacteria. Attention to skin care is extremely important for the critical care practitioner who is using antimicrobial soap and latex gloves frequently. Lotions and emollients should be used to prevent skin breakdown. If skin breakdown does occur, the employee health nurse should be consulted for possible treatment or work restriction until the condition resolves.

Skin Breakdown

Skin breakdown is a major risk with critically ill patients due to immobility, poor nutrition, invasive lines, surgical sites, poor circulation, edema, and incontinence issues. Skin can become very fragile and easily tear. Pressure ulcers can start to occur in as little as 2 hours. Healthy people are constantly repositioning themselves, even in their sleep, to relieve areas of pressure. Critically ill patients who cannot reposition themselves rely on caregivers to assist them. Pay particular attention to pressure points that are most prone to developing breakdown, namely, heels, elbows, coccyx, and occiput. Also be cognizant of equipment that may contribute to breakdown such as ET stabilizers and even bed rails if patients are positioned in constant contact with them. As the patient's condition changes, so does the risk of developing a pressure ulcer. Assessing the patient's risk routinely with a risk assessment tool alerts the caregiver to increasing or decreasing risk and therefore potential changes in interventions.

There are many simple interventions to keep skin intact: reposition the patient minimally every 2 hours, particularly if they are not spontaneously moving; use pressure-reduction mattresses on all critically ill patients; elevate heels off the bed using pillows placed under the calves; consider elbow pads; avoid long periods of sitting in a chair without reposition; inflatable cushions (donuts) should never be used for either the sacrum or the head because they can actually cause increases in pressure on surrounding skin surfaces; and use a skin care protocol with ointment barriers for patients experiencing incontinence to prevent skin denudement.

Sleep Pattern Disturbance

All critically ill patients experience altered sleep patterns. Sleep is a problem for patients because of the pain and anxiety of a critical illness within an environment that is inundated with the life-saving activities of health care providers. Table 2–2 identifies the many reasons for patients to experience sleep deprivation. The priority of sleep in the hierarchy of patient needs is often perceived to be low by clinicians. This contradicts patients' own statements about the critical care experience. Patients complain about lack of sleep as a major stressor along with the discomfort of unrelieved pain. The vicious cycle of undertreated pain, anxiety, and sleeplessness continues unless clinicians intervene to break the cycle with simple, but essential, interventions individualized to each patient.

Noise, lights, and frequent patient interruptions are common in many critical care settings, with staff able to "tune out" the disturbances after they have worked in the setting for even a short period of time. Subjecting patients to these ICU environmental stimuli and interruptions to rest/sleep quickly can lead to sleep deprivation. Psychological changes in sleep deprivation include confusion, irritability, and agitation. Physiologic changes include depressed immune and respiratory systems and a decreased pain threshold.

Enhancing patients' sleep potential in the critical care setting involves knowledge of how the environment affects the patient and where to target interventions to best promote sleep and rest. A nighttime sleep protocol where patients are

TABLE 2–2. FACTORS CONTRIBUTING TO SLEEP DISTURBANCES IN CRITICAL CARE

Illness
- Metabolic changes
- Underlying diseases (e.g., cardiovascular disease, chronic obstructive pulmonary disease)
- Pain
- Anxiety, fear
- Delirium

Medications
- Beta-blockers
- Bronchodilators
- Benzodiazepines
- Narcotics

Environment
- Noise
- Staff conversations
- Television/radio
- Equipment alarms
- Frequent care interruptions
- Lighting
- Lack of usual bedtime routine
- Room temperature
- Uncomfortable sleep surface

TABLE 2–3. EVIDENCE-BASED PRACTICE: SLEEP PROMOTION IN CRITICAL CARE

- Assess patient's usual sleep patterns[a]
- Minimize effects of underlying disease process as possible (e.g, reduce fever, eliminate pain, minimize metabolic disturbances)[a]
- Avoid medications that disturb sleep patterns[a,b,c,d]
- Mimic patients' usual bedtime routine as able[a]
- Minimize environmental impact on sleep as possible[a]
- Utilize complementary and alternative therapies to promote sleep as appropriate[a]

Source: Compiled from [a]Richards, Benham, and DeClerk (1997), [b]Betts and Alvord (1985), [c]Espinoza and co-workers (1987), and [d]Mulloy and McNicholas (1992).

closely monitored but untouched from 1 to 5 A.M. is an excellent example of eliminating the hourly disturbances to the critically ill. Encouraging blocks of time for sleep and careful assessment of the quantity and quality of sleep are important to patient well-being. The middle-of-the-night bath should not be a standard of care for any patient. Table 2–3 details basic recommendations for sleep assessment, protecting or shielding the patient from the environment, and modifying the internal and external environments of the patient. When these activities are incorporated into standard practice routines, critically ill patients receive optimal opportunity to achieve sleep.

Psychosocial Impact

Basic Tenets

Keys to maintaining psychological integrity during a critical illness include keeping stressors at a minimum; encouraging family participation in care; promoting a proper sleep–wake cycle; encouraging communication, questions, and honest and positive feedback; empowering the patient to participate in decisions as appropriate; providing patient and family education about unit expectations and rules, procedures, medications, and the patient's physical condition; ensuring pain relief and comfort; and providing continuity of care providers. It is also important to have the patient's usual sensory and physical aids available, such as glasses, hearing aids, and dentures, as they may help to prevent confusion. Encourage the family to bring something familiar or personal from home, such as a family or pet picture.

Delirium

Delirium is evidenced by disorientation, confusion, perceptual disturbances, restlessness, distractibility, and sleep–wake cycle disturbances (see the delirium assessment tool, Figure 12–2). Due to the nature of most ICUs, it is the rare patient that is not at risk for development of confusion. Causes of confusion are usually multifactorial and include metabolic disturbances, polypharmacy, immobility, infections (particularly urinary tract and upper respiratory infections), dehydration, electrolyte imbalances, sensory impairment, and

environmental challenges. Treatment of delirium is a challenge and so prevention is ideal. Delirium is most common in postsurgical and elderly patients and is the most common cause of disruptive behavior in the critically ill. Often mislabeled "ICU psychosis," delirium is not a psychosis. Sensory overload is a common risk factor that contributes to delirium in the critically ill. Medications that also may play a role in instigating delirium include prochlorperazine, diphenhydramine, famotidine, benzodiazepines, opioids, and antidysrhythmic medications.

Medication for managing delirious behavior is best reserved for those cases in which behavioral interventions have failed. Sedative-hypnotics and anxiolytics may have precipitated the delirium and can exacerbate the sleep–wake cycle disturbances, causing more confusion. The agitated patient may require low-dose neuroleptics or short-acting benzodiazepines. Restraints are discouraged because they tend to increase agitation.

External stimulation should be minimized and a quiet, restful well-lit room maintained during the day. Consistency in care providers is also important. Repeating orientation cues minimizes fear and confusion; for example, "Good morning Bill, my name is Sue. It's Monday morning in April and you are in the hospital. I'm a nurse and will stay here with you." Background noise from a television or radio often increases anxiety as the patient has trouble processing the noise and content. Explain all procedures and tests concretely. Introduce one idea at a time, slowly, and have the patient repeat the information. Repeat and reinforce as often as needed.

If the patient demonstrates a paranoid element in his or her delirium, avoid confrontation and remain at a safe distance. Accept bizarre statements calmly, with a nod, but without agreement. Explain to the family that the behaviors are symptoms that will most likely resolve with time, resumption of normal sleep patterns, and medication. Delirious patients usually remember the events, thoughts, conversations, and provider responses that occur during delirium. The recovered patients may be embarrassed and feel guilty if they were combative during their illness.

Depression

Depression occurring with a medical illness affects the long-term recovery outcomes by lengthening the course of the illness and increasing morbidity and mortality. Risk factors that predispose for depression with medical disorders include social isolation, recent loss, pessimism, financial pressures, history of mood disorder, alcohol or substance abuse/withdrawal, previous suicide attempts, and pain.

Educating the patient and family about the temporary nature of most depressions during critical illness assists in providing reassurance that this is not an unusual phenomenon. Severe depressive symptoms often respond to pharmacologic intervention, so a psychiatric consult may be warranted. Keep in mind that it may take several weeks for antidepressants to reach their full effectiveness. If you suspect a person is depressed, ask directly. Allow the patient to initiate conversation. If negative distortions about illness and treatment are communicated, it is appropriate to correct, clarify, and reassure with realistic information to promote a more hopeful outcome. Consistency in care providers promotes trust in an ongoing relationship and enhances recovery.

A patient who has attempted suicide or is suicidal can be frightening to hospital staff. Staff are often uncertain of what to say when the patient says, "I want to kill myself . . . my life no longer has meaning." Do not avoid asking if the person is feeling suicidal; you do not promote suicidal thoughts by asking the question. Many times the communication of feeling suicidal is a cover for wanting to discuss fear, pain, or loneliness. A psychiatric referral is recommended for further evaluation and intervention.

Anxiety

Medical disorders can cause anxiety and panic-like symptoms, which are distressing to the patient and family and may exacerbate the medical condition. Treatment of the underlying medical condition may decrease the concomitant anxiety. Both pharmacologic and nonpharmacologic interventions can be helpful in managing anxiety during critical illness. Pharmacologic agents for anxiety are discussed in Chapters 6 and 7. Goals of pharmacologic therapy are to titrate the drug dose so the patient can remain cognizant and interactive with staff, family, and environment; complement pain control; and assist in promoting sleep. There are also a variety of nonpharmacologic interventions to decrease or control anxiety:

- *Breathing techniques:* Breathing techniques target somatic symptoms and include deep and slow abdominal breathing patterns. It is important to demonstrate and do the breathing with patients, as their heightened anxiety decreases their attention span. Practicing this technique may decrease anxiety and promote synchrony for patients whom you anticipate may need ventilator support.
- *Muscle relaxation:* Reduce psychomotor tension with muscle relaxation. Again, the patient will most likely be unable to cue himself or herself, so this is an excellent opportunity for the family to participate as the cuing partner. Cuing might be, "The mattress under your head, elbow, heel, and back feels heavy against your body, press harder, and then try to drift away from the mattress as you relax." Commercial relaxation tapes are available but are not as useful as the cuing by a familiar voice.
- *Imagery:* Interventions targeting cognition, such as imagery techniques, depend on the patient's capacity for attention, memory, and processing. Visualization imagery involves recalling a pleasurable, relaxing situation. For example, a hot bath, lying on a warm beach, listening to waves, or hearing birds sing. Guided imagery and hypnosis are additional therapies, but require some competency to be effective; thus, a referral is suggested. Patients who practice meditation as an alternative for stress control should be encouraged to continue, but the environment may need modification to optimize the effects.
- *Preparatory information:* Providing the patient and family with preparatory information is extremely helpful in controlling anxiety. Allowing the patient and family to control some aspects of the illness process, even if only minor aspects of care, can be anxiolytic.
- *Distraction techniques:* Distraction techniques can also interrupt the anxiety cycle. Methods for distracting can be listening to familiar music or humorous tapes, watching videos, or counting backward from 200 by 2 rapidly.
- *Use of previous coping methods:* Identify how the patient and family have dealt with stress and anxiety in the past and suggest that approach if feasible. Supporting previous coping techniques may well be adaptive.

PATIENT AND FAMILY EDUCATION

Patient and family education in the critical care environment is essential to providing information regarding diagnosis, prognosis, treatments, and procedures. In addition, education provides patients and family members a mechanism by which fears and concerns can be minimized and confronted so that they can become active members in the decisions made about care.

Providing patient and family education in critical care is challenging; multiple barriers (e.g., environmental factors, patient stability, patient and family anxiety) must be overcome, or adapted, to provide this essential intervention. The importance of education, coupled with the barriers common in critical care, necessitates that education be a continuous ongoing process engaged in by all members of the team.

Education in the critical care setting is most often done informally, rather than in traditional formal settings (e.g., classrooms). Education of the patient and family is often subtle, occurring with each interaction between the patient, family, and members of the health care team.

Assessment of Learning Readiness

Assessment of the patient's and family's learning needs should focus primarily on learning readiness. *Learning readiness* refers to that moment in time when the learner is able to comprehend and synthesize the shared information. Without learning readiness, teaching may not be useful. Questions to assess learning readiness are listed in Table 2–4.

TABLE 2–4. ASSESSMENT OF LEARNING READINESS

Generic Principles

- Do the patient and the family have questions about the diagnosis, prognosis, treatments, or procedures?
- What do the patient and the family desire to learn about?
- What is the knowledge level of the individuals being taught? What do they already know about the issues that will be taught?
- What is their current situation (condition and environment) and have they had any prior experience in a similar situation?
- Does the patient or the family have any communication barriers (e.g., language, illiteracy, culture, listening/comprehension deficits)?

Special Considerations in Critical Care

- Does the patient's condition allow you to assess this information from them (e.g., physiological/psychological stability)?
- Is the patient's support system/family/significant other available or ready to receive this information?
- What environmental factors (including time) present as barriers in the critical care unit?
- Are there other members of the health care team who may possess vital assessment information?

Strategies to Address Patient and Family Education

Prior to teaching, the information gathered in the assessment is prioritized and organized into a format that is meaningful to the learner (Table 2–5). Next, the outcome of the teaching is established along with appropriate content, and then a decision should be made about how to share the information. The next step is to teach the patient, family, and significant others (Table 2–6). Although this phase often appears to be the easiest, it is actually the most difficult. It is crucial during the communication of the content, regardless of the type of

TABLE 2–5. PRINCIPLES FOR TEACHING PLANS

Generic Principles

- Establish the outcome of the teaching.
- Determine what content needs to be taught, given the assessment.
- Identify what support systems are in place to support your educational efforts (e.g., unit leadership, education department, standardized teaching plans, teaching materials such as pamphlets, brochures, videos).
- Familiarize yourself with the content and teaching materials.
- Contact resources to clarify and provide consistency in information and to also provide additional educational support and follow-up.
- Determine the most appropriate teaching strategy (video, written materials, discussion) and to whom (patient or family) it should be directed.

Special Considerations in Critical Care

- Plan the teaching strategy *carefully*. Patients and families in the critical care environment are stressed and an overload of information adds to their stress. When planning education, consider content and amount based on the assessment of the patient, nature, and severity of the patient's illness, availability of significant others, and existing environmental barriers.

TABLE 2–6. PRINCIPLES FOR EDUCATIONAL SESSIONS

Generic Principles

- Consider the time needed to convey both the information and support system availability.
- Consider the situation the patient is currently experiencing. Postponement may need to be considered.
- Be aware of the amount of content and the patient's and the family's ability to process the information.
- Be sensitive in the delivery of the information. Make sure it is conveyed at a level that the patient and the family can understand.
- Refer to, and involve, resources as appropriate.
- Convey accurate and precise information. Make sure this information is consistent with previous information given to the patient.
- Listen carefully and solicit feedback during the session to guide the discussion and clarify any potential misinterpretations.

Special Considerations in Critical Care

- Keep the time frame and content as set. Education must be episodic due to the nature of the patient's condition and the environment.
- Provide repetition of the information. Stress and the critical care environment can alter comprehension: for this reason repetition is necessary.
- Avoid details unless the patient or family specifically requests them. Often, details can cloud the information given. Details can come later in the hospitalization, if necessary.

communication vehicle used (video, pamphlet, discussion) to listen carefully to the needs expressed by the learner and to provide clear and precise responses to those needs.

Outcome Measurement

Following educational interventions, it is essential to determine if the educational outcomes have been achieved (Table 2–7). Even if the outcome appears to have been achieved, it is not unusual that the learners may not retain all the information. Patients and families experience a great deal of stress while in the critical care environment; reinforcement is often necessary and should be anticipated.

TABLE 2-7. PRINCIPLES FOR OUTCOME MONITORING

Generic Principles

- Measure the outcome. Was the outcome met? Was the outcome unmet?
- Communicate the outcome verbally and in a written format to other members of the health care team.
- Provide necessary follow-up and reinforcement of the teaching.
- Make referrals that may have been identified in or as a result of patient and family education.
- Evaluate the teaching process for barriers or problems, and then address those areas and be aware of these for future interactions.

Special Considerations in Critical Care

- Recognize that repetition of information is the rule, not the exception. Be prepared to repeat information previously given, many times if necessary.

FAMILY-FOCUSED CARE

There is a strong evidence base to support that family presence and involvement in the ICU aids in the recovery of critically ill patients. Family members can help patients cope, reduce anxiety, and provide a resource for the patient. Families, however, also need support in maintaining their strength and having needs met to be able to function as a positive influence for the patient, rather than having a negative impact.

Developing a partnership with the family and a trusting relationship is in everyone's best interest so optimal functioning can occur. Research shows that there can frequently be disagreement between the nurse and family perspectives about the type or priorities of family needs. Therefore, it is important to discuss family needs and perceptions directly with each family and tailor interventions based on those needs (Table 2–8). Research has consistently identified five major areas of family needs:

- *Receiving assurance:* Family members need reassurance that the best possible care is being given to the patient. This instills confidence and a sense of security for the family. It can also assist in either maintaining hope or can be helpful in redefining hope to a more realistic image when appropriate.
- *Remaining near the patient:* Family members need to have consistent access to their loved one. Of primary importance to the family is the unit visiting policy. Specifics to be discussed include the number of visitors allowed at one time, age restrictions, times if not flexible or open, and how to gain access to the unit (Table 2–9). There is increasing evidence to support the presence of a family member with the patient during invasive procedures, as well as during cardiopulmonary resuscitation (CPR). Although this practice may still be controversial, family members have reported a sense of relief and gratitude at being able to remain close to the patient. It is recommended that written policies be developed through an inter-

TABLE 2–8. EVIDENCE-BASED PRACTICE: FAMILY INTERVENTIONS

Planning
- Determine what the family sees as priority needs.

Interventions
- Determine spokesperson and contact person.
- Establish optimum methods to contact and communicate with family.
- Make referrals for support services as appropriate.
- Provide information according to family needs.
- Include family in direct care.
- Provide a comfortable environment.

Evaluation
- Evaluate achievement of meeting family needs through multiple methods (e.g., feedback, satisfaction surveys, care conferences, follow-up after discharge).

Source: Adapted from Leske (1997).

TABLE 2–9. EVIDENCE-BASED PRACTICE: FAMILY VISITATION IN CRITICAL CARE

- Establish ways for families to have access to the patient (e.g., open visitation, contract visitation, unit phone numbers).
- Ask patients their preferences related to visiting.
- Promote access to patients with consistent unit policies and procedures with options for individualization.
- Prepare families for visit.
- Model interaction with patient.
- Give information about the patient condition, equipment, and technology being used.
- Monitor the response of the patient and family to visitation.

Source: Titler (1997).

disciplinary approach prior to implementing family presence at CPR or procedures.

- *Receiving information:* Communication with the patient and family should be open and honest. Clinicians should keep promises (be careful about what you promise), describe expectations, not contract for secrets, elicit preferences, apologize for inconveniences and mistakes, and maintain confidentiality. Concise, simplistic explanations without medical jargon or alphabet shorthand (e.g., PEEP, IABP) facilitates understanding. Contact interpreters, as appropriate, when language barriers exist.

Evaluate your communication by asking the patient and family for their understanding of the message you sent and its content and intent. When conflict occurs, find a private place for discussion. Avoid taking the confrontation personally. Ask yourself what is the issue and what needs to occur to reach resolution. If too much emotion is present, agree to address the issue at a later time, if possible.

It is helpful to establish a communication tree so that one family member is designated to be called if there are changes in the patient's condition. Establish a time for that person to call the unit for updates. Reassure them you are there to help or refer them to other system supports. Unit expectations and rules can be conveyed in a pamphlet for the family to refer to over time. Content that is helpful includes orientation about the philosophy of care; routines such as shift changes and physician rounds; the varied roles of personnel who work with patients; and comfort information such as food services, bathrooms, waiting areas, chapel services, transportation, and lodging. Clarify what they see and hear. Mobilize resources and include them in patient care and problem solving, as appropriate. Some critical care units invite family members to medical rounds for the discussion of their loved one. Adequate communication can decrease anxiety, increase a sense of control, and assist in improving decision making by families.

- *Being comfortable:* There should be space available in or near the ICU to meet comfort needs of the family. This should include comfortable furniture, access to phones and restrooms, and assistance with finding overnight accommodations. Encourage the family to admit when they are overwhelmed, take breaks, go to meals, rest, sleep, take care of themselves, and not to abandon members at home. Helping the family with basic comfort needs helps to decrease their distress and maintain their reserves and coping. This improves their ability to be a valuable resource for the patient.
- *Having support available:* Utilize all potential resources in meeting family needs. Relying on nursing to fulfill all family needs while they are trying to care for a critically ill patient can create tension and frustration. Assess the family for their own resources that can be maximized. Utilize hospital referrals that can assist in family support such as chaplains, social workers, and child–family life departments.

For the family, the critical care setting symbolizes a variety of hopes, fears, and beliefs that range from hope of a cure to end-of-life care. A family-focused approach can promote coping and cohesion among family members and minimize the isolation and anxiety for patients. Anticipating family needs, focusing on the present, fostering open communication, and providing information are vital to promoting psychological integrity for families. By using the event of hospitalization as a point of access, critical care clinicians assume a major role in primary prevention and assisting families to cope positively with crisis and grow from the experience.

TRANSPORTING THE CRITICALLY ILL PATIENT*

Preventing common complications and maintaining physiologic and psychosocial stability is a challenge even when in the controlled environment of the ICU. It is even more challenging when the need for transporting the critically ill patient to other areas of the hospital is necessary for diagnostic and therapeutic purposes. The decision to transport the critically ill patient out of the well-controlled environment of the critical care unit elicits a variety of responses from clinicians. It's not uncommon to hear phrases like these: "She's too sick to leave the unit!" "What if something happens en route?" "Who will take care of my other patients while I'm gone?" Responses like these underscore the clinicians' understanding of the risks involved in transporting critically ill patients.

Transporting a critically ill patient involves more than putting the patient on a stretcher and rolling him or her down the hall. Safe patient transport requires thoughtful planning, organization, and interdisciplinary communication and cooperation. The goal during transport is to maintain the same level of care, regardless of the location in the hospital. The

transfer of critically ill patients always involves some degree of risk to the patient. The decision to transfer, therefore, should be based on an assessment of the potential benefits of transfer and be weighed against the potential risks.

The reason for moving a critically ill patient is typically the need for care, technology, or specialists not available in the critical care unit. Whenever feasible, diagnostic testing or simple procedures should be performed at the patient's bedside within the critical care unit. If the diagnostic test or procedural intervention under consideration is unlikely to alter management or outcome of the patient, then the risk of transfer may outweigh the benefit. It is imperative that every member of the health care team assist in clarifying what, if any, benefit may be derived from transport.

Assessment of Risk for Complications

Prior to initiating transport, a patient's risk for development of complications during transport should be systematically assessed. The switching of life support technologies in the critical care unit to portable devices may lead to undesired physiologic changes. In addition, complications may arise from environmental conditions outside the critical care unit that are difficult to control, resulting in body temperature fluctuations or inadvertent movement of invasive devices (e.g., ET, chest tubes, IV devices). Common complications associated with transportation are summarized in Table 2–10.

Respiratory Complications

Maintaining adequate ventilation and oxygenation during transport is a challenge. Patients who are not intubated prior

TABLE 2–10. POTENTIAL COMPLICATIONS DURING TRANSPORT

Pulmonary
Hyperventilation
Hypoventilation
Airway obstruction
Aspiration
Recurrent pneumothorax
Arterial blood gas changes

Cardiovascular
Hypotension
Hypertension
Arrhythmias
Decreased tissue perfusion
Cardiac ischemia
Peripheral ischemia

Neurologic
Increased intracranial pressure
Cerebral hypoxia
Cerebral hypercarbia
Paralysis

Gastrointestinal
Nausea
Vomiting
Pain

---

*Adapted from American Association of Critical-Care Nurses: *Guidelines for the Transfer of Critically Ill Patients.* Aliso Viejo, CA: AACN; 1998.

to their transfer are at risk for developing airway obstruction. This is particularly a problem in patients with decreased levels of consciousness. Continuous monitoring of airway patency is critical to ensure rapid implementation of airway strategies, if necessary. Elective intubation prior to transport may need to be considered for patients at high risk for airway problems.

For patients who are intubated, ventilation is often maintained manually during the transport itself. Delivery of the appropriate minute ventilation is difficult, because tidal volume delivery must be estimated. Hypoventilation or hyperventilation can result in pH changes, which may lead to deficits in tissue perfusion and oxygenation. Therefore, respiratory and nursing personnel who are properly trained in the mechanisms of manual ventilation need to provide ventilation during transport. Some facilities have a portable ventilator that delivers an appropriate tidal volume during the transfer. If the patient currently is requiring positive end expiratory pressure (PEEP), the percentage of inspired oxygen (FiO_2) may need to be increased during transport to balance the loss of PEEP. Increasing the FiO_2 for any patient requiring transfer may help to avoid other complications from hypoxia. The patient's ventilator may also be transported to the destination so the patient can be placed back on the ventilator during the procedure.

Cardiovascular Complications

Whether related to their underlying disease processes or the anxiety of being taken out of a controlled environment, the potential for cardiovascular complications exists in all patients being transported. These complications include hypotension, hypertension, arrhythmias, tachycardia, ischemia, and acute pulmonary edema (heart failure). Many of these complications can be avoided by adequate patient preparation with pharmacologic agents to maintain hemodynamic stability and manage pain and anxiety. Continuous infusions should be carefully maintained during transport, with special attention given to IV lines during movement of the patient from one surface to another. Additional emergency equipment may need to be taken on the transport such as hand pumps for patients on ventricular assist devices.

Neurologic Complications

The potential for respiratory and cardiovascular changes during transport increases the risk for cerebral hypoxia, hypercarbia, and intracranial pressure (ICP) changes. Patients with high baseline ICP may require additional interventions to stabilize cerebral perfusion and oxygenation prior to transport (e.g., hyperventilation, increased PaO_2, blood pressure control). In addition, patients with suspected cranial or vertebral fractures are at high risk for neurologic damage during repositioning from bed to transport carts or diagnostic tables. Proper immobilization of the spine is imperative in these situations, as is the avoidance of unnecessary repositioning of the patient. Positioning the head in the midline position with the head of the bed elevated, when not contraindicated, may decrease the risk of increases in ICP.

Gastrointestinal Complications

Gastrointestinal (GI) complications may include nausea or vomiting, which can threaten the patient's airway, as well as cause discomfort. Premedicating patients at risk for GI upset with an H_2 blocker or an antiemetic may be helpful. For patients with large nasogastric (NG) drainage, preparations to continue NG drainage during transportation or in the destination location may be necessary.

Pain

The level of pain experienced by the patient is likely to be increased during transport. Many of the diagnostic tests and therapeutic interventions in other hospital departments are uncomfortable or painful. Anxiety associated with transport may also increase the level of pain. Additional pain medication, anxiolytic drugs, or both may be required to ensure adequate pain management during the transport process. Keeping the patient and family members well informed is also helpful in decreasing anxiety levels.

Level of Care Required During Transport

During transport, there should be no interruption in the monitoring or maintenance of the patient's vital functions. The equipment used during transport, as well as the skill level of accompanying personnel, must be equivalent with the interventions required or anticipated for the patient while in the critical care unit (Table 2–11). Intermittent and continuous monitoring of physiologic status (e.g., cardiac output and rhythm, blood pressure, oxygenation, ventilation) should continue during transport and while the patient is away from the critical care unit (Table 2–12).

Questions that need to be answered to prepare for transfer include the following:

- What is the current level of care (equipment, personnel)?
- What will be needed during the transfer or at the destination to maintain that level of care?
- What additional resources may be required during transport (e.g., pain and sedation medication)?
- Do I have all the necessary equipment needed in the event of an emergency during the transport?

If you are unsure what capabilities exist at the destination, call in advance to ask the receiving area what capabilities they have for support during the patient's time there; for example, are there adequate outlets to plug in electrical equipment rather than continuing to use battery power, do they have capability for high levels of suction pressure if needed, or what specialty instructions need to be followed in magnetic resonance imaging? Will they be ready to take the patient immediately into the procedure with no waiting?

TABLE 2–11. TRANSPORT PERSONNEL AND EQUIPMENT REQUIREMENTS

Personnel

A minimum of two people should accompany the patient.

One of the accompanying personnel should be the critical care nurse assigned to the patient or a specifically trained critical care transfer nurse. This critical care nurse should have completed a competency-based orientation and meet the described standards for critical care nurses.

Additional personnel may include a respiratory therapist, registered nurse, critical care technician, or physician. A respiratory therapist should accompany all patients requiring mechanical ventilation.

Equipment

The following minimal equipment should be available.

- Cardiac monitor/defibrillator.
- Airway management equipment and resuscitation bag of proper size and fit for the patient.
- Oxygen source of ample volume to support the patient's needs for the projected time out of the ICU, with an additional 30-minute reserve.
- Standard resuscitation drugs: epinephrine, lidocaine, atropine.
- Blood pressure cuff (sphygmomanometer) and stethoscope.
- Ample supply of the IV fluids and continuous drip medications (regulated by battery-operated infusion pumps) being administered to the patient.
- Additional medications to provide the patient's scheduled intermittent medication doses and to meet anticipated needs (e.g., sedation) with appropriate orders to allow their administration if a physician is not present.
- For patients receiving mechanical support of ventilation, a device capable of delivering the same volume, pressure, and PEEP and an Fio_2 equal to or greater than that the patient is receiving in the ICU. For practical reasons, in adults an Fio_2 of 1.0 is most feasible during transfer because this eliminates the need for an air tank and air–oxygen blender. During neonatal transfer, Fio_2 should be precisely controlled.
- Resuscitation cart and suction equipment need not accompany each patient being transferred, but such equipment should be stationed in areas used by critically ill patients and be readily available (within 1 minutes) by a predetermined mechanism for emergencies that may occur en route.

From: American Association of Critical-Care Nurses: Guidelines for the transfer of critically ill patients. Aliso Viejo, CA: AACN, 1998.

Preparation

Before transfer, the plan of care for the patient during and after transfer should be coordinated to ensure continuity of care and availability of appropriate resources (Table 2–13). The receiving units should be contacted to confirm that all preparations for the patient's arrival have been completed. Communication, both written and verbal, between team members should delineate the current status of the patient, management priorities, and the process to follow in the event of untoward events (e.g., unexpected hemodynamic instability or airway problems).

After you have assessed the patient's risk for transport complications, the patient should be prepared for transfer, both physically and mentally. As you are organizing the equipment and monitors, explain the transfer process to the patient and family. The explanation should include a description of the sensations the patient may expect, how long the procedure should last, and the role of individual members

TABLE 2–12. MONITORING DURING TRANSFER

- If technologically possible, patients being transferred should receive the same physiologic monitoring during transfer that they were receiving in the ICU.
- Minimally, all critically ill patients being transferred must have continuous monitoring of ECG and pulse oximetry and intermittent measurement and documentation of blood pressure, respiratory rate, and pulse rate.
- In addition, selected patients, based on clinical status, may benefit from monitoring by capnography; continuous measurement of blood pressure, PAP, and ICP; and intermittent measurement of CVP, Pao_2, and CO.
- Intubated patients receiving mechanical support of ventilation should have airway pressure monitored. If a transfer ventilator is used, it should have alarms to indicate disconnects or excessively high airway pressures.

From: American Association of Critical-Care Nurses: Guidelines for the transfer of critically ill patients. Aliso Viejo, CA: AACN, 1998.

of the transport team. It is important to allay any patient or family anxiety by identifying current caregivers who will accompany the patient during transport. The availability of emergency equipment and drugs and how communication is handled during transportation also may be information that will reassure the patient and family.

Transport

Once preparations are complete, the actual transfer can begin. Ensure that the portable equipment has adequate battery life to last well beyond the anticipated transfer time in case of unanticipated delays. Connect each of the portable monitoring devices prior to disconnection from the bedside equipment, if possible. This enables a comparison of hemodynamic values with the portable equipment.

Once hemodynamic pressure and noninvasive oxygenation monitors are in place and values verified, disconnect the patient from the mechanical ventilator or bedside oxygen

TABLE 2–13. PRETRANSFER COORDINATION AND COMMUNICATION

- Physician-to-physician and/or nurse-to-nurse communicating reaagrding the patient's condition and treatment preceding and following the transfer should be documented in the medical record when the management of the patient will be assumed by a different team while the patient is away from the ICU.
- The area to which the patient is being transferred (x-ray, operating room, nuclear medicine, etc.) must confirm that it is ready to receive the patient and immediately begin the procedure or test for which the patient is being transferred.
- Ancillary services (e.g., security, respiratory therapy, escort) must be notified as to the timing of the transfer and the equipment and support needed.
- The responsible physician must be notified either to accompany the patient or to be aware that the patient is out of the ICU at this time and may have an acute event requiring the physician's response to provide emergency care in another area of the hospital.
- Documentation in the medical record must include the indication for transfer, the patient's status during transfer and whether the patient is expected to return to the ICU.

From: American Association of Critical-Care Nurses: Guidelines for the transfer of critically ill patients. Aliso Viejo, CA: AACN, 1998.

AT THE BEDSIDE
▶ Risk Factors During Transport

Mr. W., a 45-year-old man, was involved in a motor vehicle accident when he fell asleep on his way home from work. Mr. W. was not wearing a seat belt, and there were no air bags in the car. His injuries included chest contusions and broken ribs from the steering wheel and lacerations of his scalp from the windshield.

He was stabilized in the emergency department with the insertion of a chest tube to relieve his left pneumothorax and placement of a pulmonary artery (PA) catheter to monitor for possible cardiac tamponade. He was then admitted to the intensive care unit. Mr. W. was assigned to one of the critical care nurses, Nancy, who had two other patients. One of these patients was mechanically ventilated, having undergone repair of an abdominal aortic aneurysm yesterday, and the other was recovering from a large anterior myocardial infarction suffered after a total hip replacement.

A chest CT had been ordered for Mr. W. Nancy was aware of the possible complications he might experience during transport: respiratory, cardiovascular, or safety compromises. Possible respiratory complications included upper airway obstruction, respiratory depression, hypoxia, or hypercarbia, especially in a patient who has head and chest trauma and whose oxygenation is already compromised. Cardiovascular risks included hypotension, tachycardia due to cardiac tamponade, and decreased tissue perfusion due to decreased cardiac output and increased tissue oxygen demand during the transfer. Anxiety was another potential complication that Nancy considered, both from the activity of transfer and the uncertainty of Mr. W.'s future.

Anticipating complications, Nancy planned ahead. She asked that Mr. W. be intubated and mechanically ventilated prior to the transport. With his respiratory status under control, Mr. W. could be safely medicated for pain and anxiety, and ultimately decrease his oxygen demand. Intubating Mr. W. electively in the controlled environment of the ICU prevented an emergency situation by eliminating the possible complications of respiratory arrest and emergency intubation.

Throughout the time away from the critical care environment, it is imperative that vigilant monitoring occur regarding the patient's response not only to the transport, but also to the procedure or therapeutic intervention. Alterations in drug administration, particularly analgesics, sedatives, and vasoactive drugs, are frequently needed during the time away from the critical care unit to maintain physiologic stability. Documentation of assessment findings, interventions, and the patient's responses should continue throughout the transport process.

Following return to the critical care unit, monitoring systems and interventions are reestablished and the patient is completely reassessed. Often, some adjustment in pharmacologic therapy or ventilator support is required following transport. Allowing for some uninterrupted time for the family to be at the patient's bedside and for patient rest is another important priority following return to the unit. Documentation of the patient's overall response to the transport situation should be included in the medical record.

Interfacility Transfers

Interfacility patient transfers, although similar to transfers within a hospital, frequently can be more challenging. The biggest differences between the two are the isolation of the patient in the transfer vehicle, limited equipment and personnel, and a high complication rate due to longer transport periods and inability to control environmental conditions (e.g., temperature, atmospheric pressure, sudden movements), which may cause physiologic instability.

The primary consideration in interfacility transfer is maintaining the same level of care provided in the critical care unit. Accordingly, the mode of transfer should be selected with this in mind. The resources available in the sending facility must be made as portable as possible and must accompany the patient. For example, intraaortic balloon pump therapy and ventilation must be continued without interruption. This requirement often challenges critical care practitioners' skills and abilities, as well as the equipment resources necessary to ensure a safe transport. Detailed information regarding the planning for interfacility transfer has been developed by multidisciplinary professional groups and is summarized in Chapter 25.

source, and begin portable ventilation and oxygenation. Assess for clinical signs and symptoms of respiratory distress and changes in ventilation and oxygenation. It may be easier to transfer the patient on the bed if it will fit in elevators and spaces in the receiving area. Check IV lines, pressure lines, monitor cables, NG tubes, chest tubes, Foley catheters, or drains of any sort to ensure proper placement during transport and to guard against accidental removal during transport.

During transport, the critical care nurse is responsible for continuous assessment of cardiopulmonary status (electrocardiograph, blood pressures, respiration, oxygenation, etc.) and interventions as required to ensure stability.

TRANSITIONING TO THE NEXT STAGE OF CARE

Planning for transitioning of the patient to the next stage of care (e.g., transfer from ICU to telemetry) should begin soon after the patient is admitted to the ICU. It involves assessing minimally where and with whom the patient lives, what external resources were being used prior to admission, and what resources are anticipated to be required on transfer out of the ICU. Complex patients require extensive preplanning in achieving a successful transition. As the patient stabilizes

AT THE BEDSIDE
▶ *Preparing for Transport*

Having recognized and addressed Mr. W.'s risk factors, his nurse Nancy organized the team for the transport of Mr. W. to CT scan, making sure another nurse was able to care for her other patients while she was off the unit. Mr. W. needed a respiratory therapist during the transport. Other members of the transport team included two transporters to help manage the equipment, open doors, and hold elevators. Nancy gathered the portable equipment and connected it to Mr. W. This included a cardiac monitor, a blood pressure monitor, a pulse oximeter, and a monitor for the PA pressures. IV lines were organized so that only essential infusions were transported with Mr. W.

Other concerns that Nancy considered included: Is there a nurse in the CT suite who can care for Mr. W. once he arrives there? How long should she expect him to be gone? Are there electrical outlets for all this equipment in CT? How long will the batteries last? Is there oxygen available in CT? Will the water seal for the chest tube hang on the bed? Will he need suction? Is there suction in the CT suite? What medicines does Mr. W. need? Does he need something for pain or his next dose of antibiotic? Will he need new IV fluids while he is gone? If he is able, does he understand the procedure that he's going to have? Where is his family? Do they know what is going on?

Fortunately for Nancy, one battery-operated machine was able to monitor pressures, cardiac rhythm, and pulse oximetry. The respiratory therapist used a portable ventilator to provide ventilation and oxygenation. A ventilator was set up in the CT suite for Mr. W. The chest tube drain fit over the rail around the bed, maintaining the water seal without suction. The Foley catheter also had a special hook on the side of the bed.

Mr. W. was understandably anxious about what was going on, as was his wife. While Nancy got all the equipment together, she talked to both of them about what to expect during the transport, as well as in the CT suite. She explained how long the procedure should last, and where Mrs. W. could wait while the procedure was in progress. She allowed Mrs. W. to stay with her husband as long as possible during the transfer.

and improves, the thought of leaving the ICU can be frightening as it is perceived as moving to a level of care where there are fewer staff to monitor the patient. Reinforce the positive aspect of planning for the transition in that it is a sign that the patient is improving and making progress.

If the patient is transferring to another institution, such as an acute or subacute rehabilitation facility, consider having the family visit the facility prior to transfer. This gives them an opportunity to meet the new caregivers, ask any questions they may have, and be a positive influence on alleviating any anxiety the patient may be experiencing about the transfer. If the transfer is internal, to another patient care unit and the patient's care is complex, consider working with the receiving unit staff in advance to inform them of the anticipated plan of care and any patient preferences. Identify a primary nurse in advance from the receiving unit, if possible, who may be able to take the time to meet the patient before the transfer. Clinical nurse specialists or nurse managers may also be able to meet the patient and family, describe the receiving unit, and act as a resource after the transfer, again giving a sense of control to the patient and family.

SUPPORTING PATIENTS AND FAMILIES DURING THE DYING PROCESS

At times, transitioning of care means planning care for the patient who is dying. Caring for the dying patient and his or her family can be a most rewarding challenge. The use of advance directives provides an avenue for discussing values and beliefs associated with dying and living. Hopefully, discussions prior to a traumatic event or critical care admission have occurred so the patient is empowered to institute stopping or continuing life support measures and has designated a surrogate decision maker. If advanced directives are in place, then advocating for those wishes and promoting comfort are primary responsibilities of clinicians. If previous discussions have not taken place, as with an unexpected traumatic accident, then requesting system resources to assist the family while you attend to the patient's critical needs is appropriate. Providing for clergy to assist with spiritual needs and rituals also can help the family to cope with the crisis.

It is important to have an awareness of your own philosophical feelings about death when caring for dying persons. Be genuine in your care, touch, and presence, and do not feel compelled to talk. Take your cue from the patient. Crying or laughing with the patient and family is an acknowledgment of humanness, an existential relationship, and a rare gift in a unique encounter.

SELECTED BIBLIOGRAPHY

Family Interventions/Visitation

Lazure LL, Baun MM: Increasing patient control of family visiting in the coronary care unit. *Am J Crit Care* 1995;4:157–164.

Leske JS: Interventions to decrease family anxiety. *Crit Care Nurse* 2002;22(6):61–65.

Leske JS: Comparison of family stresses, strengths, and outcomes after trauma and surgery. *AACN Clinical Issues: Advanced Practice in Acute and Critical Care* 2003;14(1):33–41.

MacLean SL, Guzetta CE, White C, et al: Family presence during cardiopulmonary resuscitation and invasive procedures: practices of critical care and emergency nurses. *J Emerg Nurs* 2003; 29(3):208–221.

Redley B, Beanland C, Botti M: Accompanying critically ill relatives in emergency departments. *J Adv Nurs* 2003;44(1):88–98.

Roland R, Russell J, Richards KC, Sullivan SC: Visitation in critical care: Processes and outcomes of a performance improvement initiative. *J Nurs Care Quality* 2001;15(2):18–26.

Simpson T: Critical care patients' perceptions of visits. *Heart Lung* 1991;20:681–688.

York NL: Implementing a family presence protocol option. *Dimensions Crit Care Nurs* 2004;23(2):84–88.

Infection Control

Bennett JV, Brockmann PS (eds): *Hospital Infections,* 3rd ed. Boston: Little, Brown; 1994.

Soule BM (ed): *The APIC Curriculum for Infection Control Practice,* vols. 1–3. Dubuque, IA: Kendall/Hunt; 1983.

Wenzel RP (ed): *Prevention and Control of Nosocomial Infections,* 2nd ed. Baltimore: Williams & Wilkins; 1993.

Multidisciplinary Plans of Care

Renholm M, Leino-Kilpi H, Suominen T: Critical pathways. A systematic review. *J Nurs Admin* 2002;32(4):196–202.

Wall DK: *Critical Pathway Development Guide: A Team-Oriented Approach for Developing Critical Pathways.* Chicago: Precept Press; 1998.

Patient and Family Education

Redman BK: *The Process of Patient Education,* 7th ed. St. Louis, MO: CV Mosby-Year Book; 1993.

Smith CE: *Patient Education: Nurses in Partnership with Other Health Professionals.* New York: Grune & Stratton; 1987.

Psychological Problems

Barry PD: *Psychosocial Nursing: Care of Physically Ill Patients and Their Families,* 3rd ed. Philadelphia: JB Lippincott; 1996.

ICU Delirium and Cognitive Impairment Study Group. Vanderbilt University. Accessed July 23, 2004. Available from URL: www.icudelirium.org/delirirum//

Justic M: Does "ICU psychosis" really exist? *Crit Care Nurse* 2000;20(3):28–37.

Ely W, Margolin R, Francis J, et al. Evaluation of delirium in critically ill patients: Validation of the Confusion Assessment Method for the Intensive Care Unit (CAM-ICU). *Crit Care Med* 2001;29:1370–1379.

Skin Breakdown

Carlson EV, Kemp MG, Shott S: Predicting the risk of pressure ulcers in critically ill patients. *Am J Crit Care* 1999;8(4):262–269.

Sleep Deprivation

Beck-Little R, Weinrich SP: Assessment and management of sleep disorders in the elderly. *J Gerontol Nurs* 1998;24:24–29.

Honkers VL: Sleep deprivation in critical care units. *Crit Care Nurs Q* 2003;26(3):179–189.

Kahn DM, Cook TE, Carlisle CC, Nelson DL, Kramer NR, Millman RP: Identification and modification of environmental noise in an ICU setting. *Chest* 1998;114:535–540.

McDowell JA, Mion LC, Lydon TJ, Inouye SK: A nonpharmacologic sleep protocol for hospitalized older patients. *J Am Geriatric Soc* 1998;46:700–705.

Richards KC: Effect of a back massage and relaxation intervention on sleep in critically ill patients. *Am J Crit Care* 1998;7:288–299.

Richards KC, Nagel C, Markie M, Elwell J, Barone C: Use of complementary and alternative therapies to promote sleep in critically ill patients. *Crit Care Nurs Clin North Am* 2003;15(3):329–340.

Richards KC, Gibson R, Overton-McCoy AL: Effects of massage in acute and critical care. *AACN Clinical Issues* 2000;11:77–96.

Richards KC: Sleep promotion in the critical care unit. *AACN Clinical Issues* 1994;5:152–158.

Simpson T, Lee ER, Cameron C: Patients' perceptions of environmental factors that disturb sleep after cardiac surgery. *Am J Crit Care* 1996;5:173–181.

Tamburri LM, DiBrienza R, Zozula R, Redeker NS: Nocturnal care interactions with patients in critical care units. *Am J Crit Care* 2004;13(2):102–112.

Walder B, Francioli D, Meyer JJ, et al: Effects of guidelines implementation in a surgical intensive care unit to control nighttime light and noise levels. *Crit Care Med* 2000;28:2242–2247.

Wallace CJ, Robins J, Alvord CS, Walker JM: The effect of earplugs on sleep measures during exposure to simulated intensive care unit noise. *Am J Crit Care* 1999;8:210–219.

Zimmerman L, Nieveen J, Barnason S, Schmaderer M: The effects of music interventions on postoperative pain and sleep in coronary artery bypass graft (CABG) patients. *Scholarly Inquiry for Nursing Practice* 1996;10:153–170.

Evidence-Based Practice

Agency for Healthcare Research and Quality (AHRQ): *Prevention of Venous Thromboembolism After Injury.* Evidence Report/Technology Assessment Number 22. Silver Spring, MD: AHRQ; 2001.

AHRQ: *Clinical Practice Guidelines. Pressure Ulcers in Adults: Prediction and Prevention.* Accessed July 23, 2004 from URL: www.ahrq.gov

AACN VAP Practice Alert. Aliso Viejo, CA: AADN; 2004. Available from URL: http://www.aacn.org

American Association of Critical-Care Nurses (AACN): *Guidelines for the Transfer of Critically Ill Patients.* Aliso Viejo, CA: AACN; 1998.

Betts TA, Alvord C: Beta-blockers and sleep: A controlled trial. *Eur J Clin Pharmacol* 1985;28(Suppl):65–68.

Centers for Disease Control and Prevention (CDC): Guidelines for prevention of health-care-associated pneumonia, 2003: Recommendations of CDC and the Healthcare Infection Control Practices Advisory Committee. *MMWR* 2004;53:1–35.

CDC: Guidelines for the prevention of intravascular catheter-related infections. *MMWR* 2002;51;1–26.

CDC, Division of Healthcare Quality and Promotion: *Guidelines and recommendations. Prevention of healthcare-associated infections.* Accessed July 23, 2004 from URL: www.cdc.gov/ncidod/hip/Guide/guide.htm

Espinoza H, Antic R, Thornton AT, McEvoy RD: The effects of

aminophylline on sleep and sleep disordered breathing in patients with obstructive sleep apnea syndrome. *Am Rev Respir Dis* 1987; 136:80–84.

Leske JS: Family needs and interventions. In Chulay M, Molter NC (eds): *AACN Protocols for Practice: Creating a Healing Environment Series.* Aliso Viejo, CA: AACN; 1997.

Mulloy E, McNicholas WT: Theophylline in obstructive sleep apnea: A double-blind evaluation. *Chest* 1992;101:753–757.

Richards K, Benham G, DeClerk L: Promoting sleep in acute and critical care. In Chulay M, Molter NC (eds): *AACN Protocols for Practice: Creating a Healing Environment Series.* Aliso Viejo, CA: AACN; 1997.

Titler M: Family visitation and partnership in the critical care unit. In Chulay M, Molter NC (eds): *ACNN Protocols for Practice. Creating a Healing Environment Series.* Aliso Viejo, CA: AACN; 1997.

Interpretation and Management of Basic Cardiac Rhythms

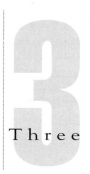

Three

Carol Jacobson

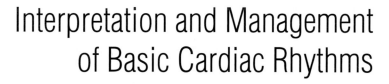

▶ Knowledge Competencies

1. Correctly identify key elements of electrocardiogram (ECG) waveforms, complexes, and intervals:
   - P wave
   - QRS complex
   - T wave
   - ST segment
   - PR interval
   - QT interval
   - RR interval
   - Rate (atrial and ventricular)

2. Compare and contrast the etiology, ECG characteristics, and management of common cardiac rhythms and conduction abnormalities:
   - Sinus node rhythms
   - Atrial rhythms
   - Junctional rhythms
   - Ventricular rhythms
   - AV blocks

3. Describe the indications for, and use of, temporary pacemakers, defibrillation, and cardioversion for the treatment of serious cardiac arrhythmias.

Continuous monitoring of cardiac rhythm in the critically ill patient is an important aspect of cardiovascular assessment. Frequent analysis of ECG rate and rhythm provides for early identification and treatment of alternations in cardiac rhythm, as well as abnormal conditions in other body systems. This chapter presents a review of basic cardiac electrophysiology and information essential to the identification and treatment of common cardiac arrhythmias. Advanced cardiac arrhythmias, as well as 12-lead ECG interpretation, are described in Chapter 18.

BASIC ELECTROPHYSIOLOGY

The sinus node is the normal pacemaker of the heart because it has the highest rate of the normal pacemaker sites. The sinus node normally fires at a regular rate of 60 to 100 beats/min. The impulse spreads from the sinus node through the atria and to the atrioventricular (AV) node, where it encounters a slight delay before it travels through the bundle of His, right and left bundle branches, and Purkinje fibers into the ventricles. The spread of this wave of depolarization through the heart gives rise to the classical surface ECG, which can be monitored continuously at the bedside.

The ECG is a graphic record of the electrical activity of the heart. Impulse formation and conduction throughout the heart produce weak electrical currents through the entire body. The difference in potential between a positive and a negative area within the body can be measured on the body surface by a *galvanometer,* an instrument consisting of a wire between the poles of an electromagnet. As current passes through the wire, the instrument is controlled by the magnetic field. The ECG machine contains a galvanometer that detects changes in surface potential, amplifies the signal, and records these body surface potential changes over time on calibrated moving paper.

By convention, if a positive electrode is placed on the side facing the advancing wave of depolarization, a positive deflection is produced (Figure 3–1A). If the poles of the galvanometer are reversed, however, a negative deflection is produced. The magnitude, or height, of the deflection represents the thickness of the muscle involved. If a positive

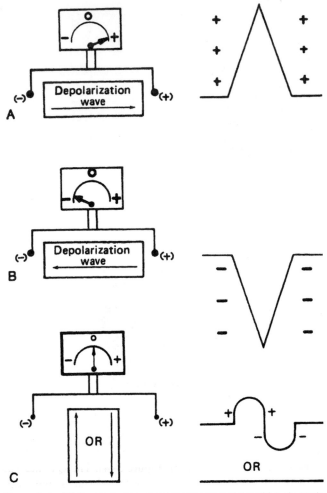

Figure 3–1. (**A**) Depolarization wave traveling toward a positive electrode results in a positive or upright deflection of the stylus. (**B**) Depolarization wave traveling away from a positive electrode results in a negative or downward deflection of the stylus. (**C**) Depolarization wave traveling in a direction that is perpendicular to the positive electrode results in a biphasic or isoelectric inscription. (*From: Gilmore SB, Woods SL: Electrocardiography and vectorcardiography. In Woods SL, Froelicher ES, Motzer SU [eds]: Cardiac Nursing, 3rd ed. Philadelphia: JB Lippincott; 1995, p. 291.*)

electrode is placed on the side from which the wave of depolarization is receding, a negative deflection results (Figure 3–1B). If an electrode is placed at right angles (perpendicular) to the wave of depolarization, a biphasic deflection or no deflection (isoelectric) occurs (Figure 3–1C).

ECG WAVEFORMS, COMPLEXES, AND INTERVALS

The ECG waves, complexes, and intervals are illustrated in Figure 3–2.

P Wave

The P wave represents atrial muscle depolarization. It is normally 2.5 mm or less in height and 0.11 second or less in duration. The voltage of positive deflections is measured from the upper portion of the baseline to the peak of the wave. The atrial repolarization (atrial T wave) is wide and of low amplitude and therefore is not seen or is buried in the QRS complex.

QRS Complex

The QRS complex (beginning of the Q wave to the end of the S wave) represents ventricular muscle depolarization. The first negative deflection is the Q wave, which is less than 0.03 second in duration and less than 25% of the R-wave amplitude; the first positive deflection is the R wave; the S wave is the first negative deflection after the R wave. The voltage of negative deflections is measured from the lower portion of the baseline to the nadir of the wave. Figure 3–3 shows examples of various QRS complex configurations. When a wave is less than 5 mm vertically, small letters (q, r, s) are used; when a wave is 5 mm or more vertically, capital letters (Q, R, S) are used. When a complex is all negative, it is called a QS complex. Not all QRS complexes have all three waveforms. The QRS complex is measured from the beginning of the Q wave, or if no Q wave is present, from the beginning of R wave, to the end of the S wave. The QRS complex is normally 0.04 to 0.10 second in duration. The QRS complex in the chest leads (V_1 to V_6) can be 0.01 to 0.02 second longer than in the limb leads.

T and U Waves

The T and U waves represent ventricular muscle repolarization. They follow the QRS complex and are usually of the same deflection as the QRS complex. If a U wave is seen, it follows the T wave. The presence of a U wave may indicate an electrolyte abnormality. It is thought to be the result of the slow repolarization of the intraventricular (Purkinje) conduction system.

ST Segment

The ST segment, which represents early repolarization of the ventricles, is from the end of the S wave (J point) to the beginning of the T wave.

PR Interval

The PR interval is measured from the beginning of the P wave to the beginning of the Q wave, or if no Q wave is present, to the beginning of the R wave, and represents the time required for the impulse to travel through the atria and conduction system to the Purkinje fibers. In adults with normal heart rates, the PR interval usually ranges from 0.12 to 0.20 second in duration. The PR segment is isoelectric and is measured from the end of the P wave to the beginning of the QRS complex.

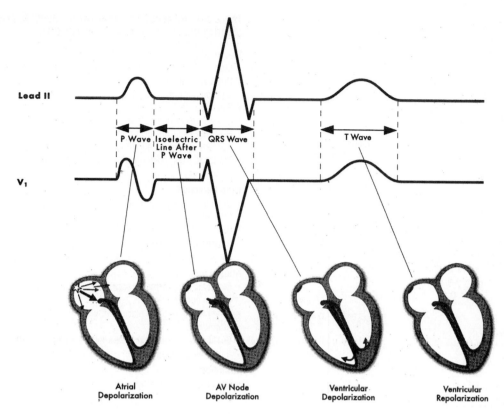

Figure 3–2. Electrocardiographic waves, complexes, and intervals in leads II and V_1.

QT Interval

The QT interval, which represents electrical systole, is measured from the beginning of the Q wave to the end of the T wave. If no Q wave is present, the beginning of the R wave is used for the QRS measurement. The QT interval varies with heart rate and must be corrected to a heart rate of 60/min (QT_c) following measurement. This correction is done by use of a nomogram (Figure 3–4). The QT interval is usually less than half the RR interval (measured from the beginning of one R wave to the beginning of the next R wave) and usually is 0.32 to 0.40 second in duration if the heart rate is 65 to 95/min. The QT_c should not exceed 0.42 second in men or 0.43 second in women. The J point is the point where the QRS complex ends and the ST segment begins.

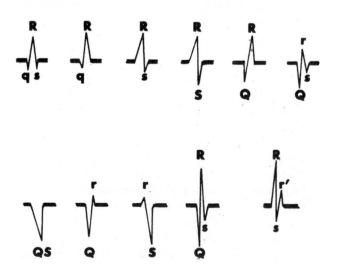

Figure 3–3. Examples of various QRS complexes and proper labeling of component waveforms. (*Source: Gilmore SB, Woods SL: Electrocardiography and vectorcardiography. In Woods SL, Froelicher ES, Motzer SU [eds]: Cardiac Nursing, 3rd ed. Philadelphia: JB Lippincott; 1995, p. 293.*)

CARDIAC MONITORING

Cardiac monitoring provides continuous observation of the patient's heart rate and rhythm and is a routine nursing procedure in all types of critical care and telemetry units as well as in emergency departments, postanesthesia recovery units, and many operating rooms. Cardiac monitoring has also become common in areas where patients receive treatments or procedures requiring conscious sedation or where the administration of certain medications could result in cardiac arrhythmias. The goals of cardiac monitoring can range from simple heart rate and basic rhythm monitoring to sophisticated arrhythmia diagnosis and ST segment monitoring for cardiac ischemia detection. Cardiac monitoring can be done using a 3-wire, 5-wire, or 10-wire cable, which connects the patient to the cardiac monitor or portable telemetry box.

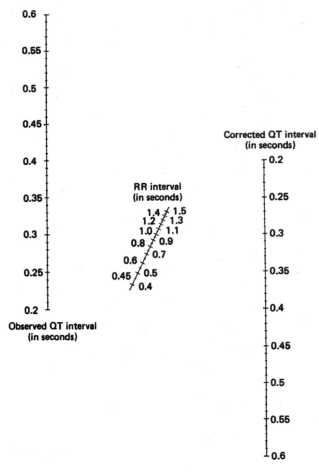

Figure 3–4. Nomogram for rate correction of QT interval. Measure the observed QT interval and the RR interval. Mark these values in the respective columns on the chart (left and middle). Place a ruler across these two points. The point at which the extension of this line crosses the third column is read as the corrected QT interval (QT$_c$). This nomogram is based on the following equation: QT$_c$ is equal to the observed QT interval divided by the square root of the RR interval. (*Source: Kissen M, et al: A nomogram for rate correction of the QT interval in the electrocardiogram. Am Heart J 1948;35:991.*)

TABLE 3–1. EVIDENCE-BASED PRACTICE: BEDSIDE CARDIAC MONITORING FOR ARRHYTHMIA DETECTION

Electrode Application
- Make sure skin is clean and dry before applying monitoring electrodes.
- Place arm electrodes on shoulder (front, top, or back) as close to where arm joins torso as possible.
- Place leg electrodes below the rib cage or on hips.
- Place V$_1$ electrode at fourth intercostal space at right sternal border.
- Place V$_6$ electrode at fifth intercostal space at left midaxillary line.
- Replace electrodes every 48 hours or more often if skin irritation occurs.
- Mark electrode position with indelible ink to ensure consistent lead placement.

Lead Selection
- Use lead V$_1$ as the primary arrhythmia monitoring lead whenever possible.
- Use lead V$_6$ if lead V$_1$ is not available.
- If using a 3-wire system, use MCL$_1$ as the primary lead and MCL$_6$ as the second choice lead.

Alarm Limits
- Set heart rate alarms as appropriate for patient's current heart rate and clinical condition.
- *Never* turn heart rate alarms off while patient's rhythm is being monitored.
- Set alarm limits on other parameters if using a computerized arrhythmia monitoring system.

Documentation
- Document the monitoring lead on every rhythm strip.
- Document heart rate, PR interval, QRS width, QT interval every shift and with any significant rhythm change.
- Document rhythm strip with every significant rhythm change:
  - Onset and termination of tachycardias.
  - Symptomatic bradycardias or tachycardias.
  - Conversion into or out of atrial flutter or atrial fibrillation.
  - All rhythms requiring immediate treatment.
- Place rhythm strips flat on page (avoid folding or winding strips into chart).

Transporting Monitored Patients
- Continue cardiac monitoring using a portable, battery-operated monitor-defibrillator if patient is required to leave a monitored unit for diagnostic or therapeutic procedures.
- Monitored patients must be accompanied by a health care provider skilled in ECG interpretation and defibrillation during transport.

Sources: Compiled from Jacobson (2005), Drew, Califf, Funk, and associates (2004), and the American Association of Critical Care Nurse (2004).

The choice of monitoring lead is based on the goals of monitoring in a particular patient population and by the patient's clinical situation. Because arrhythmias are the most common complication of ischemic heart disease and myocardial infarction (MI), monitoring for arrhythmia diagnosis is a priority in these patients. Although many arrhythmias can be recognized in any lead, research consistently shows that ventricular lead 1 (V$_1$) and V$_6$, or their bipolar equivalents Modified Chest lead 1 (MCL$_1$) and MCL$_6$ are the best leads for differentiating wide QRS rhythms (Table 3–1). The QRS morphologies displayed in these leads are useful in differentiating ventricular tachycardia (VT) from supraventricular tachycardia with aberrant intraventricular conduction and for recognizing right and left bundle branch block (see Chapter 18, Advanced ECG Concepts).

Correct placement of monitoring electrodes is critical to obtaining accurate information from any monitoring lead. Most currently available bedside monitors utilize either a 3-wire or a 5-wire monitoring cable. A 5-wire system offers several advantages over the 3-wire system (Table 3–2). With a 5-wire system, it is possible to monitor more than one lead at a time and it is possible to monitor a true unipolar V$_1$ lead, which is superior to its bipolar equivalent MCL$_1$ in differentiating wide QRS rhythms. With a 5-wire system, all 12 standard ECG leads can be obtained by selecting the desired lead on the bedside monitor and moving the one chest lead to the appropriate spot on the thorax to record the precordial leads V$_1$ through V$_6$ (see Chapter 18, Advanced ECG Concepts). Figure 3–5 illustrates correct lead placement for a

TABLE 3–2. ADVANTAGES OF COMMON MONITORING LEADS

Lead	Advantages
Preferred Monitoring Leads	
V_1 and V_6 (or MCL_1 and MCL_6 if using a 3-wire system)	Differentiate between right and left bundle branch block
	Morphology clues to differentiate between ventricular beats and supraventricular beats with aberrant conduction
	Differentiate between right and left ventricular ectopy
	Differentiate between right and left ventricular pacing
	Usually shows well-formed P waves
	Placement of electrodes keeps apex clear for auscultation or defibrillation
Other Monitoring Leads	
Lead II	Usually shows well-formed P waves
Lead III or aVF	Often best lead for identification of atrial flutter waves
Lewis Lead (negative electrode at second right intercostal space, positive electrode and fourth right intercostal space)	Usually has tall, upright QRS complex on which to synchronize machine for cardioversion
	Allows identification of retrograde P waves
	Assists in diagnosis of hemiblock
	Allow identification of retrograde P waves
	Identification of atrial flutter waves
	Best limb leads for ST segment monitoring
	Often best lead to identify P waves

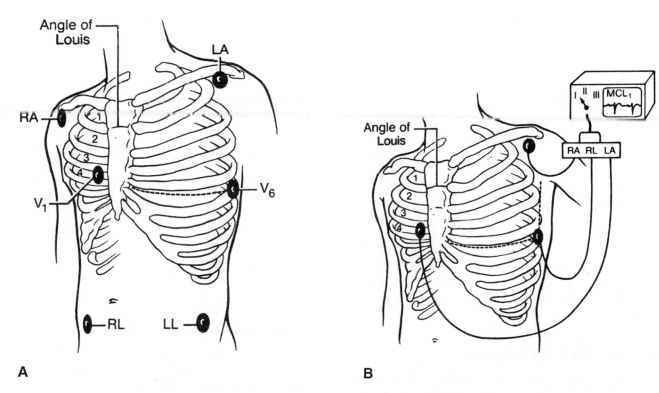

A

B

Figure 3–5. **(A)** Correct electrode placement for using a 5-wire monitoring cable. Right and left arm electrodes are placed on the shoulders and right and left leg electrodes are placed low on the thorax or on the hips. With the arm and leg electrodes placed as illustrated, leads I, II, III, aVR, aVL, and aVF can be obtained by selecting the desired lead on the bedside monitor. To obtain lead V_1 place the chest lead in the fourth intercostal space at the right sternal border and select "V" on the bedside monitor. To obtain lead V_6, place the chest lead in the fifth intercostal space at the left midaxillary line and select "V" on the bedside monitor. **(B)** Correct lead placement for obtaining MCL_1 and MCL_6 using a 3-wire lead system. Place the right arm electrode on the left shoulder; the left arm electrode in the fourth intercostal space at the right sternal border; and the left leg electrode in the fifth intercostal space at the left midaxillary line. To monitor in MCL_1, select lead I on the bedside monitor. To monitor in MCL_6, select lead II on the bedside monitor. (*Source: Adapted from Drew BJ: Bedside electrocardiogram monitoring. AACN Clinical Issues in Critical Care Nursing 1993;4:26, 28*).

5-wire system. Arm electrodes are placed on the shoulders as close as possible to where the arms join the torso. Placing the arm electrodes on the posterior shoulder keeps the anterior chest area clear for defibrillation paddles if needed, and avoids irritating the skin in the subclavicular area where an intravenous (IV) catheter might need to be placed. Leg electrodes are placed at the level of the lowest ribs on the thorax or on the hips. The desired V or precordial lead is obtained by placing the chest electrode at the appropriate location on the chest and selecting "V" on the bedside monitor. To monitor in V_1, place the chest electrode in the fourth intercostal space at the right sternal border. To monitor in V_6, place the chest electrode in the fifth intercostal space at the left midaxillary line.

When using a 3-wire monitoring system with electrodes placed in their conventional locations on the right and left shoulders and on the left hip or low thorax, leads I, II, or III can be monitored by selecting the desired lead on the bedside monitor. It is not possible to obtain a true unipolar V_1 or V_6 lead with a 3-wire system. In this case, the bipolar equivalents MCL_1 and MCL_6 can be used as substitutes for V_1 and V_6 but to obtain them requires placing electrodes in unconventional places. Figure 3–5 shows electrode placement for a 3-wire system that allows the user to monitor either MCL_1 or MCL_6. Place the right arm electrode on the left shoulder, the left arm electrode at the V_1 position (fourth intercostal space at the right sternal border), and the left leg electrode in the V_6 position (fifth intercostal space at the left midaxillary line). With electrodes in this position, select "lead I" on the monitor to obtain MCL_1 and switch to lead II on the monitor to record MCL_6.

The electrode sites on the skin should be clean, dry, and relatively flat. Shave hair, if present, and clean the skin with alcohol to remove any oils. Mildly abrade the skin with a gauze or abrading pad supplied on electrode packaging to improve transmission of the ECG signal. Apply the pregelled electrodes to the chest in the appropriate locations. Set the heart rate alarm limits based on the patient's clinical situation and current heart rate. Bedside monitoring systems have default alarms that adjust the high- and low-rate limits based on the learned heart rate. Electrodes are changed often enough to prevent skin breakdown and provide artifact-free tracings.

DETERMINATION OF THE HEART RATE

ECG paper generally moves at a speed of 25 mm/sec. Each small box horizontally is equal to 0.04 second. One large box (five small boxes) horizontally equals 0.20 second (5 × 0.04 second); one large box (five small boxes) vertically is equal to 5 mm (Figure 3–6).

Heart rate can be obtained from the ECG strip by several methods. The first, and most accurate if the rhythm is regular, is to count the number of small boxes (one small box = 0.04 second) between two R waves, and then divide that num-

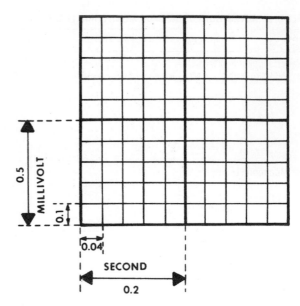

Figure 3–6. Time and voltage lines on ECG paper, at standard voltage and speed (one small box = 1 mm). Vertical measurements: 1 mm × 0.1 mV; 5 mm × 0.5 mV; 10 mm × 1 mV. Horizontal measurements: 1 mm × 0.04 second; 5 mm × 0.20 second; 25 mm × 1 second; 1500 mm × 60 seconds. (*Source: Gilmore SB, Woods SL: Electrocardiography and vectorcardiography. In Woods SL, Froelicher ES, Motzer SU [eds]: Cardiac Nursing, 3rd ed. Philadelphia: JB Lippincott; 1995, p. 291.*)

ber into 1500. There are 1500 0.04-second interval boxes in a 1-minute strip (Figure 3–7A). Another method is to count the number of large boxes (one large box = 0.20 second) between two R waves, and then divide that number into 300 or use a standardized table (Table 3–3).

The third method for computing heart rate, especially useful when the rhythm is irregular, is to count the number of RR intervals in 6 seconds and multiply that number by 10. The ECG paper is usually marked at 3-second intervals (15 large boxes horizontally) by a vertical line at the top of the paper (Figure 3–7B). The RR intervals are counted, not the QRS complexes, to avoid overestimating the heart rate.

Any of these three methods can also be used to calculate the atrial rate by using P waves instead of R waves.

DETERMINATION OF CARDIAC RHYTHM

Correct determination of the cardiac rhythm requires a systematic evaluation of the ECG. The following steps are used to determine the cardiac rhythm:

1. Calculate the atrial (P wave) rate.
2. Calculate the ventricular (QRS complex) rate.
3. Determine the regularity and shape of the P waves.
4. Determine the regularity, shape, and width of the QRS complexes.
5. Measure the PR interval.
6. Interpret the arrhythmia as described below.

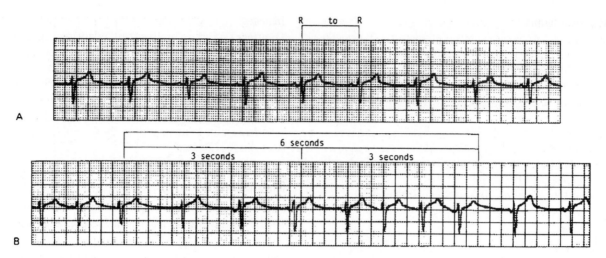

Figure 3–7. **(A)** Heart rate determination for a regular rhythm using little boxes between two R waves. One RR interval is marked at the top of the ECG paper. There are 25 little boxes between these two R waves. There are 1500 little boxes in a 60-second strip. By dividing 1500 by 25, one calculates a heart rate of 60 beats/min. Heart rate can also be determined for a regular rhythm counting large boxes between R waves. There are five large boxes between R waves. There are 300 large boxes in a 60-second strip. By dividing 300 by 5, one calculates a heart rate of 60 beats/min. **(B)** Heart rate determination for a regular or irregular rhythm using the number of RR intervals in a 6-second strip and multiplying by 10. There are seven RR intervals in this example. Multiplying by 10 gives a heart rate of 70/minute. (*Source: Gilmore SB, Woods SL: Electrocardiography and vectorcardiography. In Woods SL, Froelicher ES, Motzer SU [eds]: Cardiac Nursing, 3rd ed. Philadelphia: JB Lippincott; 1995, p. 295.*)

COMMON ARRHYTHMIAS

An *arrhythmia* is any cardiac rhythm that is not normal sinus rhythm. An arrhythmia may result from altered impulse formation or altered impulse conduction. Arrhythmias are named by the place where they originate and by their rate. Arrhythmias are grouped as follows:

1. Rhythms originating in the sinus node
2. Rhythms originating in the atria
3. Rhythms originating in the junction
4. Rhythms originating in the ventricle
5. AV blocks

The etiology, ECG characteristics, and treatment of the basic cardiac arrhythmias are presented here and summarized in Chapter 28 (Cardiac Rhythms, ECG Characteristics, and Treatment Guide).

RHYTHMS ORIGINATING IN THE SINUS NODE (Figure 3–8)

TABLE 3–3. HEART RATE DETERMINATION USING THE ELECTROCARDIOGRAM LARGE BOXES

Number of Large Boxes Between R Waves	Heart Rate (beats/min)
1	300
2	150
3	100
4	75
5	60
6	50
7	40
8	38
9	33
10	30

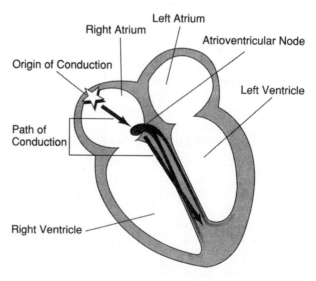

Figure 3–8. Rhythms originating in the sinus node.

Normal Sinus Rhythm

ECG Characteristics

- *Rate:* 60 to 100 beats/min
- *Rhythm:* Regular
- *P waves:* Precede every QRS complex; consistent in shape
- *PR interval:* 0.12 to 0.20 second
- *QRS complex:* 0.04 to 0.10 second
- *Conduction:* Normal through atria, AV node, bundle branches, and ventricles
- *Example of normal sinus rhythm* (Figure 3–9)

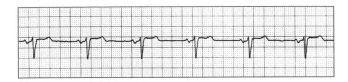

Figure 3–9. Normal sinus rhythm.

Sinus Bradycardia

All aspects of sinus bradycardia are the same as normal sinus rhythm except the rate is slower. It can be a normal finding in athletes and during sleep. Sinus bradycardia may be a response to vagal stimulation, such as carotid sinus massage, ocular pressure, or vomiting. Sinus bradycardia can be caused by inferior MI, myxedema, obstructive jaundice, uremia, increased intracranial pressure, glaucoma, anorexia nervosa, and sick sinus syndrome. Sinus bradycardia can be a response to several medications, including digitalis, beta-blockers, and some calcium channel blockers.

ECG Characteristics

- *Rate:* Less than 60 beats/min
- *Rhythm:* Regular
- *P waves:* Precede every QRS; consistent in shape
- *PR interval:* Usually normal (0.12 to 0.20 second)
- *QRS complex:* Usually normal (0.04 to 0.10 second)
- *Conduction:* Normal through atria, AV node, bundle branches, and ventricles
- *Example of sinus bradycardia* (Figure 3–10)

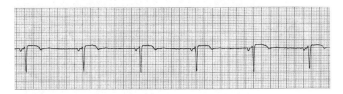

Figure 3–10. Sinus brachycardia.

Treatment

Treatment of sinus bradycardia is not required unless the patient is symptomatic. If the arrhythmia is accompanied by hypotension, confusion, diaphoresis, chest pain, or other signs of hemodynamic compromise or by ventricular ectopy, 0.5 to 1.0 mg of atropine IV is the treatment of choice. Attempts are made to decrease vagal stimulation. If the arrhythmia is due to medications, they are held until their need has been reevaluated.

Sinus Tachycardia

Sinus tachycardia is a sinus rhythm at a rate greater than 100 beats/min. Sinus tachycardia is a normal response to exercise and emotion. Sinus tachycardia that persists at rest usually indicates some underlying problem, such as fever, acute blood loss, shock, pain, anxiety, heart failure, hypermetabolic states, or anemia. Sinus tachycardia is a normal physiologic response to a decrease in cardiac output; cardiac output is the product of heart rate and stroke volume. Sinus tachycardia can be caused by the following medications: atropine, isoproterenol, epinephrine, dopamine, dobutamine, norepinephrine, nitroprusside, and caffeine.

ECG Characteristics

- *Rate:* Greater than 100 beats/min
- *Rhythm:* Regular
- *P waves:* Precede every QRS; consistent in shape; may be buried in the preceding T wave
- *PR interval:* Usually normal; may be difficult to measure if P waves are buried in T waves
- *QRS complex:* Usually normal
- *Conduction:* Normal through atria, AV node, bundle branches, and ventricles
- *Example of sinus tachycardia* (Figure 3–11)

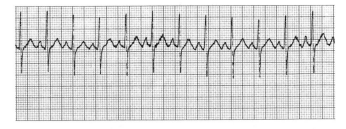

Figure 3–11. Sinus tachycardia.

Treatment

Treatment of sinus tachycardia is directed at the underlying cause. This arrhythmia is a physiologic response to a decrease in cardiac output, and it should never be ignored, especially in the cardiac patient. Because the ventricles fill with blood and the coronary arteries perfuse during diastole, persistent tachycardia can cause decreased stroke volume, decreased cardiac output, and decreased coronary perfusion secondary to the decreased diastolic time that occurs with rapid heart rates. Carotid sinus pressure may slow the heart rate temporarily and thereby help in ruling out other arrhythmias.

Sinus Arrhythmia

Sinus arrhythmia occurs when the sinus node discharges irregularly. It occurs frequently as a normal phenomenon and is commonly associated with the phases of respiration. During inspiration, the sinus node fires faster; during expiration, it slows. Digitalis toxicity may also cause this arrhythmia. Sinus arrhythmia looks like normal sinus rhythm except for the sinus irregularity.

ECG Characteristics

- *Rate:* 60 to 100 beats/min
- *Rhythm:* Irregular; phasic increase and decrease in rate, which may or may not be related to respiration
- *P waves:* Precede every QRS; consistent in shape
- *PR interval:* Usually normal
- *QRS complex:* Usually normal
- *Conduction:* Normal through atria, AV node, bundle branches, and ventricles
- *Example of sinus arrhythmia* (Figure 3–12)

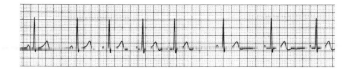

Figure 3–12. Sinus arrhythmia.

Treatment

Treatment of sinus arrhythmia usually is not necessary. If the arrhythmia is thought to be due to digitalis toxicity, then digitalis is held. Atropine increases the rate and eliminates the irregularity.

Sinus Arrest

Sinus arrest occurs when sinus node firing is depressed and impulses are not formed when expected. The result is an absent P wave at the expected time. The QRS complex is also missing, unless there is escape of a junctional or ventricular impulse (see below for description). If only one sinus impulse fails to form, this is usually called a *sinus pause*. If more than one sinus impulse in a row fails to form, this is termed a *sinus arrest*. Because the sinus node is not forming impulses regularly as expected, the PP interval in sinus arrest is not an exact multiple of the sinus cycle. Causes of sinus arrest include vagal stimulation, carotid sinus sensitivity, and MI interrupting the blood supply to the sinus

node. Drugs such as digitalis, beta-blockers, and calcium channel blockers can also cause sinus arrest.

ECG Characteristics

- *Rate:* Usually within normal range, but may be in the bradycardia range
- *Rhythm:* Irregular due to absence of sinus node discharge
- *P waves:* Present when sinus node is firing and absent during periods of sinus arrest; when present, they precede every QRS complex and are consistent in shape
- *PR interval:* Usually normal when P waves are present
- *QRS complex:* Usually normal when sinus node is functioning and absent during periods of sinus arrest, unless escape beats occur
- *Conduction:* Normal through atria, AV node, bundle branches, and ventricles when sinus node is firing; when the sinus node fails to form impulses, there is no conduction through the atria
- *Example of sinus arrest* (Figure 3–13)

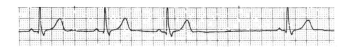

Figure 3–13. Sinus arrest.

Treatment

Treatment of sinus arrest is aimed at the underlying cause. Drugs that are thought to be responsible are discontinued and vagal stimulation is minimized. If periods of sinus arrest are frequent and cause hemodynamic compromise, 0.5 to 1.0 mg of atropine IV may increase the rate. Pacemaker therapy may be necessary if other forms of management fail to increase the rate to acceptable levels.

ARRHYTHMIAS ORIGINATING IN THE ATRIA (Figure 3–14)

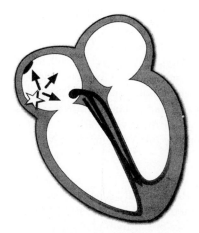

Figure 3–14. Arrhythmias originating in the atria.

Premature Atrial Complexes

A premature atrial complex (PAC) occurs when an irritable focus in the atria fires before the next sinus node impulse is due to fire. PACs can be caused by caffeine, alcohol, nicotine, congestive heart failure (CHF), pulmonary disease, interruption of atrial blood supply by myocardial ischemia or infarction, anxiety, and hypermetabolic states. PACs can also occur in normal hearts.

ECG Characteristics

- *Rate:* Usually within normal range.
- *Rhythm:* Usually regular except when PACs occur, resulting in early beats. PACs usually have a noncompensatory pause (interval between the complex preceding and that following the PAC is less than two normal RR intervals) because premature depolarization of the atria by the PAC usually causes premature depolarization of the sinus node as well, thus causing the sinus node to "reset" itself.
- *P waves:* Precede every QRS. The configuration of the premature P wave differs from that of the sinus P waves because the premature impulse originates in a different part of the atria, with atrial depolarization occurring in a different pattern. Very early P waves may be buried in the preceding T wave, altering the space of that T wave.
- *PR interval:* May be normal or long depending on the prematurity of the beat; very early PACs may find the AV junction still partially refractory and unable to conduct at a normal rate, resulting in a prolonged PR interval.
- *QRS complex:* May be normal, aberrant (wide), or absent, depending on the prematurity of the beat. If the ventricles have repolarized completely they will be able to conduct the early impulse normally, resulting in a normal QRS. If the PAC occurs during the relative refractory period of the bundle branches or ventricles, the impulse will conduct aberrantly and the QRS will be wide. If the PAC occurs very early during the complete refractory period of the bundle branches or ventricles, the impulse will not conduct to the ventricles and the QRS will be absent.
- *Conduction:* PACs travel through the atria differently from sinus impulses because they originate from a different spot; conduction through the AV node, bundle branches, and ventricles is usually normal unless the PAC is very early.
- *Example of PACs* (Figure 3–15AB)

Treatment

Treatment of PACs usually is not necessary because they do not cause hemodynamic compromise. Frequent PACs may precede more serious arrhythmias such as atrial fibrillation. Treatment is directed at the cause. Drugs such as quinidine,

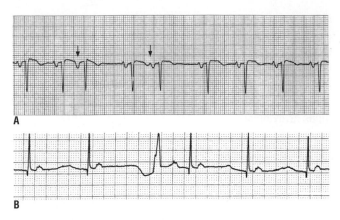

Figure 3–15. **(A)** PAC conducted normally in the ventricle. **(B)** PAC conducted aberrantly in the ventricle.

disopyramide, or procainamide can be used to suppress atrial activity if necessary.

Wandering Atrial Pacemaker

Wandering atrial pacemaker refers to rhythms that exhibit varying P wave morphology as the site of impulse formation shifts from the sinus node to various sites in the atria or into the AV junction. This occurs when two (usually sinus and junctional) or more supraventricular pacemakers compete with each other for control of the heart. Because the rates of these competing pacemakers are almost identical, it is common to have atrial fusion occur as the atria are activated by more than one wave of depolarization at a time, resulting in varying P wave morphology. Wandering atrial pacemaker can be due to increased vagal tone that slows the sinus pacemaker or to enhanced automaticity in atrial or junctional pacemaker cells, causing them to compete with the sinus node for control.

ECG Characteristics

- *Rate:* 60 to 100 beats/min; if the rate is faster than 100 beats/min, it is called *multifocal atrial tachycardia* (MAT)
- *Rhythm:* May be slightly irregular
- *P waves:* Varying shapes (upright, flat, inverted, notched) as impulses originate in different parts of the atria or junction; at least three different P wave shapes should be seen
- *PR interval:* May vary depending on proximity of the pacemaker to the AV node
- *QRS complex:* Usually normal
- *Conduction:* Conduction through the atria varies as they are depolarized from different spots; conduction through the bundle branches and ventricles is usually normal
- *Example of WAP* (Figure 3–16)

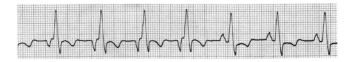

Figure 3–16. Wandering atrial pacemaker.

Treatment

Treatment of WAP usually is not necessary. If slow heart rates lead to symptoms, atropine can be given. Treatment of MAT is directed toward eliminating the cause, including hypoxia and electrolyte imbalances. Antiarrhythmic therapy is often ineffective. Beta-blockers, verapamil, flecainide, amiodarone, and magnesium may be successful.

Atrial Tachycardia (Figure 3–17)

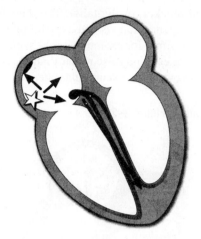

Figure 3–17. Atrial tachycardia.

Atrial tachycardia is a rapid atrial rhythm occurring at a rate of 120 to 250 beats/min. When the arrhythmia abruptly starts and terminates, it is called paroxysmal atrial tachycardia. Rapid atrial rate can be caused by emotions, caffeine, tobacco, alcohol, fatigue, or sympathomimetic drugs. Whenever the atrial rate is rapid, the AV node begins to block some of the impulses attempting to travel through it to protect the ventricles from excessively rapid rates. In normal healthy hearts the AV node can usually conduct each atrial impulse up to rates of about 180 to 200 beats/min. In patients with cardiac disease or who have taken too much digitalis, the AV node may not be able to conduct each impulse and atrial tachycardia with block occurs.

ECG Characteristics

- *Rate:* Atrial rate is 120 to 250 beats/min
- *Rhythm:* Regular unless there is variable block at the AV node
- *P waves:* Differ in shape from sinus P waves because they are ectopic. Precede each QRS complex but may be hidden in preceding T wave. When block is present, more than one P wave will appear before each QRS complex.
- *PR interval:* May be shorter than normal but often difficult to measure because of hidden P waves
- *QRS complex:* Usually normal but may be wide if aberrant conduction is present

- *Conduction:* Usually normal through the AV node and into the ventricles. In atrial tachycardia with block some atrial impulses do not conduct into the ventricles. Aberrant ventricular conduction may occur if atrial impulses are conducted into the ventricles while the ventricles are still partially refractory.
- *Example of atrial tachycardia* (Figure 3–18)

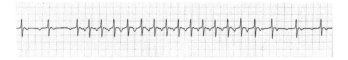

Figure 3–18. Atrial tachycardia.

Treatment

Treatment of atrial tachycardia is directed toward eliminating the cause and decreasing the ventricular rate. Sedation may terminate the rhythm or slow the rate. Vagal stimulation, either through carotid sinus massage or the Valsalva maneuver, may slow the rate or convert the rhythm to sinus rhythm. Digitalis slows the ventricular rate by increasing the block at the AV node, but it can also be the cause of atrial tachycardia with block and is discontinued if that is the case. Propranolol, verapamil, and diltiazem increase block at the AV node and may either slow the ventricular rate or terminate the tachycardia. Types IA, IC, and III antiarrhythmics may be effective in reducing the number of tachycardia episodes, but can also be proarrhythmic. Radiofrequency catheter ablation of the ectopic focus or reentry circuit is successful in many cases

Atrial Flutter (Figure 3–19)

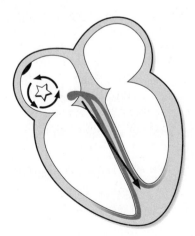

Figure 3–19. Atrial flutter.

In atrial flutter, the atria are depolarized at rates of 250 to 350 times per minute. Classic or typical atrial flutter is due to a fixed reentry circuit in the right atrium around which the impulse circulates in a counterclockwise direction, resulting in negative flutter waves in leads II and III and an atrial rate between 250 and 350 beats/min (most commonly 300 beats/min). At such rapid atrial rates, the AV node usually blocks at least half of the impulses to protect the ventricles from excessive rates. Causes of atrial flutter include rheumatic heart disease, atherosclerotic heart disease, thyrotoxicosis, heart failure, and myocardial ischemia or infarction. Because the ventricular rate in atrial flutter can be quite fast, symptoms associated with decreased cardiac output can occur. Mural thrombi may form in the atria due to the fact that there is no strong atrial contraction, and blood stasis occurs, leading to a risk of systemic or pulmonary emboli.

ECG Characteristics

- *Rate:* Atrial rate varies between 250 and 350 beats/min, most commonly 300; ventricular rate varies depending on the amount of block at the AV node, most commonly 150 beats/min and rarely 300 beats/min
- *Rhythm:* Atrial rhythm is regular; ventricular rhythm may be regular or irregular due to varying AV block
- *P waves:* F waves (flutter waves) are seen, characterized by a very regular, "sawtooth" pattern; one F wave is usually hidden in the QRS complex, and when 2:1 conduction occurs, F waves may not be readily apparent
- *FR interval (flutter wave to the beginning of the QRS complex):* May be consistent or may vary
- *QRS complex:* Usually normal; aberration can occur
- *Conduction:* Usually normal through the AV node and ventricles
- *Examples of atrial flutter* (Figure 3–20AB)

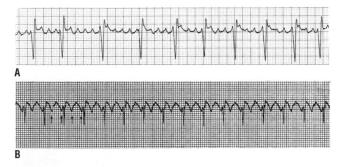

A

B

Figure 3–20. (A) Atrial flutter with 4:1 conduction. **(B)** Atrial flutter with 2:1 conduction.

Treatment

The immediate goal of treatment depends on the hemodynamic consequences of the arrhythmia. Ventricular rate control is the priority if cardiac output is significantly compromised due to rapid ventricular rates. Electrical (direct current) cardioversion may be necessary as an immediate treatment, especially if 1:1 conduction occurs. IV calcium channel blockers (verapamil or diltiazem) or beta-blockers can be used for ventricular rate control. Conversion to sinus rhythm can be accomplished by electrical cardioversion, drug therapy, or overdrive atrial pacing. Class IA (disopyramide, procainamide), type IC (flecainide, propafenone), or type III antiarrhythmics (sotalol, amiodarone, ibutilide, dofetilide) may convert flutter to sinus rhythm. These agents are also useful in maintaining sinus rhythm after conversion. Drugs that slow the atrial rate, like class IA or IC drugs, should not be used unless the ventricular rate has been controlled with an AV nodal blocking agent (a calcium channel blocker, beta-blocker, or digitalis). The danger of giving class IA or IC agents alone is that as atrial rate slows from 300 to 200 beats/min; for example, it is possible for the AV node to conduct each impulse rather than block impulses, thus leading to even faster ventricular rates.

Atrial Fibrillation (Figure 3–21)

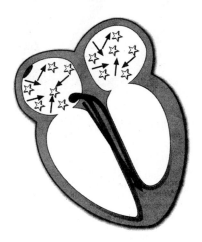

Figure 3–21. Atrial fibrillation.

Atrial fibrillation is an extremely rapid and disorganized pattern of depolarization in the atria. Atrial fibrillation is the most common rhythm seen in adults (next to sinus rhythm) and can be chronic or occur in paroxysms. Atrial fibrillation commonly occurs in the presence of atherosclerotic or rheumatic heart disease, thyrotoxicosis, CHF, cardiomyopathy, valve disease, pulmonary disease, MI, congenital heart disease, and after cardiac surgery. If the ventricular response to atrial fibrillation is very rapid, cardiac output can be reduced secondary to decreased diastolic filling time in the ventricles. Because the atria are quivering rather than contracting, atrial kick is lost, which can also reduce cardiac output. Another possible complication is mural thrombus formation in the atria due to stasis of blood as the atria quiver.

ECG Characteristics

- *Rate:* Atrial rate is 400 to 600 beats/min or faster. Ventricular rate varies depending on the amount of block at the AV node. In new atrial fibrillation, the ventricular response is usually quite rapid, 160 to

200 beats/min; in treated atrial fibrillation, the ventricular rate is controlled in the normal range of 60 to 100 beats/min.

- *Rhythm:* Irregular; one of the distinguishing features of atrial fibrillation is the marked irregularity of the ventricular response
- *P waves:* Not present; atrial activity is chaotic with no formed atrial impulses visible; irregular F waves are often seen, and vary in size from coarse to very fine
- *PR interval:* Not measurable; there are no P waves
- *QRS complex:* Usually normal; aberration is common
- *Conduction:* Conduction within the atria is disorganized and follows a very irregular pattern. Most of the atrial impulses are blocked within the AV junction. Those impulses that are conducted through the AV junction are usually conducted normally through the ventricles. If an atrial impulse reaches the bundle branch system during its refractory period, aberrant intraventricular conduction can occur.
- *Examples of atrial fibrillation* (Figure 3–22AB)

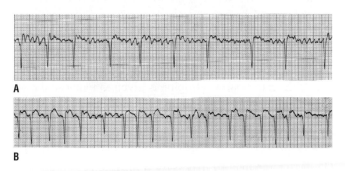

A

B

Figure 3–22. **(A)** Atrial fibrillation with a controlled ventricular response. **(B)** Atrial fibrillation with an uncontrolled ventricular response.

Treatment

Treatment of atrial fibrillation is directed toward eliminating the cause, controlling ventricular rate, restoring and maintaining sinus rhythm, and preventing thromboembolism. Electrical cardioversion may be necessary if the patient is hemodynamically unstable because of rapid ventricular rates. IV calcium channel blockers (diltiazem, verapamil) and beta-blockers are commonly used in the acute situation for ventricular rate control. Beta-blockers, calcium channel blockers, and digitalis can be used orally for long-term rate control. Atrial antiarrhythmic drugs used to convert atrial fibrillation to sinus rhythm and to maintain sinus rhythm include class IA agents (procainamide, disopyramide), class IC agents (flecainide, propafenone), and class III agents (amiodarone, sotalol, ibutilide, dofetilide). Anticoagulation with warfarin is necessary if atrial fibrillation is chronic. Nonpharmacologic therapies used for treatment of atrial fibrillation include implantable atrial defibrillators and radiofrequency catheter ablation. Atrial defibrillators detect the onset of atrial fibrillation and deliver a shock between two intra-

cardiac leads to terminate atrial fibrillation. Ablation to create linear lesions within the atria (similar to the surgical Maze procedure) may be successful, as well as focal ablations around the orifice of the pulmonary veins in the left atrium.

ARRHYTHMIAS ORIGINATING IN THE ATRIOVENTRICULAR JUNCTION (Figure 3–23)

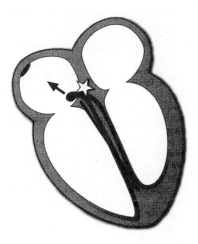

Figure 3–23. Arrhythmias originating in the AV junction.

Cells surrounding the AV node in the AV junction are capable of initiating impulses and controlling the heart rhythm. Junctional beats and junctional rhythms can appear in any of three ways on the ECG depending on the location of the junctional pacemaker and the speed of conduction of the impulse into the atria and ventricles:

- When a junctional focus fires, the wave of depolarization spreads backward (retrograde) into the atria as well as forward (antegrade) into the ventricles. If the impulse arrives in the atria before it arrives in the ventricles, the ECG shows a P wave (usually inverted because the atria are depolarizing from bottom to top) followed immediately by a QRS complex as the impulse reaches the ventricles. In this case the PR interval is very short, usually 0.10 second or less.
- If the junctional impulse reaches both the atria and the ventricles at the same time, only a QRS is seen on the ECG because the ventricles are much larger than the atria and only ventricular depolarization will be seen, even though the atria are also depolarizing.
- If the junctional impulse reaches the ventricles before it reaches the atria, the QRS precedes the P wave on the ECG. Again, the P wave is usually inverted because of retrograde atrial depolarization, and the RP interval (distance from the beginning of the QRS to the beginning of the following P wave) is short.

Premature Junctional Complexes

Premature junctional complexes (PJCs) are due to an irritable focus in the AV junction. Irritability can be due to coronary heart disease or MI disrupting blood flow to the AV junction, nicotine, caffeine, emotions, or drugs such as digitalis.

ECG Characteristics

- *Rate:* 60 to 100 beats/min or whatever the rate of the basic rhythm
- *Rhythm:* Regular except for occurrence of premature beats
- *P waves:* May occur before, during, or after the QRS complex of the premature beat and are usually inverted
- *PR interval:* Short, usually 0.10 second or less when P waves precede the QRS
- *QRS complex:* Usually normal but may be aberrant if the PJC occurs very early and conducts into the ventricles during the refractory period of a bundle branch
- *Conduction:* Retrograde through the atria; usually normal through the ventricles
- *Example of a PJC* (Figure 3–24)

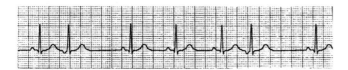

Figure 3–24. Premature junctional complexes.

Treatment

Treatment is not necessary for PJCs.

Junctional Rhythm, Accelerated Junctional Rhythm, and Junctional Tachycardia

Junctional rhythms can occur if the sinus node rate falls below the rate of the AV junctional pacemakers or when atrial conduction through the AV junction has been disrupted. Junctional rhythms commonly occur from digitalis toxicity or following inferior MI owing to disruption of blood supply to the sinus node and the AV junction. These rhythms are classified according to their rate: junctional rhythm usually occurs at a rate of 40 to 60 beats/min, accelerated junctional rhythm occurs at a rate of 60 to 100 beats/min, and junctional tachycardia occurs at rates of 100 to 250 beats/min.

ECG Characteristics

- *Rate:* Junctional rhythm, 40 to 60 beats/min; accelerated junctional rhythm, 60 to 100 beats/min; junctional tachycardia, 100 to 250 beats/min
- *Rhythm:* Regular

- *P waves:* May precede or follow QRS
- *PR interval:* Short, 0.10 second or less
- *QRS complex:* Usually normal
- *Conduction:* Retrograde through the atria; normal through the ventricles
- *Examples of junctional rhythm, accelerated junctional rhythm, and junctional tachycardia* (Figure 3–25AB)

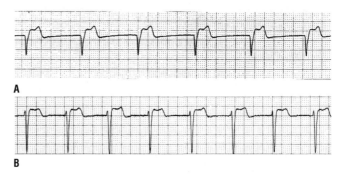

Figure 3–25. **(A)** Junctional rhythm. **(B)** Accelerated junctional rhythm.

Treatment

Treatment of junctional rhythm rarely is required unless the rate is too slow or too fast to maintain adequate cardiac output. If the rate is slow, atropine is given to increase the sinus rate and override the junctional focus or to increase the rate of firing of the junctional pacemaker. If the rate is fast, drugs such as verapamil, propranolol, or digitalis may be effective in slowing the rate or terminating the arrhythmia. Cardioversion may be necessary if the rate is so rapid that cardiac output is severely limited. Because digitalis toxicity is a common cause of junctional rhythms, the drug should be held.

ARRHYTHMIAS ORIGINATING IN THE VENTRICLES (Figure 3–26)

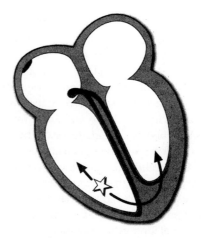

Figure 3–26. Arrhythmias originating in the ventricles.

Ventricular arrhythmias originate in the ventricular muscle or Purkinje system and are considered to be more dangerous than other arrhythmias because of their potential to severely decrease cardiac output. However, as with any arrhythmia, ventricular rate is a key determinant of how well a patient can tolerate a ventricular rhythm. Ventricular rhythms can range in severity from mild, well-tolerated rhythms to pulseless rhythms leading to sudden cardiac death.

Premature Ventricular Complexes

Premature ventricular complexes (PVCs) are caused by premature depolarization of cells in the ventricular myocardium or Purkinje system or to reentry in the ventricles. PVCs can be caused by hypoxia, myocardial ischemia, hypokalemia, acidosis, exercise, increased levels of circulating catecholamines, digitalis toxicity, caffeine, alcohol, among other causes. PVCs increase with aging and are more common in people with coronary disease, valve disease, hypertension, cardiomyopathy, and other forms of heart disease. PVCs are not dangerous in people with normal hearts but are associated with higher mortality rates in patients with structural heart disease or acute MI, especially if left ventricular function is reduced. PVCs are considered potentially malignant when they occur more frequently than 10 per hour or are repetitive (occur in pairs, triplets, or more than three in a row) in patients with coronary disease, previous MI, cardiomyopathy, and reduced ejection fraction.

ECG Characteristics

- *Rate:* 60 to 100 beats/min or the rate of the basic rhythm
- *Rhythm:* Irregular because of the early beats
- *P waves:* Not related to the PVCs. Sinus rhythm is usually not interrupted by the premature beats, so sinus P waves can often be seen occurring regularly throughout the rhythm. P waves may occasionally follow PVCs due to retrograde conduction from the ventricle backward through the atria; these P waves are inverted.
- *PR interval:* Not present before most PVCs; if a P wave happens, by coincidence, to precede a PVC, the PR interval is short
- *QRS complex:* Wide and bizarre; greater than 0.10 second in duration; may vary in morphology (size, shape) if they originate from more than one focus in the ventricles (multifocal PVCs)
- *Conduction:* Impulses originating in the ventricles conduct through the ventricles from muscle cell to muscle cell rather than through Purkinje fibers, resulting in wide QRS complexes. Some PVCs may conduct retrograde into the atria, resulting in inverted P waves following the PVC. When the sinus rhythm is undisturbed by PVCs, the atria depolarize normally.
- *Examples of a PVCs* (Figure 3–27AB)

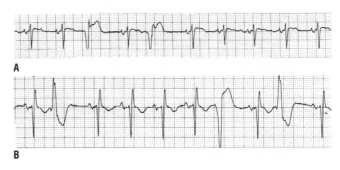

Figure 3–27. Premature ventricular complexes.

Treatment

The significance of PVCs depends on the clinical setting in which they occur. Many people have chronic PVCs that do not need to be treated, and most of these people are asymptomatic. There is no evidence that suppression of PVCs reduces mortality, especially in patients with no structural heart disease. If PVCs cause bothersome palpitations, patients are told to avoid caffeine, tobacco, other stimulants, and try stress reduction techniques. Low-dose beta-blockers may reduce PVC frequency and the perception of palpitations and can be used for symptom relief. In the setting of an acute MI or myocardial ischemia, PVCs may be precursors of more dangerous ventricular arrhythmias, especially when they occur near the apex of the T wave (R on T PVCs). Unless PVCs result in hemodynamic instability or symptomatic VT, most physicians elect not to treat them. If PVCs are to be treated, IV lidocaine is usually the recommended drug. Other antiarrhythmic agents such as procainamide or amiodarone can be used IV for acute control. Beta-blockers are often effective in suppressing repetitive PVCs and have become the drugs of choice for treating post-MI PVCs that are symptomatic. Many other drugs effectively reduce the frequency of PVCs, including quinidine, disopyramide, flecainide, mexiletine, tocainide, moricizine, propafenone, and sotalol, but are rarely used for this purpose because of the potential for proarrhythmia and increased incidence of sudden death.

Ventricular Rhythm and Accelerated Ventricular Rhythm

Ventricular rhythm occurs when an ectopic focus in the ventricle fires at a rate under 50 beats/min. This rhythm occurs as an escape rhythm when the sinus node and junctional tissue fail to fire or fail to conduct their impulses to the ventricle. Accelerated ventricular rhythm occurs when an ectopic focus in the ventricles fires at a rate of 50 to 100 beats/min. The causes of this accelerated ventricular rhythm are similar to those of VT, but accelerated ventricular rhythm commonly occurs in the presence of inferior MI when the rate of the sinus node slows below the rate of the latent ventricular pacemaker. Accelerated ventricular rhythm is a common arrhythmia after thrombolytic therapy, when reperfusion of the damaged myocardium occurs.

ECG Characteristics

- *Rate:* Less than 50 beats/min for ventricular rhythm and 50 to 100 beats/min for accelerated ventricular rhythm
- *Rhythm:* Usually regular
- *P waves:* May be seen but at a slower rate than the ventricular focus, with dissociation from the QRS
- *PR interval*: Not measured
- *QRS complex:* Wide and bizarre
- *Conduction:* If sinus rhythm is the basic rhythm, atrial conduction is normal; impulses originating in the ventricles conduct via muscle cell-to-cell conduction, resulting in the wide QRS complex
- *Examples of ventricular rhythm and accelerated ventricular rhythm* (Figure 3–28AB)

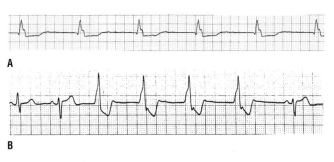

A

B

Figure 3–28. (A) Escape ventricular rhythm. **(B)** Accelerated ventricular rhythm.

Treatment

The treatment of accelerated ventricular rhythm depends on its cause and how well it is tolerated by the patient. This arrhythmia alone is usually not harmful because the ventricular rate is within normal limits and usually adequate to maintain cardiac output. Suppressive therapy is rarely used because abolishing the ventricular rhythm may leave an even less desirable heart rate. If the patient is symptomatic because of the loss of atrial kick, atropine can be used to increase the rate of the sinus node and overdrive the ventricular rhythm. If the ventricular rhythm is an escape rhythm, then treatment is directed toward increasing the rate of the escape rhythm or pacing the heart temporarily. Usually, accelerated ventricular rhythm is transient and benign and does not require treatment.

Ventricular Tachycardia

VT is a rapid ventricular rhythm at a rate greater than 100 beats/min. VT can be classified according to (1) duration, *nonsustained* (lasts <30 seconds), *sustained* (lasts >30 seconds), or *incessant* (VT present most of the time); and (2) morphology (ECG appearance of QRS complexes), *monomorphic* (QRS complexes have the same shape during tachycardia), *polymorphic* (QRS complexes vary randomly in shape), or *bidirectional* (alternating upright and negative

QRS complexes during tachycardia). The terms *salvos* and *bursts* are often used to describe short runs of VT (5 to 10 or more beats in a row). The most common cause of VT is coronary artery disease, including acute ischemia, acute MI, and prior MI. Other causes include cardiomyopathy, valvular heart disease, congenital heart disease, arrhythmogenic right ventricular dysplasia, cardiac tumors, cardiac surgery, and the proarrhythmic effects of many drugs.

ECG Characteristics

- *Rate:* Ventricular rate is faster than 100 beats/min
- *Rhythm:* Usually regular but may be slightly irregular
- *P waves:* Dissociated from QRS complexes. If sinus rhythm is the underlying basic rhythm, they are regular. P waves may be seen but are not related to QRS complexes. P waves are often buried within QRS complexes.
- *PR interval:* Not measurable because of dissociation of P waves from QRS complexes
- *QRS complex:* Wide and bizarre; greater than 0.10 second in duration
- *Conduction:* Impulse originates in one ventricle and spreads via muscle cell-to-cell conduction through both ventricles; there may be retrograde conduction through the atria, but more often the sinus node continues to fire regularly and depolarize the atria normally
- *Example of VT* (Figure 3–29)

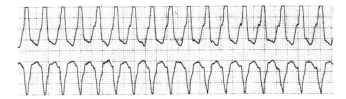

Figure 3–29. Ventricular tachycardia.

Treatment

Immediate treatment of VT depends on how well the rhythm is tolerated by the patient. The two main determinants of patient tolerance of any tachycardia are ventricular rate and underlying left ventricular function. VT can be an emergency if cardiac output is severely decreased because of a very rapid rate or poor left ventricular function. The preferred immediate treatment for severely symptomatic VT is cardioversion, but defibrillation can be performed if there is not time to synchronize the shock. If the patient is not severely symptomatic, lidocaine is often used for acute treatment of VT. IV procainamide, amiodarone, or magnesium sulfate can also be used for acute treatment. Maintenance therapy may be prescribed with the same drugs used for PVCs, with increasing emphasis on class III agents with beta-blocker effects, like amiodarone and sotalol. Some VTs can be treated with radiofrequency catheter ablation to abolish the ectopic focus. The implantable cardioverter defibrillator is frequently used for recurrent VT in patients with reduced ejection fractions or drug refractory VT.

Ventricular Fibrillation (Figure 3–30)

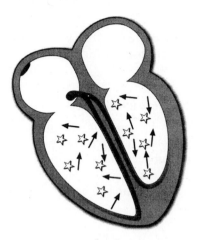

Figure 3–30. Ventricular fibrillation.

Ventricular fibrillation (VF) is rapid, ineffective quivering of the ventricles and is fatal without immediate treatment. Electrical activity originates in the ventricles and spreads in a chaotic, irregular pattern throughout both ventricles. There is no cardiac output or palpable pulse with VF.

ECG Characteristics

- *Rate:* Rapid, uncoordinated, ineffective
- *Rhythm:* Chaotic, irregular
- *P waves:* None seen
- *PR interval:* None
- *QRS complex:* No formed QRS complexes seen; rapid, irregular undulations without any specific pattern
- *Conduction:* Multiple ectopic foci firing simultaneously in ventricles and depolarizing them irregularly and without any organized pattern; ventricles are not contracting
- *Example of ventricular fibrillation* (Figure 3–31)

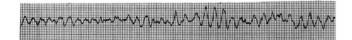

Figure 3–31. Ventricular fibrillation.

Treatment

VF requires immediate defibrillation. Synchronized cardioversion is not possible because there are no formed QRS complexes on which to synchronize the shock. Cardiopulmonary resuscitation (CPR) must be performed until a defib-

rillator is available, and then defibrillation at 200 J is recommended. If VF continues, an immediate second shock at 300 J and a third shock at 360 J, if necessary, are recommended. If VF does not convert after three shocks, CPR needs to be continued and drug therapy initiated. Antiarrhythmic agents such as lidocaine, procainamide, amiodarone, or magnesium are commonly used in an effort to convert VF. Once the rhythm has converted, maintenance therapy with IV antiarrhythmic agents is continued. Beta-blockers and amiodarone appear to be the most effective agents for long-term drug therapy options. The implantable cardioverter defibrillator is becoming the standard of care for survivors of VF that occurs in the absence of acute ischemia.

Ventricular Asystole (Figure 3–32)

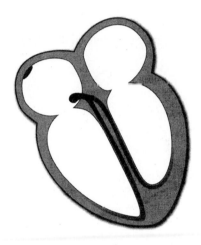

Figure 3–32. Ventricular asystole.

Ventricular asystole is the absence of any ventricular rhythm: no QRS complex, no pulse, and no cardiac output. Ventricular asystole is always fatal unless treated immediately.

ECG Characteristics

- *Rate:* None
- *Rhythm:* None
- *P waves:* May be present if the sinus node is functioning
- *PR interval:* None
- *QRS complex:* None
- *Conduction:* Atrial conduction may be normal if the sinus node is functioning; there is no conduction into the ventricles
- *Example of ventricular asystole* (Figure 3–33)

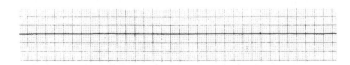

Figure 3–33. Ventricular asystole.

Treatment

CPR must be initiated immediately if the patient is to survive. IV epinephrine and atropine may be given in an effort to stimulate a rhythm. If pacing is to be used, external pacing is instituted early in the resuscitation attempt. Asystole has a very poor prognosis despite the best resuscitation efforts because it usually represents extensive myocardial ischemia or severe underlying metabolic problems.

ATRIOVENTRICULAR BLOCKS

The term *atrioventricular block* is used to describe arrhythmias in which there is delayed or failed conduction of supraventricular impulses into the ventricles. AV blocks have been classified according to location of the block and severity of the conduction abnormality.

First-Degree Atrioventricular Block (Figure 3–34)

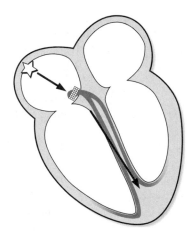

Figure 3–34. First-degree AV block.

First-degree AV block is defined as prolonged AV conduction time of supraventricular impulses into the ventricles. This delay usually occurs in the AV node, and all impulses conduct to the ventricles, but with delayed conduction times. First-degree AV block can be due to coronary artery disease, rheumatic heart disease, or administration of digitalis, beta-blockers, or calcium channel blockers. First-degree AV block can be normal in people with slow heart rates or high vagal tone.

ECG Characteristics

- *Rate:* Can occur at any sinus rate, usually 60 to 100 beats/min
- *Rhythm:* Regular
- *P waves:* Normal; precede every QRS
- *PR interval:* Prolonged above 0.20 second
- *QRS complex:* Usually normal
- *Conduction:* Normal through the atria, delayed through the AV node, and normal through the ventricles
- *Example of first-degree AV block* (Figure 3–35)

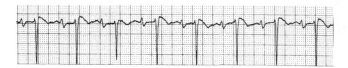

Figure 3–35. First-degree AV block.

Treatment

Treatment of first-degree AV block is usually not required, but block should be observed for progression to more severe block.

Second-Degree Atrioventricular Block

Second-degree AV block occurs when one atrial impulse at a time fails to be conducted to the ventricles. Second-degree AV block can be divided into two distinct categories: type I block, occurring in the AV node, and type II block, occurring below the AV node in the bundle of His or bundle-branch system (Figure 3–36).

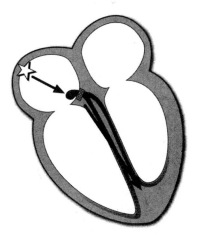

Figure 3–36. Type I second-degree AV block.

Type I Second-Degree Atrioventricular Block

Type I second-degree AV block, often referred to as *Wenckebach block,* is a progressive increase in conduction times of consecutive atrial impulses into the ventricles until one impulse fails to conduct, or is "dropped." The PR intervals gradually lengthen until one P wave fails to conduct and is not followed by a QRS complex, resulting in a pause, after which the cycle repeats itself. This type of block is commonly associated with inferior MI, coronary heart disease, aortic valve disease, mitral valve prolapse, atrial septal defects, and administration of digitalis, beta-blockers, or calcium channel blockers.

ECG Characteristics

- *Rate:* Can occur at any sinus or atrial rate
- *Rhythm:* Irregular; overall appearance of the rhythm demonstrates "group beating"

- *P waves:* Normal; some P waves are not conducted to the ventricles, but only one at a time fails to conduct to the ventricle
- *PR interval:* Gradually lengthens in consecutive beats; the PR interval preceding the pause is longer than that following the pause
- *QRS complex:* Usually normal unless there is associated bundle branch block
- *Conduction:* Normal through the atria; progressively delayed through the AV node until an impulse fails to conduct. Ventricular conduction is normal. Conduction ratios can vary, with ratios as low as 2:1 (every other P wave is blocked) up to high ratios such as 15:14 (every 15th P wave is blocked)
- *Example of second-degree AV block type I* (Figure 3–37)

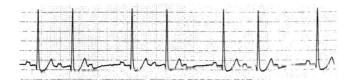

Figure 3–37. Second-degree AV block, Mobitz I.

Treatment

Treatment of type I second-degree AV block depends on the conduction ratio, the resulting ventricular rate, and the patient's tolerance for the rhythm. If ventricular rates are slow enough to decrease cardiac output, the treatment is atropine to increase the sinus rate and speed conduction through the AV node. At higher conduction ratios where the ventricular rate is within a normal range, no treatment is necessary. If the block is due to digitalis or beta-blockers, those drugs are held. This type of block is usually temporary and benign, and seldom requires pacing, although temporary pacing may be needed when the ventricular rate is slow.

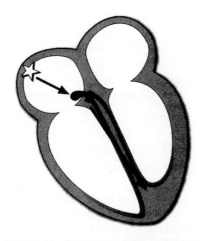

Figure 3–38. Type II second-degree AV block.

Type II Second-Degree Atrioventricular Block (Figure 3–38)

Type II second-degree AV block is sudden failure of conduction of an atrial impulse to the ventricles without progressive increases in conduction time of consecutive P waves. Type II block occurs below the AV node and is usually associated with bundle branch block; therefore, the dropped beats are usually a manifestation of bilateral bundle branch block. This form of block appears on the ECG much the same as type I block except that there is no progressive increase in PR intervals before the blocked beats. Type II block is less common than type I block, but is a more serious form of block. It occurs in rheumatic heart disease, coronary heart disease, primary disease of the conduction system, and in the presence of acute anterior MI. Type II block is more dangerous than type I because of a higher incidence of associated symptoms and progression to complete AV block

ECG Characteristics

- *Rate:* Can occur at any basic rate
- *Rhythm:* Irregular due to blocked beats
- *P waves:* Usually regular and precede each QRS; periodically a P wave is not followed by a QRS complex
- *PR interval:* Constant before conducted beats; the PR interval preceding the pause is the same as that following the pause
- *QRS complex:* Usually wide due to associated bundle branch block
- *Conduction:* Normal through the atria and through the AV node but intermittently blocked in the bundle branch system and fails to reach the ventricles. Conduction through the ventricles is abnormally slow due to associated bundle branch block. Conduction ratios can vary from 2:1 to only occasional blocked beats
- *Example of second-degree AV block type II* (Figure 3–39)

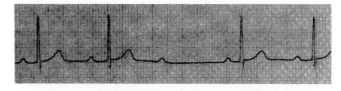

Figure 3–39. Second-degree AV block, Mobitz II.

Treatment

Treatment usually includes pacemaker therapy because this type of block is often permanent and progresses to complete block. External pacing can be used for treatment of symptomatic type II block until transvenous pacing can be initiated. Atropine is not recommended because it may result in further slowing of ventricular rate by increasing the number of impulses conducting through the AV node and bombarding the diseased bundles with more impulses than they can handle, resulting in further conduction failure.

High-Grade Atrioventricular Block

High-grade (or advanced) AV block is present when two or more consecutive atrial impulses are blocked when the atrial rate is reasonable (less than 135/min) and conduction fails because of the block itself and not because of interference from an escape pacemaker. High-grade AV block may be type I, occurring in the AV node, or type II, occurring below the AV node. The significance of high-grade block depends on the conduction ratio and the resulting ventricular rate. Because ventricular rates tend to be slow, this arrhythmia is frequently symptomatic and requires treatment.

ECG Characteristics

- *Rate:* Atrial rate less than 135 beats/min
- *Rhythm:* Regular or irregular, depending on conduction pattern
- *P waves:* Normal; present before every conducted QRS, but several P waves may not be followed by QRS complexes
- *PR interval:* Constant before conducted beats; may be normal or prolonged
- *QRS complex:* Usually normal in type I block and wide in type II block
- *Conduction:* Normal through the atria. Two or more consecutive atrial impulses fail to conduct to the ventricles. Ventricular conduction is normal in type I block and abnormally slow in type II block.
- *Example of high-grade AV block* (Figure 3–40)

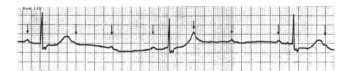

Figure 3–40. High-grade AV block.

Treatment

Treatment of high-grade block is necessary if the patient is symptomatic. Atropine can be given and is generally more effective in type I block. A transcutaneous pacemaker may be required until transvenous pacing can be initiated, and permanent pacing is often necessary in type II high-grade block.

Third-Degree Atrioventricular Block (Complete Block) (Figure 3-41)

Third-degree AV block is complete failure of conduction of all atrial impulses to the ventricles. In third-degree AV

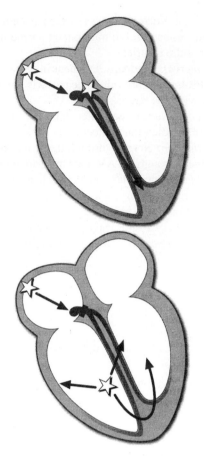

Figure 3–41. Third-degree AV block (complete block).

block, there is complete AV dissociation; the atria are usually under the control of the sinus node, although complete block can occur with any atrial arrhythmia; and either a junctional or ventricular pacemaker controls the ventricles. The ventricular rate is usually less than 45 beats/min; a faster rate could indicate an accelerated junctional or ventricular rhythm that interferes with conduction from the atria into the ventricles by causing physiologic refractoriness in the conduction system, thus causing a physiologic failure of conduction that must be differentiated from the abnormal conduction system function of complete AV block. Causes of complete AV block include coronary artery disease, MI, Lev disease, Lenègre disease, cardiac surgery, congenital heart disease, and drugs that slow AV conduction such as digitalis, beta-blockers, and calcium channel blockers.

ECG Characteristics

- *Rate:* Atrial rate is usually normal; ventricular rate is less than 45 beats/min
- *Rhythm:* Regular
- *P waves:* Normal but dissociated from QRS complexes
- *PR interval:* No consistent PR intervals because there is no relationship between P waves and QRS complexes

- *QRS complex:* Normal if ventricles controlled by a junctional pacemaker; wide if controlled by a ventricular pacemaker
- *Conduction:* Normal through the atria. All impulses are blocked at the AV node or in the bundle branches, so there is no conduction to the ventricles. Conduction through the ventricles is normal if a junctional escape rhythm occurs, and abnormally slow if a ventricular escape rhythm occurs

- *Examples of third-degree AV block* (Figure 3–42AB)

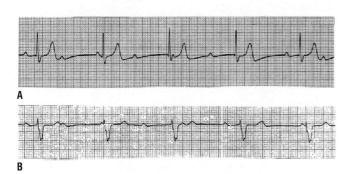

A

B

Figure 3–42. (A) Third-degree AV block with junctional escape rhythm. **(B)** Third-degree AV block with ventricular escape rhythm.

Treatment

Third-degree AV block can occur without significant symptoms if it occurs gradually and the heart has time to compensate for the slow ventricular rate. If it occurs suddenly in the presence of acute MI, its significance depends on the resulting ventricular rate and the patient's tolerance. Treatment of complete heart block with symptoms of decreased cardiac output includes transcutaneous pacing until transvenous pacing can be initiated. Atropine can be given but is not usually effective in restoring conduction. CPR should be performed until a pacemaker can be inserted if cardiac output is severely decreased.

TEMPORARY PACING

Indications

If the heart fails to generate or conduct impulses to the ventricle, the myocardium can be electrically stimulated using a cardiac pacemaker. A cardiac pacemaker has two components: a pulse generator and a pacing electrode or lead. Temporary cardiac pacing is indicated in any situation in which bradycardia results in symptoms of decreased cerebral tissue perfusion or hemodynamic compromise and does not respond to drug therapy. Signs and symptoms of hemodynamic instability are hypotension, change in mental status, angina, or pulmonary edema. Temporary pacing is also used to suppress rapid ectopic rhythms by briefly pacing the heart at a faster rate than the existing rate. Following pacing termina-

tion, return to a normal rhythm may occur if the rapid ectopic focus has been suppressed, allowing the sinus node to resume as the pacemaker. This type of pacing is termed *overdrive pacing* to distinguish it from pacing for bradycardic conditions.

Temporary cardiac pacing is accomplished by transvenous, epicardial, or external pacing methods. If continued cardiac pacing is required, insertion of permanent pacemakers is done electively. The following section presents an overview of temporary ventricular pacing principles. A more detailed explanation of pacemaker functions is covered in Chapter 18, Advanced ECG Concepts.

Transvenous Pacing

Transvenous pacing is usually done by percutaneous puncture of the internal jugular, subclavian, antecubital, or femoral vein and threading a pacing lead into the apex of the right ventricle so that the tip of the pacing lead contacts the wall of the ventricle (Figure 3–43A). The transvenous pacing lead is attached to an external pulse generator that is kept either on the patient or at the bedside. Transvenous pacing is usually necessary only for a few days until the rhythm returns to normal or a permanent pacemaker is inserted.

Epicardial Pacing

Epicardial pacing is done through electrodes placed on the atria or ventricles during cardiac surgery. The pacing electrode end of the lead is looped through or loosely sutured to the epicardial surface of the atria or ventricles and the other end is pulled through the chest wall, sutured to the skin, and attached to an external pulse generator (Figure 3–43B). A ground wire is often placed subcutaneously in the chest wall and pulled through with the other leads. The number and placement of leads varies with the surgeon.

Components of a Pacing System

The basic components of a cardiac pacing system are the pulse generator and the pacing lead. The *pulse generator* contains the power source (battery) and all of the electronic circuitry that controls pacemaker function. A temporary pulse generator is a box that is kept at the bedside and is usually powered by a regular 9-volt battery. It has controls on the front that allow the operator to set pacing rate, strength of the pacing stimulus (output), and sensitivity settings (Figure 3–43C).

The *pacing lead* is an insulated wire used to transmit the electrical current from the pulse generator to the myocardium. A unipolar lead contains a single wire and a bipolar lead contains two wires that are insulated from each other. In a unipolar lead, the electrode is an exposed metal tip at the end of the lead that contacts the myocardium and serves as the negative pole of the pacing circuit. In a bipolar lead, the end of the lead is a metal tip that contacts myocardium

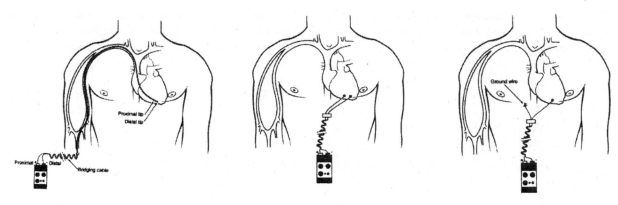

Figure 3–43. Temporary single chamber ventricular pacing. **(A)** Transvenous pacing with pacing lead in apex of right ventricle. **(B)** Bipolar epicardial pacing with two epicardial wires on ventricle. **(C)** Unipolar epicardial pacing with one wire on ventricle and one ground wire in mediastinum. (*Source: Jacobson C, Gerity D. Pacemakers and implantable defibrillators. In Woods SL, Froelicher ES, Motzer SU [eds]: Cardiac Nursing, 4th ed. Philadelphia: Lippincott; 2000, pp. 671–672.*)

and serves as the negative pole, and the positive pole is an exposed metal ring located a few millimeters proximal to the distal tip.

Basics of Pacemaker Operation

Electrical current flows in a closed-loop circuit between two pieces of metal (poles). For current to flow, there must be conductive material (i.e., a lead, muscle, or conductive solution) between the two poles. In the heart, the pacing lead, cardiac muscle, and body tissues serve as conducting material for the flow of electrical current in the pacing system. The pacing circuit consists of the pacemaker pulse generator (the power source), the conducting lead (pacing lead), and the myocardium. The electrical stimulus travels from the pulse generator through the pacing lead to the myocardium, through the myocardium, and back to the pulse generator, thus completing the circuit

Temporary transvenous pacing is done using bipolar pacing leads. Epicardial pacing can be done with either bipolar or unipolar leads. The term *bipolar* means that both of the poles in the pacing system are in or on the heart. In a bipolar system, the pulse generator initiates the electrical impulse and delivers it out the negative terminal of the pacemaker to the pacing lead. The impulse travels down the lead to the distal electrode (negative pole or cathode) that is in contact with myocardium. As the impulse reaches the tip, it travels through the myocardium and returns to the positive pole (or anode) of the system, completing the circuit. In a bipolar system, the positive pole is the proximal ring located a few millimeters proximal to the distal tip. The circuit over which the electrical impulse travels in a bipolar system is small because the two poles are located close together on the lead. This results in a small pacing spike on the ECG as the pacing stimulus travels between the two poles. If the stimulus is strong enough to depolarize the myocardium, the pacing spike is immediately followed by a P wave if the lead

is in the atrium, or a wide QRS complex if the lead is in the ventricle.

A unipolar system has only one of the two poles in or on the heart. In a temporary unipolar epicardial pacing system, a ground lead placed in the subcutaneous tissue in the mediastinum serves as the second pole. Unipolar pacemakers work the same way as bipolar systems, but the circuit over which the impulse travels is larger because of the greater distance between the two poles. This results in a large pacing spike on the ECG as the impulse travels between the two poles.

Capture and Sensing

The two main functions of a pacing system are capture and sensing. *Capture* means that a pacing stimulus results in depolarization of the chamber being paced (Figure 3–44). Capture is determined by the strength of the stimulus, which is measured in milliamperes (mA), the amount of time the stimulus is applied to the heart (pulse width), and by contact of the pacing electrode with the myocardium. Capture cannot occur unless the distal tip of the pacing lead is in contact with healthy myocardium that is capable of responding to the stimulus. Pacing in infarcted tissue usually prevents capture. Similarly, if the catheter is floating in the cavity of the ventricle and not in direct contact with myocardium, capture will not occur. In temporary pacing, the output dial on the face of the pulse generator controls stimulus strength, and can be set and changed easily by the operator. Temporary pulse generators usually are capable of delivering a stimulus of from 0.1 to 20 mA.

Sensing means that the pacemaker is able to detect the presence of intrinsic cardiac activity (Figure 3–45). The sensing circuit controls how sensitive the pacemaker is to intrinsic cardiac depolarizations. Intrinsic activity is measured in millivolts (mV), and the higher the number, the larger the intrinsic signal. For example, a 10-mV QRS com-

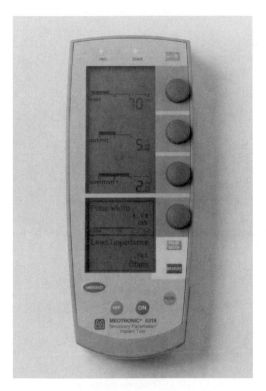

Figure 3–44. Temporary pacemaker pulse generator. (*Source: Medtronic, Inc., Minneapolis, MN*).

plex is larger than a 2-mV QRS. When pacemaker sensitivity needs to be increased to make the pacemaker "see" smaller signals, the sensitivity number must be decreased. For example, a sensitivity of 2 mV is more sensitive than one of 5 mV.

A fence analogy may help to explain sensitivity. Think of sensitivity as a fence standing between the pacemaker and what it wants to see, the ventricle, for example. If there is a 10-foot-high fence (or a 10-mV sensitivity) between the two,

the pacemaker may not see what the ventricle is doing. To make the pacemaker able to see, the fence needs to be lowered. Lowering the fence to 2 feet would probably enable the pacemaker to see the ventricle. Changing the sensitivity from 10 to 2 mV is like lowering the fence—the pacemaker becomes more sensitive and is able to "see" intrinsic activity more easily. Thus, to increase the sensitivity of a pacemaker, the millivolt number (fence) must be decreased.

Asynchronous (Fixed-Rate) Pacing Mode

A pacemaker programmed to an asynchronous mode paces at the programmed rate regardless of intrinsic cardiac activity. This can result in competition between the pacemaker and the heart's own electrical activity. Asynchronous pacing in the ventricle is unsafe because of the potential for pacing stimuli to fall in the vulnerable period of repolarization and cause VF.

Demand Mode

The term *demand* means that the pacemaker paces only when the heart fails to depolarize on its own, that is, the pacemaker fires only "on demand." In demand mode, the pacemaker's sensing circuit is capable of sensing intrinsic cardiac activity and inhibiting pacer output when intrinsic activity is present. Sensing takes place between the two poles of the pacemaker. A bipolar system senses over a small area because the poles are close together, and this can result in "undersensing" of intrinsic signals. A unipolar system senses over a large area because the poles are far apart, and this can result in "oversensing." A unipolar system is more likely to sense myopotentials caused by muscle movement and inappropriately inhibit pacemaker output, potentially resulting in periods of asystole if the patient has no underlying cardiac rhythm. The demand mode should always be used for ventricular pacing to avoid the possibility of VF.

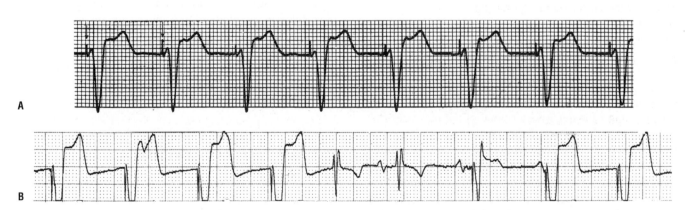

Figure 3–45. (A) Ventricular pacing with 100% capture. Arrows show pacing spikes, each one followed by a wide QRS complex indicating ventricular capture. **(B)** Rhythm strip of a ventricular pacemaker in the demand mode. There is appropriate sensing of intrinsic QRS complexes and appropriate pacing with ventricular capture when the intrinsic QRS complexes fall below the pre-set rate of the pacemaker. The seventh beat is fusion between the intrinsic QRS and the paced beat, a normal phenomenon in ventricular pacing.

ECG Characteristics of Paced Rhythms (Figure 3–46)

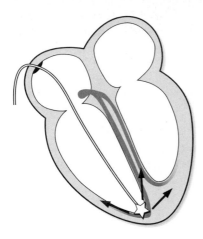

Figure 3–46. ECG characteristics of paced rhythms.

A paced ventricular beat begins with a pacing spike, which indicates that an electrical stimulus was released by the pacemaker. If the pacing stimulus is strong enough to depolarize the ventricle, the spike is followed by a wide QRS complex and a T wave that is oriented in the opposite direction of the QRS complex. Figure 3–46 illustrates ventricular pacing with 100% capture.

Figure 3–45B is the ECG of a ventricular pacemaker that is functioning correctly in the demand mode. The pacemaker generates an impulse when it senses that the heart rate has decreased below the set pacing rate. Therefore, the pacemaker senses the intrinsic cardiac rhythm of the patient and only generates an impulse when the rate falls below the preset pacing rate. Refer to Chapter 18 (Advanced ECG Concepts) for more detailed information on single and dual chamber pacing.

Initiating Transvenous Ventricular Pacing

Temporary transvenous pacing leads are bipolar and have two tails, one marked "positive" or "proximal" and the other marked "negative" or "distal," that are connected to the pulse generator. To initiate ventricular pacing using a transvenous lead (see Figure 3–43A)

1. Connect the negative terminal of the pulse generator to the distal end of the pacing lead.
2. Connect the positive terminal of the pulse generator to the proximal end of the pacing lead.
3. Set the rate at 70 to 80 beats/min or as ordered by physician.
4. Set the output at 5 mA, then determine stimulation threshold and set two to three times higher.
5. Set the sensitivity at 2 mV and adjust according to sensitivity threshold.

Initiating Epicardial Pacing

To initiate bipolar ventricular pacing (two leads on the ventricle; see Figure 3–43B)

1. Connect the negative terminal of the pulse generator to one of the ventricular leads.
2. Connect the positive terminal of the pulse generator to the other ventricular lead.
3. Set the rate at 70 to 80 beats/min or as ordered.
4. Set the output at 5 mA, then determine stimulation threshold and set two to three times higher.
5. Set the sensitivity at 2 mV and adjust according to sensitivity threshold.

To initiate unipolar ventricular pacing (one lead on the ventricle;—see Figure 3–43C)

1. Connect the negative terminal of the pulse generator to the ventricular lead.
2. Connect the positive terminal of the pulse generator to the ground lead.
3. Set the rate at 70 to 80 beats/min or as ordered by physician.
4. Set the output at 5 mA, then determine stimulation threshold and set two to three times higher.
5. Set the sensitivity at 2 mV and adjust according to sensitivity threshold.

External (Transcutaneous) Pacemakers

The emergent nature of many bradycardic rhythms requires immediate temporary pacing. Because transvenous catheter placement is difficult to accomplish quickly, external pacing is the preferred method for rapid, easy initiation of cardiac pacing in emergent situations until a transvenous pacemaker can be inserted. External pacing is done through large-surface adhesive electrodes attached to the anterior and posterior chest wall and connected to an external pacing unit (Figure 3–47). The pacing current passes through skin and chest wall structures to reach the heart; therefore, large energies are required to achieve capture. Sedation and analgesia are usually needed to minimize the discomfort felt by the patient during pacing. Transcutaneous pacing spikes are usually very large, often distorting the QRS complex. The presence of a pulse with every pacing spike confirms ventricular capture.

DEFIBRILLATION AND CARDIOVERSION

Defibrillation

Defibrillation is the therapeutic use of an electrical shock to temporarily depolarize an irregularly beating heart. Defibrillation is used immediately for VF or pulseless VT. Defibrillation completely depolarizes all myocardial cells and terminates the chaotic electrical activity, allowing the

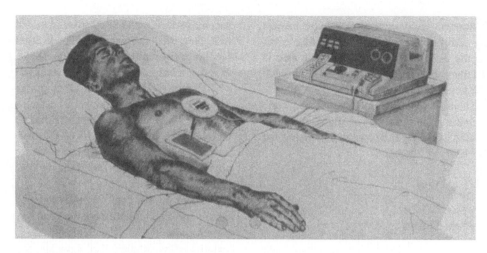

Figure 3–47. External pacemaker with adhesive pacing electrode pads on anterior and posterior chest, connected to external pacemaker at bedside. (*Source: Zoll Medical Corporation, Burlington, MA.*)

sinus node to regain control of the heart rhythm. The defibrillator paddles are placed appropriately on the chest (see below) and the defibrillator is discharged at 200 J. If the first shock does not terminate the rhythm, a second shock at 200 to 300 J is delivered, and a third shock at 360 J is delivered if the first two shocks fail. If the myocardium is anoxic or acidotic, then it may not be possible to terminate the ventricular rhythm.

The electrode paddles are applied to the anterior chest before the defibrillator is discharged. The standard electrode position for the closed-chest procedure is as follows: one paddle just to the right of the upper sternum below the right clavicle and the other paddle just to the left of the cardiac apex (Figure 3–48). To reduce skin resistance to current flow

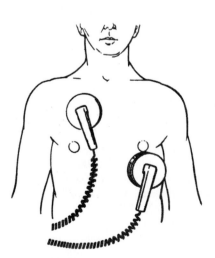

Figure 3–48. Anterior chest wall placement of paddles for cardioversion and defibrillation. (*Source: Jacobson C: Arrhythmias and conduction abnormalities. In Patrick M, et al [eds]*: Medical-Surgical Nursing: Pathophysiological Concepts, *2 ed. Lippincott: Philadelphia; 1991, p. 677.*)

and to prevent skin burns, defibrillator gel pads are used under the paddles. Care should be taken to prevent contact between the two pads because electrical bridging may occur. Self-adhesive defibrillator pads can also be used instead of the rigid metal paddles. To ensure good skin contact during defibrillation using hand-held paddles, 20 to 25 pounds of pressure should be exerted on each paddle. Make sure no one is touching the patient or the bed when the defibrillator is discharged. The electric shock is delivered by depressing both discharge buttons simultaneously. After defibrillation, the cardiac monitor and pulse are checked for signs of restored rhythm (Figure 3–49A).

Automatic External Defibrillators

An automatic external defibrillator (AED) is a device that incorporates a rhythm-analysis system and a shock advisory system for use by trained lay people in treating victims of sudden cardiac death. The American Heart Association recommends that AEDs should be available in selected areas where large gatherings of people occur and where immediate access to emergency care may be limited, such as on airplanes, in airports, sports stadiums, health and fitness facilities, and so on. It is well known that early defibrillation is the key to survival in patients experiencing VF or pulseless VT. Any delay in the delivery of the first shock, including delays related to waiting for the arrival of trained medical personnel and equipment, can decrease the chance of survival. The availability of an AED in public areas can prevent unnecessary delays in treatment and improve survival in victims of sudden cardiac death.

Operation of an AED is quite simple and can be performed by laypeople. Instructions for use are printed on the machines and voice commands also guide the operator in using the AED. Adhesive pads are placed in the standard

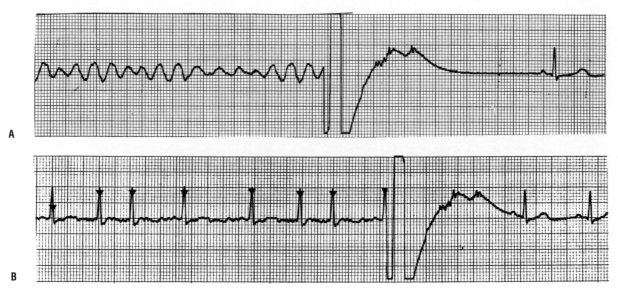

Figure 3–49. **(A)** Defibrillation of VF to sinus rhythm. **(B)** Cardioversion of atrial fibrillation to sinus rhythm. Note the synchronization mark on the QRS.

defibrillation position on the chest (see Figure 3–48), the machine is turned on, and the rhythm analysis system analyzes the patient's rhythm. If the rhythm analysis system detects a shockable rhythm, such as VF or rapid VT, a voice advises the operator to shock the patient. Delivery of the shock is a simple maneuver that only involves pushing a button. The operator is advised to "stand clear" prior to delivering the shock. After a shock is delivered, the system reanalyzes the rhythm and advises another shock if needed.

Cardioversion

Cardioversion, synchronized electrical countershock, is used to terminate arrhythmias that have QRS complexes and is usually an elective procedure. If the patient is alert and oriented, informed consent is obtained. The patient is given IV medication to promote short-acting anesthesia. The amount of voltage used varies from 50 to 200 J. The defibrillator is synchronized with the QRS complex so that an electrical impulse is discharged during ventricular depolarization, thus avoiding the vulnerable period (T wave). The discharge buttons should be held until the synchronizer fires the defibrillator. If VF occurs after cardioversion, the defibrillator is recharged immediately, and defibrillation is performed. Indications of successful response are conversion to sinus rhythm, strong peripheral pulses, and adequate blood pressure (Figure 3–49B). Airway patency should be maintained and the patient's state of consciousness assessed. Vital signs should be obtained at least every 15 minutes for 1 hour, every 30 minutes for 1 hour, and then as indicated by the patient's condition. Many cardioversions are done on an out-

patient basis and patients are discharged as soon as they are awake and vital signs are stable.

SELECTED BIBLIOGRAPHY

Cummins RO (ed): Advanced cardiac life support. Dallas: American Heart Association; 2000.

Dracup K: *Meltzer's Intensive Coronary Care,* 5th ed. Stamford, CT: Appleton & Lange, 1995.

Drew BJ, Scheinman MM: Value of electrocardiographic leads MCL1, MCL6 and other selected leads in the diagnosis of wide QRS complex tachycardia. *J Am Coll Cardiol* 1991;18:1025.

Drew BJ, Scheinman MM, Dracup K: MCL1 and MCL6 compared to V1 and V6 in distinguishing aberrant supraventricular from ventricular ectopic beats. *Pacing Clin Electrophys* 1991;14:1375.

Gilmore SB, Woods SL: Electrocardiography and vectorcardiography. In Woods SL, et al (eds): *Cardiac Nursing,* 3rd ed. Philadelphia: JB Lippincott; 1995.

Jacobson C: Arrhythmias and conduction disturbances. In Woods SL, Froelicher ES, Motzer SU (eds.) *Cardiac Nursing,* 4th ed. Philadelphia: Lippincott; 2000.

Jacobson C, Gerity D. Pacemakers and implantable defibrillators. In Woods SL, Froelicher ES, Motzer SU (eds): *Cardiac Nursing,* 4th ed. Philadelphia: Lippincott; 2000.

Kissen M, et al: A nomogram for rate correction of the QT interval in the electrocardiogram. *Am Heart J* 1948;35:991.

Marriott HJL, Conover M: *Advanced Concepts in Arrhythmias,* 3rd ed. St. Louis: CV Mosby; 1998.

Mitrani RD, Myerburg RJ, Castellanos A: Cardiac pacemakers. In Fuster V, Alexander RW, O'Rourke RA (eds): *Hurst's The Heart,* 10th ed. New York: McGraw-Hill; 2001.

Myerburg RJ, Kloosterman EM, Castellanos A: Recognition, clinical assessment, and management of arrhythmias and conduction disturbances. In Fuster V, Alexander RW, O'Rourke RA (eds): *Hurst's The Heart,* 10th ed. New York: McGraw-Hill; 2001, pp. 797–874.

Olgin JE, Zipes DP: Specific arrhythmias: Diagnosis and treatment. In Braunwald E, Zipes DP, Libby P (eds): *Heart Disease,* 6th ed. Philadelphia: W.B. Saunders; 2001, pp. 659–699.

Podrid PJ, Kowey PR (eds): *Cardiac Arrhythmia: Mechanisms, Diagnosis & Management,* 2nd ed. Philadelphia: Lippincott Williams & Wilkins; 2001.

Shanker A, Saksena S: Cardiac pacemakers. In Podrid PJ, Kowey PR (eds): *Cardiac Arrhythmia: Mechanisms, Diagnosis, and Management,* 2nd ed. Philadelphia: Lippincott Williams & Wilkins; 2001, pp. 323–356.

Evidenced-Based Practice

American Association of Critical Care Nurse (AACN). Practice Alert: Dysrhythmia Monitoring. Aliso Viejo, CA: AACN; 2004. Available from URL: http://www.aacn.org.

Drew BJ, Califf RM, Funk M, et al: Practice standards for electro-cardiographic monitoring in hospital settings. Circulation; in press, 2004.

Jacobson C: Bedside cardiac monitoring. In Chulay M, Burns S (eds): *AACN's Protocols for Practice: Technology Series.* Aliso Viejo, CA: AACN; 1996.

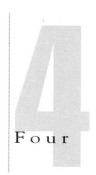

HEMODYNAMIC MONITORING

Four

Leanna R. Miller

▶ Knowledge Competencies

1. Identify the characteristics of normal and abnormal waveform pressures for the following hemodynamic monitoring parameters:
   - Central venous pressure
   - Pulmonary artery pressure
   - Arterial blood pressure
   - Cardiac output

2. Describe the basic elements of hemodynamic pressure monitoring equipment and methods used to ensure accurate pressure measurements.

3. Discuss the indications, contraindications, and general management principles for the following common hemodynamic monitoring parameters:
   - Central venous pressure
   - Pulmonary artery pressure

   - Right ventricular pressure
   - Mixed venous oxygenation
   - Arterial blood pressure
   - Cardiac output

4. Describe the use of Svo_2 monitoring in the critically ill patient.

5. Compare and contrast the clinical implications and management approaches to abnormal hemodynamic values.

6. Explain the basic elements of minimally invasive hemodynamic monitoring techniques.

Hemodynamics is the study of the interrelationship of blood pressure (BP), blood flow, vascular volumes, heart rate, ventricular function, and the physical properties of the blood. Monitoring the hemodynamic status of the critically ill patient is an integral part of critical care nursing. It is essential that critical care nurses have a working knowledge of how to obtain accurate data, analyze waveforms, and interpret and integrate the data.

Clinical examination can be a poor predictor of hemodynamics. Although noninvasive assessment techniques such as physical examination, history taking, and laboratory analysis are helpful and necessary, they do not provide the specific physiologic data available with hemodynamic monitoring. Parameters such as cardiac output (CO) and intracardiac pressures can be directly measured and monitored with special indwelling catheters. The information provided by

the catheters can provide accurate and timely information to clinicians so that appropriate interventions are ensured.

HEMODYNAMIC PARAMETERS

Cardiac Output

CO is the amount of blood pumped by the ventricles each minute. It is the product of the heart rate (HR) and the stroke volume (SV) (the amount of blood ejected by the ventricle with each contraction; Figure 4–1).

$$CO = HR \times SV$$

The normal value is 4.0 to 8.0 L/min (Table 4–1). It is important to note that these values are relative to size. Values

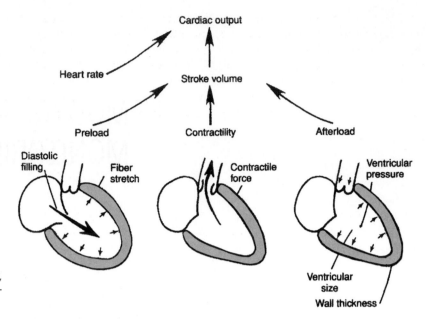

Figure 4–1. Factors affecting CO. (*Source: Price S, Wilson L.* Pathophysiology: Clinical Concepts of Disease Processes. *Philadelphia: Mosby; 1992, p. 390.*)

within the normal range for a person 5 feet tall weighing 100 pounds, may be totally inadequate for a 6-foot, 200-pound individual. Cardiac index (CI) is the CO that has been adjusted to individual body size. It is determined by dividing the CO by the individual's body surface area (BSA), which may be obtained from the Dubois body surface area chart or by pressing the CI button on the cardiac monitor. The normal value is 2.5 to 4.3 L/min/m^2 (Table 4–1).

$$CI = CO/BSA$$

TABLE 4–1. NORMAL HEMODYNAMIC AND BLOOD FLOW PARAMETERS

Parameter	Abbreviation	Formula	Normal Range
Cardiac index	CI	CO/BSA ÷ 1000	2.5–4.3 L/min/m^2
Mean arterial pressure	MAP	2(DBP) + SBP 3	70–105 mm Hg
Right atrial pressure	RAP	cm H$_2$0 = mm Hg × 1.34	2–8 mm Hg
Pulmonary artery occlusion pressure	PAOP		8–12 mm Hg
Pulmonary artery diastolic	PAD		10–15 mm Hg
Pulmonary vascular resistance	PVR	PAM–PAOP × 80 CO	100–250 dynes/sec/cm^{-5}
Pulmonary vascular resistance index	PVRI	PAM–PAOP × 80 CI	255–285 dynes/sec/m^2-cm^{-5}
Pulmonary artery mean	PAM		15–20 mm Hg
Systemic vascular resistance	SVR	MAP–RAP × 80 CO	800–1200 dynes/sec/cm^{-5}
Systemic vascular resistance index	SVRI	MAP–RAP × 80 CI	1970–2390 dynes/sec/m^2-cm^{-5}
Right ventricular stroke work index	RVSWI	(PAD–RAP) SV × 0.0138 BSA	7–12 g·m/m^2
Left ventricular stroke work index	LVSWI	(MAP–PAOP) SV × 0.0138 BSA	35–85 g·m/m^2
Oxygen delivery	DO$_2$	CaO$_2$ × CO × 10	900–1100 mL/min
Oxygen delivery index	DO$_2$I	CI × 1.38 × Hgb × Sao$_2$ × 10	360–600 mL/min/m^2
Oxygen consumption	Vo$_2$	C(a − v)O$_2$ × CO × 10	200–250 mL/min
Oxygen consumption index	Vo$_2$I	CI × 1.38(SaO$_2$ − Svo$_2$) × (Hgb)(10)	108–165 mL/min/m^2
Stroke volume	SV	SV = EDV = ESV CO/HR × 1000	50–100 mL/beat
Stroke volume index	SVI	SV/BSA CI/HR × 1000	35–60 mL/beat/m^2
Right ventricular end-diastolic volume	RVEDV	SV/EF	100–160 mL
Right ventricular end-diastolic volume index	RVEDVI	EDV/BSA	60–100 mL/m^2
Right ventricular end-systolic volume	RVESV	EDV − SV	50–100 mL
Right ventricular end-systolic volume index	RVESVI	ESV/BSA	30–60 mL/m^2
Right ventricular ejection fraction	RVEF	SV/EDV EDV − ESV/EDV	40–60%
Mixed venous saturation	Svo$_2$		60–75%
Oxygen extraction ratio	O$_2$ER	(Cao$_2$ − Cvo$_2$)/Cao$_2$ × 100	22–30%
Oxygen extraction index	O$_2$EI	Sao$_2$ − Svo$_2$/Sao$_2$ × 100	20–25%

CO measurements are used to assess the patient's perfusion status, response to therapy, and as a rapid means to evaluate the patient's hemodynamic status. As mentioned, CO is composed of heart rate and SV, or the amount of blood ejected with each contraction of the ventricle. Normal SV range is 60 to 130 mL/beat (see Table 4–1). SV depends on preload, afterload, and contractility. Therefore, CO is determined by:

1. Heart rate (and rhythm)
2. Preload
3. Afterload
4. Contractility

Low Cardiac Output/Cardiac Index

Because the SV of the left ventricle is a component used in the determination of CO, any condition or disease process which impairs the pumping (ejection) or filling of the ventricle may contribute to a decreased CO. Alterations that lead to diminished CO can be divided into two general categories: inadequate ventricular filling and inadequate ventricular emptying.

Inadequate Ventricular Filling

Factors that lead to inadequate ventricular filling include dysrhythmias, hypovolemia, cardiac tamponade, mitral or tricuspid stenosis, constrictive pericarditis, and restrictive cardiomyopathy. Each of these abnormalities leads to a decrease in preload (the amount of volume in the ventricle at end diastole), which results in a decrease in CO.

Inadequate Ventricular Ejection

Factors that lead to inadequate ventricular emptying include mitral/tricuspid insufficiency, myocardial infarction, increased afterload (hypertension, aortic/pulmonic stenosis), myocardial diseases (myocarditis, cardiomyopathy), metabolic disorders (hypoglycemia, hypoxia, severe acidosis), and use of negative inotropic drugs (beta-blockers, calcium channel blockers).

High Cardiac Output/Index

In theory, any factor that increases heart rate and contractility and decreases afterload can contribute to an increase in CO. Hyperdynamic states, such as seen in sepsis, anemia, pregnancy, and hyperthyroid crisis, may cause CO values to be increased. Increased heart rate is a major component in hyperdynamic states; however, in sepsis a profound decrease in afterload also contributes to an increased CO.

Components of Cardiac Output/Cardiac Index

Heart Rate and Rhythm

Rate

Normal heart rate is 60 to 100 beats/min. In a normal, healthy individual, an increase in heart rate can lead to an increase in CO. In a person with cardiac dysfunction, increases in heart rate can lead to a decreased CO and often

myocardial ischemia. The increase in heart rate decreases the ventricular filling time, resulting in decreased SV, which leads to decreased CO.

A lower heart rate does not necessarily result in a decrease in CO. Decreased heart rates and normal COs are often found in athletes. Their training and conditioning strengthens the myocardium such that each cardiac contraction produces an increased SV. In individuals with left ventricular (LV) dysfunction, a slow heart rate can produce a decrease in CO. This is caused by decreased contractility, as well as fewer cardiac contractions each minute.

Because CO is a product of SV times heart rate, any change in SV normally produces a change in the heart rate. If the SV is elevated, the heart rate may decrease (e.g., as seen in adaptation to exercise). If the SV falls, the heart rate normally increases. Subsequently, evaluating the cause of the tachycardia becomes an essential component of hemodynamic monitoring. Bradycardias and tachycardias are potentially dangerous because they may result in a decrease in CO. Bradycardias that develop suddenly are almost always reflective of a falling CO. The cause of tachycardia, on the other hand, must be determined because it may not reflect a low output state but rather a normal physiologic response (e.g., tachycardia with a fever). Heart rate varies between individuals and is related to many factors. Some are described below.

DECREASED HEART RATE

- Parasympathetic stimulation (vagus nerve stimulation) is a common occurrence in the critical care setting. It can occur with Valsalva maneuvers such as excessive bearing down during a bowel movement, vomiting, coughing, and suctioning.
- Conduction abnormalities, especially second- and third-degree block are often seen in patients with cardiovascular diseases. Many drugs used in the critical care setting may lead to a decreased heart rate, including digitalis, beta-blockers, calcium channel blockers, and phenylephrine (Neosynephrine).
- Athletes often have resting heart rates below 60 beats/ min without compromising CO.
- The actual heart rate is not as important as the systemic effect of the heart rate. If the patient's heart rate leads to diminished perfusion (decreased level of consciousness, decreased urinary output, hypotension, prolonged capillary refill, new-onset chest pain, etc.) treatment is initiated to increase the heart rate.

INCREASED HEART RATE

- Stress, anxiety, pain, and conditions resulting in compensatory release of endogenous catecholamines such as hypovolemia, fever, anemia, and hypotension may all produce tachycardia.
- Drugs with a direct positive chronotropic effect include epinephrine and dopamine.

Tachycardia is very common in critically ill patients. When evaluating a rapid heart rate, each of the main sources for the tachycardia are evaluated. For example, if a patient has a heart rate of 120 beats/min, the clinician rules out such factors as fever, pain, and anxiety before assuming the tachycardia is due to a reduced SV. Once these are ruled out an investigation of the cause of a low SV is accomplished. The two most common reasons for a low SV are hypovolemia and LV dysfunction. Both causes of low SV can produce an increased heart rate if no abnormality exists in regulation of the heart rate (such as autonomic nervous system dysfunction or use of drugs that interfere with the sympathetic or parasympathetic nervous system such as beta-blockers).

An increased heart rate can compensate for a decrease in SV, although this compensation is limited. The faster the heart rate, the less time exists for ventricular filling. As an increased heart rate reduces diastolic filling time, the potential exists to eventually reduce the SV. There is no specific heart rate where diastolic filling is reduced so severely that SV decreases. However, as the heart rate increases, it is important to remember that SV may be negatively affected.

Increased heart rate also has the potential to increase myocardial oxygen demand (MVO_2). The higher the heart rate, the more likely it is that the heart consumes more oxygen. Some patients are more sensitive to elevated MVO_2 than others. For example, a young person may tolerate a sinus tachycardia as high as 160 for several days, whereas a patient with coronary artery disease may decompensate and develop pulmonary edema with a heart rate in the 130s. Keeping heart rates as low as possible, particularly in patients with altered myocardial blood flow, is one way of protecting myocardial function.

Rhythm

Many of us have observed the deleterious effects produced by a supraventricular tachycardia, or a change from normal sinus rhythm to atrial fibrillation or flutter. Loss of "atrial kick" may contribute to decreased CO. Normally, the atrium contributes 20% to 40% of the ventricular filling volume. With tachycardia, that atrial contribution to SV may diminish significantly. Although those with normal cardiac function are unlikely to experience compromise, it is more likely in those with impaired cardiac function.

Stroke Volume and Stroke Volume Index

Stroke volume is the amount of blood ejected from each ventricle with each heartbeat. The right and left ventricle eject nearly the same amount, which normally is between 50 and 100 mL per heartbeat (see Table 4–1).

$$SV = (CO \times 1000)/HR$$

SV is indexed to the patient's BSA in SVI. Indexing helps to compare values regardless of the patient's size. This is calculated by most monitors. Normal SVI is 25 to 45 mL/beat/m² (see Table 4–1). Common causes of decreased stroke volume/stroke volume index (SV/SVI) in inadequate blood volume (preload), impaired ventricular contractility (strength), increased systemic vascular resistance (SVR; afterload), and cardiac valve dysfunction. High SV/SVI occurs when the vascular resistance is low (sepsis, use of vasodilators, neurogenic shock, and anaphylaxis).

Ejection Fraction

The *ejection fraction* (EF) is defined as how much blood is pumped with each contraction in relation to the volume of available blood. For example, assume the left ventricular end-diastolic volume (LVEDV is the amount of blood left in the heart just before contraction) is 100 mL. If the SV is 80 mL the EF is 80%; 80 mL of the possible 100 mL in the ventricle were ejected. A normal EF is usually over 60% (see Table 4–1).

The EF may change before the SV in certain conditions, such as LV failure and sepsis. For example, the left ventricle may dilate in response to LV dysfunction from coronary artery disease, and LVEDV increases. Although the increase in LVEDV may prevent a drop in SV, EF may not be preserved. Thus, EF and LVEDV are early indicators of ventricular dysfunction and are ideal monitoring parameters. Unfortunately, EF and LVEDV are not routinely available. SV and SI, then, are the best available measures to assess left and right ventricular dysfunction.

The SV is very important because it typically falls with hypovolemia or when the left ventricle is too weak to eject blood (LV dysfunction).

Factors Affecting Stroke Volume/Stroke Volume Index

Preload

Preload is the volume of blood that exerts a force or pressure (stretch) on the ventricles during diastole. It may also be described as the filling pressure of the ventricles at the end of diastole or the amount of blood that fills the ventricles during diastole.

According to the Frank–Starling law of the heart, the force of contraction is related to myocardial fiber stretch prior to contraction. As the fibers are stretched, the contractile force increases up to a certain point. Beyond this point, the contractile force decreases and is referred to as *ventricular failure* (Figure 4–2). With increased preload there is an increase in the volume of blood delivered to the ventricle, the myocardium is stretched and a more forceful ventricular contraction is produced. This forceful ventricular contraction yields an increase in SV, and therefore, CO. Too much preload causes the ventricular contraction to be less effective. A commonly referred to analogy uses the properties of a rubber band. The more a rubber band is stretched, the greater

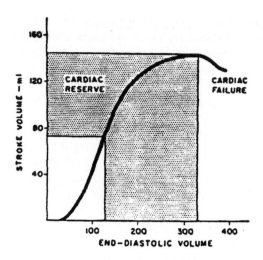

Figure 4–2. Ventricular function curve. As the end-diastolic volume increases, so does the force of ventricular contraction. The SV becomes greater up to a critical point after which SV decreases (cardiac failure). (*From Langley LF:* Review of Physiology, *3rd ed. New York: McGraw-Hill; 1971.*)

"snap" is produced when released. The rubber band may be stretched further and further, until it reaches a point where it loses its tautness and recoils.

Determinants of Preload

Preload is determined primarily by the amount of venous return to the heart. Venous constriction, venous dilation, and alterations in the total blood volume all affect preload. Preload decreases with volume changes. This can occur in hemorrhage (traumatic, surgical, gastrointestinal [GI], OB/GYN), diuresis (excessive use of diuretics, diabetic ketoaci-

dosis, diabetes insipidus), vomiting and diarrhea, third spacing (ascites, severe sepsis, congestive heart failure [CHF]), redistribution of blood flow (use of vasodilators, neurogenic shock, severe sepsis), and profound diaphoresis. Venous dilatation also results in diminished preload. Etiologies that increase venous pooling and result in decreased venous return to the heart include hyperthermia, septic shock, anaphylactic shock, and drug administration (nitroglycerin, nitroprusside) (Table 4–2).

Factors leading to increased preload include excessive administration of crystalloids or blood products and the presence of renal failure (oliguric phase). Venous constriction results in the shunting of peripheral blood to the central organs (heart and brain). The increased venous return results in an increased preload. This may occur in hypothermia, some forms of shock (hypovolemic, cardiogenic, and obstructive) and with administration of drugs that stimulate the alpha receptors (epinephrine, dopamine at doses greater than 20 μg/kg/min, norepinephrine) (see Table 4–2).

Clinical Indicators of Preload

The right ventricle pumps blood into the pulmonary circulation and the left ventricle ejects blood into the systemic circulation. Both circulatory systems are affected by preload, afterload, and contractility. These are discussed below and when appropriate the clinical indicators are differentiated by right or left heart.

RIGHT VENTRICULAR PRELOAD (CVP OR RAP)

Normal right ventricular (RV) preload is 2 to 8 mm Hg or 2 to 10 cm H_2O (see Table 4–1) (CVP = Central Venous Pressure; RAP = Right Atrial Pressure). Right atrial pres-

TABLE 4–2. HEMODYNAMIC EFFECTS OF CARDIOVASCULAR AGENTS

Drug	CO	PAOP	SVR	MAP	HR	CVP	PVR
Norepinephrine (Levophed)	↑ (slight)	↑	↑	↑	↔	↑	↑
Phenylephrine (Neosynephrine)	↔,↓	↑	↑	↑	↔,↓	↑	↑
Epinephrine	↑	↑	↑	↑	↑	↑	↑
Dobutamine (Dobutrex)	↑	↓	↓	↑ (with ↑CO)	↑ (slight)	↓	↓
Dopamine (Intropin)	↑	↑	↑	↑	↑	↑	↔
<5 μg/kg/min	↑	↑↑	(slight)	(slight)	↑	↑↑	↑
>5 μg/kg/min			↑↑	↑↑			
Digoxin (Lanoxin)	↑	↔	↔	↔	↓	↔	↔
Isoproterenol (Isuprel)	↑	↓	↓	↓	↑	↓	↓
Milrinone (Primacor)	↑	↓	↓	↔ (↓ in preload sensitive patient)	↔ (↑ in preload sensitive patient)	↓	↓
Nitroglycerine (Tridil)	↔	↓	↔	↔	↔	↓	↔
20–40 μg/min	↑	↓	↓	↓	↑	↓	↓
50–250 μg/min							
Nitroprusside (Nipride)	↑	↓	↓	↓	↑	↓	↓

sures are measured to assess right ventricular function, intravascular volume status, and the response to fluid and drug administration. CVP/RAP pressures increase because of intravascular volume overload, cardiac tamponade (effusion, blood, etc.), restrictive cardiomyopathies, and RV failure. There are three etiologies of RV failure: (1) intrinsic disease such as RV infarct or cardiomyopathies; (2) secondary to factors that increase pulmonary vascular resistance (PVR) such as pulmonary embolism, hypoxemia, chronic obstructive pulmonary disease (COPD), acute respiratory distress syndrome (ARDS), sepsis; and (3) severe LV dysfunction as seen in mitral stenosis/insufficiency or LV failure. In contrast, the only clinically significant reason for a decreased CVP/RAP is hypovolemia. CVP/RAP is a late indicator of alterations in LV function therefore limiting its value in clinical decision making.

LEFT VENTRICULAR PRELOAD (PAOP OR LAP)

Normal LV preload is 8 to 12 mm Hg (PAOP = Pulmonary artery occlusion pressure; PCWP = Pulmonary capillary wedge pressure; PAWP = Pulmonary artery wedge pressure; LAP = Left atrial pressure) Normal: 8 to 12 mm Hg (see Table 4–1). With the insertion of 1.25 to 1.50 mL of air into the balloon port of the pulmonary artery (PA) catheter, the balloon becomes lodged in a portion of the PA that is smaller than the balloon. This occludes blood flow distal to the catheter tip. The catheter tip is then exposed to the left atrial pressure. When the mitral valve is open during ventricular diastole, the pressure that is sensed is that of the left ventricle, the left ventricular end-diastolic pressure (LVEDP) or LV preload (Figure 4–3).

Pulmonary artery occlusion pressure/left arterial pressure (PAOP/LAP) increase because of intravascular volume overload, cardiac tamponade (blood, effusion, etc.), restrictive cardiomyopathies, and LV dysfunction. Common etiologies of LV dysfunction include mitral stenosis/insufficiency, aortic stenosis/insufficiency, and diminished LV compliance (ischemia, fibrosis, hypertrophy). The only clinically significant reason for a decreased PAOP/LAP is hypovolemia.

There are some conditions in which wedge and LVEDP do not correlate. LV failure with PAOP greater than 15 to 20 mm Hg and conditions with diminished LV compliance result in a PAOP less than the true LVEDP. Patients on positive end-expiratory pressure (PEEP, continuous positive airway pressure), zone 1 or 2 catheter tip placement (Figure 4–4), tachycardia (>130 beats/min), mitral stenosis/insufficiency, COPD, or pulmonary venoocclusive disease have a measured PAOP that is greater than the true LVEDP. These factors must be considered prior to therapeutic management.

The pulmonary artery diastolic (PAD) is normally 1 to 4 mm Hg higher than the LAP/PAOP due to resistance of blood flow into the pulmonary vessels; however, when the catheter is "wedged" there is no flow or resistance to flow and the number reflects LAP/PAOP. When the patient has an increased PVR the PAD and LAP/PAOP no longer correlate and cannot be used interchangeably. Conditions that cause increased PVR are hypoxemia, acidemia, massive pulmonary embolism, and pulmonary vascular disease. If the PAD and LAP/PAOP closely correlate, the PAD can be used to trend the LVEDP. This allows prolonged balloon life, and reduces the chance for pulmonary ischemia, PA damage, and rupture.

Afterload

Afterload is the resistance to ventricular emptying during systole. It is the pressure, or resistance, that the ventricles

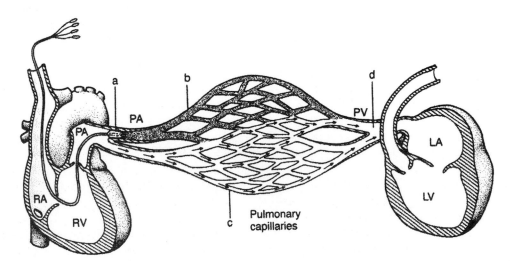

Figure 4–3. Schematic representation of the PA in the wedge position. From its position in small occluded segment of the pulmonary circulation, the PA catheter in the wedged position allows the electronic monitoring equipment to "look through" a nonactive segment of the pulmonary circulation to the hemodynamically active pulmonary veins and left atrium. (*From Darovic GO:* Hemodynamic Monitoring: Invasive and Noninvasive Clinical Application. *Philadelphia: WB Saunders; 2002, p. 207, with permission.*)

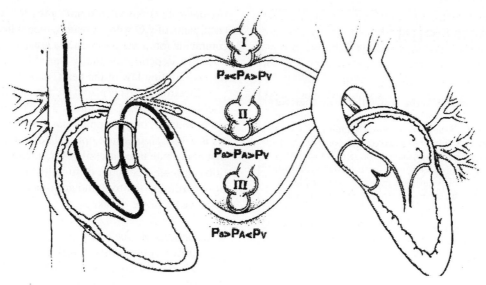

Figure 4–4. The anatomic position of a PA catheter in the PA. Zones I, II, and III characterize the relationship of alveolar (PA), arterial (Pa), and venous (Pv) pressures as described by West. (*From O'Quin R., Marinii JJ: Pulmonary artery occlusion pressure: Clinical physiology, measurement and interpretation. Am Rev Respir Dis 1983;128:319–329, with permission.*)

must overcome to open the aortic and pulmonary valves and to pump blood into the systemic and pulmonary vasculature.

Vascular resistance is determined by the length of a vessel, its diameter or radius, and the viscosity of the blood. The length of the vessel is considered to be constant. The viscosity of the blood is relatively constant except when gross volume changes occur (e.g., hemorrhage) or in polycythemia. Therefore, conditions that alter the diameter of the vessels, or the outflow tract, have a primary effect on the afterload of the ventricles.

As afterload increases (vasoconstriction or obstruction of the outflow tract) the heart must work harder to eject the volume. Afterload affects the isovolumetric contraction phase of the cardiac cycle. During this phase, the ventricular pressure rises so the ventricles are able to overcome the existing vascular resistance, open the semilunar valves, and eject the contents. Once the pressure within the ventricle is higher than the pressure in the aorta/pulmonary system the valves open and the blood is ejected from the heart. With increased afterload the heart works harder to eject the contents, leading to increased MVo_2. This is a crucial period of myocardial susceptibility to ischemic injury and is a major reason to consider afterload reduction therapies.

Common causes of increased afterload include aortic/pulmonic stenosis, hypothermia, hypertension, compensatory response to hypotension and decreased CO, classic shock states (hypovolemic, cardiogenic, and obstructive), and response to drugs that stimulate the alpha receptors (epinephrine, norepinephrine, dopamine, phenylephrine) (see Table 4–2). Decreased afterload is seen in hyperthermia, the distributive shocks (septic, anaphylactic, and neurogenic), and after administration of vasodilating drugs (nitroprusside,

nitroglycerin at higher doses, calcium channel blockers, beta-blockers, etc.) (see Table 4–2).

Clinical Indicators of Afterload

Afterload cannot be directly measured as can preload. Several hemodynamic parameters are calculated based on other measured variables. These parameters are usually referred to as *derived values*. Formulas for some common hemodynamic derived variables are listed in Table 4–1. Most bedside monitors perform the calculations necessary to achieve the values. However, it is essential for critical care nurses to know which variables are included in the calculations. This knowledge is essential to understand how hemodynamic parameters interact, to interpret the derived variables, and to select the appropriate therapy.

Systemic Vascular Resistance

Normal SVR is 800 to 1200 dynes/sec/cm^{-5} (see Table 4–1). If the SVR is elevated, the left ventricle faces an increased resistance to the ejection of blood. The SVR commonly elevates as a pathologic response to hypertension or a low CO, such as would occur in shock states. It is important for the clinician to know why the SVR is elevated. For example, if the SVR is elevated because of systemic hypertension, afterload-reducing agents are a critical part of the therapy. However, if the SVR is elevated secondary to a compensation for low CO, therapy should be directed at improving the CO more than reducing SVR.

If the SVR is low, the left ventricle faces a lower resistance to the ejection of blood. Generally, the SVR only decreases as a pathologic response to inflammatory conditions (e.g., sepsis, fever). The SVR can also be reduced in hepatic

AT THE BEDSIDE
▶ *High SVR*

A 73-year-old woman is in the unit with the diagnosis of CHF. She presently is alert and oriented but complains of severe shortness of breath. Her pulse oximeter reveals a value of 89% on a fraction of inspired oxygen content (FiO_2) of 50% via a high-humidity face mask. She has crackles throughout both lungs and has 31 pitting edema of both lower legs. She has a PA catheter inserted to aid in the interpretation of the situation. The following data are available:

BP	202/114	SVR	2674
P	74/min	PVR	191
RR	34/min		
T	37.6°C		
CO	3.9 L/min		
CI	1.9 L/min/m^2		
SI	24		
PA	43/24		
PAOP	21 mm Hg		
CVP	13 mm Hg		
SvO_2	52%		

Based on this information, the best choice for management is an afterload reducer because the SVR and blood pressure are markedly elevated. A rapid-acting agent like nitroprusside is preferable to achieve an immediate improvement in symptoms, SI, CI, and SvO_2. Caution should be used when lowering the SVR and blood pressure to avoid too rapid a change. Patients who are used to elevated blood pressures can have a decrease in organ perfusion at higher pressures than the clinician might normally expect.

disease due to increased collateral circulation or from neurogenic induced central vasodilation. Generally, if the SVR is reduced, administration of vasopressor drugs is considered. More important, treating the underlying condition is essential. If the underlying condition is not treated, the use of vasopressors provides only short-term success.

Pulmonary Vascular Resistance
PVR is lower in comparison to SVR. Normal PVR is about 100 to 250 dynes/sec/cm^{-5} (see Table 4–1). Generally, only an elevated PVR is considered a problem, because it produces a strain on the right ventricle. If this strain in unrelieved, the right ventricle eventually fails. Failure of the right ventricle results in less blood entering the lungs and the left ventricle. Systemic hypotension follows due to RV dysfunction. The most common causes of an increase in PVR include pulmonary hypertension, hypoxia, end-stage COPD (cor pulmonale), and pulmonary emboli.

Contractility
Contractility is the strength of the myocardial contraction, or the degree of myocardial fiber shortening with contraction.

Contractility contributes significantly to CO. If the other determinants of CO were constant, then a heart with a greater contractile force would produce a greater CO. However, contractility depends on many variables including preload (Frank–Starling law of the heart) and afterload.

Electrolyte levels also have a major impact on the contractility of the heart. Monitoring and treating abnormal calcium, sodium, magnesium, potassium, and phosphorus levels is essential to ensure optimal contractility. Other factors that contribute to contractility include myocardial oxygenation (ischemia), amount of functional myocardium (infarction, cardiomyopathy), and administration of positive and negative inotropic drugs.

Clinical Indicators of Contractility
Myocardial contractility is reflected indirectly in the SVI, which is the SV adjusted according to body size, and the right and left stroke work index (RVSWI and LVSWI). The normal value for SVI is 35 to 60 mL/beat/m^2; RVSWI is 7 to 12 g·m/m^2, and LVSWI is 35 to 85 g·m/m^2 (see Table 4–1) These are not direct indicators of contractility, but can be used to identify patients' at risk for poor contractility and to monitor the effects of therapeutic management.

BASIC COMPONENTS OF HEMODYNAMIC MONITORING SYSTEMS

The basic components of a hemodynamic monitoring system include an indwelling catheter connected to a pressure transducer and flush system and a bedside monitor. All components that come in contact with the vascular system must be sterile, with meticulous attention paid to maintaining a closed sterile system during use.

Pulmonary Artery Catheter
The PA catheter is a multilumen catheter inserted into the PA (Figure 4–5). Each lumen or "port" has specific functions (Table 4–3). The PA catheter typically is inserted through an introducer sheath (large-diameter, short catheter with a diaphragm) placed in a major vein. Veins used for PA catheter insertion include the internal jugular, subclavian, femoral, and less commonly, the brachial vein.

Arterial Catheter
The arterial catheter, or "A-line," has only one lumen, which is used for measuring arterial pressures and for drawing arterial blood samples (Figure 4–6). Arterial catheters are inserted in any major artery, with the most common sites being the radial and femoral arteries.

Pressure Tubing
The pressure tubing is a key component of any hemodynamic monitoring system (see Figure 4–6). It is designed to

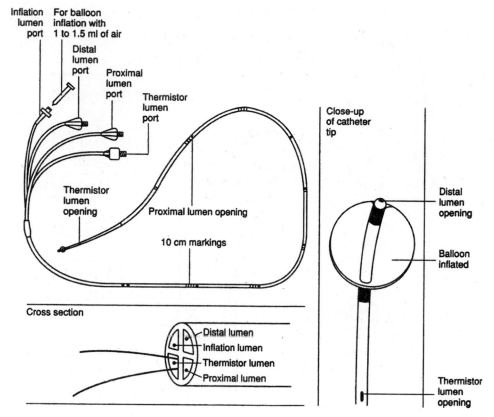

Figure 4–5. Flow-directed PA catheter (Swan-Ganz). (*From: Visalli F, Evans P: The Swan-Ganz catheter: A program for teaching safe, effective use.* Nursing *81 1981;11:1.*)

be a stiff (noncompliant) tubing to ensure accurate transfer of intravascular pressures to the transducer. The pressure tubing connects the intravascular catheter to the transducer. Many pressure tubings have stopcocks in line to facilitate blood sampling and zeroing the transducer (see below). Normally, the pressure tubing is kept as short as possible (no more than

3 to 4 feet), with a minimal number of stopcocks, to increase the accuracy of pressure measurements.

Pressure Transducer

The pressure transducer is a small electronic sensor that has the ability to convert a mechanical pressure (vascular pres-

TABLE 4–3. PULMONARY ARTERY (PA) PORT FUNCTIONS

Type of Port	Functions
Distal tip port	Measures pressure at the tip of the catheter in the PA. With proper inflation of the balloon, measures the pulmonary capillary wedge pressure (PCWP).
	Used to sample Svo_2 levels and for other blood sampling needs.
Proximal lumen port	Measures pressure 30 cm from the distal tip, usually in the right atrium (RA). Central venous pressure (CVP) and RA pressure (RAP) are synonymous terms.
	Injection site for cardiac output (CO) determinations.
	Used to draw blood samples for laboratory tests requiring venous blood. If coagulation studies are drawn, completely remove heparin from line prior to obtaining sample.
	Used for IV fluids and drug administration, if necessary.
Balloon inflation port	Inflated periodically with <1.5 mL of air to obtain PCWP tracing.
Ventricular port (on selected models of PA catheters)	Measures right ventricle (RV) pressure.
	Used for insertion of a temporary pacemaker electrode in the RV.
Ventricular infusion port (on selected models of PA catheters)	An additional lumen for IV fluid or drug administration. Located close to the proximal lumen exit area.
	May be used for CO determinations or CVP measurements, if necessary.
Cardiac output port (thermistor lumen)	Measures blood temperature near the distal tip when connected to the cardiac output computer.
	May be used to monitor body (core) temperature continuously.

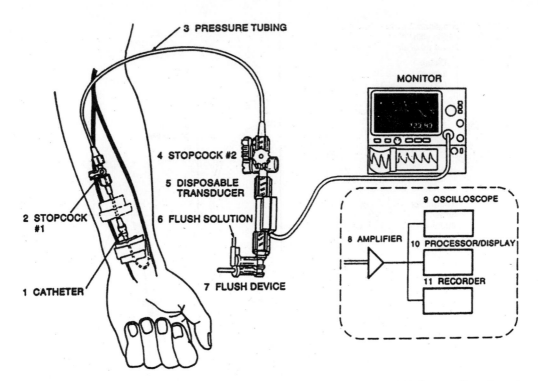

Figure 4–6. Components of a hemodynamic monitoring system. (*From: Gardner R, Hollingsworth K: Electrocardiography and pressure monitoring: How to obtain optimal results. In Shoemaker WC, Ayers S, Grenvik A, Holbrook P [eds]: Textbook of Critical Care, 3rd ed. Philadelphia: WB Saunders; 1995, p. 272.*)

sure) into an electrical signal (see Figure 4–6). This electrical signal can then be displayed on the pressure amplifier.

Pressure Amplifier

The pressure amplifier, or "bedside monitor," augments the signal from the transducer and displays the converted vascular pressure as an electrical signal (see Figure 4–6). This signal is used to display a continuous waveform on the oscilloscope of the monitor and to provide a numerical display of the pressure measurement. Most bedside monitors also have a graphic recorder to print out the pressure waveform.

Pressure Bag and Flush Device

In addition to being attached to the pressure amplifier, the transducer is connected to an intravenous (IV) solution, which is placed in a pressure bag (Figure 4–7). The IV solution is normally 500 to 1000 mL of normal saline (NS), although 5% dextrose in water (D_5W) can be used. The IV solution is placed under 300 mm Hg of pressure to provide a slow, continuous infusion of fluid through the vascular catheter.

The IV solution is placed under pressure for another reason. Included in most pressure systems is a flush device (see Figure 4–7). The flush device regulates fluid flow through the pressure tubing at a slow, continuous rate to prevent occlusion of the vascular catheter. Normally, the flush device restricts fluid flow to approximately 2 to 4 mL/h. If the flush device is activated, normally by squeezing or pulling

the flush device, a rapid flow of fluid enters the pressure tubing. Flush devices are activated for two reasons: to rapidly clear the tubing of air or blood and to check the accuracy of the tubing/catheter system (square wave test). Measuring the fluid in the IV solution should be done on every shift to determine the amount of fluid infused from the pressure bag. Depending on hospital procedures, heparin may be added to the IV solution to aid in keeping the system patent. If this is done, generally about 1 unit of 1:1000 heparin is added for every cubic centimeter (cc) of the IV solution.

Alarms

Bedside monitors have alarms for each of the hemodynamic pressures being monitored. Normally, every parameter that is being monitored has high and low alarms, which can be set to detect variations from the current value. Alarm limits are generally set to detect significant decreases or increases in pressures or rates, typically ±10% of the current values.

OBTAINING ACCURATE HEMODYNAMIC VALUES

The information obtained from hemodynamic monitoring technology must be verified for accuracy by the bedside clinician.

Zeroing the Transducer

A fundamental step in obtaining accurate hemodynamic values is to zero the transducer amplifier system. *Zeroing* is the

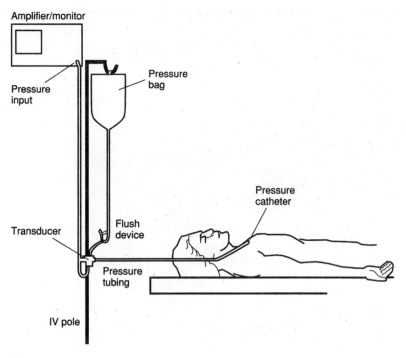

Figure 4–7. Pressure bag and flush device connected to a pressure transducer and monitoring system. (*From: Ahrens TS, Taylor L: Hemodynamic Waveform Analysis. Philadelphia: WB Saunders; 1992, p. 210.*)

act of electronically compensating for any offset (distortion) in the transducer. This is normally done by exposing the transducer to air and pushing an automatic zero button on the bedside monitor. This step is performed at least once before obtaining the first hemodynamic reading after catheter insertion. Because it is an electronic function, it normally has to be performed only once when the transducer and amplifier are first attached to the in situ catheter.

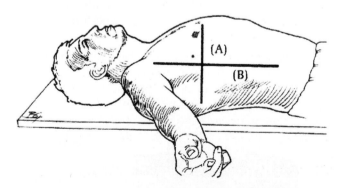

Figure 4–8. Referencing and zeroing the hemodynamic monitoring system in a supine patient. The phlebostatic axis is determined by drawing an imaginary vertical line from the fourth ICS on the sternal border to the right side of the chest **(A)**. A second imaginary line is drawn horizontally at the level of the midpoint between the anterior and posterior surface of the chest **(B)**. The phlebostatic axis is located at the intersection of points A and B. (*From Keckeisen M, Chulay M, Gawlinski A [eds]: Pulmonary artery pressure monitoring. In Hemodynamic Monitoring Series. Aliso Viejo, CA: AACN; 1998, p. 11.*)

Leveling the Transducer to the Catheter Tip

Leveling is the process of aligning the tip of the vascular catheter horizontal to a zero reference position, usually a stopcock in the pressure tubing close to the transducer. The reference point is the phlebostatic axis and is found at the intersection between the fourth intercostal space (ICS) and half the AP diameter of the chest (Figure 4–8 and Table 4–4).

There are two basic methods for leveling. When the transducer and stopcocks are mounted on a pole close to the bed, the pole height is adjusted to have the stopcock opening

---

TABLE 4–4. EVIDENCED-BASED PRACTICE: PULMONARY ARTERY PRESSURE MEASUREMENT

- Verify the accuracy of the transducer–patient interface by performing a square waveform test at the beginning of each shift.[a,b]
- Position the patient supine prior to PAP/RAP (CVP)/PAOP measurements. Head of bed elevation can be at any angle from 0° (flat) to 60°.[a,b]
- Level the transducer air–fluid interface to the phlebostatic axis (4th ICS/½ AP diameter of the chest) with the patient in a supine position prior to PAP/RAP/PAOP measurements.[a,b]
- Obtain PAP/RAP/PAOP measurements from a graphic (analog) tracing at end-expiration.[a,b]
- Use a simultaneous ECG tracing to assist with proper PAP/RAP/PAOP waveform identification.[a,b]
- PA catheters can be safely withdrawn and removed by competent registered nurses.[a,b]

Data from: [a]American Association of Critical-Care Nurses (2004). [b]Keckeisen (1998).

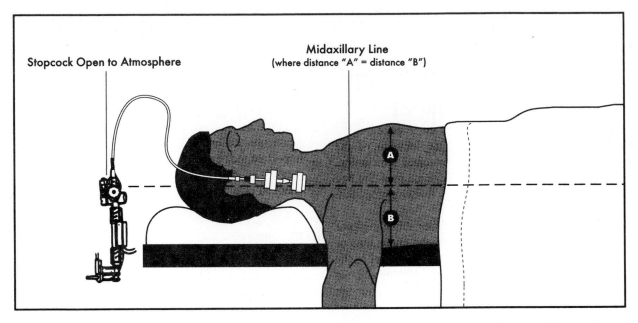

Figure 4–9. Typical leveling of PA catheter with stopcock attached to the transducer for mounting on a pole. The stopcock close to the transducer is opened to atmospheric pressure (air) horizontal to the fourth ICS at the midaxillary line.

horizontal to the external reference location of the catheter tip (Figure 4–9). To ensure horizontal positioning, a carpenter's level is usually necessary. Each time the bed height or patient position is altered, this leveling procedure must be repeated (Figure 4–10).

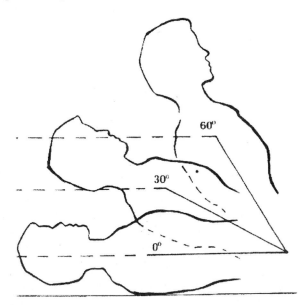

Figure 4–10. The level of the phlebostatic axis as the patient moves flat to a higher level of backrest. The level of the axis for referencing and zeroing the air–fluid interface rotates on the axis and remains horizontal as the patient moves from flat to increasingly higher backrest positions. For accurate hemodynamic pressure readings at difference backrest elevations, the air–fluid interface must be at the level of the phlebostatic axis. (*From Bridges EJ, Woods SL: Pulmonary artery pressure measurement: State of the art.* Heart Lung *1993;22[2]:101.*)

The other method for leveling places the transducer and stopcock at the correct location on the chest wall or arm (Figure 4–11). Taping or strapping the transducer to the appropriate location on the body eliminates the need for repeating the leveling procedure when bed heights are changed. As long as the transducer/stopcock position remains horizontal to the external reference location, no releveling is required.

Leveling must be performed when obtaining the first set of hemodynamic information and any time the transducer is no longer horizontal to the external reference location. When obtaining the first set of readings, zeroing and leveling are frequently performed simultaneously. After this initial combined effort, zeroing does not need to be performed when leveling is done.

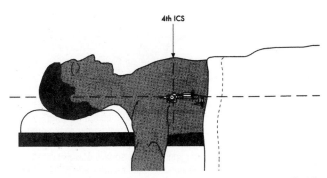

Figure 4–11. Leveling a transducer for mounting on the chest wall at the fourth ICS at the midaxillary line.

Calibration of the Transducer/Amplifier System

If the transducer/amplifier system is suspected of being in-accurate, calibration can be performed. Calibration is less important today because all disposable transducers are pre-calibrated by the manufacturer. If calibration needs to be checked prior to use, or if a reading is in doubt, a simple static pressure check can be done before the transducer is attached to the patient. Detailed descriptions of how to perform static pressure checks are found in most hemodynamic monitoring texts.

Ensuring Accurate Waveform Transmission

For hemodynamic monitoring to provide accurate information, the vascular pressure must be transmitted back to the transducer unaltered and then converted accurately into an electrical signal. For this waveform to be transmitted unaltered, no obstructions or distortions to the signal should be present along the transmission route. Distortion of the waveform leads to inaccurate pressure interpretations. A variety of factors can cause distortions to the waveform, including catheter obstructions (e.g., clots, catheter bending, blood or air in tubing), excessive tubing or connectors, and transducer damage. Verification of an accurate transmission of the waveform to the transducer is checked by the bedside nurse by performing a square wave test. This occurs at the beginning of each shift (see Table 4–4).

Square Wave Test

The square wave test is performed on all hemodynamic pressure systems before assuming that the waveforms and pressures obtained are accurate. The square wave test is performed by recording the pressure waveform while fast flushing the catheter (Figure 4–12). The fast-flush valve is pulled or squeezed, depending on the model, for at least 1 second and then rapidly released. The tracing should show a rapid rise in the waveform to the top of the graph paper, with a square pattern. Release of the flush device should show a rapid decrease in pressure below the baseline of the pressure waveform (undershoot), followed immediately by a small increase above the baseline (overshoot) prior to re-sumption of the normal pressure waveform. Square wave tests with these characteristics are called *optimally damped tests* and represent an accurate waveform transmission. The square wave test is the best method available to the clinician to check the accuracy of hemodynamic monitoring equipment. For example, if an arterial line is to be examined for accuracy, a square wave test should be done. Do not compare the arterial line pressure with an indirect blood pressure reading with a sphygmomanometer, because the indirect method is usually less accurate than the direct method (arterial line pressure). If the square wave test indicates optimal damping, then the arterial line pressure is accurate.

Two problems may exist with waveform transmissions, and are referred to as *overdamping* and *underdamping* (Table 4–5).

Overdamping

If something absorbs the pressure wave (like air or blood in the tubing, stopcocks, or connections), it is said to be *over-damped.* Overdamping decreases systolic pressures and increases diastolic pressures. An overdamped square wave test reflects the obstruction in waveform transmission. Characteristics of overdamping include a loss of the undershoot and overshoot waves after release of the flush valve and a slurring of the downstroke (Figure 4–13).

Underdamping

If something accentuates the pressure wave (like excessive tubing), it is said to be *underdamped.* Underdamping increases systolic pressures and decreases diastolic pressures (Figure 4–14). An underdamped square wave test reflects the amplification of pressure waves and includes large under-shoot and overshoot waves after the release of the flush valve. Table 4–6 summarizes the methods of assessing and ensuring the accuracy of hemodynamic monitoring systems.

Care of the Tubing/Catheter System

Nosocomial infections related to the tubing/catheter system are usually caused by the entry of organisms through stop-cocks. Stopcocks are opened for blood sampling and zero-ing the transducer only when necessary. Closed, needleless systems are used whenever feasible to decrease the risks to the patient and clinician.

Tubing changes, including flush device, transducer, and flush solution, should occur every 72 hours. The frequency of catheter device changes is controversial, but must occur whenever the catheter is suspected as a source of an IV infection or by institutional policy.

Some clinicians believe it is safe to leave intravascular catheters in place until some sign of inflammation or infection develops. This approach may be safe, but it assumes more risk of developing catheter-related infection than the routine 4- to 5-day change guideline. Considering that the development of a single catheter-related infection can substantially increase the length of stay, it may be worthwhile to routinely change intravascular catheters. However, there is still a widespread variation in the practice of changing intravascular catheters at this time.

INSERTION AND REMOVAL OF CATHETERS

Pulmonary Artery Catheters

PA catheters are frequently inserted to assess cardiac and respiratory function, as well as to guide fluid and vasoactive drug administration in the critically ill patient.

TABLE 4–5. ASSESSING DAMPING CONCEPTS FROM SQUARE WAVE TEST

Square Wave Test	Clinical Effect	Corrective Action
Optimally damped	Produces accurate waveform and pressure.	None required.

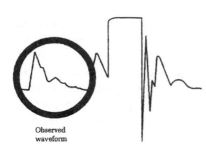

Figure 4–12. Optimally Damped System. When the fast flush of the continuous flush system is activated and quickly released, a sharp upstroke terminates in a flat line at the maximal indicator on the monitor and hardcopy. This is followed by an immediate and rapid downstroke extending below the baseline with just 1 or 2 oscillations within 0.12 second (minimal ringing) and a quick return to baseline. The patient's pressure waveform is also clearly defined with all components of the waveform, such as the dicrotic notch on an arterial waveform, clearly visible. Intervention: There is no adjustment in the monitoring system required. (*Reprinted from Darovic GO, Vanriper S, Vanriper J: Fluid-filled monitoring systems. In: Darovic GO.* Hemodynamic Monitoring: Invasive and Noninvasive Clinical Application, *3rd ed. Philadelphia PA: WB Saunders Co; 1995:161–162. Used with permission.*)

Square Wave Test	Clinical Effect	Corrective Action
Overdamped	Produces a falsely low systolic and high diastolic value.	Check the system for air, blood, loose connections or kinks in the tubing or catheter. Verify extension tubing has not been added.

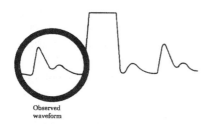

Figure 4–13. Overdamped System. The upstroke of the square wave appears somewhat slurred, the waveform does not extend below the baseline after the fast flush, and there is no ringing after the flush. The patient's waveform displays a falsely decreased systolic pressure and a false high diastolic pressure as well as poorly defined components of the pressure tracing such as a diminished or absent dicrotic notch on arterial waveforms. Interventions: To correct the problem, (1) check for the presence of blood clots, blood left in the catheter following blood sampling, or air bubbles at any point from the catheter tip to the transducer and eliminate them as necessary. (2) Use low compliance (rigid), short (less than 3 to 4 feet) monitoring tubing. (3) Ensure there are no loose connections. (4) Check for kinks in the line. (*Reprinted from Darovic GO, Vanriper S, Vanriper J: Fluid-filled monitoring systems. In: Darovic GO.* Hemodynamic Monitoring: Invasive and Noninvasive Clinical Application, *3rd ed. Philadelphia PA: WB Saunders Co; 1995:161–162. Used with permission.*)

Square Wave Test	Clinical Effect	Corrective Action
Underdamped	Produces a falsely high systolic and low diastolic value.	Remove unnecessary tubing and stopcocks. Add a damping device.

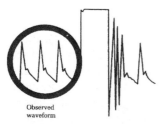

Figure 4–14. Underdamped System. The waveform is characterized by numerous amplified oscillations above and below the baseline following the fast flush. The monitored pressure wave displays false high systolic pressure (overshoot), possibly false low diastolic pressures, and "ringing" artifacts on the waveform. Intervention: To correct the problem, remove all air bubbles in the fluid system. Use large bore, shorter tubing, or use a damping device. (*Reprinted from Darovic GO, Vanriper S, Vanriper J: Fluid-filled monitoring systems. In: Darovic GO.* Hemodynamic Monitoring: Invasive and Noninvasive Clinical Application, *3rd ed. Philadelphia PA: WB Saunders Co; 1995:161–162. Used with permission.*)

TABLE 4–6. SUMMARY OF METHODS FOR ASSESSING AND ENSURING ACCURACY OF HEMODYNAMIC MONITORING SYSTEMS[a]

Method	When Performed
Zero transducer	Should only be performed once. If the transducer zeros properly, a waveform should be visible on the monitor.
Level the tansducer	Leveling should be done prior to each pressure reading and with any substantive change in pressures.
Square wave test	Should be performed prior to every reading and after blood has been withdrawn from the catheter.
Calibration	Calibration should be performed once prior to using the transducer.

[a]If a transducer has been zeroed, leveled, and calibrated and has an optimally damped square wave test, the monitor display is accurate.

Insertion

PA catheters can be inserted into most large-diameter veins, with the internal jugular vein being the most common insertion site. Typically, the PA catheter is placed into a percutaneously inserted introducer sheath with a sterile sleeve to maintain the sterility of the PA catheter after insertion (Figure 4–15). As the catheter is advanced into the right atrium, the balloon at the tip of the catheter is inflated with 1.25 to 1.50 mL of air. Inflation of the balloon during insertion

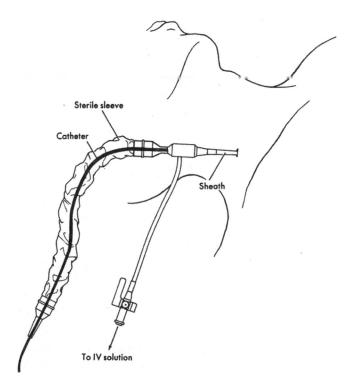

Figure 4–15. PA catheter inserted through an introducer sheath in the right internal jugular vein. The sterile sleeve of the introducer allows advancement of the PA catheter after insertion, if necessary. The side port of the sheath is connected to an IV to reduce clotting around the sheath and permit fluid administration. (*From: Daily E, Schroeder J:* Techniques in Bedside Hemodynamic Monitoring, *3rd ed. St. Louis, MO: CV Mosby; 1985, p. 93.*)

allows blood flow through the heart to direct, or pull, the catheter up into the PA (Figure 4–16). Following proper placement of the catheter within the PA, the balloon is deflated.

Pressure at the tip of the PA catheter is monitored continuously as the catheter is advanced through the right heart and into the PA. Changes in pressure and waveform configurations allow clinicians to identify the location of the PA catheter as it is directed into the right atrium, through the tricuspid valve into the right ventricle, through the pulmonic valve, and into the PA (Table 4–7). Normal pressures for each of the chambers are summarized in Tables 4–1 and 4–7. Occasionally, bedside fluoroscopy also is needed to assist with proper insertion of the catheter.

Following insertion, the PA pressure waveform is monitored continuously to identify migration of the catheter tip into a small branch of the PA, obstructing blood flow to distal lung tissue or backward into the right ventricle. A chest x-ray is obtained after insertion to verify proper location and rule out presence of pneumothorax, kinking of the catheter, or other complications.

Removal

Removing the PA catheter is a clinical decision based on the assessment that the data from the catheter are no longer critical to monitor. This decision may be made anywhere from a few hours to several days after insertion. The removal of the PA catheter is normally performed by a physician, although in some institutions nurses perform this task (see Table 4–4).

Following the discontinuance of IV fluids, all stopcocks to the patient are turned off to avoid air entry into the venous system during catheter removal. The balloon of the catheter is deflated and the patient is placed in a supine position with the head of the bed flat. While the catheter is being gently withdrawn, the patient is instructed to exhale or hold his or her breath to further decrease the chance of air embolus. Resistance during catheter withdrawal may indicate catheter knotting and/or entrapment in a valve leaflet or chordae tendineae. A chest x-ray is necessary to confirm the problem and special removal procedures are performed to avoid structural damage to the heart.

Complications

Complications associated with PA catheters include those associated with insertion, maintenance, and removal of the device (Table 4–8). During insertion, the most common complication is ventricular ectopy (premature ventricular contractions [PVCs], ventricular tachycardia or fibrillation) from catheter irritation of the ventricular wall. Similar to complications associated with central venous catheters, pneumothorax or air emboli may occur during insertion or removal of a PA catheter. Introduction of microorganisms and subsequent infection are always a risk. A rare but serious complication is damage to the tricuspid or pulmonic valves.

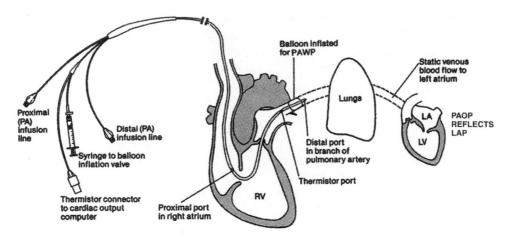

Figure 4–16. PA catheter inserted into the PA.

Pulmonary hemorrhage or infarct may also occur during inadvertent migration of the PA catheter into small-diameter branches of the PA or from balloon rupture. Prevention and treatment strategies are summarized in Table 4–8 for each of these complications.

Arterial Catheters

Blood pressure measurement with the indirect method (sphygmomanometer) is not as accurate as direct blood pressure measurement, particularly during conditions of abnormal blood flow (high or low CO states), SVR, or body temperature. The prevalence of these conditions in critically ill patients may necessitate insertion of an arterial catheter to directly measure blood pressure.

Insertion

Arterial catheters are short (<4 inches) catheters that can be inserted into radial, brachial, axillary, femoral, or pedal arteries. The most common site is the radial artery. Arterial catheters can be placed by cut down or with percutaneous insertion techniques, the latter being the most common insertion method.

General insertion steps for percutaneous insertion are similar to IV catheter insertion. Prior to insertion of a radial artery catheter, however, an Allen test is performed to verify the adequacy of circulation to the hand in the event of radial artery thrombosis. The Allen test is performed by completely obstructing blood flow to the hand by compressing the radial and ulnar arteries for a minute or two. If adequate collateral blood flow exists, there will be rapid return of color to the hand upon release of the ulnar artery (Figure 4–17).

During insertion, care is exercised not to damage the arterial vessel by excessive probing or movement of the needle. Bleeding into the tissues occurs quite easily if the vessel is damaged, causing obstruction to distal blood flow and nerve pressure. Following artery cannulation, the catheter is connected to the pressure transducer and a high-pressure infusion system to prevent blood from backing up into the tubing and fluid container (see Figure 4–6).

Removal

The removal of the arterial catheter is warranted when an accurate blood pressure can be obtained via noninvasive methods, the blood pressure is no longer labile, or when frequent arterial blood samples are no longer indicated. Removal of arterial catheters is commonly performed by the nurse using procedures similar to IV catheter removal, but because they are in an artery greater attention to achieving hemostasis is required. Following catheter removal, firm pressure is maintained over the site for at least 5 minutes or until hemostasis occurs. This prevents bleeding and hematoma formation. For patients with coagulation abnormalities, manual pressure may need to be applied for 10 minutes or longer. Pressure dressings, rather than manual pressure, at the site are not recommended as a means to achieve hemostasis. Once hemostasis is achieved, a pressure dressing may be used but is generally not needed.

Frequent assessment of the site after catheter removal is recommended to identify rebleeding and thrombosis of the artery. Checking the extremity for the presence of pulses, circulation, and bleeding is recommended for a few hours after catheter removal.

Complications

A variety of complications are associated with arterial catheters (Table 4–9). The most serious are related to bleeding from the arterial catheter and loss of arterial flow to the extremity from thrombus formation. Loose connections in the arterial system can lead to rapid and massive blood loss. The morbidity and mortality associated with these complications require stringent safeguards (Luer-lock connections, minimum number of stopcocks, pressure alarm system activated at all times) to prevent bleeding and to rapidly iden-

TABLE 4–7. PRESSURE WAVEFORMS OBSERVED DURING PULMONARY ARTERY (PA) CATHETER INSERTION

Location	Pressure Waveform	Normal Pressures
Right atrium		2–8 mm Hg
Right ventricle		Systolic, 20–30 mm Hg Diastolic, 0–5 mm Hg
Pulmonary artery		Systolic, 20–30 mm Hg Diastolic, 10–15 mm Hg
Pulmonary artery wedge		8–12 mm Hg

With permission from: Boggs R, Wooldridge-King M: AACN procedure manual, *3rd ed. Philadelphia: WB Saunders, 1993, pp. 308, 324, 326, 334.*

TABLE 4–8. PROBLEMS ENCOUNTERED WITH PULMONARY ARTERY (PA) CATHETERS[a]

Problem	Cause
Phlebitis or local infection at insertion site	Mechanical irritation or contamination.
Ventricular irritability	Looping of excess catheter in right ventricle. Migration of catheter from PA to RV. Irritation of the endocardium during catheter passage.
Apparent wedging of cathether with balloon deflated	Forward migration of catheter tip caused by blood flow, excessive loop in RV, or inadequate suturing of catheter at insertion site.
Pulmonary hemorrhage or infarction, or both	Distal migration of catheter tip. Continuous or prolonged wedging of catheter. Overinflation of balloon while catheter is wedged. Failure of balloon to deflate.
"Overwedging" or damped PAW	Overinflation of balloon. Frequent inflation of balloon.
PA balloon rupture	Overinflation of balloon. Frequent inflations of balloon. Syringe deflation, damaging wall of balloon.
Infection	Nonsterile insertion techniques. Contamination via skin. Contamination through stopcock ports or catheter hub. Fluid contamination from transducer through cracked membrane of disposable dome. Prolonged catheter placement.
Heart block during insertion of catheter	Mechanical irritation of His bundle in patients with preexisting left bundle branch block

[a]PAW, pulmonary artery wedge; RV, right ventricle; PA, pulmonary artery. *From: Daily E, Schroeder J: Techniques in bedside hemodynamic monitoring, 5th ed. St. Louis, MO; CV Mosby. 1994, pp. 134–136.*

Prevention	Treatment
Prepare skin properly before insertion. Use sterile technique during insertion and dressing change. Insert smoothly and rapidly. Use Teflon-coated introducer. Attach silver-impregnated cuff to introducer. Change dressings, stopcocks, and connecting tubing every 24–48 hours. Remove catheter or change insertion site every 4 days.	Remove catheter. Apply warm compresses. Give pain medication as necessary.
Suture catheter at insertion site; check chest film. Position catheter tip in main right or left PA. Keep balloon inflated during advancement; advance gently.	Reposition catheter; remove loop. Inflate balloon to encourage catheter flotation out to PA. Advance rapidly out to PA.
Check catheter tip by fluoroscopy; position in main right or left PA. Check catheter position on x-ray film if fluoroscopy is not used. Suture catheter in place at insertion site.	Aspirate blood from catheter; if catheter is wedged, sample will be arterialized and obtained with difficulty. If wedged, slowly pull back catheter until PA waveform appears. If not wedged, gently aspirate and flush catheter with saline; catheter tip can partially clot, causing damping that resembles damped PAW waveform.
Check chest film immediately after insertion and 12–24 hours later; remove any catheter loop in RA or RV. Leave balloon deflated. Suture catheter at skin to prevent inadvertent advancement. Position catheter in main right or left PA. Pull catheter back to pulmonary artery if it spontaneously wedges. Do not flush catheter when in wedge position. Inflate balloon slowly with only enough air to obtain a PAW waveform. Do not inflate 7-Fr catheter with more than 1–1.5 mL of air. Do not inflate if resistance is met.	Deflate balloon. Place patient on side (catheter tip down). Stop anticoagulation. Consider "wedge" angiogram. Intubate with double-lumen ET. Recommend surgery, if severe hemorrhage.
Watch waveform during inflation; inject only enough air to obtain PAW pressure. Do not inflate 7-Fr catheter with more than 1–1.5 mL of air. Check inflated balloon-shape before insertion.	Deflate balloon; reinflate slowly with only enough air to obtain PAW pressure. Deflate balloon; reposition and slowly reinflate.
Inflate slowly with only enough air to obtain a PAW pressure. Monitor PAD pressure as reflection of PAW and LVEDP. Allow passive deflation of balloon. Remove syringe after inflation.	Remove syringe to prevent further air injection. Monitor PAD pressure.
Use sterile techniques. Use sterile catheter sleeve. Prepare skin with effective antiseptic (chlorhexidine). Apply iodophor ointment and sterile gauze dressing daily. Do not use clear semipermeable dressing. Inspect site daily. Reassess need for catheter after 3 days. Avoid internal jugular approach. Use sterile dead-end caps on all stopcock ports. Change IV solution, stopcock, and tubing every 24–48 hours. Do not use IV solution that contains glucose. Check transducer domes for cracks. Change transducers every 48 hours. Change disposable dome after countershock. Do not use IV solution that contains glucose. Change catheter insertion site every 4 days.	Remove catheter. Use antibiotics.
Insert catheter expeditiously with balloon inflated. Insert transvenous pacing catheter before PA catheter insertion.	Use temporary pacemaker or flotation catheter with pacing wire.

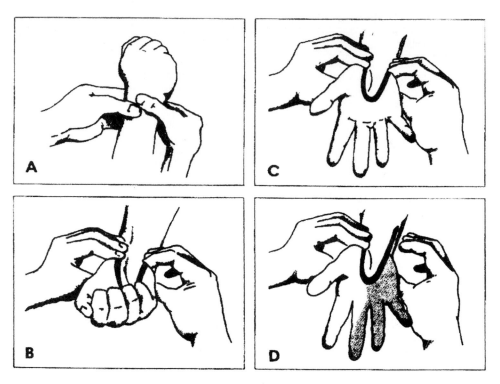

Figure 4–17. Allen's test. (*From DeGroot KD, Damato MB: Monitoring intra-arterial pressure.* Crit Care Nurs *1986;6[1]:74–78.*)

tify disruptions in the arterial system. The catheters are removed as early as possible to prevent the potential for thrombus formation.

OBTAINING AND INTERPRETING HEMODYNAMIC WAVEFORMS

To obtain hemodynamic values, interpretation of hemodynamic waveforms is necessary. A multichannel strip recorder, which provides both an electrocardiographic (ECG) and pressure tracing are required elements (Figure 4–18). Many institutions also use respiratory pressure waveforms, graphed simultaneously with the ECG and hemodynamic waveforms, to ensure accurate identification of end expiration.

The larger the scale, the easier is the interpretation of the wave. All waveforms are easily obtained simply by activating the record function of the bedside monitor. When obtaining waveforms for interpretation, make sure the calibration scales on the left side of the paper are properly aligned with the paper grid. Improperly aligned calibration marks increase the difficulty in reading the waveform and increase potential errors in interpretation.

Patient Positioning

The patient is placed in the supine position, with the backrest elevated anywhere from 0° to 60° (see Figure 4–10). Generally, data should not be obtained if the patient is on his or her side, because it is difficult to identify the location of the

catheter tip for purposes of leveling (Figure 4–19). Improper leveling distorts atrial and venous pressure readings.

It is important to remember that patient comfort is a key issue when obtaining hemodynamic waveform readings. Do not position a spontaneously breathing patient with dyspnea flat for the sole reason of obtaining hemodynamic readings. It is best to obtain values in the position in which the patient is most comfortable.

Interpretation

Correct interpretation of hemodynamic waveforms involves careful assessment of venous and arterial pressure waveforms. Normal values for each of the hemodynamic pressures are listed in Table 4–1. In addition, Chapter 26, Hemodynamic Monitoring Troubleshooting Guide, lists common problems and approaches to hemodynamic monitoring systems.

Atrial and Venous Waveforms

Pressures in the atrial and venous systems are significantly lower than in the ventricular and arterial systems. The two primary atrial/venous pressures measured in critically ill patients are the CVP (also called the RAP), and the PAOP. These pressures are used to estimate ventricular pressures because, at the time of ventricular end diastole, the mitral and tricuspid valves are open (see Figure 4–3). This allows a clear communication between the ventricles and the atrium, with equilibration of pressures in the two chambers. Ideally, ventricular pressures are better measures of ventricular function than atrial estimates; however, direct ventricular pressure measurement

TABLE 4–9. PROBLEMS ENCOUNTERED WITH ARTERIAL CATHETERS

Problem	Cause	Prevention	Treatment
Hematoma after withdrawal of needle	Bleeding or oozing at puncture site.	Maintain firm pressure on site during withdrawal of catheter and for 5–15 minutes (as necessary) after withdrawal. Apply elastic tape (Elastoplast) firmly over puncture site. For femoral arterial puncture sites, leave a sandbag on site for 1–2 hours to prevent oozing. If patient is receiving heparin, discontinue 2 hours before catheter removal.	Continue to hold pressure to puncture site until oozing stops. Apply sandbag to femoral puncture site for 1–2 hours after removal of catheter.
Decreased or absent pulse distal to puncture site	Spasm of artery. Thrombosis of artery.	Introduce arterial needle cleanly, nontraumatically. Use 1 unit heparin to 1 mL IV fluid.	Inject lidocaine locally at insertion site and 10 mg into arterial catheter. Arteriotomy and Fogarty catheterization both distally and proximally from the puncture site result in return of pulse in more than 90% of cases if brachial or femoral artery is used.
Bleedback into tubing, dome, or transducer	Insufficient pressure on IV bag. Loose connections.	Maintain 300 mm HG pressure on IV bag. Use Luer-Lock stopcocks; tighten periodically.	Replace transducer. "Fast-flush" through system. Tighten all connections.
Hemorrhage	Loose connections.	Keep all connecting sites visible. Observe connecting sites frequently. Use built-in alarm system. Use Luer-Lock stopcocks.	Tighten all connections.
Emboli	Clot from catheter tip into bloodstream	Always aspirate and discard before flushing. Use continuous flush device. Use 1 unit heparin to 1 mL IV fluid. Gently flush <2–4 mL.	Remove catheter.
Local infection	Forward movement of contaminated catheter. Break in sterile technique. Prolonged catheter use.	Carefully suture catheter at insertion site. Always use aseptic technique. Remove catheter after 72–96 hours. Inspect and care for insertion site daily, including dressing change and antibiotic or iodophor ointment.	Remove catheter. Prescribe antibiotic.
Sepsis	Break in sterile technique. Prolonged catheter use. Bacterial growth in IV fluid.	Use percutaneous insertion. Always use aseptic technique. Remove catheter after 72–96 hours. Change transducer, stopcocks, and tubing every 96 hours. Do not use IV fluid containing glucose. Use sterile dead-end caps on all ports of stopcocks. Carefully flush remaining blood from stopcocks after blood sampling.	Remove catheter. Prescribe antibiotic.

From: Daily E, Schroeder J: Techniques in bedside hemodynamic monitoring, 5th ed. St. Louis, MO; CV Mosby, 1994, pp. 165–166.

is not always available. Atrial pressures are then used as a substitute. If ventricular waveforms are available, they should be used in place of atrial pressures. CVP and PAOP are the clinical measurements commonly performed to assess "preload" of the right and left ventricles, respectively.

Central Venous Pressure

The CVP is important because it is used to approximate the right ventricular end-diastolic pressure (RVEDP). Ventricular end-diastolic pressures, both right and left, are used to estimate the cardiac function and fluid status. The RVEDP is used to assess RV function and general fluid status.

A normal CVP is between 2 and 8 mm Hg. Low CVP values typically reflect hypovolemia or decreased venous

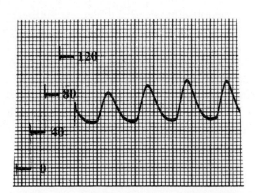

Figure 4–18. Graphic tracing of an arterial waveform preceded by calibration scale markings (0/40/80/120 mm Hg). Note how the scale markers line up with the heavy line of the tracing paper. Each 1-mm line represents 4 mm Hg in this scale.

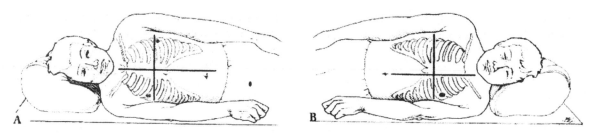

Figure 4–19. Referencing and zeroing the hemodynamic monitoring system in a patient in the lateral position. **(A)** For the right lateral position, the reference point is at the intersection of the fourth ICS and the midsternum. **(B)** For the left lateral position, the reference point is the intersection of the fourth ICS and the left parasternal border. (*From Keckeisen M, Chulay M, Gawlinski A [eds]: Pulmonary artery pressure monitoring. In* Hemodynamic Monitoring Series. *Aliso Viejo, CA: AACN; 1998, p. 12.*)

return. High CVP values reflect overhydration, increased venous return, or right-sided cardiac failure. If the CVP and SV are low, hypovolemia is assumed. If the CVP is high and the SV is low, RV dysfunction is likely.

CVP is obtained from the proximal port of the PA catheter or the tip of central venous catheter. Measurement of CVP is done simultaneously with the ECG. Using the ECG allows the identification of the point where the CVP best correlates with the RVEDP.

The CVP is read by one of two techniques. The first technique is to take the mean (average) of the a wave of the CVP waveform (Figure 4–20). Although three waves normally exist on atrial waveforms (a, c, and v waves), the mean of the a wave most closely approximates ventricular end-diastolic pressure. The a wave of the CVP waveform starts just after the P wave on the ECG is observed and represents atrial contraction. By taking the reading at the highest point of the a wave, adding it to the reading at the lowest

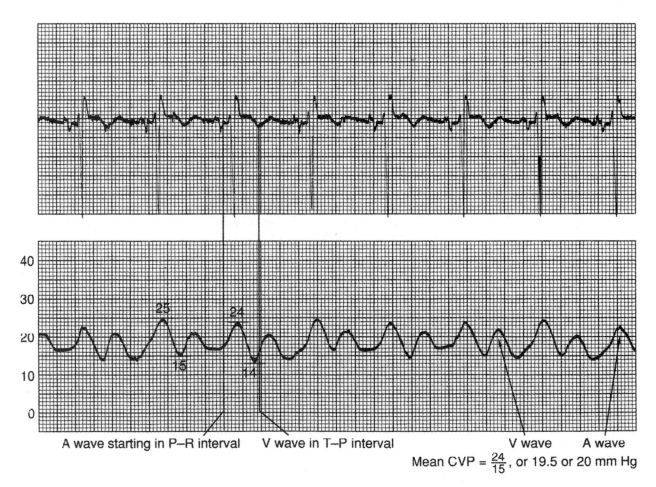

A wave starting in P–R interval   V wave in T–P interval   V wave   A wave

Mean CVP = $\frac{24}{15}$, or 19.5 or 20 mm Hg

Figure 4–20. Reading a CVP waveform by averaging the A wave. (*From: Ahrens TS, Taylor L:* Hemodynamic Waveform Analysis. *Philadelphia: WB Saunders; 1992, p. 31.*)

point of that a wave, and dividing by 2, the average or mean CVP reading is obtained (generally a line is drawn though the middle of the a waves to derive a number).

A second method, the Z-point technique, also can be used to estimate ventricular end-diastolic pressures (Figure 4–21). The Z-point is taken just before the closure of the tricuspid valve. This point is located on a CVP tracing in the mid to late QRS complex area. The Z-point technique is especially useful when an a wave does not exist, for example, in atrial fibrillation when atrial contraction is absent.

By isolating the a wave or using the Z-point technique, atrial pressures can reasonably estimate ventricular end-diastolic pressure. It is helpful to read these values off a multichannel strip recorder and not the digital display on the bedside monitor. Monitor values tend to be accurate in simple waveforms but become less reliable when the waveforms are complex (see Table 4–4).

Central Venous Pressure: Abnormal Venous Waveforms

Two types of abnormal CVP waveforms are common. Large a waves (also called *cannon a waves*) occur when the atrium contracts against a closed tricuspid value (Figure 4–22). This occurs most commonly with arrhythmias like PVCs or third-degree heart block. Giant v waves are common in conditions such as tricuspid insufficiency or ventricular failure. Using the z-point for CVP readings prevents incorrect interpretations associated with the use of large a or v waves.

Pulmonary Artery Occlusion Pressure (Wedge Pressure)

Although the CVP is useful in assessing RV function, the assessment of LV function is generally more important. In LV dysfunction (e.g., with myocardial infarction or cardiomyopathies), a threat to tissue oxygenation and survival

may exist due to low CO. The PAOP is used to assess LV function and provide appropriate therapy.

Interpreting the PAOP is very similar to interpreting a CVP waveform with the obvious exception that the PAOP assesses LVEDP, not RVEDP. The LVEDP is used to assess LV function and systemic fluid status.

A normal PAOP is 8 to 12 mm Hg. Low values reflect hypovolemia, with high values indicating hypervolemia and/or LV failure. Mitral valve abnormalities also cause elevations in PAOP. When PAOP and SV are normal normovolemia and acceptable LV function is assumed. If the PAOP and SV are low hypovolemia is likely. When PAOP is high (usually greater than 18 mm Hg) but SV is low, LV dysfunction is assumed.

A PAOP waveform is obtained from the distal port of the PA catheter when the balloon on the catheter is inflated. Inflation of the balloon is performed for only a few seconds (8 to 15 seconds) to avoid a disruption in pulmonary blood flow. When inflating the balloon, inflate only to the volume necessary to obtain the PAOP waveform (1.25 to 1.50 mL). Record how much air it takes to inflate the balloon. If it takes less air to obtain a PAOP value than at a previous inflation, the catheter may have migrated further into the pulmonary artery. If it takes more air to obtain a PAOP, the catheter may have moved back. If no resistance is felt when the balloon is inflated and no PAOP tracing occurs, notify the physician of a possible balloon rupture. When deflating the balloon, allow air to leave the balloon passively. Actively aspirating the air out of the balloon damages the balloon and is not necessary for complete emptying.

The characteristics and interpretation of PAOP and CVP waveforms are similar. The difference between interpreting a CVP and a PAOP waveform mainly centers on the

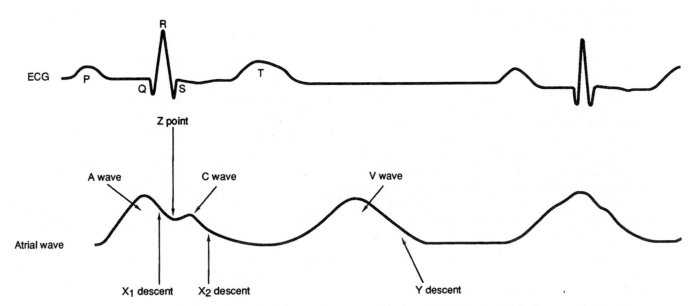

Figure 4–21. Use of the Z-point to read a CVP waveform. (*From: Ahrens TS:* Hemodynamic Waveform Analysis, *p. 24. Philadelphia: WB Saunders; 1992, p. 24.*)

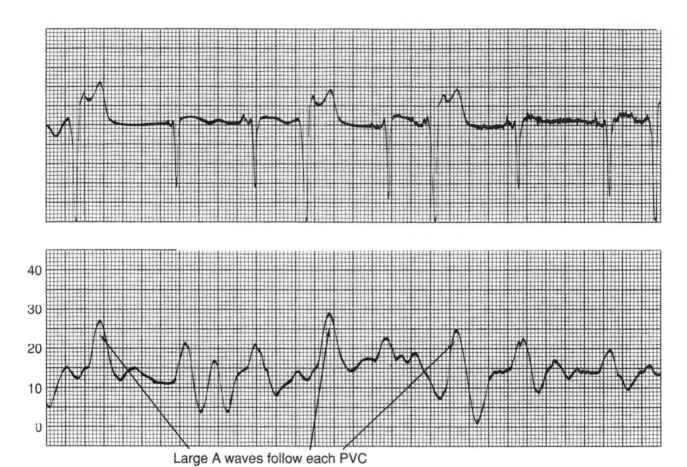

Figure 4–22. Giant A waves with loss of atrioventricular synchrony. (*From Ahrens TS:* Hemodynamic Waveform Analysis. *Philadelphia: WB Saunders; 1992, p. 54.*)

Large A waves follow each PVC

delay in waveform correlation with the ECG (Figure 4–23). This delay occurs because the tip of the PA catheter is further away from the left atrium. On a PAOP waveform, the a wave begins near the end of the QRS complex. Averaging the a wave's highest and lowest values, as previously described for CVP readings, is one method for obtaining the PAOP. If the Z-point is to be used for a PAOP reading, this point is found at the end or immediately after (about 0.08 second) the QRS complex (Figure 4–24).

Assessment of LV function is commonly performed with the PAOP. The use of the PAOP to estimate LVEDP is based on the assumption that a measurement from an obstructed pulmonary capillary reflects an uninterrupted flow of blood to the left atrium because no valves exist in the PA system. A second assumption is that when the mitral valve is open, left atrial pressures reflect LVEDP. As long as these assumptions are accurate, the use of the PAOP to estimate LVEDP is acceptable.

Pulmonary Artery Occlusion Pressure: Abnormal Waveforms
Similar abnormal PAOP waveforms occur as with CVP measurements. Large a waves are observed when the left atrium contracts against a closed mitral valve. Large v waves are ob-

served during mitral valve insufficiency and left heart failure (see Figures 4–22 and 4–24).

Arterial and Ventricular Waveforms
An arterial waveform, such as seen in systemic and PA tracings, has three common characteristics: rapid upstroke; dicrotic notch; and progressive diastolic runoff (Figure 4–25). Diastole is read near the end of the QRS complex with systole read before the peak of the T wave. The mean arterial pressure can be calculated (see Table 4–1) or obtained from the digital display on the bedside monitor.

A ventricular waveform also has three common characteristics: rapid upstroke, rapid drop in pressure, and terminal diastolic rise (Figure 4–26). Systole and diastole are read in the same manner as for an arterial waveform. LV waveforms are not available in the clinical area, but can be obtained during cardiac catheterization. Normally, RV waveforms are only observed during insertion of the PA catheter or if an extra lumen is present on the catheter which exists into the RV (see Table 4–7). If an RV waveform is present during monitoring, it is important to verify the location of the catheter. The catheter may have mi-

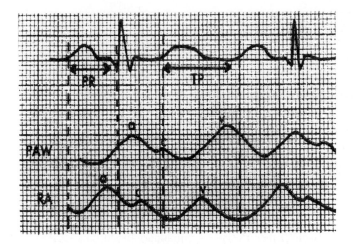

Figure 4–23. PAOP and RA waveforms illustrating the difference in timing of waveform components relative to the ECG. (*From Daily EK: Hemodynamic waveform analysis.* J Cardiovasc Nurs *2001;15[2]:6–22.*)

grated out of the PA and into the RV. A catheter that is floating free in the ventricle tends to cause ventricular ectopy (PVC) if the catheter comes into contact with the ventricular wall. In addition, assessment of PA pressures is not possible.

If the RAP/CVP is high (over 6 mm Hg), particularly if the SV is low, some ventricular dysfunction is suspected. If the RAP/CVP is low (<2 mm Hg) and the SV is low, hypovolemia is suspected. Hypovolemia is also possible if the PAOP is low (<8 mm Hg) and the SV is reduced. If the PAOP is high (over 18 mm Hg) and SV is reduced, LV dysfunction may be present.

PA Waveforms

PA pressures are obtained from a flow-directed PA catheter (see Figure 4–5). The PA pressure is typically low in comparison to the systemic pressure. The PA pressure is determined by the RV CO and the PVR. PA blood pressure is generally in the region of 20 to 30 mm Hg systolic and 10 to 15 mm Hg diastolic (Figure 4–27). PA pressure reading is measured from the distal port of the PA catheter.

The low-pressure pulmonary system is critical to adequate gas exchange in the lungs. If the pressure in the pulmonary vasculature elevates, the capillary hydrostatic pressure exceeds capillary osmotic pressure and forces fluid out of the vessels. If the pulmonary lymphatic drainage capability is exceeded, interstitial and alveolar flooding occur, with resulting interference in oxygen and carbon dioxide exchange.

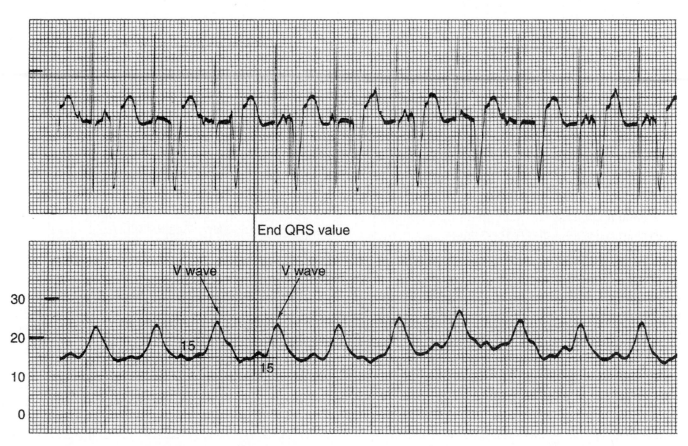

Figure 4–24. Use of the Z-point to read a CVP waveform (PAOP, 15 mm Hg). (*From: Ahrens TS, Taylor L:* Hemodynamic Waveform Analysis. *Philadelphia: WB Saunders; 1992, p. 320.*)

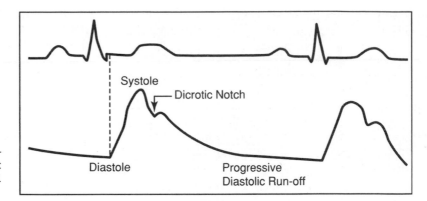

Figure 4–25. Characteristics of an arterial waveform. (*From: Ahrens TS, Prentice D:* Critical Care: Certification Preparation and Review, *3rd ed. Stamford, CT: Appleton & Lange, 1993, p. 82.*)

Normally, the PA pressure is high enough to ensure blood flow through the lungs to the left atrium. Subsequently, blood pressure in the pulmonary arteries only needs to be high enough to overcome the resistance in the left atrium. The mean PA pressure must always be higher than left atrial pressure or blood flow through the lungs is not possible. As a practical guideline, the PAD pressure is higher than the mean left atrial pressure (the mean left atrial pressure is generally estimated by PAOP). If the PAD value is less than the left atrial or wedge pressure, either a very low pulmonary blood flow state exists or the waveforms have been misinterpreted.

Measurement of PA pressures can be helpful in diagnosing many clinical conditions. Elevated PA pressures occur in pulmonary hypertension, chronic pulmonary disease, mitral valve disease, LV failure, hypoxia, and pulmonary emboli. Below-normal PA pressures occur primarily in conditions that produce hypovolemia. If blood volumes are reduced, less resistance to ventricular ejection occurs,

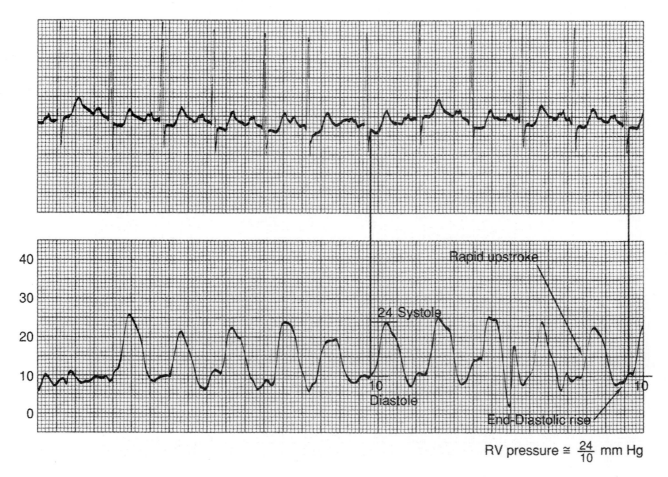

Figure 4–26. Characteristics of a ventricular waveform. (*From: Ahrens TS, Taylor L:* Hemodynamic Waveform Analysis. *Philadelphia: WB Saunders; 1992, p. 98.*)

resulting in a drop in arterial pressures. In this situation, the PAD pressure is also close to the left atrial pressure.

Systemic Arterial Pressures

Direct measurement of systemic arterial pressures is obtained from the tip of an arterial catheter and leveled to the phlebostatic axis (see Figure 4–11), with pressure waveforms interpreted as described. Normal pressures are generally in the region of 100 to 120 mm Hg systolic, 60 to 80 mm Hg diastolic, and 70 to 105 mm Hg mean (see Table 4–1).

Systemic arterial pressures are not interpreted without other clinical information. In general, however, hypotension is assumed if the mean arterial pressure drops below 60 mm Hg. Hypertension is assumed if the systolic blood pressure (SBP) is greater than 140 to 160 mm Hg or the diastolic pressure exceeds 90 mm Hg.

The arterial pressure is one of the most commonly used parameters for assessing the adequacy of blood flow to the tissues. Blood pressure is determined by two factors, CO and SVR. Blood pressure does not reflect early clinical changes in hemodynamics because of the interaction with CO and SVR.

In addition, the CO is comprised of heart rate and SV. These two interact to maintain a normal CO. Subsequently, if the SV begins to fall due to loss of volume (hypovolemia) or dysfunction (LV failure), the heart rate increases to offset the decrease in SV. The net effect is to maintain the CO at near normal levels. If the CO does not change, then there is no change in the blood pressure.

A key point for the nurse to consider is that because of these compensatory mechanisms, blood pressure may not signal early clinical changes in hemodynamic status. If a patient begins to bleed postoperatively, the blood pressure generally does not reflect this change until compensation is no longer possible. And, in fact hypotension is sometimes difficult to evaluate. It is possible that true hypotension exists only when tissue hypoxia is present and end organs are affected. Although tradition dictates that we identify hypotension using predefined levels of blood pressure, other measures such as mixed venous saturation of hemoglobin (SvO_2) and lactate levels may be better indicators. SvO_2 monitoring is described later in this chapter.

Although studies identify the role of hypertension in circulatory damage, the specific level of hypertension that results in the damage is unclear. Therefore, any SBP over 140 is considered potentially injurious to the vasculature.

Artifacts in Hemodynamic Waveforms: Respiratory Influence

Respiration can physiologically change hemodynamic pressures. Spontaneous breathing augments venous return and slightly increases resistance to left ventricle filling. Mechanical ventilation does the opposite, potentially reducing venous return and reducing the resistance on the heart. The effect of respiration on waveforms is noted in Figures 4–28 and 4–29.

A spontaneous breath or a triggered ventilator breath produces a drop in the waveform because of the decrease in pleural pressure (Figure 4–30). A ventilator breath produces an upward distortion of the baseline, due to an increase in pleural and intrathoracic pressure (Figures 4–31 and 4–32). The key to reading the waveform correctly is to isolate the point where pleural pressure is closest to atmospheric pressure. This point is usually at end expiration, just prior to inspiration (Figure 4–33).

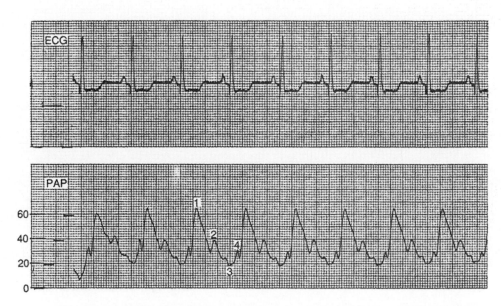

Figure 4–27. PA waveform and components. 1, PA systole; 2, dichrotic notch; 3, PA end diastole; 4, anacrotic notch of PA valve opening. (*From Boggs R, Wooldridge-King M:* AACN Procedure Manual for Critical Care, *3rd ed. Philadelphia: WB Saunders; 1993, p. 316.*)

Cardiac Output

Perhaps the most important information obtained from the PA catheter is the measurement of blood flow parameters such as CO and SV. Understanding these parameters is critical to assessing the adequacy of cardiac function. Flow parameters like CO and SV are the first parameters assessed when monitoring hemodynamic data. Descriptions of the parameters are found at the beginning of this chapter.

If flow parameters are adequate, tissue oxygenation is generally maintained. If flow parameters are abnormal, the clinician must suspect a threat to tissue oxygenation and consider interventions aimed at improving cardiac function. Keep in mind that blood flow can fluctuate with many conditions. If hypovolemia is present (e.g., from GI bleeding or postoperative complications), blood flow drops. If LV failure is present (e.g., from myocardial infarction or CHF), blood flow drops. The bedside nurse detects these changes and intervenes appropriately. Although noninvasive CO and other bioimpedance devices may be helpful in assessing blood flow, the gold standard continues to be the hemodynamic monitoring with a PA catheter.

Although changes in blood flow may at times be obvious (the patient loses pulses, changes level of consciousness, decreases urine output), the measures are nonspecific and are often late signs of compromise. The most important component of tissue oxygenation is blood flow. Hemodynamic monitoring is an accurate and important means of assessing the adequacy of tissue oxygen delivery.

Measurement of Cardiac Output

CO measurements using a PA catheter are obtained by one of two methods: the intermittent thermodilution technique or the continuous technique. Both types of measures rely on measuring changes in blood temperatures. The most commonly used technique is the intermittent thermodilution technique (Figure 4–34). The technique is based on injecting a known volume of fluid at a given temperature into the blood. As the blood temperature changes to near the injectate temperature, a sensor near the distal tip of the PA catheter measures this change. CO is then computed based on the temperature change and the time it takes the injected volume to pass the thermistor. The calculation of CI is automatically done by most CO computers if body surface information is available

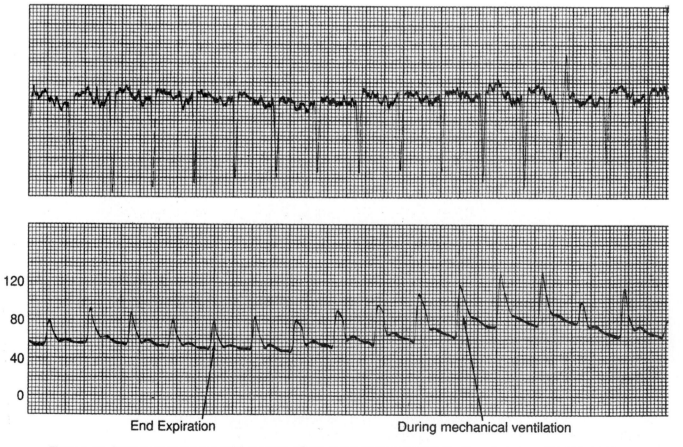

Figure 4–28. Effect of respiration on arterial pressures. (*From:* Ahrens TS: Hemodynamic Waveform Analysis, *p. 161. Philadelphia: WB Saunders; 1992, p. 161.*)

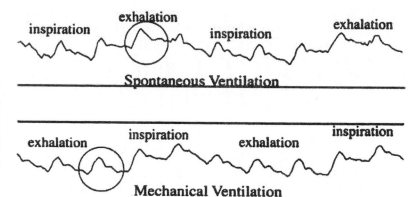

Figure 4–29. A PA waveform demonstrating respiratory effects. During spontaneous ventilation, hemodynamic pressures fall during inspiration and rise during exhalation. With mechanical ventilation, pressures rise during inspiration and fall during exhalation. The circled waveforms identify end expiration in each ventilatory mode. (*From Daily EK: Hemodynamic waveform analysis.* J Cardiovasc Nurs *2001;15[2]:6–22.*)

(see Table 4–1). The temperature change during injection can be graphically displayed on the CO computer or bedside monitor as a CO curve (Figure 4–35A). If the CO is low, the curve is small and the tail of the curve is long reflecting the slow change in temperature past the thermistor (Figure 4–35B). If the CO is high, the curve is high and the tail of the curve is short reflecting the rapid change in temperature sensed by the thermistor (Figure 4–35C).

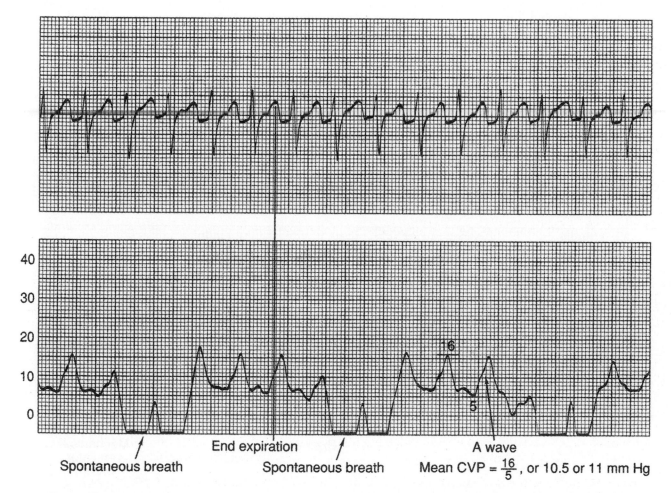

Figure 4–30. Effect of a spontaneous breath on a CVP waveform. (*From: Ahrens TS:* Hemodynamic Waveform Analysis. *Philadelphia: WB Saunders; 1992, p. 165.*)

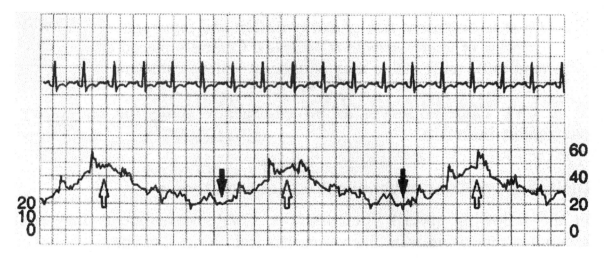

Figure 4–31. Right atrial waveform, from a PA catheter with simultaneously recorded ECG from a head-injured patient with neurogenic pulmonary edema. The patient is being maintained on controlled mechanical ventilation with 30 cm H_2O PEEP. Peak inspiratory pressure are 100 cm H_2O. The open arrows indicate the positive-pressure (ventilator) breaths and the solid arrows indicate end expiration. It is at this point that the RAP is recorded. Note that the end-expiratory pressure measurement is approximately 20 mm Hg. This grossly elevated value should not be considered to be a "true" indication of intravascular volume or RV function. Rather, the pressure measurement is spuriously elevated as a result of the excessively high intrathoracic pressure surrounding the heart and blood vessels. (*Darovic GO:* Hemodynamic Monitoring, Invasive and Noninvasive Clinical Application, *3rd ed. Philadelphia: WB Saunders; 1995.*)

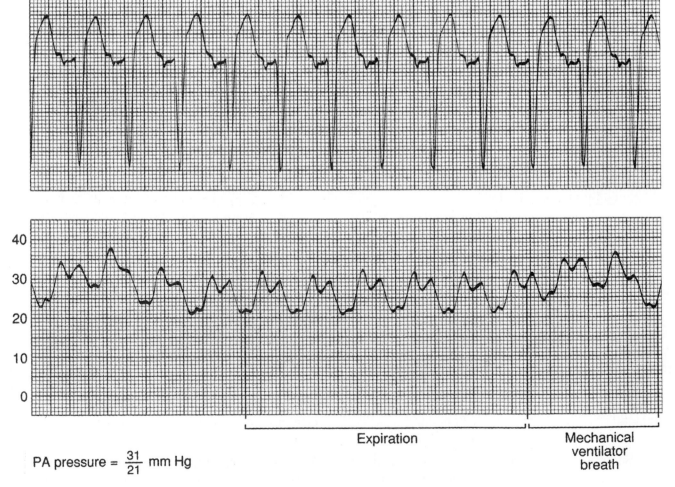

PA pressure = $\frac{31}{21}$ mm Hg

Figure 4–32. Effect of a mechanical ventilator breath on PA waveform. (*From: Ahrens TS:* Hemodynamic Waveform Recognition. *Philadelphia: WB Saunders; 1993, p. 92.*)

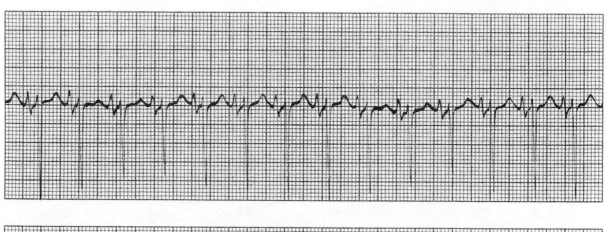

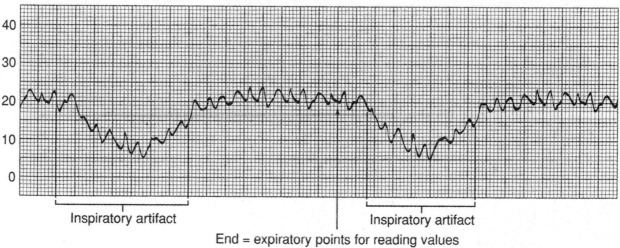

Inspiratory artifact   Inspiratory artifact

End = expiratory points for reading values

Mean PCWP = 20 mm Hg

Figure 4–33. Reading end expiration before a spontaneous breath. (*From: Ahrens TS, Taylor L:* Hemodynamic Waveform Analysis. *Philadelphia: WB Saunders; 1992, p. 170.*)

Key Concepts in Measuring Cardiac Output

To correctly measure the CO, the nurse needs to program the bedside CO computer with the following information:

- *Type of PA catheter.* Different companies may have different catheter configurations. This requires a slightly different computation by the computer. The manufacturer provides the correct computation constant to be programmed into the CO computer.
- *Volume of injectate.* Normally, 5 or 10 mL of D_5W or NS is used.
- *Temperature of the injectate.* Either cold (also called iced) or room-temperature injectate can be used. When using cold injectate, the injectate solution must be placed in a container of ice water (Figure 4–34A). Room-temperature injectate has an advantage in that it avoids the cumbersome cooling system necessary with iced injectate. Whichever technique is used, the system should be a closed system to prevent increased risk of IV nosocomial infections.

- *Computation constant.* The manufacturer of the CO system provides the correct computation constant to use based on the specific solution volume and temperature used for CO measurements. This information is programmed into the CO computer before performing CO measurements.

FACTORS AFFECTING ACCURACY

For thermodilution CO to be accurate, several factors should be present. These factors include a functioning tricuspid value, no ventricular septal defect, and a stable cardiac rhythm. The presence of cardiac valve or rhythm abnormalities causes the thermodilution CO measurement to be inaccurate. Chapter 26, Hemodynamic Troubleshooting Guide, identifies common problems associated with measurement of CO.

Interpreting Cardiac Output and Cardiac Index

The CI is a critical parameter to monitor because blood flow is the key to adequate oxygen delivery. If a threat to blood

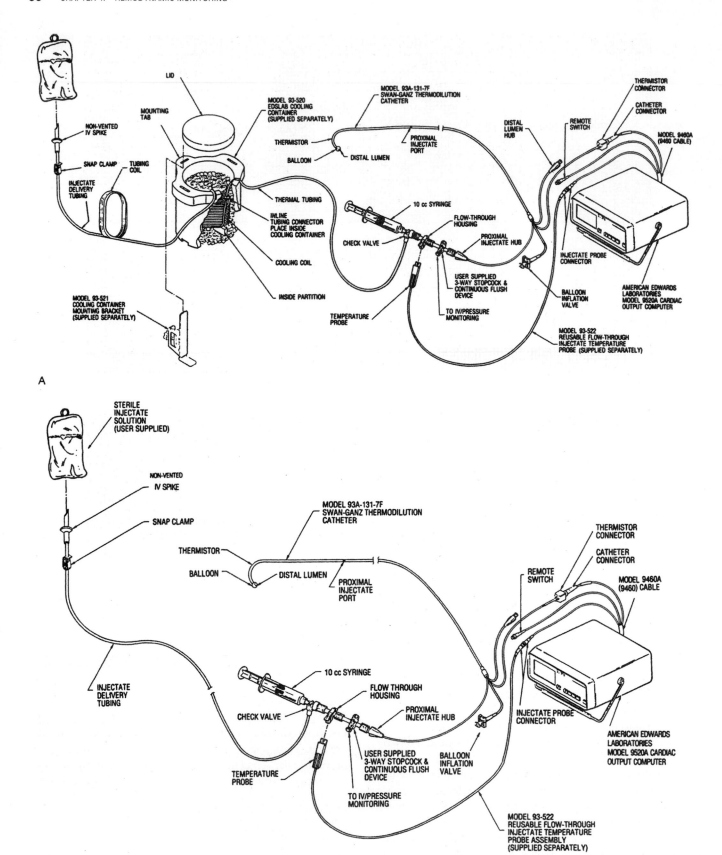

Figure 4–34. Closed thermodilution CO setup. **(A)** Iced injectable setup. **(B)** Room-temperature injectate setup. (*From: Baxter Healthcare Corporation, Edwards Critical Care Division, Santa Ana, CA.*)

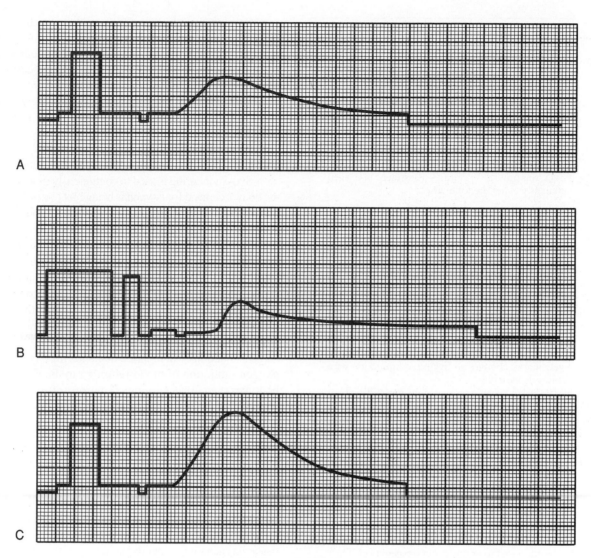

Figure 4–35. (**A**) Normal CO curve. (**B**) Low CO curve. (**C**) High CO curve.

flow occurs, tissue oxygenation is immediately placed at risk. If adequate blood flow is present, as measured with the CO or CI, generally one can assume the patient does not have a major disturbance in oxygenation.

There is no one CI that requires intervention. However, CI below 2.5 L/min/m^2 is considered circulatory compromise and further assessment is warranted. If the CI drops below 2.2 L/min/m^2, the investigation becomes urgent. However, some patients tolerate low CI without clinical problems. Tracking trends in CI values is generally more useful than monitoring single data points because temporary changes in values may not be clinically significant. In any event, with drops in CI circulatory compromise and tissue hypoxia may ensue. Using both CI and tissue oxygenation parameters, such as Svo_2, increase the accuracy in identifying a clinically dangerous event (Table 4–10).

CONTINUOUS MIXED VENOUS OXYGEN MONITORING (Svo_2)

Svo_2 Monitoring Principles

The PA catheter allows clinicians many monitoring capabilities that help to guide therapeutic interventions in the critically ill. One such option is the continuous monitoring of mixed venous oxygenation. Svo_2 catheters are different from

TABLE 4–10. TISSUE OXYGENATION PARAMETERS

Svo_2	60–75%
Lactate	1–2 mEq/L
pH	7.35–7.45
Pyruvate	0.1–0.2 mEq/L
HCO_3	22–26 mEq/L

AT THE BEDSIDE
▶ Sv_{O_2}

A 35-year-old woman with pancreatitis and ARDS experiences a progressively worsening oxygenation status. The care team decided to replace her PA catheter with an Sv_{O_2} catheter to better monitor and manage the patient. Once the Sv_{O_2} catheter was in place and calibrated, it was noted that her Sv_{O_2} was only 55%. A quick assessment of oxygen supply variables yielded the following:

Hct	22%
CO	6 L/min
PAOP	18 mm Hg
Sa_{O_2}	91% on an Fi_{O_2} of 0.6, PEEP of 15 cm H_2O

Given the high level of ventilatory support already in place, the team felt that augmentation of oxygen-carrying capacity with transfusions of packed red blood cells (PRBC) would provide the greatest boost to oxygenation. Following the infusion of 2 units of PRBC, the Sv_{O_2} increased to 70%. Over the course of the next few days, ventilatory support was gradually decreased by monitoring the effect of ventilatory changes on Sv_{O_2} in conjunction with other supply-side variables.

On day 6, she became increasingly agitated and her Sv_{O_2} decreased to 60%. She was febrile and her sputum was noted to be purulent appearing. Sputum cultures were obtained and other reasons the agitation were also considered. A STAT chest radiograph was obtained to rule out pneumothorax (it was ruled out), and an arterial blood gas was obtained. AGB revealed a pH of 45 mm Hg, and a Pa_{O_2} of 55 mm Hg. Her ventilator settings were IMV of 12/min (spontaneous rate was 10 above the ventilation), Fi_{O_2} or 0.45, PEEP of 5 cm H_2O, Hct of 29%, and CO of 6 L/min.

The team recognized that both supply and demand needed to be addressed to optimize her oxygenation. Thus, ventilatory settings were increased as follows:

Fi_{O_2}	0.60
PEEP	10 cm H_2O
IMV	20/min

Because CO and Hct were considered adequate, the team then considered the patient's demand requirements. Their assessment indicated that agitation and fever were both increasing demand, so both sedatives and antipyretics were ordered in conjunction with fluids and antibiotics. Sv_{O_2} increased to 75% following these interventions.

Continuous Sv_{O_2} monitoring is used as a diagnostic and therapeutic management tool. It provides early warning of alterations in hemodynamic status and a continuous monitor of the relationship between oxygen delivery and consumption. Many therapeutic strategies are added and adjusted in response to the changes in the Sv_{O_2}. If a blood pressure is considered low (mean arterial pressure <70 mm Hg) but the Sv_{O_2} is above 60%, then the blood pressure is not contributing to a decrease in tissue perfusion. However, if the blood pressure and Sv_{O_2} are low, interventions to improve perfusion are essential.

Sv_{O_2} monitoring is used to continuously monitor how well the body's demand for oxygen is being met under different clinical conditions. To understand this concept, an understanding of how the tissues are supplied with oxygen is necessary.

Blood leaves the left heart 100% saturated with oxygen and is transported to the tissues for cellular use based on the amount of perfusion (CO). Under normal conditions, only about 25% of the oxygen available on the hemoglobin is extracted by the tissues, with blood returning to the right heart with approximately 75% of the hemoglobin saturated with oxygen. Normal values for oxygen saturation are 70% to 80%.

In situations where tissue demands for oxygen increase, oxygen saturation of blood returning to the right heart will be lower than 70%. Clinical situations of increased tissue demand for oxygen include fever, pain, anxiety, infection, seizures, and some "routine" nursing activities like turning and suctioning. In contrast, hypothermia dramatically decreases oxygen consumption by the tissues. Interventions, then, are directed at decreasing or increasing the oxygen requirements as needed.

The concept of oxygen utilization is often referred to as *supply and demand* (or more accurately *consumption*) and is the essential concept inherent in Sv_{O_2} monitoring. Because tissue oxygenation depends on hemoglobin level, saturation of hemoglobin, oxygen consumption, and CO, the saturation of blood returning to the PA tells us much about the interaction of these four variables and can be used to assess the adequacy of interventions.

Selected Examples of Clinical Applications

Sv_{O_2} and Low Cardiac Output

In low output states, hemoglobin is moved more slowly through the body, so there is a decrease in oxygen delivery (supply). There also is more time for oxygen extraction at the tissue level. Sv_{O_2} levels in someone with cardiogenic shock are typically low (below 70%) due to slow perfusion and high tissue extraction of oxygen. The addition of an inotropic agent such as dobutamine may increase the CO and thus increase the Sv_{O_2}. Conversely, decreases in Sv_{O_2} may be observed as inotropic agents are weaned, indicating decreases in CO. Sv_{O_2} values between 30% and 49% have been associated with disruptions in the ability to produce adenosine triphosphate. This appreciably increases the rate of anaerobic metabolism and can contribute to an elevated lactate level.

other PA catheters in that they have two special fiber optic bundles within the catheter that determine the oxygen saturation of hemoglobin by measuring the wavelength (color) of reflected light. Light is transmitted down one bundle and is reflected off the oxygen-saturated hemoglobin, returning up the other bundle. This information is quantified by the bedside computer and numerically displayed as the percentage of saturation of the mixed venous blood.

Sv_{O_2} and High Output States

In sepsis, CO is often very high (>10 L/min). In this hyper-metabolic, hyperdynamic output state, blood moves very quickly past the tissues and extraction is less than optimal. Sv_{O_2} levels are frequently above normal (>80%), indicating that extraction of oxygen at the tissue level is low. Despite the availability of oxygen, tissue hypoxia exists and is confirmed with lactic acid measurements (although this is a late sign of tissue hypoxia).

Sv_{O_2} and Blood Loss

In acute blood loss, hemoglobin is decreased and the body extracts more from the available hemoglobin. Sv_{O_2} levels decrease and are an early indication of acute blood loss. Transfusions (providing they are adequate in number and rate) result in an increase in Sv_{O_2}.

To enhance oxygen delivery and decrease consumption the components of supply and demand are considered. Oxygen supply may be increased by improving CO (fluids followed by inotropes), increasing saturation (FiO_2 level, PEEP, etc.), and by increasing hemoglobin (transfusion of red cells). Examples of how demand may be lowered include decreasing activity, controlling patient–ventilator dys-synchrony, preventing agitation and thrashing, and avoiding shivering, The Sv_{O_2} catheter may be used to rapidly calculate and assess oxygen supply and consumption (Table 4–11) and direct therapies.

Troubleshooting the Sv_{O_2} Catheter

The instructions for calibration of the Sv_{O_2} catheter must be followed if readings are to be accurate. It is also important that measurements be compared periodically with co-oximeter measurements of Sv_{O_2} drawn slowly from the distal port of the PA. The Sv_{O_2} monitor can be recalibrated if saturations vary. This is referred to as an *in vivo calibration*.

It is also important that the catheters be free floating in the PA and not have fibrin or clots attached to the end, which might affect the fiber optic measurement of saturation. A guide for this is called *light intensity* and refers to the amount of transmitted light required to obtain a suitable reflected signal back to the monitor. Guidelines for the levels of light intensity help the clinician to assess the accuracy of the Sv_{O_2} readings. The size and position of the light intensity signal help the nurse to detect such complications as a catheter in wedge position or clot formation.

TABLE 4–11. SUPPLY AND CONSUMPTION CALCULATION

A. Arterial side (supply) =
   [(Hbg × arterial oxygen saturation × 1.34*) × cardiac output] × 10**
B. Venous side (return) =
   [(Hbg × venous oxygen saturation × 1.34) × cardiac output] × 10**
C. Consumption = A − B***   Normal = 250 mL/min

*A constant reflecting the amount of oxygen in milliliters that the hemoglobin can hold.
**A constant to convert the unit of measurement to milliliters.
***Simplified calculation omitting the negligible contribution of oxygen dissolved in plasma.

Sv_{O_2} catheters can be helpful in the assessment of oxygenation in the critically ill patient. An additional benefit may be a reduction in the need for frequent CO measurements, arterial blood gas parameters, and hemoglobin levels. However, as with any tool, the successful application of Sv_{O_2} monitoring depends on user familiarity and a comprehensive knowledge of essential concepts.

RIGHT VENTRICULAR EJECTION FRACTION CATHETERS

Monitoring Principles

The amount of blood in the ventricle at end diastole that is ejected during systole is the EF. It is a key indicator of the contractile force of the heart. A catheter has been designed with a rapid-responding thermistor that detects temperature changes between contractions to identify the EF. The catheter consists of two intracardiac electrodes that sense R-wave activity and a fast-response thermistor that senses changes in PA temperature. A known amount of injectate at a known temperature is injected into the right atrium. The injectate mixes with blood and is propelled by the RV into the PA. The thermistor, located in the PA, senses changes in temperature resulting from the bolus of injectate. EF is dependent on a beat-to-beat change in temperature. To determine the right ventricular ejection fraction (RVEF), the thermistor senses changes of temperature and correlates the change in temperature with an R wave, allowing the computer to calculate EF or percent of blood ejected with each beat. Once EF is obtained, the computer determines the SV and calculates end-diastolic volume (EDV = SV/EF). The SVI divided by the EF provides the ventricular end-diastolic volume index, which is a better indicator of volume status (preload) than PAOP or RAP.

The RV volumes and RVEF can be used to determine the optimal preload of the right ventricle. The end-diastolic volume (EDV) represents the amount of volume in the ventricle at the end of diastole or the amount of volume available for the ventricle to eject. The preload value of the RV normally is 100 to 160 mL (see Table 4–1). The end-systolic volume is the volume of blood remaining in the ventricle after systole or the residual amount of blood that remains in the ventricle after contraction and normally is 50 to 100 mL (see Table 4–1). As the RV afterload acutely increases or contractility decreases, the ventricles are unable to pump as effectively and this value increases (Table 4–12).

Troubleshooting

The catheter must be positioned properly to interpret volume and blood flow. Assessing the RA and PA waveforms and noting the volume required to produce a "wedge" waveform ensures the catheter is properly positioned and free floating to maximize accuracy.

TABLE 4–12. FACTORS THAT ALTER RIGHT VENTRICULAR PARAMETERS

Parameter	Increase	Decrease
RV end-diastolic volume	Volume Increased RV afterload Decreased RV contractility Decreased HR	Diuretics Decreased RV afterload Increased RV contractility Increased HR
RV end-systolic volume	Volume Increased RV afterload Decreased RV contractility	Diuretics Decreased RV afterload Increased RV contractility
RV ejection fraction	Decreased RV afterload Increased RV contractility	Increased RV afterload Decreased RV contractility

Any condition that causes wide fluctuations in temperature can cause inaccuracies in the values. Large changes in venous return, administration of large volumes of fluid, and rapid changes in core temperature lead to variations in the values. Heart rates above 150 beats/min alter the patient's R-R interval and lead to unreliable measurements.

MINIMALLY INVASIVE HEMODYNAMIC MONITORING

Thoracic Bioimpedance

The resistance of current flow (impedance) across the chest is inversely related to the thoracic fluid. Using a current that flows from outer electrode (transmit current) to inner sensor (Figure 4–36), the SV can be determined. Changes in impedance occur with changes in blood flow and velocity through the ascending aorta. The impedance changes reflect aortic flow, which is directly related to ventricular function (contractility).

Variables that change the bioimpedance and alter the relationship between impedance and SV are changes in hematocrit, lung water, lead contact, shivering, mechanical ventilation, and rhythm changes. Thoracic bioimpedance is a useful method for trend analysis but is not accurate enough for diagnostic interpretation. Its major application has been outside the critical care setting (CHF clinics, emergency department, pacemaker clinics). Management of acutely ill patients in the outpatient setting may be the most important contribution of this technology.

Esophageal Doppler Cardiac Output

The color esophageal Doppler uses sound to measure the aortic blood flow velocity. The red blood cells moving toward the Doppler appear red and the red blood cells moving away from the Doppler appear blue. The speed of the blood intensifies the color. A waveform is used to interpret "capture" of the blood flow. Doppler CO provides immediate measures of blood flow, unlike delayed measurements achieved with the PA catheter.

A transducer probe is lubricated and inserted into the esophagus to a depth of 35 to 40 cm. It is positioned to mea-sure blood flow in the descending thoracic aorta (Figure 4–37). Reassessment of probe placement (monitoring the waveform) is crucial to accurate measurement. A beam is directed at the red blood cells flowing into the descending aorta and their movement is depicted as a waveform of blood velocity versus flow time. From this information CO and SV are determined as well as information of preload, afterload, and contractility.

Contraindications for the use of transesophageal Doppler monitoring include coarctation of the aorta, esophageal pathology, coagulopathies, and patients with intra-aortic balloon pumps. Sedation is required for the entire time the probe is in place.

Carbon Dioxide Rebreathing

A modified Fick equation is used to predict CO:

$$CO = V_{CO_2}/C_{vCO_2} - C_{aCO_2}.$$

Mixed venous CO_2 is estimated through a rebreathing technique using a special device. This monitoring technique is relatively new in the United States and has several limitations when used to assess the critically ill. End-tidal CO_2 (P_{etCO_2}) is used to replace arterial CO_2 values. Exhaled air is obtained from a rebreathing circuit attached to the ventilator. The CO can be measured by noting the change in exhaled CO_2 during normal breathing and rebreathing.

One of the major limitations to CO_2 rebreathing is that it does not measure the intracardiac pressures. Patients must be on controlled mechanical ventilation (no spontaneous ventilations). Other variables that alter the accuracy of this method are rapidly fluctuating CO, changes in dead space and dysrhythmias. Patients with $\dot{V}/\dot{Q}$ matching diseases have altered CO_2 production that alters the exhaled CO_2 and leads to less accurate interpretation of CO.

Gastric Tonometry (pHi)

When stressed the body shunts perfusion toward vital organs (brain and heart) at the expense of less vital areas (splanchnic circulation). Mucosal tonometry is an indirect monitor of regional blood flow and metabolic balance. A special nasogastric tube is placed (Figure 4–38). CO_2 diffuses from the

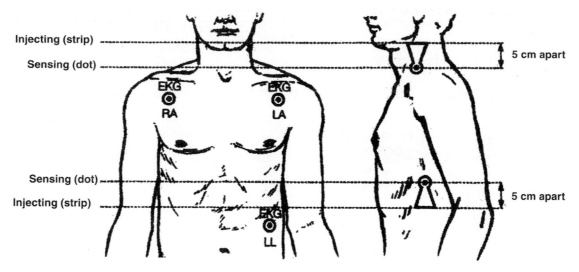

Figure 4–36. Electrode placement for thoracic electrical bioimpedance. (*From Von Reuden K, Turner MA, Lynn CA: A new approach to hemodynamic monitoring. RN 1999;62[8]:53–58.*)

mucosa into the lumen of the stomach and across the silicone balloon of the tonometer. The balloon is permeable to CO_2 and the gas diffuses from the gastric mucosa into the saline solution within the gastric balloon. This should closely reflect the P_{CO_2} of the gastric mucosa. Gastric tonometry (pHi) is then used as a marker of perfusion abnormality and the adequacy of resuscitation.

Gastric enteral feedings usually cause gastric hypersecretion and lower the pHi, which leads to inaccurate values. This conflicts with the trend to early enteral feedings for improved patient outcomes. Placement of a postpyloric tube and close monitoring of residual can eliminate this limitation. Accurate measurement is totally dependent on complete blockade of gastric secretion of acid requiring drug administration.

Sublingual Capnometry ($P_{SL}CO_2$)

Esophageal tissue and proximal gastric intestinal mucosa (sublingual) respond similarly to decreased blood flow as does the gastric mucosa. Increase in $P_{SL}CO_2$ directly correlates with a decrease in sublingual blood flow. It is a noninvasive method of identifying regional abnormalities in blood flow.

It consists of a disposable P_{CO_2} sensor, a fiberoptic cable that connects to a blood gas analyzer and a blood gas monitoring instrument (Figure 4–39). The optical fiber is coated with a silicone membrane with a CO_2-sensitive dye that is permeable to CO_2. The CO_2 passes through the membrane and comes into contact with the dye. A signal is transmitted and converted to a numeric CO_2 value displayed on the handheld blood gas analyzer. The $P_{SL}CO_2$ measurements are obtained by placing the disposable sensor under the tongue with the sensor facing the sublingual mucosa. Within 5 minutes, a $P_{SL}CO_2$ measurement is recorded.

The technology has been used to diagnose and quantify the severity of circulatory shock, with a predictive value of 100%. It has also been used to validate the endpoints of resuscitation. A $P_{SL}CO_2$ lower than 45 mm Hg accurately predicts hemodynamic stability. The only significant limitation with the method is noncontinuous data collection.

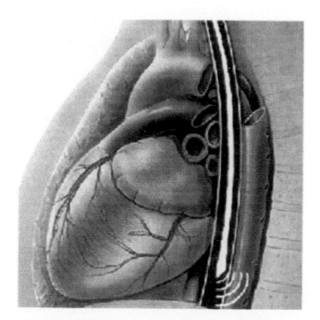

Figure 4–37. Esophageal Doppler monitor probe placement. (*Used with permission for Deltex Medical, Inc., Severna Park, MD.*)

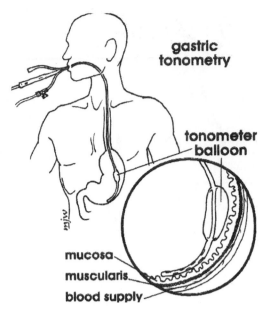

Figure 4–38. Gastric tonometry. (*From Boswell SA, Scalea TM: Sublingual capnometry. AACN Clinical Issues 2003;14[2]:180 [Illustration by Mark Wieber]*).

APPLICATION OF HEMODYNAMIC PARAMETERS

Low Cardiac Output States

Hemodynamic disturbances present as either a high or low blood flow state. Initially, compensatory mechanisms may present to keep blood flow normal, but eventually the out-

---

AT THE BEDSIDE
▶ *Hypovolemia*

A 67-year-old woman is admitted to the unit with the diagnosis of hypotension of unknown origin. She presently is unresponsive but is breathing spontaneously and is not intubated. Breath sounds are clear, urine output is 15 mL in 8 hours, and her skin is cool. A PA catheter is inserted to aid in the interpretation of the situation. The following data are available:

BP	86/54	SI	16 mL/m^2
P	118/min	PA	24/10
RR	30/min	PAOP	6 mm Hg
T	37.3°C	CVP	3 mm Hg
CI	1.9 L/min/m^2	SvO$_2$	50%

Note the low blood flow (CI and SI below normal) and low intracardiac pressures (pulmonary capillary wedge pressure). This combination of low flows and intracardiac pressures is consistent with hypovolemia. In addition, the SvO$_2$ is low, indicating that a threat to tissue oxygenation is likely.

The exact cause of the hypovolemia cannot be discerned from the hemodynamics. Further investigation to isolate the exact problem, such as GI bleeding, dehydration, or other forms of blood loss, is necessary to diagnose the underlying cause of the hypovolemia.

---

put becomes either too high or too low. The most common situation is the development of a low CO state.

Low CO states fall into two categories: hypovolemia or LV dysfunction. Although many conditions can cause

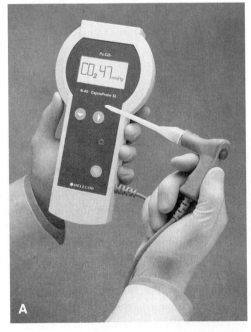
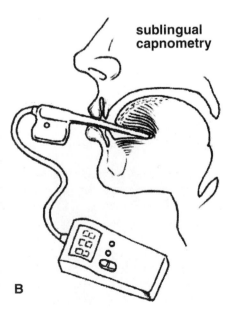

Figure 4–39. Sublingual capnometry. The CapnoProbe Sublingual System. (*From Boswell S, Scalea T: Sublingual capnometry. AACN Clinical Issues 2003;14[2]:181. Reprinted with permissions of Nellcor Puritan Bennett, Inc., Pleasanton, CA* **[A]** *and Mark Wieber* **[B]**.)

either hypovolemia or LV dysfunction, all produce a low CO state. Before the CO falls, however, the SV decreases. Therefore, the SV or SI is an earlier warning sign of impending low-flow states. As such, it should be examined before the CO or index. When SV can no longer be compensated (by heart rate), the total blood flow (CO) decreases. From a tissue oxygenation perspective, the drop in SV does not harm oxygen delivery as long as the total blood flow (CO) is maintained. Parameters such as SvO_2 remain normal as long as total blood flow is unchanged. Because SV decreases in both hypovolemia and LV dysfunction, without necessarily changing CO or SvO_2 levels, it is important to assess SVI first when examining hemodynamic parameters.

Identifying the cause of the low-flow state (e.g., hypovolemia or LV dysfunction) is based on a combination of clinical and hemodynamic information. For example, the patient's physical assessment and history might reveal the presence of a pathologic clinical condition such as LV failure. From a hemodynamic monitoring perspective, the use of intracardiac pressures (PAOP, CVP) is the most common method of differentiating the cause of the low blood flow state. Management of low CO states begins by treating problems of either LV dysfunction or hypovolemia.

Left Ventricular Dysfunction

Low CO states that are caused by LV dysfunction are managed with a variety of therapies to decrease LV work and improve performance: improvement of contractility, preload reduction, and afterload reduction. Generally, pharmacologic therapies are used to treat the dysfunctional left ventricle. However, a few physical interventions are available, such as allowing the patient to sit up, attempting to reduce anxiety, as well as mechanical supports, such as intraaortic balloon pumping and ventricular assist devices (see Chapter 19, Advanced Cardiovascular Concepts). Improvement of LV function, however, relies heavily on pharmacologic support (see Table 4–2).

Improvement of Contractility

If a patient presents with symptoms of LV dysfunction, relief is obtained by improving LV function. Inotropic therapy commonly is employed during an acute episode of LV dysfunction. Inotropic therapy increases the strength of the cardiac contraction, thereby increasing EF, SV, CO, and tissue oxygenation.

Three common inotropic drugs are used in acute care to improve ventricular contractility: dobutamine (Dobutrex), dopamine, and milrinone (Primacor) (Table 4–13). Although other agents are used occasionally, by far the most common drug used in acute treatment is dobutamine. Dobutamine acts as a sympathetic stimulant, increasing the stimulation of beta cells of the sympathetic nervous system. This stimulation produces a positive inotropic (contractile) response, as well as a positive chronotropic (heart rate) response. Dobutamine also has a slight vasodilator effect due to B_2 stimulation, causing a slight reduction in preload and afterload. Based

---

AT THE BEDSIDE
▶ *Left Ventricular Dysfunction*

A 76-year-old man is admitted to the unit with the diagnosis of acute inferior wall myocardial infarction and a history of COPD. During the shift he begins to complain of shortness of breath. He has crackles one-third the way up his posterior lobes along with expiratory wheezing. He has an S_3 (gallop) and a II/VI systolic murmur. The following hemodynamic information was obtained on admission:

BP	100/58	PA	38/23
P	112/min	PAOP	21 mm Hg
CI	2.1 L/min/m^2	CVP	13 mm Hg
CO	4.6 L/min	SvO_2	49%
SI	19		

This patient presents with low blood flow (CI and SI) and high intracardiac pressures (PAOP, CVP). The combination of low blood flow and high filling pressures suggests LV and RV dysfunction. The low SvO_2 level suggests a serious disturbance in tissue oxygenation. Intervention to support CO is required. Further investigation to isolate the exact problem, such as CHF, myocardial infarction, or cardiomyopathy, is necessary.

---

on these effects, dobutamine is an ideal first choice to pharmacologically increase the CO and SV.

If dobutamine is not effective, milrinone may be used because its action is different from dobutamine. Dobutamine may not be effective in cases where sympathetic stimulation has already achieved its maximal impact. Milrinone is a phosphodiesterase inhibitor, increasing the availability of intracellular calcium. Although milrinone is associated with coagulopathic side effects (decreases platelet count), it is a logical alternative to dobutamine or dopamine.

Dopamine also can be used to improve the contractile state of the heart. Because dopamine also stimulates alpha cells of the sympathetic nervous system, afterload also increases, a situation that is not always desired in low CO states. The net effect is an improvement in blood pressure and possibly CO and SV, but the cost in terms of myocardial oxygen consumption is higher than with the other two inotropes. As such, dopamine is not a first-line drug to treat acute LV dysfunction unless hypotension is present.

The potential negative effect of inotropic therapy is the increase in myocardial oxygen consumption that accompanies the increased contractile state. Unfortunately, it is not easy to measure myocardial oxygenation. Because of this potential problem, many clinicians prefer to use agents that either reduce preload or afterload, neither of which increases myocardial oxygen consumption.

Preload Reduction

Reduction of preload is thought to be beneficial in the patient with LV dysfunction by decreasing the distention of over-

AT THE BEDSIDE
▶ *Inotropic Therapy*

A 71-year-old man is admitted to the ICU with hypotension of unknown origin. He presently has a fiberoptic PA catheter in place to determine the origin of the hypotension. At 1800 hours, he is unresponsive with a Glasgow Coma score of 4. His vital signs and PA catheter reveal the following information:

BP	102/68
P	101/min
CO	3.9 L/min
CI	2.3 L/min/m^2
SI	23
PA	42/22
PAOP	18 mm Hg
CVP	12 mm Hg
SvO$_2$	51%

Dobutamine is added to the patient's management regime. One hour after the dobutamine, a repeat set of hemodynamics reveals the following:

BP	104/66
P	106/min
CO	4.4 L/min
CI	2.6 L/min/m^2
SI	25
PA	40/20
PAOP	14 mm Hg
CVP	13 mm Hg
SvO$_2$	57%

Based on the slight improvement in SI, CI, and SvO$_2$, as well as the decrease in PAOP, there has been a mild improvement in the hemodynamic parameters. Further titration of dobutamine should be considered because SvO$_2$ is not within normal limits.

stretched myocardial muscle fibers. Many therapies have been designed for preload reduction, although they generally fall into one of two groups: drugs that reduce blood volume (diuretics) and those that promote vasodilation (nitrates, calcium channel blockers, and beta-blockers) (Table 4–14).

TABLE 4–13. COMMON INOTROPIC THERAPIES IN TREATING ABNORMAL HEMODYNAMICS

Drug	Dosage	Onset of Action	Route
Dobutamine (Dobutrex)	1–20 µg/kg/min	1–2 min	IV
Dopamine (Intropin)	2–10 µg/kg/min	1–2 min	IV
Milrinone (Primacor)	Loading 0.75 mg/kg, then 5–10 µg/kg/min	<5 min	IV
Digoxin (normally not used in acute LV failure)	0.5 mg at first; then 0.25 every 6 hours until desired effect, then 0.125–0.25 mg/d	1–2 h	IV

TABLE 4–14. COMMON PRELOAD REDUCERS FOR ABNORMAL HEMODYNAMICS

Drug	Dosage	Onset of Action	Route
Diuretic Agents			
Furosemide (Lasix)	20 mg or higher	<5 min	IV/PO
Bumetanide (Bumex)	0.5–10 mg/d	<5 min	IV/PO
Ethacrynic Acid (Edecrin)	50–100 mg/d	<5 min	IV/PO
Chlorothiazide (Diuril)	500–2000 mg/d	1–2 h	IV/PO
Metolazone (Zaroxolyn)	2.5–20 mg/d	1 h	PO
Mannitol	12.5–200 g/d	<5 min	IV
Vasodilating Agents			
Dopamine	1–2 µg/kg/min	<5 min	IV
Nitroglycerine (Tridil, Nitrostat IV)	5–400 µg	1–2 min	IV

The most common approach to reduce preload is diuretic therapy. Diuretics are preferred because they eliminate excess fluid. As the left ventricle begins to fail, blood flow is decreased to the kidneys. This reduced blood flow is interpreted by the kidneys as insufficient blood volume. The kidneys then increase the reabsorption of water, producing an increase in intravascular volume. This increase contributes to venous engorgement and dependent edema in CHF.

The most common diuretics used to reduce preload are the loop diuretics. Loop diuretics work by blocking the reabsorption of sodium and water in the loop of Henle. The subsequent loss of sodium and water allows for a reduction in vascular volume. The reduction in vascular volume theoretically reduces the amount of blood returning to the heart and reduces the tension on myocardial muscle. The reduced tension allows the heart to return to a more normal contractile state.

Other preload reducers, such as nitroglycerine, act by promoting vasodilation. The result of vasodilation is to reduce the amount of blood returning to the heart. The net effect is to reduce preload and improve the LV contractile state. In clinical practice, it is common to use either form of preload reduction or both. Preload reducers such as nitroglycerine have the added benefit of improving myocardial blood flow. However, they do not contribute to diuresis.

Afterload Reduction

The cornerstone of long-term LV dysfunction management is the use of drugs to reduce afterload (resistance to ejection of blood). Short-term reduction of afterload, such as one sees in the acutely ill patient with LV dysfunction, is important, but is used only after ensuring the presence of an adequate SV. When afterload reduction should be used in acute care is not universally agreed upon. However, it may be beneficial to lower blood pressure or SVR to decrease afterload because doing so reduces LV work, improves LV contractility, and reduces myocardial oxygen consumption.

In an acutely ill patient with LV dysfunction, afterload reduction is employed when the patient is hypertensive

AT THE BEDSIDE
▶ *Preload Reduction*

A 77-year-old woman is in the unit following an episode of angina that precipitated an episode of CHF. She has a PA catheter in place, which reveals her initial set of information. Also, she has a second set of hemodynamics that indicates her status following the initiation of nitroglycerine. Based on these data, was the nitroglycerine effective in improving her hemodynamics?

	Initial Values	Postnitroglycerine Values
BP	114/76	112/72
P	106/min	92/min
CI	2.4 L/min/m^2	2.6 L/min/m^2
SI	23	28
PA	40/23	35/20
PAOP	22 mm Hg	17 mm Hg
CVP	12 mm Hg	9 mm Hg
SvO$_2$	56%	65%

Based on the increase in SI and SvO$_2$, as well as a decrease in PAOP, this therapy appears to have been effective. Even though the CO did not change markedly, the increase was enough to improve tissue oxygenation. This example illustrates the need to evaluate more than one parameter (such as the PAOP).

or has a high SVR. Generally, afterload reducers are used initially only if the blood pressure or high SVR is considered to be the cause of the LV dysfunction. Otherwise, afterload reducers are added after inotropic therapy and preload reduction.

In acute management of an increased afterload, the most common afterload reducer is nitroprusside (Table 4–15). This arterial dilating agent works very fast (within 2 minutes) and has only a short-acting half-life (about 2 minutes). The disadvantage of nitroprusside is that it breaks down into thiocyanate, a precursor to cyanide. Toxic levels of thio-

cyanate can accumulate within 2 days of administration. The antidote for thiocyanate poisoning is sodium thiosulfate.

Other rapid afterload-reducing agents are available, including newer calcium channel- and beta-blocking agents. Keep in mind that these agents might act as negative inotropes and actually weaken the heart. Their use in acute management of LV dysfunction is controversial, although their long-term use in managing CHF is well established.

Other common agents to reduce afterload are the angiotensin-converting enzyme inhibitors. Generally, these drugs are used for the chronic management of afterload in an oral form, although some IV forms are available (enalapril). See Chapter 7, Pharmacology, for additional information on drug therapy.

Hypovolemia

If the underlying cause of the low CO state is hypovolemia, two key approaches are used: preload augmentation and identification of the optimal type of preload agent. Identifying when to treat a patient who is potentially hypovolemic is greatly enhanced with hemodynamic monitoring. It is critical to use the guidelines outlined to avoid common errors in interpretation of hemodynamic monitoring data. For example, in the patient who is hypovolemic, the SV or SVI changes when vascular volume has been significantly altered. This change in SV is frequently accompanied by reduced cardiac pressures (e.g., PAOP, CVP). However, the key parameter to monitor is SV. Keep in mind that cardiac pressures do not necessarily reflect changes in volume, due to ventricular compliance. To avoid errors in interpreting hypovolemia, always examine if a low SV is present before examining the cardiac pressures.

Perhaps one of the most controversial areas in the treatment of hypovolemia is the choice of the agent to use in improving vascular volume. There are three major categories of agents to be considered: blood, crystalloids, and colloids. Blood solutions such as packed cells or whole blood are in somewhat of a special category. They are not restricted to the patient who has a low SV, unlike the other categories. Blood

TABLE 4–15. COMMON AFTERLOAD REDUCING AGENTS

Drug	Dose	Onset of Action	Route
Smooth Muscle Relaxants and Alpha Inhibitors			
Nitroprusside (Nipride)	0.5–10 μg/kg/min	1–2 min	IV
Nitroglycerine (Tridil, Nitrostat IV)	5–400 μg	1–2 min	IV
Diazoxide (Hyperstat IV)	50–150 mg	1–2 min	IV
Hydralazine (Apresoline)	10–40 mg	10–20 min	IV/IM
Methyldopa (Aldomet)	250 mg–1 g	2 h	IV
Trimethaphan (Arfonad)	3–6 mg/min	1–2 min	IV
Phentolamine (Regitine)	0.1–2 mg/min	<1 min	IV
Angiotension-Converting Enzyme Inhibitors			
Captopril (Capoten)	25–400 mg/d in 2–3 doses	15–30 min	PO
Enalapril/Enalaprilat (Vasotec/Vasotec IV)	2.5–4.0 mg/d	15 min	PO/IV
Lisinopril (Zestril)	10–40 mg/d	1 h	PO

is used when hemoglobin levels are less than 7 g/dL, regardless of any other clinical sign. This approach is necessary due to the potential decrease in oxygen-carrying capacity.

Crystalloids are solutions such as normal saline and lactated Ringer's solution. They obtain their benefit primarily through the sodium in the solution. Sodium levels in crystalloid solutions are generally near blood levels (approximately 140 mEq). Colloids are solutions such as blood products (albumin) or synthetic solutions (hetastarch, a glucose polymer). Their fluid-retaining effect is due to the large molecules (protein or glucose polymers) in the solution.

There are several advantages of crystalloid solutions. They are inexpensive and do not produce immunologic responses. The key clinical advantage is that they expand into all fluid compartments (vascular, interstitial, and intracellular) because most of the solution does not remain in just the vascular bed. For example, if 1000 mL of normal saline is given, less than 200 mL is believed to stay in the vascular bed. The rest diffuses into the other fluid compartments. This makes crystalloids ideal for treating patients who have chronic hypovolemia or dehydration. This advantage is also a limitation in some cases. If a rapid vascular expansion is required, it takes large volumes of crystalloids because most of the solution is not staying in the vascular system.

Colloids have one key advantage over crystalloids in that they rapidly expand the vascular volume. Virtually all the colloid solution infused remains in the vascular bed, at least initially. This allows for a much more rapid treatment of hypovolemia, frequently necessary in conditions such as trauma and postoperative bleeding. One disadvantage to colloids is their expense. Controversy does exist, however, about whether colloids are any more effective than crystalloids. Concerns have been raised that colloids may potentially cause harm in conditions with capillary leak syndromes (e.g., sepsis and ARDS). In these conditions, the leakage of fluid through damaged capillaries is exacerbated if large proteins (or glucose polymers) leak through the capillaries because they pull large amounts of fluid along with them.

Although crystalloids appear to be generally as effective as colloids, the best agent is still controversial. Each has its own benefits and limitations. Regardless of which is to be used, its effect should be measured on how well it improves tissue oxygenation, SV, SVI, and intracardiac pressures.

AT THE BEDSIDE
▶ *Hypovolemia*

A 62-year-old man is in the unit with the diagnosis of ruptured diverticula. He presently is unresponsive and is being prepared for surgery. Breath sounds are clear, urine output is 20 mL in 9 hours, and his skin is cool and dry. A PA catheter is inserted to aid in the interpretation of the situation. The following data are available:

BP	82/58
P	111/min
RR	33/min
T	38.4°C
CI	1.7 L/min/m²
SI	15
PA	23/11
PAOP	7 mm Hg
CVP	2 mm Hg
SvO_2	53%

The most important parameters to treat are the low SI, CI, and SvO_2. A threat to tissue oxygenation clearly exists based on these parameters. Immediate supportive therapy includes a fluid bolus of normal saline or lactated Ringer's solution. Blood products (whole blood, albumin) or other colloids (hetastarch or pentastarch) could also be considered until the patient is taken to surgery.

High Cardiac Output States

CO values can be elevated as well as lowered. In healthy people, COs elevate secondary to increased oxygen demand (e.g., exercise) or psychological stimulation (fear, anxiety). In clinical practice, three reasons exist for an increased CO: response to a systemic inflammation (e.g., sepsis, systemic inflammatory response syndrome), hepatic disease, or neurogenic-mediated vasodilation (Table 4–16). The most common reason for the CO to elevate is systemic inflammation. Inflammation, which is common in conditions such as sepsis, causes SVR to decrease. This decrease in resistance produces a compensatory increase in CO. The increase in CO might be minimal or marked. The key point to remember is that the CO elevation is a sign of a problem

---

TABLE 4–16. HEMODYNAMIC PROFILES IN SHOCK

Parameters	Hypovolemic Shock	Cardiogenic Shock	Neurogenic Shock	Anaphylactic Shock	Septic Shock Early	Septic Shock Late	Obstructive Shock
RAP	↓	↑	↓	↓	↓	↑	↑
PAOP	↓	↑	↓	↓	↓	↑	↑
CO/CI	↓	↓	N↓	↓	N↑	↓	↓
BP	↓	↓	↓	↓	↓	↓	↓
PAP	N↓↑	↑	N↓	N↓↑	N↓	↑	↑
SVR	↑	↑	↓	↓	↓	↑	↑

Abbreviation: N, normal.

rather than the problem. If the problem is treated, the CO will return to normal.

When a patient has high COs in sepsis, it does not mean the heart is functioning normally. Because of the release of myocardial depressant factors, the EF normally is depressed in sepsis. The method by which the SV is maintained is through an increase in EDV. This increase in EDV allows SV to be maintained even though the EF is reduced.

If the hemodynamic problem appears to be a low SVR, initial treatment centers on increasing afterload (SVR), augmenting preload, and administration of inotropic therapy. None of these therapies for managing low SVR states is curative, and the underlying cause of the low SVR (such as infection) must be corrected. The following section only addresses the management of low SVR states, because preload and inotropic therapy have been discussed.

Increasing the afterload/SVR is usually accomplished by administering an alpha-stimulating drug. Three common agents used for this purpose: norepinephrine (Levophed), dopamine (Intropin), and phenylephrine. Norepinephrine and dopamine have a combination of alpha and beta stimulation, producing both vasoconstriction and increased cardiac stimulation (inotropic and chronotropic responses). This makes the heart beat both stronger and faster. These two agents have a greater likelihood of increasing blood pressure and SVR due to this combined cardiac and vascular effect. Phenylephrine is only an alpha stimulant, which has some advantages. Because it only causes alpha stimulation, there is less direct effect on the heart. Although the SVR and blood pressure might not be increased as quickly with phenylephrine, it does avoid some of the direct increase of myocardial oxygen consumption that is seen with norepinephrine and dopamine. Clinically, any of these agents may be used to increase the SVR. Because they are strong alpha stimulants, their use should be considered with a degree of caution.

Direct alpha stimulants can cause severe vasoconstriction. These agents are so strong that if they infiltrate into normal tissue, the resulting vasoconstriction might cause local tissue death. As a precaution, these drugs are only given in large, central veins. From an assessment perspective, if these drugs are effective, the SVR should increase as well as the blood pressure. However, it is critical to remember that when these drugs are used tissue oxygenation as well as SVR and blood pressure must be assessed. If the SVR or blood pressure increases, parameters such as SvO_2 also increase. SVR and blood pressure do not always directly correlate with blood flow, which makes the addition of tissue oxygenation parameters (like SvO_2) an essential part of assessing the effect of vasopressors like norepinephrine, dopamine, and phenylephrine.

Fluid administration with crystalloids (or colloids) is common because the low SVR produces a pseudohypovolemia from vasodilation. Fluid is administered to the same end points as in the case of the patient with hypovolemia.

Inotropic therapy can be given to try to increase CO and oxygen delivery. Administration of inotropic therapy might

---

AT THE BEDSIDE
▶ *Low SVR*

A 65-year-old man is in the unit after developing hypotension on the floor. He had femoral-popliteal bypass surgery 4 days earlier and was doing well until yesterday. He began to complain of generalized malaise with the following vital signs:

BP	122/78	RR	27/min
P	110/min	T	38.1°C

His wound site is reddened but has no drainage. This morning, he was less oriented and was hypotensive (BP 88/54, P 114/min), prompting a transfer to the unit. He does not complain of any discomfort or shortness of breath. His lung sounds are clear and he has a pulse oximeter value of 99%. A flow-directed PA catheter is inserted to assist in the assessment of the cause of hypotension. The following data are available from the PA catheter:

CO	10.5 L/min	SVR	475
CI	6.0 L/min/m²	PVR	51
PA	22/11	CVP	2 mm Hg
PAOP	8 mm Hg	SvO_2	84%

Based on this information, a systemic inflammation appears to be developing, producing a low SVR. In addition, the vasodilation is also producing low cardiac pressures. The most likely immediate therapies are fluid therapies (normal saline or lactated Ringer's solution) and perhaps vasopressors (norepinephrine, phenylephrine, or vasopressin). Obviously, none of these therapies is curative and a more definitive therapy (such as appropriate antibiotics and identification of source of septic trigger) needs to be applied.

---

seem unusual in a patient with a high CO. However, some investigators believe that oxygen delivery needs to be increased to supranormal levels to help improve patient outcome. Supranormal oxygen delivery can be achieved by such methods as fluid administration and inotropic therapy. Whether this concept is valid or not has not been clarified in the literature.

One of the reasons for suspecting that supranormal amounts of oxygen are required is the microcapillary shunting and diminished cellular oxygenation that occurs in low SVR states like sepsis (Figure 4–40). The result is tissue hypoxia. SvO_2 levels are paradoxically high, reflecting the regional maldistribution of blood flow. Because of a lack of blood flow to some regions, oxygen delivery is forced to supranormal levels in an attempt to force oxygen into these threatened areas.

Whether this therapy is effective is still being investigated. If the problem is simply microcapillary shunting, increasing oxygen delivery might be sufficient. However, if the problem is diminished cellular oxygenation or an inability to effectively use oxygen, then increased oxygen delivery alone is unlikely to be helpful.

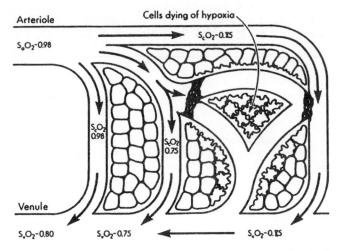

Figure 4–40. Microcapillary shunting due to obstruction at the capillary level. (*From: Ahrens TS, Rutherford KA:* Essentials of Oxygenation, *p. 108. Boston: Jones & Bartlett; 1993.*)

SELECTED BIBLIOGRAPHY

Hemodynamic Monitoring

Ahrens TS: Airway pressure measurement as an aid in hemodynamic waveform interpretation. *Crit Care Nurse* 1992;12: 44–48.

Ahrens TS: *Hemodynamic Waveform Recognition.* Philadelphia: WB Saunders; 1993.

Ahrens TS, Taylor L: *Hemodynamic Waveform Analysis.* Philadelphia: WB Saunders; 1992.

Bigatello LM, George E. Hemodynamic monitoring. *Minerva Anesthesiology* 2000;68(4):219–225.

Cilley RE, Sharenberg AM, Bongiorno PF, et al: Low oxygen delivery produced by anemia, hypoxia, and low cardiac output. *J Surgical Res* 1991;51:425–433.

Connors AF, Speroff T, Sawson NV: The effectiveness of right heart catheterization in the initial care of critically ill patients. *JAMA* 1996;276(11):889–897.

Cruz K, Franklin C: The pulmonary artery catheter: uses and controversies. *Crit Care Clin* 2001;17(2):271–291.

Daily EK: Hemodynamic waveform analysis. *J Cardiovascular Nurs* 2001;15(2):6–22.

Daily EK, Schroeder JS. *Techniques in Bedside Hemodynamic Monitoring.* St. Louis: Mosby; 1994.

Dalen JE, Bone RC: Is it time to pull the pulmonary artery catheter? *JAMA* 1996;276(11):916–918.

Darivuc DO: *Hemodynamic Monitoring: Invasive and Noninvasive Clinical Application.* Philadelphia: Saunders; 2002.

Della Rocca G, Costa MG: Hemodynamic–volumetric monitoring. *Minerva Anesthesiology* 2004;70(4):229–232.

Gawlinski A: Cardiac output monitoring. In Chulay M, Gawlinski A (eds): *Hemodynamic Monitoring Series.* Aliso Viejo, CA: AACN; 1998.

Imperial-Perez F, McRae M: Arterial pressure monitoring. In Chulay M, Gawlinski Λ (eds): *Hemodynamic Monitoring Series.* Aliso Viejo, CA:AACN; 1998.

Keckeisen M: Pulmonary artery pressure monitoring. In Chulay M, Gawlinski A (eds): *Hemodynamic Monitoring Series.* Aliso Viejo, CA: AACN; 1998.

Kohli-Seth R, Oropello JM: The future of bedside monitoring. *Crit Care Clin* 2000;16(4):557–578.

Kupeli I, Satwicz PR: Mixed venous oximetry. *Intl Anesthesiol Clin* 1989;27:176–183.

Leeper B: Monitoring right ventricular volumes. *AACN Clinical Issues* 2003;14(2):208–219.

Monnet X, Richard C, Teboul JL: The pulmonary artery catheter in critically ill patients. Does it change outcomes? *Minerva Anesthesiology* 2004;70(4):219–224.

Ott K, Johnson K, Ahrens T: New technologies in the assessment of hemodynamic parameters. *J Cardiovasc Nurs* 2001;15(2):41–55.

Pinsky MR: Hemodynamic monitoring in the intensive care unit. *Clin Chest Med* 2003;24(4):549–560.

Pittman JA, Ping JS, Mark JB: Arterial and central venous pressure monitoring. *Intl Anesthes Clin* 2004;42(1):13–30.

Prentice D, Ahrens T: Controversies in the use of the pulmonary artery catheter. *J Cardiovascular Nurs* 2001;15(2):1–5.

Quaal SJ: Improving the accuracy of pulmonary artery catheter measurement. *J Cardiovasc Nurs* 2001;15(2):71–82.

Sandham JD: Pulmonary artery catheter use—Refining the question. *Crit Care Med* 2004;32(4):1070–1071.

Vender JS, Franklin M: Hemodynamic assessment of the critically ill patient. *Intl Anesthesiol Clin* 2004;42(1):31–58.

Minimally Invasive Hemodynamic Monitoring

Akamatsu S, Oda A, Terazawa E: Automated cardiac output measurement by transesophageal color Doppler echocardiography. *Anesthes Analges* 2004;98(5):1232–1238.

Boswell SA, Scalea TM: Sublingual capnometry. *AACN Clinical Issues* 2003;14(2):176–184.

Cottis R, Magee N, Higgins DJ: Haemodynamic monitoring with pulse-induced contour cardiac output (PiCCO) in critical care. *Intens Crit Care Nurs* 2003;19:301–307.

Heard SO: Gastric tonometry: the hemodynamic monitor of choice. *Chest* 2003;123(5 Suppl):469S–474S.

Hett DA, Jonas MM: Non-invasive cardiac output monitoring. *Intens Crit Care Nurs* 2004;20(2):103–108.

L'E Orme RM, Pigott DW, Mihm FG: Measurement of cardiac output by transpulmonary arterial thermodilution using a long radial artery catheter. A comparison with intermittent pulmonary artery thermodilution. *Anaesthesia* 2004;59(6):590–594.

Martins S, Soares RM, Branco L: Non-invasive monitoring of pulmonary capillary wedge pressure in heart failure. *Eur J Heart Fail* 2001;3(1):41–46.

Odenstedt H, Stenqvist O, Lundin S: Clinical evaluation of a partial CO_2 rebreathing technique for cardiac output monitoring in critically ill patients. *Acta Anaesthesiol Scand* 2002;46(2):152–159.

Pearse RM, Ikram K, Barry J: Equipment review: An appraisal of the LiDCO trade mark plus method of measuring cardiac output. *Crit Care* 2004;8(3):190–195.

Peyton PJ, Robinson JB, McCall PR: Noninvasive measurement of intrapulmonary shunting. *J Cardiothorac Vasc Anesth* 2004;18(1):47–52.

Silver MA, Cianci P, Brennan S: Evaluation of impedance cardiography as an alternative to pulmonary artery catheterization in critically ill patients. *Congestive Heart Failure* 2004;10 (Suppl 2):17–21.

Summers RL, Parrott CW, Quale C: Use of noninvasive hemodynamics to aid decision making in the initiation and titration of neurohormonal agents. *Congestive Heart Failure* 2004;10(Suppl 2):28–31.

Turner MA: Doppler-based hemodynamic monitoring. *AACN Clinical Issues* 2003;14(2):220–231.

Yung GL, Fedullo PF, Kinninger K: Comparison of impedance cardiography to direct Fick and thermodilution cardiac output determination in pulmonary arterial hypertension. *Congestive Heart Failure* 2004;10(Suppl 2):7–10.

Therapeutics

Adams KF: Guiding heart failure care by invasive hemodynamic measurements: Possible or useful? *J Cardiac Fail* 2002;8(2):71–73.

Brazdzionyte J, Macas A, Sirvinskas E: Application of methods for hemodynamic monitoring in critical cardiac pathology (an experimental model for assessment of hemodynamics). *Medicina* 2002;38(8):835–842.

Di Giantomasso D, Morimatsu H, May CN: Increasing renal blood flow: Low-dose dopamine or medium-dose norepinephrine. *Chest* 2004;125(6):2260–2267.

Faybik P, Hetz H, Baker A: Iced versus room temperature injectate for assessment of cardiac output, intrathoracic blood volume, and extravascular lung water by single transpulmonary thermodilution. *J Crit Care* 2004;19(2):103–107.

Jain M, Canham M, Upadhyay D: Variability in interventions with pulmonary artery catheter data. *Intens Care Med* 2003;29(11): 2059–2062.

Khot UN, Novaro GM, Popovic ZB: Nitroprusside in critically ill patients with left ventricular dysfunction and aortic stenosis. *N Engl J Med* 2003;348(18):1756–1763.

Kumar A, Anel R, Bunnell E: Pulmonary artery occlusion pressure and central venous pressure fail to predict ventricular filling volume, cardiac performance, or the response to volume infusion in normal subjects. *Crit Care Med* 2004;32(3):691–699.

Leuchte IIII, Schwaiblmair M, Baumgartner RA: Hemodynamic response to sildenafil, nitric oxide, and iloprose in primary pulmonary hypertension. *Chest* 2004;125(2):580–586.

Papp A, Uusaro A, Parviainen I: Myocardial function and haemodynamics in extensive burn trauma: Evaluation by clinical signs, invasive monitoring, echocardiography and cytokine concentrations. A prospective clinical study. *Acta Anaesthesiol Scand* 2003;47(10):1257–1263.

Shoemaker WC, Wo CC, Yu S: Invasive and noninvasive hemodynamic monitoring of acutely ill sepsis and septic shock patients in the emergency department. *Eur J Emerg Med* 2000; 7(3):169–175.

Szokol JW, Murphy GS: Transesophageal echocardiographic monitoring of hemodynamics. *Intl Anesthesiol Clin* 2004;42(1): 59–81.

Evidence-Based Practice Guidelines

AACN Hemodynamic Monitoring Practice Alert. Aliso Viejo, CA: AACN; 2004 Available from URL: http://www.aacn.org

American Association of Critical-Care Nurses (AACN): *Practice Alert: Pulmonary Artery Pressure Measurement.* Aliso Viejo, CA: AACN; 2004. Available from URL: http://www.aacn.org.

Gawlinski A: *AACN Protocol for Practice: Cardiac Output Monitoring.* Aliso Viejo, CA: AACN; 1998.

Imperial-Perez F, McRae M: *AACN Protocol for Practice: Arterial Pressure Monitoring.* Aliso Viejo, CA: AACN; 1998.

Jesurum JT: *AACN Protocol for Practice: SvO$_2$ Monitoring.* Aliso Viejo, CA: AACN; 1998.

Keckeisen M: *AACN Protocol for Practice: Pulmonary Artery Pressure Monitoring.* Aliso Viejo, CA: AACN; 1998.

Pulmonary Artery Continuing Education Project (PACEP). Available from URL: http://www.pacep.org

Airway and Ventilatory Management

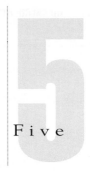

Five

Robert E. St. John

▶ Knowledge Competencies

1. Interpret normal and abnormal arterial blood gas results and common management strategies for treatment.
2. Identify indications, complications, and management strategies for artificial airways, oxygen delivery, and monitoring devices.
3. Identify indications, principles of operation, complications, and management strategies for mechanical ventilation.

RESPIRATORY ASSESSMENT TECHNIQUES, DIAGNOSTIC TESTS, AND MONITORING SYSTEMS

Arterial Blood Gas Monitoring

Arterial blood gas (ABG) monitoring is frequently performed in critically ill patients to assess acid–base balance, ventilation, and oxygenation. An arterial blood sample is analyzed for oxygen tension (PaO_2), carbon dioxide tension ($PaCO_2$), and pH using a blood gas analyzer. From these measurements, several other parameters are calculated by the blood gas analyzer, including base excess (BE), bicarbonate (HCO_3^-), and oxygen saturation (SaO_2). Arterial SaO_2 can be directly measured if a cooximeter is available. Normal ABG values analysis are listed in Table 5–1.

ABG samples are obtained by direct puncture of an artery, usually the radial artery, or by withdrawing blood through an indwelling arterial catheter system. A heparinized syringe is used to collect the sample to prevent clotting of the blood prior to analysis. Blood gas samples are kept on ice until analyzed to prevent the continued transfer of CO_2 and O_2 in and out of the red blood cells. ABG analysis equipment is often kept in or near the critical care unit to maximize accuracy and decrease the time for reporting of results. Regardless of the method used to obtain the ABG sample, practitioners should wear gloves and follow universal precautions to prevent exposure to blood during the sampling procedure.

New indwelling devices are available for the continuous monitoring of ABG values by insertion of special probes into arterial catheters. These probes are then connected to a bedside analysis machine that continuously displays ABG values. These devices are infrequently used in critical care units at this time because of their cost.

Techniques

Indwelling Arterial Catheters

All the pressure monitoring systems used with indwelling arterial catheters have sites where samples of arterial blood can be withdrawn for ABG analysis or other laboratory testing (Figure 5–1). Using the stopcock closest to the catheter insertion site, or the indwelling syringe or reservoir of the needleless systems, a 3- to 5-mL sample of blood is withdrawn to clear the catheter system of any flush system fluid. A 1-mL sample for ABG analysis is then obtained in a heparinized syringe. Any air remaining in the syringe is then removed, an airtight cap is placed on the end of the syringe, and the sample is placed on ice to ensure accuracy of the measurement. The arterial catheter system is then flushed to clear the line of any residual blood.

TABLE 5–1. LABORATORY AND CALCULATED RESPIRATORY VALUES

Parameter	Value
Arterial Blood Gases	
pH	7.35–7.45
$Paco_2$	35–45 mm Hg
HCO_3	22–26 mEq/L
Base Excess	−2–+2 mEq/L
Pao_2	70–95 mm Hg (normals vary with age and altitude)
Sao_2	>95% (normals vary with age and altitude)
Mixed Venous Blood Gases	
pH	7.33–7.43
$Pavco_2$	35–45 mm Hg
$Pavo_2$	35–40 mEq/L
Sao_2	70–80%
Respiratory Parameters	
Tidal volume (Vt)	6–8 mL/kg
Respiratory rate	8–16/min
Respiratory static compliance	70–100 mL/cm H_2O
Inspiratory force (IF)	≥20 cm H_2O
Respiratory Calculations	
Alveolar gas equation (Pao_2)	$Pao_2 = \dfrac{Fio_2(P_{ATM} - P_{H_2O}) - Paco_2}{\text{Respiratory quotient (RQ)}}$
Static compliance	$\dfrac{Vt}{(\text{Plateau pressure} - PEEP)}$

Complications associated with this technique for obtaining ABG samples include infection and hemorrhage. Any time an invasive system is used, the potential exists for contamination of the sterile system. The use of needleless systems on indwelling catheter systems decreases patients' risk for infection, as well as the critical care practitioners' risk for accidental needlestick injuries, and should be used whenever feasible. Hemorrhage is a rare complication, occurring when stopcocks are inadvertently left in the wrong position after blood withdrawal. This complication can be avoided by carefully following the proper technique during blood sampling, limiting sample withdrawal to experienced critical care practitioners, and keeping the pressure alarm system of the bedside monitoring system activated at all times.

Arterial Puncture

When indwelling arterial catheters are not in place, ABG samples are obtained by directly puncturing the artery with a needle and syringe. The most common sites for arterial puncture are the radial, brachial, and femoral arteries. Similar to venipuncture, the technique for obtaining an ABG sample is relatively simple, but success in obtaining the sample requires experience.

An Allen's test is performed prior to obtaining an ABG by puncture and prior to the insertion of an arterial line into the radial artery. The Allen's test requires that the ulnar and radial pulses be occluded for a brief period of time with the forearm held upward to facilitate blood emptying the hand. Once blanching of the hand is observed, the forearm is placed in a downward position, the ulnar artery is released, and the hand is observed for flushing. If the hand flushes, it is clear that the ulnar artery is capable of supplying blood to the fingers should the radial artery be damaged.

Following location of the pulsating artery and antiseptic preparation of the skin, the needle is inserted into the artery at a 45° angle with the bevel facing upward. The needle is slowly advanced until arterial blood appears in the syringe barrel or the insertion depth is below the artery location. If blood is not obtained, the needle is pulled back to just below the skin and relocation of the pulsating artery is verified prior to advancing the needle again.

As soon as the 1-mL sample of arterial blood is obtained, the syringe is withdrawn and firm pressure quickly applied to the insertion site with a sterile gauze pad. Handheld pressure is maintained for at least 5 minutes and the site inspected for bleeding or oozing. If present, pressure should be reapplied until all evidence of oozing has stopped. Pressure dressings are not applied until hemostasis has been achieved.

As described, all air must be removed from the ABG syringe and an airtight cap applied to the end (remove the needle first). Given the importance of maintaining pressure at the puncture site, it is sometimes helpful to have another practitioner assisting during arterial puncture to ensure appropriate handling of the blood sample.

Complications associated with arterial puncture include arterial vessel tears, air embolism, hemorrhage, arterial obstruction, loss of extremity, and infection. Using proper technique during sampling can dramatically decrease the incidence of these complications. Damage to the artery may be decreased by using a small diameter needle (21 to 23 gauge in adults) and by avoiding multiple attempts at the same site. After one or two failed attempts at entering the artery, a different site should be selected or another experienced practitioner enlisted to attempt the ABG sampling.

Hemorrhage can occur easily into the surrounding tissues if adequate hemostasis is not achieved with direct pressure. Bleeding into the tissue can range from small blood loss with minimal local damage to large blood loss with loss of distal circulation and even exsanguination. Large blood loss is more commonly seen with femoral punctures and is often the result of inadequate pressure on the artery following needle removal. Bleeding from the femoral artery is difficult to visualize, so significant blood loss can occur before practitioners are alerted to the problem. For this reason, the femoral site is the least preferred site for ABG sampling and is used only when other sites are not accessible.

The need for frequent ABG sampling for ventilation and oxygenation assessment and management may require the insertion of an arterial catheter and monitoring system to decrease the risks associated with repetitive arterial punctures.

Analysis

The best approach to analyzing the results of ABGs is a systematic one. Analysis is accomplished by evaluating acid–

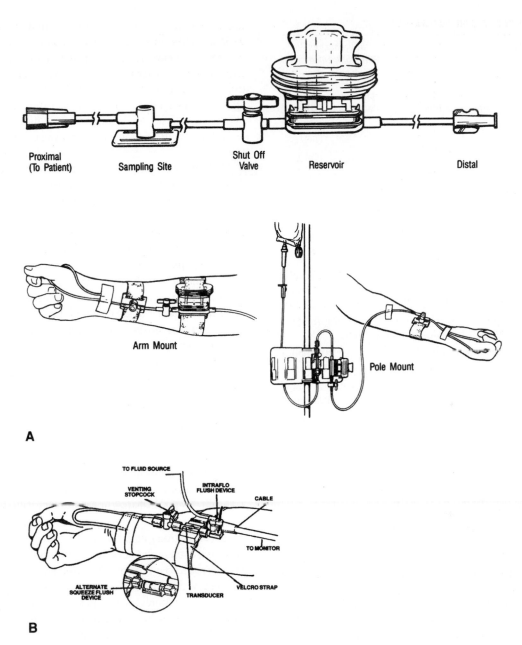

Figure 5–1. Examples of indwelling arterial catheter systems for blood gas analysis. **(A)** Closed blood withdrawal system. **(B)** Open blood withdrawal system. (*Courtesy of: Edwards Lifesciences* [*A*], *and Hospira Critical Care Systems, North Chicago, IL* [*B*].)

base and oxygenation status. Upon receipt of ABG results, the practitioner first identifies any abnormal values (see Table 5–1). Then a systematic evaluation of acid–base and oxygenation status is done.

Acid–Base Analysis

Optimal cellular functioning occurs when the pH of the blood is between 7.35 and 7.45. Decreases in pH below 7.35 are termed *acidemia,* and increases in pH above 7.45 are termed *alkalemia.* When the amount of acids or bases in the body increases or decreases, the pH changes if the ratio of acids to bases is altered. For example, if acid production increases, and there is no change in the amount of base pro-

duction, pH decreases. If the base production were to increase as well, as a response to increased acid production, then no change in pH would occur because the ratio of acids to bases would be maintained. Because the body functions best at a pH in the 7.35 to 7.45 range, there are strong systems in place to maintain the balance between acids and bases, even if one of those components is functioning abnormally. Although a variety of regulatory systems are involved in acid–base balance, the bicarbonate (HCO_3^-) and carbon dioxide (CO_2) levels are the primary regulators.

- *Metabolic component:* HCO_3^- levels are controlled primarily by the kidneys and have been termed the

TABLE 5–2. ACID–BASE ABNORMALITIES

Acid–Base Abnormality	Primary ABG Abnormalities			ABG Changes With Compensation (*if present*)	
	pH	Paco$_2$	HCO$_3^-$	Respiratory (Paco$_2$)	Metabolic (HCO$_3^-$)
Alkalemia					
Metabolic	↑		↑	↑	
Respiratory	↑	↓			↓
Acidemia					
Metabolic	↓		↓	↓	
Respiratory	↓	↑			↑

metabolic component of the acid–base system. By increasing or decreasing the amount of HCO$_3^-$ excreted in the kidneys, the pH of the blood can be increased or decreased. Changes in HCO$_3^-$ excretion may take up to 24 hours or longer to accomplish, but can be maintained for prolonged periods.

- *Respiratory component:* CO$_2$ levels are controlled primarily by the lungs and are termed the *respiratory component* of the acid–base system. By increasing or decreasing the amount of CO$_2$ excreted by the lungs, the pH of the blood can be increased or decreased. Changes in CO$_2$ excretion can occur rapidly, within a minute, by increasing or decreasing respiration (minute ventilation). Compensation by the respiratory system is difficult to maintain over long periods of time (>24 hours).
- *Acid–base abnormalities:* A variety of conditions may result in acid–base abnormalities (Tables 5–2 and 5–3).

Metabolic alkalemia is present when the pH is above 7.45 and the HCO$_3^-$ is above 26 mEq/L. In metabolic alkalosis there is either a primary increase in hydrogen ion (H$^+$) loss or HCO$_3^-$ gain. The respiratory system attempts to compensate for the increased pH by decreasing the amount of CO$_2$ eliminated from the body (alveolar hypoventilation). This compensatory attempt by the respiratory system results

in a change in pH, but rarely to a normal value. Clinical situations or conditions that cause metabolic alkalemia include loss of body acids (nasogastric suction of HCl, vomiting, excessive diuretic therapy, steroids, hypokalemia) and ingestion of exogenous bicarbonate or citrate substances. Management of metabolic alkalosis is directed at treating the underlying cause, decreasing or stopping the acid loss (e.g., use of antiemetic therapy for vomiting), and replacing electrolytes.

Metabolic acidemia is present when the pH is below 7.35 and the HCO$_3^-$ is below 22 mEq/L. In metabolic acidosis there is excessive loss of HCO$_3^-$ from the body by the kidneys or the accumulation of acid. The respiratory system attempts to compensate for the decreased pH by increasing the amount of CO$_2$ eliminated (alveolar hyperventilation). This compensatory attempt by the respiratory system results in a change in pH toward normal. Clinical situations or conditions that cause metabolic acidosis include increased metabolic formation of acids (diabetic ketoacidosis, uremic acidosis, lactic acidosis), loss of bicarbonate (diarrhea, renal tubular acidosis), hyperkalemia, toxins (salicylates overdose, ethylene and propylene glycol, methanol, paraldehyde), and adrenal insufficiency. Management of metabolic acidosis is directed at treating the underlying cause, decreasing acid formation (e.g., decreasing lactic acid production by improving cardiac output [CO] in shock), decreasing bicarbonate losses (e.g., treatment of diarrhea), removal of toxins through dialysis or cathartics, or administering sodium bicarbonate (NaHCO$_3$) in extreme metabolic acidemia states.

Respiratory alkalemia occurs when the pH is above 7.45 and the Paco$_2$ is below 35 mm Hg. In respiratory alkalosis, there is an excessive amount of ventilation (alveolar hyperventilation) and removal of CO$_2$ from the body. If these ABG changes persist for 24 hours or more, the kidneys attempt to compensate for the elevated pH by increasing the excretion of HCO$_3^-$ until normal or near-normal pH levels occur. Clinical situations or conditions that cause respiratory alkalosis include neurogenic hyperventilation, interstitial lung diseases, pulmonary embolism, asthma, acute anxiety/stress/fear, hyperventilation syndromes, excessive mechanical ventilation, and severe hypoxemia. Management

TABLE 5–3. EXAMPLES OF ARTERIAL BLOOD GAS RESULTS

ABG Analysis	pH	Paco$_2$ (mm Hg)	HCO$_3^-$ (mEq/L)	Base Excess	Pao$_2$ (mm Hg)	Sao$_2$ (%)
Normal ABG	7.37	38	24	−1	85	96
Respiratory acidosis, no compensation, with hypoxemia	7.28	51	25	−1	63	89
Metabolic acidosis, no compensation, normal oxygenation	7.23	33	14	−12	92	97
Metabolic alkalosis, partial compensation, normal oxygenation	7.49	48	37	+11	84	95
Respiratory acidosis, full compensation, with hypoxemia	7.35	59	33	+6	55	86
Respiratory alkalosis, no compensation, with hypoxemia	7.52	31	24	0	60	88
Metabolic acidosis, partial compensation, wth hypoxemia	7.30	29	16	−9	54	85
Laboratory error	7.31	32	28	0	92	96

of respiratory alkalosis is directed at treating the underlying cause and decreasing excessive ventilation if possible.

Respiratory acidemia occurs when the pH is below 7.35 and the $PaCO_2$ is above 45 mm Hg. In respiratory acidosis there is an inadequate amount of ventilation (alveolar hypoventilation) and removal of CO_2 from the body. If these ABG changes persist for 24 hours or more, the kidneys attempt to compensate for the decreased pH by increasing the amount of HCO_3^- in the body (decreased excretion of HCO_3^- in the urine) until normal or near-normal pH levels occur. Clinical situations or conditions that cause respiratory acidosis include overall hypoventilation associated with respiratory failure (e.g., acute respiratory distress syndrome [ARDS], severe asthma, pneumonia, chronic obstructive pulmonary diseases, sleep apnea), pulmonary embolism, pulmonary edema, pneumothorax, respiratory center depression, and neuromuscular disturbances in the presence of normal lungs, and inadequate mechanical ventilation. Management of respiratory acidosis is directed at treating the underlying cause and improving ventilation.

Mixed (combined) disturbance is the simultaneous development of a primary respiratory and metabolic acid–base disturbance. For example, metabolic acidosis may occur from diabetic ketoacidosis, with respiratory acidosis occurring from respiratory failure associated with aspiration pneumonia. Mixed acid–base disturbances create a more complex picture when examining ABGs and are beyond the scope of this text.

Oxygenation

After determining the acid–base status from the ABG, assessment of the adequacy of oxygenation is assessed. Normal values for $PaCO_2$ depend on age and altitude. Lower levels of $PaCO_2$ are acceptable as normal with increasing age and altitude levels. In general, $PaCO_2$ levels between 80 and 100 mm Hg are considered normal.

SaO_2 levels are also affected by age and altitude, with values above 95% considered normal. Hemoglobin saturation with oxygen is primarily influenced by the amount of available oxygen in the plasma (Figure 5–2). The S shape to the oxyhemoglobin curve emphasizes that as long as $PaCO_2$ levels are above 60 mm Hg, 90% or more of the hemoglobin is bound or saturated with O_2. Factors that can shift the oxyhemoglobin curve to the right and left include temperature, pH, $PaCO_2$, and abnormal hemoglobin conditions. In general, shifting the curve to the right decreases the affinity of oxygen for hemoglobin, resulting in an increase in the amount of oxygen released to the tissues. Shifting of the curve to the left increases the affinity of oxygen for hemoglobin, resulting in a decreased amount of oxygen released to the tissues.

A decrease in $PaCO_2$ below normal values is *hypoxemia.* A variety of conditions cause hypoxemia:

- *Low inspired oxygen:* Usually, the fraction of inspired oxygen concentration (FiO_2) is reduced at high

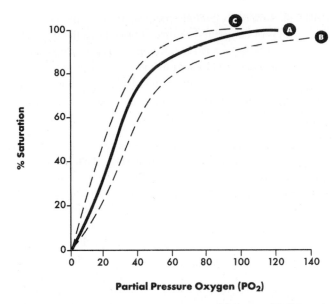

Figure 5–2. Oxyhemoglobin dissociation curve. **(A)** Normal. **(B)** Shift to the right. **(C)** Shift to the left.

altitudes or when toxic gases are inhaled. Inadequate or inappropriately low FiO_2 administration may contribute to hypoxic respiratory failure in patients with other cardiopulmonary diseases.

- *Overall hypoventilation:* Decreases in tidal volume (Vt), respiratory rate, or both reduce minute ventilation and cause hypoventilation. Alveoli are underventilated, leading to a fall in alveolar oxygen tension ($PaCO_2$) and decreased $PaCO_2$ levels. Causes of hypoventilation include respiratory center depression from drug overdose, anesthesia, excessive analgesic administration, neuromuscular disturbances, and fatigue.

- *Ventilation–perfusion mismatch:* When the balance between adequately ventilated and perfused alveoli is altered, hypoxemia develops. Perfusion of blood past underventilated alveoli decreases the availability of oxygen for gas exchange, leading to poorly oxygenated blood in the pulmonary vasculature. Examples of this include bronchospasm, atelectasis, secretion retention, pneumonia, pulmonary embolism, and pulmonary edema.

- *Diffusion defect:* Thickening of the alveolar–capillary membrane decreases oxygen diffusion and leads to hypoxemia. Causes of diffusion defects are chronic disease states such as fibrosis and sarcoidosis. Hypoxemia usually responds to supplemental oxygen in conditions of diffusion impairment (e.g., interstitial lung disease).

- *Shunt:* When blood bypasses or shunts past the alveoli, gas exchange cannot occur and blood returns to the left side without being oxygenated. Shunts caused anatomically include pulmonary arteriovenous fistulas or congenital cardiac anomalies of the heart and great vessels, such as tetralogy of Fallot. Physiologic shunts are caused by a variety of conditions that result in closed, nonventilated alveoli such as seen in ARDS.

- *Low mixed venous oxygenation:* Under normal conditions, the lungs fully oxygenate the pulmonary arterial blood and mixed venous oxygen tension (PvO_2) does not affect PaO_2 significantly. However, a reduced PvO_2 can lower the PaO_2 significantly when either ventilation–perfusion mismatch or intrapulmonary shunting is present. Conditions that can contribute to low mixed venous oxygenation include low CO, anemia, hypoxemia, and increased oxygen consumption. Improving tissue oxygen delivery by increasing CO or hemoglobin usually decreases oxygen extraction and improves mixed venous oxygen saturation (SvO_2).

Venous Blood Gas Monitoring

Analysis of oxygen and carbon dioxide levels in the venous blood provides additional information about the adequacy of perfusion and oxygen use by the tissues. Venous blood gas analysis, also referred to as a *mixed venous blood gas sample,* is done in the same manner as an ABG analysis, but with a venous blood sample. The venous sample can be obtained from the distal tip of a pulmonary artery (PA) catheter or from a central venous pressure (CVP) catheter. If the distal tip of the PA catheter is used, withdrawal of the blood should be done slowly over a 20-second period to avoid arterialization of the PA blood. This approach is not important when sampling through a CVP catheter. Normal values for venous blood gas values are listed in Table 5–1. Continuous mixed venous saturation (SvO_2) can be done with a special PA catheter. More information on SvO_2 monitoring is found in Chapter 4, Hemodynamic Monitoring.

Pulse Oximetry

Pulse oximetry is a common method for the continuous, noninvasive monitoring of SaO_2. A sensor is applied to skin over areas with strong arterial pulsatile blood flow, typically one of the peripheral fingers or toes (Figure 5–3). Alternative sites include the bridge of the nose, ear, and more recently introduced, the forehead (Figure 5–4). The forehead sensor is a reflectance sensor and provides a central monitoring site location. The SaO_2 sensor is connected to a pulse oximeter monitor unit via a cable. Light-emitting diodes on one side of the sensor transmit light of two different wavelengths (infrared and red) through arterial blood flowing under the sensor. Depending on the level of oxygen saturation of hemoglobin in the arterial blood, different amounts of light are detected on the other side of the sensor (transmission)

AT THE BEDSIDE
▶ *Respiratory Failure*

A 73-year-old woman with a long history of asthma was admitted to the intermediate care unit with viral pneumonia. Vital signs and laboratory tests on admission were:

Temperature	38.1°C (oral)
Heart rate	110/min, slightly labored
BP	148/90 mm Hg

ABGs on room air were:

pH	7.33
$PaCO_2$	46 mm Hg
HCO_3^2	26 mEq/L
BE	0 mEq/L
PaO_2	53 mm Hg

She was begun on oxygen therapy at 28% O_2, using a Venturi mask to ensure accurate O_2 delivery. Within 2 hours her BP, heart rate, and respiratory rate had decreased to normal values, with improvement in her PaO_2 level (68 mm Hg).

Two days after admission, she became progressively more dyspneic, with heart rate, BP, and respiratory rate increases. ABGs at that time revealed a respiratory acidosis with partial compensation and hypoxemia on 35% O_2 by Venturi mask:

pH	7.31
$PaCO_2$	55 mm Hg
HCO_3^2	29 mEq/L
BE	22 mEq/L
PaO_2	48 mm Hg

The patient was intubated with a 7.5-mm oral ET tube without difficulty, and placed on a microprocessor ventilator (mode, SIMV; rate, 15/min; Vt, 600 mL; FiO_2, 0.5; PEEP, 5 cm H_2O). Immediately after intubation and initiation of mechanical ventilation, her BP decreased to 90/64 mm Hg. Following a 500-mL bolus of IV fluids, BP returned to normal values (118/70). ABGs 15 minutes after ventilation were:

pH	7.36
$PaCO_2$	50 mm Hg
HCO_3^2	29 mEq/L
BE	12 mEq/L
PaO_2	65 mm Hg

---

or via scattered light on the same side of the light emitters (reflectance). This photodetection aspect of the sensor transmits information to the microprocessor within the monitor, which when uses various internal software algorithms for calculation and digital display of the oxygen saturation and pulse rate.

When blood perfusion is adequate and SaO_2 levels are greater than 70%, depending on the type of sensor being used and monitoring site, there is generally a close correla-

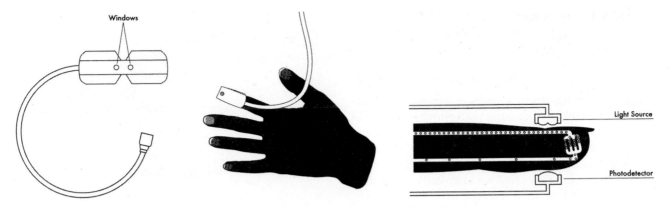

Figure 5–3. Pulse oximeter. **(A)** Sensor. **(B)** Schematic of sensor operation on finger.

tion between the saturation reading from the pulse oximeter (SpO_2) and SaO_2 directly measured from ABGs. In situations where perfusion to the sensor is markedly diminished (e.g., peripheral vasoconstriction due to disease, drugs, or hypothermia), the ability of the pulse oximeter to detect a signal may be less than under normal perfusion conditions. Newer generation pulse oximeters have the ability to detect signals during most poor perfusion conditions as well as during excessive motion, which was previously recognized as a common source of artifact interference.

Pulse oximetry has several advantages for respiratory monitoring. The ability to have continuous information on the SaO_2 level of critically ill patients without the need for an invasive arterial puncture decreases infection risks and blood loss from frequent ABG analysis. In addition, these monitors are easy to use, well tolerated by most patients, and portable enough to use during transport.

The major disadvantage of pulse oximeters for assessing oxygen status is that accuracy depends on adequate arterial signal. Clinical situations that decrease the accuracy of the device include:

- Hypotension
- Low CO states
- Vasoconstriction or vasoactive drugs
- Hypothermia
- Movement of the sensor and/or poor skin adherence

Because these conditions commonly occur in critically ill patients, caution is exercised when using pulse oximetry in critical care units. Proper use (Table 5–4) and periodic validation of the accuracy of the devices with ABG analysis utilizing a CO oximeter instrument is essential to avoid erroneous patient assessment.

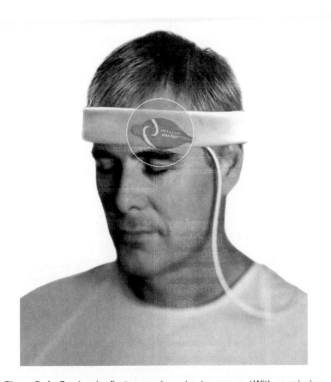

Figure 5–4. Forehead reflectance pulse oximeter sensor. (*With permission, Nellcor Puritan Bennett Inc., Pleasanton, CA.*)

TABLE 5–4. TIPS TO MAXIMIZE SAFETY AND ACCURACY OF PULSE OXIMETRY

- Apply sensor to dry finger of nondominant hand according to manufacturer's directions and observe for adequate pulse wave generation on microprocessing unit.
- Avoid tension on the sensor cable.
- Rotate application sites and change sensor according to manufacturer's directions whenever adherence is poor.
- In children and elderly patients, assess application sites more often and carefully assess skin for heat damage from sensor light source.
- Verify adequacy of pulse wave generation prior to obtaining readings.
- If pulse wave generation is inadequate, check for proper adherence to skin and position. Apply a new sensor to another site, if necessary.
- Compare pulse oximeter SaO_2 values with arterial blood gases periodically, when changes in the clinical condition may decrease accuracy and/or when values do not fit the clinical situation.

Assessing Pulmonary Function

A variety of measurements beside ABG analysis can assist the practitioner to further evaluate the respiratory system in the critically ill patient.

Measurement of selected lung volumes can be easily accomplished at the bedside. Vt, minute ventilation, and inspiratory force (IF) are measured with portable, handheld equipment (spirometer and IF meter, respectively). Lung compliance and alveolar oxygen content can be calculated with standard formulas (see Table 5–1). Frequent trend monitoring of these parameters provides an objective evaluation of the patient's response to interventions.

End-Tidal Carbon Dioxide Monitoring

CO_2 is a byproduct of cellular metabolism and is transported in the venous blood to the lungs where it is eliminated via the lungs during exhalation. End-tidal CO_2 is the amount of CO_2 present at the end of exhalation and is expressed either as a percentage (PetCO$_2$%) or partial pressure (PetCO$_2$). The normal range for PetCO$_2$ is typically 1 to 4 mm Hg less than the arterial carbon dioxide tension or PaCO$_2$. For this reason, clinicians have sought to use this noninvasive monitoring method for assessing ventilation status over time. Thus, under conditions of normal ventilation and perfusion ($\dot{V}/\dot{Q}$) matching, the relationship between PetCO$_2$ and PaCO$_2$ is relatively close. However, in critical illness where $\dot{V}/\dot{Q}$ relationships are frequently abnormal, this gradient may be as high as 20 mm Hg or more, thus limiting the use of this technology to accurately reflect alveolar ventilation.

Currently available end-tidal CO_2 monitoring devices fall into one of several categories; colorimetric, capnometric (numeric display only), or capnographic (numeric and graphical display). Colorimetric devices are pH-sensitive colored paper strips that change color in response to different concentrations of carbon dioxide (Figure 5–5). They are typically used for either initial or intermittent monitoring purposes such as verifying endotracheal tube (ET) placement in the trachea following intubation or in some cases, to rule out inadvertent pulmonary placement of enteral feeding tubes following insertion. A capnometer provides a visual analog or digital display of the concentration of the PetCO$_2$. Capnography includes both capnometry plus the addition of a calibrated graphic recording of the exhaled CO_2 on a breath-by-breath basis and is perhaps the most common instrument used for continuous monitoring. Figure 5–6 demonstrates the various phases of a normal carbon dioxide waveform during exhalation.

Capnography devices measure exhaled carbon dioxide using one of several different techniques: infrared spectrography, Raman spectrography, mass spectrometry, or a laser-based technology called molecular correlation spectroscopy as the infrared emission source. The laser creates an infrared emission precisely matching the absorption rate spectrum of CO_2 and eliminates the need for moving parts. A capnogra-

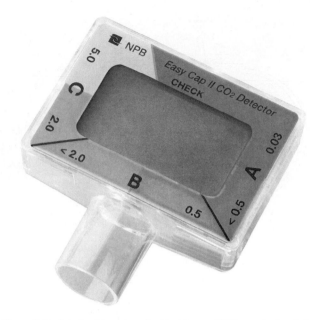

Figure 5–5. Colorimetric carbon dioxide detector. (*With permission, Nellcor Puritan Bennett Inc., Pleasanton, CA.*)

phy device using this technology is shown in Figure 5–7. All capnographs sample and measure expired gases either directly at the patient–ventilator interface (mainstream analysis) or collected and transported via small bore tubing to the sensor in the monitor (sidestream analysis). Each technique has advantages and disadvantages and the user should strictly follow manufacturer recommendations for optimal performance.

Clinical application of capnography includes assessment of endotracheal or tracheostomy tube placement, gastric or small bowel tube placement, pulmonary blood flow, and, as noted, alveolar ventilation, providing $\dot{V}/\dot{Q}$ relationships are normal. Assessment of the capnographic waveform alone can yield useful information in detecting ventilator malfunction, response to changes in ventilator settings and weaning attempts, and depth of neuromuscular blockade. It should be noted that although capnography is commonly used in patients with artificial airways, this monitoring technique can also be used in nonintubated patients via a modified nasal cannula.

AIRWAY MANAGEMENT

Maintaining an open and patent airway is an important aspect of critical care management. Patency can be ensured through conservative techniques such as coughing, head and neck positioning, and alignment. If conservative techniques fail, insertion of an oral or nasal airway or ET may be required.

Oropharyngeal Airway

The oropharyngeal airway, or oral bite block, is used to relieve upper airway obstruction caused by tongue relaxation

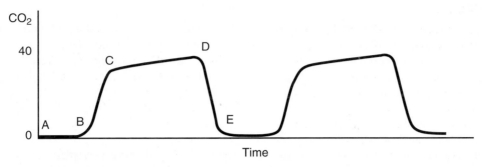

Figure 5–6. Capnogram waveform phases. *Phase A to B:* Early exhalation. This represents anatomic dead space and contains little carbon dioxide. *Phase B to C:* Combination of dead space and alveolar gas. *Phase C to D:* Exhalation of mostly alveolar gas (alveolar plateau). *D:* End-tidal point, that is exhalation of carbon dioxide at maximum point. *Phase D to E:* Inspiration begins and carbon dioxide concentration rapidly falls to baseline or zero. (*With permission, Oridion Systems Ltd., Jerusalem, Israel.*)

(e.g., postanesthesia or during unconsciousness), secretions, seizures, or biting down on oral ETs (Figure 5–8A). Oral airways are made of rigid plastic or rubber material, semicircular in shape, and available in sizes ranging from infants to adults. The airway is inserted with the concave curve of the airway facing up into the roof of the mouth. The oral airway is then rotated down 180° during insertion to fit the curvature of the tongue and ensure the tongue is not obstructing the airway. The tip of the oropharyngeal airway rests near the posterior pharyngeal wall. For this reason, oral airways are not recommended for use in alert patients because they may trigger the gag reflex and cause vomiting. Oropharyngeal airways are temporary devices for achieving airway patency.

Management of oropharyngeal airways includes frequent assessment of the lips and tongue to identify pressure areas. The airway is removed at least every 12 hours to check for pressure areas and to provide oral hygiene.

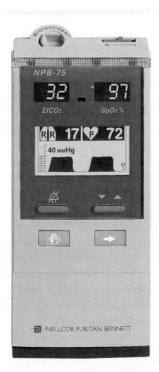

Figure 5–7. Combined capnography (sidestream) and pulse oximetry instrument. (*With permission, Nellcor Puritan Bennett Inc., Pleasanton, CA.*)

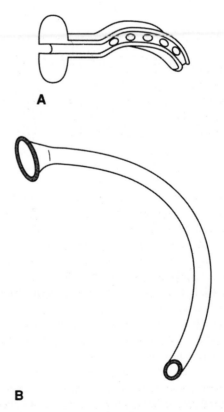

Figure 5–8. (A) Oropharyngeal and **(B)** nasopharyngeal airways.

Nasopharyngeal Airway

The nasopharyngeal airway, or nasal trumpet, is another device to maintain airway patency, especially in the semiconscious patient (Figure 5–8B). The nasopharyngeal airway is also used to facilitate nasotracheal suctioning. Made of soft malleable rubber or soft plastic, the nasal airway ranges in sizes from 26 to 35 Fr. Prior to insertion, a topical anesthetic (e.g., viscous lidocaine), based on hospital policy, may be applied to the nares prior to insertion. The nasopharyngeal airway, lubricated with a water-soluble gel, is gently inserted into one of the nares. The patency of the airway is assessed by listening for, or feeling with your hand, air movement during expiration. A small piece of tape should be used to secure the airway to the nose to prevent displacement. Complications of these airways include bleeding, sinusitis, and erosion of the mucous membranes.

Care of the patient with a nasal airway includes frequent assessment for pressure areas and occlusion of the airway with dried secretions. Sinusitis has been documented as a complication. The continued need for the nasal airway is assessed daily and rotation of the airway from nostril to nostril is done on a daily basis. When performing nasotracheal suctioning through the nasal airway, the suction catheter is lubricated with a water-soluble gel to ease passage. Refer to the following discussion on suctioning for additional standards of care.

Laryngeal Mask Airway

The laryngeal mask airway (LMA) is an ET with a small mask on one end that can be passed orally over the larynx to provide ventilatory assistance and prevent aspiration. Placement of the LMA is easier than intubation using a standard ET. Commonly used as the primary airway device in the operating room for certain types of surgical procedures, it should, however, only be considered a temporary airway for patients who require prolonged ventilatory support.

Combitube

The Combitube is an esophageal/tracheal double-lumen airway that allows for rapid airway establishment through either esophageal or tracheal placement. It is used primarily for difficult or emergency intubation and its design permits blind placement without the need for a laryngoscope. The Combitube design permits positive-pressure ventilation, but an ET or tracheostomy is eventually needed. The primary advantages to using the Combitube are less training required to use than standard intubation, no special equipment required, and the cuff provides some protection against aspiration of gastric contents. The tube is contraindicated in responsive patients with intact gag reflexes, patients with known esophageal pathology, patients who have ingested caustic substances, and patients under 5 feet in height.

Artificial Airways

Artificial airways (oral and nasal endotracheal tubes, tracheostomy tubes) are used when a patent airway cannot be maintained with an adjunct airway device for mechanical ventilation or to manage severe airway obstruction. The artificial airway also protects the lower airway from aspiration of oral or gastric secretions and allows for easier secretion removal.

Types of Artificial Airways and Insertion

Endotracheal tubes are made of either polyvinyl chloride or silicone and are available in a variety of sizes and lengths (Figure 5–9A). Standard features include a 15-mm adapter at

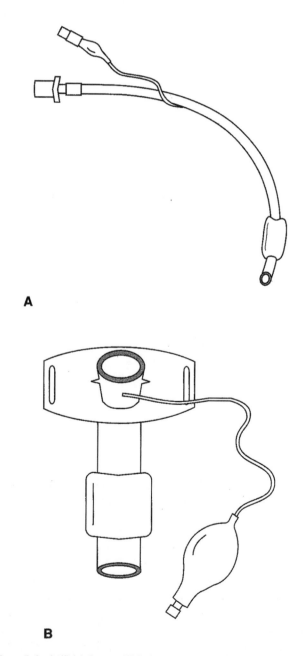

A

B

Figure 5–9. Artificial airways. **(A)** Endotracheal tube. **(B)** Tracheostomy tube.

the end of the tube for connection to various life support equipment such as mechanical ventilation circuits, closed-suction catheter systems, swivel adapters, or a manual resuscitation bag (MRB). Tubes may be cuffed or uncuffed. For cuffed tubes, air is manually injected into the cuff located near the distal tip of the ET tube through a small one-way pilot valve and inflation lumen. Distance markers are located along the side of the tube for identification of tube position. A radiopaque line is also located on all tubes so as to aid in determining proper position radiographically.

ET tubes are inserted into the patient's trachea either through the mouth or nose (Figures 5–10 and 5–11). Orally inserted endotracheal tubes are more common than the nasal route because nasal intubation is associated with sinus infections and are considered an independent risk factor for developing ventilator-associated pneumonia (VAP). With use of the laryngoscope, the upper airway is visualized and the tube is inserted through the vocal cords into the trachea, 2 to 4 cm above the carina. The presence of bilateral breath sounds, along with equal chest excursion during inspiration and the absence of breath sounds over the stomach, preliminarily confirms proper tube placement. The use of an end-tidal CO_2 monitor or colorimetric carbon dioxide detector may also be a useful assessment tool in determining tracheal placement. A portable chest x-ray verifies proper tube placement. Once proper placement is confirmed, the tube is anchored to prevent movement with either tape or a special ET fixation device (Figure 5–12). The centimeter marking of the ET tube at the lip is documented and checked each shift to monitor proper tube placement.

Endotracheal tube sizes are typically identified by the tubes internal diameter in millimeters (mm ID). The size of the tube is printed on the tube and generally also on the outside packaging. Knowledge of the tube ID is critical; the smaller the mm ID, the higher the resistance to breathing through the tube, thus increasing the work of breathing. The most common ET sizes used in adults is 7.0 to 9.0 mm ID.

ET tubes can be safely left in place for up to several weeks, but tracheostomy is often considered following 10 to 14 days of intubation. If the need for an artificial airway is anticipated for an extended period of time, a tracheostomy tube may be indicated earlier, but the decision is always individualized. Complications of ET intubation are numerous and include laryngeal and tracheal damage, laryngospasm, aspiration, infection, discomfort, sinusitis, and subglottic injury.

The majority of tracheostomy tubes used in critically ill patients are made of medical-grade plastic or silicone and come in a variety of sizes (Figure 5–9B). As with ET tubes, a standard 15-mm adapter at the proximal end ensures universal connection to MRBs and ventilator circuits. Tracheostomy tubes may be inserted as an elective procedure using a standard open surgical technique in the operating room or at the bedside via a percutaneous insertion. This technique involves a procedure in which a small incision is

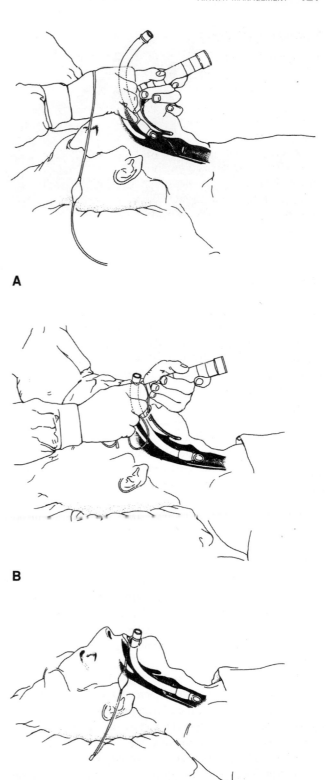

A

B

C

Figure 5–10. Oral intubation with an endotracheal (ET) tube. **(A)** Insertion of ET tube through the mouth with the aid of a laryngoscope. **(B)** ET tube advanced through the vocal cords into the trachea. ET tube positioned with the cuff below the vocal cords. (*From Boggs R, Wooldridge-King M:* AACN Procedure Manual for Critical Care, *3rd ed, pp. 34–36. Philadelphia: WB Saunders; 1993.*)

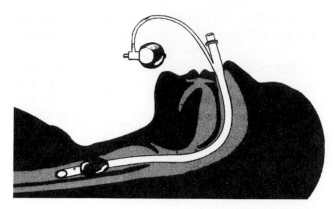

Figure 5–11. Nasal endotracheal tube. (*With permission, Nellcor Puritan Bennett, Inc., Pleasanton, CA.*)

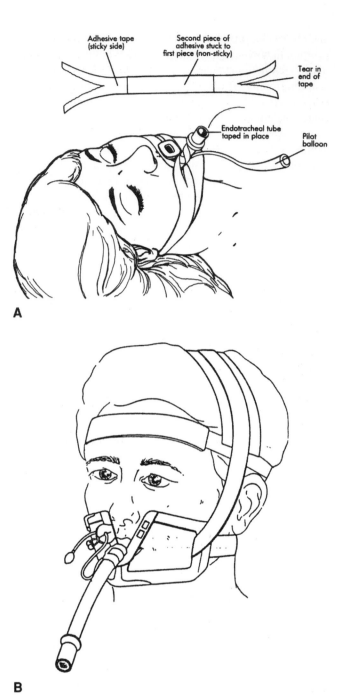

Figure 5–12. Methods for anchoring an endotracheal tube to prevent movement. **(A)** Taping of an oral ET tube. (*From Boggs R, Wooldridge-King M: AACN Procedure Manual for Critical Care, 3rd ed, p. 108. Philadelphia: WB Saunders; 1993.*) **(B)** Use of a special fixation device. (*From: Kaplow R, Bookbinder M: A comparison of four endotracheal tube holders.* Heart Lung *1994;23[1]:60.*)

made in the neck and a series of dilators are manually passed into the trachea over a guide wire creating a stoma opening through which the tracheostomy tube is inserted into place. Bedside placement obviates the need for patient transport outside the ICU with its associated risks and some feel that the procedure costs are less because operating room charges are avoided.

Tracheostomies are secured with cotton twill tape or latex-free Velcro latching tube holders attached to openings on the neck flange or plate of the tube. Many tracheostomy tubes have inner cannulae that can be easily removed for periodic cleaning (reusable) or replacement (disposable). Tracheostomy tubes, in general, are better tolerated by patients than oral or nasal ET tubes in terms of comfort. Further, there are more nutrition and communication options available to patients with tracheostomy tubes than with endotracheal tubes.

Complications of tracheostomies include hemorrhage from erosion of the innominate artery; tracheal stenosis, malacia, or perforation; laryngeal nerve injury; aspiration; infection; air leak; and mechanical problems. Most complications rarely occur with proper management.

Cuff Inflation

Following insertion of an endotracheal or tracheostomy tube, the cuff of the tube is inflated with just enough air to create an effective seal. The cuff is typically inflated with the lowest possible pressure that prevents air leak during mechanical ventilation and decreases the risk of pulmonary aspiration. Cuff pressure is maintained under 25 mm Hg. Excessive cuff pressure causes tracheal ischemia, necrosis, and erosion, as well as overinflation-related obstruction of the distal airway from cuff herniation. It is important to recognize that even a properly inflated cuffed artificial airway does not protect the patient from aspiration of liquids.

There are two common techniques to ensure proper cuff inflation without overinflation: the minimal leak and minimal occlusive volume techniques. The minimal leak technique involves listening over the larynx during positive pressure breaths with a stethoscope while inflating the tube cuff in 1- to 2-mL increments. Inflation continues until only a small air leak, or rush of air, is heard over the larynx during peak inspiration. The minimal leak technique should result in no more than a 50- to 100-mL air loss per breath during mechanical ventilation. The cuff pressure and amount of air instilled into the cuff are recorded following the maneuver.

The minimal occlusive volume cuff inflation technique is similar to the minimal leak technique. Cuff inflation continues, however, until the air leak completely disappears. The amount of air instilled and the cuff pressure are recorded during cuff inflation and periodically to ensure an intracuff pres-

sure of less than 25 mm Hg. Manual palpation of the tube pilot balloon does not ensure optimal inflation assessment.

Cuff Pressure Measurement

The connection of a stopcock to the cuff lumen allows for the simultaneous measurement of pressure during inflation or periodic checking (Figure 5–13). However, more common is

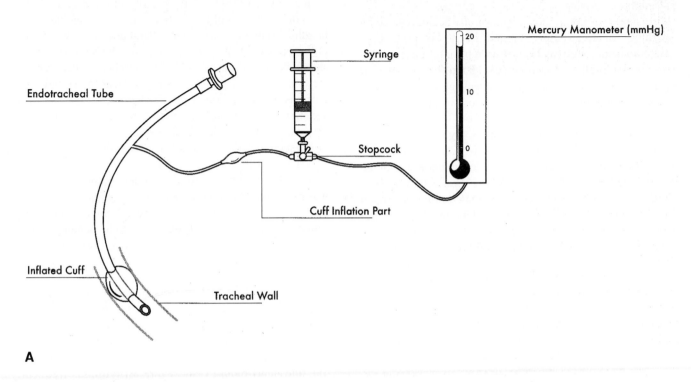

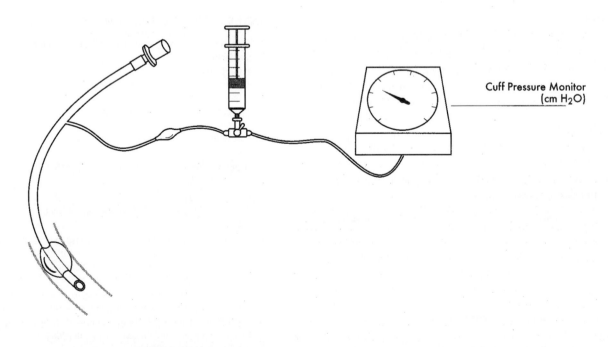

Figure 5–13. Measurement of cuff pressure with **(A)** bedside mercury manometer or **(B)** cuff pressure monitor.

the use of a manual hand-held cuff inflator. The need for pressures greater than 25 mm Hg to properly seal the trachea may indicate the ET tube diameter is too small for the trachea. In this case the cuff is inflated to properly seal the trachea until the appropriately sized ET tube can be electively reinserted.

Endotracheal Suctioning

Pulmonary secretion removal is normally accomplished by coughing. An effective cough requires a closed epiglottis so intrathoracic pressure can be increased prior to sudden opening of the epiglottis and secretion expulsion. The presence of an artificial airway such as an ET prevents glottic closure and effective coughing, necessitating the use of periodic endotracheal suctioning to remove secretions.

Currently, two methods are commonly used for ET suctioning: the closed and open methods. *Closed suctioning* means the ventilator circuit remains closed while suctioning is performed, whereas *open suctioning* means the ventilator circuit is opened, or removed, during suctioning. The open method requires disconnection of the ET tube from the mechanical ventilator or oxygen therapy source and insertion of a suction catheter each time the patient requires suctioning. The closed method refers to a closed suction catheter system device that remains attached to the ventilator circuit, allowing periodic insertion of the suction catheter through a diaphragm to suction without removing the patient from the ventilator. Following suctioning, the catheter is withdrawn into a plastic sleeve of the in-line device until the next suctioning procedure. Recommendations for use of the open and closed techniques in various clinical situations are summarized in Table 5–5.

Indications

The need for ET suctioning is determined by a variety of clinical signs and symptoms, such as coughing, increased inspiratory pressures on the ventilator, and the presence of adventitious sounds (rhonchi, gurgling) during chest auscultation. Suctioning may also be performed periodically to ensure airway patency. Suctioning is only done when there is a clinical indication and never on a routine schedule.

TABLE 5–5. CLINICAL INDICATIONS FOR USE OF CLOSED AND OPEN CATHETER SUCTIONING SETUPS

Closed Method	Open Method
• Suctioning frequency every hour or less	• Intubated <24 hours
• Copious amounts of secretions	• Small to moderate secretions
• High levels of PEEP (>10 cm H_2O)	• Suctioning frequency every 2 hours
• Decreases in Sao_2 or hemodynamic compromise during suctioning	
• Highly contagious respiratory infections (TB, MRSA)	
• Blood in secretions	

Procedure

Hyperoxygenation with 100% O_2 is provided with each suctioning episode, whether using an open or closed technique (Table 5–6). Hyperoxygenation helps to prevent decreases in arterial oxygen levels after suctioning. Hyperoxygenation can be achieved by increasing the O_2 delivered via the mechanical ventilator or by using an MRB to deliver 100% O_2. At least two or three breaths of 100% O_2 are given before and after each pass of the suction catheter. In spontaneously breathing patients, encourage several deep breaths of 100% O_2 before and after each suction pass. The Vt of the breaths should be at least the usual Vt. The number of suction passes are limited to only those necessary to clear the airway of secretions—usually two or three. The mechanical act of inserting the suction catheter into the trachea can stimulate the vagus nerve and result in bradycardia or asystole. Each pass of the suction catheter should be 10 seconds or less.

The instillation of 5 to 10 mL of normal saline is no longer advocated during routine ET suctioning. This practice was previously thought to decrease secretion viscosity and increase secretion removal during ET suctioning. Bolus saline instillation has not been shown to be beneficial and is associated with Sao_2 decreases and bronchospasm.

Complications

A variety of complications are associated with ET suctioning. Decreases in Pao_2 have been well documented when no hyperoxygenation therapy is provided with suctioning. Serious cardiac arrhythmias occur occasionally with suctioning, and include bradycardia, asystole, ventricular tachycardia, and heart block. Less severe arrhythmias frequently

TABLE 5–6. STEPS FOR SUCTIONING THROUGH AN ARTIFICIAL AIRWAY

1. Determine the need for suctioning. Clinical indicators of the need for suctioning include
   • Coughing
   • Increase in ventilator airway pressures
   • Respiratory distress
   • Decrease in arterial oxygen levels
   • Decreased breath sounds
   • Adventitious sounds during chest auscultation or noisy respirations
   • Assessment of airway patency
2. Hyperoxygenate with 100% oxygen using MRB or ventilator before and after each suction pass.
3. Limit suction passes to two or three at most, with suction duration limited to 10 seconds or less. Use sterile technique in hospitalized patients.
4. Continuously monitor the patient's response to suctioning (cardiac rhythm, Sao_2, color, heart rate, respiratory rate, MAP, ICP, and the patient's subjective response). Stop suctioning and hyperoxygenate immediately if signs of intolerance occur.
5. Once the airway is cleared, document the patient's tolerance of the procedure along with a description of the secretions removed. Remember to compare your findings with the report from the previous shift. Changes in secretion color or volume indicate a change in the patient's pulmonary condition.

occur with suctioning and include premature ventricular contractions, atrial contractions, and supraventricular tachycardia. Other complications associated with suctioning include increases in arterial pressure and intracranial pressure, bronchospasm, tracheal wall damage, and nosocomial pneumonia. Many of these complications can be minimized by using sterile technique, vigilant monitoring during and after suctioning, and hyperoxygenation before and after each suction pass.

Extubation

The reversal or significant improvement of the underlying condition(s) that led to the use of artificial airways usually signals the readiness for removal of the airway. Common indicators of readiness for artificial airway removal include the ability to

- maintain spontaneous breathing and adequate ABG values with minimal to moderate amounts of O_2 administration (FiO_2 <0.50);
- protect the airway; and
- clear pulmonary secretions.

Removal of an artificial airway usually occurs following weaning from mechanical ventilatory support (see the discussion on weaning later). Preparations for extubation include an explanation to the patient and family of what to expect, the need to cough, medication for pain, setting up the appropriate method for delivering O_2 therapy (e.g., face mask, nasal cannula), and positioning the patient with the head of the bed elevated at 30° to 45° to improve diaphragmatic function. Suctioning of the artificial airway is performed prior to extubation if clinically indicated. Obtaining a baseline cardiopulmonary assessment also is important for later evaluation of the response to extubation. Usually, extubation is performed earlier in the day, when full ancillary staff are available to assist if reintubation is required.

Hyperoxygenation with 100% O_2 is provided for 30 to 60 seconds prior to extubation in case respiratory distress occurs immediately after extubation and reintubation is necessary. The artificial airway is then removed following complete deflation of the ET or tracheostomy cuff, if present. Immediately apply the oxygen delivery method and encourage the patient to take deep breaths.

Monitor the patient's response to the extubation. Significant changes in heart rate, respiratory rate, and/or blood pressure of more than 10% of baseline values may indicate respiratory compromise, necessitating more extensive assessment and possible reintubation. Pulmonary auscultation is also performed.

Complications associated with extubation include aspiration, bronchospasm, and tracheal damage. Coughing and deep breathing are encouraged while monitoring vital signs and the upper airway for stridor. Inspiratory stridor occurs from glottic and subglottic edema and may develop immediately or take several hours. If the patient's clinical status

permits, treatment with 2.5% racemic epinephrine (0.5 mL in 3 mL of normal saline) is administered via an aerosol delivery device. If the upper airway obstruction persists or worsens, reintubation is generally required. A reattempt at extubation is usually delayed for 24 to 72 hours following reintubation for upper airway obstruction.

OXYGEN THERAPY

Oxygen is used for any number of clinical problems (Table 5–7). The overall goals for oxygen use include increasing alveolar O_2 tension (PaO_2) to treat hypoxemia, decreasing the work of breathing, and maximizing myocardial and tissue oxygen supply.

Complications

As with any drug, oxygen should be used cautiously. The hazards of oxygen misuse can be as dangerous as the lack of appropriate use. Alveolar hypoventilation, absorption atelectasis, and oxygen toxicity can be life threatening.

Alveolar Hypoventilation

Alveolar hypoventilation is underventilation of alveoli, and is a side effect of great concern in patients with chronic obstructive pulmonary disease (COPD) with carbon dioxide retention. As the patient with COPD adjusts to chronically high levels of $PaCO_2$, the chemoreceptors in the medulla of the brain lose responsiveness to high $PaCO_2$ levels. Hypoxemia, then, becomes the primary stimulus for ventilation. However, correction of hypoxemia in the patient with COPD

TABLE 5–7. COMMON INDICATIONS FOR OXYGEN THERAPY

- Decreased cardiac performance
- Increased metabolic need for O_2 (fever, burns)
- Acute changes in level of consciousness (restlessness, confusion)
- Acute shortness of breath
- Decreased O_2 saturation
- PaO_2 <60 mm Hg or SaO_2 <90%
- Normal PaO_2 or SaO_2 with signs and symptoms of significant hypoxia
- Myocardial infarction
- Carbon monoxide (CO) poisoning
- Methemoglobinemia (a form of hemoglobin where ferrous iron is oxidized to ferric form, causing a high affinity for O_2 with decreased O_2 release at tissue level)
- Acute anemia
- Cardiopulmonary arrest
- Reduced cardiac output
- Consider in the presence of hypotension, tachycardia, cyanosis, chest pain, dyspnea, and acute neurologic dysfunction
- During stressful procedures and situations, especially in high-risk patients (e.g., endotracheal suctioning, bronchoscopy, thoracentesis, PA catheterization, travel at high altitudes)

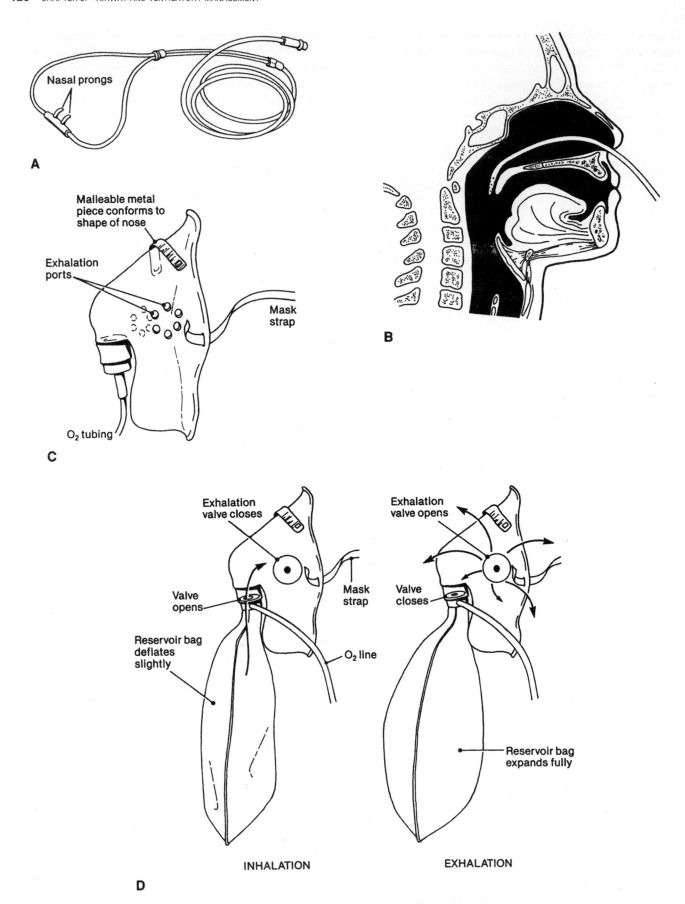

Figure 5–14. Noninvasive and invasive methods for O_2 delivery. **(A)** Nasal prongs. **(B)** Nasal catheter. **(C)** Face mask. **(D)** Nonrebreathing mask. (*From: Kersten L:* Comprehensive Respiratory Nursing, *pp. 608, 609. Philadelphia: WB Saunders; 1989.*)

remains important with a target PaO_2 of 55 to 60 mm Hg ($SaO_2 \geq 89\%$), despite the presence of hypercapnia.

Absorption Atelectasis

Absorption atelectasis results when high concentrations of O_2 (>90%) are given for long periods of time and nitrogen is washed out of the lungs. The nitrogen in inspired gas is approximately 79% of the total atmospheric gases. The large partial pressure of nitrogen in the alveoli helps to maintain open alveoli because it is not absorbed. Removal of nitrogen by inspiring 90% to 100% O_2 results in alveolar closure because oxygen readily diffuses into the pulmonary capillary.

Oxygen Toxicity

The toxic effects of oxygen are targeted primarily to the pulmonary and central nervous systems (CNS). CNS toxicity usually occurs with hyperbaric oxygen treatment. Signs and symptoms include nausea, anxiety, numbness, visual disturbances, muscular twitching, and grand mal seizures. The physiologic mechanism is not understood fully but is felt to be related to subtle neural and biochemical changes that alter the electric activity of the CNS.

Pulmonary oxygen toxicity is due to prolonged exposure to high FiO_2 levels that may lead to ARDS or bronchopulmonary dysplasia. Two phases of lung injury result. The first phase occurs after 1 to 4 days of exposure to higher O_2 levels and is manifested by decreased tracheal mucosal blood flow and tracheobronchitis. Vital capacity decreases due to poor lung expansion and progressive atelectasis persists. The alveolar capillary membrane becomes progressively impaired, decreasing gas exchange. The second phase occurs after 12 days of high exposure. The alveolar septa thickens and an ARDS picture develops, with high associated mortality (see Chapter 13, Hematology and Immune Systems).

Caring for the patient who requires high levels of oxygen requires astute monitoring by the critical care nurse. Monitor those patients at risk for absorption atelectasis and oxygen toxicity. Signs and symptoms include nonproductive cough, substernal chest pain, general malaise, fatigue, nausea, and vomiting.

An oxygen concentration of 100% ($FiO_2 = 1.0$) is regarded as safe for short periods of time (<24 hours). Oxygen concentrations greater than 50% for more than 24 to 48 hours may damage the lungs and worsen respiratory problems. Oxygen delivery levels are decreased as soon as PaO_2 levels return to clinically acceptable levels (>60 mm Hg).

Oxygen Delivery

Noninvasive Devices

Face masks and nasal cannulas are standard oxygen delivery devices for the spontaneously breathing patient (Figure 5–14). Oxygen can be delivered with a high- or low-flow device, with the concentration of O_2 delivered ranging from less than 21% to approximately 80% (Table 5–8). An example of a high-flow device is the Venturi mask system that can deliver precise concentrations of oxygen (Figure 5–16A). The usual FiO_2 values delivered with this type of mask are 24%, 28%, 31%, 35%, 40%, and 50%. Often, Venturi masks are useful in patients with COPD and hypercapnia because the clinician can titrate the PaO_2 to minimize carbon dioxide retention. An example of a low-flow system is the nasal cannula or prongs. Nasal prongs flow rate ranges are limited to 5 L/min. The main advantage of nasal prongs is that the patient can drink, eat, and speak during oxygen administration. Their disadvantage is that the exact FiO_2 delivered is unknown, because it is influenced by the patient's peak inspiratory flow demand and breathing pattern. As a general guide, 1 L/min of O_2 flow is an approximate equivalent to an FiO_2 of 24%, and each additional liter of oxygen flow increases the FiO_2 by approximately 4%. Nonrebreathing masks can achieve higher oxygen concentrations (approximately 80% to 90%) than partial rebreathing systems. A one-way valve placed between the mask and reservoir bag with a nonrebreathing system prevents exhaled gases from entering the bag, thus maximizing the delivered FiO_2.

Invasive Devices

Manual Resuscitation Bags

MRBs provide 40% to 100% O_2 at adult Vt and respiratory rates to an ET or tracheostomy tube (Figure 5–15B).

Mechanical Ventilators

The most common method for delivering oxygen invasively is with a mechanical ventilator. Oxygen delivery can be accurately delivered from 21% to 100% O_2. Mechanical ventilation is discussed below in more detail.

TABLE 5–8. APPROXIMATE OXYGEN DELIVERY WITH COMMON NONINVASIVE AND INVASIVE OXYGEN DEVICES[a]

Device	% O_2
Nasal Prongs/Catheter	
2 L/min	28
4 L/min	36
5 L/min	40
Face Mask	
5 L/min	30
10 L/min	50
Nonbreathing Mask	80–90
Venturi Mask	
24%	24
28%	28
35%	35
Manual Resuscitation Bag (MRB)	
PMR-2	20–80
Laerdal	100
Disposable MRB	Dependent on model

[a]Actual delivery dependent on minute ventilation rates except for Venturi mask.

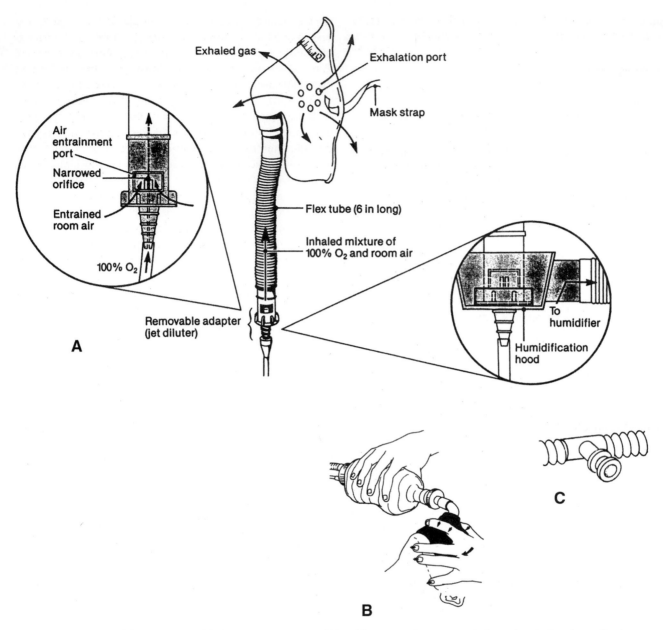

Air
entrainment
port

Narrowed
orifice

Entrained
room air

100% O_2

Exhaled gas

Exhalation port

Mask strap

Flex tube (6 in long)

Inhaled mixture of
100% O_2 and room air

To
humidifier

Humidification
hood

Removable adapter
{ (jet diluter)

A

B

C

Figure 5–15. **(A)** Venturi device. **(B)** Manual resuscitation bag (MRB). **(C)** T-piece. (*From: Kersten L:* Comprehensive Respiratory Nursing, *pp. 611, 629. Philadelphia: WB Saunders; 1989.*)

Tracheal Gas Insufflation

Tracheal gas insufflation (TGI) is a new technique that may improve alveolar ventilation when used as an adjunct to conventional mechanical ventilation. A small catheter (2.2 mm) is passed down the ET to just above the carina and low flows of oxygen (2 to 4 L/min) are delivered. This technique is reserved for selected patients in whom traditional ventilatory modes have not provided optimal oxygenation and ventilation. To date, few data are available on the efficacy of TGI; thus, it is not recommended for widespread use.

Transtracheal Oxygen Therapy

Transtracheal oxygen therapy is a method of administering continuous oxygen to patients with chronic hypoxemia. The therapy requires the percutaneous placement of a small plastic catheter into the trachea. The catheter is inserted directly into the trachea above the suprasternal notch under local anesthesia in an outpatient setting. This device allows for low O_2 flow rates (<1 to 2 L/min) to treat chronic hypoxemia. Advantages of this method for chronic O_2 delivery include improved mobility and patient esthetics because the tubing and catheter, unlike the nasal cannula or face mask, can often be hidden from view, avoidance of nasal and ear irritation from nasal cannulas, decreased O_2 requirements, and correction of refractory hypoxemia.

Typically, these patients are managed in the outpatient setting, but occasionally they may be in critical care. It is important to maintain the catheter unless specifically ordered to discontinue its use. The stoma formation process takes several weeks and if the catheter is removed, the stoma is likely to close. The catheter is cleaned daily to prevent the formation of mucous plugs. Refer to the manufacturer's guidelines for further recommendations on care of the catheter while the patient is hospitalized.

T-Piece

Oxygen can also be provided directly to an ET or tracheostomy tube with a T-piece, or blow by, in spontaneously breathing patients who do not require ventilatory support (Figure 5–15C). The T-piece is connected directly to the ET tube, providing 21% to 80% O_2.

BASIC VENTILATORY MANAGEMENT

Indications

Mechanical ventilation is indicated when noninvasive management modalities fail to adequately support oxygenation and/or ventilation. The decision to initiate mechanical ventilation is based on the ability of the patient to support their oxygenation and/or ventilation needs. The inability of the

patient to maintain clinically acceptable CO_2 levels and acid–base status is referred to as *respiratory failure* and is a common indicator for mechanical ventilation intervention. *Refractory hypoxemia,* which is the inability to establish and maintain acceptable oxygenation levels despite the administration of oxygen-enriched breathing environments, is also a common reason for mechanical ventilation. Table 5–9 presents a variety of physiologic indicators for initiating mechanical ventilation. By monitoring these indicators, it is possible to differentiate stable or improving values from continuing decompensation. The need for mechanical ventilation may then be anticipated to avoid emergent use of ventilatory support.

Depending on the underlying cause of the respiratory failure, different indicators may be assessed to determine the need for mechanical ventilation. Many of the causes of respiratory failure, however, are due to inadequate alveolar ventilation and/or hypoxemia, with abnormal ABG values and physical assessment as the primary indicators for ventilatory support.

General Principles

Mechanical ventilators are designed to partially or completely support ventilation. Two different categories of ventilators are available to provide ventilatory support. Negative-pressure ventilators decrease intrathoracic pressure by applying negative pressure to the chest wall, typically with a shell placed around the chest (Figure 5–16A). The decrease in intrathoracic pressure causes atmospheric gas to be drawn

TABLE 5–9. INDICATIONS FOR MECHANICAL VENTILATION

Basic Physiologic Impairment	Best Available Indicators	Approximate Normal Range	Values Indicating Need for Ventilatory Support
Inadequate alveolar ventilation (acute ventilatory failure)	$Paco_2$, mm Hg	36–44	Acute increase from normal or patient's baseline
	Arterial pH	7.36–7.44	<7.25–7.30
Hypoxemia (acute oxygenation failure)	Alveolar-to-arterial Po_2 gradient breathing 100% O_2, mm Hg	25–65	>350
	Intrapulmonary right-to-left shunt fraction, percentage	<5	>20–25
	Pao_2/Fio_2, mm Hg	350–400	<200
Inadequate lung expansion	Tidal volume, mL/kg	5–8	<4–5
	Vital capacity	60–75	<10
	Respiratory rate, breaths/min (adults)	12–20	>35
Inadequate respiratory muscle strength	Maximum inspiratory force, cm H_2O	−80 to −100	≤25
	Maximum voluntary ventilation, L/min	120–180	<2 × resting ventilatory requirement
	Vital capacity, mL/kg	60–75	<10–15
Excessive work of breathing	Minute ventilation necessary to maintain normal $Paco_2$, L/min	5–10	>15–20
	Dead space ratio, percentage	0.25–0.40	>0.60
	Respiratory rate, breaths/min (adults)	12–20	>35
Unstable ventilatory drive	Breathing pattern; clinical setting		

From: Luce J, Pierson D (eds.): Critical Care Medicine. *Philadelphia: WB Saunders; 1988, p. 219.*

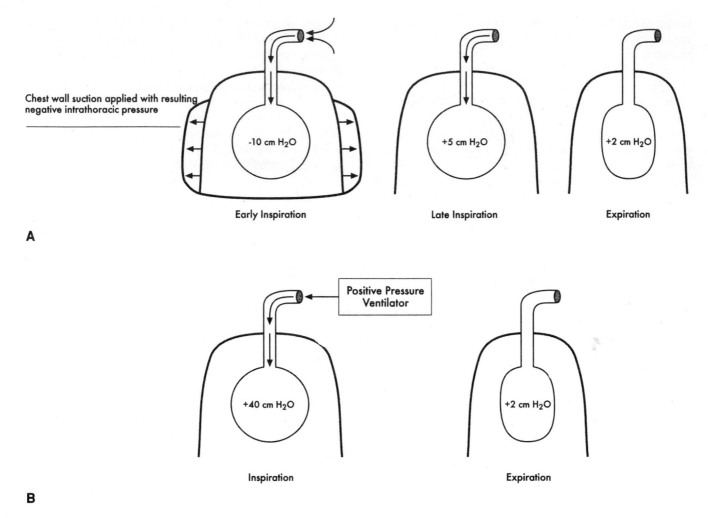

Chest wall suction applied with resulting
negative intrathoracic pressure

-10 cm H₂O

Early Inspiration

+5 cm H₂O

Late Inspiration

+2 cm H₂O

Expiration

A

Positive Pressure
Ventilator

+40 cm H₂O

Inspiration

+2 cm H₂O

Expiration

B

Figure 5–16. Principles of mechanical ventilation as provided by **(A)** negative-pressure and **(B)** positive-pressure ventilators.

into the lungs. Positive-pressure ventilators deliver pressurized gases into the lung during inspiration (Figure 5–16B). Positive-pressure ventilators can dramatically increase intrathoracic pressures during inspiration, potentially decreasing venous return and CO.

Negative-pressure ventilators are rarely used to manage acute respiratory problems in critical care. These devices are typically used for long-term noninvasive ventilatory support when respiratory muscle strength is inadequate to support unassisted, spontaneous breathing. Since the emergence of other, noninvasive modes of positive pressure (e.g., Bi-PAP), negative pressure ventilators are infrequently selected (refer to Chapter 20, Advanced Respiratory Concepts). This chapter focuses only on the use of positive-pressure ventilators for ventilatory support.

Patient-Ventilator System

Positive-pressure ventilatory support can be accomplished invasively or noninvasively. Invasive mechanical ventilation is still widely used in most hospitals for supporting ven-

tilation, although noninvasive technologies, which do not require the use of an artificial airway, are becoming more popular. To provide invasive positive-pressure ventilation, intubation of the trachea is required via an ET or tracheostomy tube. The ventilator is then connected to the artificial airway with a tubing circuit to maintain a closed delivery system (Figure 5–17). During the inspiratory cycle gas from the ventilator is usually directed through a heated humidifier prior to entering the lungs through the ET or tracheostomy tube. At the completion of inspiration, gas is passively exhaled through the expiratory side of the tubing circuit.

Ventilator Tubing Circuit

The humidifier located on the inspiratory side of the circuit is necessary to overcome two primary problems. First, the presence of an artificial airway allows gas entering the lungs to bypass the normal upper airway humidification process. Second, the higher flows and larger volumes typically administered during mechanical ventilation require additional

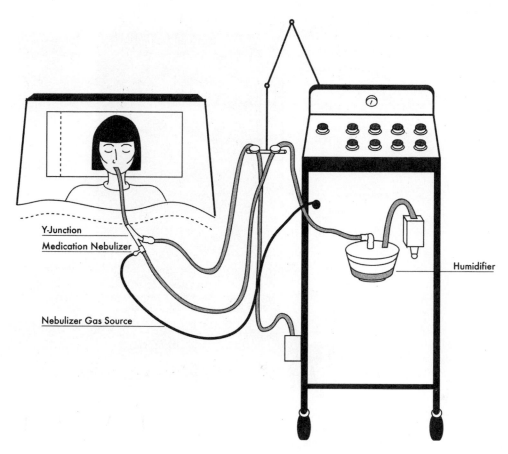

Figure 5–17. Typical setup of a ventilator, closed system tubing circuit, and humidifier connected to an ET tube.

humidification to avoid excessive intrapulmonary membrane drying.

Pressure within the ventilator tubing circuit is continuously monitored to alert clinicians to excessively high or low airway pressures. Airway pressure is dynamically displayed on the front of the ventilator control panel.

Traditionally ventilator circuits have incorporated special water collection cups in the tubing to prevent the condensation from humidified gas from obstructing the tubing. Recently, however, it has become common to use ventilator circuits containing heated wires that run through the inspiratory and expiratory limbs of the circuit. These wires maintain the temperature of the gas at or close to body temperature, significantly reducing the condensation and rainout of humidity in the gas, eliminating the need for in-line water traps. Certain medications, such as bronchodilators or steroids, also can be nebulized into the lungs through an aerosol-generating device located in the inspiratory side of the circuit.

The ventilator tubing circuit is maintained as a closed circuit as much as possible to avoid interrupting ventilation and oxygenation to the patient, as well as to decrease the potential for nosocomial pneumonias. Avoiding frequent changes of the ventilator circuit may also decrease the risk of nosocomial pneumonias (see Chapter 10, Respiratory System).

Ventilator Control Panel

The user interface or control panel of the ventilator usually incorporates three basic sections or areas: (1) control settings for the type and amount of ventilation and oxygen delivery, (2) alarm settings to specify desired high and low limits for key ventilatory measurements, and (3) visual displays of monitored parameters (Figure 5–18). The number and configuration of these controls and displays vary from ventilator model to model, but their function and principles remain essentially the same.

Control Settings

The control settings area of the user interface allows the clinician to set the mode of ventilation, volume, pressure, respiratory rate, FiO_2, positive end-expiratory pressure (PEEP) level, inspiratory trigger sensitivity or effort, and a variety of other breath delivery options (e.g., inspiratory flow rate, inspiratory waveform pattern).

Alarm Settings

Alarms, which continuously monitor ventilator function, are essential to ensure safe and effective mechanical ventilation. Both high and low alarms are typically set to identify when critical parameters vary from the desired levels. Common

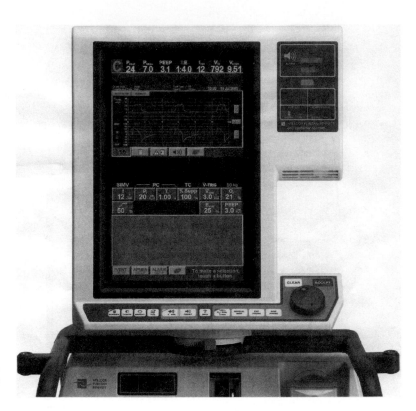

Figure 5-18. Ventilator display control panel. (*With permission Nellcor Puritan Bennett, Inc. Pleasanton, CA.*)

alarms include exhaled Vt, exhaled minute volume, Fio_2 delivery, respiratory rate, and airway pressures.

Visual Displays

Airway pressures, respiratory rate, exhaled volumes, and the inspiratory to expiratory (I:E) ratio are among the most common visually displayed breath to breath values on the ventilator. Airway pressures are monitored during inspiration and exhalation and are often displayed as Peak Pressure, Mean Pressure, and End-Expiratory Pressure. A breath delivered by the ventilator produces higher airway pressures than an unassisted, spontaneous breath by the patient (Figure 5-19). The presence of PEEP is identified by a positive value at the end of expiration rather than 0 cm H_2O. Careful observation of the airway pressures provides the clinician with a great deal of information about the patient's respiratory effort, coordination with the ventilator, and changes in lung compliance.

The display of the patient's exhaled Vt reflects the amount of gas that is returned to the ventilator via the expiratory tubing with each respiratory cycle. Exhaled volumes are measured and displayed with each breath. The patient's total exhaled minute volume is also often displayed. Exhaled Vts for ventilator-assisted mandatory breaths should be similar ($\pm 10\%$) to the desired Vt setting selected on the control panel. The Vt of spontaneous breaths, or partially ventilator-supported breaths, however, may be different from the Vt control setting.

Modes

The *mode* of ventilation refers to one of several different methods that a ventilator uses to support ventilation. These modes generate different levels of airway pressures, volumes, and patterns of respiration and, therefore, different levels of support. The greater the level of ventilator support, the less muscle work performed by the patient. This "work of breathing" varies considerably with each of the modes of ventilation (see Chapter 20, Advanced Respiratory Concepts).

The different modes of ventilation used to support ventilation depend on the underlying respiratory problem and clinical preferences. A brief description of the basic modes of mechanical ventilation follows. Applications of modes of ventilation and more complex modes are discussed in Chapter 20, Advanced Respiratory Concepts.

Control Ventilation

The control mode of ventilation ensures that patients receive a predetermined number and volume of breaths each minute. No deviations from the respiratory rate or Vt settings are desired with this mode of ventilation. Generally the patient is heavily sedated and/or paralyzed with neuromuscular blocking agents to achieve the goal (see Chapter 6, Pain, Sedation, and Neuromuscular Blockade Management). The airway pressures, Vt delivery, and pattern of breathing typically observed with control ventilation are shown in Figure 5-20A.

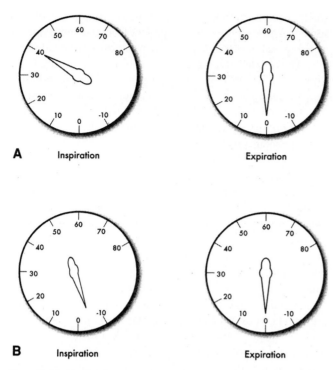

A Inspiration   Expiration

B Inspiration   Expiration

Figure 5–19. Typical airway pressure gauge changes during a **(A)** ventilator-assisted breath and a **(B)** spontaneous breath (cm H_2O).

All the inspiratory waveforms appear in a regular pattern and appear the same in configuration. The lack of waveform deflections prior to inspiration indicates the breath was initiated by the ventilator and not by the patient.

Assist-Control Ventilation

The assist-control mode of ventilation ensures that a predetermined number and volume of breaths is delivered by the ventilator each minute should the patient not initiate respirations at that rate or above. If the patient attempts to initiate breaths at a rate greater than the set minimum value, the ventilator delivers the spontaneously initiated breaths at the prescribed Vt; the patient may determine the total rate (Figure 5–20B). Work of breathing with this mode is variable (see Chapter 20, Advanced Respiratory Concepts).

Assist-control ventilation is often used when the patient is initially intubated (because minute ventilation requirements can be determined by the patient), for short-term ventilatory support such as postanesthesia, and as a support mode when high levels of ventilatory support are required. Excessive ventilation can occur with this mode in situations where the patient's spontaneous respiratory rate increases for nonrespiratory reasons (e.g., pain, CNS dysfunction). The increased minute volume may result in potentially dangerous

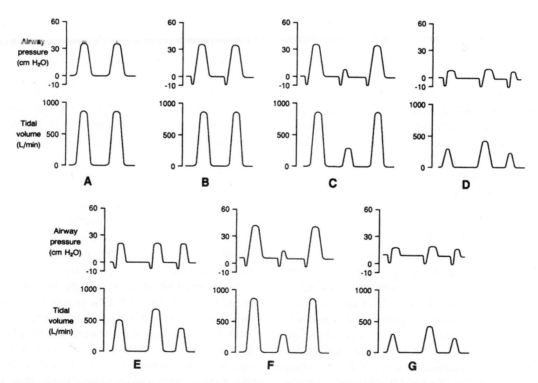

Figure 5–20. Airway pressures, tidal volumes (Vt), and patterns of breathing for different modes of mechanical ventilation. **(A)** Controlled ventilation. **(B)** Assist-control ventilation. **(C)** SIMV. **(D)** Spontaneous breathing. **(E)** Pressure support. **(F)** PEEP with SIMV. **(G)** CPAP. (*From: Dossey B, Guzzetta C, Kenner C:* Critical Care Nursing: Body-Mind-Spirit, *p. 225. Philadelphia: JB Lippincott; 1992.*)

respiratory alkalosis. Changing to a different mode of ventilation or employing sedation may be necessary in these situations.

Synchronized Intermittent Mandatory Ventilation

The synchronized intermittent mandatory ventilation (SIMV) mode of ventilation ensures (or mandates) that a predetermined number of breaths at a selected Vt are delivered each minute. Any additional breaths initiated by the patient are allowed but, in contrast to the assist-control mode, these breaths are not delivered by the ventilator. The patient is allowed to spontaneously breathe at the depth and rate desired until it is time for the next ventilator-assisted, or mandatory, breath. Mandatory breaths are synchronized with the patient's inspiratory effort, if present, to optimize patient–ventilator synchrony. The spontaneous breaths taken during SIMV are at the same Fio_2 as the mandatory breaths (Figure 5–20C).

The SIMV mode is a commonly used mode of mechanical ventilation. Originally designated as a ventilator mode for the gradual weaning of patients from mechanical ventilation, the use of a high-rate setting of SIMV can provide total ventilatory support. Reduction of the number of mandatory breaths allows the patient to slowly resume greater and greater responsibility for spontaneous breathing. SIMV can be used for similar indications as the assist-control mode, as well as for weaning the patient from mechanical ventilatory support.

The work of breathing with this mode of ventilation depends on the Vt and rate of the spontaneous breaths. When the mandatory, intermittent breaths provide the majority of minute volume, the work of breathing by the patient may be less than when spontaneous breathing constitutes a larger proportion of the patient's total minute volume.

Although strong clinician and institutional biases exist regarding whether to use SIMV or other modes for ventilatory support, little data exist to clarify which mode of ventilation is best. Close observation of the physiologic and psychological response to the ventilatory mode is required, and consideration is given to trials on alternative modes if warranted.

Spontaneous Breathing

Many ventilators have a mode that allows the patient to breathe spontaneously without ventilator support (Figure 5–20D). This is similar to placing the patient on a T-piece or blow-by oxygen setup, except it does have the benefit of providing continuous monitoring of exhaled volumes, airway pressures, and other parameters. All the work of breathing is performed by the patient during spontaneous breathing. Use of the ventilator rather than the T-piece during spontaneous breathing actually may slightly increase the work of breathing. This occurs because of the additional inspiratory muscle work that is required to trigger flow delivery for each spontaneous breath. The amount of additional work required varies with different ventilator models. In some situations, removing the patient from the ventilator for weaning may result in a decrease in the work of breathing.

This mode of ventilation is often identified as CPAP, flow-by, or SPONT on the ventilator. Continuous positive airway pressure (CPAP) is a spontaneous breathing setting with the addition of PEEP during the breathing cycle (see below). If no PEEP has been applied, the CPAP setting is similar to spontaneous breathing.

Pressure Support

Pressure support (PS) is a spontaneous breath type, available in SIMV and SPONT modes, which maintains a set positive pressure during the spontaneous inspiration (Figure 5–20E). The volume of a gas delivered by the ventilator during each inspiration varies depending on the level of pressure support and the demand of the patient. The higher the pressure support level, the higher the amount of gas delivered with each breath. Higher levels of pressure support can augment the spontaneous Vt and decrease the work of breathing associated with spontaneous breathing. At low levels of support, it is primarily used to overcome the airway resistance caused by breathing through the artificial airway and the breathing circuit. The airway pressure achieved during a pressure support breath is the result of the pressure support setting plus the set PEEP level.

PEEP/CPAP

PEEP is used in conjunction with any of the ventilator modes to help stabilize alveolar lung volume and improve oxygenation (Figure 5–20FG). The application of positive pressure to the airways during expiration may keep alveoli open and prevent early closure during exhalation. Lung compliance and ventilation–perfusion matching are often improved by prevention of early alveolar closure. If alveolar "recruitment" is not needed and excessive PEEP/CPAP is applied, it may result in adverse hemodynamic or respiratory compromise.

PEEP/CPAP is indicated for hypoxemia, which is secondary to diffuse lung injury (e.g., ARDS, interstitial pneumonitis). PEEP/CPAP levels of 5 cm Hg or less are often used to provide "physiologic PEEP." The presence of the artificial airway allows intrathoracic pressure to fall to zero, which is below the usual level of intrathoracic pressure at end expiration ($+2$ or $+3$ cm H_2O).

Use of PEEP may increase the risk of barotrauma due to higher mean and peak airway pressures during ventilation, especially when peak pressures are greater than 40 cm H_2O. Venous return and CO may also be affected by these high pressures. If CO decreases with PEEP/CPAP initiation and oxygenation is improved, a fluid bolus may correct hypovolemia. Other complications from PEEP/CPAP are increases in intracranial pressure, decreased renal perfusion, hepatic congestion, and worsening of intracardiac shunts.

Complications

Significant complications can arise from the use of mechanical ventilation and can be categorized as those associated with the patient's response to mechanical ventilation or those arising from ventilator malfunctions. Although the approach to minimizing or treating the complications of mechanical ventilation relate to the underlying cause, it is critical that frequent assessment of the patient, ventilator equipment, and the patient's response to ventilatory management be accomplished. Many clinicians participate in activities to assess the patient and ventilator, but the ultimate responsibility for ensuring continuous ventilatory support of the patient falls to the critical care nurse. Critically evaluating clinical indicators such as pH, $PaCO_2$, PaO_2, SpO_2, heart rate, BP, and so on, in conjunction with patient status and ventilatory parameters, is essential to decrease complications associated with this highly complex technology.

Patient Response

Hemodynamic Compromise

Normal intrathoracic pressure changes during inspiration and expiration fluctuate between -3 and -5 cm H_2O during inspiration and $+3$ and $+5$ cm H_2O during expiration. The use of positive-pressure ventilation dramatically increases intrathoracic pressures during inspiration, commonly to $+30$ cm H_2O or higher. These high airway pressures impede venous return to the right atrium, thus decreasing CO. In some patients, this decrease in CO can be clinically significant, leading to increased heart rate and decreased blood pressure and perfusion to vital organs.

Whenever mechanical ventilation is instituted, or when ventilator changes are made, it is important to assess the patient's cardiovascular response. Approaches to managing hemodynamic compromise include increasing the preload of the heart (e.g., fluid administration), decreasing the airway pressures exerted during mechanical ventilation by ensuring appropriate airway management techniques (suctioning, positioning, etc.), and by judiciously applying ventilator adjuncts can increase ventilating pressures. Ventilation strategies employing different modes and breath types may be helpful in managing airway pressures and are discussed in Chapter 20, Advanced Respiratory Concepts.

Barotrauma and Volutrauma

Barotrauma describes damage to the pulmonary system due to alveolar rupture from excessive airway pressures or overdistention of alveoli. Alveolar gas enters the interstitial pulmonary structures causing pneumothorax, pneumomediastinum, pneumoperitoneum, or subcutaneous emphysema. The potential for pneumothorax and cardiovascular collapse requires prompt management of pneumothorax and should be considered whenever airway pressure rises acutely, breath sounds are diminished unilaterally, or blood pressure falls abruptly. *Volutrauma* describes alveolar damage that results from high pressures resulting from large-volume ventilation in patients with ARDS. Different from barotrauma, this damage results in alveolar fractures and flooding (non-ARDS ARDS; see Chapter 20, Advanced Respiratory Concepts).

Patients with obstructive airway diseases (e.g., asthma, bronchospasm), unevenly distributed lung disease (e.g., lobar pneumonia), or hyperinflated lungs (e.g., emphysema) are at high risk for barotrauma. Techniques to decrease the incidence of barotrauma include the use of small Vts, cautious use of PEEP, and the avoidance of high airway pressures and development of auto-PEEP in high-risk patients.

Auto-PEEP occurs when a delivered breath is incompletely exhaled before the onset of the next inspiration. This gas trapping increases overall lung volumes, inadvertently raising the end-expiratory pressure in the alveoli. The presence of auto-PEEP increases the risk for complications from PEEP. Ventilator patients with COPD (e.g., asthma, emphysema) or high respiratory rates are at increased risk for the development of auto-PEEP.

Auto-PEEP, also termed *intrinsic PEEP,* is difficult to diagnose because it cannot be observed on the airway pressure display at end expiration. The technique for assessment for auto-PEEP varies with different ventilatory models and modes, but typically involves measuring the airway pressure close to the artificial airway during occlusion of the expiratory ventilator circuit during end expiration. Auto-PEEP can be minimized by

- maximizing the length of time for expiration (e.g., increasing inspiratory flow rates);
- decreasing obstructions to expiratory flow (e.g., using larger diameter ET tubes, eliminating bronchospasm and secretions); and
- avoiding overventilation.

Ventilator-Associated Pneumonia

VAP is a frequent complication, and is associated with increased patient morbidity and mortality. Prevention is aimed at avoiding colonization and subsequent aspiration of bacteria into the lower airway. Elevation of the head of the bed and avoiding excessive gastric distention are thought to help minimize the occurrence of aspiration. A specially designed ET (Figure 5–21) incorporates a dedicated suction lumen over the ET cuff, which permits continuous or intermittent suctioning of subglottic secretions pooled above the cuff. Removal of the accumulated secretions may be particularly helpful before cuff deflation or manipulation. Recent studies have demonstrated that the application of continuous aspiration of subglottic secretions may prevent or delay the onset of VAP (see Table 5–10).

Positive Fluid Balance and Hyponatremia

Hyponatremia with total body sodium excess is a common occurrence following the institution of mechanical ventilation and develops from several factors, including applied

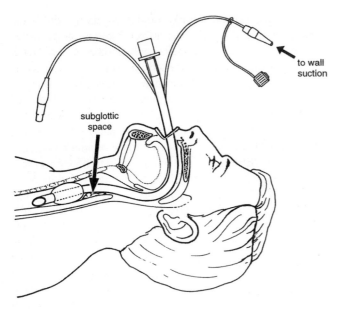

Figure 5–21. Cuffed endotracheal tube with dedicated lumen for continuous aspiration of subglottic secretions accumulated immediately above the tube cuff. (*With permission Nellcor Puritan Bennett Inc., Pleasanton, CA.*)

PEEP, humidification of inspired gases, hypotonic fluid administration and diuretics, and increased levels of circulating antidiuretic hormone.

Upper Gastrointestinal Hemorrhage

Upper gastrointestinal (GI) bleeding may develop secondary to ulceration or gastritis. The prevention of stress bleeding requires ensuring hemodynamic stability and the administration of proton-pump inhibitors, H_2 receptor antagonists, antacids, or cytoprotective agents as appropriate (see Chapter 7, Pharmacology for in-depth discussion of GI prophylaxis).

Ventilator Malfunction

Problems related to the proper functioning of mechanical ventilators, although rare, may have devastating consequences for patients. Many of the alarm systems on ventilators are designed to alert clinicians to improperly functioning ventilatory systems. These alarm systems must be activated at all times if ventilator malfunction problems are to be quickly identified and corrected, and untoward patient events avoided.

Many of the "problems" identified with ventilatory equipment are actually related to inappropriate setup or use of the devices. Ventilator circuits that are not properly connected, alarm systems that are set improperly, or inadequate ventilator settings for a particular clinical condition are examples of some of these operator-related occurrences.

There are occasions, however, when ventilator systems do not operate properly. Examples of ventilator malfunctions include valve mechanisms sticking and obstructing gas flow, inadequate or excessive gas delivery, electronic

circuit failures in microprocessing-based ventilators, failures with complete shutdown, and power failures or surges in the institution.

The most important approach to ventilator malfunction is to maintain a high level of vigilance to determine if ventilators are performing properly. Ensuring that alarm systems are set appropriately at all times, providing frequent routine assessment of ventilator functioning, and the use of experienced support personnel to maintain the ventilator systems are some of the most crucial activities necessary to avoid patient problems. In addition, whenever ventilator malfunction is suspected, the patient should be immediately removed from the device and temporary ventilation and oxygenation provided with an MRB or another ventilator until the question of proper functioning is resolved. Any sudden change in the patient's respiratory or cardiovascular status alerts the clinician to consider potential ventilator malfunction as a cause. Chapter 27, Ventilatory Troubleshooting Guide, details common approaches to equipment- and patient-related problems during mechanical ventilation.

Weaning From Short-Term Mechanical Ventilation

The process of transitioning the ventilator-dependent patient to unassisted spontaneous breathing is *weaning from mechanical ventilation.* This is a period of time where the level of ventilator support for oxygenation and ventilation is decreased, either gradually or abruptly, while monitoring the patient's response to the resumption of spontaneous breathing. Weaning is considered to be complete, or successful, when the patient is able to spontaneously breathe for 24 to 48 hours. Often, removal of the artificial airway occurs before that time if clinicians are optimistic that the patient's respiratory status will not deteriorate. The vast majority of patients intubated and ventilated for short periods of time (<72 hours) are successfully weaned over a 2- to 8-hour period. Approximately 20% of patients, however, require extended time periods to successfully complete the weaning process, with some being unable to breathe without mechanical ventilation. Chapter 20, Advanced Respiratory Concepts, presents information on weaning the patient requiring long-term mechanical ventilation.

Weaning proceeds when the underlying pulmonary disorder that led to mechanical ventilation has sufficiently resolved, and the patient is alert and able to protect the airway. Unnecessary delays in weaning from mechanical ventilation increase the likelihood of complications such as ventilator-induced lung injury, pneumonia, discomfort, and increases in hospitalization costs. Thus, aggressive and timely weaning trials are encouraged.

Steps in the Weaning Process

Assessment of Readiness

Readiness to wean from short-term mechanical ventilation (STMV) may be assessed with a wide variety of criteria (see

TABLE 5–10. STRATEGIES TO FACILITATE WEANING

- Explain the weaning process to the patient/family and maintain open communication throughout weaning.
- Position to maximize ventilatory effort (sitting upright in bed or chair).
- Administer analgesics to relieve pain and sedatives to control anxiety, if appropriate.
- Remain with the patient during the weaning trial and/or provide a highly vigilant presence.
- Frequently assess the patient's response to the weaning trial.
- Avoid unnecessary physical exertion, plainful procedures, and/or transports during the weaning trials.
- Maximize the physical environment to be conducive to weaning (e.g., temperature, noise, distractions).

Chapter 20, Advanced Respiratory Concepts). However, in most institutions, assessment of readiness to wean includes just three or four criteria for most short-term ventilator patients. Some examples are:

- ABGs within normal limits on minimal to moderate amounts of ventilatory support (FiO_2 ≤0.50, minute ventilation ≤10 L/min, PEEP ≤5 cm H_2O)
- Negative inspiratory pressure ≤20 cm H_2O
- Spontaneous Vt ≥5 mL/kg
- Vital capacity ≥10 mL/kg
- Respiratory rate <30 breaths/min
- Spontaneous rapid-shallow breathing index <100 to 105

Following selection of the method for weaning (see the discussion below), the actual weaning trial can begin. It is important to prepare both the patient and the critical care environment properly to maximize the chances for weaning success (Table 5–10). Interventions include appropriate explanations of the process to the patient, positioning and medication to improve ventilatory efforts, and the avoidance of unnecessary activities during the weaning trial. Throughout the weaning time, continuous monitoring for signs and symptoms of respiratory distress or fatigue is essential (Table 5–11). Many of these indicators are subtle, but careful monitoring of baseline levels before weaning progresses and throughout the trial provides objective indicators of the need to return the patient to previous levels of ventilator support.

TABLE 5–11. CLINICAL INDICATORS OF THE NEED TO STOP WEANING TRIAL

- Dyspnea
- Increased respiratory rate, heart rate, or BP
- Shallow breaths or decreased spontaneous Vt
- Accessory muscle use
- Anxiety
- Deterioration if PaO_2 or $PaCO_2$, SpO_2 and/or ↓pH

The need to temporarily stop the weaning trial is not viewed as, or termed, a *failure*. Instead it simply suggests that more time needs to be provided to ensure success. A full evaluation of the multiple reasons for inability to wean is necessary, however. Assessment and evaluation of patients requiring mechanical ventilation longer than 72 hours is discussed in detail in Chapter 20, Advanced Respiratory Concepts.

Weaning Trials

Generally, weaning trials for patients ventilated short term are accomplished with spontaneous breathing trials (SBT) on T-piece or CPAP. The SBT duration is generally at least 30 minutes but no more than 120 minutes. Some prefer low levels of pressure support ventilation for trials. A decision to extubate is made with the conclusion of a successful trial. The need for reintubation is not uncommon and is associated with increased mortality. Thus, premature attempts at extubation are to be avoided. Some suggest that noninvasive positive-pressure ventilation via face or nasal mask may be useful for patients with respiratory failure following extubation. However, a recent international, multicenter study demonstrated that this therapy does not prevent the need for reintubation or reduce mortality in these cases.

Methods

A variety of methods are available for weaning patients from mechanical ventilation. To date, research on these techniques has not clearly identified any one method as optimal for weaning from short-term mechanical ventilation. Most institutions, however, use one or two approaches routinely. A number of recently published randomized controlled trials demonstrated that the outcomes of patients managed under protocols driven by nonphysician clinicians were better than those managed with standard physician-directed care. Most experts on weaning believe that, with short-term ventilator-dependent patients, the actual method used to wean the patient is less important to weaning success than using a consistently applied protocol strategy that is individualized.

- *SIMV:* One of the most popular methods of weaning patients in the past uses the SIMV mode. By progressively decreasing the number of mandated breaths delivered by the ventilator, the patient performs more and more of the work of breathing by increasing spontaneous breathing. Advantages to the SIMV mode are the presence of built-in alarms to alert clinicians when ventilation problems occur and the guarantee of a minimum amount of minute ventilation. The disadvantage of SIMV is that each spontaneous breath requires some additional work of breathing to open the valve of the demand reservoir for gas. Depending on the type of ventilator, this increased work of breathing is felt to be relatively minor and to not interfere with most short-term weaning attempts. SIMV is used either alone or in conjunction with pressure support (SIMV + PS).

- *T-Piece or Blow By:* The T-piece method of weaning involves removing the patient from the mechanical ventilator and attaching an oxygen source to the artificial airway with a "T" piece for a SBT (see Figure 5–16C). No ventilatory support occurs with this device, with the patient completely breathing spontaneously the entire time this device is connected. The advantage of this method of weaning is that the resistance to breathing is low, because no special valves need to be opened to initiate gas flow. Rapid assessment of the patient's ability to spontaneously breathe is another purported advantage. Limitations of this SBT are that it may cause ventilatory muscle overload and fatigue. When this occurs, it usually appears early in the SBT, so the patient must be closely monitored during the initial few minutes. Other disadvantages with the T-piece are that PEEP therapy cannot be maintained and there are few alarm or backup systems to support the patient should ventilation be inadequate. It is critical to recognize that this technique relies on the clinician to monitor for signs and symptoms of respiratory difficulty and fatigue. Frequently, the FiO_2 is increased by at least 10% over the FiO_2 setting on the ventilator to prevent hypoxemia from the lower Vt of spontaneous breaths. Patients who fail a SBT should receive a stable, nonfatiguing, comfortable form of ventilatory support for rest following the trial.
- *CPAP:* The use of the ventilator to allow spontaneous breathing periods without mandated breaths, similar to the T-piece, can be done with the CPAP mode. With this approach, ventilator alarm systems can be used to monitor spontaneous breathing rates and volumes, and a small amount of continuous pressure (5 cm H_2O) can be applied if needed. The disadvantage of this approach, similar to the SIMV mode, is that the work of breathing resulting from the need to open the demand valve to receive gas flow for the breath is higher than with the T-piece. For most patients, this slight additional work of breathing is not likely to be a critical factor to their weaning success or failure unless the trial is unduly long. If needed, a low level of pressure support (e.g., 5 to 7 cm H_2O) may also be added to offset this workload (CPAP + PS)
- *Pressure Support:* Another method for weaning from ventilation is the use of PS ventilation. With this method, patients can spontaneously breathe on the ventilator with a small amount of ventilator "support" to augment their spontaneous breaths. This technique overcomes some of the resistance to breathing associated with ET tubes and demand valves. The main disadvantage with this approach is that clinicians may underestimate the degree of support to spontaneous breathing provided with this method and prematurely

stop the weaning process. See Chapter 20, Advanced Respiratory Concepts, for a more detailed explanation of PS ventilation and weaning.

Troubleshooting Ventilators

The complexity of ventilators and the dynamic state of the patient's clinical condition, as well as the patient's response to ventilation, create a variety of common problems that may occur during mechanical ventilation. It is crucial that critical care clinicians be expert in the prevention, identification, and management of ventilator-associated problems in critically ill patients. Chapter 27, Ventilatory Troubleshooting Guide, details specific causes and intervention and prevention strategies for common ventilator-related problems.

During mechanical ventilation, sudden changes in the clinical condition of the patient, particularly respiratory distress, as well as the occurrence of ventilator alarms or abnormal functioning of the ventilator, require immediate assessment and intervention. A systematic approach to each of these situations prevents or minimizes untoward ventilator events (Figure 5–22).

The first step is to determine the presence of respiratory distress or hemodynamic instability. If either is present the patient is removed from the mechanical ventilator and manually ventilated with a MRB and 100% O_2 for a few minutes.

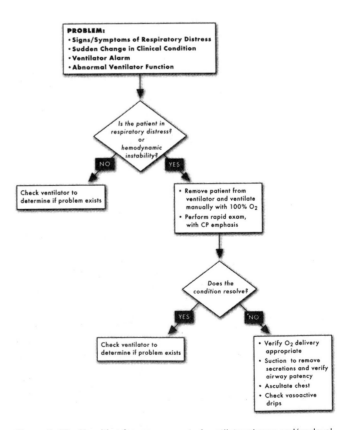

Figure 5–22. Algorithm for management of ventilator alarms and/or development of acute respiratory distress.

During manual ventilation, a quick assessment of the respiratory and cardiovascular system is made, noting changes from previous status. Clinical improvement rapidly following removal from the ventilator suggests a ventilator problem. Manual ventilation is continued while another clinician corrects the ventilator problem (e.g., tubing leaks or disconnections, inaccurate gas delivery) or replaces the ventilator. Continuation of respiratory distress after removal from the ventilator and during manual ventilation suggests a patient-related cause.

Communication

Mechanically ventilated patients are unable to speak and communicate verbally due to the presence of a cuffed ET or tracheostomy tube. The inability to speak is frustrating for the patient, nurse, and members of the health care team. Impaired communication results in patients experiencing anxiety and fear, symptoms that can have a deleterious effect on their physical and emotional conditions. Patients interviewed after extubation reveal how isolated and alone they felt because of their inability to speak.

Common Communication Problems

Patients' perceptions of communication difficulties related to mechanical ventilation include (1) inability to communicate, (2) insufficient explanations, (3) inadequate understanding, (4) fears related to potential dangers associated with the inability to speak, and (5) difficulty with communication methods. Except for the problem of inability to vocalize, all of the problems cited by ventilated patients may be resolved easily by critical care practitioners. For instance, "insufficient explanations" and "inadequate understanding" can be remedied by frequent repetition of all plans and procedures in language that is understandable to a nonmedical person and that takes into account that attention span and cognitive abilities, especially memory, are frequently diminished due to the underlying illness or injury, effects of medications and anesthesia, and the impact of the critical care environment.

Although most messages the ventilated patient needs to communicate lie within a narrow range ("pain," "hunger," "water," and "sleep"), communicating these basic needs is often difficult. Most adults are accustomed to attending to their own basic needs, but in the intensive care unit, not only are they unable to physically perform certain activities, they also cannot communicate their needs effectively. Basic needs include such activities as bathing, brushing teeth, combing hair, urinating and defecating, eating, drinking, and sleeping. Other examples include simple requests or statements such as "too hot," "too cold," "turn me," "up," "down," "straighten my legs," "my arm hurts," "I can't breathe," and "moisten my lips."

Patients have described difficulties with communication methods while being mechanically ventilated. This also can be avoided by assessing the patient's communication

abilities. Is the patient alert and oriented? Can the patient answer simple yes and no questions? Does the patient speak English? Can the patient use at least one hand to gesture? Does the patient have sufficient strength and dexterity to hold a pen and write? Are the patient's hearing and vision adequate? Knowledge of the patient's communication abilities assists the clinician to identify appropriate communication methods.

Once the most successful communication methods have been identified for a particular patient, they should be written into the plan of care. Critical care units are very busy places, so it is easy to forget about the ventilated patient's need for communication. Continuity among health care professionals in their approach to communication with nonvocal patients improves the quality of care and increases patient satisfaction.

Methods to Enhance Communication

A variety of methods for augmenting communication are available and can be classified into two categories: nonvocal treatments (gestures, lip reading, mouthing words, paper and pen, alphabet/numeric boards, flashcards, etc.) and vocal treatments (talking tracheostomy tubes and speaking valves). The best way to communicate with the patient who has an artificial airway or who is being mechanically ventilated is still unknown.

Nonvocal Treatments

Individual patient needs vary and it is recommended that the nurse use a variety of nonvocal treatments (e.g., gestures, alphabet board, and paper and pen). Success with communication interventions varies with the diagnosis, age, type of injury or disease, type of respiratory assist devices, and psychosocial factors. For instance, lip reading can be successful in patients who have tracheostomies because the lips and mouth are visible, but in the endotracheally intubated patient, where tape and tube holders limit lip movement and visibility, lip reading may be less successful.

Writing

Typically the easiest, most common method of communication readily available is the paper and pen. However, the supine position is not especially conducive to writing legibly. The absence of proper eyeglasses, an injured or immobilized dominant writing hand, or lack of strength also can make writing difficult for mechanically ventilated patients. Writing paper should be placed on a firm writing surface (e.g., clipboard) with an attached felt-tipped pen that writes in any position. Strength, finger flexibility, and dexterity are required to grasp a pen. Many patients prefer to use a Magic Slate (Western Publishing Co., Racine, WI) or a Magna Doodle (Tyco Industries, Mount Laurel, NJ). These pressure-sensitive, inexpensive toy screens can be purchased at any department store; with them messages can be easily erased, maintaining the privacy of a written message.

A phenomenon of decoding exists between patient's written words (which often look like scribbling) and the nurse's ability to read what the patient wrote. The majority of the time, the nurse can read the writing of the patient even when it seems indistinguishable to a casual observer. This is due in part to the fact that over 65% of all communication is nonverbal and many contextual cues exist to assist in understanding and communicating effectively.

Gesturing

Another nonvocal method of communication that can be very effective is the deliberate use of gestures. Gestures are best suited for the short-term ventilated patient who is alert and can move at least one hand, even if only minimally. Generally, well-understood gestures are emblematic, have a low level of symbolism, and are easily interpreted by most people.

For example, ventilated patients often indicate that they need suctioning by curving an index finger (to resemble a suction catheter), raising a hand toward the ET tube, and moving their hand back and forth. This is known as an idiosyncratic gesture, a gesture that is used by a particular community, namely, the nurse and the ventilated patient. Other idiosyncratic gestures include "ice chips," "moisten my mouth," "spray throat," "fan," and "doctor."

One important aspect of communicating by gesture is to "mirror" the gesture(s) back to the patient, at the same time verbalizing the message or idea conveyed by the patient's gesture. This mirroring ensures accuracy in interpretation and assists the clinician and patient to form a repertoire to be used successfully in future gestural conversations. When observing a patient's gestures, stand back from the bed, and watch his or her arms and hands. Most gestures are easily understood, especially those most frequently used by patients (e.g., the head nod, indicating "yes" or "no"). Practitioners should ask simple yes-and-no questions, but avoid playing "twenty questions" with ventilated patients because this can be very frustrating. Before trying to guess the needs of ventilated patients, give them the opportunity to use gestures to communicate their needs.

Alphabet Board/Picture Board

For patients who do not speak English, a picture board is sometimes useful along with well-understood gestures. Picture boards have images of common patient needs (e.g., bedpan, glass of water, medications, family, doctor, nurse) that the patient can point to. Picture boards, although commercially available, can be made easily and laminated to more uniquely meet the needs of a specific critical care population.

Another approach is the use of flash cards that can be purchased or made. Language flash cards contain common words or phrases in English or foreign languages.

Vocal Treatments

If patients with tracheostomy tubes in place have intact organs of speech, they may benefit from vocal treatment strategies like pneumatic and electrical devices, fenestrated tracheostomy tubes, talking tracheostomy tubes, and tracheostomy speaking valves. Several conditions preclude use of vocalization devices, such as neurologic conditions that impair vocalization (e.g., Guillain-Barré syndrome), severe upper airway obstruction (e.g., head/neck trauma), or vocal cord adduction (e.g., presence of an ET tube).

Two vocal treatments for tracheostomized patients are the one-way speaking valve and the fenestrated tracheostomy tube (Figure 5–23). These tubes allow air to leak through fenestration points or holes in the outer cannula of the tracheostomy tube. There have been reported incidences

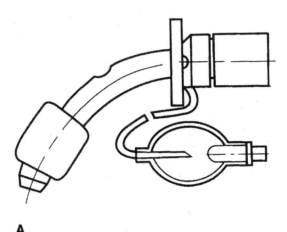

A

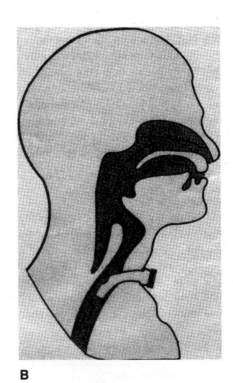

B

Figure 5–23. (A) Fenestrated tracheostomy tube. **(B)** Opening above the cuff site allowing gas flow past the vocal cords during inspiration and expiration. (*With permission Nellcor Puritan Bennett Inc, Pleasanton, CA.*)

of granuloma tissue development at the site adjacent to the fenestration, which resolves after removal of the tube. In addition, fenestrated ports often become clogged with secretions, again preventing voicing.

Another vocal treatment is the talking tracheostomy (e.g., Portex Talk Trach) tube, which is designed to provide a means of verbal communication for the ventilator-dependent patient (Figure 5–24). It operates by gas flowing (4–6 L/min) through an airflow line, which has a fenestration just above the tracheostomy tube cuff. The air flows through the glottis, thus supporting vocalization if the patient is able to form words with their mouth. Under most circumstances, vocalization is heard as a soft whisper. The cuff remains inflated with these tubes so that a closed ventilation system is maintained. However, an outside air source must be provided, which is usually not humidified and the trachea can become dry and irritated. The line for this air source requires diligent cleaning and flushing of the air port to prevent it from becoming clogged. The patients must be able to manually divert air through the tube via a thumb port control, which requires manual dexterity and coordination. The voice quality produced with this device ranges from that of a soft whisper or hoarse sounding. Patients who were otherwise considered to be "unweanable" have been reported to take a renewed interest in the weaning process and some successfully wean upon hearing their own voice.

Teaching Communication Methods

The critical care environment presents many teaching and learning challenges. Patients and families are under a considerable amount of stress, so the nurse must be a very creative teacher and offer communication techniques that are simple, effective, and easy to learn. The desire to communicate with loved ones, however, often makes the family very willing to learn. Frequently, it is the family who makes up large-lettered communication boards, or purchases a Magic Slate for the patient to use. Suggesting that families do this is usually very well received, because loved ones want so desperately to help in some way.

All patients should be informed prior to intubation that they will be unable to speak during the intubation period. A flipchart illustrating what an endotracheal or tracheostomy tube is like, with labeling in simple words, may be shown to patients who will be electively intubated (e.g., for planned surgery). Practicing with a few nonverbal communication techniques before intubation (e.g., gestures, alphabet boards, flash cards) is also beneficial. Another important point to emphasize with patients is that being unable to speak is usually temporary, just while the breathing tube is in place. If preintubation explanations are not feasible or possible, provide these explanations to the intubated patient.

Principles of Management

The majority of interventions related to mechanical ventilation focus on maximizing oxygenation and ventilation, and preventing complications associated with artificial airways and the sequelae of assisting the patient's ventilation and oxygenation with an invasive mechanical device.

Maximizing Oxygenation and Ventilation

Ensure Synchrony of Respiratory Patterns

- Provide frequent explanations of the purpose of the ventilator.
- Monitor the patient's response to ventilator therapy and for signs that the patient is out of phase with the ventilator respiratory pattern.

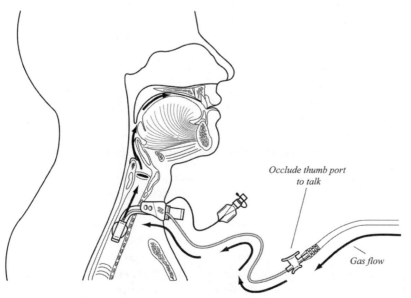

Occlude thumb port to talk

Gas flow

Figure 5–24. Tracheostomy tube with side port to facilitate speech. (*With permission, Smith Medical, Keen, NH.*)

- Consider ventilator setting changes to maximize synchrony (e.g., changes in flow rates, respiratory rates, sensitivities, and/or modes).
- Administer sedative agents as required to prevent asynchrony with the ventilator. Avoid the use of neuromuscular blocking agents unless absolutely necessary.

Maintain a Patent Airway

- Suction only when clinically indicated according to patient assessment (see Table 5–6).
- Decrease secretion viscosity by maintaining adequate hydration, humidification of all inhaled gases, and administration of mucolytic agents as appropriate.
- Monitor for signs and symptoms of bronchospasm and administer bronchodilator therapy as appropriate (see Chapter 9, Cardiovascular System).
- Prevent obstruction of oral ET tubes by using an oral bite block if necessary.

Monitor Oxygenation and Ventilation Status Frequently

- ABG analysis as appropriate (e.g., after some ventilator changes, with respiratory distress or cardiovascular instability, or with significant changes in clinical condition).
- Continuous noninvasive monitoring of SpO_2. Validate noninvasive measures with periodic ABG analysis (see Table 5–4).
- Observe for signs and symptoms of decreases in PaO_2, increases in $PaCO_2$, and respiratory distress. Development of respiratory distress requires immediate intervention (see Figure 5–22).
- Reposition frequently to improve ventilation–perfusion relationships and prevent atelectasis.
- Aggressively manage pain, particularly chest and upper abdominal pain, to increase mobility, deep breathing, and coughing (see Chapter 6, Pain, Sedation, and Neuromuscular Blockade Management).

Physiotherapy and Monitoring

- Administer chest physiotherapy for selected clinical conditions (e.g., large mucous production, lobar atelectasis).
- Monitor oxygenation status closely during chest physiotherapy for signs and symptoms of arterial desaturation.

Maintain Oxygenation and Ventilatory Support at All Times

- Ensure proper operation of the mechanical ventilator by activation of appropriately set alarms and frequent assessment of device function (usually, check every 1 to 2 hours).
- During even brief periods of removal from mechanical ventilation, maintain ventilation and oxygenation with MRB. During intrahospital transport, verify adequacy of ventilatory support equipment, particularly the maintenance of PEEP (when >10 cm H_2O is required) as well as ensuring adequate portable oxygen supply tank pressure.
- Emergency sources of portable oxygen should be readily available in the event of loss of wall oxygen capabilities.

Preventing Complications

1. Maintain ET or tracheostomy cuff pressures less than 25 mm Hg.
2. Maintain artificial airway position by securing with a properly fitting holder device or selected tapes. Frequently verify proper ET position by noting ET marking at lip or nares placed after intubation.
3. Ensure tape or devices used to secure the artificial airway are properly applied and are not causing pressure areas or skin breakdown. Periodic repositioning of ET tubes may be required to prevent skin integrity problems.
4. Use a bite block with oral ET tubes if necessary to prevent accidental biting of the tube.
5. Provide frequent mouth care and assess for development of pressure areas from ET tubes. Move the ET from one side of the mouth to the other daily or more frequently if necessary.
6. Assess for signs and symptoms of sinusitis with nasal ET tube use (e.g., pain in sinus area with pressure, purulent drainage from nares, fever, increased white blood cell count).

Maximizing Communication

1. Assess communication abilities and establish at least a method for nonverbal communication (see the discussion of communication below). Assist family members in using that approach with the patient.
2. Anticipate patient needs and concerns in the planning of care.
3. Ensure that call lights, bells, or other methods for notifying unit personnel of patient needs are in place at all times.
4. Frequently repeat information about communication limitations and how to use different nonverbal communication methods.

Reducing Anxiety and Providing Psychosocial Support

1. Maintain a calm, supportive environment to avoid unnecessary escalation of anxiety. Provide brief explanations of activities and procedures. The vigilance and presence of health care providers during anxiety periods is crucial to avoid panic by patients and visiting family members.
2. Teach the patient relaxation techniques to control anxiety.

3. Administer mild doses of anxiolytics (e.g., lorazepam or diazepam) that do not depress respiration (see Chapter 6, Pain, Sedation, and Neuromuscular Blockade, and Chapter 9, Cardiovascular System).
4. Encourage the family to stay with the patient as much as desired and to participate in caregiver activities as appropriate. Presence of a family member provides comfort to the patient and assists the family member to better cope with the critical illness.

SELECTED BIBLIOGRAPHY

General Critical Care

Ackerman MH, Mick DJ: Instillation of normal saline before suctioning in patients with pulmonary infections: A prospective randomized controlled trial. *Am J Crit Care* 1998;7(4):261–266.

American Association of Critical-Care Nurses (AACN): *Practice alert: Ventilator Associated Pneumonia.* Aliso Viejo, CA: AACN; 2004. Available from URL: www.aacn.org

Burton GG, Hodgkin JE, Ward JJ: *Respiratory Care: A Guide to Clinical Practice.* Philadelphia: JB Lippincott; 1991.

Centers for Disease Control and Prevention: Guidelines for preventing health-care-associated pneumonia, 2003: Recommendations of CDC and the Health Care Infection Control Practices Advisory Committee. *MMWR* 2004;53(No. RR-3):1–35.

Dossey BM, Guzzetta CE, Kenner, CV: *Critical Care Nursing: Body, Mind, Spirit.* Philadelphia: JB Lippincott; 1992.

DuPuis YG: *Ventilators: Theory and Clinical Application*, 2nd ed. St. Louis: CV Mosby; 1992.

Fernandez R, Blanch L, Mancebo J, et al: Endotracheal tube cuff pressure assessment: Pitfalls of finger estimation and need for objective measurement. *Crit Care Med* 1990;18(12):1423–1426.

Kersten D: *Comprehensive Respiratory Nursing.* Philadelphia: WB Saunders; 1989.

Kollef MH: Prevention of hospital-associated pneumonia and ventilator associated pneumonia. *Crit Care Med* 2004;32:1396–1405.

Luce J, Pierson D, Tyler M: *Intensive Respiratory Care*, 2nd ed. Philadelphia: WB Saunders; 1993.

McPherson S: *Respiratory Therapy Equipment*, 4th ed. St. Louis, MO: CV Mosby; 1990.

Sole ML, Byers JF, Ludy JE, et al: A multisite survey of suctioning techniques and airway management practices. *Am J Crit Care* 2003;12(3):220–232.

Stauffer JL: Complications of endotracheal intubation and tracheotomy. *Respir Care* 1999;44(7):828–844.

St John RE: Advances in artificial airway management. *Crit Care Nurs Clin North Am* 1999;11(1):7–17.

St John R, Seckel M: Airway Management. In: Burns SM (series ed.): *AACN Protocols for Practice: Care of the Mechanically Ventilated Patient Series.* Aliso Viejo, CA: AACN; 2005.

Wilkins R, Stoller JK, Scanlan CL, et al: *Fundamentals of Respiratory Care*, 8th ed. St. Louis: Mosby; 2003.

Zeitoun SS, de Barros AL, Diccini S: A prospective, randomized study of ventilator-associated pneumonia in patients using a closed vs. open suction system. *J Clin Nurs* 2003;12(4):484–489.

Ventilator Management

Aguilar J, Fernandez R, Blanch L: Recruitment maneuvers during lung protective ventilation in acute respiratory distress syndrome. *Am J Respir Crit Care Med* 2002;165:165–170.

Ahrens T, Sona C: Capnography application in acute and critical care. *AACN Clin Issues* 2003;14:123–132.

Branson R, Davis B, Davis K, et al: A comparison of reflective and transmission oximetry in patients with poor perfusion. *Respir Care* 2003;48:1086 (abstract).

Burton GG, Hodgkin JE, Wark JJ: *Respiratory Care: A Guide to Clinical Practice*, 3rd ed. Philadelphia: JB Lippincott; 1993.

Dries DJ, McGonigal MD, Malian MS, et al: Protocol-driven ventilator weaning reduces use of mechanical ventilation, rate of early reintubation, and ventilator-associated pneumonia. *J Trauma* 2004;56:943–952.

Esteban A, Frutos-Vivar F, Ferguson ND, et al: Noninvasive positive-pressure ventilation for respiratory failure after extubation. *N Engl J Med* 2004;350:2452–2460.

Esteban A, Frutos F, Tobin MJ, et al: A comparison of four methods of weaning patients from mechanical ventilation. *N Engl J Med* 1995;332:345–350.

Grap MJ: Pulse oximetry. In Burns S (ed): *AACN's Protocols for Practice: Care of the Mechanically Ventilated Patient Series.* Aliso Viejo, CA: AACN; 1999.

Burns SM: Weaning from mechanical ventilation. In Burns S (ed): *AACN Protocols for Practice: Care of the Mechanically Ventilated Patient Series.* Aliso Viejo, CA: AACN; 2005.

Hanneman SG, Ingersoll GL, Knebel AR, et al: Weaning from short-term mechanical ventilation: A review. *Am J Crit Care* 1994;3(6):421–441.

Knebel A, Shekleton M, Burns S, et al: Weaning from mechanical ventilation. *Am J Crit Care* 1994;3(6):416–420.

Kollef MH, Shapiro SD, Silver P, et al: A randomized controlled trial of protocol-directed versus physician-directed weaning from mechanical ventilation. *Crit Care Med* 1997;25:567–574.

MacIntyre NR: Evidence-based ventilator weaning and discontinuation. *Respir Care* 2004;49:830–836.

MacLeod DB, Cortinez LI, Keifer J, et al: Pulse oximeter response profiles under hypoxic and hypothermic conditions in healthy volunteers. *Anesthesiology* 2003;99:A1057.

Petrucci N, Iacovelli W: Ventilation with smaller tidal volumes: A quantitative systematic review of randomized controlled trials. *Anesth Analg* 2004;99:193–200.

Pierson DJ, Kacmarek RM: *Foundations of Respiratory Care.* New York: Churchill Livingstone; 1992.

St. John RE: End-tidal CO_2 monitoring. In Chulay M, Burns S (eds): *AACN's Protocols for Practice: Care of the Mechanically Ventilated Patient Series.* Aliso Viejo, CA: AACN; 1999.

St. John R: End-tidal CO_2 monitoring. In Burns SM (series ed.): *AACN's Protocols for Practice: Non-Invasive Monitoring Series.* Aliso Viejo, CA: AACN: 2005.

Tobin M: *Principles and Practice of Mechanical Ventilation.* New York: McGraw-Hill; 1994.

Communication

Buckwalter K, Cusack D, Sidles E, et al: Increasing communication ability in aphasic/dysarthric patients. *West J Nurs Res* 1989; 11(6):736–747.

Connolly M: *Temporarily Nonvocal Trauma Patients and Their Gestures: A Descriptive Study.* Dissertation Abstracts International, University Microfilm, 1992.

Connolly M: Nonvocal treatments for short and long-term ventilator patients. In Mason M (ed): *Speech Pathology for Tracheostomized and Ventilator Dependent Patients.* Newport Beach, CA: Voicing, Inc.; 1993.

Connolly M, Shekleton M: Communicating with ventilator dependent patients. *Dimensions Crit Care Nurs* 1991;10(2):115–122.

Dowden PA, Honsinger MJ, Beukelman DR: Serving nonspeaking patients in acute care settings: An intervention approach. *Augmentative Altern Communication* 1986:25–33.

Lawless C: Helping patients with endotracheal and tracheostomy tubes communicate. *Am J Nurs* 1975;75:2151–2158.

Mitsuda PM, Baarslag-Benson R, Hazel K, et al: Augmentative communication in intensive and acute care unit settings. In Yorkston KM (ed): *Augmentative Communication in the Medical Setting*, pp 5–56. Tucson, AZ: Communication Skill Builders, Inc.; 1992.

Pain, Sedation, and Neuromuscular Blockade Management

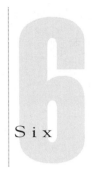

Six

Joan Michiko Ching and Suzanne M. Burns

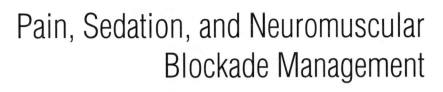

▶ **Knowledge Competencies**

1. Describe a multilevel approach to pain management.
2. Compare and contrast pain-relieving therapies for the critically ill:
   - Nonsteroidal anti-inflammatory drugs.
   - Opioids, including patient-controlled analgesia.
   - Epidural analgesia with opioids and/or local anesthetics.
   - Nonpharmacologic therapies: distraction, cutaneous stimulation, imagery, and relaxation techniques.
3. Recognize the interactions among relaxation, sedation, and pain control and describe nonpharmacologic and

pharmacologic interventions to promote relaxation and comfort in the critically ill.

4. Describe special considerations for pain management in vulnerable populations.
5. Identify the need for sedation, common sedative drugs, and how to monitor and manage the patient requiring sedation.
6. Describe the method for monitoring neuromuscular blockade in the critically ill patient.

Pain management is central to the care of the critically ill or injured patient. Patients identify physical care that promotes pain relief and comfort as an important element of their hospitalization and recovery, especially while in the critical care environment. Providing optimum pain relief for critically ill patients not only enhances their psychoemotional well-being, but also can help to avert additional physiologic injury for a patient who is already physiologically compromised. This chapter explores a multilevel approach to pain management in critically ill patients based on the physiologic mechanisms of pain transmission and human responses to pain. Within the multilevel approach, specific pharmacologic and nonpharmacologic pain management techniques are described, including the integral relationships among relaxation, sedation, and pain relief. Strategies also are presented that promote comfort and are easy to incorporate into a plan of care for critically ill patients. Finally, special considerations are delineated for vulnerable populations within the critical care setting.

PHYSIOLOGIC MECHANISMS OF PAIN

Peripheral Mechanisms

The pain response is elicited with tissue injuries, whether actual or potential. Undifferentiated free nerve endings, or *nociceptors,* are the major receptors signaling tissue injury (Figure 6–1). Nociceptors are polymodal and can be stimulated by thermal, mechanical, and chemical stimuli. Nociception refers to the transmission of impulses by sensory nerves, which signal tissue injury.

At the site of injury, the release of a variety of neurochemical substances potentiates the activation of peripheral nociceptors. Many of these substances are also mediators of the inflammatory response and include histamine, kinins, prostaglandins, serotonin, and leukotrienes (Figure 6–2).

The nociceptive impulse travels to the spinal cord via specialized, afferent sensory fibers. Small, myelinated A-delta fibers conduct nociceptive signals rapidly to the spinal cord.

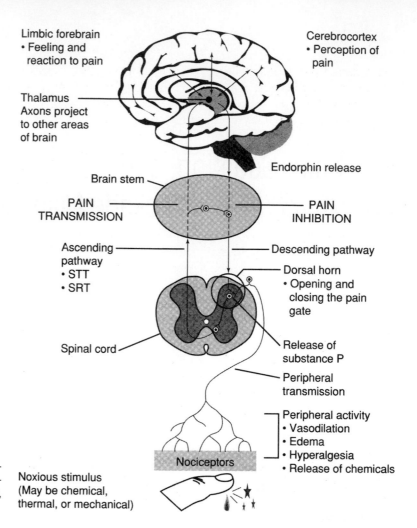

Figure 6–1. Physiologic pathway of pain transmission. (*From: Wild LR, Evans L: Pain. In Copstead L [ed]: Perspectives on Pathophysiology, p. 934. Philadelphia: WB Saunders; 1995.*)

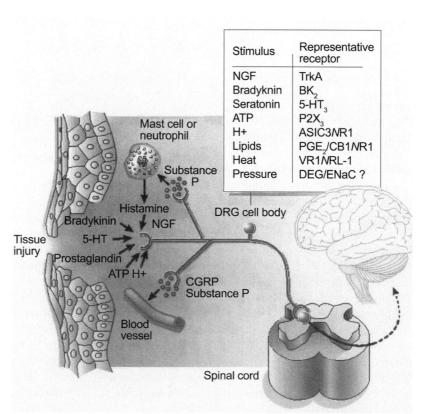

Stimulus	Representative receptor
NGF	TrkA
Bradyknin	BK_2
Seratonin	$5\text{-}HT_3$
ATP	$P2X_3$
H+	ASIC3/VR1
Lipids	PGE_2/CB1/VR1
Heat	VR1/VRL-1
Pressure	DEG/ENaC ?

Figure 6–2. Peripheral nociceptors and the inflammatory response at the site of injury. (*From Julius D, Basbaum AI: Molecular mechanisms of nociception.* Nature *2001;413:203–210.*)

The A-delta fibers transmit sensations that are generally localized and sharp in quality. In addition to A-delta fibers, smaller, unmyelinated C fibers also transmit nociceptive signals to the spinal cord. Because C fibers are unmyelinated, their conduction speed is much slower than their A-delta counterparts. The sensory quality of signals carried by C fibers tends to be dull and unlocalized (Figure 6–3).

Spinal Cord Integration

Sensory afferent fibers enter the spinal cord via the dorsal nerve, synapsing with cell bodies of spinal cord interneurons in the dorsal horn (see Figure 6–1). Most of the A-delta and C fibers synapse in laminae I through V, in an area referred to as the *substantia gelatinosa*. Numerous neurotransmitters (e.g., substance P, glutamate, and calcitonin gene-related peptide) and other receptor systems (e.g., opiate, alpha-adrenergic, and serotonergic receptors) modulate the processing of nociceptive inputs in the spinal cord.

Central Processing

Following spinal cord integration, nociceptive impulses travel to the brain via specialized, ascending somatosensory pathways (see Figure 6–1). The spinothalamic tract conducts nociceptive signals directly from the spinal cord to the thalamus. The spinoreticulothalamic tract projects signals to the reticular formation and the mesencephalon in the midbrain, as well as to the thalamus. From the thalamus, axons project to somatosensory areas of the cerebrocortex and limbic forebrain. The unique physiologic, cognitive, and emotional responses to pain are determined and modulated by the specific areas to which the somatosensory pathways project. For example, the thalamus regulates the neurochemical response to pain, and the cortical and limbic projections are responsible for the perception of pain and aversive response to pain, respectively. Similarly, the reticular activating system regulates the heightened state of awareness that accompanies pain. The modulation of pain by activities in these specific areas of the brain is the basis of many of the analgesic therapies available to treat pain.

RESPONSES TO PAIN

Human responses to pain can be both physical and emotional. The physiologic responses to pain are the result of hypothalamic activation of the sympathetic nervous system associated with the stress response. Sympathetic activation leads to

- blood shifts from superficial vessels to striated muscle, the heart, the lungs, and the nervous system;
- dilation of the bronchioles to increase oxygenation;
- increased cardiac contractility;
- inhibition of gastric secretions and contraction; and
- increases in circulating blood glucose for energy.

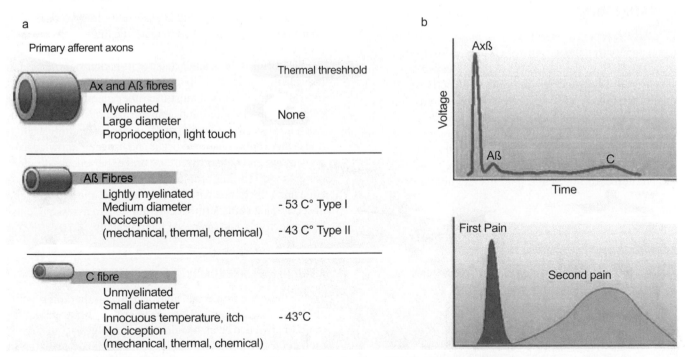

Figure 6–3. Nociceptor transmission differs in speed and type of pain. (*From Julius D, Basbaum AI: Molecular mechanisms of nociception.* Nature *2001;413:203–210.*)

Signs and symptoms of sympathetic activation frequently accompany nociception and pain:

- Increased heart rate
- Increased blood pressure
- Increased respiratory rate
- Pupil dilation
- Pallor and perspiration
- Nausea and vomiting

Although patients experiencing acute pain often exhibit signs and symptoms such as these, it is critical to note that the absence of any or all of these signs and symptoms does not negate the presence of pain. In fact, some patients, especially those who are critically ill and with little or no compensatory reserves, may have a shock-like clinical picture in the presence of pain.

Critically ill patients also express pain both verbally and nonverbally. The expressions can take many forms, some of which are subtle cues that could easily be overlooked (Table 6–1). Any signs that may indicate pain warrant further exploration and assessment.

Although physiologic and behavioral correlates of acute pain have been described, each person's response to pain is unique. Also, it is important to remember that patients who are receiving neuromuscular blocking agents (e.g., pancuronium, vecuronium, or atracurium) may be unable to exhibit even subtle signs of discomfort because of the therapeutic paralysis. Neuromuscular blocking agents do not affect sensory nerves and have no analgesic qualities.

PAIN ASSESSMENT

Pain assessment is a core element of ongoing surveillance of the critically ill patient. Self-report of pain intensity and distress should be used whenever possible, especially for patients who can talk or communicate effectively. Regular documentation of pain assessment not only helps to monitor the efficacy of analgesic therapies, but also helps to ensure communication among caregivers regarding patients' pain. A variety of tools to assess pain intensity are available. Three commonly used scales are shown in Table 6–2. With the Numeric Rating Scale, patients use numbers between

TABLE 6–1. EXAMPLES OF PAIN EXPRESSION IN CRITICALLY ILL PATIENTS

Verbal Cues	Facial Cues	Body Movements
Moaning	Grimacing	Splinting
Crying	Wincing	Rubbing
Screaming	Eye signals	Rocking
Silence		Rhythmic movement of extremity
		Shaking or tapping bed rails
		Grabbing the nurse's arm

TABLE 6–2. PAIN ASSESSMENT TOOLS COMMONLY USED IN CRITICALLY ILL PATIENTS

Numeric Rating Scales (NRS)

NRS Verbal (*0 to 10 scale*)	NRS-101 (*0 to 100 scale*)
0 = no pain	0 = no pain
10 = worst pain imaginable	100 = worst pain imaginable

Verbal Descriptive Scale

None   Mild   Moderate   Severe

Visual Analog Scale

no pain _____ worst pain imaginable

0 and 10 or 0 and 100 to describe their pain intensity. Some patients find it easier to use adjectives to describe their pain. The Verbal Descriptive Scale offers patients a standardized list of adjectives to describe their pain intensity. With the Visual Analogue Scale (VAS), patients indicate their pain intensity by drawing a vertical line, bisecting a 10-cm baseline. The baseline is anchored at either end by the terms no pain and worst pain imaginable. A numeric conversion is done by measuring the line from the left anchor to the patient's mark, in centimeters.

Any of these scales can be used with patients who are intubated and unable to speak. For example, patients can be asked to use their fingers to indicate a number between 0 and 10; similarly, patients can be asked to indicate by nodding their head or pointing to the appropriate adjective or number as they either hear or read the list of choices. With the VAS, the line can be printed on a sheet of paper or marker board and the patients asked to mark the line to indicate their level of pain.

Unfortunately, some critically ill patients are unable to indicate their pain intensity either verbally or nonverbally. In these situations, nurses must use other clues to assess their patient's pain. In addition to monitoring physiologic parameters, nurses can also anticipate and recognize clinical situations where pain is likely to occur and use their knowledge of physiology and pathophysiology and experience with other patients with similar problems. By combining their knowledge and experience with well-developed interviewing and observational skills, critical care nurses can assess patients' pain effectively and intervene appropriately.

A MULTILEVEL APPROACH TO PAIN MANAGEMENT

Today there are numerous approaches and therapies available to treat acute pain. Whereas pharmacologic techniques traditionally have been the mainstay of analgesia, other complementary or nonpharmacologic methods are growing in their acceptance and use in clinical practice. Most therapies used in the treatment of acute pain can be used effectively

TABLE 6–3. EVIDENCED-BASED PRACTICE: PAIN MANAGEMENT

- Regularly assess and document pain and response to therapy using a scale appropriate for your patient ("0–10" numeric rating scale is recommended).[a,b,c]

- For patients who cannot communicate, assess pain-related behaviors (movement, facial expression, posturing) and physiologic indicators (heart rate, blood pressure, respiratory rate) and the change in these parameters following analgesic therapies.[b,c]

- To ensure consistent analgesia, use scheduled opioid doses or a continuous infusion rather than an "as needed" regimen.[b,c]

- Use NSAIDs or acetaminophen as adjuncts to opioids in selected patients. However, limit ketorolac therapy to 5 days, with close monitoring for the development of renal insufficiency or GI bleeding.[b,c]

- Incorporate nonpharmacologic therapies such as the application of heat/cold, positioning, distraction, or relaxation into the treatment plan as tolerated by your patient.[c]

Data compiled from: [a]Society of Critical Care Medicine, American Society of Health-System Pharmacists (2002). [b]Society of Critical Care Medicine, American Society of Health-System Pharmacists (2002). [c]Stanik-Hutt (1998).

in the critically ill. Evidenced-based practice guidelines to maximize analgesia in critically ill patients are summarized in Table 6–3.

One of the central goals of pain management is to combine therapies that target as many of the processes involved in nociception and pain transmission as possible. Analgesic therapies, both pharmacologic and nonpharmacologic, exert their effects by altering nociception at specific structures within the peripheral or central nervous system (CNS; i.e., the peripheral nociceptors, the spinal cord, or the brain) or by altering the transmission of nociceptive impulses between these structures (Figure 6–4). By understanding where analgesic therapies work, nurses can more effectively select a combination of therapies working at different sites to best treat the source or type of pain patients experience and, subsequently, help patients achieve optimal analgesia.

To assist nurses to select and maximize analgesic therapies, for each of the analgesic therapies presented here, there is a brief description of where and how the selected therapy works, clinical situations where it can be used most effectively, and strategies for titrating the therapy. Finally, because few therapies exert a singular effect, a summary of secondary or side effects commonly associated with the therapies and strategies to minimize their occurrence are also addressed.

NONSTEROIDAL ANTI-INFLAMMATORY DRUGS

Nonsteroidal anti-inflammatory drugs (NSAIDs) target the peripheral nociceptors. The NSAIDs exert their effect by modifying or reducing the amount of prostaglandin produced at the site of injury by inhibiting the formation of the enzyme cyclooxygenase, which is responsible for the breakdown of arachidonic acid and formation of the neurotransmitter prostaglandin. As prostaglandin inhibitors, the NSAIDs have been shown to have opioid-sparing effects and are very effective in managing pain associated with inflammation, trauma to peripheral tissues (e.g., soft tissue injuries), bone pain (e.g., fractures, metastatic disease), and pain associated with indwelling tubes and drains (e.g., chest tubes).

One of the NSAIDs commonly used in the critical care setting is ketorolac tromethamine (Toradol). Ketorolac is currently the only parenteral NSAID preparation available in the United States and can be administered safely by either the intravenous (IV) or the intramuscular (IM) route. Recommended dosing for ketorolac is a 30-mg loading dose followed by 15 mg every 6 hours. Like all NSAIDs, ketorolac has a ceiling effect where administration of higher doses offers no additional therapeutic benefit yet significantly increases the risk of toxicity.

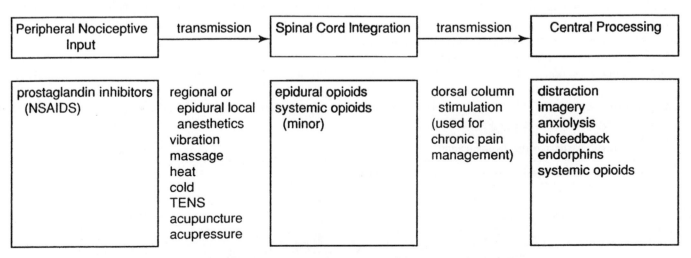

Figure 6–4. A multilevel approach to pain management.

Side Effects

The side effects associated with the use of NSAIDs relate to the function of prostaglandins in physiologic processes in addition to nociception. For example, gastrointestinal (GI) irritation and bleeding may result from NSAID use because prostaglandins are necessary for maintaining the mucous lining of the stomach. Similarly, the enzyme cyclooxygenase is needed for the eventual production of thromboxane, a key substance involved in platelet function. As a result, when NSAIDs are used chronically or in high doses, platelet aggregation may be altered, leading to bleeding problems. NSAID use can also lead to renal toxicity. Cross-sensitivities with other NSAIDs have also been documented (e.g., ibuprofen, naproxen, indomethacin, piroxicam, aspirin). For these reasons, ketorolac and other NSAIDs should be avoided for patients who have a history of gastric ulceration, renal insufficiency, and coagulopathies or a documented sensitivity to aspirin or other NSAIDs. The severity of all NSAID-related side effects increases with high doses or prolonged use. For this reason, ketorolac is designed for short-term therapy only and should not be used for more than 5 days.

OPIOIDS

The principal modality of pain management in the critical care setting continues to be opioids. Traditionally referred to as *narcotics,* opioids produce their analgesic effects primarily by binding with specialized opiate receptors throughout the CNS and thereby altering the perception of pain. Opiate receptors are located in the brain, spinal cord, and GI tract. Although opioids work primarily within the CNS, they also have been shown to have some local or peripheral effects.

Opioids are well tolerated by most critically ill patients and can be administered by many routes including IV, IM, oral, buccal, nasal, rectal, transdermal, and intraspinal. Morphine sulfate is still the most widely used opioid and serves as the gold standard against which others are compared. Other opioids commonly used in the care of the critically ill include hydromorphone (Dilaudid), fentanyl (Sublimaze), and meperidine (Demerol). One of the key aspects of opioid therapy is that each potentially produces the same degree of pain relief; none is inherently more likely to produce analgesia than another. Table 6–4 summarizes the equi-

analgesic IV doses and special considerations for commonly used opioids.

Side Effects

Patients' responses to opioids, both analgesic responses and side effects, are highly individualized. Just as all the opioid agents have similar pain-relieving potential, all opioids currently available share similar side effect profiles. When side effects do occur, it is important to remember that they are primarily the result of opioid pharmacology, as opposed to the route of administration.

Nausea and Vomiting

Nausea and vomiting are distressing side effects often related to opioids that, unfortunately, many patients experience. Generally, nausea and vomiting result from stimulation of the chemoreceptor trigger zone (CTZ) in the brain and/or from slowed GI peristalsis. Nausea and vomiting often can be managed effectively with anti-emetic therapy. Metoclopramide (Reglan), a procainamide derivative, works both centrally at the CTZ and at the GI level to increase gastric motility. Most patients will benefit from a 10-mg IV dose every 4 to 6 hours.

The vestibular system also sends input to the CTZ. For this reason, opioid-related nausea frequently is exacerbated by movement. If patients complain of movement-related nausea, the application of a transdermal scopolamine patch can help prevent and treat opioid-induced nausea. The use of transdermal scopolamine is best avoided in patients older than 60 years because the drug has been reported to increase the incidence and severity of confusion in older patients.

Other anti-emetics such as the phenothiazines (prochlorperazine [Compazine], 2.5 to 10 mg IV) and the butyrophenones (droperidol [Inapsine], 0.625 mg IV) treat nausea through their effects at the CTZ. The serotonin antagonist ondansetron (Zofran) is also effective for treatment of opioid-related nausea. The doses required for postoperative or opioid-related nausea are significantly smaller doses (4 mg IV) than those used with emetogenic chemotherapy.

Pruritus

Pruritus is another opioid-related side effect commonly reported by patients. The actual mechanisms producing opioid-related pruritus are unknown. Although antihistamines can

TABLE 6–4. COMMONLY USED INTRAVENOUS OPIODS

Drug	Equianalgesic Dose	Onset (min)	Duration (h)	Special Considerations
Morphine	1 mg	2–5	4	
Hydromorphone	0.15 mg	2–5	2–4	
Fentanyl	10–25 μg	1–2	1–1.5	Highly lipid soluble; muscle rigidity has been reported with high doses
Meperidine	10 mg	2–5	2–3	Active metabolite (normeperidine) which can accumulate resulting in CNS excitation and seizures; tachyarrhythmias can result

provide symptomatic relief for some patients, the role of histamine in opioid-related pruritus is unclear. One of the drawbacks of using antihistamine agents, such as diphenhydramine (Benadryl), is the sedation associated with their use. Similar to other opioid side effects, the incidence and severity of pruritus is dose related and tends to diminish with ongoing use.

Constipation

Constipation, another common side effect, results from opioid binding at opiate receptors in the GI tract and decreased peristalsis. Whereas the incidence of constipation may be low in critically ill patients, it is important to remember that it is likely to be a problem for many patients after the critical phase of their illness or injury. The best treatment for constipation is prevention by ensuring adequate hydration, as well as by administering stimulant laxatives and stool softeners, as needed.

Urinary Retention

Urinary retention can result from increased smooth muscle tone caused by opioids, especially in the detrussor muscle of the bladder. Opioids have no effect on urine production and neither cause nor worsen oliguria. Urinary retention is generally not a problem for critically ill patients because many have indwelling urinary catheters to facilitate and measure bladder drainage.

Respiratory Depression

Opioid therapy can result in respiratory depression through its effects on the respiratory centers in the brain stem. Both respiratory rate and depth of breathing can decrease as a result of opioids, usually in a dose-dependent fashion. Patients at increased risk for respiratory depression include the elderly, those with preexisting cardiopulmonary diseases, and those who receive large doses. Frequently, the earliest sign of respiratory depression is an increased level of sedation, making this an important component of patient assessment. Other signs and symptoms of respiratory depression include decreased depth of breathing, often combined with slowed respiratory rate, constriction of pupils, and hypercapnia ($Paco_2$ >45 mm Hg).

Clinically significant respiratory depression is usually treated with IV naloxone (Narcan). Naloxone is an opioid antagonist; it binds with opiate receptors, temporarily displacing the opioid and suspending its pharmacologic effects. As with other medications, naloxone should be administered in very small doses and titrated to the desired level of alertness (Table 6–5). It should be emphasized that the half-life of naloxone is short—approximately 30 to 45 minutes. Because of its short half-life, additional doses of naloxone may be needed. Naloxone should be used with caution in patients with underlying cardiovascular disease; the acute onset of

TABLE 6–5. ADMINISTRATION OF NALOXONE

1. Support ventilation.
2. Dilute 0.4 mg (400 μg) ampule of naloxone with normal saline to constitute a 10-mL solution.
3. Administer in 1-mL increments, every 2–5 min, titrating to desired effect. Onset of action: approximately 2 min.
4. Continue to monitor patient; readminister naloxone as needed. Duration of action: approximately 45 min.
5. For patients requiring ongoing doses, consider naloxone infusion: administer at 50–250 μg/h, titrating to desired response.

hypertension, pulmonary hypertension, and pulmonary edema with naloxone administration has been reported. Also, naloxone should be avoided in patients who have developed a tolerance to opioids since as an opioid antagonist it can precipitate withdrawal or acute abstinence syndrome.

Intravenous Opioids

Because many critically ill patients are unable to use the oral route and pain management needs often fluctuate, the IV route is used most often. One of the advantages of IV opioids is their rapid onset of action, allowing for easy titration. Loading doses of IV opioids should be administered to achieve an adequate blood level of the drug; additional doses can then be administered intermittently to maintain analgesic levels.

Many critically ill patients can benefit from the addition of a continuous IV opioid infusion. For example, patients who may not be able to communicate their pain management needs effectively, including those who are receiving neuromuscular blocking agents, are good candidates for continuous opioid infusions. The continuous infusion not only helps achieve the appropriate blood levels, but also can be easily titrated to maintain consistent blood levels. Patients who experience significant fluctuations in analgesia or side effects related to opioid administration may also benefit from the constant blood levels provided by continuous infusions. Whenever possible, the maintenance dose for the infusion should be based on patients' previous opioid requirements.

Patient-Controlled Analgesia

Patient-controlled analgesia (PCA) pumps can also be used effectively in the critical care setting to administer opioids. With PCA, patients self-administer small doses of an opioid infusion using a programmable pump. PCA prescriptions typically include an incremental or bolus dose of the selected drug, a lockout or delay interval, and either a 1- or 4-hour limit; many of the PCA devices also can be programmed to deliver a basal or background infusion. The *incremental dose* refers to the amount of the drug the patient receives following pump activation. The initial dose usually ranges between 0.5 and 2.0 mg of morphine, or its equivalent (see Table 6–4). The lockout or delay interval typically ranges between 5 and 10 minutes, which is enough time for the prescribed drug to circulate and take effect, yet allows the patient to easily titrate the medication over time. The 1- or 4-hour limit serves as an additional safety feature by regulating the amount of medication the patient can receive over this period of time.

Assessing whether a critically ill patient is capable of using PCA is critical to the success of this analgesic therapy. PCA should not be prescribed for the patient who is unable to reliably self-administer pain medication (e.g., a patient with a decreased level of consciousness). A patient, however, who is cognitively intact but unable to activate the PCA button due to lack of manual dexterity or strength may utilize a PCA device that has been ergonomically adapted to suit the patient with impaired motor abilities (e.g., a pressure switch pad). Lastly, if PCA is prescribed, patients, family members, and visitors should be educated that the patient is the only person to activate the PCA device. Family members and friends may think they are helping by activating the PCA device for the patient and not realize this can produce life-threatening sedation and respiratory depression.

Titrating PCA

As with nurse-administered IV opioid boluses, PCA is most effective when patients can titrate the amount of medication they receive to meet their analgesic needs by maintaining consistent blood levels. Patients usually find a dose and frequency that balances pain relief with other medication-related side effects such as sedation. It is best to start PCA therapy after the patient has received loading doses to achieve adequate blood levels of the prescribed opioid. For patients who continue to experience pain while using the PCA pump, the first step in titration is to increase the incremental or bolus dose, usually by 50%. If patients continue to have pain in spite of the increased dose, the lockout interval or delay should then be reduced, if possible.

Patients who report problems with awakening in pain and feeling "behind" with their analgesia may benefit from the addition of a low-dose, continuous infusion. A continuous infusion is also recommended for patients who have pre-existing opioid tolerance. In this way, the continuous infusion maintains their baseline opioid requirements, and the patient-controlled incremental doses are available to help manage any new pain they experience. The hourly dose of the continuous infusion should be equi-analgesic to and calculated from patients' preexisting opioid requirements.

Switching From IV to Oral Opioid Analgesia

Most often switching from IV to oral opioids is accomplished when acute pain subsides and the patient is able to tolerate oral or enteral nutrition. Patients who receive anal-

---

AT THE BEDSIDE
Epidural Catheter Pain Management

A 59-year-old man was admitted to the surgical ICU following a thoracotomy with wedge resection of the left lung for small-cell lung cancer. On his second postoperative day, he continued to be mechanically ventilated with extubation planned for later in the day. He had two left pleural chest tubes in place with moderate amounts of drainage and a continuing air leak. He was alert, responsive, and able to communicate his needs by writing notes and gesturing. He had a thoracic epidural catheter in place (T7–8) with a bupivacaine (0.625 mg/mL) and fentanyl (5 µg/mL) combination infusing at 6 mL/h. When asked about his pain level, he wrote that it was 4 on a scale of 0 (no pain) to 10 (worst pain imaginable).

After he was extubated, his nurse noticed he was reluctant to cough and seemed to have some difficulty taking a deep breath. She also noticed his oxygen saturation was slowly drifting downward from 97% to 95%. His respiratory rate was increasing, as was his heart rate. When she listened to his breath sounds, they were bilateral and equal, but diminished throughout with scattered gurgles. When she asked him about his pain, he said his pain was still a 4 as long as he did not move or cough. He also indicated that he tried to avoid taking a deep breath because it would make him cough and that made the pain go to an 8 or 10.

The nurse knew it would be important for this patient to breathe deeply and cough to clear his lungs, but his pain and discomfort were limiting his ability to perform those maneuvers. She discussed strategies to help minimize the pain associated with activity. First, she found an extra pillow for him to use as a splint to support not only his incision and chest wall, but also to stabilize his chest tubes.

Next, the nurse assessed the level of sensory blockade provided by the epidural LA. When she found his sensory level to extend bilaterally from T-10 to T-6, while his incision extended to T-4, she called the anesthesiologist to confer about increasing the rate of the bupivacaine infusion to increase the distribution of the LA to cover the incisional area. She also inquired about adding ketorolac to his analgesic regimen to help with pain associated with the chest tubes.

The addition of the pillows for splinting especially helped the patient to take deep breaths. The anesthesiologist prescribed an increase in the infusion rate to 10 mL/h and added ketorolac, 15 mg, IV every 6 hours. Over the course of the next 2 hours, the sensory block extended from T-11 to T-4 and the patient was able to cough more effectively, with less pain. His oxygen saturation returned to 97%.

---

gesics by mouth or via the enteral route can experience comparable pain relief to parenteral analgesia with less risk of infection and at lowered cost. Calculating the equi-analgesic dose increases the likelihood that the transition to the oral route will be made without loss of pain control. A creative way to wean PCA is to substitute oral or enteral opioid (like morphine or oxycodone) for the amount of drug given by

AT THE BEDSIDE
▶ *Chemical Dependence*

A 22-year-old woman was admitted to the cardiovascular ICU (CVICU) following a tricuspid valve replacement related to recurrent subacute bacterial endocarditis. She has a self-reported history of heroin use (approximately 2 g/d).

She was extubated within the first 24 hours after surgery, but remained in the CVICU for stabilization of fluid balance. During change-of-shift report the off-going nurse commented that ". . . she is a constant whine. She refuses to do anything. All she wants is to go out for a smoke and more drugs. She had 10 mg of IV morphine from the PCA pump."

When the nurse came into this patient's room to make her initial assessment, the patient said, "I can't take much more of this pain." The nurse probed further and asked her to use some numbers to describe her pain. She replied, "It's at 10!"

The nurse noticed that the patient was reluctant to move and refused to cough. Her vital signs were:

Heart rate	130/min
BP	150/85 mm Hg
Temperature	38.5°C (orally)
Respiration rate	26/min, shallow

The nurse was concerned that because of this patient's preoperative use of heroin, she might not be receiving adequate doses of morphine. She consulted the clinical nurse specialist for assistance in calculating an equivalent dose of morphine based on the usual heroin use. Using an estimated equivalence of heroin of 1 g = 10 to 15 mg morphine, the nurse calculated that the patient would need approximately 20 to 30 mg of morphine per day to account for her preexisting opioid tolerance; analgesic needs related to her surgery would need to be in addition to this baseline need. The primary nurse approached the surgical team to discuss the potential benefits of using a PCA pump in addition to a continuous infusion of morphine. "By doing this," the nurse explained, "She could receive her baseline opioid requirements related to her tolerance by the continuous infusion, while using the patient-controlled boluses to treat her new surgical pain. The PCA could also offer her some control during a time in her recovery when there are few avenues to maintain it." In addition to starting the PCA with a continuous infusion, the surgical team and the primary nurse also discussed using other nonopioid agents such as NSAIDs to augment her analgesia.

In addition to the changes in the medications, the primary nurse worked with the patient to use relaxation techniques. The nurse explained that relaxation techniques could be thought of as "boosters" to her pain medications and were something that she could do to control the pain. They also agreed to try massage in the evening to try to promote sleep and relaxation.

continuous infusion plus one-half of the total dosage of PCA demand doses. Over the next 24 hours, reducing PCA consumption by increasing the lockout period or reducing the bolus size may help to transition the patient and narrow the

"analgesic gap" between different routes. Controlled-release preparations of morphine and oxycodone, designed to be taken less frequently than their immediate-release counterparts, should not be crushed, halved, or administered into enteral feeding tubes to prevent opioid overdosage.

EPIDURAL ANALGESIA

Over the past decade the use of epidural analgesia has grown rapidly, especially in the critical care setting. The advantages of epidural analgesia include improved pain control with less sedation, lower overall opioid doses, and generally longer duration. Epidural analgesia has been associated with a lower morbidity and mortality in critically ill patients. Both opioids and local anesthetics (LAs), either alone or in combination, commonly are administered via the epidural route. Epidural analgesia may be administered by several methods, including intermittent bolus dosing, continuous infusion or PCA technology. The mechanisms of action and the resultant clinical effects produced by epidurally administered opioids and LAs are distinct. For this reason, these agents not only are discussed separately, but also should be distinguished when used in clinical practice.

Epidural Opioids

When opioids are administered epidurally, they diffuse into the cerebrospinal fluid and into the spinal cord (Figure 6–5). There, the opioids bind with opiate receptors in the substantia gelatinosa, preventing the release of the neurotransmitter, substance P, and subsequently alter the transmission of nociceptive impulses from the spinal cord to the brain. Because the opioid is concentrated in the areas of high opiate receptor density and where nociceptive impulses are entering the spinal cord, lower doses offer enhanced analgesia, with few, if any, supraspinal effects such as drowsiness.

A variety of opioids are commonly used for epidural analgesia including morphine, fentanyl, meperidine, and hydromorphone. Preservative-free (PF) preparations are usually preferred because some preservative agents can have neurotoxic effects. The opioids can be administered either by intermittent bolus or continuous infusion depending on the pharmacokinetic activity of the selected agent. For example, fentanyl is generally administered via continuous infusion due to its high lipid solubility, resulting in a short duration of action. In contrast, the low lipid solubility of PF morphine results in a delayed onset of action (30 to 60 minutes) and a prolonged duration of action (6 to 12 hours). Because of this, PF morphine can be administered effectively as an intermittent bolus.

Side Effects

The side effects associated with epidural opioids are the same as those described for oral opioids. It is important to remember that side effects are related more closely to the drug

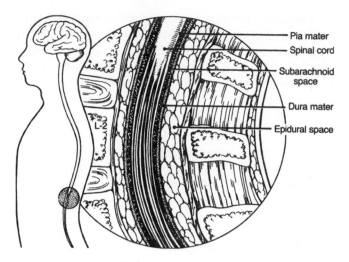

Pia mater
Spinal cord
Subarachnoid space
Dura mater
Epidural space

Figure 6–5. Epidural space for catheter placement.

administered than by the route of administration. For example, the incidence of nausea and vomiting with epidural morphine is similar to that associated with IV morphine. Although epidural opioids were once feared to be associated with a higher risk of respiratory depression, clinical studies and experience have not confirmed this risk. The incidence of respiratory depression has been reported as being no higher than 0.2%. Risk factors for respiratory depression are similar to those seen with IV opioids: increasing age, high doses, underlying cardiopulmonary dysfunction, and the use of perioperative or supplemental parenteral opioids in addition to epidural opioids.

Epidural Local Anesthetics

Epidural opioids can also be combined with dilute concentrations of LAs. When administered in combination, these agents work synergistically, reducing the amount of each agent that is needed to produce analgesia. Whereas epidurally administered opioids work in the dorsal horn of the spinal cord, epidural LAs exert work primarily at the dorsal nerve root by blocking the conduction of afferent sensory fibers. The extent of the blockade is dose related. Higher LA concentrations block more afferent fibers within a given region, resulting in an increased density of the blockade. Higher infusion rates of LA-containing solutions increase the extent or spread of the blockade because more afferent fibers are blocked over a broader region.

Bupivacaine is the LA most commonly used for epidural analgesia and is usually administered in combination with either fentanyl or PF morphine as a continuous infusion. The concentration of bipuvicaine used for epidural analgesia usually ranges between 1/16% (0.065 mg/mL) and 1/8% (1.25 mg/mL). These concentrations are significantly lower than those used for surgical anesthesia, which usually

range between 1/4% and 1/2% bipuvicaine. The type and concentration of opioid used in combination with bipuvicaine vary by practitioner and organizational preferences, but usually range between 2 and 5 μg/mL fentanyl or between 0.02 and 0.04 mg/mL PF morphine.

Side Effects

The side effects accompanying LAs are a direct result of the conduction blockade produced by the agents. Unfortunately, the LA agents are relatively nonspecific in their capacity to block nerve conduction. That is, LAs not only block sensory afferent fibers, but also can block the conduction of motor efferent and autonomic nerve fibers within the same dermatomal regions. Side effects associated with epidural LAs include hypotension—especially postural hypotension from sympathetic blockade—and functional motor deficits from varying degrees of efferent motor fiber blockade. Sensory deficits, including changes in proprioception in the joints of the lower extremities, can accompany epidural LA administration due to the blockade of non-nociceptive sensory afferents.

The extent and type of side effects that can be anticipated with epidural LAs depend on three primary factors: the location of the epidural catheter, the concentration of the LA administered, and the volume or rate of infusion. For example, if a patient has an epidural catheter placed within the midthoracic region, one can anticipate signs of sympathetic nervous blockade, such as postural hypotension, because the sympathetic nerve fibers are concentrated in the thoracic region. In contrast, a patient with a lumbar catheter may experience a mild degree of motor weakness in the lower extremities because the motor efferent and nerves exit the spine in the lumbar region. This usually presents clinically as either heaviness in a lower extremity or an inability to "lock" the knee in place when standing.

Also, as noted, both the concentration and infusion rate of the LA influence the severity and extent of side effects. The density of the blockade and intensity of observed side effects may be increased with high LA concentrations. With higher infusion volumes, greater spread of the LA can be anticipated which can, in turn, lead to a greater number or extent of side effects. If side effects occur, the dose of the LA often is reduced either by decreasing the concentration of the solution or by decreasing the rate.

Titrating Epidural Analgesia

To maximize epidural analgesia, doses may need to be adjusted. With opioids alone, the dose needed to produce effective analgesia is best predicted by the patient's age as opposed to body size. Older patients typically require lower doses to achieve pain relief than those who are younger. Small bolus doses of fentanyl (50 μg) can help to safely titrate the epidural dose or infusion to treat pain. Similarly, a small bolus dose of fentanyl can also help to treat breakthrough pain that may occur with increased patient activity or procedures. For patients receiving combinations of LAs and opioids, a small bolus dose of the prescribed infusate in conjunction with an increased rate can help to titrate pain relief. Recall, however, that increasing the rate of the LA infusion increases the spread of the drug to additional dermatomes, whereas increasing the LA concentration increases the depth or intensity of the blockade and subsequent analgesia.

CUTANEOUS STIMULATION

One of the primary nonpharmacologic techniques for pain management used in the critical care setting is cutaneous stimulation. Cutaneous stimulation produces its analgesic effect by the altering conduction of sensory impulses as they move from the periphery to the spinal cord through the stimulation of the largest sensory afferent fibers, known as the A-alpha and A-beta fibers. The sensory information transmitted by these large fibers is conducted more rapidly than that carried by their smaller counterparts (A-delta and C fibers). As a result, nociceptive input from the A-delta and C fibers is believed to be "preempted" by the sensory input from the non-noxious cutaneous stimuli. Examples of cutaneous stimulation include the application of heat, cold, vibration, or massage. Transcutaneous electrical nerve stimulation units produce similar effects by electrically stimulating large sensory fibers.

Cutaneous stimulation can produce potent analgesia whether used as a complementary therapy with other pharmacologic treatments or as an independent treatment modality. Nurses can integrate these therapies easily and safely into analgesic treatment plans for the critically ill, especially for patients who may be unable to tolerate higher opioid doses. To apply or administer cutaneous stimulation, one simply needs to stimulate sensory fibers anywhere between the site of injury and the spinal cord, but within the sensory dermatome (Figure 6–6). Massage, especially back massage, has additional analgesic benefits; it has been shown to promote relaxation and sleep, both of which can influence patients' responses to pain.

DISTRACTION

Distraction techniques such as music, conversation, television viewing, laughter, and deep breathing for relaxation can be valuable adjuncts to pharmacologic therapies. These techniques produce their analgesic effects by sending intense stimuli through the thalamus, midbrain, and brain stem, which can increase the production of modulating substances such as endorphins. Also, because the brain can process only a limited amount of incoming signals at any given time, the input provided by distraction techniques "competes" with nociceptive inputs. This is particularly true for the reticular activating system.

When planning for and using distraction techniques, keep in mind that they are most effective when activities are interesting to the patient (e.g., their favorite type of music, television program, or video) and when they involve multiple senses such as hearing, vision, touch, and movement. Activities should be consistent with patients' energy levels and, most of all, be flexible to meet changing demands.

IMAGERY

Imagery is another technique that can be used effectively with critically ill patients, particularly during planned procedures. Imagery alters the perception of pain stimuli within the brain, promotes relaxation, and increases the production of endorphins in the brain. Patients can use imagery independently or use guided imagery where either a care provider, family member, or friend helps to "guide" the patient in painting an imaginary picture. The more details that can be pictured with the image, the more effective it can be. As with distraction techniques, tapping into multiple sensations is beneficial. Some patients prefer to involve the pain in their picture and imagine it melting or fading away. Other patients may prefer to paint a picture in their mind of a favorite place or activity. Strategies to help guide patients include the use of details to describe the imaginary scene (e.g., "smell the fresh scent of the ocean air" or "see the intense red hue of the sun setting beyond the snow-capped mountains") and the use of relaxing sensory terms such as *floating, smooth, dissolving, lighter,* or *melting.* If the patients are able to talk, it can be helpful to have them describe the image they see using appropriate detail, although some patients will prefer not to talk and instead focus on their evolving image. Again, it is important to be flexible in the approach to imagery to maximize its benefits.

RELAXATION AND SEDATION TECHNIQUES

Because critically ill patients experience numerous stressors, most patients benefit from the inclusion of relaxation or anxiolytic therapies. The use of relaxation techniques can help to interrupt the vicious cycle involving pain, anxiety, and muscle tension that often develops when pain goes unrelieved. The physiologic response associated with relaxation includes decreased oxygen consumption, respiratory rate, heart rate, and muscle tension; blood pressure may either normalize or decrease.

A wide variety of pharmacologic and nonpharmacologic techniques can be used safely and effectively with critically ill patients to achieve relaxation and/or sedation. Relaxation techniques are simple to use and can be particularly useful in situations involving brief procedures such as turning or minor dressing changes, and following coughing or endotracheal suctioning or other stressful events.

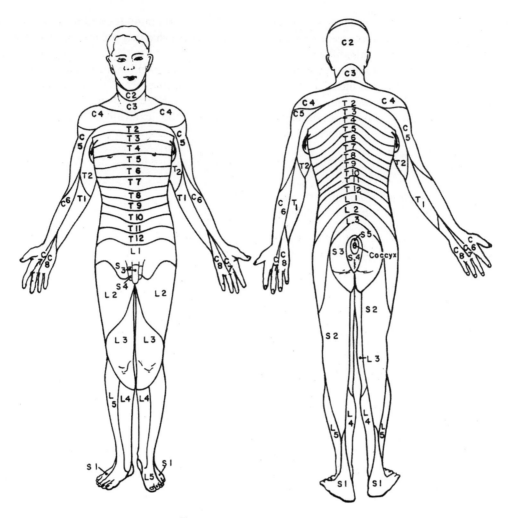

Figure 6–6. Sensory dermatomes.

Deep Breathing and Progressive Relaxation

Guided deep breathing and progressive relaxation can be incorporated easily into a plan of care for the critically ill patient. Nurses can coach patients with deep breathing exercises by helping them to focus on and guide their breathing patterns. As patients begin to control their breathing, nurses can work with them to begin progressive relaxation of their muscles. To do this, the nurse can say to the patient as he or she just begins to exhale, "Now begin to relax, from the top of your head to the tips of your toes." Change the pitch of the voice to be higher for "top of your head," lower for "tips of your toes," and be timed such that the final phrase ends as the patient completes exhalation. This procedure capitalizes on the positive aspects of normal body functions, as the body tends to relax naturally during exhalation. This process can and should be "practiced" during nonstressful periods to augment its efficacy. In fact, teaching and coaching patients to use deep breathing exercises helps to equip them with a life-long skill that can be used any time stressful or painful situations arise.

Presence

Probably the single most important aspect of promoting comfort in the critically ill or injured is the underlying relationship between the patient and his or her care providers. *Presence* not only refers to physically "being there," but also refers to psychologically "being with" a patient. Although presence has not been well-defined as an intervention protocol, patients regularly describe the importance of the support that their nurses render simply by "being there" and "being with" them.

SPECIAL CONSIDERATIONS FOR PAIN MANAGEMENT IN THE ELDERLY

The pain experience of elderly patients has often been shadowed by myths and misperceptions. Some believe that older patients have less pain because their extensive life experiences have equipped them to cope with discomfort more effectively. Although this may be true for some individuals, to accept this generalization as truth for all elderly patients is short sighted. In fact, the incidence of and morbidity associated with pain is higher in the elderly than in the general population. Many elderly patients continue to experience chronic pain in addition to any acute pain associated with their critical illness or injury. Major sources of underlying pain in the elderly include low back pain, arthritis, headache, chest pain, and neuropathies.

Assessment

Elderly patients often report pain very differently from younger patients due to physiologic, psychological, and cultural changes accompanying age. Some patients may fear loss of control or being labeled as a "bad patient" if they report pain-related concerns. Also, for some patients the presence of pain may be symbolic of impending death, especially in the critical care setting. In such cases, a patient may be reticent to report his or her pain to a care provider or family member as if to deny pain is to deny death. For reasons such as these, it is important for nurses not only to assure patients about the nature of their pain and the importance of reporting any discomfort, but also to use a variety of pain assessment strategies to incorporate behavioral or physiologic indicators of pain.

Similar strategies are often needed to assess pain in persons who are cognitively impaired. Preliminary reports from ongoing work among nursing home patients suggest that many patients with moderate to severe cognitive impairment are able to report acute pain reliably at the time they are asked. For these patients, pain recall and integration of pain experience over time may be less reliable.

Interventions

Critically ill elderly patients can benefit from any of the analgesic therapies discussed. It is important to recall that for some elderly patients, medication requirements may be reduced due to the decreased clearance with varying degrees of renal insufficiency that accompanies aging. However, as with all patients, regardless of age, analgesic requirements are highly individualized and doses should be carefully titrated to achieve pain relief.

SEDATION

The critical care environment can be uncomfortable and anxiety provoking for patients and families. Critically ill patients, especially those requiring mechanical ventilation, often require sedation to decrease awareness of noxious stimuli, ensure tolerance of medical therapies, and protect from inadvertent self-harm. Manifestations of intolerance include behaviors such as agitation, thrashing, ventilator dyssynchrony, and the inability to rest or sleep. Because all of these behaviors can be manifestations of pain or discomfort,

it is important that appropriate analgesia be administered prior to the provision of sedatives. Occasionally, even high-dose infusions of analgesics and anxiolytics are not adequate to ensure a safe and tolerant state. In these instances neuromuscular blockade (NMB) may be necessary.

To ensure that appropriate and adequate anxiolysis is achieved in the critically ill patient, the nurse must be able to identify the need for sedation, the drugs most commonly used, the level of sedation required, and how to monitor and manage the sedated patient. Clear identification of the reason for sedation is the first step in the process. To ensure that the choice of sedative and goals for sedation administration are appropriate, it is important to identify the reason for sedation.

Reasons for sedation
Amnesia
One of the most common reasons for sedative use is to ensure amnesia. Many of the procedures and interventions performed in critical care may potentially cause pain and anxiety. In anticipation of this, sedatives are proactively administered, often concomitantly with analgesics.

Ventilator Tolerance
Ineffective, dys-synchronous, and excessive respiratory effort results in increased work of breathing and increased oxygen consumption. Sedative use in these conditions may be life saving. Also, in severe respiratory failure conditions, such as acute respiratory distress syndrome (ARDS) or acute asthma, the use of protective lung strategies (i.e., low tidal volume ventilation) and selected modes of ventilation (i.e., inverse ratio ventilation) result in acid–base abnormalities and nonphysiologic respiratory patterns that are not well-tolerated in the conscious patient. To ensure tolerance in these cases sedatives are necessary and often combined with paralytic agents to assure the goal (see Chapter 20, Advanced Respiratory Concepts).

Anxiety and Fear
Anxiety and fear are symptoms that can be experienced by critically ill patients who are conscious. These symptoms, though, are often difficult to assess in critically ill patients because many cannot adequately communicate their feelings secondary to the underlying condition or the presence of artificial airways. When the patient can identify anxiety or fear (the most severe level of anxiety and one associated with extreme fight or flight behaviors), the treatment goals are clear. However, in the patient who cannot, the presence of behaviors and signs that are associated with anxiety and/or fear are used as evidence and are the reason sedatives are provided. They include nonspecific signs of distress such as agitation, thrashing, diaphoresis, facial grimacing, blood pressure elevation, and increased heart rate. Unfortunately, these

nonspecific signs may also be indicative of pain. Pain management requirements must be addressed prior to the administration of sedation in such cases. In most cases both analgesia and sedation are provided to ensure comfort.

Patient Safety and Agitation

Agitation includes any activity that appears unhelpful or potentially harmful to the patient. The patient may be aware of the activity and be able to communicate the reason for the activity; more commonly they are not aware, making it difficult to identify the reason for the agitation. The patient appears distressed and the associated activity includes episodic or continuous nonpurposeful movements in the bed, severe thrashing, attempts to remove tubes, efforts to get out of bed, or other behaviors which may threaten patient or staff safety. Reasons for agitation include pain and anxiety, preexisting conditions that require pharmacologic interventions (i.e., preexisting psychiatric history), withdrawal from certain medications such as benzodiazepines (especially if they have been on them for a long time), and delirium tremens. Patients who experience inadequately controlled agitation face a high risk of morbidity and mortality.

Sleep Deprivation

Sleep deprivation is common among critically ill patients. Although patients may appear restful, physiologically they may never experience those stages of sleep that ensure a "rested" state (i.e., rapid eye movement sleep, stages 3 and 4). These restorative stages of sleep are adversely affected by many factors, including medications. Sleep deprivation is also common among those with pain, discomfort, and anxiety. Additionally, sleep deprivation may be a result of the increased auditory, tactile, and visual stimuli ubiquitous to the critical care environment.

Delirium

Delirium appears to be more prevalent in critically ill patients than previously assumed. Often called *intensive care unit (ICU) psychosis,* delirium is frequently a diagnosis of exclusion. Agitation is the most common physical manifestation, and other causes must be ruled out first. The condition is associated with disorientation, disorganized thinking, altered sleep–wake cycles, illusions, and hallucinations (see Figure 12–2). Risk factors include medications such as steroids or sensory overload or underload.

Drugs for Sedation

After ensuring that the presence of pain is either ruled out or addressed with the appropriate administration of analgesics, sedatives may be selected based on patient-specific factors such as the level and duration of sedation required. Sedative category summaries follow and comprehensive descriptions of the drugs are found in Chapter 7, Pharmacology.

Short-Term Duration Sedatives

These sedatives have a rapid onset of action and a short duration of effect.

- *Midazolam* is a popular benzodiazepine that fits in this category. It can be administered intermittently in a bolus IV form or as a continuous infusion. Long-term infusions (>24 hours) of midazolam are discouraged because the drug has an active metabolite that may accumulate in the presence of drugs, renal disease, liver disease, or old age.
- *Propofol* is an IV *general* anesthetic designed for use as a continuous infusion. This drug is often preferred for short-term sedation use (<24 hours) and in those patients who may need a few days of sedation but in whom a very rapid offset of effect is desired. An example is the patient requiring frequent neurologic assessments. The drug is lipid based and serves as a source of calories. It should be used cautiously in those with high triglycerides. Frequent changes of the containers and tubing are required to prevent potential growth of microorganisms.
- *Dexmedetomadine* is an alpha-2 receptor agonist that has been approved only for very short term use (<24 hours) in the ICU setting. Two of the reasons the drug may be an attractive choice include the drug's ability to either eliminate or decrease the need for other analgesic medications such as opioids, and the fact that it does not produce respiratory depression. Further, patients on the drug are rapidly arousable and alert when stimulated.
- *Ketamine* is an IV general anesthetic that produces analgesia, anesthesia, and amnesia without loss of consciousness. It may be given in an IV bolus form, intranasally, or orally. Although contraindicated in those with elevated intracranial pressure, its bronchodilatory properties make it a good choice in those with asthma. A well-known side effect of ketamine is hallucinations; however, these may be prevented with concurrent use of benzodiazepines. It is rarely a first-line sedative of choice, but is commonly used in patients requiring painful, frequent skin debridement procedures.

Intermediate-Term Sedatives

These drugs have an intermediate onset of action and duration of effect. However, when given as infusions they may last much longer as they are lipophilic.

- *Lorazepam* is the most commonly used benzodiazepine in critical care and can be administered orally and IV as an intermittent bolus or continuous infusion. When given orally or in a bolus intermittent form, the drug effect is intermediate; however, when used as a continuous infusion (>24 hours), its effect is more long term (and it should be considered as such) because awakening may take hours to days to accomplish. Lorazepam may accumulate in those with decreased metabolic function such as the elderly or those with hepatic dysfunction; however, there is less risk overall because there is minimal active metabolite accumulation with the drug.

Long-Acting Sedatives

- *Diazepam and chlordiazpoxide*, long-acting benzodiazepines, are rarely used in critical care; however, they may be selected for treatment of severe alcohol withdrawal. They may be given orally or as an IV bolus.

Drugs for Delirium

The drug of choice for management of ICU delirium is haloperidol. Haloperidol sedates without significant respiratory suppression and is associated with little potential for the development of tolerance or dependence. It does, however, have potential adverse side effects that must be closely monitored. Extrapyramidal reactions such as dystonia and the potential for neuroleptic malignant syndrome are possible. Another is the effect of haloperidol on QTc intervals; QTc interval monitoring is essential and required when using the drug.

Goals of Sedation, Monitoring, and Management

The goal of sedation administration is important to identify (anxiety, sleep, ventilator tolerance, amnesia, etc.) and once accomplished, a level of sedation may be determined. For example, in the patient who is anxious and unable to sleep, the goal is very different than if the patient is unstable, on a ventilator, and suffering from profound hypoxemia. Sedation scales have been developed in an effort to assist with the management of sedation and are helpful tools for the bedside clinician.

Sedation Scales: Goals and Monitoring

Sedation scales allow the nurse to select a level of sedation for the patient in collaboration with the health care team. Descriptors of each level of sedation are provided so that the sedative may be adjusted appropriately. Sedation monitoring is done at least hourly and the level of sedation achieved is recorded. Use of a valid and reliable sedation assessment scale is recommended (Tables 6–6 and 6–7), rather than scales that are institutionally developed and lack proper testing.

One of the major concerns related to the use of sedation scales is that they do not promote the aggressive withdrawal of the sedative drugs. This is important because recent studies have linked the use of sedative infusions to prolonged ventilator duration, and ICU and hospital lengths

of stay. Additional criticisms of scales include a lack of differentiation of domains for sedation assessment (e.g., safety, sleep, dys-synchrony), the nondirectional nature of the scales (they do not help the caregiver to evaluate other conditions such as pain or delirium), and a confusing combination of subjective and objective discriminators.

Sedation Management

Management of sedation is an essential step in attaining positive outcomes for critically ill patients. Many patients require sedatives for the treatment of mild to moderate anxiety while in the critical care unit. Treatment of such anxiety is appropriate and rarely results in adverse effects. Generally the sedatives are provided orally and occasionally as an IV bolus. The doses are adjusted to prevent excessive drowsiness or respiratory depression (Figure 6–7). Appropriately dosed, use of the sedatives does not interfere with clinical progress such as weaning or rehabilitation. In contrast, it is especially important to consider the effects associated with sedation infusions on outcomes.

In patients who require high levels of sedation to prevent self-harm and or to ensure that lung protective strategies may be used, sedation infusions and/or frequent IV bolus sedation are essential care elements. To avoid excessive sedation, current recommendations include the use of sedation management algorithms and periodic, usually daily, interruptions of sedation therapy to reassess the needed level of sedation. Approaches such as these have been shown to decrease sedation duration, and length of mechanical ventilation and hospital stay.

NEUROMUSCULAR BLOCKADE

The use of NMB in the critical care unit is generally confined to those severe situations where aggressive management of analgesics and sedatives, in addition to ventilator parameter manipulations, are not enough to ensure patient ventilator synchrony and the patient's safety. In these cases, the patient's muscular movements contribute to hemodynamic and pulmonary instability. NMB may also be necessary, as previously noted, when protective lung strategies are employed. The strategies used to manage patients with ARDS and acute asthma, for example, result in hypercarbia and acidosis (permissive hypercarbia), which may be poorly tolerated (see Chapter 20, Advanced Respiratory Concepts). In these cases, the use of neuromuscular blocking agents may be life saving and are an important part of care. The use of NMB agents is also associated with prolonged neuropathies and myopathies, especially when used in conjunction with steroids. In addition, the evaluation of neurologic status is difficult and may obviate the use of the agents. Thus, NMB agents should be used sparingly and only in the most severe situations as described.

TABLE 6–6. FOUR DIFFERENT SEDATION ASSESSMENT SCALES WITH VALIDITY AND RELIABILITY IN ADULT PATIENTS

Ramsay Scale[a]	Sedation-Agitation Scale[b]	Motor Activity Assessment Scale[c]	Richmond Agitation Sedation Scale[d]
6 No response	1 Unarousable (minimal or no response to noxious stimuli, does not communicate or follow commands)	0 Unresponsive (does not move with noxious stimuli)	−5 Unresponsive (no response to voice or physical stimulation)
5 Patient asleep with a sluggish response to a light glabellar tap	2 Very sedated (arouses to physical stimuli but does not communicate or follow commands; may move spontaneously)	1 Responsive only to noxious stimuli (opens eyes or raises eyebrows or turns head toward stimulus or moves limb with noxious stimulus)	−4 Deep sedation (no response to voice, but any movement to physical stimulation
4 Patient asleep with a brisk response to a light glabellar tap	3 Sedated (difficult to arouse, awakens to verbal stimuli or gentle shaking but drifts off again, follows simple commands)	2 Responsive to touch or name (open eyes or raises eyebrows or turns head toward stimulus or moves limb when touched or name is loudly spoken)	−3 Moderate sedation (any movement, but no eye contact to voice)
3 Patient responds to commands only	4 Calm and cooperative (calm, awakens easily, follows commands)	3 Calm and cooperative (no external stimulus is required to elicit movement purposefully and follows command)	−2 Light sedation (briefly, <10 sec, awakening with eye contact to voice)
2 Patient cooperative, oriented, and tranquil	5 Agitated (anxious or mildly agitated, attempting to sit up, calms down to verbal instructions)	4 Restless and cooperative (no external stimulus is required to elicit movement and patient is picking at sheets or tubes or uncovering self and follows commands)	−1 Drowsy (not fully alert, but has sustained, >10 sec, awakening with eye contact to voice)
1 Patient anxious, agitated, or both	6 Very agitated (does not calm, despite frequent verbal reminding of limits; requires physical restraints, biting ET tube)	5 Agitated (No external stimulus is required to elicit movement and attempting to sit up or moves limbs out of bed and does not consistently follow commands)	0 Alert and calm
	7 Dangerous agitation (pulling at ET tube, trying to remove catheter, climbing over bed rail, striking at staff, thrashing side to side)	6 Dangerously agitated, uncooperative (no external stimulus is required to elicit movement and patient is pulling at tubes or catheters or thrashing side to side or striking at staff or trying to climb out of bed and does not calm down when asked)	1 Restless (anxious or apprehensive but movements not aggressive or vigorous)
			2 Agitated (frequent nonpurposeful movement or patient–ventilator dysynchrony)
			3 Very agitated (pulls on or removes tubes or catheters or has aggressive behavior toward staff)
			4 Combative (overly combative or violent; immediate danger to staff)

Data compiled from: [a]Ramsay et al (1974), [b]Riker et al (1994); [c]Devlin et al (1999), and [d]Sessler et al (2002).

Neuromuscular Blocking Agents

The most common neuromuscular blocking agents used in critical care are the nondepolarizing agents (see Chapter 7, Pharmacology, for a comprehensive discussion of chemical paralytic agents). The agents block the transmission of nerve impulses by blocking cholinergic receptors; muscle paralysis results. The degree of blockade varies depending on the dose and the amount of receptor blockade.

Short-Acting NMB

Mivacurium is rapid acting and has a short duration of action (15 minutes). It may be given as an IV bolus initially but then is provided by infusion. Mivacurium is metabolized by pseudocholinesterase.

Intermediate-Acting NMB

These agents may be administered via an IV bolus, at least initially (i.e., intubation), but then are provided by infusion because they are rapidly metabolized (20 to 50 minutes). *Vecuronium,* a steroid-based agent, is metabolized by the liver and excreted renally. The combination of steroids and this steroid-based agent may contribute to myopathies. *Atracurium* and *cis-atricurium* are metabolized in the plasma by Hofmann elimination. There is minimal to no histamine release with the drug.

Long-Acting NMB

Pancuronium, a steroid-based agent, is generally given by intermittent IV bolus. Although labor intensive (the bolus is

TABLE 6–7. EVIDENCED-BASED PRACTICE: SEDATION MANAGEMENT

- Provide adequate analgesia and treat underlying physiological disturbances like hypoxemia, hypoglycemia, and hypotension before administering sedatives.[a,b]
- Use a validated sedation assessment scale like the Riker Sedation-Agitation Scale or Motor Activity Assessment Scale to regularly assess sedation and response to therapy.[a,b]
- Use sedation guidelines, an algorithm or a protocol to help guide selection and titration of a sedative.[a]
- To minimize prolonged sedative effects, titrate sedative doses to a defined endpoint and systematically taper sedative doses over time or interrupt therapy daily. Reinstitute as needed.[a,c]
- Watch for opioid, benzodiazepine, or propofol withdrawal if patients have received high doses or more than 7 days of continuous therapy and taper doses systematically to prevent withdrawal symptoms.[a,c]
- Promote better sleep by minimizing noise, modifying ambient light, and using nonpharmacologic interventions like relaxation, music therapy, or massage in combination with sedative therapy.[a,c]
- Use NMB to manage ventilation, manage increased intracranial pressure, treat muscle, spasms and decrease oxygen consumption only when all other means have been tried without success.[a,b]
- Before initiating NMB, medicate the patient with sedative and analgesic drugs to provide adequate sedation and analgesia according to physician orders.[b]
- Assess your patient's level of NMB both clinically and by train of four monitoring with the goal of adjusting the degree of NMB to achieve one or two twitches.[a,b]
- For patients receiving neuromuscular blocking agents and corticosteroids (or drugs that affect neuromuscular transmission), discontinue blocking agents as soon as possible to prevent prolonged recovery or complications.[a,b]

Data compiled from: [a]Society of Critical Care Medicine, American Society of Health-System Pharmacists (2002). [b]Consensus Conference on Sedation Assessment (2004). [c]Jacobi J, Fraser G, Coursin D, et al. (2002).

often required hourly), the intermittent dosing does allow for frequent reassessment. Pancuronium is vagolytic and can cause tachycardia; it may be contraindicated in patients with cardiovascular disease. Pancuronium is metabolized by the liver and is renally excreted.

Monitoring and Management

Monitoring NMB is accomplished with the use of a peripheral nerve stimulator or by monitoring airway pressure waveforms. The goal is to provide the least amount of the drug so that recovery is rapid when the drug is discontinued. How these aspects of care and others are managed are essential to ensuring good outcomes.

Peripheral Nerve Stimulation

Peripheral nerve stimulators (PNSs) are devices that deliver a series of electrical stimuli via electrodes to nerves under the skin (Figure 6–8). The electrical stimuli cause muscular contractions if the neuromuscular junction is functioning properly. Typically, peripheral nerve stimulation is performed on the ulnar nerve at the wrist, with the temple area of the head as another potential site for nerve stimulation. When electrical stimuli are applied to the ulnar nerve, the

thumb abducts and the fingers flex if the neuromuscular junction is intact.

The stimulator technique most commonly used to assess NMB is the Train of Four. With this technique, four small electrical stimuli are given every half second. The degree of NMB can be assessed by observing or palpating the number of muscle twitches elicited during the series of four electrical stimuli (see Figure 6–8). When no NMB is present, four twitches of similar intensity, or height, are noted. Following the administration of a nondepolarizing neuromuscular blocking agent, many of the neuromuscular junctions are blocked. This produces minimal response to the four delivered stimuli. As the level of NMB decreases over time, the number of twitches observed increases until four strong, equal twitches are observed, indicating that no NMB is present.

The degree of NMB is approximately 90% when one small twitch is palpated, 80% with two small twitches, and about 75% with three small twitches. Typically, in critical care patients, a moderate blockade level of 75% to 80% is usually sufficient to achieve respiratory muscle relaxation and improved gas exchange. The presence of two or three twitches in response to the Train of Four stimulation indicates a reasonable level of NMB for most critically ill patients. At this level of blockade, stimulation of the nerve does not result in excessive muscular contraction but saturation (100% block) has not occurred.

Although the PNS is helpful in the short term, it may be less reliable in patients requiring NMB for days. This is especially true when anasarca is present because the increase in edema decreases stimulus transmission. It is important to remember that the technique is somewhat uncomfortable and frequent assessments using the PNS should be avoided.

Airway Pressure Monitoring

Most ventilators today provide respiratory waveform graphic displays. Even if they do not, the simplest of the waveforms, airway pressure, can be readily adapted for display on existing bedside monitoring systems. The airway pressure waveform may be used to monitor patient generated respiratory activity (Figure 6–9). For example, regardless of the mode of ventilation, if chemical paralysis is adequate, there is an absence of spontaneous respiratory effort. If a spontaneous effort is noted on the waveform (a negative deflection), the NMB agents are increased. The airway pressure monitoring technique is especially helpful when initiating NMB and to assess withdrawal of the drug.

Management

Patients who are paralyzed may still experience pain, anxiety, and fear. To that end, it is essential that patients receiving NMB agents are provided with analgesics and sedatives. With virtually no exceptions, sedation and analgesia should be used in combination for those receiving NMB agents.

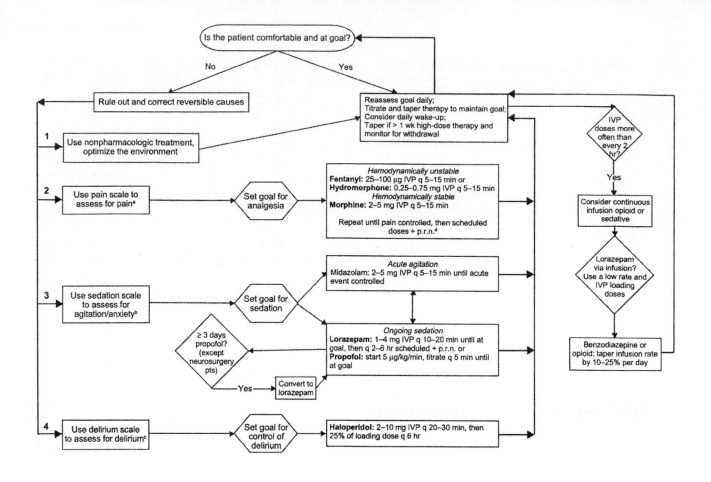

Figure 6–7. Algorithm for the sedation and analgesia of mechanically ventilated patients.[a]Numeric rating scale or other pain scale. [b]Riker Sedation-Agitation Scale or other sedation scale. [c]Confusion Assessment Method for the ICU. (*From: Clinical practice guidelines for the sustained use of sedatives and analgesics in the critically ill adult.* Crit Care Med *2002;30:124; used with permission*).

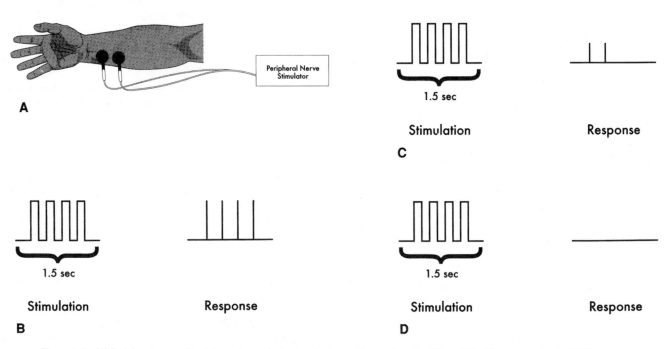

Figure 6–8. **(A)** Peripheral nerve stimulator and graphic display of a train of four pattern for **(B)** no NMB, **(C)** moderate block (80%), and **(D)** complete block.

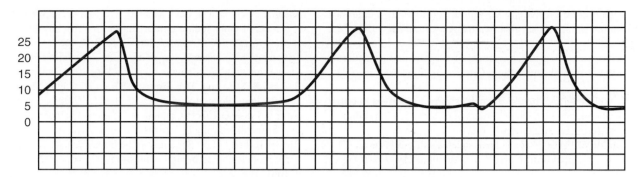

Figure 6–9. Example of spontaneous effort on assist-control volume ventilation. Note negative deflection prior to volume breath indicating inadequate level of NMB. (*From: Burns S: Continuous airway pressure monitoring. In Chulay M, Burns S [eds]: AACN Protocols for Practice: Care of the Mechanically Ventilated Patient. Aliso Viejo, CA: AACN; 1996, with permission*).

Amnesia is a desired outcome; no patient should experience a "trapped in body" state.

In addition, because patients are unable to move or breathe on their own, the nurse must be extremely vigilant about those situations that potentially could affect the patient's safety (ventilator disconnect, harm from external forces). Physical care interventions are extremely important as well, and include the use of eye lubricants, frequent turning, and the use of prophylactic agents such as heparin to prevent deep vein thrombosis. Because the patient cannot communicate yet may hear, it is important to verbally reassure the patient and provide frequent explanations about what is happening throughout the course of the day and night.

Determining whether NMB agents need to be continued may be very difficult. One practical method is to stop the infusions of NMB agents daily to assess the need for continuation. Then, if signs of intolerance such as rapid oxygen desaturation occur with the intervention, the sedatives and narcotics may be increased first. Tolerance of sedatives and analgesics is common and to be expected; increasing doses of the drugs may be necessary. If intolerance is still noted, the NMB agents may be resumed. Regardless of the method used, it is clear that the goal should be to use the agents for as short a time as possible.

SELECTED BIBLIOGRAPHY

Pain Management

American Pain Society: *Principles of Analgesic Use in the Treatment of Acute Pain and Cancer Pain,* 5th ed. Glenview, IL: American Pain Society; 2003.

Beyer JE: *The Oucher: A User's Manual and Technical Report.* Evanston, IL: Hospital Play Equipment; 1984.

Burke DF, Dunwoody CJ: Naloxone: A word of caution. *Orthopaedic Nursing* 1990;9(4):44–46.

Cook J, Rideout E, Browne G: The prevalence of pain complaints in a general population. *Pain* 1984;2:49–53.

Faucett J: Care of the critically ill patient in pain: The importance of nursing. In Puntillo KA (ed): *Pain in the Critically Ill.* Gaithersburg, MD: Aspen; 1991.

Gardner DL: Presence. In Bulechek GM, McCloskey JC (eds): *Nursing Interventions: Essential Nursing Treatments,* pp. 316–324. Philadelphia: WB Saunders; 1992.

Julius D, Basbaum AI: Molecular mechanisms of nociception. *Nature* 2001;413:203–210.

Maxam-Moore VA, Wilkie DJ, Woods SL: Analgesics for cardiac surgery patients in critical care: Describing current practice. *Am J Crit Care* 1994;3:31–39.

McCaffery M, Pasero C: *Pain: Clinical Manual,* 2nd ed. St. Louis: Mosby; 1999.

McGrath P, Johnson G, Goodman J, et al: CHEOPS: A behavioral scale for rating postoperative pain in children. *Advances Pain Res Ther* 1985;9:395–402.

Pettigrew J: Intensive nursing care: The ministry of presence. *Crit Care Nurs Clin North Am* 1990;2(3):503–508.

Puntillo K: Pain experience in intensive care patients. *Heart Lung* 1990;19:526–533.

Puntillo K: Advances in management of acute pain: Great strides or tiny footsteps? *Capsules Comments Crit Care Nurs* 1995;3:97–100.

Puntillo K, Weiss SJ: Pain: Its mediators and associated morbidity in critically ill cardiovascular surgical patients. *Nurs Res* 1994;43:31–36.

Puntillo KA, Morris AB, Thompson CL, et al: Pain behaviors observed during six common procedures: Results from Thunder Project II. *Crit Care Med* 2004;32(2):421–427.

Puntillo KA, White C, Morris AB, et al: Patients' perceptions and responses to procedural pain: Results from Thunder Project II. *Am J Crit Care* 2001;10(4):238–251.

Puntillo KA, Wild LR, Morris AB, et al: Practices and predictors of analgesic interventions for adults undergoing painful procedures. *Am J Crit Care* 2002;11(5):415–429.

Rakel B, Herr K: Assessment and treatment of postoperative pain in the older adult. *J Perianesthesia Nurs* 2004;19(3):194–208.

Ready LB, Chadwick HS, Ross B: Age predicts effective epidural morphine dose after abdominal hysterectomy. *Anesthes Analges* 1987;66:1215–1218.

Ready LB, Loper KA, Nessly M, Wild L: Postoperative epidural morphine is safe on surgical wards. *Anesthesiology* 1991;75: 452–456.

Summer G, Puntillo K: Management of surgical and procedural pain in the critical care setting. *Crit Care Clin North Am* 2001; 13:233–242.

Sun X, Weissman C: The use of analgesics and sedatives in critically ill patients: Physicians' orders versus medications administered. *Heart Lung* 1994;23:169–176.

Tittle M, McMillan SC: Pain and pain-related side effects in an ICU and on a surgical unit: Nurses' management. *Am J Crit Care* 1994;3:25–39.

Thompson C, White C, Wild L, et al: Translating research into practice. *Crit Care Nurs Clin North Am* 2001;13:541–546.

US Department of Health and Human Services: *Acute Pain Management: Operative or Medical Procedures and Trauma. Clinical Practice Guidelines*. Rockville, MD: Agency for Health Care Policy and Research, Public Health Service, US Department of Health and Human Services; 1992.

Wong DL, Baker CM: Pain in children: Comparison of assessment scales. *Pediatr Nurs* 1988;14(1):9–17.

Yeager MP, Glass DD, Neff RK, Brinck-Johnsen T: Epidural anesthesia and analgesia in high-risk surgical patients. *Anesthesia* 1987;66:729–736.

Sedation and Neuromuscular Blockade

Belleville J, Ward D, Bloor B, et al: Effects of intravenous dexmedetomidine in humans. Sedation, ventilation, and metabolic rate. *Anesthesia* 1992;77:1125–1133.

Brook AD, Ahrens TS, Schaff R, et al: Effect of a nursing-implemented sedation protocol on the duration of mechanical ventilation. *Crit Care Med* 1999;27:2609–2615.

DeJonge B, Cook D, Appere-De-Vecchi C, et al: Using and understanding sedation scoring systems: A systematic review. *Intens Care Med* 2000;26:275–285.

Devlin JW, Boleski G, Miynarek M, et al: Motor Activity Assessment Scale: A valid and reliable sedation scale for use with mechanically ventilated patients in an adult surgical intensive care unit. *Crit Care Med* 1999;27:1271–1275.

Ely W, Truman B, Shintani A, et al: Monitoring sedation status over time in ICU patients: Reliability and validity of the Richmond Agitation-Sedation Scale (RASS). *JAMA* 2003;22(289): 2983–2991.

Hall E, Uhrich T, Barney J, et al: Sedative amnesic, and analgesic properties of small-dose dexmedetomidine infusions. *Anesth Analg* 2000;90:699–705.

Kress JP, Pohlman, O'Connor MF, Hall JB: Daily interruption of sedative infusions in critically ill patients undergoing mechanical ventilation. *N Engl J Med* 2000;342:1471–1477.

Kress JP, Pohlman AS, Hall JB: Sedation and Analgesia in the Intensive Care Unit. *Am J Respir Crit Care Med* 2002;166:1024–1028.

Kress JP, Gehlbach B, Lacy M, et al: The long-term psychological effects of daily sedative interruption on critically ill patients. *Am J Respir Crit Care Med* 2003;168:1457–1461.

Ostermann M, Keenan S, Seiferling R, et al: Sedation in the intensive care unit: A systematic review. *JAMA* 2000;283:1451–1459.

Ramsay MA, Savege TM, Simpson BR, et al: Controlled sedation with alphaxalone-alphadolone. *Br Med J* 1974;2:656–659.

Riker R, Fraser G, Cox P: Continuous infusion of haloperidol controls agitation in critically ill patients. *Crit Care Med* 1994;22:433–440.

Riker RR, Fraser GL: Sedation in the intensive care unit: refining the models and defining the questions. *Crit Care Med* 2002;30: 1661–1663.

Riker, RR, Picard JT, Fraser GL: Prospective evaluation of the Sedation-Agitation Scale for adult critically ill patients. *Crit Care Med* 1999; 27:1271–1275.

Sessler C, Gosnet M, Grap MJ: The Richmond Agitation-Sedation Scale: Validity and reliability in adult intensive care unit patients. *Am J Respir Crit Care Med* 2002;166:1338–1344.

Venn RM, Newman PJ, Grounds RM: A phase II study to evaluate the efficacy of dexmedetomidine for sedation in the medical intensive care unit [on-line version]. *Intens Care Med* November 2002.

Weinert CR, Chlan L, Gross C: Sedating critically ill patients: Factors affecting nurses' delivery of sedative therapy. *Am J Crit Care* 2001;10(3):156–165.

Evidence-Based Practice Guidelines

Burns S: Continuous airway pressure monitoring. In Burns S (ed): *AACN Protocols for Practice: Care of the Mechanically Ventilated Patient*. Aliso Viejo, CA: AACN; 2005.

Jacobi J, Fraser G, Coursin D, et al: Clinical practice guidelines for the sustained use of sedatives and analgesics in the critically ill adult. *Crit Care Med* 2002;30(1):119–141.

Luer J: Sedation and neuromuscular blockade. In Chulay M, Burns S (eds): *AACN Protocols for Practice: Care of the Mechanically Ventilated Patient*. Viejo, CA: AACN; in press.

Members of the Abbott/AACN/Saint Thomas Sedation Expert Panel (alphabetically): Bader MK, Burns SM, Campbell M, Chulay M, DeJong M, Fontaine D, Luer J, Vollman K, Wild L. Consensus conference on sedation assessment: A collaborative venture by Abbott Laboratories, American Association of Critical-Care Nurses, and Saint Thomas Health System. *Crit Care Nurse* 2004;24:33–41.

Society of Critical Care Medicine, American Society of Health-System Pharmacists: Clinical practice guidelines for sustained neuromuscular blockade in the adult critically ill patient. *Crit Care Med* 2002;30(1):142–156.

Society of Critical Care Medicine, American Society of Health-System Pharmacists: Sedation, analgesia, and neuromuscular blockade of the critically ill adult: Revised clinical practice guidelines for 2002. *Crit Care Med* 2002;30(1):117–118.

Stanik-Hutt J: Pain management in the acutely ill. In Chulay M, Molter N (eds): *AACN's Protocols for Practice: Creating a Healing Environment Series*. Aliso Viejo, CA: AACN; 1998.

Pharmacology

Earnest Alexander

Seven

> ▶ **Knowledge Competencies**
>
> 1. Discuss advantages and disadvantages of various routes for medication delivery in critically ill patients.
>
> 2. Identify indications for use, mechanism of action, administration guidelines, side effects, and contraindications for drugs commonly administered in critical illness.

Critically ill patients often receive multiple medications during their admissions to an intensive care unit. These patients may be at risk for increased pharmacologic or adverse effects from their medications because of altered metabolism and elimination. Decreased organ function or drug interactions may produce increased serum drug concentrations resulting in enhanced or adverse pharmacologic effects. Therefore, it is important to be familiar with each patient's medications, including the drug's metabolic profile, drug interactions, and adverse effect profile. This chapter reviews medications commonly used in intensive care units and discusses their mechanisms of action, indications for use, common adverse effects, contraindications, and usual doses. A summary of intravenous (IV) medication information is provided in Chapter 23, Pharmacology Tables.

MEDICATION ADMINISTRATION METHODS

Intravenous

Intravenous (IV) administration is the preferred route for medications in critically ill patients because it permits complete and reliable delivery. Depending on the indication and the therapy, medications may be administered by IV push, intermittent infusion, or continuous infusion. Typically, *IV push* refers to administration of a drug over 3 to 5 minutes; *intermittent infusion* refers to 15-minute to 2-hour drug administration several times per day, and *continuous infusion* administration occurs over a prolonged period of time.

Intramuscular or Subcutaneous

Intramuscular (IM) or subcutaneous (SC) administration of medications should be restricted in critically ill patients because the onset of drug action may be prolonged, lack of adequate muscle or subcutaneous fat tissue may not permit these injections, hypotensive or hypovolemic patients may exhibit inadequate or altered peripheral perfusion, or inadequate perfusion may occur in areas of the body where medications have been injected in patients who are medically paralyzed. These routes of administration may result in incomplete, unpredictable, or erratic drug absorption. If medication is not absorbed from the injection site, a depot of medication can develop. Once perfusion is restored, allowing drug absorption, a supratherapeutic or toxic effect may occur from the absorption of the accumulated stores of the drug. Patients with thrombocytopenia or who are receiving thrombolytic agents or anticoagulants may develop hematomas and bleeding complications. Finally, administering frequent IM injections may also be inconvenient and painful for patients.

Oral

Oral (PO) administration of medication can also result in incomplete, unpredictable, or erratic absorption. This may be caused by the presence of an ileus impairing drug absorption, or to diarrhea decreasing gastrointestinal (GI) tract transit time and time for drug absorption. Diarrhea may have a pronounced effect on the absorption of sustained-release preparations such as theophylline, procainamide, or calcium channel blocking agents, resulting in a suboptimal serum drug concentration or clinical response. Several medications such as fluconazole and the fluoroquinolones have been shown to exhibit excellent bioavailability when orally administered to critically ill patients. The availability of an oral suspension for some of these agents makes oral administration a reliable and cost-effective alternative for patients with limited IV access.

In patients unable to swallow, tablets are often crushed and capsules opened for administration through nasogastric tubes. This practice is time consuming and often results in blockage of the tube, necessitating removal of the clogged tube and insertion of a new tube. If enteral nutrition is being administered through the tube, it often has to be stopped for medication administration, resulting in inadequate nutrition for patients. Also, several medications (e.g., phenytoin, carbamazepine, and warfarin) have been shown to compete, or interact, with enteral nutrition solutions. This interaction results in decreased absorption of these agents, or complex formation with the nutrition solution leading to precipitation and clogging of the feeding tube.

Liquid medications may circumvent the need to crush tablets or open capsules, but have their own limitations. Many liquid dosage forms contain sorbitol as a flavoring agent or as the primary delivery vehicle. Sorbitol's hyperosmolarity is a frequent cause of diarrhea in critically ill patients, especially in patients receiving enteral nutrition. Potassium chloride elixir is extremely hyperosmolar and requires dilution with 120 to 160 mL of water before administration. Administering undiluted potassium chloride elixir can result in osmotic diarrhea.

Lastly, sustained-release or enteric-coated preparations are difficult to administer to critically ill patients. When sustained-release products are crushed, the patient absorbs the whole dose immediately as opposed to gradually over a period of 6, 8, 12, or 24 hours. This results in supratherapeutic or toxic effects soon after the administration of the medication, with subtherapeutic effects at the end of the dosing interval. Sustained-release preparations must be converted to equivalent daily doses of immediate-release dosing forms and administered at more frequent dosing intervals. Enteric-coated dosage forms that are crushed may be inactivated by gastric juices or may cause stomach irritation. Enteric-coated tablets are specifically formulated to pass through the stomach intact so that they can enter the small intestine before they begin to dissolve.

Sublingual

Because of the high degree of vascularity of the sublingual mucosa, sublingual administration of medication often produces serum concentrations of medication that parallel IV administration, and an onset of action that is often faster than orally administered medications.

Traditionally, nitroglycerin has been one of the few medications administered sublingually (SL) to critically ill patients. Several oral and IV medications, however, have been shown to produce therapeutic effects after sublingual administration. Captopril has been shown to reliably and predictably lower blood pressure in patients with hypertensive urgency. Oral lorazepam tablets have been administered SL to treat patients in status epilepticus; preparations of oral triazolam and IV midazolam have been shown to produce sedation after sublingual administration.

Intranasal

Intranasal administration is becoming a popular way to effectively administer sedative and analgesic agents. The high degree of vascularity of the nasal mucosa results in rapid and complete absorption of medication. Agents that have been administered successfully intranasally include meperidine, fentanyl, sufentanil, butorphanol, ketamine, and midazolam.

Transdermal

Transdermal administration of medication is of limited value in critically ill patients. Although nitroglycerin ointment is extremely effective as a temporizing measure before IV access is established in the acute management of patients with angina, congestive heart failure (CHF), pulmonary edema, or hypertension, nitroglycerin transdermal patches are of limited benefit. Transdermal patches are limited by their slow onset of activity and their inability for dose titration. Also, patients with decreased peripheral perfusion may not sufficiently absorb transdermally administered medications to produce the desired therapeutic effect. Transdermal preparations of clonidine, nitroglycerin, or fentanyl may be beneficial in patients who have been stabilized on IV or oral doses, but require chronic administration of these agents. Chronic use of nitroglycerin transdermal patches is further complicated by the development of tolerance. However, the development of tolerance can be avoided by removing the patch at bedtime, allowing for an 8- to 10-hour "nitrate-free" period.

A eutectic mixture of local anesthetic (EMLA) is a combination of lidocaine and prilocaine. This local anesthetic mixture can be used to anesthetize the skin before insertion of IV catheters or the injection of local anesthetics that may be required to produce deeper levels of topical anesthesia.

Although transdermal administration of medications is an infrequent method of drug administration in critically ill patients, its use should not be overlooked as a potential cause of adverse effects in this patient population. Extensive application to burned, abraded, or denuded skin can result in significant systemic absorption of topically applied medications. Excessive use of viscous lidocaine products or mouthwashes containing lidocaine to provide local anesthesia for mucositis or esophagitis also can result in significant systemic absorption of lidocaine. Lidocaine administered topically to the oral mucosa has resulted in serum concentrations capable of producing seizures. The diffuse application of topical glucocorticosteroid preparations also can lead to absorption capable of producing adrenal suppression. This is especially true with the high-potency fluorinated steroid preparations such as betamethasone dipropionate, clobetasol propionate, desoximetasone, or fluocinonide.

CENTRAL NERVOUS SYSTEM PHARMACOLOGY

Sedatives

Sedatives can be divided into four main categories: benzodiazepines, barbiturates, neuroleptics, and miscellaneous agents. Benzodiazepines are the most commonly used sedatives in critically ill patients. Neuroleptics typically are used in patients who manifest a psychological or behavioral component to their sedative needs, and barbiturates are reserved for patients with head injuries and increased intracranial pressure. Propofol is a short-acting IV general anesthetic that is approved for use as a sedative for mechanically ventilated critically ill patients. Dosing of sedatives should be guided by frequent assessment of the level of sedation with a valid and reliable sedation assessment scale (see Chapter 6, Pain, Sedation, and Neuromuscular Blockade Management).

Benzodiazepines

Benzodiazepines are the most frequently used agents for sedation in critically ill patients. These agents provide sedation, decrease anxiety, have anticonvulsant properties, possess indirect muscle relaxant properties, and induce antegrade amnesia. Benzodiazepines bind to gamma-aminobutyric acid (GABA) receptors located in the central nervous system, modulating this inhibitory neurotransmitter. These agents have a wide margin of safety as well as flexibility in their routes of administration.

Benzodiazepines are frequently used to provide short-term sedation and amnesia during imaging procedures, other diagnostic procedures, and invasive procedures such as central venous catheter placement or bronchoscopy. A common long-term indication for using benzodiazepines is sedation and amnesia during mechanical ventilation.

Benzodiazepines are associated with minimal adverse effects. Excessive sedation and confusion can occur with initial doses, but these effects diminish as tolerance develops during therapy. Elderly and pediatric patients may exhibit a paradoxical effect manifested as irritability, agitation, hostility, hallucinations, and anxiety. Respiratory depression may be seen in patients receiving concurrent narcotics, as well as in elderly patients and patients with chronic obstructive pulmonary disease (COPD).

Monitoring Parameters

Mental status, level of consciousness, respiratory rate, and level of comfort should be monitored in any patient receiving a benzodiazepine. Signs and symptoms of withdrawal reactions should be monitored for patients receiving short-acting agents (i.e., midazolam).

Midazolam

Midazolam is a short-acting water-soluble benzodiazepine that may be administered IV, IM, SL, PO, or rectally. Clearance of midazolam has been shown to be extremely variable in critically ill patients; patients with liver disease, shock, or concurrently receiving enzyme inhibiting drugs such as erythromycin or fluconazole; and hypoalbuminemia, with its elimination half-life increased by as much as 6 to 12 hours. Midazolam's two primary metabolites, 1-hydroxymidazolam and 1-hydroxymidazolam glucuronide, have been shown to accumulate in critically ill patients contributing additional pharmacologic effects. Geriatric patients demonstrate prolonged half-lives secondary to age-related reduction in liver function.

Dose

- *IV bolus:* 0.025 to 0.035 mg/kg
- *Continuous infusion:* 0.5 to 5.0 mcg/kg/min

Lorazepam

Lorazepam is an intermediate-acting benzodiazepine that offers the advantage of not having its metabolism affected by impaired hepatic function, age, or interacting drugs. Glucuronidation in the liver is the route of elimination of lorazepam. Because lorazepam is relatively water insoluble, it must be diluted in propylene glycol, and it is propylene glycol that is responsible for the hypotension that may be seen after bolus IV administration. Recently, administration of lorazepam by continuous IV infusion has been advocated. However, this method of administration is hampered by the relative water insolubility of lorazepam. Large volumes of fluid are required to maintain the drug in solution, so that only 20 to 40 mg can be safely dissolved in 250 mL of dextrose-5%-water (D_5W). In-line filters are recommended when administering lorazepam by continuous infusion because of the potential for the drug to precipitate. Finally, lorazepam's long elimination half-life of 10 to 20 hours limits its dosing flexibility by continuous infusion. Patients requiring high-dose infusions may be at risk for developing propylene glycol toxicity, which is manifested as a hyperosmolar state with a metabolic acidosis.

Dose

- *IV bolus:* 0.5 to 2.0 mg q1–4h
- *Continuous infusion:* 0.06 mg/kg/h

Diazepam

Diazepam is a long-acting benzodiazepine with a faster onset of action than lorazepam or midazolam. Although its duration of action is 1 to 2 hours after a single dose, it displays cumulative effects because its active metabolites contribute to its pharmacologic effect. Desmethyldiazepam has a half-life of approximately 150 to 200 hours, so it accumulates slowly and then is slowly eliminated from the body after diazepam is discontinued. Diazepam metabolism is reduced in patients with hepatic failure and in patients receiving drugs that inhibit hepatic microsomal enzymes. Diazepam may be used for one or two doses as a periprocedure anxiolytic and amnestic, but should not be used for routine sedation of mechanically ventilated patients.

Dose

- *IV bolus:* 2.5 to 5.0 mg q2–4h
- *Continuous infusion:* Not recommended

Benzodiazepine Antagonist

Flumazenil

Flumazenil is a specific benzodiazepine antagonist indicated for the reversal of benzodiazepine-induced moderate sedation, recurrent sedation, and benzodiazepine overdose. It should be used with caution in patients who have received benzodiazepines for an extended period of time to prevent the precipitation of withdrawal reactions.

Dose

- *Reversal of conscious sedation:* 0.2 mg IV over 2 minutes, followed in 45 seconds by 0.2 mg repeated every minute as needed to a maximum dose of 1 mg. Reversal of recurrent sedation is the same as for conscious sedation, except doses may be repeated every 20 minutes as needed.
- *Benzodiazepine overdose:* 0.2 mg over 30 seconds followed by 0.3 mg over 30 seconds; repeated doses of 0.5 mg can be administered over 30 seconds at 1-minute intervals up to a cumulative dose of 3 mg. With a partial response after 3 mg, additional doses up to a total dose of 5 mg may be administered. In all of the above-mentioned scenarios, no more than 1 mg should be administered at any one time, and no more than 3 mg in any 1 hour. *Continuous infusion:* 0.1 to 0.5 mg/h (for the reversal of long-acting benzodiazepines or massive overdoses).

Monitoring Parameters

- Level of consciousness and signs and symptoms of withdrawal reactions.

Neuroleptics

Haloperidol

Haloperidol is a major tranquilizer commonly used for the management of agitated or delirious patients who fail to respond adequately to nonpharmacologic interventions or other sedatives. This agent has the advantage of limited respiratory depression and little potential for the development of tolerance or dependence. Although its exact mechanism of action is unknown, it probably involves dopaminergic receptor blockade in the central nervous system, resulting in central nervous system depression at the subcortical level of the brain.

Intravenous haloperidol is the most frequently used neuroleptic for controlling agitation in critically ill patients. Initial doses of 2 to 5 mg may be doubled every 15 to 20 minutes until the patient is adequately sedated. Single IV doses as large as 150 mg have been safely administered to patients, as well as total daily doses of approximately 1000 mg. As soon as the patient's symptoms are controlled, the total dose required to calm the patient should be divided into four equal doses and administered every 6 hours on a regularly scheduled basis. When the patient's symptoms are stable, the daily dose should be rapidly tapered to the smallest dose that controls the patient's symptoms. Continuous IV infusions have also been advocated to allow flexible dosing to control patient's symptoms. High doses of haloperidol may prolong the QTc interval in patients, especially those patients receiving haloperidol continuous infusions. Monitoring the QTc interval is mandatory for all patients receiving haloperidol by continuous infusion.

The major side effect of haloperidol is its extrapyramidal reactions, such as akathisia and dystonia. These reactions usually occur early in therapy and may resolve with dose reduction or discontinuation of the drug. However, in more severe cases, diphenhydramine, 25 to 50 mg IV, or benztropine, 1 to 2 mg IV, may be required to relieve the symptoms. Extrapyramidal reactions appear to be more common after oral haloperidol than after IV haloperidol administration. Neuroleptic malignant syndrome may also be seen with this agent, manifested by hyperthermia, severe extrapyramidal reactions, altered mental status, and autonomic instability. Treatment involves supportive care and the administration of dantrolene. Cardiovascular side effects include hypotension.

Dose

- *IV bolus:* 1 to 10 mg (titrated up as clinically indicated)
- Continuous infusion: 10 mg/h (not generally recommended)

Monitoring Parameters

- Mental status, blood pressure, electrocardiogram (ECG), and electrolytes (especially with continuous infusions)

Barbiturates

Barbiturates are primarily used to reduce intracranial pressure in head injury patients after conservative therapy has failed. Barbiturates decrease cerebral oxygen consumption, decrease cerebral blood flow, and potentially scavenge free oxygen radicals.

The general central nervous system depression associated with the use of barbiturates may cause excessive sedation as well as respiratory depression. Barbiturates produce direct myocardial depression, reducing cardiac output as well as increasing venous capacitance. Rapid IV administration can result in arrhythmias and hypotension.

Pentobarbital

Pentobarbital continuous infusions are commonly used to induce barbiturate coma. The infusion should be titrated to maintain intracranial pressure less than 20 mm Hg and cerebral perfusion pressure greater than 60 mm Hg. The mean arterial pressure should be maintained in a range that provides an adequate cerebral perfusion pressure. Therapeutic serum pentobarbital concentrations are 20 to 50 mg/L.

Dose

- *IV bolus*: 5 to 10 mg/kg infused over 2 hours
- *Continuous infusion*: 0.5 to 4 mg/kg/h

Monitoring Parameters

- Level of consciousness, intracranial pressure, cerebral perfusion pressure, blood pressure, and serum pentobarbital concentration

Miscellaneous Agents

Propofol

Propofol is an IV general anesthetic that has become popular for sedation of mechanically ventilated patients. Propofol use is typically limited to fewer than 3 days because of the rapid development of tolerance or is used as the primary sedative in daily awakening protocols. The advantages of propofol are its rapid onset and short duration of action compared to the benzodiazepines. Propofol has been associated with hypotension in critically ill patients, especially those who are hypotensive or hypovolemic. Hypotension can be avoided by limiting bolus doses to 0.25 to 0.50 mg/kg and the initial infusion rate to 5 mcg/kg/min. The fat emulsion vehicle of propofol has been shown to support the growth of microorganisms. The manufacturer recommends changing the IV tubing of extemporaneously prepared infusions every 6 hours, or every 12 hours if the infusion bottles are used. Propofol is formulated in a fat emulsion vehicle that provides 1.1 calories/mL and its infusion rate must be accounted for when determining a patient's nutrition support regimen because the fat emulsion base can be considered as a calorie source. High infusion rates can be a cause of hypertriglyceridemia. Propofol is available in 50- and 100-mL infusion vials. To decrease waste, 50-mL vials should be used when changing vials in patients who are scheduled for IV line changes, extubation from mechanical ventilation, and low infusion rates.

Dose

- *IV bolus*: 0.25 to 0.50 mg/kg
- *Continuous infusion*: 5 to 50 mcg/kg/min

Monitoring Parameters

- Level of consciousness, blood pressure, and serum triglyceride level, especially at high infusion rates.

Ketamine

Ketamine is an analog of phencyclidine that is commonly used as an IV general anesthetic. It is an agent that produces analgesia, anesthesia, and amnesia without the loss of consciousness. The onset of anesthesia after a single 0.5- to 1.0-mg/kg bolus dose is within 1 to 2 minutes and lasts approximately 5 to 10 minutes. Ketamine causes sympathetic stimulation that normally increases blood pressure and heart rate while maintaining cardiac output. This may be important in patients with hypovolemia. Ketamine is useful in patients who require repeated painful procedures such as wound debridement. The bronchodilatory effects of ketamine may be beneficial in patients experiencing status asthmaticus. However, ketamine increases intracranial pressure and should be avoided in patients with head injuries, space-occupying lesions, or any other conditions that may cause an increase in intracranial pressure. Emergence reactions or hallucinations, commonly seen after ketamine anesthesia, may be prevented with the concurrent use of benzodiazepines.

Dose

- *IV bolus*: 1 to 4.5 mg/kg
- *Continuous infusion*: 5 to 45 mcg/kg/min
- *Oral*: 10 mg/kg diluted in 1 to 2 ounces of juice
- *Intranasal*: 5 mg/kg

Monitoring Parameters

- Levels of sedation and analgesia, heart rate, blood pressure, and mental status

Dexmedetomidine

Dexmedetomidine is a relatively selective alpha$_2$-adrenergic agonist with sedative properties indicated for the short-term ($<$24 h) sedation of intubated and mechanically ventilated patients. Dexmedetomidine is not associated with respiratory depression but has been associated with reductions in heart rate and blood pressure. Some patients may complain of increased awareness while receiving the drug in the intensive care unit. Dexmedetomidine has minimal amnestic properties and most patients require breakthrough doses of sedatives and analgesics while receiving the drug. The agent has been evaluated for longer term sedation, up to 7 days in a limited number of mechanically ventilated patients. In this setting a reduction of the loading infusion is advised to minimize cardiovascular depression. However, a higher maintenance infusion may be required compared to short-term postoperative sedation.

Dose

- *IV bolus:* 1 mcg/kg over 10 minutes
- *Continuous infusions:* 0.2 to 0.7 mcg/kg/h

Monitoring Parameters

- Levels of sedation and analgesia, heart rate, and blood pressure

Analgesics

Narcotics

Narcotics produce their effects by reversibly binding to the mu, delta, kappa, and sigma opiate receptors located in the central nervous system. Mu-1 receptors are associated with analgesia, and mu-2 receptors are associated with respiratory depression, bradycardia, euphoria, and dependence. Delta receptors have no selective agonist and modulate mu receptor activity. Kappa receptors function at the spinal and supraspinal levels and are associated with sedation. Sigma receptors are associated with dysphoria and psychotomimetic effects.

Monitoring Parameters

- Level of pain or comfort, blood pressure, renal function, and respiratory rate

Morphine

Morphine is the most commonly used narcotic analgesic. Morphine is hepatically metabolized to several metabolites, including morphine-6-glucuronide (M6G), which is approximately 5 to 10 times more potent than morphine. M6G is renally eliminated and after repeated dosing can accumulate in patients with reduced renal function, producing enhanced pharmacologic effects. Morphine's clearance is reduced in critically ill patients due to increased protein binding, decreased hepatic blood flow, or reduced hepatocellular function. Morphine possesses vasodilatory properties due to either direct effects on the vasculature or histamine release.

Dose

- *IV bolus:* 2 to 5 mg
- *Continuous infusion:* 2 to 5 mg/h

Patient-Controlled Analgesia (PCA)

- *IV bolus:* 0.5 to 3.0 mg
- *Lockout interval:* 5 to 20 minutes

Meperidine

Meperidine is a short-acting opioid that has one-seventh the potency of morphine. It is hepatically metabolized to normeperidine, which is renally eliminated, and is also a neurotoxin. Normeperidine can accumulate in patients with reduced renal function, resulting in seizures. Meperidine should be avoided in patients taking monoamine oxidase inhibitors because of the potential for development of a hypertensive crisis when these agents are administered concurrently.

Dose

- *IV bolus:* 25 to 100 mg
- *Continuous infusion:* 5 to 35 mg/h

PCA

- *IV bolus:* 5 to 30 mg
- *Lockout interval:* 5 to 15 minutes

Fentanyl

Fentanyl is an analog of meperidine that is 100 times more potent than morphine. After single doses, its duration of action is limited by its rapid distribution into fat tissue. However, after repeated dosing or continuous infusion administration, fat stores become saturated, thereby prolonging its terminal elimination half-life to more than 24 hours. Unlike morphine, fentanyl does not cause histamine release.

Dose

- *IV bolus:* 25 to 75 mcg q1–2h
- *Continuous infusion:* 50 to 100 mcg/h
- *Transdermal:* Patients not previously on opioids: 25 mcg/h
- *Opioid-tolerant patients:* 25 to 100 mcg/h

PCA

- *IV bolus:* 25 to 100 mcg
- *Lockout interval:* 5 to 10 minutes

Opioid Antagonist

Naloxone

Naloxone is a pure opiate antagonist that displaces opioid agonists from the mu, delta, and kappa receptor binding sites. Naloxone reverses narcotic-induced respiratory depression, producing an increase in respiratory rate and minute ventilation, a decrease in arterial P_{CO_2}, and normalization of blood pressure if reduced. Narcotic-induced sedation or sleep is also reversed by naloxone. Naloxone reverses analgesia, increases sympathetic nervous system activity, and may result in tachycardia, hypertension, pulmonary edema, and cardiac arrhythmias. Because its duration of action is generally shorter than that of opiates, the effect of opiates may return after the effects of naloxone dissipate. Naloxone administration produces withdrawal symptoms in patients who have been taking narcotic analgesics chronically. Diluting and slowly administering naloxone in incremental doses can prevent the precipitation of acute withdrawal reactions as well as prevent the increase in sympathetic stimulation that may accompany the reversal of analgesia. One 0.4-mg ampule should be diluted with 0.9% NaCl (saline) to 10 mL to produce a concentration of 0.04 mg/mL. Sequential doses of 0.04 to 0.08 mg should be administered slowly until the desired response is obtained.

Dose

- *Postoperative opiate depression:* Initial dose: 0.1 to 0.2 mg given at 2- to 3-minute intervals until the desired response is obtained. Additional doses may be necessary depending on the response of the patient and the dose and duration of the opiate administered.
- *Continuous infusion:* 3 to 5 mcg/kg/h
- *Known or suspected opiate overdose:* Initial dose: 0.4 to 2.0 mg administered at 2- to 3-minute intervals if necessary. If no response is observed after a total of 10 mg has been administered, other causes of the depressive state should be determined.
- *Continuous infusion:* Loading dose: 0.4 mg, followed by 2.5 to 5 mcg/kg/h and titrated to the patient's response.

Monitoring Parameters

- Signs and symptoms of withdrawal reactions, respiratory rate, blood pressure, mental status, level of consciousness, and pupil size

Nonsteroidal Anti-Inflammatory Drugs

Ketorolac

Ketorolac is a nonsteroidal anti-inflammatory drug (NSAID) that is indicated for the short-term treatment of moderately severe acute pain that requires analgesia at the opioid level. The drug exhibits anti-inflammatory, analgesic, and antipyretic activities. Its mechanism of action is thought to be due to inhibition of prostaglandin synthesis by inhibiting cyclooxygenase, an enzyme that catalyzes the formation of endoperoxidases from arachidonic acid. NSAIDs are more efficacious in the treatment of prostaglandin-mediated pain. Ketorolac is the only currently available NSAID approved for IM, IV, and oral administration, and it is often used in combination with other analgesics because pain often involves multiple mechanisms. Combination therapy may be more efficacious than single-drug regimens, and combinations with narcotics can decrease narcotic requirements, minimizing narcotic side effects.

Ketorolac is associated with the same adverse effects as orally administered NSAIDs, such as reversible platelet effects, GI bleeding, and reduced renal function. Ketorolac is contraindicated in patients with advanced renal failure and in patients at risk for renal failure due to volume depletion. Therefore, volume depletion should be corrected before administering ketorolac. Because of the potential for significant adverse effects, the maximum combined duration of parenteral and oral use is limited to 5 days.

Dose

- *Loading dose:* <65 years: 60 mg; >65 years or <50 kg: 30 mg
- *Maintenance dose:* <65 years: 30 mg q6h; >65 years or <50 kg: 15 mg q6h

Monitoring Parameters

- Renal function and volume status

Neuromuscular Blocking Agents

Neuromuscular blocking agents (NMBA; see Table 23–2) are primarily used to obtain, protect, and maintain a safe secure airway and to assist with mechanical ventilation. These agents have no sedative, amnestic, anesthetic, or analgesic properties. The indications for using NMBA in critically ill patients can be divided into short- and long-term indications. Short-term indications include endotracheal intubation, stability during patient transport, hemodynamic monitoring, radiologic procedures, dressing changes, and minor surgical procedures. The primary long-term indications are optimizing mechanical ventilation, decreasing oxygen consumption, controlling increased intracranial pressure, and managing muscle spasms associated with tetanus. Neuromuscular blocking agents are categorized as either depolarizing or nondepolarizing agents.

Depolarizing Agents

Succinylcholine

Succinylcholine is the only depolarizing agent available for clinical use and is the agent of choice for rapid intubation of the trachea. Succinylcholine binds to acetylcholine receptors causing a persistent depolarization of the muscle endplate resulting in paralysis.

Succinylcholine may increase serum potassium approximately 0.5 mEq/L after a standard intubating dose of 1 to 2 mg/kg. Critically ill patients with burns, spinal cord injury, and trauma with extensive skeletal muscle damage, upper and lower motor neuron disease, and prolonged bed rest are predisposed to the development of hyperkalemia after a dose of succinylcholine because of the development of nonfunctional extrajunctional acetylcholine receptors. These receptors bind succinylcholine without causing paralysis, but depolarize the muscle cells, releasing potassium and increasing serum potassium concentrations into the supratherapeutic or toxic range. Although hyperkalemia can occur within the first 24 hours after injury, patients are most at risk during the period from 7 days after injury until 9 months later. Therefore, succinylcholine is contraindicated in these patients. In situations where succinylcholine is contraindicated, a short-acting or intermediate-acting nondepolarizing agent may be used. Succinylcholine is rapidly hydrolyzed by pseudocholinesterase; however, patients with atypical pseudocholinesterase may experience prolonged blockade. Other conditions associated with prolonged blockade resulting from reduced cholinesterase activity include pregnancy, liver disease, acute infections, carcinomas, uremia, and burns.

Dose

- See Table 23–3.

Monitoring Parameters

- Renal function, electrolytes (especially potassium), acid–base status, and level of paralysis

Nondepolarizing Agents

Nondepolarizing agents are competitive antagonists of acetylcholine at the acetylcholine receptor. Nondepolarizing agents are subdivided according to chemical class either aminosteroid (pancuronium, rocuronium, vecuronium) or benzylisoquinolinium (atracurium, cisatracurium, doxacurium, mivacurium). These agents are further classified according to duration of action: short (mivacurium), intermediate (atracurium, cisatracurium, rocuronium, vecuronium), and long (doxacurium, pancuronium).

Nondepolarizing agents can be used for short- or long-term indications in critically ill patients. Short-term indications include intubation, stability during intrahospital transport, and immobility during procedures. Long-term indications include mechanical ventilation after optimal doses of sedatives and analgesics have not been able to prevent a patient from "fighting the ventilator."

Selecting an Agent

Several factors should be considered when selecting the most appropriate agent for a patient. The onset and duration of paralysis should match that required by the procedure. Short procedures (i.e., endotracheal intubation) may require a short-acting agent with rapid onset, such as succinylcholine. Bolus doses of intermediate- or long-acting agents may be selected for longer procedures (i.e., dressing changes, radiologic scans). Long-term indications such as mechanical ventilation may require intermittent doses of long-acting agents or continuous infusions of intermediate-acting agents. The patient's underlying pathophysiology also must be considered when selecting a neuromuscular blocking agent. Succinylcholine should be avoided in patients at risk for developing hyperkalemia. Pancuronium's vagolytic effect can increase heart rate and blood pressure and should be used with caution in patients with unstable coronary artery disease. Vecuronium and pancuronium are metabolized to 3-hydroxy metabolites that have 50% of the activity of the parent compounds. These metabolites are renally eliminated and have been shown to accumulate in patients with renal dysfunction producing prolonged periods of paralysis. Monitoring patients and adjusting doses, dosing intervals, or continuous infusion rates with the aid of a peripheral nerve stimulator to maintain one or two twitches of a Train-of-Four (TOF) stimulation can usually prevent

this adverse effect from occurring (see Chapter 6, Pain and Sedation Management). Atracurium or cisatracurium should be considered for patients in multisystem organ failure because of their independence on organ function for metabolism and elimination.

Neuromuscular blocking agents should be used for management of an adult ICU patient only when all other means to manage the patient have been tried without success. The majority of critically ill patients can be managed effectively with pancuronium. For patients for whom vagolysis is contraindicated (e.g., cardiovascular disease), NMBAs other than pancuronium may be used. For patients with significant hepatic or renal disease, cisatracurium or atracurium is recommended. Patients receiving neuromuscular blocking agents should be assessed both clinically and by TOF monitoring with a goal of adjusting the neuromuscular blocking agent to achieve one to two twitches. Patients receiving NMBA therapy should also be medicated to provide adequate sedation and analgesia.

Side Effects

Although adverse effects are minimal, several can be significant. Atracurium and mivacurium can cause histamine release after rapid IV bolus injection, resulting in hypotension and flushing. Injecting each agent over at least 60 seconds can prevent this adverse effect. Laudanosine, atracurium's primary metabolite, has been shown to produce seizures in dogs after it achieves high concentrations in the cerebral spinal fluid. However, there are no reports of critically ill patients experiencing adverse central nervous system events from the accumulation of laudanosine.

The steroid-based agents, pancuronium and vecuronium are metabolized to 3-hydroxy metabolites that have 50% of the activity of the parent compounds. These metabolites are renally eliminated and have been shown to accumulate in patients with renal dysfunction, producing prolonged periods of paralysis. Monitoring patients and adjusting doses, dosing intervals, or continuous infusion rates with the aid of a peripheral nerve stimulator to maintain one or two twitches of a TOF stimulation can usually prevent this adverse effect from occurring (see Chapter 6).

A more serious complication associated with the use of nondepolarizing agents is the development of a prolonged disuse atrophy syndrome. This syndrome has been shown to occur after the extended administration of steroid-based and benzylisoquinolinium agents and cannot be prevented with peripheral nerve stimulation monitoring. Patients receiving steroids may be predisposed to developing this complication; however, this association remains to be conclusively proven.

Tolerance or the need to increase doses to maintain a stable level of paralysis is often encountered in patients receiving these agents for an extended duration. Tolerance may be attributed to the proliferation of nonfunctional extrajunctional receptors that bind drug but do not cause paralysis, increased volume of distribution resulting in lower serum concentrations at the neuromuscular junction, and binding to acute phase reactant proteins, decreasing the free, pharmacologically active fraction. An additional consideration for patients requiring NMBAs is the use of prophylactic eye care to prevent corneal abrasions. For patients receiving NMBA and corticosteroids, every effort should be made to discontinue the neuromuscular blocking agents as soon as possible.

Dose

• See Table 23–2.

Monitoring Parameters

• Level of paralysis (peripheral nerve stimulation), renal function, and liver function

Anticonvulsants

Hydantoins

Phenytoin

Phenytoin is the primary anticonvulsant used for the acute control of generalized tonic clonic seizures, following the administration of benzodiazepines, and for maintenance therapy once the seizure has been controlled. Phenytoin stabilizes neuronal cell membranes and decreases the spread of seizure activity. Phenytoin may inhibit neuronal depolarizations by blocking sodium channels in excitatory pathways and prevent increases in intracellular potassium concentrations and decreases in intracellular calcium concentrations.

The bioavailability of oral phenytoin is approximately 90% to 100%. Dissolution is the rate-limiting step in phenytoin absorption with peak serum concentrations occurring 3 to 12 hours after a dose. The rate of absorption is dose dependent, with increasing times to peak concentration with increasing doses. In addition, the dissolution and absorption rate depend on the phenytoin formulation administered. The Dilantin Kapseal brand of phenytoin capsules has the dissolution characteristics of an extended-release preparation, whereas generic phenytoin products possess rapid-release characteristics and are absorbed more quickly. Extended-release and rapid-release products are not interchangeable, and only extended-release products may be administered in a single daily dose.

Phenytoin is 90% to 95% bound to albumin. In critically ill patients the pharmacologically free fraction is highly variable and ranges between 10% and 27% of the total serum concentration. The free fraction has been shown to increase by more than 100% from baseline during the first week of illness and is generally associated with a significant reduction in serum albumin concentration. Alterations in albumin binding also may be seen in hypoalbuminemia (<2.5 g/dL), major trauma, sepsis, burns, malnutrition, and surgery, as well as liver or renal disease, and may result in an increase in a free concentration with potentially toxic effects. Significant

alterations in phenytoin metabolism usually do not occur until the serum albumin falls below 2.5 g/dL. Equations used to normalize the phenytoin concentration in patients with hypoalbuminemia are usually unreliable, and direct measurement of the free phenytoin concentration should be used to adjust therapy.

Phenytoin is metabolized by the cytochrome P450 enzyme system to its inactive primary metabolite 5-(p-hydroxyphenyl)-5-phenylhydantoin, which is glucuronidated and renally eliminated. Phenytoin undergoes dose-dependent metabolism such that proportional increases in the dose may result in greater than proportional increases in the serum concentration. It is difficult to predict the concentration at which a patient's metabolism will become saturated, so that any changes in dose above 400 to 500 mg/d need to be carefully monitored. Because phenytoin displays nonlinear metabolism, *half-life* is an inappropriate term to describe phenytoin elimination. Phenytoin metabolism is usually referred to as the time it takes to eliminate 50% (t_{50}) of a given daily dose. In normal patients taking 300 mg/d, the t_{50} is about 22 hours. As the dose is increased, the t_{50} increases, with the time to reach steady-state becoming progressively longer. The time to steady-state may vary from several days to several weeks depending on the dose and the patient's ability to metabolize the drug. Phenytoin metabolism can be affected by drugs that induce or inhibit its metabolic pathway. The effects of enzyme induction can occur within 2 days to 2 weeks after starting an agent. Inhibition usually occurs within 1 to 2 days after a drug is started and its effects usually last until the inhibiting drug is eliminated from the body. Phenytoin clearance is increased in critically ill patients resulting in serum concentrations less than 10 mg/L. The mechanism for the increase in clearance is unclear, but may be caused by changes in protein binding, induction in phenytoin metabolism, or a stress-related transient increase in hepatic metabolic function.

The recommended phenytoin loading dose of 15 to 20 mg/kg produces serum concentrations between 20 and 30 mg/L. Loading doses of 18 to 20 mg/kg are recommended for treating status epilepticus, and loading doses of 15 to 18 mg/kg are recommended for seizure prophylaxis after head injury or neurosurgery. The serum concentration increases approximately 1.4 mg/L for each 1 mg/kg of phenytoin administered.

The maintenance dose should be started 8 to 12 hours after the loading dose. The usual adult maintenance dose is 5 to 6 mg/kg per day, although critically ill patients or patients with neurotrauma may require doses of 6.0 to 7.5 mg/kg per day. Intravenous maintenance doses should be administered every 6 to 8 hours to maintain therapeutic serum concentrations.

Phenytoin precipitates in dextrose-containing solutions and should only be mixed in 0.9% sodium chloride solutions. To prevent phlebitis, the maximum concentration for peripheral administration is 10 mg/mL; a final concentration of 20 mg/mL may used if the dose is being administered through a central venous catheter. Phenytoin solution must be administered through an in-line 1.2- or 5.0-μ filter to prevent the administration of phenytoin crystals into the systemic circulation. Phenytoin doses should not be administered at a rate faster than 50 mg/min because hypotension and arrhythmias may occur because of its propylene glycol diluent. The infusion rate should be decreased by 50% if hypotension or arrhythmias develop.

Oral administration is not usually recommended in critically ill patients because of the risk of erratic or incomplete absorption. Phenytoin oral suspension may adhere to the inside walls of oro- or nasogastric tubes, reducing the dose delivered to the patient. If phenytoin is administered through a feeding tube, the tube should be flushed with 30 to 60 mL of 0.9% sodium chloride before and after administering the dose. After the dose is administered the feeding tube should be clamped for 1 hour before restarting the feeding solution. Oral absorption may be impaired by concomitant administration with enteral nutrition solutions, reducing its bioavailability and resulting in erratic serum concentrations with seizures occurring as a result of subtherapeutic serum concentrations. Phenytoin oral solution must be shaken prior to use to ensure uniformity in the distribution of the phenytoin particles throughout the suspension. If the suspension is not shaken before obtaining a dose, the phenytoin powder settles to the bottom of the bottle producing subtherapeutic doses when the bottle is first opened and toxic doses as the bottle is used.

Hemodialysis and hemofiltration have no effect on phenytoin clearance. Agents known to inhibit or enhance this enzymatic pathway may affect phenytoin's clearance. Early adverse effects that may be associated with increasing serum concentrations are nystagmus (>20 mg/L), ataxia (>30 mg/L), and lethargy, confusion, and impaired cognitive function (>40 mg/L).

The normal therapeutic range for the total phenytoin serum concentration is 10 to 20 mg/L with the free fraction therapeutic range of 1 to 2 mg/L. Serum concentration of 20 to 30 mg/L may be required in patients who are having seizures. Phenytoin serum concentrations can be obtained 30 to 60 minutes after the loading dose is infused to assess the adequacy of the dose. Trough concentrations should be monitored 2 to 3 times a week, particularly after the first week of therapy. Measurement of free phenytoin concentrations may be indicated in critically ill patients, patients with serum albumin concentrations less than 2.5 g/dL, renal failure, or receiving drugs known to displace phenytoin from albumin binding sites. Other monitoring parameters include the patient's seizure activity and medication profile for agents known to alter phenytoin's metabolism.

Dose

- *Loading dose:* 15 to 20 mg/kg IV
- *Maintenance dose:* 5 mg/kg/d IV or PO

Monitoring Parameters
- Seizure activity, electroencephalogram (EEG), serum phenytoin concentration (free phenytoin concentration if applicable), albumin, liver function, infusion rate, blood pressure, ECG with IV administration, and IV injection site

Fosphenytoin

Fosphenytoin is a phenytoin prodrug with good aqueous solubility that was developed to be a water-soluble alternative to phenytoin. In patients unable to tolerate oral phenytoin, equimolar doses of fosphenytoin have been shown to produce equal or greater plasma phenytoin concentrations. Although phenytoin sodium 50 mg is equal to fosphenytoin sodium 75 mg, phenytoin should be converted to fosphenytoin on a milligram-per-milligram basis (e.g., phenytoin 300 mg should be converted to fosphenytoin 300 mg).

Fosphenytoin, administered IM or IV, is rapidly and completely converted to phenytoin in vivo, resulting in essentially 100% bioavailability. The conversion half-life to phenytoin is about 33 minutes following IM administration and about 15 minutes after IV infusion. After IM administration, peak plasma fosphenytoin concentrations occur approximately 30 minutes postdose, with peak phenytoin concentrations occurring in about 3 hours. Fosphenytoin's peak concentration following IV administration occurs at the end of the infusion, with peak phenytoin concentrations occurring in approximately 40 to 75 minutes. In patients with renal or hepatic dysfunction or hypoalbuminemia, there is enhanced conversion to phenytoin without an increase in clearance. Fosphenytoin is 90% to 95% bound to plasma proteins and is saturable with the percent of bound fosphenytoin decreasing as the fosphenytoin dose increases.

The maximum total phenytoin concentration increases with increasing fosphenytoin doses, but the total phenytoin concentration is less affected by increasing fosphenytoin infusion rates. Maximum free phenytoin concentrations are nearly constant at infusion rates up to 50 mg phenytoin equivalents (PE)/min, whereas they increase with faster infusion rates secondary to phenytoin displacement from albumin binding sites in the presence of high fosphenytoin concentrations.

For the treatment of status epilepticus, the recommended loading dose of IV fosphenytoin is 15 to 20 PE/kg, and it should not be administered faster than 150 mg PE/min because of the risk of hypotension. Fosphenytoin 15 to 20 mg PE/kg infused at 100 to 150 mg PE/min yields plasma-free phenytoin concentrations over time that approximate those achieved when an equimolar dose of IV phenytoin is administered at 50 mg/min. In the treatment of status epilepticus, total phenytoin concentrations greater than 10 mg/L and free phenytoin concentrations greater than 1 mg/mL are achieved with 10 to 20 minutes after starting the infusion. Intramuscular fosphenytoin should not be used in the treatment of status epilepticus because therapeutic phenytoin concentrations are not achieved as quickly as with IV administration.

In nonemergent situations, loading doses of 10 to 20 PE/kg administered IV or IM is recommended. In nonemergent situations, IV administration of infusion rates of 50 to 100 mg PE/min may be acceptable, but results in slightly lower and delayed maximum free phenytoin concentrations as compared with administration at higher infusion rates. The initial daily maintenance dose is 4 to 6 mg PE/kg per day. Dosing adjustments are not required when IM fosphenytoin is substituted temporarily for oral phenytoin. However, patients switched from once-daily extended-release phenytoin capsules may require twice-daily or more frequent administration of fosphenytoin to maintain similar peak and trough phenytoin concentrations.

The incidence of adverse effects tends to increase as both dose and infusion rate are increased. At doses above 15 mg PE/kg and infusion rates higher than 150 mg PE/min, transient pruritis, tinnitus, nystagmus, somnolence, and ataxia occur more frequently than at lower doses or infusion rates. Severe burning, itching, and paresthesias of the groin are commonly associated with infusion rates greater than 150 mg PE/min. Slowing or temporarily stopping the infusion can minimize the frequency and severity of these reactions. Continuous cardiac rate and rhythm, blood pressure, and respiratory function should be monitored throughout the fosphenytoin infusion and for 10 to 20 minutes after the end of the infusion.

Following fosphenytoin administration, phenytoin concentrations should not be monitored until the conversion to phenytoin is complete. This occurs within 2 hours after the end of an IV infusion and 5 hours after an IM injection. Prior to complete conversion, commonly used immunoanalytic techniques such as fluorescence polarization and enzyme-mediated assays may significantly overestimate plasma phenytoin concentrations because of cross-reactivity with fosphenytoin. Blood samples collected before complete conversion to phenytoin should be collected in tubes containing EDTA as an anticoagulant to minimize the ex vivo conversion of fosphenytoin to phenytoin. Monitoring is similar to phenytoin. In critically ill patients with renal failure receiving fosphenytoin, one or more metabolites of adducts of fosphenytoin accumulate and display significant cross-reactivity with several phenytoin immunoassay methods. The AxSYM, TDx phenytoin II, ACS:180, and Vitros assays display falsely increased phenytoin concentrations, up to 20 times higher than high-pressure liquid chromatography (HPLC) methods.

Barbiturates

Pentobarbital

Pentobarbital is a barbiturate mainly used to control intracranial pressure in patients with head injuries. Pentobarbital may also be used in patients with status epilepticus who are refractory to other anticonvulsants. The central nervous system protective effect of pentobarbital may be attributed to decreased cerebral oxygen consumption allowing a proportionate decrease in cerebral blood flow and potentially scavenging free oxygen radicals. Its anticonvulsant effects are similar to phenobarbital. Pentobarbital produces a dose-dependent depression of the central nervous system beginning with sedation and ending with coma and death. At high serum concentrations, pentobarbital suppresses the respiratory drive necessitating mechanical ventilation during therapeutic pentobarbital coma.

Pentobarbital has a greater affinity for adipose tissue than phenobarbital. Its lipophilicity causes it to cross the blood–brain barrier faster than phenobarbital to produce its central nervous system effects. Pentobarbital is hepatically metabolized with an average half-life of 22 hours. In head injured patients pentobarbital's clearance is faster with its half-life averaging 15 to 19 hours. Alterations in hepatic microsomal enzymes can be expected to alter its clearance and half-life.

The usual loading dose required to induce pentobarbital coma is 5 to 10 mg/kg infused over 2 hours. Each 1 mg/kg increases the serum concentration approximately 1 mg/L. The maintenance infusion is begun at a rate of 1 mg/kg per hour and can be adjusted in increments of 0.5 to 1.0 mg/kg per hour to a final infusion rate that achieves an appropriate reduction in intracranial pressure. Typical maintenance infusion rates range from 0.5 to 4.0 mg/kg per hour producing serum concentrations between 20 and 50 mg/L. The usual dose for control of status epilepticus is an initial loading dose of 5 to 10 mg/kg followed by a maintenance infusion of 0.5 to 1.0 mg/kg per hour. Rapid administration of pentobarbital may result in hypotension and arrhythmias secondary to its propylene glycol diluent. If the systolic blood pressure drops 10 to 20 mm Hg, the infusion rate should be reduced by 50%, and if the systolic blood pressure drops more than 20 mm Hg, volume resuscitation and vasopressors may be required for blood pressure support. The IV administration of pentobarbital also may cause respiratory depression, apnea, laryngospasm, or hypotension, particularly if injected too rapidly.

The infusion may be discontinued after 72 hours of intracranial pressure control or if there is deterioration in the cardiovascular status of the patient. The infusion should be tapered over 48 to 72 hours by decreasing the infusion rate by 25% every 12 hours. The patient should be monitored during this time for increases in intracranial pressure or the development of seizures.

Serum concentrations should be obtained 1 to 2 hours after the loading infusion and then daily. The serum concentration within 24 hours after starting therapy does not reflect steady-state conditions. If the 24-hour concentration has changed from the post-loading dose by 33% to 50% and is less than 20 mg/L or greater than 50 mg/L, the infusion should be increased or decreased by 0.5 to 1.0 mg/kg per hour. Serum concentrations should be monitored in conjunction with the patient's physiologic parameters such as brain stem reflexes, intracranial pressure, systemic blood pressure, EEG, and hemodynamic parameters. Acceptable therapeutic endpoints include a mean arterial pressure of 70 to 80 mm Hg, cerebral perfusion pressure of greater than 60 mm Hg, intracranial pressure of greater than 20 mm Hg, EEG showing a 30- to 60-second burst suppression pattern, and an absence of muscular movement and brainstem reflexes on neurologic examination. However, deeper levels of sedation may not be needed if seizures are controlled, or intracranial pressure is less than 20 mm Hg.

Phenobarbital

Phenobarbital may be added for patients who have not responded to IV benzodiazepines and phenytoin. Phenobarbital depresses excitatory postsynaptic seizure discharge and increases the convulsive threshold for electrical and chemical stimulation. This effect is due to the inhibiting effects of GABA.

Phenobarbital is 90% to 100% bioavailable with peak concentrations occurring in 0.5 to 4 hours after an oral or IM dose. Peak brain concentrations occur approximately 20 to 40 minutes after an administered dose. Phenobarbital is primarily hepatically metabolized by the cytochrome P450 microsomal enzyme system with approximately 25% of a dose excreted unchanged in the urine. The half-life of phenobarbital is 96 hours with steady-state conditions being achieved in about 2 to 3 weeks.

The usual loading dose of phenobarbital is 20 mg/kg and achieves a serum concentration of about 20 mg/L. Each 1 mg/kg dose increment increases the serum concentration by about 1.5 mg/L. The loading dose has the potential to decrease respiratory drive in patients who have received other central nervous system depressants. The maximum IV infusion rate is 50 mg/min or less. Infusion rates above 50 mg/min may cause hypotension because of its propylene glycol diluent. Blood pressure should be monitored during the loading infusion, and the infusion rate should be decreased by 50% if hypotension develops.

The maintenance dose should be started within 24 hours after the loading dose. The typical adult maintenance dose of 2 to 4 mg/kg per day produces serum concentrations in the range of 10 to 30 mg/L. Each 1 mg/kg per day increase in the maintenance dose increases the serum concentration about 10 mg/L. Lower doses should be used in elderly patients, patients with renal failure, and patients with liver dysfunction because of their reduced abilities to eliminate the drug. The maintenance dose should be administered as a single daily dose because of its long half-life, with this dose usually given at bedtime because of phenobarbital's sedative properties. In cases of excessive sedation, the daily dose may be administered as smaller doses two to three times per day. Tolerance usually develops to sedation with long-term administration.

Hemodialysis removes a significant amount of phenobarbital. Posthemodialysis serum concentrations should be monitored and supplemented doses administered after hemodialysis to maintain the serum concentration within the therapeutic range.

Phenobarbital serum concentrations can be monitored 30 to 60 minutes after the end of the loading infusion to assess the adequacy of the dose. Maintenance doses should be monitored every 3 to 4 days in patients with changing hemodynamic status, because the patients may have alterations in their ability to eliminate the drug resulting in increased or decreased serum concentrations. If the serum concentrations are fluctuating, they should be monitored daily to prevent excessive rises in the serum concentrations and toxicity or subtherapeutic serum concentrations and seizures. The serum concentration may be monitored once a week if stable. Trough concentrations are typically monitored, but because of its long half-life, there is minimal peak to trough variation in the serum concentration so that a drug level can be drawn anytime during the dosing interval. When patients regain consciousness, serum levels may not be needed if the patients are not having seizures.

Dose

- *Loading dose:* 20 mg/kg IV (1 mg/kg increases the serum concentration 1 mg/L)
- *Maintenance dose:* 3 to 5 mg/kg/d IV or PO

Monitoring Parameters

- Seizure activity, EEG, serum phenobarbital concentration, infusion rate, blood pressure, and ECG with IV administration

Benzodiazepines

Benzodiazepines are the primary agents in the management of status epilepticus. These agents suppress the spread of seizure activity but do not abolish the abnormal discharge from a seizure focus. Although IV diazepam has the fastest onset of action, lorazepam or midazolam are equally efficacious in controlling seizure activity. They are the agents of choice to temporarily control seizures and to gain time for the loading of phenytoin or phenobarbital. Phenytoin may also be used prophylactically in patients who are at risk for seizures after neurosurgery or following head injuries.

Monitoring Parameters

- Seizure activity, EEG, and respiratory rate and quality

CARDIOVASCULAR SYSTEM PHARMACOLOGY

Miscellaneous Agents

Nesiritide

Nesiritide is a recombinant human b-type natriuretic peptide, which is a cardiac hormone that regulates cardiovascular homeostasis and fluid volume during states of volume and pressure overload. The agent is effective in reducing pulmonary capillary wedge pressure and improving dyspnea symptoms in patients with acutely decompensated CHF who have dyspnea at rest or with minimal activity. The most common adverse effects include hypotension, tachycardia, and/or bradycardia.

Dose

- *IV bolus:* 2 mcg/kg
- *Continuous infusion:* 0.01 mcg/kg/min

Monitoring Parameters

- Blood pressure, heart rate, urine output, and hemodynamic parameters

Fenoldopam

Fenoldopam is a benzapine derivative with selective dopamine-1 receptor agonist properties, similar to dopamine. This dopaminergic stimulation results in a decrease in systemic blood pressure with an increase in natriuresis and urine output. The primary use of fenoldopam is in the management of severe hypertension, particularly in patients with renal impairment.

Dose

- *Continuous infusion:* 0.1 to 1.6 mcg/kg/min

Monitoring Parameters

- Blood pressure, urine output, and hemodynamic parameters

Parenteral Vasodilators (see Chapter 23)

Nitrates

Sodium Nitroprusside

Sodium nitroprusside is a balanced vasodilator affecting the arterial and venous systems. Blood pressure reduction occurs within seconds after an infusion is started, with a duration of action of less than 10 minutes once the infusion is discontinued. Sodium nitroprusside is considered the agent of choice in acute hypertensive conditions such as hypertensive encephalopathy, intracerebral infarction, subarachnoid hemorrhage, carotid endarterectomy, malignant hypertension, microangiopathic anemia, and aortic dissection, and after general surgical procedures, major vascular procedures, or renal transplantation.

If sodium nitroprusside is used for longer than 48 hours, there is the risk of thiocyanate toxicity. However, this may only be a concern in patients with renal dysfunction. In this setting, thiocyanate serum concentrations should be monitored to ensure that they remain below 10 mg/dL. Other potential side effects include methemoglobinemia and cyanide toxicity. Nitroprusside should be used with caution in the setting of increased intracranial pressure, such as head trauma or postcraniotomy, where it may cause an increase in cerebral blood flow. Nitroprusside's effects on intracranial pressure may be attenuated by a lowered $PaCO_2$ and raised PaO_2. In pregnant women, nitroprusside should be reserved only for refractory hypertension associated with eclampsia, because of the potential risk to the fetus.

Dose

- *Continuous infusion:* 0.5 to 10.0 mcg/kg/min

Monitoring Parameters

- Blood pressure, renal function, thiocyanate concentration (prolonged infusions), acid–base status, and hemodynamic parameters

Nitroglycerin

Nitroglycerin is a preferential venous dilator affecting the venous system at low doses, but relaxes arterial smooth muscle at higher doses. The onset of blood pressure reduction after starting a nitroglycerin infusion is similar to sodium nitroprusside, approximately 1 to 3 minutes, with a duration of action of less than 10 minutes. Headaches are a common adverse effect that may occur with nitroglycerin therapy and can be treated with acetaminophen. Tachyphylaxis can be seen with the IV infusion, similar to what is seen after the chronic use of topical nitroglycerin preparations. In patients receiving heparin in addition to nitroglycerin, increased doses of heparin may be required to maintain a therapeutic partial thromboplastin time (PTT). The mechanism by which nitroglycerin causes heparin resistance is unknown. However, the PTT should be closely monitored in patients receiving nitroglycerin and heparin concurrently.

Nitroglycerin is the preferred agent in the setting of hypertension associated with myocardial ischemia or infarction because its net effect is a reduction in oxygen consumption.

Dose

- *Continuous infusion:* 10 to 300 mcg/min

Monitoring Parameters

- Blood pressure, heart rate, signs and symptoms of ischemia, hemodynamic parameters (if applicable), and PTT (in patients receiving heparin concurrently)

Arterial Vasodilating Agents

Hydralazine

Hydralazine reduces peripheral vascular resistance by directly relaxing arterial smooth muscle. Blood pressure reduction occurs within 5 to 20 minutes after an IV dose and lasts approximately 2 to 6 hours. Common adverse effects include headache, nausea, vomiting, palpitations, and tachycardia. Reflex tachycardia may precipitate anginal attacks.

Dose

- 10 to 25 mg IV q2–4h

Monitoring Parameters

- Blood pressure and heart rate

Diazoxide

Diazoxide is a nondiuretic that reduces peripheral vascular resistance by directly relaxing arterial smooth muscle. Side effects such as hypotension, nausea and vomiting, dizziness, weakness, hyperglycemia, and reflex tachycardia have been associated with the use of the higher 300-mg dosing regimen. Using lower dose regimens produces similar but less severe side effects. Caution should be used when diazoxide is administered with other antihypertensive agents because excessive hypotension may result.

Blood pressure reduction occurs within 1 to 2 minutes and lasts 3 to 12 hours after a dose. Blood pressure should be monitored frequently until stable, and then monitored hourly.

Dose

- *IV bolus:* 50 to 150 mg q5min
- *Continuous infusion:* 7.5 to 30.0 mg/min

Monitoring Parameters

- Blood pressure, heart rate, and serum glucose

Ganglionic Blocking Agents

Trimethaphan

Trimethaphan is the only IV ganglionic blocking agent available. The onset of blood pressure reduction is within minutes after starting an infusion, with a duration of action of up to 20 minutes after stopping the infusion. However, hypotension may persist for several hours after the administration of higher doses. Adverse effects that have been associated with the use of trimethaphan include ileus, urinary retention, and mydriasis.

Trimethaphan in combination with a beta-blocker may be used as an alternative to nitroprusside in the setting of an acute aortic dissection. Trimethaphan should be avoided in hypertension associated with eclampsia and renal vasculature disorders.

Dose

- *Continuous infusion:* 0.5 to 5.0 mg/min

Monitoring Parameters

- Blood pressure, heart rate, bowel sounds, GI tract function, and bladder function

Alpha- and Beta-Adrenergic Blocking Agents

Labetalol

Labetalol is a combined alpha- and beta-adrenergic blocking agent with a specificity of beta receptors to alpha receptors of approximately 7:1. Labetalol may be administered parenterally by escalating bolus doses or by continuous infusion. The onset of action after the administration of labetalol is within 5 minutes with a duration of effect from 2 to 12 hours. Because labetalol possesses beta-blocking properties, it may produce bronchospasm in individuals with asthma or reactive airway disease. It also may produce conduction system disturbances or bradycardia in susceptible individuals, and its negative inotropic properties may exacerbate symptoms of CHF.

Labetalol may be considered as an alternative to sodium nitroprusside in the setting of hypertension associated with head trauma or postcraniotomy, spinal cord syndromes, transverse lesions of the spinal cord, Guillain-Barré syndrome, or autonomic hyperreflexia, as well as hypertension associated with sympathomimetics (e.g., cocaine, amphetamines, phencyclidine, nasal decongestants, or certain diet pills) or withdrawal of centrally acting antihypertensive agents (e.g., beta-blockers, clonidine, or methyldopa). It also may be used as an alternative to phentolamine in the setting of pheochromocytoma because of its alpha- and beta-blocking properties.

Dose

- *IV bolus:* 20 mg over 2 minutes, then 40 to 80 mg IV q10 min to a total of 300 mg
- *Continuous infusion:* 1 to 4 mg/min and titrate to effect

Monitoring Parameters

- Blood pressure, heart rate, ECG, and signs and symptoms of heart failure or bronchospasm (if applicable)

Alpha-Adrenergic Blocking Agents

Phentolamine

Phentolamine is an alpha-adrenergic blocking agent that may be administered parenterally by bolus injection or continuous infusion. Onset of action is within 1 to 2 minutes, with a duration of action of 3 to 10 minutes. Potential adverse effects that may occur with phentolamine include tachycardia, GI stimulation, and hypoglycemia.

Phentolamine is considered the drug of choice for the treatment of hypertension associated with pheochromocytoma because of its ability to block alpha-adrenergic receptors. Also, it is the primary agent used to treat acute hypertensive episodes in patients receiving monoamine oxidase inhibitors.

Dose

- *IV bolus:* 5 to 10 mg q5–15min
- *Continuous infusion:* 1 to 10 mg/min

Monitoring Parameters

- Blood pressure and heart rate

Beta-Adrenergic Blocking Agents

Beta-adrenergic blocking agents available for IV delivery include propranolol, esmolol, metoprolol, and atenolol. Propranolol and metoprolol may be administered by bolus injection or continuous infusion. Atenolol typically is administered by bolus injection, and esmolol is administered by continuous infusion. A continuous infusion of esmolol may or may not be preceded by an initial bolus injection.

Esmolol has the fastest onset and shortest duration of action, approximately 1 to 3 minutes and 20 to 30 minutes, respectively. Propranolol and metoprolol have similar onset times, but durations of action vary between 1 and 6 hours. The duration of action after a bolus dose of atenolol is approximately 12 hours.

All agents may produce bronchospasm in individuals with asthma or reactive airway disease and may produce conduction system disturbances or bradycardia in susceptible individuals. Also, because of their negative inotropic properties, they may exacerbate symptoms of CHF.

Beta-blocking agents typically are used as adjuncts with other agents in the treatment of acute hypertension. They may be used with sodium nitroprusside or trimethaphan in the treatment of acute aortic dissections. They should be administered to patients with hypertension associated with pheochromocytoma only after phentolamine has been given. Also, they are the agents of choice in patients who have been maintained on beta-blocking agents for the chronic management of hypertension but who have abruptly stopped therapy.

Beta-blocking agents should be avoided in patients with hypertensive encephalopathy, intracranial infarctions, or subarachnoid hemorrhages because of their central nervous system depressant effects. They also should be avoided in patients with acute pulmonary edema because of their negative inotropic properties. Finally, beta-blocking agents should be avoided in hypertension associated with eclampsia and renal vasculature disorders.

Dose

- *Atenolol:* IV bolus: 5 mg over 5 minutes, followed by 5 mg IV 10 minutes later
- *Esmolol:* IV bolus 500 mcg/kg; continuous infusion: 50 to 400 mcg/kg/min
- *Metoprolol:* IV bolus: 5 mg IV q2min × 3 doses
- *Propranolol:* IV bolus: 0.5 to 1.0 mg q5–15min; continuous infusion: 1 to 4 mg/h

Monitoring Parameters

- Blood pressure, heart rate, ECG, and signs and symptoms of heart failure or bronchospasm (if applicable)

Angiotensin-Converting Enzyme Inhibitors

Angiotensin-converting enzyme (ACE) inhibitors competitively inhibit angiotensin-converting enzyme, which is responsible for the conversion of angiotensin I to angiotensin II. In addition, these agents inactivate bradykinin and other vasodilatory prostaglandins, resulting in an increase in plasma renin concentrations and a reduction in plasma aldosterone concentrations. The net effect is a reduction in blood pressure in hypertensive patients and a reduction in afterload in patients with CHF.

ACE inhibitors are indicated in the management of hypertension and CHF. Adverse effects associated with ACE inhibitors include rash, taste disturbances, and cough. Initial-dose hypotension may occur in patients who are hypovolemic, hyponatremic, or who have been aggressively diuresed. Hypotension may be avoided or minimized by starting with low doses or withholding diuretics for 24 to 48 hours. Worsening of renal function may occur in patients with bilateral renal artery stenosis.

Enalapril

Enalapril is a prodrug that is converted in the liver to its active moiety, enalaprilat, a long-acting ACE inhibitor. Enalapril is available in an oral dosage form, and enalaprilat is available in the IV form. Following an IV dose of enalaprilat, blood pressure lowering occurs within 15 minutes and lasts 4 to 6 hours.

Dose

- *Enalaprilat:* IV bolus: 0.625 to 1.250 mg over 5 minutes q6h; continuous infusion: not recommended
- *Enalapril:* oral: 2.5 to 40.0 mg qd

Monitoring Parameters

- Blood pressure, heart rate, renal function, and electrolytes

Calcium Channel Blocking Agents

Calcium channel blocking agents may be used as alternative therapy in the treatment of hypertension resulting from hypertensive encephalopathy, myocardial ischemia, malignant hypertension, or eclampsia, or after renal transplantation.

Nicardipine

Nicardipine is an IV calcium channel blocking agent that is primarily indicated for the treatment of hypertension. Onset is within 5 minutes with duration of approximately 30 minutes. Nicardipine also is available in an oral dosage form so that patients started on IV therapy can convert to oral therapy when indicated.

Dose

- *Continuous infusion:* 5 mg/h, increase every 15 minutes to a maximum of 15 mg/h
- *Oral:* 20 to 40 mg q8h

Monitoring Parameters

- Blood pressure and heart rate

Central Sympatholytic Agents

Clonidine

Clonidine is an oral agent that stimulates alpha$_2$-adrenergic receptors in the medulla oblongata, causing inhibition of sympathetic vasomotor centers. Although clonidine typically is used as maintenance antihypertensive therapy, it can be used in the setting of hypertensive urgencies or emergencies. Its antihypertensive effects may be seen within 30 minutes and last 8 to 12 hours. Once blood pressure is controlled, oral maintenance clonidine therapy may be started.

Centrally acting sympatholytics rarely are indicated as first-line agents except when hypertension may be due to the abrupt withdrawal of one of these agents.

Dose

- *Hypertensive urgency:* 0.2 mg PO initially, then 0.1 mg/h PO (to a maximum of 0.8 mg)
- *Transdermal:* TTS-1 (0.1 mg/d) to TTS-3 (0.3 mg/d) topically q1week

Monitoring Parameters

- Blood pressure, heart rate, and mental status

Antiarrhythmics

Antiarrhythmic agents are divided into five classes. Dosage information for individual antiarrhythmic agents is listed in Chapter 23 (see Table 23–4).

Class I Agents

Class I agents are further divided into four subclasses: Ia (procainamide, quinidine, disopyramide), Ib (lidocaine, tocainide, mexiletine), Ic (flecainide, propafenone), and others (moricizine). All class I agents block sodium channels in the myocardium and inhibit potassium repolarizing currents to prolong repolarization.

Class Ia Agents

Class Ia agents inhibit the fast sodium channel (phase 0 of the action potential), slow conduction at elevated serum drug concentrations, and prolong action potential duration and repolarization. Class Ia agents can cause proarrhythmic complications by prolonging the QT interval or by depressing conduction and promoting reentry.

Monitoring Parameters

- ECG (QRS complex, QT interval, arrhythmia frequency)

Class Ib Agents

Class Ib agents have little effect on phase 0 depolarization and conduction velocity, but shorten the action potential duration and repolarization. QT prolongation typically does not occur with class Ib agents. Class Ib agents act selectively on diseased or ischemic tissue where they block conduction and interrupt reentry circuits.

Monitoring Parameters

- ECG (QT interval, arrhythmia frequency)

Class Ic Agents

Class Ic agents inhibit the fast sodium channel and cause a marked depression of phase 0 of the action potential and slow conduction profoundly, but have minimal effects on repolarization. The dramatic effects of these agents on conduction may account for their significant proarrhythmic effects, which limit their use in patients with supraventricular arrhythmias and structural heart disease.

Monitoring Parameters

- ECG (PR interval and QRS complex, arrhythmia frequency)

Class Ib/Ic Agents

Moricizine is a phenothiazine derivative that possesses electrophysiologic effects similar to class Ib and Ic agents. It slows atrioventricular nodal and intraventricular conduction without affecting the action potential duration or repolarization. Its use is limited to patients with life-threatening ventricular arrhythmias resistant to other agents.

Monitoring Parameters

- ECG (PR interval and QRS complex, arrhythmia frequency)

Class II Agents

Beta-blocking agents inactivate sodium channels and depress phase 4 depolarization and increase the refractory period of the atrioventricular node. These agents have no effect on repolarization. Beta-blockers competitively antagonize catecholamine binding at beta-adrenergic receptors.

Beta-blocking agents can be classified as selective or nonselective agents. *Nonselective agents* bind to beta-1 receptors located on myocardial cells and beta-2 receptors located on bronchial and skeletal smooth muscle. Stimulation of beta-1 receptors causes an increase in heart rate and contractility, whereas stimulation of beta-2 receptors results in bronchodilation and vasodilation. Selective beta-blocking agents block beta-1 receptors in the heart at low or moderate doses, but they become less selective with increasing doses.

Class II agents are used for the prophylaxis and treatment of both supraventricular arrhythmias and arrhythmias associated with catecholamine excess or stimulation, slowing the ventricular response in atrial fibrillation, lowering blood pressure, decreasing heart rate, and decreasing ischemia. Esmolol is useful especially for the rapid, short-term control of ventricular response in atrial fibrillation or flutter.

Nonselective beta-blocking agents should be avoided or used with caution in patients with CHF, atrioventricular nodal blockade, asthma, COPD, peripheral vascular disease,

Raynaud's phenomenon, and diabetes. Beta-1 selective beta-blocking agents should be used with caution in these populations.

Monitoring Parameters

- ECG (heart rate, PR interval, arrhythmia frequency)

Class III Agents

Class III agents (amiodarone, bretylium, and sotalol) lengthen the action potential duration and effective refractory period and prolong repolarization. Additionally, amiodarone possesses alpha- and beta-blocking effects and calcium channel blocking properties and inhibits the fast sodium channel. Bretylium is taken up into sympathetic nerve endings, causing a release of norepinephrine followed by a depletion of norepinephrine in the nerve ending. Sotalol possesses nonselective beta-blocking properties. These agents usually are reserved for arrhythmias refractory to other antiarrhythmic agents. Although torsades de pointes is relatively rare with amiodarone, precautions should be taken to prevent hypokalemia- or digitalis-toxicity–induced arrhythmias. Sotalol may be associated with proarrhythmic effects in the setting of hypokalemia, bradycardia, high sotalol dose, and QT-interval prolongation, and in patients with preexisting CHF.

Monitoring Parameters

- *Amiodarone:* ECG (PR and QT intervals, arrhythmia frequency)
- *Sotalol:* ECG (QT interval, QRS complex, arrhythmia frequency)

Class IV Agents

Calcium channel blocking agents inhibit calcium channels within the atrioventricular node and sinoatrial node, prolong conduction through the atrioventricular and sinoatrial nodes, and prolong the functional refractory period of the nodes, as well as depress phase 4 depolarization. Class IV agents are used for the prophylaxis and treatment of supraventricular arrhythmias and to slow the ventricular response in atrial fibrillation, flutter, and multifocal atrial tachycardia.

Monitoring Parameters

- ECG (PR interval, arrhythmia frequency)

Class V Agents

Adenosine, digoxin, and atropine possess different pharmacologic properties but ultimately affect the sinoatrial node or atrioventricular node. Adenosine decreases conduction through the atrioventricular node by increasing potassium conductance, causing hyperpolarization and a decrease in calcium channel conduction in myocardial cells within the atrioventricular node. Digoxin slows the sinoatrial node rate of depolarization and conduction through the atrioventricular node primarily through vagal stimulating effects.

The primary arrhythmias seen in critically ill patients include multifocal atrial tachycardia, supraventricular tachycardias including atrial fibrillation and atrial flutter and atrial, and ventricular ectopy. Multifocal atrial tachycardia is usually attributed to the underlying illness and rarely requires pharmacologic intervention. Atrial and ventricular ectopy, including tachyarrhythmias, may be associated with the underlying illness, electrolyte abnormalities, or medications (catecholamines). These usually respond to the correction of the underlying cause and rarely require pharmacologic intervention. Hemodynamically stable atrial fibrillation and atrial flutter can usually be treated pharmacologically. Hemodynamically unstable atrial fibrillation and atrial flutter should be treated with electrical cardioversion. Ventricular rate control has typically been achieved with digoxin, diltiazem, or beta-blocker with conversion to normal sinus rhythm being attempted with a class Ia antiarrhythmic agent (procainamide, quinidine). Class Ia agents are problematic in certain patients (post-myocardial infarction [MI]) and are being replaced as first-line therapy by newer agents such as ibutilide, amiodarone, sotalol, and propafenone.

Ibutilide

Ibutilide is a class III antiarrhythmic agent indicated for the conversion of recent-onset atrial fibrillation and atrial flutter to normal sinus rhythm. Ibutilide causes the prolongation of the refractory period and action potential duration, with little or no effect on conduction velocity or automaticity. Its electrophysiologic effects are predominantly derived from activation of a slow sodium inward current. Ibutilide can cause slowing of the sinus rate and atrioventricular node conduction, but has no effect on heart rate, PR interval, or QRS interval. The drug is associated with minimal hemodynamic effects with no significant effect on cardiac output, mean pulmonary arterial pressure, or pulmonary capillary wedge pressure. Ibutilide has not been shown to lower blood pressure or worsen CHF.

Ibutilide has been shown to be more effective than procainamide and sotalol in terminating atrial fibrillation and atrial flutter. In addition, ibutilide has been shown to decrease the amount of joules required to treat resistant atrial fibrillation and atrial flutter during cardioversion. Depending on the duration of atrial fibrillation or flutter, ibutilide has an efficacy rate of 22% to 43% and 37% to 76%, respectively, for terminating these arrhythmias. Ibutilide is only available as an IV dosage form and cannot be used for the long-term maintenance of normal sinus rhythm.

Sustained and nonsustained polymorphic ventricular tachycardia is the most significant adverse effect associated with ibutilide. The overall incidence of polymorphic ventricular tachycardia diagnosed as torsades de pointes was 4.3%, including 1.7% of patients in whom the arrhythmia was sustained and required cardioversion. Ibutilide administration should be avoided in patients receiving other agents that prolong the QTc interval, including class Ia or III antiarrhythmic agents, phenothiazines, antidepressants, and some antihistamines. Before ibutilide administration, patients should be screened carefully to exclude high-risk individuals, such as those with a QTc interval greater than 440 ms or bradycardia. Serum potassium and magnesium levels should be measured and corrected before the drug is administered. The ibutilide infusion should be stopped in the event of nonsustained or sustained ventricular tachycardia or marked prolongation in the QTc interval. Patients should be monitored for at least 4 hours after the infusion or until the QTc returns to baseline, with longer monitoring if nonsustained ventricular tachycardia develops.

Amiodarone

Amiodarone is a class II antiarrhythmic agent with some calcium channel blocking and beta-blocking properties. Its antiarrhythmic effect is due to the prolongation of the action potential duration and refractory period, and secondarily through alpha-adrenergic and beta-adrenergic blockade. In patients with recent onset (<48 hours) atrial fibrillation or atrial flutter, IV amiodarone has been shown to restore normal sinus rhythm within 8 hours in approximately 60% to 70% of treated patients. Although IV amiodarone has been associated with negative inotropic effects, minimal side effects are associated with its short-term administration. Amiodarone is recommended as an option for the treatment of wide complex tachycardia; stable, narrow complex supraventricular tachycardia; stable, monomorphic or polymorphic ventricular tachycardia; atrial fibrillation and flutter; ventricular fibrillation; and pulseless ventricular tachycardia.

Other Agents

Propafenone and sotalol are two additional agents that have been shown to be effective in converting recent onset atrial fibrillation and atrial flutter to normal sinus rhythm.

DOFETILIDE

Dofetilide is a recently FDA approved class III antiarrhythmic (potassium channel blocker) agent for rhythm conversion in patients with atrial fibrillation. The agent has been approved with substantial restrictions, such as initiation of drug therapy only in hospital with continuous ECG monitoring and dosing using a prespecified dosing algorithm. Proarrhythmic events and sudden cardiac death are the most substantial adverse events associated with dofetilide administration leading to these restrictions. The dose should be adjusted according to QT prolongation and creatinine clearance. If the QTc is greater than 400 msec, dofetilide is contraindicated.

Dose

- Modified based on creatinine clearance and QT or QTc interval. The usual recommended oral dose is 250 mcg bid.

ADENOSINE

Adenosine depresses sinus node automaticity and atrioventricular nodal conduction. Adenosine is indicated for the acute termination of atrioventricular nodal and reentrant tachycardia, and for supraventricular tachycardias, including Wolff-Parkinson-White syndrome.

ATROPINE

Atropine increases the sinus rate and decreases atrioventricular nodal conduction time and effective refractory period by decreasing vagal tone. The major indications for the use of atropine include symptomatic sinus bradycardia, sinus arrest, sinoatrial block, and type I second-degree atrioventricular block.

DIGOXIN

Digoxin is indicated for the treatment of supraventricular tachycardia and for controlling ventricular response associated with supraventricular tachycardia.

Monitoring Parameters

- ECG (heart rate, PR interval, ST segment, T wave, arrhythmia frequency)

Thrombolytic Agents

Thrombolytic agents are beneficial in all types of MIs, including in patients with previous MIs and regardless of age. The 1999 American College of Cardiology/American Heart Association guidelines for thrombolytic agents in the treatment of acute MI include the following recommendations in order from most supported by published literature (Class I) to least supported (Class III).

Class I Recommendations

- Elapsed time from onset of infarctive symptoms <12 hours
- ST segment elevation >1 mm in two contiguous leads
- <75 years of age, or a new bundle branch block with a history suggesting acute MI

Class IIa Recommendations

- ST segment elevation
- >75 years of age

Class IIb Recommendations

- ST segment elevation
- Time to therapy between 12 and 24 hours, or
- Blood pressure >180 mm Hg systolic and/or >110 mm Hg diastolic associated with high-risk MI

Class III Recommendations

- ST segment elevation
- Time to therapy >24 hours
- Ischemic pain resolved or ST segment depression only

Absolute contraindications to the use of thrombolytic agents include any active or recent bleeding, suspected aortic dissection, intracranial or intraspinal neoplasm, arteriovenous malformation or aneurysms, neurosurgery or significant closed head injury within the previous 3 months, ischemic stroke within the previous 3 months (except acute ischemic stroke within 3 hours), or facial trauma in the preceding 3 months. Relative contraindications include acute or chronic severe uncontrolled hypertension, ischemic stroke more than 3 months prior, traumatic or prolonged cardiopulmonary resuscitation greater than 10 minutes in duration, major surgery within the previous 3 weeks, internal bleeding within 2 to 4 weeks, noncompressible vascular punctures, prior allergic reaction to thrombolytics, pregnancy, active peptic ulcer, and current anticoagulation (risk increasing with increasing INR).

Adverse effects include bleeding from the GI or genitourinary tracts, as well as gingival bleeding and epistaxis. Superficial bleeding may occur from trauma sites such as those for IV access or invasive procedures. Intramuscular injections, as well as noncompressible arterial punctures, should be avoided during thrombolytic therapy.

Monitoring Parameters

- *For short-term thrombolytic therapy of MI:* ECG, signs and symptoms of ischemia, and signs and symptoms of bleeding at IV injection sites (laboratory monitoring is of little value)
- *Continuous infusion therapy:* thrombin time, activated PTT, and fibrinogen, in addition to above-mentioned monitoring parameters

Streptokinase

Streptokinase is indicated in the treatment of acute MI, deep venous thrombosis, and pulmonary embolism. Streptokinase works indirectly by forming a streptokinase–plasminogen activator complex, thus activating other plasminogen and converting it to the proteolytic enzyme plasmin. Plasmin hydrolyzes fibrin, fibrinogen, factors II, V, VIII, complement, and kallikreinogen. The duration of action is immediate after IV administration and lasts approximately 6 to 8 hours after the infusion is discontinued. Occasional allergic reactions may occur including fever, urticaria, itching, flushing, and musculoskeletal pain. Although anaphylaxis is rare, transient hypotension may occur.

Dose

- *Acute MI:* 1.5 million U IV over 1 hour
- *Deep venous thrombosis:* 250,000-U IV bolus over 30 to 60 minutes, followed by 100,000 U/h for 2 to 3 days
- *Pulmonary embolism:* 250,000-U IV bolus over 30 to 60 minutes, followed by 100,000 U/h for 12 to 24 hours

Alteplase

Alteplase (recombinant tissue-type plasminogen activator) has a high affinity for fibrin-bound plasminogen, allowing activation on the fibrin surface. Most plasmin formed remains bound to the fibrin clot, minimizing systemic effects. Alteplase is non-antigenic and should be considered in patients who have received streptokinase or anistreplase in the previous 6 to 9 months. The risk of an intracerebral bleed is approximately 0.5%.

Dose

- *Acute MI:* 100 mg IV over 3 hours (10 mg IV over 2 minutes, then 50 mg over 1 hour, and then 40 mg over 2 hours)
- *Pulmonary embolism:* 100 mg IV over 2 hours

Tenecteplase

Tenecteplase (recombinant TNK-tissue type plasminogen activator) has a longer elimination half-life (20 to 24 minutes) and is more resistant to inactivation by plasminogen activator inhibitor-1 than alteplase. Tenecteplase appears more fibrin specific than alteplase, which may account for a lower rate of noncerebral bleeding comparatively. However, there have been reports of antibody development to tenecteplase. Tenecteplase and alteplase have similar clinical efficacy for thrombolysis after MI.

Dose

- *Acute MI:* 30 to 50 mg (based on weight) IV over 5 seconds

Reteplase

Reteplase is a recombinant plasminogen activator for use in acute MI and pulmonary embolism as a thrombolytic agent. Reteplase has a longer half-life (13 to 16 minutes) than that of alteplase, allowing for bolus administration. The dosing regimen requires double bolus doses.

Dose

- *Acute MI and pulmonary embolism:* two 10-U IV bolus doses, infused over 2 minutes via a dedicated line; the second dose is administered 30 minutes after the initiation of the first injection

Vasoconstricting Agents

Dopamine is recommended as a first-line agent for increasing blood pressure in patients with clinical signs of septic shock and hypotension not initially responsive to fluid. Dopamine and norepinephrine are both effective for increasing blood pressure. Dopamine raises cardiac output more than norepinephrine, but its use may be limited by tachyarrhythmias. Norepinephrine may be a more effective vasopressor in some patients. Phenylephrine is an alternative, especially in patients experiencing tachyarrhythmias. Epinephrine should be considered for refractory hypotension. The use of epinephrine has been associated with elevated serum lactate levels. The routine use of low-dose dopamine (<5 mcg/kg/min) to maintain renal function is not recommended, although low-dose dopamine may increase renal blood flow in some patients when added to norepinephrine (see Table 23–3).

Dobutamine is the first choice for patients with low cardiac index (<2.5 L/min/m^2) after fluid resuscitation and an adequate mean arterial pressure. In patients with evidence of tissue hypoxia, the addition of dobutamine may be helpful to increase cardiac output and improve organ perfusion. Increasing cardiac index to "supranormal" levels (>4.4 L/min/m^2) has not been shown to improve outcome. Norepinephrine and dobutamine can be titrated separately to maintain both blood pressure and cardiac output. Epinephrine and dopamine can be used to increase cardiac output, but mesenteric perfusion may decrease with epinephrine, and gastric mucosal perfusion may be decreased with dopamine.

Dopamine is both an indirect-acting and a direct-acting agent. Dopamine works indirectly by causing the release of norepinephrine from nerve terminal storage vesicles as well as directly by stimulating alpha and beta receptors. Dopamine is unique in that it produces different pharmacologic responses based on the dose infused. At doses less than 5 mcg/kg per minute, dopamine stimulates dopaminergic receptors in the kidneys. Doses between 5 and 10 mcg/kg per minute are typically associated with an increase in inotropy resulting from stimulation of beta receptors in the heart, and doses above 10 mcg/kg per minute stimulate peripheral alpha-adrenergic receptors, producing vasoconstriction and an increase in blood pressure. Doses above 20 to 30 mcg/kg per minute usually produce no added response, so that if doses in this range do not produce the desired increase in blood pressure, alternative agents such as norepinephrine, phenylephrine, or epinephrine should be instituted.

Renal-dose dopamine, doses less than 5 mcg/kg per minute, is commonly used with other vasoactive agents (i.e., norepinephrine, phenylephrine, dobutamine) to improve or maintain urine output. The benefit of this practice remains to be proven in humans and its use for this purpose should be questioned. Dopamine increases urine output through a diuretic effect by increasing sodium excretion.

Norepinephrine is a direct-acting vasoactive agent. It possesses alpha- and beta-adrenergic agonist properties producing mixed vasoconstrictor and inotropic effects. As a vasoconstrictor it is useful when dopamine has produced an inadequate increase in blood pressure. Norepinephrine's effect on the heart includes a more pronounced effect on inotropy than on heart rate.

Phenylephrine is a pure alpha-adrenergic agonist. It produces vasoconstriction without a direct effect on the heart, although it may cause a reflex bradycardia. Phenylephrine may be useful when dopamine, dobutamine, norepinephrine, or epinephrine cause tachyarrhythmias and when a vasoconstrictor is required.

Epinephrine possesses alpha- and beta-adrenergic effects, increasing heart rate, contractility, and vasoconstriction with higher doses. Epinephrine's use is reserved for when other, less potent, vasoconstrictors are inadequate. Adverse effects include tachyarrhythmias; myocardial, mesenteric, renal, and extremity ischemia; and hyperglycemia.

Vasopressin is an emerging therapeutic agent for the hemodynamic support of septic and vasodilatory shock. The hormone mediates vasoconstriction via V1-receptor activation on vascular smooth muscle. During septic shock, vasopressin levels are particularly low. Exogenous vasopressin administration is based on the theory of hormone replacement. Vasopressin infusions of 0.01 to 0.04 U/min are advocated in patients with septic and/or vasodilatory shock to minimize harmful vasoconstriction of the gut vasculature. Currently this agent is still considered as second-line therapy to high-dose dopamine or norepinephrine.

Dose

- See Table 23–3.

Monitoring Parameters

- Blood pressure, heart rate, ECG, urine output, and hemodynamic parameters

Inotropic Agents (see Table 23–3)

Catecholamines

Dobutamine
Dobutamine produces pronounced beta-adrenergic effects such as increases in inotropy and chronotropy along with vasodilation. Dobutamine is useful especially for the acute management of low cardiac output states. Adverse effects associated with the use of dobutamine include tachyarrhythmias and ischemia.

Dopamine
Dopamine in the range of 5 to 10 mcg/kg per minute typically produces an increase in inotropy and chronotropy. Doses above 10 mcg/kg per minute typically produce alpha-adrenergic effects.

Isoproterenol
Isoproterenol is a potent pure beta receptor agonist. It has potent inotropic, chronotropic, and vasodilatory properties. Its use typically is reserved for temporizing life-threatening bradycardia. Adverse effects associated with isoproterenol include tachyarrhythmias, myocardial ischemia, and hypotension.

Epinephrine
Epinephrine produces pronounced effects on heart rate and contractility and is used when other inotropic agents have not resulted in the desired pharmacologic response. Epinephrine is associated with tachyarrhythmias; myocardial, mesenteric, renal, and extremity ischemia; and hyperglycemia.

Dose

- See Table 23–3.

Monitoring Parameters

- Blood pressure, heart rate, ECG, urine output, and hemodynamic parameters

Phosphodiesterase Inhibitors

Inamrinone and Milrinone

Inamrinone and milrinone produce increases in contractility and heart rate, as well as vasodilation. The mechanism of action of these agents is thought to be due to the inhibition of myocardial cyclic adenosine monophosphate phosphodiesterase (AMP) activity resulting in increased cellular concentrations of cyclic AMP. Increased tissue concentrations of cyclic AMP may result in the alteration of extracellular and intracellular calcium concentrations, thereby affecting the availability of calcium to contractile proteins by prolonging the release of calcium into the sarcoplasmic reticulum and increasing the rate of calcium sequestration. These agents are useful in the setting of low-output heart failure and can be combined with dobutamine to increase cardiac output. Inamrinone is formerly known as amrinone. The product was renamed because of potential to confuse with amiodarone. Inamrinone has been associated with thrombocytopenia as well as a flulike syndrome. Both inamrinone and milrinone can produce tachyarrhythmias, ischemia, and hypotension.

Dose

- *Inamrinone:* loading dose: 0.75 to 3.00 mg/kg; maintenance dose: 5 to 20 mcg/kg/min
- *Milrinone:* loading dose: 50 mcg/kg; maintenance dose: 0.375 to 0.750 mcg/kg/min

Monitoring Parameters

- Blood pressure, heart rate, ECG, urine output, hemodynamic parameters, and platelet count (especially inamrinone)

Activated Protein C

Drotrecogin Alfa

Drotrecogin alfa (activated) is the first agent demonstrated to decrease mortality in severely septic patients during the PROWESS trial. The active component of drotrecogin alfa is activated protein C, an endogenously produced protein, which is suppressed during severe sepsis. Activated protein C has three primary properties in the body: anti-inflammatory, antithrombotic, and profibrinolytic. These properties are thought to lead to decreased end-organ failure secondary to impaired microthrombi formation in severely septic patients. The most significant adverse effects associated with drotrecogin alfa use are serious bleeding events (e.g., intracranial hemorrhage, procedural bleeding).

Dose

- *Continuous infusion:* 24 mcg/kg/h for 96 hours administered through a dedicated line or a dedicated lumen of a multilumen catheter

Monitoring Parameters

- Signs and symptoms of bleeding

ANTI-INFECTIVE PHARMACOLOGY

Aminoglycosides

Gentamicin, tobramycin, and amikacin are the most commonly used aminoglycoside antibiotics in critically ill patients. These agents are typically used with antipseudomonal penicillins or third- or fourth-generation cephalosporins for additional gram-negative bacteria coverage. Occasionally they are added to vancomycin or a penicillin for synergy against staphylococcal or enterococcal organisms.

Aminoglycosides are not metabolized but are cleared from the body through the kidney by glomerular filtration with some proximal tubular reabsorption occurring. The clearance of aminoglycosides parallels glomerular filtration, and a reduction in glomerular filtration results in a reduction in clearance with elevation in serum concentrations. Additional factors accounting for the reduced aminoglycoside clearance in critically ill patients include the level of positive end-expiratory pressure and the use of vasoactive agents to maintain blood pressure and perfusion. Aminoglycosides are removed from the body by hemodialysis, peritoneal dialysis, continuous renal replacement therapy (CRRT), extracorporeal membrane oxygenation, exchange transfusion, and cardiopulmonary bypass.

The major limiting factors in the use of aminoglycosides are drug-induced ototoxicity and nephrotoxicity. Ototoxicity results from the loss of sensory hair cells in the cochlea and vestibular labyrinth. Gentamicin is primarily vestibulotoxic, amikacin causes primarily cochlear damage, and tobramycin affects vestibular and cochlear function equally. Symptoms of ototoxicity typically appear within the first 1 to 2 weeks of therapy but may be delayed as long as 10 to 14 days after stopping therapy. Early damage may be reversible, but it may become permanent if the agent is continued. Vestibular toxicity may be manifested by vertigo, ataxia, nystagmus, nausea, and vomiting, but these symptoms may not be apparent in a sedated or paralyzed critically ill patient. Cochlear damage occurs as subclinical high-frequency hearing loss that is usually irreversible and may progress to deafness even if the drug is discontinued. It is difficult to diagnose hearing loss in the absence of pretherapy audiograms. Risk factors for ototoxicity include advanced age, duration of therapy more than 10 days, total dose, previous aminoglycoside therapy, and renal impairment.

Nephrotoxicity has been estimated to occur in up to 30% of critically ill patients and typically develops 2 to 5 days after starting therapy. An increase in serum creatinine of 0.5 mg/dL above baseline has been arbitrarily defined as significant and as possible evidence of nephrotoxicity. Nephrotoxicity is associated with a reduction in glomerular filtration rate, impaired concentrating ability, increased serum creatinine, and increased urea nitrogen. In most cases, the renal insufficiency is nonoliguric and reversible. The mechanism of nephrotoxicity is possibly related to the inhibition of intracellular phospholipases in lysosomes of tubular cells in the proximal tubule resulting in rupture or dysfunction of the lysosome, leading to proximal tubular necrosis. Risk factors for the development of aminoglycoside nephrotoxicity include advanced age, prolonged therapy, preexisting renal disease, preexisting liver disease, volume depletion, shock, and concurrent use of other nephrotoxins such as amphotericin B, cyclosporine, or cisplatin.

Aminoglycosides are effectively removed during hemodialysis. However, there is a rebound in the serum concentration within the first 2 hours after the completion of hemodialysis as the serum and tissues reach a new equilibrium. Therefore, a serum concentration should be drawn at least 2 hours after a dialysis treatment. Typically a dose of 1 to 2 mg/kg of gentamicin or tobramycin (amikacin 4 to 8 mg/kg) is sufficient to increase the serum level into the therapeutic range after dialysis. Continuous hemofiltration is also effective at removing aminoglycosides. Up to 35% of a dose can be removed during a 24-hour period of CRRT. Initially, several blood samples may be required to determine the drug's pharmacokinetic profile for dosing regimen adjustments. If the hemofiltration rate remains constant, aminoglycoside clearance should remain stable, permitting the administration of a stable dosing regimen. In this setting, drug concentration monitoring may only be required two to three times a week.

Vancomycin

Vancomycin is a glycopeptide antibiotic active against gram-positive and certain anaerobic organisms. It exerts its antimicrobial effects by binding with peptidoglycan and inhibiting bacterial cell wall synthesis. In addition, the antibacterial effects of vancomycin also include alteration of bacterial cell wall permeability and selective inhibition of RNA synthesis.

Vancomycin is minimally absorbed after oral administration. After single or multiple doses, therapeutic vancomycin concentrations can be found in ascitic, pericardial, peritoneal, pleural, and synovial fluids. Vancomycin penetrates poorly into cerebrospinal fluid (CSF), with CSF penetration being directly proportional to vancomycin dose and degree of meningeal inflammation. Vancomycin is eliminated through the kidneys primarily via glomerular filtration with a limited degree of tubular secretion. Nonrenal

elimination occurs through the liver and accounts for about 30% of total clearance. The elimination half-life of vancomycin is 3 to 13 hours in patients with normal renal function and increases in proportion to decreasing creatinine clearance. In acute renal failure, nonrenal clearance is maintained but eventually declines approaching the nonrenal clearance in chronic renal failure. In critically ill patients with reduced renal function, the increase in half-life may be due to a reduction in clearance as well as an increase in the volume of distribution.

Vancomycin is removed minimally during hemodialysis with cuprophane filter membranes, so that dosage supplementation after hemodialysis is not necessary. Vancomycin's half-life averages 150 hours in patients with chronic renal failure. With the newer high-flux polysulfone hemodialysis filters, vancomycin is removed to a greater degree, resulting in significant reductions in vancomycin serum concentrations. However, there is a significant redistribution period that takes place over the 12-hour period after the high-flux hemodialysis procedure with postdialysis concentrations similar to predialysis concentrations. Therefore, dose supplementation should be based on concentrations obtained at least 12 hours after dialysis.

Vancomycin is removed very effectively by CRRT resulting in a reduction in half-life to 24 to 48 hours. Up to 33% of a dose can be eliminated during a 24-hour hemofiltration period. Supplemental doses of vancomycin may need to be administered every 2 to 5 days in patients undergoing CRRT.

The most common adverse effect of vancomycin is the "red-man syndrome," which is a histamine-like reaction associated with rapid vancomycin infusion and characterized by flushing, tingling, pruritus, erythema, and a macular papular rash. It typically begins 15 to 45 minutes after starting the infusion and abates 10 to 60 minutes after stopping the infusion. It may be avoided or minimized by infusing the dose over 2 hours or by pretreating the patient with diphenhydramine, 25 to 50 mg, 15 to 30 minutes before the vancomycin infusion. Other rare, but reported, adverse effects include rash, thrombophlebitis, chills, fever, and neutropenia.

Other Antibiotics

Linezolid

Linezolid is an oxazolidinone derivative approved for the treatment of vancomycin-resistant enterococcal infections, nosocomial or community-acquired pneumonia secondary to resistant gram-positive organisms (i.e., methicillin resistant), complicated skin and skin structure infections including diabetic foot infections (without concomitant osteomyelitis), and uncomplicated skin and skin structure infections. Pharmacokinetic studies have documented that linezolid has excellent penetration into epithelial lung fluid and soft tissue.

The most troublesome adverse effect is myelosuppression including anemia, leukopoenia, and thrombocytopenia, typically occurring with prolonged administration of longer than 14 days duration. Linezolid is a monoamine oxidase inhibitor. Monoamine oxidase is an enzyme that breaks down amine neurotransmitters (i.e., epinephrine, norepinephrine, dopamine, and serotonin). Inhibition of monoamine oxidase results in increased concentrations of amine neurotransmitters resulting in increased sympathetic outflow. Linezolid's ability to inhibit monoamine oxidase degradation of serotonin results in increased serotonin levels and the development of the serotonin syndrome, which is manifested by hypertension, an altered mental status manifested by confusion, delirium, tremors, and fatigue. This interaction is important because selective serotonin reuptake inhibitors are among the most widely prescribed antidepressants in the United States.

PULMONARY PHARMACOLOGY

Theophylline

Theophylline is a phosphodiesterase inhibitor which produces bronchodilatation possibly by inhibiting cyclic AMP phosphodiesterase, inhibition of cellular calcium translocation, inhibition of leukotriene production, reduction in the reuptake or metabolism of catecholamines, and blockade of adenosine receptors. The use of theophylline for bronchospastic or lung disease has declined over the past decade. Most clinicians no longer use it as standard therapy for patients admitted to the hospital with bronchospasm; however, occasional patients may benefit from theophylline therapy. Theophylline should be used with caution in critically ill patients for several reasons. First, theophylline is metabolized in the liver and illnesses such as low cardiac output heart failure or hepatic failure may impair the ability of the liver to metabolize theophylline, resulting in increased serum concentrations. Second, antibiotics and anticonvulsants routinely administered to critically ill patients are known to alter theophylline's metabolism.

In patients without a recent history of theophylline ingestion, the parenteral administration of 6 mg/kg of IV aminophylline (aminophylline = 85% theophylline) produces a serum theophylline concentration of approximately 10 mg/L. In patients with a recent history of theophylline ingestion, a serum theophylline concentration should be obtained before administering a loading dose. Once the serum concentration is known, a partial loading dose may be administered to increase the concentration to the desired level. Each 1.2 mg/kg aminophylline (theophylline 1.0 mg/kg) increases the theophylline serum concentration approximately 2 mg/L. The loading dose should be administered over 30 to 60 minutes to avoid the development of tachycardia or arrhythmias.

The maintenance infusion should be started following the completion of the loading dose and should be adjusted according the patient's underlying clinical status (smokers: 0.9 mg/kg/h; nonsmokers: 0.6 mg/kg/h; liver failure or CHF: 0.3 mg/kg/h). These infusion rates are designed to achieve a serum concentration of approximately 10 mg/L. In most patients, concentrations above 10 mg/L are rarely indicated and may be associated with adverse effects.

When an IV regimen is converted to an oral regimen, the total daily theophylline dose should be calculated and divided into two to four equal doses depending on the theophylline product selected for chronic administration. When switching to a sustained-release product, the IV infusion should be discontinued with administration of the first sustained-release dose to maintain constant serum theophylline concentrations. Overlapping of the oral dose and IV infusion is not recommended because of the increase in serum theophylline concentrations and the potential development of toxicity resulting from the absorption of the sustained-release product.

Adverse effects occur more frequently at serum concentration above 20 mg/L and include anorexia, nausea, vomiting, epigastric pain, diarrhea, restlessness, irritability, insomnia, and headache. Serious arrhythmias and convulsions usually occur at serum concentrations above 35 mg/L, but have occurred at lower concentrations and may not be preceded by less serious toxicity.

Theophylline concentrations should be determined daily until they are stable. In addition, theophylline concentrations should be obtained daily in unstable patients and in whom interacting drugs are started or stopped. Levels may be measured once or twice weekly if the patient, theophylline level, and drug regimen are stable.

Dose

- *Loading dose:* 6 mg/kg IV or PO (each 1.2 mg/kg aminophylline increases the theophylline serum concentration 2 mg/L)
- *Continuous infusion:* smokers: 0.9 mg/kg/h; nonsmokers: 0.6 mg/kg/h; liver failure, CHF: 0.3 mg/kg/h

Monitoring Parameters

- Serum theophylline concentration, signs and symptoms of toxicity such as tachycardia, arrhythmias, nausea, vomiting, and seizures

Albuterol

Albuterol is a selective beta-2 agonist, used to treat or prevent reversible bronchospasm. Adverse effects tend to be associated with inadvertent beta-1 stimulation leading to cardiovascular events including tachycardia, premature ventricular contractions, and palpitations.

Monitoring Parameters

- Heart rate, pulmonary function tests

Levalbuterol

Levalbuterol is the active enantiomer of racemic albuterol. Dose ranging studies in stable ambulatory asthmatics and patients with COPD have documented that levalbuterol 0.63 mg and albuterol 2.5 mg produced equivalent increases in the magnitude and duration of FEV_1. There are no studies evaluating the efficacy of levalbuterol in hospitalized or critically ill patients. One study assessing the tachycardic effects of these agents in critically ill patients showed a clinically insignificant increase in heart rate following the administration of either agent.

Monitoring Parameters

- Heart rate, pulmonary function tests

GASTROINTESTINAL PHARMACOLOGY

Stress Ulcer Prophylaxis

Stress ulcers are superficial lesions commonly involving the mucosal layer of the stomach that appear after stressful events such as trauma, surgery, burns, sepsis, or organ failure. Risk factors for the development of stress ulcers include coagulopathy, patients requiring mechanical ventilation for more than 48 hours, patients with a history of GI ulceration or bleeding within the past year, sepsis, an ICU stay longer than 1 week, occult bleeding lasting more than 6 days, and the use of high dose steroids (>250 mg of hydrocortisone or the equivalent). Numerous studies support the use of antacids, H_2-receptor antagonists, and sucralfate. There are limited prospective comparative studies supporting the use of proton pump inhibitors (PPI) for preventing stress ulcer formation in critically ill patients. PPIs have not been shown to prevent the development of stress ulcers, maintain the gastric pH above 4, or prevent gastric bleeding. Simplified lansoprazole and omeprazole suspensions have been compounded with sodium bicarbonate for administration through feeding or nasogastric tubes for stress ulcer prophylaxis in critically ill patients unable to take medications by mouth. Simplified omeprazole suspensions have been documented to release the total daily dose immediately after administration rather than over 24 hours resulting in limited acid suppression. The routine use of oral or IV PPI for stress ulcer prophylaxis should be limited until prospective comparative studies with standard agents are completed.

Antacids

Antacids once were considered the primary agents for the prevention of stress gastritis. Their main attributes were their effectiveness and low cost. However, this was offset by the need to administer 30- to 120-mL doses every 1 to 2 hours. Large doses of antacids had the potential to produce large gastric residual volumes, resulting in gastric distention and bloating, as well as increasing the risk for aspiration.

Magnesium-containing antacids are associated with diarrhea and can produce hypermagnesemia in patients with renal failure. Aluminum-containing antacids are associated with constipation and hypophosphatemia. Large, frequent doses of antacids prevent the effective delivery of enteral nutrition. Finally, antacids are known to impair the absorption of digoxin, ciprofloxacin, and captopril. Also, alkalinization of the GI tract may predispose patients to nosocomial pneumonias with gram-negative organisms that originate in the GI tract.

Dose

- 30 to 120 mL PO, NG q1–4h

Monitoring Parameters

- Nasogastric aspirate pH, serum electrolytes, bowel function (diarrhea, constipation, bloating), hemoglobin, hematocrit, and nasogastric aspirate and stool guaiac

H_2 Antagonists

Ranitidine, cimetidine, and famotidine essentially have replaced antacids as therapy for the prevention of stress gastritis. These agents have the benefit of requiring administration only every 6 to 12 hours or may be delivered by continuous infusion. When they are administered by continuous infusion, they may be added to parenteral nutrition solutions, decreasing the need for multiple daily doses. Each agent has been associated with thrombocytopenia and mental status changes. Mental status changes typically occur in elderly patients or in patients with reduced renal function in whom the doses have not been adjusted to account for the reduction in renal function. Cimetidine also has been shown to inhibit hepatic microsomal enzymes, thus impairing the metabolism of agents such as theophylline and lidocaine. Also, similar to antacids, alkalinization of the GI tract with H_2 antagonists may predispose patients to nosocomial pneumonias with gram-negative organisms that originate in the GI tract.

Dose

- *Ranitidine:* intermittent IV: 50 mg q8h; continuous infusion: 6.25 mg/h
- *Cimetidine:* intermittent IV: 300 mg q6h; continuous infusion: 37.5 mg/h
- *Famotidine:* intermittent IV: 20 mg q12h; continuous infusion: not recommended

Monitoring Parameters

- Nasogastric aspirate pH, platelet count, hemoglobin, hematocrit, and nasogastric aspirate and stool guaiac

Other Agents

Sucralfate

Sucralfate is an aluminum disaccharide compound that has been shown to be safe and effective for the prophylaxis of stress gastritis. Sucralfate may work by increasing bicarbonate secretion, mucus secretion, or prostaglandin synthesis to prevent the formation of stress ulcers. Sucralfate has no effect on gastric pH. It can be administered either as a suspension or as a tablet that can be partially dissolved in 10 to 30 mL of water and administered orally or through a nasogastric tube. Although sucralfate is free from systemic side effects, it has been reported to cause hypophosphatemia, constipation, and the formation of bezoars. Because sucralfate does not increase gastric pH, it lacks the ability to alkalinize the gastric environment and may decrease the development of gram-negative nosocomial pneumonias. Sucralfate is an effective alternative to H_2 antagonists in patients with thrombocytopenia or mental status changes. Also, it may be a useful alternative in patients receiving medications whose metabolism may be inhibited by cimetidine.

Dose

- 1 g PO, NG q6h

Monitoring Parameters

- Hemoglobin, hematocrit, nasogastric aspirate, and stool guaiac

Acute Peptic Ulcer Bleeding

Proton Pump Inhibitors
Proton pump inhibitors have demonstrated efficacy in preventing rebleeding and reducing transfusion requirements in several randomized controlled trials. The rationale for adjunctive acid suppressant therapy is based on in vitro data demonstrating clot stability and platelet aggregation enhancement at high gastric pHs (>6). High-dose IV PPI therapy in conjunction with therapeutic endoscopy is the most cost-effective approach for the management of hospitalized patients with acute peptic ulcer bleeding.

Pantoprazole is available as an oral tablet and IV injection, and lansoprazole, omeprazole, and esomeprazole are available as oral capsules. It is advisable to transition to oral/enteral PPI therapy, if possible, after 72 hours of IV continuous infusion. The 72-hour time period for continuous infusions is the longest duration that has been studied.

Dose

- *Pantoprazole:* IV bolus 80 mg; continuous infusion: 8 mg/h for 72 hours

Variceal Hemorrhage

Upper GI bleeding is a common problem encountered in the intensive care unit. Its mortality remains around 10%. Vasoactive drugs to control bleeding play an important role in the immediate treatment of acute upper GI bleeding associated with variceal hemorrhage.

Vasopressin
Vasopressin is still one of the most commonly used agents for this purpose. Vasopressin is a nonspecific vasoconstrictor that reduces portal pressure by constricting the splanchnic bed and reducing blood flow into the portal system. Vasopressin is successful in stopping bleeding in about 50% of patients. Many of the adverse effects of vasopressin are caused by its relative nonselective vasoconstrictor effect. Myocardial, mesenteric, and cutaneous ischemia have been reported in association with its use. Drug-related adverse effects have been reported in up to 25% of patients receiving vasopressin. The use of transdermal or IV nitrates with vasopressin reduces the incidence of these adverse effects.

Dose

- 0.3 to 0.9 units/min

Monitoring Parameters

- Hemoglobin, hematocrit, nasogastric aspirate, stool guaiac, ECG, signs and symptoms of ischemia, blood pressure, and heart rate

Octreotide
Octreotide, the longer acting synthetic analog of somatostatin, reduces splanchnic blood flow and has a modest effect on hepatic blood flow and wedged hepatic venous pressure with little systemic circulation effects. Although octreotide produces the same results as vasopressin in the control of bleeding and transfusion requirements, it produces significantly fewer adverse effects. Continuous infusion of octreotide has been shown to be as effective as injection sclerotherapy in control of variceal hemorrhage.

Dose

- *Initial bolus dose:* 100 mcg, followed by 50-mcg/h continuous infusion

Monitoring Parameters

- Hemoglobin, hematocrit, nasogastric aspirate, and stool guaiac

Propranolol
Propranolol has been shown to reduce portal pressure both acutely and chronically in patients with portal hypertension by reducing splanchnic blood flow. The primary use of propranolol has been in the prevention of variceal bleeding. Propranolol or other beta-blockers should be avoided in patients experiencing acute GI bleeding, because beta-blocking agents may prevent the compensatory tachycardia needed to maintain cardiac output and blood pressure in the setting of hemorrhage.

Monitoring Parameters

- Hemoglobin, hematocrit, heart rate, and blood pressure

RENAL PHARMACOLOGY

Diuretics

Diuretics may be categorized in a number of ways, including site of action, chemical structure, and potency. Although many diuretics are available for oral and IV administration, intravenously administered agents typically are given to critically ill patients because of their guaranteed absorption and more predictable responses. Therefore, the primary agents used in intensive care units are the intravenously administered loop diuretics, thiazide diuretics, and osmotic agents. However, the oral thiazidelike agent, metolazone, is used commonly in combination with loop diuretics to maintain urine output for patients with diuretic resistance.

Monitoring Parameters

- Urine output, blood pressure, renal function, electrolytes, weight, fluid balance, and hemodynamic parameters (if applicable)

Loop Diuretics

Loop diuretics (furosemide, bumetanide, torsemide) act by inhibiting active transport of chloride and possibly sodium in the thick ascending loop of Henle. Administration of loop diuretics results in enhanced excretion of sodium, potassium, hydrogen, magnesium, ammonium, and bicarbonate. Chloride excretion exceeds sodium excretion. Maximum electrolyte loss is greater with loop diuretics than with thiazide diuretics. Furosemide, bumetanide, and torsemide have some renal vasodilator properties that reduce renal vascular resistance and increase renal blood flow. Additionally, these three agents decrease peripheral vascular resistance and increase venous capacitance. These effects may account for the decrease in left ventricular filling pressure that occurs before the onset of diuresis in patients with CHF.

Loop diuretics typically are used for the treatment of edema associated with CHF, the management of hypertension complicated by CHF or renal failure, in combination with hypotensive agents in the treatment of hypertensive crisis, especially when associated with acute pulmonary edema or renal failure, and in combination with 0.9% sodium chloride to increase calcium excretion in patients with hypercalcemia.

Common adverse effects associated with loop diuretic administration include hypotension from excessive reduction in plasma volume, hypokalemia and hypochloremia resulting in metabolic alkalosis, and hypomagnesia. Reduction in these electrolytes may predispose patients to the development of supraventricular and ventricular ectopy. Tinnitus, with reversible or permanent hearing impairment, may occur with the rapid administration of large IV doses. Typically, IV bolus doses of furosemide should not be administered faster than 40 mg/min.

Dose

- *Furosemide:* IV bolus: 10 to 100 mg q1–6h; continuous infusion: 1 to 15 mg/h
- *Bumetanide:* IV bolus: 0.5 to 2.5 mg q1–2h; continuous infusion: 0.08 to 0.30 mg/h
- *Torsemide:* IV bolus: 5 to 20 mg qd

Thiazide Diuretics

Thiazide (IV chlorothiazide) and thiazidelike (PO metolazone) diuretics enhance excretion of sodium, chloride, and water by inhibiting the transport of sodium across the renal tubular epithelium in the cortical diluting segment of the nephron. Thiazides also increase the excretion of potassium and bicarbonate.

Thiazide diuretics are used in the management of edema and hypertension as monotherapy or in combination with other agents. They have less potent diuretic and antihypertensive effects than loop diuretics. Intravenously administered chlorothiazide or oral metolazone is often used in combination with loop diuretics in patients with diuretic resistance. By acting at a different site in the nephron, this combination of agents may restore diuretic responsiveness. Thiazide diuretics decrease glomerular filtration rate, and this effect may contribute to their decreased efficacy is patients with reduced renal function (glomerular filtration rate <20 mL/min). Metolazone, unlike thiazide diuretics, does not substantially decrease glomerular filtration rate or renal plasma flow and often produces a diuretic effect even in patients with glomerular filtration rates less than 20 mL/min.

Adverse effects that may occur with the administration of thiazide diuretics include hypovolemia and hypotension, hypochloremia and hypokalemia resulting in a metabolic alkalosis, hypercalcemia, hyperuricemia, and the precipitation of acute gouty attacks.

Dose

- *Chlorothiazide:* 500 to 1000 mg IV q12h
- *Metolazone:* 2.5 to 20.0 mg PO qd

Osmotic Diuretics

Mannitol

Mannitol is an osmotic diuretic commonly used in patients with increased intracranial pressure. Mannitol produces a diuretic effect by increasing the osmotic pressure of the glomerular filtrate and preventing the tubular reabsorption of water and solutes. Mannitol increases the excretion of sodium, water, potassium, and chloride, as well as other electrolytes.

Mannitol is used to treat acute oliguric renal failure, reduce intracranial pressure, and reduce intraocular pressure. The renal protective effects of mannitol may be due to its ability to prevent nephrotoxins from becoming concentrated in the tubular fluid. However, its ability to prevent or reverse acute renal failure may be due to restoring renal blood flow, glomerular filtration rate, urine flow, and sodium excretion. To be effective in preventing or reversing renal failure, mannitol must be administered before reductions in glomerular filtration rate or renal blood flow have resulted in acute tubular damage. Mannitol is useful in the treatment of cerebral edema, especially when there is evidence of herniation or the development of cord compression.

The most severe adverse effect of mannitol is overexpansion of extracellular fluid and circulatory overload, producing acute CHF and pulmonary edema. This effect typically occurs in patients with severely impaired renal function. Therefore, mannitol should not be administered to individuals in whom adequate renal function and urine flow have not been established.

Dose

- 0.25 to 0.50 g/kg, then 0.25 to 0.50 g/kg q4h

Monitoring Parameters

- Urine output, blood pressure, renal function, electrolytes, weight, fluid balance, hemodynamic parameters (if applicable), serum osmolarity, and intracranial pressure (if applicable)

HEMATOLOGIC PHARMACOLOGY

Anticoagulants

Heparin

Heparin consists of a group of mucopolysaccharides derived from the mast cells of beef lung or porcine intestinal tissues. It binds with antithrombin III, accelerating the rate at which antithrombin III neutralizes coagulation factors II, VII, IX, X, XI, and XII. Heparin is used for prophylaxis and treatment of venous thrombosis and pulmonary embolism, atrial fibrillation with embolization, and treatment of acute disseminated intravascular coagulation.

Subcutaneously administered heparin is absorbed slowly and completely over the dosing interval. The total amount of heparin required to achieve the same degree of anticoagulation over the same time period does not appear to differ whether the heparin is administered subcutaneously or intravenously. The apparent volume of distribution of heparin is directly proportional to body weight, and it has been suggested that the dose should be based on ideal body weight in obese patients. Others suggest that in obese patients the dose should be normalized to total body weight.

The metabolism and elimination of heparin involves the process of depolymerization and desulfation. Enzymes reported to be involved in heparin metabolism include heparinase and desulfatase, which cleave heparin into oligosaccharides. The half-life of heparin ranges from 0.4 to 2.5 hours. Patients with underlying thromboembolic disease have been

shown to have shorter elimination half-lives, faster clearance, and require larger doses to maintain adequate thrombotic activity.

Traditionally, heparin therapy has been initiated with a standard 5000-U loading dose followed by a continuous infusion of 1000 U/h. The use of weight-based nomograms utilizing an 85-U/kg loading dose followed by a continuous infusion of 18 U/kg per hour and scheduled activated PTT monitoring has been shown to achieve a therapeutic PTT sooner than traditional methods. However, the use of weight-based nomograms has not been shown to decrease thrombotic events or bleeding complications.

The main adverse effects may be attributed to excessive anticoagulation. Bleeding occurs in 3% to 20% of patients receiving short-term, high-dose therapy. Bleeding is increased threefold when the PTT is 2.0 to 2.9 times above control and eightfold when the PTT is more than three times the control value. Heparin-induced thrombocytopenia may occur in 1% to 5% of patients receiving the drug.

The PTT is the test used to monitor and adjust heparin doses. Although heparin is typically administered as a continuous infusion, it is important that samples are collected as close to steady state as possible. After starting heparin therapy or adjusting the dose, PTT values should be drawn at least 6 to 8 hours after the change. Samples drawn too early are misleading and may result in inappropriate dose adjustments. Once the heparin dose has been determined, daily monitoring of the PTT for minor adjustments in the heparin dose is indicated. Large variations in subsequent coagulation tests should be investigated to ensure that the patient's condition has not changed or the patient is not developing thrombocytopenia.

Platelet counts should be monitored every 2 to 3 days while a patient is receiving heparin to assess for heparin-induced thrombocytopenia, thrombosis, or hemorrhage. Hemoglobin and hematocrit should be monitored every 2 to 3 days to assess for the presence of bleeding. Additionally sputum, urine, and stool should be examined for the presence of blood. Patients should be examined for signs of bleeding at IV access sites and for the development of hematomas and ecchymosis. In addition, IM injections should be avoided in patients receiving heparin and elective invasive procedures should be avoided or rescheduled.

Dose

- *Full therapy:* standard 5000-U bolus, followed by a continuous infusion of 1000 U/h
- *Individualized dosing:* bolus: 80 U/kg followed by a continuous infusion of 18 U/kg/h; infusion rates should be adjusted to maintain a PTT between 1.5 to 2.0 times the control value

Monitoring Parameters

- PTT, hemoglobin, hematocrit, and signs of active bleeding

Low-Molecular-Weight Heparins

Low-molecular-weight heparin may be an alternative to unfractionated heparin for the treatment of deep venous thrombosis, pulmonary embolism, and acute MI. Low-molecular-weight heparin may be less time consuming for nurses and laboratories and more comfortable for patients by allowing them to be discharged earlier from the hospital. The use of a fixed-dose regimen avoids the need for serial monitoring of the PTT and follow-up dose adjustments. Enoxaparin is the most studied low-molecular-weight heparin. Its dose for the treatment of deep venous thrombosis, pulmonary embolism, and acute MI is 1 mg/kg q12h. Dalteparin is another agent that has been shown to be as effective as unfractionated heparin in the treatment of thromboembolic disease and acute MI. Dalteparin 200 U/kg once daily is the typical dose used for the treatment of thromboembolic disease; 120 U/kg followed by 120 U/kg 12 hours later has been used in patients with acute MI receiving streptokinase. Warfarin can be started with the first dose of enoxaparin or dalteparin. Enoxaparin or dalteparin should be continued until two consecutive therapeutic International Normalized Ratio (INR) values are achieved, typically in about 5 to 7 days. Low-molecular-weight heparin has been shown to be as efficacious as unfractionated heparin with half of the bleeding complications.

Both dalteparin and enoxaparin are primarily renally eliminated with the potential for drug accumulation in patients with renal impairment. The subsequent risk of over-anticoagulation in these patients has prompted a number of pharmacokinetic studies that have been performed in renally impaired patients both with and without renal replacement therapy. These studies have provided conflicting data regarding the need to decrease dose, extend dosing interval, or avoid low-molecular-weight heparin therapy in this group of patients. Because these agents work by inhibiting factor Xa activity, it is possible to monitor their anticoagulation by measuring anti-factor Xa levels. This is a useful monitoring tool, particularly when compared with serum drug levels. Based on a lack of clear dosing adjustment guidelines for renal impairment, most clinicians adjust dosing based on anti-factor Xa levels in patients with significant renal impairment (i.e., creatinine clearance <30 mL/min) or simply avoid using these agents. The dosing adjustment for enoxaparin in patients with creatinine clearances less than 30 mL/min is to extend the dosing interval from 12 hours to 24 hours in both prophylaxis and treatment of thrombosis. No such dosage adjustment guideline has been approved for dalteparin.

Several studies have documented that critically ill patients have significantly lower anti-Xa levels in response to single daily doses when compared to patients on general medical wards. Factor Xa activity may need to be monitored in critically ill patients to adjust doses to ensure adequate anticoagulation to prevent deep venous clots from developing.

Warfarin

Warfarin prevents the conversion of vitamin K back to its active form from the vitamin K epoxide, impairing the formation of vitamin K–dependent clotting factors VII, IX, X, prothrombin, and protein C. Warfarin in indicated in the treatment of venous thrombosis or pulmonary embolism following full-dose heparin therapy. Warfarin is also used for chronic therapy to reduce the risk of thromboembolic episodes in patients with chronic atrial fibrillation.

Warfarin is rapidly and extensively absorbed from the GI tract. Peak plasma concentrations occur between 60 and 90 minutes after an oral dose with bioavailability ranging between 75% and 100%. Albumin is the principal binding protein with 97.5% to 99.9% of warfarin being bound.

Warfarin's metabolism is stereospecific. The R-isomer is oxidized to 6-hydroxywarfarin and further reduced to 9S, 11R-warfarin alcohols. The S-isomer is oxidized to 7-hydroxywarfarin and further reduced to 9S, 11R-warfarin alcohols. The stereospecific isomer alcohol metabolites have anticoagulant activity in humans. The warfarin alcohols are renally eliminated. The elimination half-lives of the two warfarin isomers differ substantially. The S-isomer half-life is approximately 33 hours and the R-isomer half-life is 45 hours.

Warfarin therapy may be started on the first day of heparin therapy. Traditionally, warfarin 5 mg daily is started for the first 2 to 3 days then adjusted to maintain the desired prothrombin time (PT) or INR. The timing of INR measurements relative to changes in daily dose is important. After the administration of a warfarin dose, the peak depression of coagulation occurs in about 36 hours. It is important to select an appropriate time during a given dosing interval and perform coagulation tests consistently at that time. After the first four to five doses, the fluctuation in the INR over a 24-hour dosing interval is minimal. The time course of stabilization of warfarin plasma concentrations and coagulation response during continued administration of maintenance doses is less clear. A minimum of 10 days appears to be necessary before the dose–response curve shows interval-to-interval stability. During the first week of therapy two INR measurements should be determined to assess the impact of warfarin accumulation on INR. Several factors should be assessed when evaluating an unexpected response to warfarin. Laboratory results should be verified to exclude inaccurate or spurious results. The medication profile should be reviewed to exclude drug–drug interactions including changes in warfarin product, and the patient should be evaluated for disease–drug interactions, nutritional–drug interactions, and noncompliance.

Bleeding is the major complication associated with the use of warfarin, occurring in 6% to 29% of patients receiving the drug. Bleeding complications include ecchymoses, hemoptysis, and epistaxis, as well as fatal or life-threatening hemorrhage.

Dose

- 10 mg PO qd × 3 days, then adjusted to maintain the INR between 2 and 3
- To prevent thromboembolism associated with prosthetic heart valves, the dose should be adjusted to maintain an INR between 2.5 and 3.5

Monitoring Parameters

- INR, hemoglobin, hematocrit, and signs of active bleeding

Direct Thrombin Inhibitors

Bivalirudin

Bivalirudin is an anticoagulant with direct thrombin inhibitor properties. Bivalirudin, when given with aspirin, is indicated for use as an anticoagulant in patients with unstable angina undergoing coronary angioplasty. It has been used as a substitute for heparin; potential advantages over heparin include activity against clot-bound thrombin, more predictable anticoagulation, and no inhibition by components of the platelet release reaction. One study has suggested the efficacy of SC bivalirudin in preventing deep vein thrombosis in orthopedic surgery patients. The place in therapy of bivalirudin will be determined by further comparisons with heparin, low-molecular-weight heparins, and recombinant hirudin.

Dose

- *Bolus:* 1 mg/kg
- *Continuous infusion:* 2.5 mg/kg/h × 4 hours, if necessary 0.2 mg/kg/h for up to 20 hours

Monitoring Parameters

- Activated PTT, activated clotting time (ACT), hemoglobin, hematocrit, and signs of active bleeding

Lepirudin

Lepirudin is a recombinant hirudin direct thrombin inhibitor indicated for the treatment of heparin-induced thrombocytopenia type II. It has also been studied in the treatment of acute coronary syndromes, MI, and other thromboembolic disorders mandating parenteral antithrombotic therapy such as disseminated intravascular coagulation.

Dose

- *Bolus:* 0.4 mg/kg
- *Continuous infusion:* 0.15 mg/kg/h for up to 10 days

Monitoring Parameters

- Activated PTT, hemoglobin, hematocrit, and signs of active bleeding

Argatroban

Argatroban is a selective thrombin inhibitor indicated for the prevention or treatment of thrombosis in heparin-induced thrombocytopenia and for use in percutaneous coronary interventions (PCIs). It has also shown effectiveness in ischemic stroke and as an adjunct to thrombolysis in patients with acute MI. Further studies are needed to establish effectiveness for other indications. Argatroban is dosed as a continuous infusion that is titrated based on activated PTT, similar to heparin. During PCI, the ACT may be used. A notable drug-laboratory value interaction is the increase in PT and INR values that occurs with argatroban therapy, which may complicate the monitoring of warfarin therapy once oral anticoagulation is initiated.

Dose

- *Bolus:* 350 mcg/kg
- *Continuous infusion:* 25 mcg/kg/min

Monitoring Parameters

- Activated PTT, ACT, PT, INR, hemoglobin, hematocrit, and signs of active bleeding

Glycoprotein IIb/IIIa Inhibitor

Glycoprotein IIb/IIIa inhibitors are recommended, in addition to aspirin and heparin, in patients with acute coronary syndrome awaiting PCI. If the glycoprotein IIb/IIIa inhibitor is started in the catheterization laboratory just before PCI, abciximab is the agent of choice.

Dose

- *Abciximab:* Bolus: 0.25 mg/kg over 10 to 60 minutes; continuous infusion: 0.125 mcg/kg/min for 12 hours (maximum infusion of 10 mcg mcg/min)
- *Tirofiban:* Bolus infusion: 0.4 mcg/kg/min over 30 minutes; continuous infusion: 0.1 mcg/kg/min for 12 to 24 hours after angioplasty or artherectomy.
- *Eptifibatide:* Bolus: 180 mcg/kg; continuous infusion: 2 mcg/kg/min until discharge or coronary artery bypass grafting (maximum of 72 hours).

Monitoring Parameters

- Platelet count, hemoglobin, hematocrit, and signs of active bleeding

IMMUNOSUPPRESSIVE AGENTS

Cyclosporine

Cyclosporine is used to prevent allograft rejection after solid organ transplantation and graft-versus-host disease in bone marrow transplant patients. Unlike other immunosuppressive agents, cyclosporine does not suppress bone marrow function. Cyclosporine inhibits cytokine synthesis and receptor expression needed for T-lymphocyte activation by interrupting signal transduction. Cyclosporine binds to cyclophilin and the calcium-dependent phosphatase, calcineurin. Calcineurin is required for the proper assembly of a transcription factor, which binds to the interleukin-2 (IL-2) gene and enhances IL-2 synthesis. The complex of cyclosporine, cyclophilin, and calcineurin inhibits the activation of this transcription factor, resulting in decreased IL-2 production. A lack of cytokine disrupts the activation and proliferation of the helper and cytotoxic T-cells that are essential for rejection.

Cyclosporine is poorly absorbed from the GI tract with bioavailability averaging 30%. Its absorption is influenced by the type of organ transplant, time from transplantation, presence of biliary drainage, liver function, intestinal dysfunction, and the use of drugs that alter intestinal function. Cyclosporine is metabolized by cytochrome p450 isoenzyme 3a to numerous metabolites with more than 90% of the dose excreted into the bile and eliminated in the feces. The kidneys eliminate less than 1% of the dose. There is no evidence that the metabolites have significant immunosuppressive activity compared with cyclosporine and none of the metabolites are known to cause nephrotoxicity.

The initial IV dose is 3 mg/kg per day infused over 2 to 12 to 24 hours to minimize the renal effects of the drug. Intravenous cyclosporine is diluted in Cremophor EL and must be diluted in 20 to 250 mL of D_5W or 0.9% sodium chloride before administration. Cremophor is associated with side effects such as flushing, shortness of breath, tachycardia, and hypotension.

The standard oral dose of cyclosporine is 10 mg/kg per day divided into two doses. Because of poor oral absorption, the oral dose is three times the IV dose. When converting from IV to oral administration, it is important to increase the oral dose by a factor of three to maintain stable cyclosporine concentrations. The oral solution can be administered diluted with chocolate milk or juice and administered through a nasogastric tube. The tube should be flushed before and after cyclosporine is administered to ensure complete drug delivery and optimal absorption.

The newer microemulsion formulation of cyclosporine capsules and solution has increased bioavailability compared to the original formulation of cyclosporine capsules and solution. These formulations are not bioequivalent and cannot be used interchangeably. Converting from cyclosporine capsules and solution for microemulsion to cyclosporine capsules and oral solution using as 1:1 mg/kg per day ratio may result in lower cyclosporine blood concentrations. Conversion between formulations should be made utilizing increased monitoring to avoid toxicity due to high concentrations or possible organ rejection due to low concentrations.

Nephrotoxicity is cyclosporine's major adverse effect. Three types of nephrotoxicity have been shown to occur. The first is an acute reversible reduction in glomerular filtration; second, tubular toxicity with possible enzymuria and aminoaciduria; and third, irreversible interstitial fibrosis and arteriopathy. The exact mechanism of cyclosporine nephro-toxicity is unclear, but may involve alterations in the various vasoactive substances in the kidney. Other side effects include a dose-dependent increase in bilirubin that occurs within the first 3 months after transplantation. Hyperkalemia can develop secondary to cyclosporine nephrotoxicity. Cyclosporine-induced hypomagnesemia can cause seizures. Neurotoxic effects such as tremors and paresthesias may occur in up to 15% of treated patients. Hypertension occurs frequently and may be due to the nephrotoxic effects or renal vasoconstrictive effects of the drug.

Tacrolimus (FK506)

Tacrolimus is a macrolide antibiotic produced by the fermentation broth of *Streptomyces tsukubaensis*. Although it bears no structural similarity to cyclosporine, its mode of action parallels cyclosporine. Tacrolimus exhibits similar in vitro effects to cyclosporine, but at concentrations 100 times lower than those of cyclosporine.

Tacrolimus is primarily metabolized in the liver by the cytochrome P450 isoenzyme 3A4 to at least 15 metabolites. There is also some evidence to suggest that tacrolimus may be metabolized in the gut. The 13-O-Demethyl-tacrolimus appears to be the major metabolite in patient blood. Less than 1% of a dose is excreted unchanged in the urine of liver transplant patients. Renal clearance accounts for less than 1% of total body clearance. The mean terminal elimination half-life is 12 hours but ranges from 8 to 40 hours. Patients with liver impairment have a longer tacrolimus half-life, reduced clearance, and elevated tacrolimus concentrations. The elevated tacrolimus concentrations are associated with increased nephrotoxicity in these patients. Because tacrolimus is primarily metabolized by the cytochrome p450 enzyme system, it is anticipated that drugs known to interact with this enzyme system may affect tacrolimus disposition.

The usual initial IV dose is 50 to 100 mcg/kg per day and should be administered no sooner than 6 hours after transplantation. In most cases, IV therapy can be switched to oral therapy within 2 to 4 days after starting therapy. The oral dose should start 8 to 12 hours after the IV infusion has been stopped. The usual initial oral dose is 150 to 300 mcg/kg per day, administered in two divided doses every 12 hours.

Nephrotoxicity is the most common adverse effect associated with the use of tacrolimus. Nephrotoxicity occurs in up to 40% of transplant patients receiving tacrolimus. Other side effects observed during tacrolimus therapy include headache, tremor, insomnia, diarrhea, hypertension, hyperglycemia, and hyperkalemia.

Sirolimus (Rapamycin)

Sirolimus is an immunosuppressive agent used to the prophylaxis of organ rejection in patients receiving renal transplants. It typically is used in regimens containing cyclosporine and corticosteroids. Sirolimus inhibits T-lymphocyte activation and proliferation that occurs in response to antigenic and cytokine stimulation. Sirolimus also inhibits antibody production.

Sirolimus is administered orally once daily. The initial dose of sirolimus should be administered as soon as possible after transplantation. A loading dose of 6 mg is usually followed by a maintenance dose of 2 mg/d. Maintenance doses should be reduced by approximately one third in patients with hepatic impairment. The loading dose does not need to be adjusted and the dosage does not have to be reduced in patients with renal impairment. It is recommended that sirolimus be taken 4 hours after cyclosporine modified oral solution or capsules.

Routine therapeutic drug level monitoring is not required in most patients. Sirolimus levels should be monitored in patients with hepatic impairment, during concurrent administration of cytochrome p450 cyp3a4 inducers and inhibitors, or when cyclosporine dosing is reduced or discontinued. Mean sirolimus whole blood trough concentrations, as measured by immunoassay, are approximately 9 ng/mL for the 2-mg/d dose and 17 ng/mL for the 5-mg/d dose. Results from other assays may differ from those with an immunoassay. On average, chromatographic methods such as HPLC or mass spectroscopy yields results that are 20% lower than immunoassay whole blood determinations.

SPECIAL DOSING CONSIDERATIONS

Continuous Renal Replacement Therapy

The techniques used to provide renal support to critically ill patients have changed considerably during the last 15 years. Continuous renal replacement therapies such as continuous arteriovenous hemofiltration (CAVH) or continuous venovenous (CVVH) hemofiltration, are replacing conventional hemodialysis in critically ill patients. Recommendations for drug dosage adjustments in conventional dialysis cannot be applied to these newer techniques because of their continuous character and lower clearance rates. Clinical studies on the influence of CRRT on drug elimination are limited.

Hemofiltration alone typically produces an effective glomerular filtration rate of approximately 20 mL/min, and the addition of dialysis increases the effective glomerular filtration rate to 30 to 40 mL/min. Increasing the dialysis flow rate from 1 to 2 L/h further increases the effective glomerular filtration rate. Several points should be remembered when selecting drug doses in patients receiving CRRT. First, drugs that are less than 80% protein bound, have a volume of distribution less than 1 L/kg, and a renal clearance greater than 35% will be removed during CRRT. Second, medication removal is highest with CVVH with dialysis, next highest with CVVH, and lowest with CAVH. Shorter dosing intervals should be chosen for patients being treated with hemofiltration with dialysis, and longer dosing intervals should be selected for patients on hemofiltration alone, especially

CAVH. Third, the following guidelines may be used for dosage adjustments during CRRT in the absence of published recommendations. The manufacturer's dosage recommendations for creatinine clearances <20 mL/min may be used in patients receiving hemofiltration alone. In patients receiving hemofiltration with dialysis, the manufacturer's dosage recommendations for creatinine clearances below 30 to 40 mL/min may be used. Fourth, serum concentration monitoring should be used to adjust the doses of aminoglycoside antibiotics and vancomycin. Finally, drugs such as catecholamines, narcotics, and sedatives are minimally removed during CRRT. The doses of these drug classes should be titrated based on the patient's clinical response.

Drug Disposition in the Elderly

The elderly population is the fastest growing segment of the population in the United States. Older patients consume nearly three times as many prescription drugs as younger patients and therefore are at risk for experiencing significantly more drug–drug interactions and adverse drug events. The most common risk factors that contribute to adverse events include polypharmacy, low body mass, preexisting chronic disease, excessive length of therapy, organ dysfunction, and prior history of drug reaction. Special attention must be paid on the part of healthcare professionals when dosing medications in these patients with low body mass and potentially impaired metabolism and clearance of drug secondary to age-related organ dysfunction (e.g., renal or hepatic impairment). Agents that are of particular interest in this population include sedatives, antihypertensives, narrow therapeutic index drugs, and anti-infectives. These agents often require a decrease in dose or the extension of the dosing interval to facilitate drug clearance and minimize the likelihood of toxicity.

Therapeutic Drug Monitoring

Therapeutic drug monitoring is the process of using drug concentrations, pharmacokinetic principles, and pharmacodynamics to optimize drug therapy (see Table 23–5). The goal of therapeutic drug monitoring is to maximize the therapeutic effect while avoiding toxicity. Drugs that are toxic at serum concentrations close to those required for therapeutic effect are the drugs most commonly monitored. The indications for therapeutic drug monitoring include narrow therapeutic range, no clinically observable endpoint, unpredictable dose–response relationship, serious consequences of toxicity or lack of efficacy, correlation between serum concentration and efficacy or toxicity, and the availability of serum drug concentrations.

There are multiple indications for obtaining serum drug concentrations. The specific indication is important, because it affects the timing of the sample. Timing of sample collection depends on the question being asked. The indications for obtaining serum drug concentrations include therapeutic confirmation, limited objective monitoring parameters, poor

---

AT THE BEDSIDE
► *Tips for Calculating IV*
Medication Infusion Rates

Information Required to Calculate IV Infusion Rates to Deliver Specific Medication Doses

- Dose to be infused (e.g., mg/kg/min, mg/min, mg/h)
- Concentration of IV solution (e.g., dopamine 400 mg in D_5W 250 mL = 1.6 mg/mL; nitroglycerin 50 mg in D_5W 250 mL = 200 mcg/mL)
- Patient's weight

1. Calculate the IV infusion rate in milliliters per hour for a 70-kg patient requiring dobutamine 5 mcg/kg/min using a dobutamine admixture of 500 mg in D_5W 250 mL.

   - Dose to be infused: 5 mcg/kg/min
   - Dobutamine concentration: 500 mg/250 mL = 2 mg/mL or 2000 mcg/mL
   - Patient weight: 70 kg

Calculation:

5 mcg/kg/min × 70 kg = 350 mcg/min

350 mcg/min × 60 min/h = 21,000 mcg/h

21,000 mcg/h ÷ 2000 mcg/mL = 10.5 mL/h

Answer: Setting the infusion pump at 10.5 mL/h will deliver dobutamine at a dose of 5 mcg/kg/min.

2. Calculate the IV infusion rate in milliliters per hour for a 70-kg patient requiring nitroglycerin 50 mcg/min using a nitroglycerin admixture of 50 mg in D_5W 250 mL.

   - Dose to be infused: 50 mcg/min
   - Nitroglycerin concentration: 50 mg/250 mL = 0.2 mg/mL or 200 mcg/mL
   - Patient weight: 70 kg

Calculation:

50 mcg/min × 60 min/h = 3000 mcg/h

3000 mcg/h ÷ 200 mcg/mL = 15 mL/h

Answer: Setting the infusion pump at 15 mL/h will deliver nitroglycerin at a dose of 50 mcg/min.

3. Calculate the IV loading dose and infusion rate in milliliters per hour for a 70-kg patient requiring aminophylline 0.6 mg/kg per hour using an aminophylline admixture of 1 g in D_5W 500 mL. The loading dose should be diluted in D_5W 100 mL and infused over 30 minutes.

   - Desired dose: Loading dose: 6 mg/kg
     Maintenance infusion: 0.6 mg/kg/h
   - Aminophylline concentration:
     Aminophylline vial: 500 mg/20 mL = 25 mg/mL
     Aminophylline infusion: 1 g/500 mL = 2 mg/mL
   - Patient weight: 70 kg

Calculation:

Loading dose: 6 mg/kg × 70 kg = 420 mg

420 mg ÷ 25 mg/mL = 16.8 mL

Infusion rate: Aminophylline 16.8 mL + D_5W 100 mL = 116.8 mL

116.8 mL ÷ 0.5/h = 233.6 mL/h

Answer: Setting the infusion pump at 234 mL/h will infuse the aminophylline loading dose over 1/2 hour

Maintenance dose: 0.6 mg/kg/h × 70 kg = 42 mg/h

42 mg/h ÷ 2 mg/mL = 21 mL/h

Answer: Setting the infusion pump at 21 mL/h will deliver the aminophylline maintenance dose at 42 mg/h, or 0.6 mg/kg/h.

---

patient response, suspected toxicity, identification of drug interactions, determination of individual pharmacokinetic parameters, and changes in patient pathophysiology or disease state.

The timing of serum drug concentrations is critical for the interpretation of the results. The timing of peak serum drug concentrations depends on the route of administration and the drug product. Peak serum drug concentrations occur soon after an IV bolus dose, whereas they are delayed after IM, SC, or oral doses. Oral medications can be administered as either liquid or rapid- or slow-release dosage forms (e.g., theophylline). The absorption and distribution phases must be considered when obtaining a peak serum drug concentration. The peak serum concentration may be much higher and occur earlier after a liquid or rapid-release dosage form compared to a sustained-release dosage form. Trough concen-

trations usually are obtained just prior to the next dose. Drugs with long half-lives (e.g., phenobarbital) or sustained-release dosage forms (e.g., theophylline) have minimal variation between their peak and trough concentrations. The timing of the determination of serum concentrations may be less critical in patients taking these dosage forms. Serum drug concentrations may be drawn at any time after achieving a steady state in a patient who is receiving a drug by continuous IV infusion. However, in patients receiving a drug by continuous infusion, the serum specimen should be drawn from a site away from where the drug is infusing. If toxicity is suspected, serum drug concentrations can be obtained at any time during the dosing interval.

Appropriate interpretation of serum concentrations is the step that requires an understanding of relevant patient factors, pharmacokinetics of the drug, and dosing regimen.

Misinterpretation of serum drug concentrations can result in ineffective and, at worst, harmful dosage adjustments. Interpreting serum concentrations includes an assessment of whether the patient's dose is appropriate, if the patient is at a steady state, the timing of the blood samples, an assessment of whether the time of blood sampling is appropriate for the indication, and an evaluation of the method of delivery to assess the completeness of drug delivery. Serum drug concentrations should be interpreted within the context of the individual patient's condition. Therapeutic ranges serve as guidelines for each patient. Doses should not be adjusted on the basis of laboratory results alone. Individual dosage ranges should be developed for each patient as various patients may experience therapeutic efficacy, failure, or toxicity within a given therapeutic range.

SELECTED BIBLIOGRAPHY

General

Knoben JE, Anderson PO (eds): *Handbook of Clinical Drug Data.* Hamilton, IL: Drug Intelligence Publications; 1998.

Park G, Shelly M (eds): *Pharmacology of the Critically Ill Patient.* London: BMJ Books; 2001.

Susla GM, Masur H, Cunnion RE, et al: *Handbook of Critical Care Drug Therapy,* 2nd ed. New York: Churchill Livingston; 2000.

Townsend P (ed): Applied pharmacokinetics. In Rippe JM, Irwin RS, Alpert JS, Fink MP (eds): *Intensive Care Medicine,* 3rd ed. Boston: Little Brown; 2003.

Evidence-Based Practice Guidelines

Chulay M, Susla GM (eds): *AACN Protocols for Practice: Medication Administration Series.* Aliso Viejo, CA: AACN; 1999.

The American Heart Association in collaboration with the International Liaison Committee on Resuscitation (ILCOR): Guidelines 2000 for cardiopulmonary resuscitation and emergency cardiovascular care. Part 6: Advanced cardiovascular life support. *Circulation* 2000;102(Suppl I, Part 6):1–143.

Sedation and Analgesia Task Force: Clinical practice guidelines for the sustained use of sedatives and analgesics in the critically ill adult. *Am J Health Syst Pharm* 2002;59:150–178.

Trujillo MH, Bellorin-Font E: Drugs commonly administered by intravenous infusion in intensive care units: A practical guide. *Crit Care Med* 1990;18:232–238.

Vincent JL, International Sepsis Forum: Hemodynamic support in septic shock. *Intensive Care Med* 2001;27:S80–S92.

Ethical and Legal Considerations

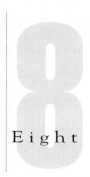

Eight

Juanita Reigle

> ▶ Knowledge Competencies
>
> 1. Characterize the nurse's role as patient advocate in upholding the doctrine of informed consent.
> 2. Describe the elements that determine decision-making capacity.
> 3. Identify the purpose and use of advance directives in guiding care for the incompetent patient.

As new ethical issues in critical care continue to emerge, practitioners in critical care must develop skills in moral reasoning. An ethical dilemma occurs when two (or more) morally acceptable courses of action are present and to choose one prevents selecting another. The dilemma is further complicated as either choice can be supported by an ethical principle, yet there are consequences for either choice. Competence in moral decision making evolves throughout one's professional career. However, there are general moral principles and guidelines that direct ethical reasoning and provide a standard to which professional nurses are held. Beginning clinicians, as well as more experienced nurses, should be familiar with the moral expectations and ethical accountability embedded in the nursing profession. This chapter introduces the elements that serve as a foundation for moral decision making. Ethical principles and rules, the ethic of care, patient advocacy, and other issues of ethical concern to critical care nurses are discussed.

THE FOUNDATION FOR ETHICAL DECISION MAKING

Professional Codes and Standards

The purpose of professional codes is to identify the moral requirements of a profession and the relationships in which they engage. The Code for Nurses developed by the American Nurses Association (ANA) articulates the essential values, principles, and obligations that guide nursing actions. The ANA Code identifies common moral themes that arise in nursing practice and provides a framework for moral inquiry.

In addition to a code of ethics, nurses function in accordance with particular standards of practice. *Standards of nursing practice* are delineated by professional organizations and statutory bodies that govern the practice of nursing in various jurisdictions. Derived from nursing's contract with society, professional nursing standards define the criteria for the assessment and evaluation of nursing practice. External bodies, such as state boards of nursing, impose certain regulations for licensure, regulate the practice of nursing, and evaluate and monitor the actions of professional nurses. Many organizations also delineate standards of practice for registered nurses practicing in a defined area of specialty. For example, the American Association of Critical-Care Nurses (AACN) has established standards and expectations of performance for nurses practicing in critical care.

Standards of practice outlined by statutory bodies and specialty organizations are not confined to clinical skills and knowledge. Nurses are expected to function within the profession's code of ethics and are held morally and legally accountable for unethical practice. When allegations of unsafe, illegal, or unethical practice arise, the regulatory body serves to protect the public by investigating and disciplining the culpable professional. Although specialty organizations do not have authority to retract professional licensure, issues of professional misconduct are reviewed and may result in revocation of certification and notification of external parties.

Position Statements and Guidelines

In an effort to address specific issues in clinical practice, many professional organizations develop position statements or guidelines. The purpose of position statements is to apply the values, principles, and rules described in the Code for Nurses to particular contemporary ethical issues. Familiarity with the AACN and ANA position statements helps the critical care nurse to clarify and articulate a position consistent with the professional values of nursing.

In the case example, the critical care nurse is asked to intentionally hasten a patient's death. The Code for Nurses and ANA position statements on assisted suicide and active euthanasia clarify the nurse's role when such requests are made. In addition, the ANA position statement on pain management and control of distressing symptoms in dying pa-

---

AT THE BEDSIDE
▶ *Making the Right Decision*

A 72-year-old grandmother has been in the coronary care unit for 4 weeks following a large anterolateral myocardial infarction. She has suffered from CHF, pulmonary edema, and hypotension, and now has developed ARDS. Her family is very supportive and visits her often. The physicians have communicated with the family, and, because the patient does not have an advance directive, the family has entrusted the physicians with making the "right decisions."

Currently, she requires maximal ventilator support to maintain adequate oxygenation. Her cardiac output and blood pressure are maintained at an adequate level with IV vasopressors and inotropic agents. Attempts to keep her pain free are sometimes thwarted by a drop in her blood pressure when she receives morphine and other medications. The nurses believe that it is inappropriate to continue treating her aggressively and that the patient does not want such extensive treatment. They believe that she is able to make decisions regarding her life, even though she cannot speak. She appropriately gestures to the nurses and maintains eye contact when the nurses talk to her. She is weak, and her writing is often difficult to read.

When the nurse asks the physician to please ask the patient what she wants before they begin new treatments, the physician responds that the patient is "not competent because of her illness and prolonged stay in the CCU." The physician states that the family told him to make the "right decisions" and that gives him the authority to decide what is best for this patient. The nurse is uncomfortable providing aggressive care based on the physician's perspective rather than a clear understanding of the patient's values and goals regarding continued treatment.

AT THE BEDSIDE
▶ *Refusing Further Treatment*

A 68-year-old man is admitted to the coronary care unit following exacerbation of heart failure secondary to dilated cardiomyopathy. Despite aggressive treatment, his cardiac index remains at 1.9 with an SVR of 600. His ABGs were pH 7.30, $PaCO_2$ 56 mm Hg, and PaO_2 60 mm Hg on 100% nonrebreather. The patient refused intubation and any further treatments. He openly discussed his fear of prolonged suffering and asked the nurse to accelerate his death with a lethal dose of morphine.

---

tients provides guidance for addressing the physical and emotional needs of patients at the end of life. In this case, the nurse and physician should explore the patient's request for an accelerated death and explain the legal and moral boundaries of his request. The option to withdraw treatment and provide aggressive palliative care should be offered and examined with the patient. A treatment plan that reflects the patient's underlying needs (a comfortable death) should be developed so that compassionate and humane care is provided.

Institutional Policies

Because critical care nurses practice within organizations, institutional policies and procedures affect and direct their practice. Institutional guidelines for assessing decision-making capacity or policies for the determination of brain death guide individuals employed by, or practicing within, the organization. These policies usually reflect ethical expectations congruent with the professional codes of ethics. However, in some circumstances, organizations may assume a particular position or value and therefore expect the employees to uphold this position. For example, some hospitals endorse particular religious positions and may prohibit professional practices that violate these positions. Ideally, the nurse and institution have complementary values and beliefs about professional responsibilities and obligations.

Institutions often provide internal resources to help clinicians resolve difficult ethical issues. Institutional ethics committees provide consultation on ethical situations and institutional policies outlining the procedures of case review should be available to all employees.

Legal Standards

Public policies and state and federal laws directed at health care influence the practice of health care professionals. Policies from agencies such as the Centers for Disease Control and Prevention or the Department of Health and Human Services (DHHS) generate changes in practice and in the actions of health professionals. For example, the DHHS established regulations for institutional review boards regarding the protection of human research subjects. State and federal laws often complement public policies and reinforce the position set forth. Additionally, state and federal laws outline expected behaviors or actions, such as the federal recommendations in the Patient Self-Determination Act (PSDA).

Critical care nurses must understand legislation that directly influences clinical practice, such as state laws influencing advance directives. Beyond this immediate need, clinicians should rely on resources within the institution and professional organizations to interpret and clarify relevant policies and laws affecting practice.

Principles of Ethics

One of the dominant and most influential perspectives in biomedical ethics is that of principle ethics. Inherent in this viewpoint is the belief that some basic moral principles serve to define, describe, and interpret the essence of ethical obligations in human society. These basic principles, and derivative imperatives or rules, are considered prima facie or binding. Therefore, to breach a principle is wrong unless there are prevailing and compelling reasons that outweigh the necessary infringement. The principles and rules are binding, but not absolute.

Because many approaches to ethics integrate the rules and principles outlined by the principle-oriented approach, understanding the fundamental concepts of principle-based ethics is helpful to the critical care nurse. The primary principles used are nonmaleficence, beneficence, utility, justice, and respect for persons (or autonomy). The derivative principles or rules include privacy, confidentiality, veracity, and fidelity.

The principles are not ordered in a particular hierarchy, but their application and interpretation are based on the specific features of the dilemma. In other words, once the underlying principles in conflict are identified, values of the decision makers influence which principle takes precedence over other moral claims.

Nonmaleficence

The principle of nonmaleficence imposes the duty to do no harm. This injunction suggests that the nurse should not knowingly inflict harm and is responsible if negligent actions result in detrimental consequences. In general, a critical care nurse preserves the principle of nonmaleficence by maintaining competence and practicing within accepted standards of care.

Although the principle of nonmaleficence appears straightforward and easily preserved, there are some situations in which the nurse may inflict harm with the intent of providing for a greater good to be realized. The concept that supports this reasoning is called the *principle of double effect*. For example, some of the harmful consequences of pain medication, such as respiratory depression, may be outweighed by the greater good of easing a terminally ill patient's pain at the end of life. The use of pain medication in this case is justified because a greater good, that of comfort, is recognized by the patient and caregivers as more desirable than the avoidance of respiratory depression. The patient and decision makers make this decision by considering the benefits and burdens of the proposed treatments and considering the consequences of the decision.

Beneficence

The ethical principle of beneficence affirms an obligation to prevent harm, remove harm, and promote good by actively helping others to advance and realize their interests. Intrinsic to this principle is action. The nurse moves beyond the concept of not inflicting harm (nonmaleficence) by actively preventing and removing harm, providing safe and competent care, and by promoting the well-being of others.

When the patient's safety or well-being is threatened by the actions of others, the nurse is obligated to remove and prevent harm. Knowledge of unsafe, illegal, or unethical practice by any health care provider obligates the nurse both morally and legally to intervene. The nurse must remove the immediate danger and communicate the infringement to the appropriate sources to prevent further harm. The nurse should turn to institutional policies and state nurse practice acts for guidance in the appropriate process of reporting.

To optimize the patient's well-being and prevent harm, nurses must practice with the essential knowledge and skills required of the clinical setting. Nurses are expected to practice according to established standards of practice, to continue professional learning to improve clinical practice, and to refrain from providing care measures in which they are not proficient.

Beyond the provision of safe nursing care, the promotion of the patient's well-being requires that the patient's perspective be known and valued. Therefore, the nurse must gain an understanding of the patient's underlying value structure to ensure that the care provided is consistent with the patient's wishes. The duty to do good requires that the health care team understand the patient's interpretation of what is "good."

Critical care nurses may find the balance between the patient's beliefs and the duty to promote good is difficult and confusing. In the critical care setting it is often unclear what actions or course of treatment will most benefit the patient physiologically and which plan best reflects the patient's values. This lack of certainty may result in fragmented discussions with the patient or surrogate and a treatment plan that reflects the values of the health care team rather than the patient. The nurse's moral obligation is to continue to promote the patient's interests by pursuing an accurate representation of the patient's beliefs and values, and to raise concerns of conflicting interpretations to appropriate members of the health care team.

Utility

As any critical care nurse knows, avoiding all harms and producing only good effects is often impossible. The concept of utility or proportionality advocates for a positive balance of benefits over burdens. *Benefits* contribute to the patient's well-being by improving the patient's health, such as through eradication of disease or symptom management. Benefits also are realized when the patient's quality of life is enhanced. *Burdens,* on the other hand, produce no measurable improvement in health or quality of life and may increase the patient's suffering or debilitation.

The benefit–burden analysis is advanced as a morally appropriate process to delineate and evaluate treatment choices. When provided with complete, comprehensive information regarding approaches to treatment, patients weigh the benefits and burdens of the proposed plans. Although a proposed course of treatment may be recommended by health care providers, it is the patient's analysis of the risks and benefits that guides the treatment plan. However, if the patient is incapable of participating in the decision-making process, the designated surrogate examines the options and determines the course of treatment based on an understanding of the patient's underlying values and beliefs.

Respect for Persons (Autonomy)

The principle of respect for persons or autonomy affirms the freedom and right of an individual to make decisions and choose actions based on that individual's personal values and beliefs. In other words, an autonomous choice is an informed decision made without coercion that reflects the individual's underlying interests and values.

To respect a person's autonomy is to recognize that patients may hold certain views and take particular actions that are incongruent with the values of the health care providers. Often this concept is difficult for health care providers to accept and endorse, particularly when the patient's choice conflicts with the caregivers' view of what is best in this situation. As an advocate, the nurse appreciates this diversity and continues to provide care as long as the patient's choice is an informed decision and does not infringe on the autonomous actions of others.

Patients in the critical care setting often have varying degrees of autonomy. The capacity of critically ill patients to participate in the decision-making process often is compromised and constrained by internal factors such as the effects of pharmacologic agents, the emotional elements associated with a sudden acute illness, and the physiologic factors related to the underlying illness. External factors, such as the intensive care environment, also influence the patient's potential to make autonomous choices. The critical care nurse advocates for the patient by promoting, as much as possible, the factors that constrain the patient's freedom to make autonomous choices. In this way the nurse supports the principle of respect for personal autonomy and upholding the ethical duty of beneficence.

Justice

The principle of humanitarian justice requires that similar cases be treated in similar ways and that all persons are to be treated according to their needs. Patients are to be treated equally regardless of disease state, socioeconomic status, gender, age, religious beliefs, or moral convictions. Treating patients equally does not mean treating all patients in the same manner. Instead, the health care needs of the patient, rather than other nonrelevant factors, determine the amount of health care resources received. For example, individuals in a community may have equal access to a critical care unit when they are critically ill. However, once patients are admitted to critical care, essential resources are allocated to patients based on individual needs. For example, a patient with a myocardial infarction receives antiarrhythmic therapy, and a patient with respiratory distress is supported by mechanical ventilation.

The principle of justice is complex, includes several characteristics, and can be interpreted in divergent and controversial ways. One concept underlying the principle of justice that is important to nursing is that of fair distribution. When resources are limited, the benefits and burdens of health care must be distributed fairly within society. This theory is evident in discussions encompassing issues of organ transplantation. The manner in which patients are placed on waiting lists, the limited availability of organs, the cost of transplantation, and the responsibility of society to meet the health care requirements of patients in need of transplantation are several issues involving fair distribution.

Critical care nurses allocate nursing resources to patients, other members of the health care team, and other areas within the institution. The complex and competing demands for nursing resources can lead to chaotic and random decisions. The principle of justice argues for a comprehensive, thoughtful plan that outlines a decision-making process in times of opposing claims.

Privacy and Confidentiality

Privacy and confidentiality are associated, but distinct, concepts that are derived from the principles of respect for autonomy, beneficence, and nonmaleficence. *Privacy* refers to the right of an individual to be free from unjustified access by others.

In the critical care setting the patient's privacy often is disregarded. The design of many critical care units includes easy visualization of patients from the nurses' station, and open access to the patient is presumed by most caregivers. This suggests a breach of individual privacy. Critical care practitioners should be particularly attentive to requesting permission from the patient for any bodily intrusion or physical exposure. The casual infringement of an individual's privacy erodes the foundation for establishing a trusting and caring practitioner–patient relationship.

Confidentiality is described in terms of the protection of information. When the patient shares information with the nurse or a member of the health care team, the information should be treated as confidential and discussed only with those directly involved in the patient's care. Exceptions to confidentiality include quality improvement activities, mandatory disclosures to public health agencies, reporting abuse, or required disclosure in a judicial setting. When an exception exists, the individual should be informed that the required reporting will occur. Most other disclosures of information obtained in a confidential manner should be shared with appropriate persons only when strong and compelling reasons to do so exist. Again, the patient should be informed of the impending disclosure, and ideally the patient should authorize the disclosure.

Violations of patient confidentiality occur in many subtle ways. The computerization of medical records and the use of facsimile distribution of personal medical information is common practice in many institutions. Persons unrelated to the patient's medical care who have access to the computers or facsimile may view confidential information without the individual's permission. Other ways in which confidentiality is unprotected include casual conversations in hallways or elevators in which patient information is shared within earshot of strangers, the unauthorized release of patient information to friends or the media, and health care professionals within the institution taking the liberty to view a coworker's medical record.

Nurses may feel conflicted when a patient discloses confidential information. The profession of nursing strongly values the principle of respect for persons and highly regards the concept of protecting confidential information. Therefore, decisions to break a patient's confidentiality must be well considered and require balancing competing obligations and claims. For example, a nurse may consider breaking a patient's confidentiality if there is a clear indication that, without doing so, harm may come to another individual or identifiable others. Clearly, this decision should not be made in isolation, and the nurse should seek advice when confronted with this difficult situation.

Veracity

The rule of veracity simply means that one should tell the truth and not lie or deceive others. Derived from the principle of respect for persons and the concept of fidelity, veracity is fundamental to relationships and society. The nurse–patient relationship is based on truthful communication and the expectation that each party will adhere to the rules of veracity. Deception, misrepresentation, or inadequate disclosure of information undermines and erodes the patient's trust in health care providers.

Patients expect that information about their condition will be relayed in an open, honest, and sensitive manner. Without truthful communication, patients are unable to assess the options available and make fully informed decisions. However, the complex nature of critical illness does not always manifest as a single truth with clear boundaries. Un-

certainty about the course of the illness, the appropriate treatment, or the plan of care is common in critical care and a single "truth" may not exist. As emphasized in a model of shared decision making, patients or surrogate decision makers must be kept informed of the plan of care and areas of uncertainty should be openly acknowledged. Disclosure of uncertainty enables the patient or surrogate to realistically examine the proposed plan of care and reduces the likelihood that the health care team will proceed in a paternalistic manner.

Fidelity

Fidelity is the obligation to be faithful to commitments and promises and uphold the implicit and explicit commitments to patients, colleagues, and employers. The nurse portrays this concept by maintaining a faithful moral relationship with the patient, communicating honestly, and meeting the obligations to oneself, the profession of nursing, other health care professionals, and the employer.

The concept of fidelity is particularly important in critical care. The vulnerability of critically ill patients increases their dependency on the relationship with the nurse, thus making the nurse's faithfulness to that relationship essential. Nurses demonstrate this faithfulness by fulfilling the commitments of the relationship, which include the provision of competent care and advocacy on the patient's behalf.

In addition, the nurse is obligated to demonstrate fidelity in relationships with colleagues and employers. In this way, the principle of fidelity can be difficult to uphold as institutions may have policies, such as those related to resource utilization, that the nurse finds are in conflict with the patient's best interests. When confronted with such situations, the nurse is wise to carefully weigh the ethical principles involved, to seek guidance if necessary, and to consider a role as a moral agent of change if appropriate.

Care

The ethic of care is viewed as an alternative to the principled approach in bioethics. Rather than distinguish the ethical problem as a conflict of principles, the ethic of care invites the analysis of relationships and the associated obligations.

The ethic of care begins from an attached, involved, and interdependent position. From this standpoint, morality is viewed as caring about others, developing relationships, and maintaining connections. Moral problems result from disturbances in interpersonal relationships and disruptions in the perceived responsibilities within relationships. The resolution of moral issues emerges as the involved parties examine the contextual features and embrace the relevance of the relationship and the related responsibilities.

In contrast, a principle-oriented or justice approach typically originates from a position of detachment and individuality. This approach recognizes the concepts of fairness, rights, and equality as the core of morality. Therefore, dilemmas arise when these elements are compromised. From this perspective, the approach to moral resolution is a reliance on formal logic, deductive reasoning, and a hierarchy of principles.

For nursing, the ethic of care provides a useful approach to moral analysis. Traditionally, nursing is a profession that necessitates attachment, caring, attention to context, and the development of relationships. To maintain this position, nurses develop proficiency in nurturing and sustaining relationships with patients and within families. The ethic of care legitimizes and values the emotional, intuitive, and informal interpretation of moral issues. This perspective expands the sphere of inquiry and promotes the understanding and resolution of moral issues.

Patient Advocacy

Both the ethic of care and the ethical principles support the nurse's role as a patient advocate. Although there are many models for defining and interpreting the relationship between the nurse and patient and no model can thoroughly describe its complexity and uniqueness, the patient advocacy role offers a familiar and typical description of the moral nature of this relationship.

The advocacy role reflects a model in which the nurse acknowledges and encourages an equal relationship with the patient. The patient's values, beliefs, and rights are respected and endorsed as significant and central to the decision-making process. This interpretation is a blend of the value-based decisions model and the respect-for-persons model. In the value-based decisions model, the nurse helps the patient gain the necessary information to make an informed choice. The nurse may guide the patient or surrogate through value clarification, the identification of interests, and the process of communicating decisions. The nurse does not speak for the patient or impose particular values or preferences. Instead, the patient or surrogate is empowered to guide and direct the health care plan.

The respect-for-persons model augments the value-based model by including the expectation that nurses uphold and protect the basic human rights of patients. In this model, the nurse acts to sustain the patient's welfare by seeking the appropriate information or support for the patient. In the event the patient is unable to speak for himself or herself and no surrogate is available, the nurse protects the patient's best interests. The principle of fidelity plays an important role in this model of advocacy because the nurse's actions reflect the underlying commitment and loyalty to advancing the patient's welfare.

Assuming the role of patient advocate is not without risk. Nurses may find that obligations to oneself, the patient, the patient's family, other members of the health care team, or the institution are in conflict and have competing claims on nursing resources. These situations are intensely troubling

to nurses; the support of colleagues is essential when engaging in the analysis of difficult moral issues. In circumstances of conflict, nurses should clarify the nature and significance of the moral problem, engage in a systematic process of moral decision making, communicate concerns openly, and seek mutually acceptable resolutions. A framework within which to identify and compare options provides the necessary structure to begin the process of moral resolution.

THE PROCESS OF ETHICAL ANALYSIS

When faced with an ethical problem, the nurse is expected to implement an intellectual and reasonable process that promotes resolution. A structured approach to ethical dilemmas provides consistency, eliminates the risks of overlooking relevant contextual features, and invites thoughtful reflection on moral problems. A stepwise method that mirrors the nursing process provides the necessary elements for a comprehensive evaluation. The following steps are involved in case analysis.

Assessment

- *Identify the problem.* Clarify the competing ethical claims, the conflicting obligations, and the personal and professional values in contention. Acknowledge the emotional components and communication issues.
- *Gather the data.* Distinguish the morally relevant facts. Identify the medical, nursing, legal, social, and psychological facts. Clarify the patient's and family's religious and philosophical beliefs and values.
- *Identify the individuals involved in the dilemma.* Clarify who is involved in the problem's development and who should be involved in the decision-making process. Identify who should make the final decision, and discern what factors may impede that individual's ability to make the decision.

Plan

- *Consider* all options, and avoid restricting choices to the most obvious.
- *Identify* the harms and goods likely to arise from each option.
- *Analyze* each plan according to ethical theories and principles.
- *Search* for institutional procedures or guidelines that address this issue.

Implementation

- *Choose* a plan and act.
- *Anticipate* objections.

Evaluation

- *Outline the results of the plan.* Identify what harm or good occurred as a result of the action.
- *Identify* the necessary changes in institutional policy or other strategies to avoid similar conflicts in the future.

This stepwise process of ethical analysis incorporates ethical principles and rules, relevant medical and nursing facts, and specific contextual features, and reflects a model of shared decision making. This ideology is essential if current and future moral issues are to be addressed and negotiated.

CONTEMPORARY ETHICAL ISSUES

Informed Consent

As a patient advocate, the critical care nurse recognizes the patient's or surrogate's central role in decision making. Patients must make informed decisions based on accurate and appropriate information. By uncovering the patient's primary values and beliefs, the nurse empowers patients and surrogates to articulate their preferences. Therefore, the nurse does not speak for the patient, but instead maintains an environment in which the patient's autonomy and right to self-determination are respected and preserved.

The doctrine of informed consent encompasses four elements: disclosure, comprehension, voluntariness, and competence. The first two of these elements are related because the patient's comprehension often depends on how the information is disclosed. Information must be provided in a manner that promotes the patient's understanding of the current medical status, the proposed interventions (including the nature of the therapy and its purpose, risks, and benefits), and the reasonable alternatives to the proposed treatment.

The overriding goal of the treatment, rather than just the procedure, should be discussed with the patient and the goals should reflect the desirable and likely outcomes for this individual. The nurse can contribute significantly to the comprehension portion of the consent process by clarifying the patient's or surrogate's perception of the situation. Questions such as, "What additional information do you need to help you make this decision?" or "What do you understand are the goals of this treatment?" help to highlight the patient's interests and comprehension of the situation.

Decisions must be reached voluntarily, and any threat of coercion, manipulation, duress, or deceit is unethical. Voluntary decisions uphold the principle of respect for persons and supports the concept of self-determination. In addition, the patient must be capable of making decisions about medical care. *Competence* is a legal term and reflects judicial involvement in the determination of a patient's decision-making capacity. *Capacity* reflects a medical decision regarding the patient's functional ability to participate in the decision-making process. Determining capacity is discussed in the next section.

The intent of the informed consent process is based on the principle of autonomy. In theory, the consent process provides an individual with the necessary information to compare options and make a reasoned choice. In reality, the consent process is handled more as an event than a process. The focus is to "get consent" rather than to help the patient gain an understanding of the proposed treatment. The critical care nurse must be sensitive to the timing of such discussions and should attempt to optimize the environment and enhance the patient's ability to participate in the decision-making process. Interactions should be uninterrupted, free from distractions, during intervals when the patient is fully awake, and, if desired by the patient, in the presence of loved ones.

Nurses have both a moral and a legal duty in the consent process. Incorrect information given with the intent to deceive or mislead the patient must be reported according to institutional guidelines and in some states may qualify as professional misconduct to be reported to the profession's state board. The Code for Nurses portrays the nurse's role during the consent process as a patient advocate upholding the patient's right to self-determination. Therefore, the nurse must respect the competent patient's choice and support the patient's decisions even if the decision is contrary to the judgments of the health care team.

Determining Capacity

Patients are presumed to possess decision-making capacity unless there are clear indications that the individual's choices are harmful or inconsistent with previously stated wishes. Questioning another's ability to engage in the decision-making process should be executed with caution. Value-laden judgments of an individual's competence, such as restricting involvement based on mental illness or advanced age, should be prohibited. In addition, evaluations of capacity based on the presumed outcome of the decision are equally unjust. Capacity to make decisions is based on the patient's physical and mental health and the ability to be consistent in addressing issues. Capacity is not based on the ability to concur with health care providers or family members. Instead, a functional standard to evaluate capacity is recommended.

The functional standard of determining capacity focuses on the patient's abilities as a decision maker rather than on the condition of the patient or the projected outcome of the decision. The three elements necessary for a patient to meet the functional standard are the abilities to comprehend, to communicate, and to form and express a preference.

The ability to comprehend implies that the patient understands the information relevant to the decision. A patient must exhibit abilities sufficient to understand only the facts pertinent to the prevailing issue. Therefore, orientation to person, place, and time does not guarantee or preclude the patient's ability to understand and comprehend the relevant information.

Decision-making capacity requires a communication of the decision between the patient and health care team. Communication with critically ill patients often is compromised by pharmacologic or technological interventions. The critical care nurse should attempt to remove barriers to communication and advance the patient's opportunity to engage in the decision-making process.

The final component essential for evaluating functional capacity is evidence of the patient's ability to reason about his or her choices. An individual's choices should reflect the person's own goals, values, and preferences. To evaluate this aspect, comments such as "Tell me about some of the most difficult health care decisions that you had to make in the past," or "Describe how you reached the decision you did," are useful. The patient should recount a pattern of reasoning that is consistent with personal goals and that reflects an accurate understanding of the consequences of the decision.

When the patient lacks decision-making capacity, and attempts to control factors and return the patient to an autonomous state are unsuccessful, the health care team must rely on other sources for direction in approximating the patient's preferences. Advance directives and surrogate decision makers are two ways in which the patient's choices can be understood.

Advance Directives

The PSDA, effective December 1, 1991, is a federal law that requires health care institutions receiving Medicare or Medicaid funds to inform patients of their legal rights to make health care decisions and execute advance directives. The purpose of the PSDA is to preserve and protect the rights of adult patients to make choices regarding their medical care. The PSDA also requires institutions to inform individuals of relevant state laws surrounding the preparation and execution of advance directives.

Advance directives are statements made by an individual with decision-making capacity that describe the care or treatment he or she wishes to receive when no longer competent. Most states recognize two forms of advance directives, the treatment directive, or "living will,' and the proxy directive. The treatment directive enables the individual to specify in advance his or her treatment choices and which interventions are desired. Usually treatment directives focus on cardiopulmonary resuscitation (CPR), mechanical ventilation, nutrition and hydration, and other life-sustaining technologies.

Proxy directives, also called the durable power of attorney for health care, expand the sphere of decision making by identifying an individual to make treatment decisions when the patient is unable to do so. The appointed individual, a relative or close friend, assumes responsibility for health care decisions as soon as the patient loses the capacity

to participate in the decision-making process. Treatment decisions by the health care proxy are based on a knowledge and understanding of the patient's values and wishes regarding medical care. Most states have statutory provisions that recognize the legal authority of the health care proxy, and this individual is given complete authority to accept or refuse any procedure or treatment.

Although most adults should complete both a treatment and proxy directive, the proxy directive has some important advantages over a treatment directive. Many treatment directives are valid only under certain conditions. Terminal illness or an imminent death are common limitations required before the patient's treatment directive is enacted. Such restrictions are not relevant in proxy directives, and the sole requirement before the proxy assumes responsibility on the individual's behalf is that the patient lack decisional capacity. Furthermore, the proxy directive enables the authorized decision maker to consider the contextual and unique features of the specific situation before arriving at a decision. In this way, the benefits and burdens of proposed interventions are considered in partnership with the knowledge and understanding of the patient's preferences and values.

If a patient lacks decision-making capacity and has not previously designated a proxy decision maker in an advance directive, the health care team must identify an appropriate surrogate to make decisions on the patient's behalf. Generally, family members have the patient's best interests in mind, and many state statutes identify a hierarchy of relatives as appropriate surrogate decision makers.

Regardless of whether the decision maker is a designated proxy or family member, the process of making decisions on behalf of the incapacitated patient is difficult and arduous. If the patient left no written treatment directive, the surrogate decision maker and the designated proxy follow the same guidelines for making decisions. The decisions are made based on either the substituted judgment standard or the best interest standard.

Substituted Judgment

When a patient previously has expressed his or her wishes regarding medical care, the surrogate decision maker invokes the standard of *substituted judgment*. The patient's goals, beliefs, and values serve to guide the surrogate in constructing and shaping a decision that is congruous with the patient's expressed wishes. An ideal interpretation of substituted judgment is that the patient, if competent, would arrive at the same decision as the surrogate. This standard originates in the belief that when we know someone well enough, we often are able to determine how he or she would have reacted to a particular situation, and therefore can make decisions on that person's behalf.

Best Interests

The *best interest standard* is used when the patient's values, ideals, attitudes, or philosophy are not known. For example, a patient who never gained decision-making capacity and lacked competence throughout his or her life would not have the opportunity to articulate wishes and beliefs about health care. Using the best interest standard, the surrogate decision maker determines the course of treatment based on what would be in the patient's best interests, considering the needs, risks, and benefits to the affected person. This burden–benefit analysis includes considering the relief of suffering, restoration of function, likelihood of regaining capacity, and quality of an extended life.

Although neither the best interest standard nor the substituted judgment standard is problem free, when possible the decision maker for an incapacitated patient should follow the principles of substituted judgment. Knowledge of the patient's underlying values should guide the surrogate and will most likely result in a decision reflective of the patient's interests and well-being.

End-of-Life Issues

Decisions to Forego Life-Sustaining Treatments

Decisions to forego life-sustaining treatments are made almost daily in the hospital setting. The prevalence of these decisions does not diminish the difficulty that patients, families, nurses, and physicians face when considering this treatment decision. The model for this decision-making process should reflect a collaborative and enduring approach that promotes the patient's interests and well-being.

The patient's interests are best served when information is shared among the caregivers, patient, and family in an open and honest manner. Through this process, a plan of care that reflects the patient's goals, values, and interests is developed. Continued collaboration is essential to ensure that the plan promotes the patient's well-being and reflects the patient's preferences. However, the patient may determine that the current plan imposes treatments that are more burdensome than beneficial, and may choose to forego new or continued therapies.

Grounded in the right to noninterference, patients with capacity have the moral and legal right to forego life-sustaining treatments. The right of a capable patient to refuse treatment, even beneficial treatment, must be upheld if the elements of informed consent are met and innocent or third parties are not injured by the refusal. Ongoing dialogue among the health care team, family, and patient is appropriate so that mutually satisfactory goals are adopted. Patients must understand that refusal of treatment will not lead to inadequate care or abandonment by members of the health care team.

In patients without decisional capacity, the determination to withdraw or withhold treatments is made by the identified surrogate. If the wishes and values of the patient are known, the surrogate makes treatment decisions based on this framework. If, however, the patient's values or wishes

---

AT THE BEDSIDE
▶ *The Patient's Wishes*

An 86-year-old widower resides in an elderly care facility. He has one adult daughter who lives out of town and regularly visits him twice a month. One morning the care providers at the geriatric facility find him unresponsive with shallow respirations and a bradycardic pulse. A note, written by Mr. Johnson, is attached to his body and states that he intentionally took a lethal overdose and that he does not wish to be resuscitated. Empty bottles of levodopa and amitriptyline are found in his room next to a glass partially filled with alcohol. Residents of the geriatric facility said that Mr. Johnson had continued to express sadness over the loss of his wife 2 years ago and that progression of the Parkinson disease also was troubling to him. The providers at the geriatric facility call the rescue squad, and he is rapidly transported to the hospital.

The patient is hypotensive and unresponsive on admission to the medical intensive care unit. Laboratory tests reflecting his renal and hepatic function are grossly abnormal. Gastric lavage and activated charcoal are initiated to remove the drugs.

The patient's daughter requests that everything be done to save her father. The health care team respects the daughter's wishes as surrogate, but are concerned that this is not what the patient wanted. They believe that the likelihood of a full recovery is remote and he should be allowed a peaceful death.

---

are unknown, or the patient never had capacity to express underlying beliefs, the decision maker must consider and weigh the benefits and burdens imposed by the particular treatments. Any treatment that inflicts undue burdens on the patient without overriding benefits or that provides no benefit may be justifiably withdrawn or withheld. If the benefits outweigh the burdens, the obligation is to provide the treatment to the patient.

In cases where the identified surrogate is not acting in the patient's best interests, health care professionals have a moral obligation to negotiate an acceptable resolution to the problem. Critical care nurses should intervene when the best interest of the patient is in question. If extensive attempts to resolve the differences through the use of internal and external resources are unsuccessful in facilitating an acceptable solution, the health care professional should seek the appointment of an alternative surrogate. Often, the burden of proof is on the health care professional to justify the need for an alternative decision maker. In situations in which the patient's life is threatened and the refusal of treatment by the surrogate would jeopardize the patient's safety, the health care team must seek an alternative surrogate without prolonged discussion with the identified surrogate. This situation arises when parents who are Jehovah's Witnesses refuse a life-saving blood transfusion for their child. The health care team can rapidly acquire court approval to transfuse the minor. In less emergent situations, attempts to convince the surrogate of the need for treatment and to reach a satisfactory settlement may take more time.

In the case exploring the patient's wishes, members of the health care team interpreted the patient's actions as a decision made by a competent individual. They realized that even after aggressive treatment the patient would most likely be dependent on hemodialysis, and therefore his independence and living environment would change. On the other hand, his daughter saw her father's act as a reflection of his depression from Parkinson disease and the loss of his wife. His daughter believed that additional antidepressant medications and more frequent psychiatric evaluations would renew her father's desire to live. In this case, both parties believe they are advancing the patient's best interests. Reflection on the patient's life, work, actions, religion, and beliefs help all parties to clarify the patient's values, and may help in the development of an acceptable resolution.

Conflicts regarding the withdrawal of life-sustaining treatments often reflect differences in values and beliefs. Typically, health care professionals value life and health. When patients or surrogates choose to forego treatments that have minimal benefit, relinquishing the original goal of restoring health is difficult. This dilemma is particularly apparent in the intensive care setting, where actions and interventions are aggressive, dramatic, and often life saving. Shifting from this model to a paradigm that advocates for a calm and peaceful death requires the critical care nurse and health care team to relinquish control and to change the treatment goals to promote comfort and support the grieving process. The intensity required to support the patient and family during the process of withdrawal of treatment must also be valued and appreciated by health care professionals in critical care.

In some circumstances, surrogate decision makers insist on treatment that members of the health care team believe is burdensome and nonbeneficial for the patient. Frequently, the request for futile treatment reflects the surrogate or patient's desire to be assured that "everything" is being done to eradicate the disease or restore health. Fears of abandonment, impending death, pain, discomfort, and suffering may motivate individuals to pursue nonbeneficial, and even harmful, treatments. If patients and surrogates are kept fully informed of the goals and the successes and failures throughout the course of treatment, the request for futile therapies is less likely. If, after numerous discussions, the patient or surrogate continues to request futile treatment, eliciting help from an uninvolved party, such as an ethics committee, can facilitate discussions. Health care institutions often have policies that delineate the responsibilities of the caregiver and the resources within the institution to resolve these un-

usual situations. In rare circumstances, judicial involvement is necessary to determine the outcome of the case.

Nutrition and Hydration

To many nurses, the provision of nutrition and hydration exemplifies compassion and comfort, and is fundamental to patient care. Therefore, nurses may be distressed when the withdrawal of nutrition and hydration are considered. However, any treatment or therapy, including the provision of nutrition and hydration, may in some circumstances be judged to be more burdensome than beneficial. Medical nutrition and hydration are administered through intravenous access, nasogastric and duodenal feeding tubes, or via gastrostomy. The image of gently spoon feeding a dying patient is replaced with the reality of meeting the nutritional requirements through invasive and uncomfortable technologies.

Provision of medical nutrition and hydration should occur following a careful burden–benefit analysis. If medical nutrition and hydration support and expedite the patient's return to an acceptable level of functioning (as defined by the patient or surrogate), then provision of the therapy is beneficial. When uncertainty exists, the presumption should be to provide nutrition and hydration. On the other hand, when continued provision of nutrition and hydration is futile and will not restore an adequate nutritional status, the treatment may be discontinued. If the patient's underlying condition will not change by the provision of nutrition and hydration (as is the case with patients in persistent vegetative states or irreversible coma), or the treatment is more burdensome than beneficial to the patient, the treatment justifiably may be withheld or withdrawn.

Because the provision of food and fluids imparts important symbolic images, decisions to withdraw or withhold nutrition and hydration are difficult for caregivers and families. However, in some situations the provision of nutrition and hydration may be more harmful than good.

Pain Management

When decisions to forego life-sustaining treatments in a critically ill patient arise, issues regarding the aggressive management of pain and comfort develop. Although palliation or relief of troubling symptoms is a priority in the care of critically ill patients, once the decision to forego life-sustaining measures is made, an aggressive approach to palliation is warranted. In some circumstances, patients experience distressing symptoms despite the availability of pharmacologic agents to manage the uncomfortable effects of chronic and terminal illness. Whether due to a lack of knowledge or time, or a deliberate unwillingness to prescribe the necessary medication, inadequate symptom management is unethical. Nurses are obligated to ensure that patients receive care and treatments that are consistent with their choices. There are few patients in whom adequate pain management cannot be achieved. The ANA Position Statement on pain management and control of distressing symptoms in dying patients delineates the role of the nurse in the assessment and management of pain.

When patients require large doses of medications, such as narcotics, to effectively alleviate their symptoms, providers may be concerned that the side effects of such doses may hasten the patient's death. The ANA Code for Nurses helps to clarify this concern for nurses by affirming that nurses "should provide interventions to relieve pain and other symptoms in the dying patient even when those interventions entail risks of hastening death." The essential element in this situation is the nurse's intent in providing the medication. Because the intent is to relieve pain and suffering, and not to deliberately hasten death, the action is morally justified.

Resuscitation Decisions

Critically ill patients are susceptible to sudden and unpredictable changes in cardiopulmonary status. Most hospitalized patients presume that, unless discussed otherwise, resuscitation efforts will be instituted immediately upon cardiopulmonary arrest. In-hospital resuscitation is moderately successful, and delay in efforts significantly reduces the chance of the victim's survival. The emergent nature, the questionable effectiveness, and the presumed provision of CPR contribute to the ethical dilemmas that surround this intervention.

Do Not Resuscitate Orders

"Do not resuscitate" (DNR) or "no code" are orders to withhold CPR. Other medical or nursing interventions are not influenced directly by a DNR order. In other words, the decision to forego CPR is not a decision to forego all other interventions to sustain life. The communication surrounding this decision is one of the most important elements in designing a mutually acceptable treatment plan for a particular patient.

Appropriate discussions with the patient or surrogate must occur before a resuscitation decision is made. Conversations about resuscitation status and the overall treatment goals should occur with the patient or surrogate, physician, nurse, and other appropriate members of the health care team. Open communication and a shared understanding of the treatment plan are essential to understanding and responding to the patient's interests and preferences.

Once a decision is made regarding resuscitation status, the physician must document the discussion and decision in the medical record according to the institution's policy. When the issue of resuscitation status is not addressed with the patient or surrogate or the decision is not documented or communicated with caregivers, issues such as partial codes or slow codes result.

Slow Codes or Partial Codes

The failure to define the DNR status and other treatment or nontreatment decisions often reflects the absence of an overall treatment goal. This terminology (slow code, partial code) leads to confusion, misunderstanding, inconsistencies, or worse among members of the health care team and the patient's family. The underlying message of a slow code directive is for the caregivers to perform an intervention somewhere between an all-out effort and no effort at all. If a successful resuscitation is desired, then the appropriate attempt should be instituted. If the resuscitation is not appropriate, then no attempt should be made. To do so only confuses the family and forces caregivers to perform aggressive interventions that are not beneficial and even harmful.

Institutions should develop policies that address the process of writing and implementing a DNR order. In addition to documenting the decision, physicians also should document the process of arriving at the decision. The critical care nurse should document his or her participation in the discussion and perception of the patient's or surrogate's comprehension. In addition, the nurse must continue ongoing dialogue with the patient or surrogate, answering any questions that arise and communicating any misunderstandings with the health care team.

Patients or their surrogates must be involved in decisions surrounding resuscitation. Although some individuals believe that decisions to withhold CPR can be made without involving patients or surrogates, such decisions violate the principle of patient autonomy. Just as patients consent to other interventions in the plan of care, including decisions to omit particular treatments, the provision or withholding of CPR is based on discussions with the patient and family.

BUILDING AN ETHICAL ENVIRONMENT

Values Clarification

One of the most useful and essential skills offered by nurses is that of assisting the patient and family in values clarification. This process helps families in the burdens and benefits assessment and provides them with a framework of the patient's preferences and interests. Additionally, families are less encumbered during the bereavement process, when reflecting on the patient's hospitalization, if they feel the decisions they made for the patient reflect the patient's values.

Provide Information and Clarify Issues

Patients and families rely on nurses to clarify medical information and support the exploration and meaning of different treatment decisions. The trusting relationship that develops is based on the nurse's abilities to communicate and understand the patient's needs. Questions that help to unveil patients' families' perceptions of the situation include: "What information do you need to make this decision?" "What do you understand of your (or your loved one's) condition?" and "What are your fears about being sick?"

The information provided to patients and surrogates must be more than simply disclosing facts. The dialogue must be ongoing, open, honest, and expressed with concern. Because the understanding of new knowledge is often rooted in past learning, the nurse begins by assessing the patient's or surrogate's prior experiences with the health care system. Patients and families often draw conclusions or create relationships based on incomplete or inaccurate interpretations of information. Nurses play a key role in facilitating communication and translating discrepancies in perceptions.

Recognize Moral Distress

Moral distress refers to the suffering that occurs when individuals feel compelled to act in ways they think are unethical. Nurses often feel trapped between institutional constraints, medical directives, patient and family wishes, and personal beliefs, duties, and values. Although all moral dilemmas are challenging, situations that result in moral distress are particularly troubling because they may have lasting effects on the individual's professional and personal life. Recognizing situations that contribute to moral distress and developing strategies to preserve moral integrity are essential tools for the critical care nurse. The AACN booklet *4 A's to Rise Above Moral Distress* provides an approach to addressing situations of moral concern.

Engage in Collaborative Decision Making

Nursing offers a distinct perspective that is grounded in humanistic and caring values. Nurses recognize, interpret, and react to the patient's and family's response to health problems. Factors such as the patient's ability to adapt to changes in health, cope with a diagnosis, or adjust to a treatment are valuable contributions to a model of shared decision making. Because nursing embraces this viewpoint, nurses must have a consistent presence on the health care team. Patients and families expect and need nurses to be actively involved in planning and implementing the plan of care.

In a collaborative model, the nurse's contributions and perspectives are valued, pursued, and acknowledged. When nurses are absent from the circle of decision making, clinical and moral dilemmas arise and communication falters. Every critical care nurse must remain involved, attached, and committed to the process of shared decision making and collaborative interaction.

SELECTED BIBLIOGRAPHY

Ahronheim J, Moreno JC, Zuckerman C: *Ethics in Clinical Practice,* 2nd ed. Gaithersburg, MD: Aspen; 2000.

Beauchamp TL, Childress JF. *Principles of Biomedical Ethics,* 5th ed. New York: Oxford University Press; 2001.

Burkhardt MA, Nathaniel AK. *Ethics and Issues in Contemporary Nursing,* 2nd ed. Independence, KY: Delmar Thomson Learning; 2001.

Campbell GM, Delgado S, Heath JE, et al: *The 4A's to Rise Above Moral Distress.* Wavra T (ed). Aliso Viejo, CA: AACN; 2004.

Coughennower M: Physician assisted suicide. *Gastroenterol Nurs* 2003;26(2):55–59.

Campbell ML: Foregoing life-sustaining therapy. Aliso Viejo, CA: AACN; 1998.

Davis AJ, Aroskar MA, Liaschenko J, Drought TS: *Ethical Dilemmas and Nursing Practice,* 4th ed. Stamford, CT: Appleton & Lange; 1997.

Fry ST, Killen AR, Robinson EM: Care-based reasoning, caring, and the ethic of care: A need for clarity. *J Clin Ethics* 1996; 7(1):41–47.

Fry ST, Veatch RM: *Case Studies in Nursing Ethics,* 2nd ed. Boston: Jones & Bartlett Publishers, 2000.

Lo B: *Resolving Ethical Dilemmas: A Guide for Clinicians,* 2nd ed. Philadelphia: Lippincott Williams & Wilkins; 2000.

Matzo M, Sherman D, Penn B, Ferrell B: The End of Life Nursing Education Consortium (ELNEC) Experience. *Nurse Educator* 2003;28(6):266–270.

Georges J-J, Grypdonck M: Moral problems experienced by nurses when caring for terminally ill people: A literature review. *Nurs Ethics* 2002;9:155–178.

Grisso T, Applebaum PS: *Assessing Competence to Consent to Treatment: A Guide for Physicians and Other Health Professionals.* New York: Oxford University Press; 1998.

Ivy SS: Ethical considerations in resuscitation decisions: a nursing ethics perspective. *J Cardiovasc Nurs* 1996;10(4):47–58.

Naden D, Eriksson K: Understanding the importance of values and moral attitudes in nursing care in preserving human dignity. *Nurs Sci Q* 2004;17(1):86–91.

National Consensus Project for Quality Palliative Care: *Clinical Practice Guidelines for Quality Palliative Care.* Brooklyn, NY: National Consensus Project for Quality Palliative Care; 2004.

Oberle K, Hughes D: Doctors' and nurses' perceptions of ethical problems in end-of-life decisions. *J Advanced Nurs* 2001;33(6): 707–715.

Professional Codes, Standards, and Position Statements

American Association of Critical-Care Nurses: *Mission, Values and Ethic of Care.* Aliso Viejo, CA: AACN.

American Nurses' Association: *Position Statement on Foregoing Nutrition and Hydration.* Washington, DC: ANA; 1992.

American Nurses Association: *Position Statement on Active Euthanasia.* Washington, DC: ANA; 1994.

American Nurses' Association: *Position Statement on Assisted Suicide.* Washington, DC: ANA; 1994.

American Nurses' Association: *Position Statement on Discrimination and Racism in Health Care.* Washington, DC: ANA; 1998.

American Nurses' Association: *Position Statement on Privacy and Confidentiality.* Washington, DC: ANA; 1999

American Nurses' Association: *Code for Nurses with Interpretive Statements.* Washington, DC: ANA; 2001.

American Nurses' Association: *Position Statement on Nursing Care and Do-Not-Resuscitate (DNR) Decisions.* Washington, DC: ANA; 2003.

American Nurses' Association: *Position Statement on Pain Management and Control of Distressing Symptoms in Dying Patients.* Washington, DC: ANA; 2003.

Evidence-Based Guidelines

Puntillo K, Medina J, Rushton C, et al: End-of-life and palliative care issues in critical care. In Chulay M, Medina J (eds): *Protocols for Practice: End of Life and Palliative Care Issues in Critical Care.* Aliso Viejo, CA: AACN; 2004.

Pathologic Conditions

Two

Cardiovascular System

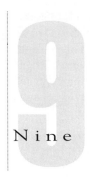

Nine

Barbara Leeper

▶ Knowledge Competencies

1. Identify indications for, complications of, and nursing management of patients undergoing coronary angiography and percutaneous coronary interventions.
2. Describe the etiology, pathophysiology, clinical presentation, patient needs, and principles of management of patients with ischemic heart disease.
3. Discuss the etiology, pathophysiology, clinical presentation, patient needs, and principles of management of patients in shock, heart failure, and hypertensive crisis.

SPECIAL ASSESSMENT TECHNIQUES, DIAGNOSTIC TESTS, AND MONITORING SYSTEMS

Assessment of Chest Pain

Obtaining an accurate assessment of chest pain history is an important aspect of differentiating cardiac chest pain from other sources of pain (e.g., musculoskeletal, respiratory, anxiety). Ischemic chest pain, caused by lack of oxygen to the myocardium, must be quickly identified for therapeutic interventions to be effective. The most important descriptors of ischemic pain include precursors of pain onset, quality of the pain, pain radiation, the severity of the pain, what relieves the pain, and timing of onset of the current episode of pain that brought the patient to the hospital. Each of these descriptors can be assessed using the "PQRST" nomogram (Table 9–1). This nomogram prompts the clinician to ask a series of questions which help clarify the characteristics of the cardiac pain.

Coronary Angiography

Coronary angiography is a common and effective method for visualizing the anatomy and patency of the coronary arteries. This procedure, also known as cardiac catheterization, is used to diagnose atherosclerotic lesions or thrombus in the coronary vessels. Cardiac catheterization is also used for evaluation of valvular disease, including stenosis or insufficiency, septal defects, congenital anomalies, and cardiac wall motion abnormalities (Table 9–2).

Procedure

Prior to cardiac catheterization the patient should be NPO for at least 6 to 12 hours, in the event that emergency intubation is required during the procedure. NPO may indicate everything except medications. Typically, if the patient is taking glucophage, the dose is reduced by one half the day of the procedure. Benadryl may be administered prior to beginning the procedure as a precautionary measure against allergic reaction to the dye. Aspirin or other platelet inhibitor agents may be administered to prevent catheter-induced platelet aggregation during the procedure. Typically, patients remain awake during the procedure, allowing them to facilitate the catheterization process by controlling respiratory patterns (e.g., breath holding during injection of radiopaque dye to improve the quality of the image). An anxiolytic agent, such as diazepam, is frequently administered during the procedure to decrease anxiety or restlessness.

An intracoronary catheter is inserted through a "sheath" or vascular introducer placed in a large artery, most commonly the femoral artery (Figure 9–1A). The catheter is then

TABLE 9–1. CHEST PAIN ASSESSMENT

	Ask the Question	Examples
P (Provoke)	What *provokes* the pain or what precipitates the pain?	Climbing the stairs, walking; or may be unpredictable—comes on at rest
Q (Quality)	What is the *quality* of the pain?	Pressure, tightness; may have associated symptoms such as nausea, vomiting, diaphoresis
R (Radiation)	Does the pain *radiate* to locations other than the chest?	Jaw, neck, scapular area, or left arm
S (Severity)	What is the *severity* of the pain (on a scale of 1 to 10)?	On a scale of 1 to 10, with 10 being the worst, how bad is your pain?
T (Timing)	What is the *time of onset* of this episode of pain that caused you to come to the hospital?	When did this episode of pain that brought you to the hospital start? Did this episode wax and wane or was it constant? For how many days, months, or years have you had similar pain?

advanced into the ascending abdominal aorta, through the aortic arch, and into the coronary arterial orifice located at the base of the aorta (Figure 9–1B). Ionic dye, visible to the observer or operator under fluoroscopy (x-ray), is then injected into the coronary arterial tree via the catheter. If the cardiac valves, septa, or ventricular wall motion is being evaluated, the catheter is advanced directly into the left ventricle, followed by injection of dye (Figure 9–1C). In a right heart catheterization, the catheter is inserted into the venous system via the inferior vena cava, passed through the right ventricle, and advanced into the pulmonary artery.

Interpretation of Results

The coronary vascular tree consists of a left and a right system (Figure 9–2). The left system consists of two main branches, the left anterior descending artery and the left circumflex artery. The right system has one main branch, the right coronary artery. Both systems have a number of smaller vessels that branch off these three primary arterial vessels. A clinically significant stenosis is considered to be an obstruction of 75% or greater in a major coronary artery or one of its major branches. If there is significant disease of only one of the major arteries, the patient is said to have single-

TABLE 9–2. INDICATIONS FOR CARDIAC CATHETERIZATION

Right Heart
- Measurement of right-sided heart pressures:
  suspected cardiac tamponade
  suspected pulmonary hypertension
- Evaluation of valvular disease (tricuspid or pulmonic)
- Evaluation of atrial or ventricular septal defects
- Measurement of AVo_2 difference

Left Heart
- Diagnosis of obstructive coronary artery disease
- Identification of lesion location prior to CABG surgery
- Measurement of left-sided heart pressures
  suspected left heart failure or cardiomyopathy
- Evaluation of valvular disease (mitral or aortic)
- Evaluation of atrial or ventricular septal defects

vessel disease. If two major vessels are affected, there is two-vessel disease, and if significant disease exists in all three major coronary arteries, then the patient has three-vessel disease. Frequently, the microvasculature, or smaller vessels branching off the major coronary artery, may also have blockages. It is common, however, to refer to these multiple lesions as single-vessel disease.

A ventriculogram is obtained by radiographic imaging during the injection of dye after advancing the catheter from the aorta, through the aortic valve, and into the left ventricle (see Figure 9–1C). A cineventriculogram provides information on ventricular wall motion, ejection fraction, and the presence and severity of mitral regurgitation and aortic regurgitation. Ejection fraction, or the percentage of blood volume ejected from the left ventricle with each contraction, is the gold standard for determining left ventricular function and is helpful in selecting treatment strategies. Left ventricular ejection fractions (LVEF) below 55% to 60% are considered to be normal. The LVEF is one of the most important predictors of long-term outcome following acute myocardial infarction (AMI). Patients with ejection fractions less than 20% have nearly 50% 1-year mortality.

Complications

During cardiac catheterization, a number of complications may occur, including dysrhythmia; coronary vasospasm; coronary dissection; allergic reaction to the dye; atrial or ventricular perforation resulting in pericardial tamponade; embolus to an extremity, a lung, or, rarely, the brain; acute closure of the left main coronary; myocardial infarction (MI); or death. Common management and prevention strategies for catheterization complications are summarized in Table 9–3.

Percutaneous Coronary Interventions

Percutaneous coronary interventions (PCIs) include percutaneous transluminal coronary angioplasty (PTCA), insertion of one or more stents, and coronary atherectomy. PTCA, also termed *angioplasty* or *balloon angioplasty,* is a cardiac catheterization with the addition of a balloon apparatus on the tip of the catheter for revascularizing the myocardium

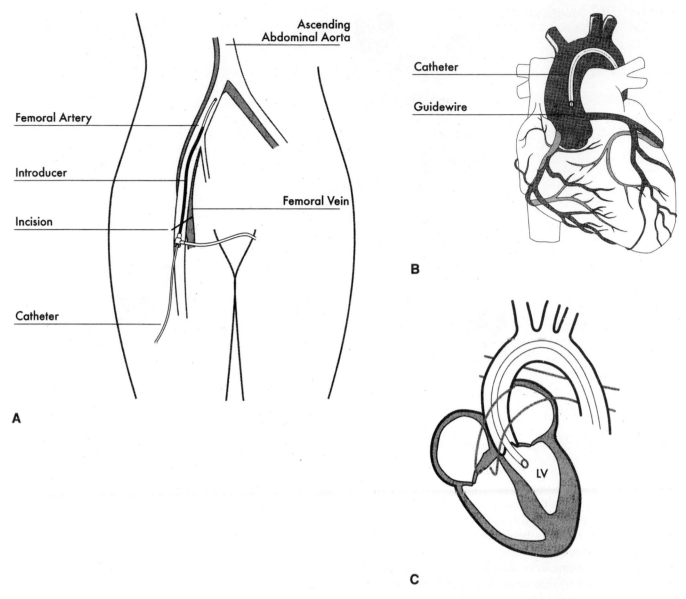

Figure 9–1. Coronary angiography. **(A)** Insertion of the coronary catheter into the femoral artery through a percutaneously inserted introducer sheath. **(B)** Coronary catheter advancement into the aorta and the left coronary artery. **(C)** Catheter advancement into the left ventricle.

(Figure 9–3). The catheter tip is advanced, generally over a guidewire, into the coronary artery until the balloon is positioned across the atherosclerotic lesion in the vessel. Once properly positioned, the balloon is inflated to stretch the vessel wall, resulting in fracture and compression of the atherosclerotic plaque and reduction of the degree of stenosis. The enlarged lumen allows a higher rate and volume of blood flow through the vessel, which translates clinically into fewer symptoms of angina and better exercise tolerance.

Complications

Angioplasty is associated with the same complications found during cardiac catheterization. In addition, complications related to manipulation of the coronary artery itself may also occur. The most common serious complications include a 2% to 10% incidence of complete occlusion of the vessel ("abrupt closure"), AMI (1% to 5% incidence), and the need for emergency coronary artery bypass surgery (1% to 2% incidence). The most important predictor of complications of MI and abrupt vessel closure is reduced coronary flow through the lesion prior to the procedure. A universal scale, the TIMI Scale, is used to quantify this rate of coronary flow (Table 9–4).

Other Percutaneous Coronary Interventions

In addition to routine balloon angioplasty, a number of other devices are now commonly used for percutaneous coronary revascularization. Intracoronary stents are small metallic

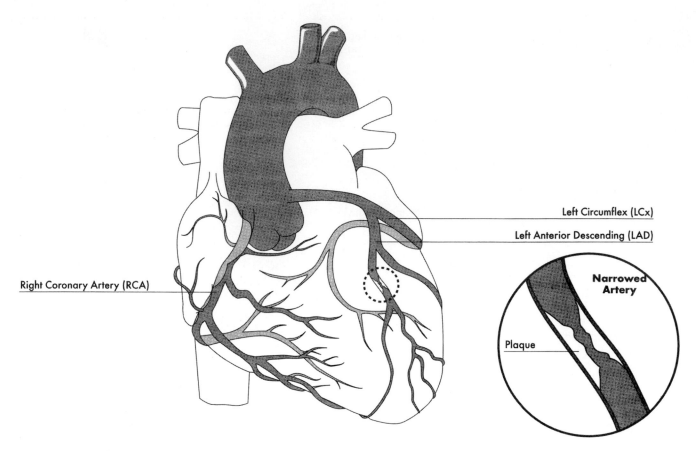

Figure 9–2. Coronary artery circulation with a coronary vessel narrowed with plaque formation.

mesh tubes placed across the stenotic area and expanded with an angioplasty balloon (Figure 9–4). Once expanded, the tube is permanently anchored in the vessel wall. Stents are effective in decreasing the rate of abrupt vessel closure seen with traditional PTCA. Some stents are coated with a drug that is bonded to a material on the stent causing the drug to be released over several months to years directly onto the arterial wall. These drug-coated stents have been shown to significantly reduce the restenosis rate associated with metal stents. Atherectomy catheters and lasers are used infrequently; however, patient outcomes are not significantly better than those achieved with traditional balloon catheters and stent deployment and may result in higher rates of complication, including AMI. Each of these devices may offer advantages over traditional balloon angioplasty catheters in situations involving specific vascular anatomy (e.g., ostial lesions) or lesion morphology (e.g., high degree of calcified plaque).

PATHOLOGIC CONDITIONS

Acute Ischemic Heart Disease

Myocardial ischemia is the lack of adequate blood supply to the heart, resulting in an insufficient supply of oxygen to

meet the demands of the heart muscle. This supply–demand mismatch, known as *ischemia,* is most often caused by thrombus formation at a site of atherosclerotic plaque rupture within a coronary artery. Decreased oxygen supply to myocardial tissue may cause a variety of symptoms such as chest discomfort (angina), shortness of breath, diaphoresis, and nausea. *Unstable angina,* defined as angina that is of new onset, increasing in frequency, or occurring at rest, and AMI are referred to as the *acute coronary syndromes* (ACS), which form the spectrum of acute ischemic heart disease.

Etiology and Pathophysiology

Intracoronary thrombus formation, and the resulting obstruction of coronary blood flow, is the pathophysiologic mechanism of acute ischemic heart disease. Preexisting atherosclerosis and spasm of the smooth muscle wall of the coronary arteries, termed *fixed obstructions,* may also contribute to reduced flow. In some situations, coronary artery spasm may play a major role, unrelated to underlying atherosclerosis. These occurrences are rare and are sometimes associated with cocaine abuse seen in MI in young patients.

The formation of a thrombus in coronary arteries is initiated by the fissuring and rupture of atherosclerotic plaque

AT THE BEDSIDE
► *Unstable Angina*

A 62-year-old man presents to the emergency department with complaints of pain in his chest and jaw. The pain, originally occurring only with exertion and resolving with rest, became increasingly persistent over the past 2 to 3 days. On the evening of his arrival, the patient experienced a 15-minute episode of severe pain while watching television. This episode he characterized as a "tight, burning feeling in my chest, and an aching in my jaw" that did not vary with respiratory effort and was accompanied by diaphoresis, nausea, and shortness of breath.

On arrival to the ED, his pain and nausea had resolved, pulse oximetry showed oxygen saturation of 98% on room air, and his vital signs were:

BP	148/86 mm Hg
HR	90 beats/min
RR	18 breaths/min
T	37.6°C orally

On physical examination heart sounds were normal, without S$_3$, S$_4$, or murmurs. Initial diagnostic tests revealed:

- ECG: Normal sinus rhythm with nonspecific ST-T wave changes
- Chest x-ray: Normal cardiac silhouette, clear lungs

A more detailed assessment of his history revealed increasing dyspnea on exertion and fatigue for the previous 6 months. Despite these symptoms, he had continued his daily 2.5-mile walking routine, sometimes experiencing shortness of breath several times during the walk. The patient reported smoking cigarettes in the past, one pack per day for 20 years, but quit 25 years ago. No ankle swelling, nocturnal dyspnea, or orthopnea were reported, nor was he aware of any family history of cardiac problems, coronary artery disease, diabetes, or hypertension.

He was started on aspirin based on his history and the likelihood of underlying coronary artery disease. He was then admitted for observation and evaluation of cardiac enzymes.

	CK Total	CK MB
ED	169 mcg/L	5 ng/mL
4 hours later	163 mcg/L	5 ng/mL

Six hours after presenting to the ED, the patient had recurrent tightness in his chest. An ECG showed T-wave inversion in the anterior leads. Sublingual nitroglycerin 0.4 mg was administered every 5 minutes with complete relief of the pressure following the second tablet. A heparin drip was started. Subsequent cardiac enzymes showed:

	CK Total	CK MB
8 hours	159 mcg/L	4 ng/mL
12 hours	152 mcg/L	4 ng/mL

Other laboratory results were normal with the exception of elevated cholesterol and triglycerides on the lipid panel. Following receipt of these results, he was scheduled for an exercise tolerance test.

The ECG recorded a heart rate of 118 beats/min after 6 minutes of exercise. Onset of chest tightness during the last minute of exercise was described as similar to that which brought him to the hospital and correlated with 1.5-mm ST depression in leads V$_4$ to V$_6$. A cardiac catheterization was scheduled.

Coronary angiography showed a 75% obstruction of the LAD artery and 90% obstruction of the diagonal branch of the same artery. LVEF was 55%. A coronary angioplasty (PTCA) was performed on both lesions.

---

in the vessel wall of the coronary artery (Figure 9–5). A continuous, dynamic process occurs whereby plaque may become unstable, for example, during periods of active accumulation of more lipid into the core of the plaque. The plaque then ruptures, dispelling its contents into the lumen of the coronary artery and causing activation of clotting factors at the site of plaque rupture. The rupture of plaque and resultant thrombus formation may eventually occlude the coronary artery.

Although most people have some degree of atherosclerotic plaque formation by age 30, the vast majority of these plaques are considered "stable." They are covered by smooth fibrous caps allowing adequate blood flow through the coronary arteries, and they are not prone to the events leading to unstable angina or MI. In young growing plaques, the fibrous cap may thin and rupture, resulting in unstable angina, ischemia, or MI.

A variety of factors predispose a plaque to fissure and rupture. Characteristics of plaque at increased risk for rupture include:

- *Location of the lesion in the vascular tree.* Areas of greater turbulence of flow and dynamic activity during the cardiac cycle are at higher risk.
- *Size of the lipid pool within the plaque.* A large amount of lipid inside the plaque core is more likely to be associated with plaque disruption.
- *Infiltration of the plaque with macrophages.* Macrophages are thought to weaken the integrity of the fibrous cap of the plaque, making it more susceptible to fissuring.

Although these characteristics determine the likelihood of plaque rupture, they are not easily identified by clinical

TABLE 9–3. CARDIAC CATHETERIZATION: COMMON COMPLICATIONS AND NURSING INTERVENTIONS

Complication	Intervention
Local bleeding due to catheter site artery damage (hematoma, hemorrhage, pseudoaneurysm)	Keep patient flat; head of bed (HOB) <30°. Discontinue heparin infusion if present. Compress the artery just above the incision (pedal pulse should be faint). Monitor for hypotension, tachycardia, or dysrhythmia. Embolectomy or vascular repair may be deemed necessary following groin ultrasound.
Coronary artery dissection	Stent will typically be placed during procedure. Monitor for dysrhythmia or tamponade. Administer heparin.
Tamponade due to perforation of the heart	Typically this will be evident in the catheter lab at the time of perforation. Monitor patient for equalization of cardiac pressures. Emergency surgery may be required for repair.
Peripheral thromboembolism	Extremity will exhibit pain, pallor, pulselessness, paresthesias, and paralysis; may also be cool to touch. Heparin or other anticoagulant should be continued. Thrombolytic therapy may be administered directly to the clot using a tracking catheter. Surgical intervention may be necessary.
Thromboembolism: CVA due to embolus	Monitor for signs and symptoms of neurologic compromise including speech patterns, orientation, vision, equal grips and pedal pushes, and sensation.
Pulmonary embolism	Provide supplemental O_2. Monitor for adequate arterial oxygen saturation and respiratory rate. Continue administration of heparin or other anticoagulant IV. Direct thrombolytic therapy may be administered using a tracking catheter; direct extraction of the clot may also be attempted. Ventilation–perfusion scan or pulmonary arteriograms may be done to verify thrombus location.
Arrhythmia	Direct irritation of the ventricular wall by the catheter tip poses the greatest risk; postprocedure risk is extremely low. Monitor the patient in lead V_1.
Infection	Use aseptic technique for all dressing changes. Monitor catheter insertion sites for erythema, inflammation, heat, or exudate. Monitor patient temperature trends.
Pulmonary edema due to recumbent position, stress of angiographic contrast, or poor left ventricular function	Elevate HOB 30°. Administer diuretics as necessary. Consider use of flexible sheath or brachial access.
Acute tubular neurosis and renal failure	Hydrate patient well prior to and following procedure with continuous infusion of normal saline (typically 8 hours before and 8 hours after at 100 mL/h). Monitor urine specific gravity trends and continue to infuse normal saline until specific gravity returns to within normal limits. Monitor for elevations in serum creatinine.
Vasovagal reaction	Administer pain medications prior to sheath removal. Monitor BP and heart rate before and after sheath removal, then every 15 minutes for four times after removal.

assessment, stress testing, or cardiac catheterization. A plaque may be caused to fissure or rupture by a number of environmental or hormonal factors, known as *triggers* (Table 9–5). These triggers may disrupt the plaque and precipitate an acute coronary event. Some of the triggers for atherosclerotic plaque rupture can be manipulated or controlled, such as blood pressure, blood glucose level, and stress. In the clinical setting, management of these variables may decrease the risk for AMI, reinfarction, and reocclusion, and should be closely monitored.

When these triggers combine to cause plaque rupture, the lipid pool is exposed and a rough surface on the intima of the vessel wall occurs, stimulating the local effects of hormonal and immune factors and initiating thrombus formation. At the same time, the fibrinolytic system is stimulated, creating a dynamic process of simultaneous attempts to form and dissolve the clot. Because of the dynamic nature of the clotting process, the thrombus may be completely or only partially obstructive, or may fluctuate intermittently between the two stages. Regardless of the maturity of the clot, the process of thrombus formation may lead to obstruction of blood flow, diminishing oxygen delivery to distal myocardium and creating a mismatch between the supply of and demand for oxygen.

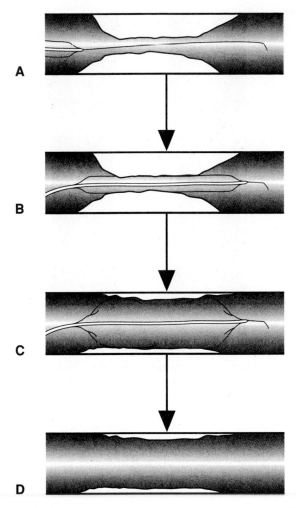

Figure 9–3. Percutaneous transluminal coronary angioplasty (PTCA). **(A)** PTCA catheter being advanced into the narrowed coronary artery over a guidewire. **(B)** Catheter position prior to balloon inflation. **(C)** Balloon inflation. **(D)** Coronary vessel following catheter removal.

TABLE 9–4. TIMI SCALE FOR QUANTIFYING CORONARY BLOOD FLOW

	Grade	Definition
0	No perfusion	There is no antegrade flow beyond the point of occlusion.
1	Penetration without perfusion	Contrast material passes beyond area of obstruction but "hangs up" and fails to opacify entire coronary bed distal to obstruction for duration of cineangiographic filming sequence.
2	Partial perfusion	Contrast material passes across obstruction and opacifies coronary bed distal to obstruction at a slower rate than its entry into or clearance from comparable areas not perfused by previously occluded vessel, e.g., the opposite coronary artery or coronary bed proximal to obstruction.
3	Complete perfusion	Antegrade flow into bed distal to obstruction occurs as promptly as antegrade flow into bed proximal to obstruction, and clearance of contrast material from the involved bed is as rapid as clearance from an uninvolved bed in same vessel or opposite artery.

From. The TIMI Study Group. The thrombolysis in myocardial infarction (TIMI) trial. Phase I findings. N Engl J Med 1985;312:932.

Clinical Presentation

Clinical presentation across the spectrum of ACS is similar, with clinical presentation differing slightly depending on the involved vessels (Table 9–6).

1. Pain or discomfort, usually in the chest (see Table 9–1)
   - Pressure or tightness in the chest
   - Jaw or neck pain
   - Left arm ache or pain
   - Epigastric discomfort
   - Scapular back pain
2. Nausea/vomiting
3. Hemodynamic instability
   - Hypotension (systolic BP >90 mm Hg or 20 mm Hg below baseline)
   - Cardiac index (CI) (<2.0 L/min/m^2)
   - Elevated pulmonary artery diastolic (PAD) and/or pulmonary capillary wedge pressure (PCWP)
   - Skin cool, clammy, diaphoretic
4. Dyspnea
5. Dysrhythmia
   - Left bundle branch block (LBBB)
   - Tachycardia/bradycardia
   - Frequent premature ventricular contractions
   - Ventricular fibrillation
6. Anxiety, sense of impending catastrophe
7. Denial

Some patient populations are predictably different in their description of chest pain, such as women and diabetics.

Because the underlying pathology of the ischemia-related diagnoses is the same (plaque rupture and thrombus formation), ischemic heart disease encompasses the entire spectrum of ischemic coronary events that are referred to as the *acute coronary syndromes* (ACS). ACS represents a continuum of clinical events that may result from the supply–demand mismatch including unstable angina, non–Q-wave MI, or Q-wave MI (Figure 9–6).

Following a decrease in oxygen supply to the myocardium, the cell membranes of "hypoxic" myocytes develop increased permeability. The cell is no longer able to regulate its internal and external environment, and the cell dies, releasing cytotoxic substances into the bloodstream. Cardiac myocytes release significant amounts of myoglobin, troponin I and T as well as cardiac-specific creatine kinase (CK-MB) when they die, causing elevation in these laboratory values and confirming the MI diagnosis.

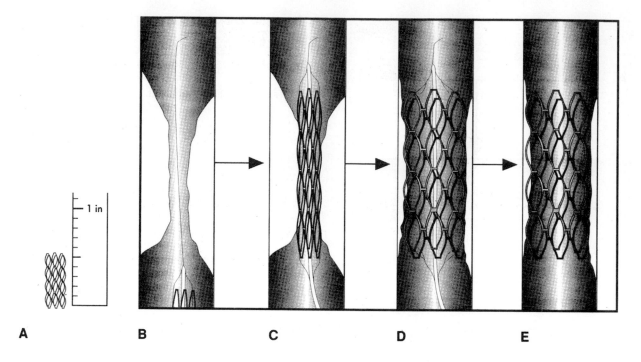

Figure 9–4. Intracoronary stent. **(A)** Size of stent device when fully deployed. **(B)** Insertion of stent into a narrowed area of a coronary artery on a balloon-inflatable catheter. **(C)** Inflation of the balloon catheter to expand the stent. **(D)** Inflation complete with stent fully expanded. **(E)** Stent following removal of balloon catheter.

Women frequently present with symptoms that are more vague than those listed such as feeling tired, short of breath, and lacking in energy. Women may be prone to deny chest pain for longer periods of time than men, delaying their arrival to the emergency department and often rendering them ineligible for thrombolytic therapy. In addition, women are typically postmenopausal when signs and symptoms of atherosclerotic disease become apparent. This predominantly older patient population may pose problems of its own such as anxiety, fear of the inability to care for oneself following MI, and other concerns to geriatric patient populations, which must be considered.

Diabetics are another patient population with predictable differences in symptomatic presentation. Diabetics have atypical pain secondary to neuropathies, and early development of atherosclerotic disease. Coronary artery disease in this patient population is diffuse, and poor distal vascular anatomy is common. Lesion morphology in diabetic patients is also more difficult to revascularize, either using percutaneous or surgical methods.

Diagnostic Tests

Unstable Angina

1. *12-Lead electrocardiogram (ECG):* Transient changes may occur and resolve; most commonly T-wave inversion or ST-segment depression.

2. *Cardiac enzymes* (Troponin [I or T], myoglobin, and CK-MB): Normal (Figure 9–7).

3. *Cardiac catheterization:* Not recommended in the acute setting, except in the case of continued pain without relief with nitroglycerin. Report is normal, or with visible atherosclerotic disease, but without complete occlusion or thrombus.

Myocardial Infarction

1. *12-Lead ECG:* Thirty-five percent of patients with AMI have ST-segment elevation (see Chapter 18, Advanced ECG Concepts). Approximately 65% of those with AMI have no ECG or other diagnostic changes.

2. *Creatine kinase* (CK and CK-MB) (see Figure 9–7)
   - Total CK >150 to 180 mcg/L
   - MB band >10 ng/mL or >3% of total
   - Peaks at 12 hours after symptom onset
   - CK-MB isoforms have better sensitivity and specificity for detecting MI within the first 6 hours

3. *Troponin T:* >0.1 to 0.2 ng/mL
   - Begins to increase 3 to 5 hours after symptom onset
   - Remains elevated for 14 to 21 days

4. *Troponin I:* >0.4 ng/mL
   - Begins to increase 3 hours after onset of myocardial ischemia onset
   - Peaks at 14 to 18 hours
   - Remains elevated for 5 to 7 days

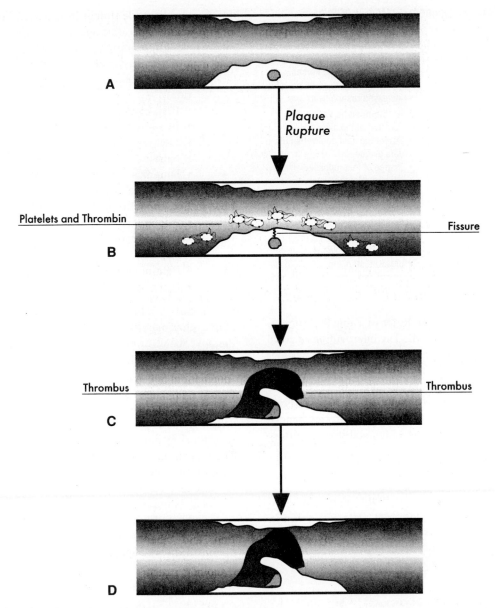

Figure 9–5. Atherosclerotic plaque formation. **(A)** Stable plaque. **(B)** Plaque with cap disruption. **(C)** Moderate amount of layered thrombus. **(D)** Occlusive thrombus.

5. *Myoglobin:* Present in serum
   - Released from myocardium within 2 hours of coronary occlusion
   - Peaks in 6 to 7 hours
   - Better marker for early detection of MI; better negative indicator if negative
6. *Cardiac catheterization:* Ventricular wall motion abnormalities (also may be seen by echocardiography); total occlusion of one or more coronary arteries.

Principles of Management of Acute Ischemic Heart Disease

Because most complications of acute ischemic heart disease directly result from reduced coronary flow, a primary ob-

jective in patient management is to optimize blood flow to the myocardium. Additional goals are to prevent complications of ischemia and infarction, alleviate angina, and reduce anxiety.

Optimize Blood Flow to the Myocardium

Regardless of whether a patient presents with unstable angina or AMI, restoration and maintenance of coronary blood flow is important to improve patient outcomes. Interventions to optimize blood flow to the myocardium include pharmacologic measures, such as antiplatelet or antithrombin agents, and mechanical measures, such as percutaneous coronary revascularization (e.g., angioplasty, stent, or other) or coronary

TABLE 9–5. HORMONAL AND ENVIRONMENTAL TRIGGERS OF PLAQUE RUPTURE

Acute	Chronic
Hemodynamic Reactivity	**Basal Hemodynamic Forces**
• Morning increase in blood pressure	• Increased resting blood pressure
• Morning increase in heart rate	• Increased resting heart rate
• Physical exertion	**Basal Hemostatic Variables**
• Emotional stress	• Location of the plaque
• Exposure to cold	• Size of the lipid pool within the core plaque
Hemostatic Reactivity	• Degree of macrophage infiltration of the plaque
• Increased coronary blood flow velocity	**Chronic Risk Factors**
• Increased viscosity of blood	• Gender (male > female)
• Decreased tPA activity	• Increasing age
• Increased platelet aggregation	• Diabetes mellitus
Vasoreactivity	• Hypercholesterolemia
• Increased plasma epinephrine	• Cigarette smoking
• Increased plasma cortisol	

artery bypass grafting (CABG). Refer to Table 9–7 for evidenced-based guidelines for AMI. The intervention selected and the optimal timing of the intervention depend on whether the occlusion of the artery is total or partial. This determination must be made as accurately and as quickly as possible, as a totally occluded artery will soon result in tissue necrosis or MI (Figure 9–8). All unstable arteries benefit from the following interventions which stabilize the artery and optimize coronary arterial flow.

MEDICAL MANAGEMENT

1. Decrease activity of coagulation system with pharmacologic therapy (Figure 9–9):
   • Antiplatelet agents: aspirin, GP IIb/IIIa receptor blocking agents (e.g., abciximab [Reopro],

eptifbatide [Integrilin], and tirofiban [Aggrastat]), thienopyridine agents (e.g., clopidogrel [Plavix])
   • Antithrombin agents: Indirect (e.g., heparin, low-molecular-weight heparin), direct (e.g., bivalirudin)
2. Increase ventricular filling time (decrease heart rate):
   • Beta-blockers
   • Bed rest for 24 hours
3. Decrease preload
   • Nitrates
   • Diuretics
   • Morphine sulfate
4. Decrease afterload
   • Angiotensin-converting enzyme (ACE) inhibitors
   • Hydralazine
5. Decrease myocardial oxygen consumption (MV_{O_2})
   • Beta-blockers
   • Bed rest for 24 hours

Totally occluded arteries require, in addition to the above pharmacologic interventions, further reperfusion therapy, such as fibrinolysis, angioplasty, or CABG, to effectively restore blood flow to the coronary artery. In the event of left main coronary artery stenosis or three-vessel disease, acute CABG is usually considered. In the acute setting, fibrinolytic therapy is often the fastest, most universally available method for reperfusion if a catheterization laboratory is not available or operational 24 hours a day. The indications, contraindications, and common complications of fibrinolytic therapy are listed in Tables 9–8 and 9–9. In those settings where the catheterization laboratory is operational 24 hours per day, primary PCI is indicated. Studies have indicated that primary PCI may be associated with slightly better outcomes and fewer complications than the use of fibrinolytic agents.

Surgical Management
CABG is one method of revascularization generally used in patients with atherosclerosis of three or more coronary vessels or in the case of significant left main coronary artery disease. CABG is performed both electively, as well as emergently, and may be performed either prior to or following an MI. The CABG procedure requires "induction" with general anesthesia, and possible initiation of cardiopulmonary bypass (blood is diverted outside of the body to a pump that mechanically oxygenates the blood before returning it to the arterial circulation) and placement of a graft into the coronary arterial tree (Figure 9–10). Technological advances have resulted in the development of stabilizer devices permitting CABG to be performed without placing the patient on cardiopulmonary bypass. The heart continues to beat while the surgeon places a device over the coronary artery site where the bypass graft is to be anastomosed, which stabilizes the small area allowing for suturing to occur. This is often referred to as *beating heart surgery*. The graft, gener-

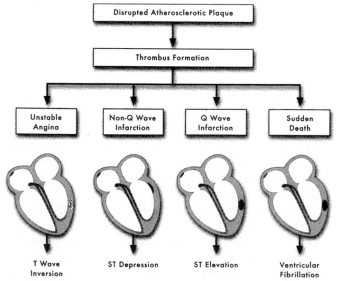

Figure 9–6. Pathophysiologic steps leading to acute coronary events.

ally a leg vein, left internal mammary artery, or radial artery, is inserted past the distal end of the blockage in the coronary artery and, in the case of a leg vein graft and radial artery graft, anastomosed to the aorta. Multiple grafts may be inserted based on the number of blockages present and the availability of viable insertion sites in the patient's native coronary tree.

INDICATIONS

The indications for CABG and long-term patient outcome following this procedure have been intensively reviewed over the past decade. In general, patients with three-vessel disease, poor LVEF ($<35\%$), or significant disease in the left main coronary artery have lower long-term morbidity and mortality with surgical revascularization (CABG) compared to medical therapy or percutaneous interventions such as angioplasty or stent. CABG may also be indicated as an emergent "rescue" procedure in patients whose coronary artery severely dissects or fractures during an attempted percutaneous procedure.

CONTRAINDICATIONS

Several populations of patients may be considered poor candidates for coronary bypass, including the very elderly, debilitated patients, patients with severely diseased distal coronary vasculature (e.g., some diabetics), and patients with extremely poor LVEF (e.g., $<10\%$ to 15%). Patients with low ejection fractions often have difficulty being weaned from cardiopulmonary bypass following the procedure. Other contraindications are those related to general anesthesia risk, including severe chronic obstructive pulmonary disease, pulmonary edema, or pulmonary hypertension.

POSTOPERATIVE MANAGEMENT

The following is a general overview of the early postoperative management of CABG patients.

1. *Maintain hemodynamic stability*: A variety of cardiac drugs are administered to maintain hemodynamic stability in the first 24 hours postoperatively. The following hemodynamic values may serve as guides for vasopressor administration and intravascular fluid therapy. In general, values greater or lower than the following require intervention:
   - Mean arterial pressure: 70 to 80 mm Hg
   - CI: 2.0 to 3.5 L/min/m^2
   - PAD/PCWP: 10 to 12 mm Hg (used primarily to evaluate need for volume replacement)
   - Central venous pressure (CVP): 5 to 10 mm Hg (used primarily to evaluate need for volume replacement)
   - HR: Intrinsic or paced rhythm in range of 80 to 100/min to keep CI ≥ 2.0
2. *Maintain ventilation and oxygenation:* Ventilation and oxygenation are maximized in the early postoperative period with mechanical ventilation. Within

2 to 12 hours, most patients have recovered from the anesthesia effects and are sufficiently stable to allow weaning from mechanical ventilation. Individuals with preexisting pulmonary problems may require longer periods of intubation until weaning can be successfully accomplished. Following weaning and extubation, supplemental O_2 therapy usually is required for 1 to 2 days to maintain PaO_2 or SaO_2 in normal ranges. Postoperative atelectasis is a common occurrence after cardiopulmonary bypass, usually requiring frequent pulmonary interventions (e.g., coughing and deep breathing, incentive spirometry, ambulation) to maintain ventilation and oxygenation.
3. Prevention of postoperative complications
   A. *Bleeding from vascular graft anastomosis sites:* Frequent monitoring of mediastinal tube drainage, hematocrit, and coagulation status; avoidance of even brief periods of hypertension.
   B. *Cardiac tamponade:* Frequent assessment for signs and symptoms of tamponade (pulsus paradoxus; increased CVP and decreased mediastinal tube drainage; increased CVP, PAD, and PAP, decreased heart sounds, blood pressure [BP], and cardiac output).
   C. *Infection:* Antibiotics are used prophylactically for 24 hours; temperature spike within 24 hours postoperatively is not abnormal (usually related to pulmonary atelectasis).
   D. *Cardiac dysrhythmias:* ECG monitoring, treat unstable rhythms, maintain K^+ and Mg^+ within normal limits with IV replacement.
   E. *Relief of postoperative pain and anxiety:* Analgesic administration is typically required to ensure pain relief, especially to facilitate ambulation, coughing, and deep breathing.

Preventing Complications Associated with Coronary Obstruction

Complications associated with acute ischemic syndromes include recurrent ischemia, infarction or reinfarction, onset of congestive heart failure (CHF), and arrhythmias.

1. *Prevent recurrent ischemia, infarction, or reinfarction*: Continue pharmacologic interventions to inhibit prothrombotic events, including ischemia and infarction (e.g., antiplatelet and antithrombin agents). Assess for recurrent angina with frequent chest pain assessment and serial 12-lead ECG and ST-segment ischemia monitoring.
2. *Continuously monitor for dysrhythmias*: Monitor, if possible, for 24 to 72 hours following an ischemic episode.
3. *Minimize potential for CHF:* Minimize myocardial oxygen consumption with the administration of beta-blockers, limit physical activity (bed rest), and avoid increases in metabolic rate (e.g., fever). Decrease

TABLE 9–6. CLINICAL PRESENTATION OF MYOCARDIAL ISCHEMIA AND INFARCTION

Type MI	Arterial Involvement	Muscle Area Supplied	Assessment
Anteroseptal wall	LAD	Anterior LV Wall, Anterior LV septum Apex LV Bundle of His Bundle branches	↓ LV function → ↓ CO, ↓ BP ↑ PAD, ↑ PCWP S_3 and S_4, with CHF Rales with pulmonary edema
Posterior septal lateral	RCA circumflex branches (right and left)	Posterior surface of LV SA node 45% AV node 10% Left atrium Lateral wall of LV	Murmurs indicating VSD (septal) PA catheter to assess R to L shunt in VSD Signals/symptoms of LV aneurysm with lateral Displaced PMI leading to signs and symptoms of mitral regurgitation
Inferior or "diaphragmatic"	RCA	RV, RA SA node 50% AV node 90% RA, RV Inferior LV Posterior IV septum Posterior LBBB Posterior LV	Symptomatic bradycardia: ↓ BP LOC changes diaphoresis ↓ CO ↑ PAD ↑ PCWP Murmurs: associated with papillary muscle dysfunction mid/holosystolic rates, pulmonary edema, nausea
Right ventricular infarction	RCA	RA, RV, inferior LV SA node AV node Posterior IV septum	Kussmaul sign JVD Hypotension ↑ SVR, ↓ PCWP, ↑ CVP S_3 with noncompliant RV Clear breath sounds initially Hepatomegaly, peripheral edema, cool clammy pale skin

ECG Changes	Likely Dysrhythmias	Possible Complications
Indicative ST elevation with or without abnormal Q waves in $V_{1,2,3,4}$ Loss of R waves in precordial leads **Reciprocal** ST depression in II, III, AVF.	RBBB, LBBB AV blocks Atrial fibrillation or flutter Ventricular tachycardia (VT) Tachycardia (septal)	Cardiogenic shock VSD Myocardial rupture Heart blocks may be permanent (LBBB) High mortality associated with this location of MI
Lateral Indicative ST elevation I, AVL, $V_{5,6}$ Loss of R wave and ↑ ST in I, AVL, V_{5-6} **Posterior Indicative** Tall, broad R waves (>0.04 sec) in V_{1-3} ↑ ST V_4R (right-sided 12 lead, V_4 position) **Posterior Reciprocal** ST depression in $V_{1,2}$, upright T wave in $V_{1,2}$	Bradycardia Mobitz I (posterior)	RV involvement Aneurysm development Papillary muscle dysfunction Heart blocks frequently resolve
Indicative ↑ ST segments in II, III, AVF Q waves in II, III, AVF **Reciprocal** ST depression in I, AVL, $V_{1,2,3,4}$	AV blocks; often progress to CHB which may be transient or permanent; Wenchebach; bradyarrhythmias	Hiccups Nausea/vomiting Papillary muscle dysfunction MR Septal rutpture (0.5–1.0%) RV involvement associated with atrial infarcts especially with atrial dysrhythmias
Indicative 1- to 2-mm ST segment elevation in V_4R ST- and T-wave elevation in II, III, AVF Q waves in II, III, AVF ST-elevation decreases in amplitude over V_{1-6}	First-degree AV block Second-degree AV block, type I Incomplete RBBB Transient CHB Atrial fibrillation VT/VF	Hypotension requiring large volumes initially to maintain systemic pressure. Once RV contractility improves fluids will mobilize, possibly requiring diuresis

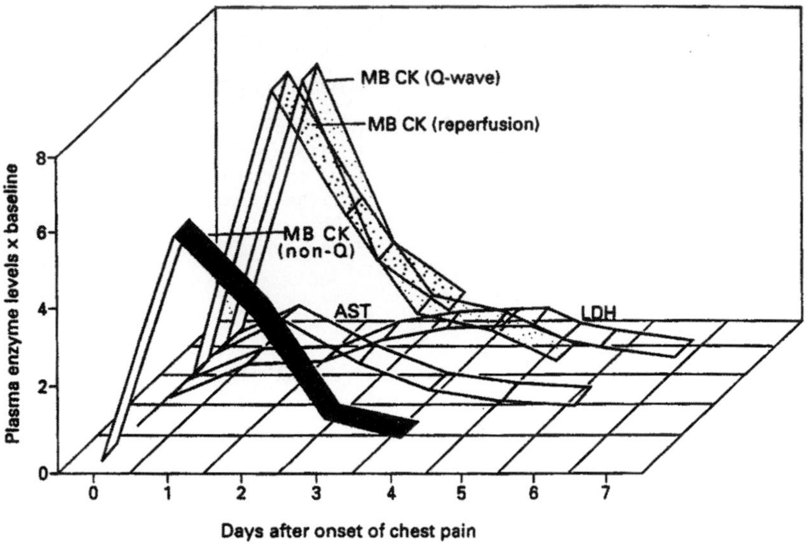

Figure 9–7. Typical plasma profiles for the MB isoenzymes of creatine kinase (MB-CK), aspartate amino transferase (AST), and lactate dehydrogenase (LDH) activities following onset of acute myocardial infarction. (*Used with permission, Alexander R, Pratt C: Diagnosis and management of acute myocardial infarction. In Fuster V, Alexander R, O'Rouke R [eds]: Hurst's The Heart, 10th ed. New York: McGraw-Hill; 2001.*)

TABLE 9–7. EVIDENCED-BASED PRACTICE: ACS—ST ELEVATION MI AND NON–ST ELEVATION MI

Diagnosis
- Diagnosis of AMI is based on two of three findings:[a,b]
  1. History of ischemic-like symptoms
  2. Changes on serial ECGs
  3. Elevation and fall in level of serum cardiac biomarkers
- Of AMI patients, 50% do not present with ST-segment elevation. Other indicators:[a,b]
  1. ST segment depression may indicate NSTEMI
  2. New LBBB
  3. ST-segment depression that resolves with relief of chest pain
  4. T-wave inversion in all chest leads may indicate NSTEMI with a critical stenosis in the proximal LAD

Acute Management
- Optimal time for initiation of therapy is within 1 hour of symptom onset. Rarely feasible due to delay in treatment seeking behavior.[a,b]
- Initial ECG should be obtained within 10 minutes of emergency department arrival[a,b]
- Oxygen, nitroglycerine and aspirin should be administered if not contraindicated[a,b]
- Reperfusion strategy: STEMI only[a,b]
  - Fibrinolytic agent should be initiated within 30 minutes of arrival if no contraindication
  - If primary PCI to be done, culprit vessel should be opened within 90 minutes of arrival
- Reperfusion Strategy for NSTEMI[a,b]
  - Fibrinolytics not recommended
  - PCI to be done within 24 hours of arrival
- Weight-based heparin or low-molecular-weight heparin[a,b]
- IV beta-blocker should be given within 12 hours of arrival[a,b]
- Lipid-lowering agent should be initiated[a,b]

Data compiled from: [a]Antman, et al. (2004). [b]Casey (2002).

left ventricular afterload with the administration of ACE inhibitors and hydralazine.

Alleviating Pain
Pain relief improves coronary flow by decreasing the level of circulating catecholamines, thereby decreasing blood pressure (afterload) and heart rate (myocardial oxygen consumption). Nitrates typically relieve anginal pain by dilating coronary arteries and increasing flow, thereby improving myocardial oxygenation and directly treating the source of the pain. Another pharmacologic intervention commonly used to relieve pain in ischemia is morphine sulfate. Although morphine is a potent narcotic that has been criticized for masking cardiac pain, it is also a potent vasodilator and effectively vasodilates coronary as well as peripheral arteries, resulting in mild afterload reduction. Severe pain, unable to be relieved with nitrates or a combination of nitrates and morphine, is typically an indication for immediate PCI if available, or transfer to a referring institution for emergency PCI.

Reducing Anxiety
The reduction of anxiety in ischemic heart disease is important for a number of reasons. The most important physiologically is the reduction of catecholamine secretion and decrease in sympathetic tone following relaxation in the anxious patient. This effect has been shown to decrease the incidence of dysrhythmias and promote vasodilation and afterload reduction. Decreasing anxiety should also increase the patient's ability to process new information regarding his or her diagnosis, and to better understand instructions for tests or procedures that will be done.

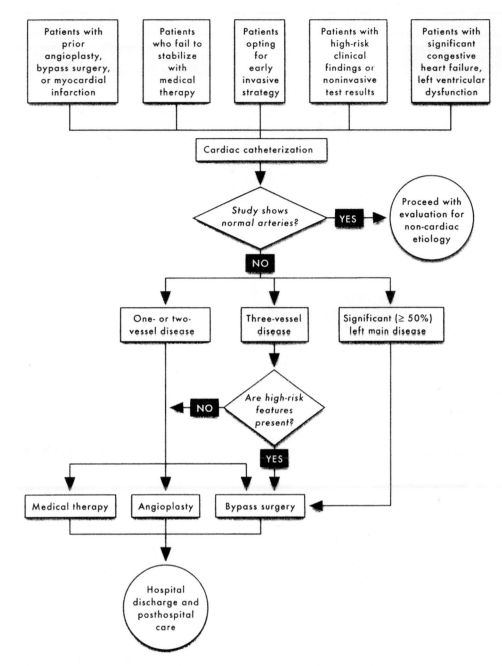

Figure 9–8. Treatment decision tree for coronary revascularization. (*Source: U.S. Department of Health and Human Services:* Unstable Angina: Diagnosis and Management [*AHCPR Pub No. 94-0602. Clinical Practice Guideline No. 10*]. *Washington, DC: DHHS; May 1994.*)

Relief of pain typically is most effective in reducing patient anxiety. In the event that pain is not relieved with nitroglycerin, or fibrinolytics in the initial treatment of ischemia, pain relievers such as morphine sulfate or anxiolytics such as lorazepam (Ativan) (short-acting) are usually effective.

A number of interventions may be done at the bedside to promote relaxation, including specific relaxation and imagery techniques, meditation, music therapy, and the use of relaxation tapes. Providing the patient and family with adequate information regarding unfamiliar surroundings, when the physician may be available to speak with them, possible "unknowns" such as tests or procedures, and important expectations such as visitation guidelines helps to provide a sense of security and facilitates relaxation by increasing the patient's level of comfort with the situation. Anxiety can also be decreased by offering the patient opportunities for control in the acute setting. Examples include the timing of simple activities such as visitor presence, bathing, and eating.

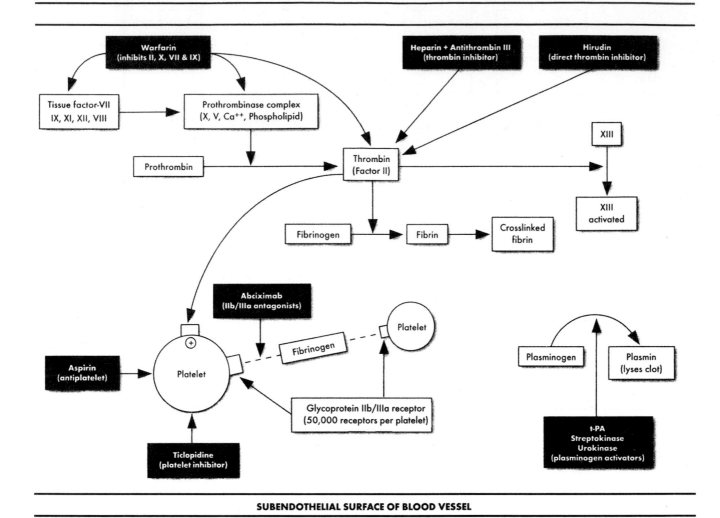

Figure 9–9. Coagulation sequence and site of antithrombotic/antiplatelet drug activity.

TABLE 9–8. INDICATIONS AND CONTRAINDICATIONS FOR THROMBOLYTIC THERAPY

Indications
- Chest pain >20 min, but typically <12 hours
- ST elevation ≥1 mm in two contiguous leads
- LBBB
- High-risk patients with chest pain >12 hours in duration may still be candidates if pain persists

Absolute Contraindications
- Active internal bleeding
- History of intracranial bleeding, cerebral neoplasm, or other intracranial pathology
- Stroke or head trauma within 6 months
- Known allergy to the drug chosen

Relative Contraindications
- Major surgery or GI bleeding within 2 months
- Traumatic puncture of noncompressible vessel
- Pregnancy or 1 month postpartum
- Uncontrolled hypertension (systolic >200 or diastolic >110)
- Trauma within 2 weeks, including CPR with rib fracture

Congestive Heart Failure

CHF is a broad term referring to the inability of the heart to pump sufficient blood to meet the oxygen and nutrient requirements of the body. A number of underlying disease processes may contribute to this "weak pump" syndrome, with coronary atherosclerosis, valvular heart disease, hypertension, and cardiomyopathy as the most common causes. Although the underlying causes are diverse, the progressive process which occurs in response to one of these initiating events is the same.

Etiology, Risk Factors, and Pathophysiology

Although CHF may result from a number of underlying etiologies, those causing left ventricular systolic dysfunction are the most common contributors. The pathophysiology of CHF is a three-stage process, beginning with an initial insult to the myocardium (phase I), followed by a response phase (phase

TABLE 9–9. COMPLICATIONS OF FIBROLYTIC THERAPY

Complication	Percentage Occurrence
Groin bleeding, local (compressible external)	25–45
Intracerebral bleeding	1.45
Retroperitoneal bleeding (noncompressible internal)	1
Gastrointestinal bleeding	4–10
Genitourinary bleeding	1–5
Other bleeding	1–5

II), and resulting in the clinical syndrome known as CHF, characterized by exhaustion of compensatory mechanisms (phase III) (Figure 9–11). Regardless of the precipitating event, the physiologic progression of the syndrome, once initiated, is the same.

Phase I

Phase I of CHF is characterized by an initiating event (e.g., MI, viral infection, chemotherapeutic agents, valvular heart disease, hypertension, idiopathic cardiomyopathy), which causes loss of myocytes. This cell loss or permanent damage to the myocytes can be either localized or diffuse, resulting in compromised ventricular function. To date, over 700 initiating factors, such as acute ischemic damage, viruses, and

toxins, have been isolated as contributors to myocardial insult and heart failure.

• *Result of phase I:* Decreased stroke volume secondary to an initial insult to the myocardium.

Phase II

A number of adaptive mechanisms occur in response to the initial insult in an effort to maintain adequate cardiac output to meet the body's needs. This phase is sometimes referred to as the *compensatory phase* (Figures 9–11 and 9–12). These compensatory mechanisms or responses include the Frank–Starling response, myocardial remodeling, and the neurohormonal response.

FRANK–STARLING RESPONSE

As cardiac output decreases and the sympathetic nervous system is activated, alpha-1 receptors are stimulated, resulting in arteriolar and venous vasoconstriction. This adaptive response initially results in increased venous return to the ventricle, increased ventricular end-diastolic volume, stretching of the ventricular myocytes, and improved stroke volume. Later, as overstretching of the ventricle occurs, this compensatory mechanism is lost, resulting in left ventricular decompensation and myocardial hypertrophy (Figure 9–13). Additionally, there is increased expression of granules in the left ventricle causing an increased release of brain

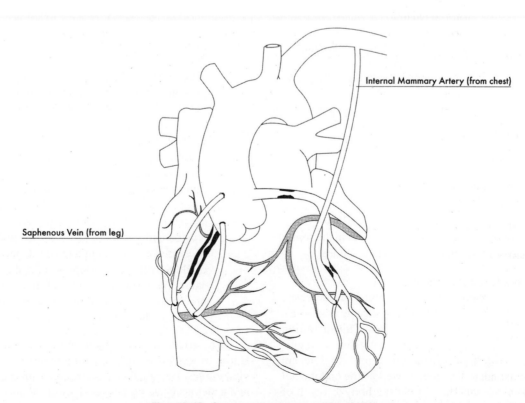

Figure 9–10. Coronary artery bypass grafting (CABG).

AT THE BEDSIDE
▶ *Congestive Heart Failure*

A 75-year-old man presents to the emergency department with diaphoresis and severe dyspnea. Initial assessment revealed the following:

RR	32/min
BP	110/90
HR	110 beats/min, irregular
JVD	Bilateral 7-mm elevation
Lungs	Bibasilar rales throughout the lower lobes
Cardiovascular	S_1, S_2 with an S_3

A pulse oximeter revealed 83% oxygen saturation. Lab work, including an arterial blood gas sample, was done with the following results:

PaO_2	60 mm Hg
$PaCO_2$	28 mm Hg
pH	7.51
SaO_2	93%

Oxygen was initiated at 40% by face mask. An ECG was done and showed left ventricular hypertrophy, left bundle and branch block, and Q waves. His chest x-ray showed an enlarged cardiac silhouette and bilateral infiltrates. A pulmonary artery catheter was placed and the following parameters were found:

RA	10 mm Hg
PA	41/35 mm Hg
PCWP	32 mm Hg
CO	3.8 L/min
CI	1.9 L/min/m^2

A dobutamine drip was started at 2.5 mcg/kg/min, and furosemide 40 mg IV was given. Cardiac catheterization was performed the next morning with the following findings:

LAD	95%
RCA	50%
LCX	75%
EF	28%
Severe asyneresis	

natriuretic peptide (BNP). Increased BNP levels in the serum are used as markers of severity of ventricular failure.

MYOCARDIAL HYPERTROPHY (REMODELING)

In response to increased vascular volume and decreased myocardial function (loss of the Frank–Starling response), the left ventricle dilates and hypertrophies. This distortion of the normal left ventricular anatomy causes mitral regurgitation and further left ventricular dilatation. Angiotensin II, produced in the adrenal cortex as well as the endothelial cells of the blood vessels throughout the body (a result of renin–angiotensin system activation), directly induces myo-

cyte hypertrophy as well. The result of these factors is decreased left ventricular reserve (stretch), increased preload (high residual volume in the ventricle following systole), and further mitral regurgitation.

NEUROHORMONAL RESPONSE

In response to decreased stroke volume and decreased renal perfusion, several neurohormonal systems are activated, each of which acts to compensate for the decrease in stroke volume. These include:

1. *Adrenergic nervous system:* Adrenergic nervous system activity is heightened in the setting of impaired ventricular function as a direct result of baroreceptor stimulation. These baroreceptors mediate the sympathetic nervous system, which in turn stimulates the beta-1 receptors. This results in an increase in heart rate and contractility.

2. *Renin–angiotensin–aldosterone system:* Decreased renal perfusion stimulates the release of renin, increasing the production of angiotensin I and II and the release of aldosterone. This causes arteriolar vasoconstriction, decreased cardiac output, increased arterial blood pressure and peripheral resistance, increased ventricular filling pressures, sodium and potassium retention (imbalance), increased volume overload, increased left ventricular wall stress, increased ventricular dilation and hypertrophy, and increased sympathetic nervous system arousal.

3. *Arginine vasopressin (AVP) system:* AVP is a potent vasoconstrictor that is normally inhibited by stretch receptors in the atria during atrial distension. In heart failure, these receptors are less sensitive, causing a decrease in AVP inhibition. This results in systemic vasoconstriction, further increasing afterload (the pressure against which the ventricle must pump to get blood out of the ventricle). Increases in AVP availability also lead to an inability to excrete free water, hypo-osmolarity, and, in general, inability to autoregulate further AVP production.

4. *Atrial natriuretic peptide (ANP):* ANP is a counter-regulatory hormone that opposes all three of the above systems, resulting in vasodilation and sodium excretion. ANP is produced in response to atrial distension and results in decreased formation of renin, decreased effects of angiotensin II, decreased release of aldosterone and vasopressin, and enhanced renal excretion of sodium and water. In chronic heart failure, the levels of ANP remain elevated, but are less so than in the acute phase (phase II).

The effects of the compensatory mechanisms in phase II lead to an increase in circulating volume and perfusion to vital organs. Eventually, these mechanisms are self-limiting and a vicious cycle of increased afterload and volume overload results. The neurohormonal response is no longer ben-

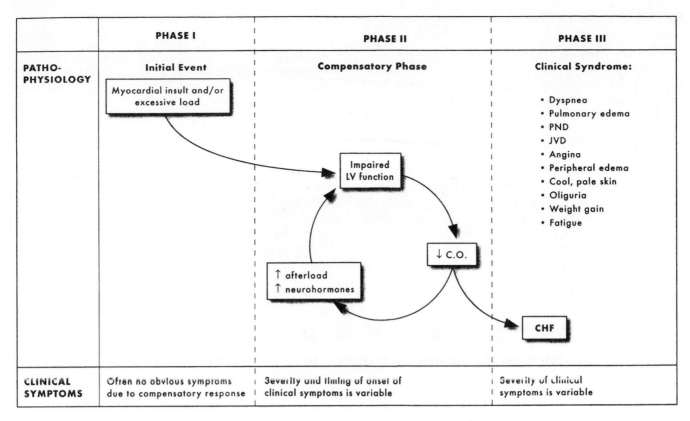

Figure 9–11. Pathophysiology of heart failure during phases I, II, and III.

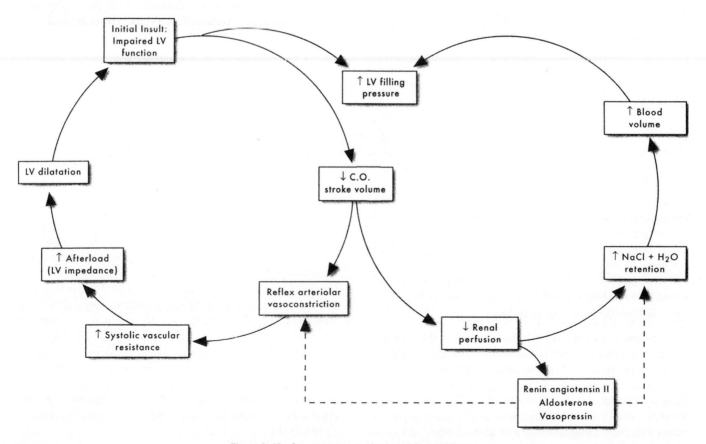

Figure 9–12. Compensatory mechanisms of heart failure.

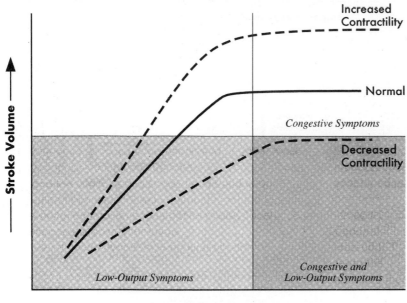

Figure 9–13. Frank–Starling curve.

eficial in the chronic state but, as seen in phase III, becomes detrimental leading to changes in the myocyte DNA resulting in programmed cell death (apoptosis) and further loss of myocytes.

- *Result of phase II:* Ventricular hypertrophy, weakened myocytes, increased arteriolar resistance, increased vascular volume, and increased ventricular wall stress occur in an effort to maintain adequate cardiac output.

Phase III

When the adaptive mechanisms of phase II fail, the clinical syndrome of heart failure follows. This third phase of heart failure is extremely variable in onset and presentation. The clinical expression and course of the disease is determined by the extent of the initial insult and myocyte damage, the severity of hemodynamic burden (volume overload), and the patient's individual neurohormonal response to these changes. Phase III is characterized by a progressive deterioration of cardiovascular functioning due to the relationship between compromised left ventricular function and excessive cardiac afterload (Figure 9–14).

- *Result of phase III:* Clinical signs and symptoms of heart failure are evident, resulting in decreased functional status and activity intolerance for the patient.

Clinical Presentation

Regardless of the underlying cause of the weak pump, patients with heart failure present with clinical signs and symptoms of intravascular and interstitial volume overload, as well as manifestations of inadequate tissue perfusion. Common findings in CHF include:

- Dyspnea (especially with exertion, commonly severe in the acute setting)
- Postural nocturnal dyspnea
- Pulmonary edema (pronounced crackles)
- Jugular venous distension (JVD)
- Chest discomfort or tightness
- Peripheral edema
- Cool, pale, cyanotic skin
- Oliguria
- Reported weight gain
- Fatigue

More specific physical signs and symptoms may vary in individuals depending on the ventricle which is primarily involved. A summary of clinical findings specific to left and right ventricular failure is presented in Table 9–10.

Because subjective assessment of symptoms and their severity may vary from clinician to clinician, a classification system is commonly used to standardize symptom severity in CHF. One system, the Killip Classification, is used primarily at initial evaluation to predict severity of illness. A second system, known as the New York Heart Association Functional Classification System, is used to provide systematic assessment of patient status and to benchmark improvement or deterioration from initial evaluation (Table 9–11).

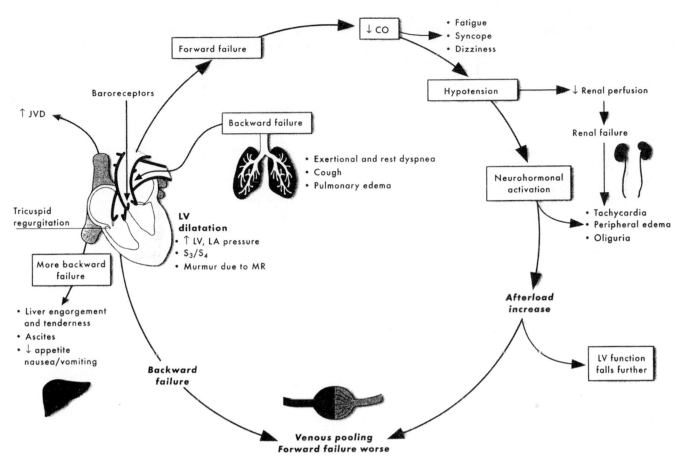

Figure 9–14. Clinical features of heart failure.

A number of conditions, both cardiac and noncardiac, are similar to heart failure in their clinical presentation and should be ruled out as possible diagnoses in the initial assessment. These conditions include MI, pulmonary disease, dysrhythmias, anemia, renal failure, nephrotic syndrome, and thyroid disease.

Diagnostic Tests

- *12-Lead ECG:* Acute ST-T wave changes, low voltage, left ventricular hypertrophy, atrial fibrillation or other tachyarrhythmias, bradyarrhythmias, Q waves from previous MI, LBBB

TABLE 9–10. CLINICAL SIGNS AND SYMPTOMS SPECIFIC TO RIGHT- AND LEFT-SIDED HEART FAILURE

Right Heart Failure	Left Heart Failure
Signs and Symptoms of Hepatic Congestion	**Signs and Symptoms of Pulmonary Congestion**
JVD	JVD
Liver enlargement and tenderness	Pulmonary edema
Positive hepatojugular reflex (pressure on liver increases JVD)	Rales
Dependent edema	Atrial fibrillation or other atrial arrhythmias secondary to atrial distension
Ascites	Pulsus alternans (every other beat diminished)
Decreased appetite, nausea, vomiting	Dyspnea
Cardiac Pressures	Cough
Increased RV pressure	Hyperventilation
Increased RA pressure	Dizziness, syncope, fatigue
Heart Sounds	**Cardiac Pressures**
S_3 (early sign)	Increased LV and LA pressure
S_4 (may also present)	Increased pulmonary artery pressures
Wide split S_2	**Heart Sounds**
Pansystolic murmur at lower left sternal border secondary to stretching of tricuspid ring	S_3 and (occasionally) S_4
	Pansystolic murmur at apex secondary to mitral regurgitation

TABLE 9–11. CLASSIFICATION OF CARDIOVASCULAR DISABILITY

Killip Classification

Class

I	Asymptomatic
II	Basilar rales, S_3
III	Pulmonary edema
IV	Shock

New York Heart Association Functional Classification

Class

I	Patients with cardiac disease but without resulting limitations of physical activity. Ordinary physical activity does not cause undue fatigue, palpitation, dyspnea, or anginal pain.
II	Patients with cardiac disease resulting in slight limitation of physical activity. They are comfortable at rest. Ordinary physical activity results in fatigue, palpitation, dyspnea, or anginal pain.
III	Patients with cardiac disease resulting in marked limitation of physical activity. They are comfortable at rest. Less than ordinary physical activity causes fatigue, palpitation, dyspnea, or anginal pain.
IV	Patient with cardiac disease resulting in inability to carry on any physical activity without discomfort. Symptoms of cardiac insufficiency or of the anginal syndrome may be present even at rest. If any physical activity is undertaken, discomfort is increased.

- *Chest x-ray:* Cardiomegaly, cardiothoracic ratio >0.5
- *Complete blood count:* Low red cell count (anemia)
- *Urinalysis:* Proteinuria, red blood cells, or casts
- *Creatinine:* Elevated
- *Albumin:* Decreased
- *Serum sodium and potassium:* Decreased
- *PAP:* Elevated
- *CI:* <2.0 L/min/m^2
- *Echocardiography:* Dilated left ventricle, right ventricle, or right atria; hypertrophied left ventricle; AV valve incompetence; diffuse or segmental hypocontractility; atrial thrombus; pericardial effusion; LVEF <40%
- *Radionuclide ventriculography:* More precise measure of right ventricular dysfunction and LVEF

Principles of Management for Congestive Heart Failure

Acute management of CHF has changed dramatically over the past decade, from an emphasis on the micromanagement of hemodynamic parameters, primarily using positive inotropes, to an emphasis on functional capacity and long-term survival with the use of neurohormonal blocking agents. This shift is due to a better understanding of the neurohormonal response and the dependence of the body on these mechanisms for compensation in low output states. Goals of patient management in CHF revolve around four general principles: (1) treatment of the underlying cause (e.g., ischemia, valvular dysfunction), (2) management of fluid volume overload, (3) improvement of ventricular function, and (4) patient and family education.

Limiting the Initial Insult and Treating the Underlying Cause
The most effective, but often the most difficult, management strategy for CHF is to limit the damage done by the initial insult. This limitation of myocardial damage and cell loss maximizes the amount of viable ventricular muscle, myocardial contractility, and overall ventricular function.

- Administer fibrinolytic therapy as soon as possible for eligible patients in the setting of AMI or facilitate immediate transfer to the cardiac catheterization laboratory for primary PCI (see the previous section on acute ischemic heart disease).
- Revascularization may be warranted in patients with persistent ischemia as a preventive measure against eventual tissue necrosis.
- Valve replacement or repair or other surgical corrections (ventricular reconstruction surgery) should be undertaken as soon as possible to prevent prolonged overstretching of the ventricular myocardium.

Management of Fluid Volume Overload
Decrease preload by the use of diuretic therapy, limitation of dietary sodium, and restriction of free water.

- Diuretics should be initiated according to the severity of the patient's signs and symptoms. More severe symptoms require intravenous therapy and loop diuretics, and less severe symptoms may be managed adequately on loop diuretics. Thiazide diuretics may be added later if the patient does not respond to the loop diuretics.
- Sodium and fluid restriction should be monitored carefully, with sodium intake not exceeding 2 g/d and free water not exceeding 1500 mL in a 24-hour period.
- Serum sodium and potassium should be monitored on a regular basis to prevent inadvertent electrolyte imbalances (each day or two in the acute setting, depending on the aggressiveness of therapy).

Improvement of Left Ventricular Function
Improvement in left ventricular function is accomplished by decreasing the workload on the heart with preload and afterload reduction and by augmenting ventricular contractility. Ventricular function is often measured directly in the acute setting by monitoring CI. As has been demonstrated by a number of large clinical trials, traditional micromanagement of hemodynamic variables, such as CI with inotropic drugs, may be detrimental to long-term patient outcome. Current recommendations do not advocate this as an initial management strategy.

- Decrease preload (see above).
- Decrease afterload by administration of pharmacologic therapy, including ACE inhibitors and vasodilators. ACE inhibitors are recommended in all heart failure patients unless otherwise contraindicated.

Contraindications to ACE therapy include previous intolerance, potassium >5.5 mEq/L, hypotension with systolic blood pressure less than 90 mm Hg, and serum creatinine greater than 3.0 mg/dL. Cautious initiation of low-dose therapy in patients with contraindications may still be considered. Vasodilators may also be used in conjunction with diuretics and ACE inhibitors if further afterload reduction is necessary. Especially in the case of underlying atherosclerotic disease, still the largest single contributor to heart failure, nitrates are often used concomitantly with ACE inhibitors and diuretics to augment afterload reduction.

- To increase myocardial contractility, ACE inhibitors should be considered as the first-line drug, with digoxin recommended for severe heart failure due to left ventricular systolic dysfunction and in mild to moderate cases of failure when optimal doses of ACE inhibitors and diuretics have failed to relieve patient symptoms.

- A relatively new recommendation is the use of beta-blockers. Specifically, carvedilol has been found to be associated with better outcomes than other drugs in this class. Caution should still be taken when initiating this therapy in patients with significant respiratory compromise or hypotension. Anticoagulation therapy is also recommended for prevention of pulmonary embolism in patients with atrial or ventricular septal stasis, a history of atrial fibrillation, or prior pulmonary embolism.

- BNP (nesiritide [Natrecor]) has been another recent addition to the management of decompensated heart failure. Nesiritide's effects include promoting diuresis and vasodilation thereby decreasing ventricular preload and afterload. The agent may also inhibit angiotensin II as well as some of the other neuro-endocrine compensatory mechanisms associated with heart failure. Initially recommended for acutely decompensated ventricular failure, the agent is being used as an intermittent infusion in heart failure outpatient settings.

- Dual chamber biventricular pacemaker/implantable cardioverter defibrillator (ICD). Approximately 60% of patients with dilated cardiomyopathy develop LBBB. In the presence of LBBB, the right and left ventricles no longer contract simultaneously but in a series causing the intraventricular septum to shift inappropriately, interfering with the aortic and mitral valve functioning. There have been several studies recently demonstrating significantly improved outcomes (quality of life, survival rates, etc.) with the use of a dual chamber biventricular pacemaker. This technology stimulates both ventricles simultaneously, causing both to contract at the same time resulting in a narrowing of the QRS complex and improved myo-

cardial contractility and cardiac output. Often the pacing technology is combined with an ICD because sudden cardiac death related to ventricular tachycardia/fibrillation is the most common cause of death in these patients.

- Cardiac assist devices (left ventricular, right ventricular, or both) can provide temporary maintenance or preservation of ventricular function, especially as a bridge to recovery, bridge to cardiac transplantation, or as destination therapy (discharge to home). These devices are inserted percutaneously or surgically using the medial sternotomy or thoracotomy approach (see Chapter 19, Advanced Cardiovascular Concepts). Left ventricular apical cannulation allows ambulation and physical rehabilitation. Technological developments have contributed to the development of small pumps allowing many to be implanted with the drive line (power source) exiting the skin. Risks related to insertion of these devices include infection, peripheral embolization including stroke, and, for some, long-term weaning difficulties in the event that an organ donor is not available. Those devices approved for destination therapy (a replacement for heart transplant) include the Heart Mate and Debakey devices.

1. *Intra-aortic balloon pump (IABP):* Femoral or brachial artery cannulation with the IABP allows for ventricular support, but restricts the patient to bed rest (femoral primarily) and compromises arterial flow to the cannulated limb.

2. *Ventricular reconstruction:* Many patients with end-stage heart failure have a previous history of coronary artery disease and MI resulting in the development of a ventricular aneurysm on the anterior wall of the left ventricle. A surgical procedure (Dor procedure) can be performed removing the aneurysm, reducing the size of the ventricle resulting in increased contractility and cardiac output. Studies have shown that patients experience improvement in physical functioning and NYHA Functional Class following this procedure.

3. *Myoplasty:* The insertion of autologous skeletal muscle (generally latissimus dorsi) into the ventricular wall via removal of the third rib. This procedure requires a 2-month "muscle training" process once the transplant is in place and therefore requires a relatively stable heart failure candidate. This procedure is rarely performed in the United States but continues to be investigated outside the United States.

Patient Education

Patients who present with CHF to the critical care unit have high acuity levels, require more intensive interventions, and have an increased need for emotional support surrounding the serious nature of the hospital admission. Previous admissions for CHF make patients more aware of the serious nature of acute episodes. Patient education, which is appropriately addressed in the acute care setting includes the following.

1. Crisis intervention is necessary, both with the patient and the family. Include encouragement to verbalize fears related to role adaptations or changes in family responsibility, lifestyle alterations and limitations, and death and dying. The completion of advanced directives and living wills should be initiated if not previously addressed.
2. Family involvement in the critical care phase should be strongly encouraged, including assistance with activities of daily living such as bathing, and "patterning" of daily activities to allow for frequent periods of rest and spacing of exertional activity. In addition, family involvement in reading or other leisure activity with the patient is often restful and relaxing, and may be useful as a diversional activity. If possible, the family should also be present for reinforcement of patient teaching regarding the medical regimen, the importance of fluid and sodium restriction, and the need for daily weights.

Shock

Shock is the inability of the circulatory system to deliver enough blood to meet the oxygen and nutrient requirements of body tissues. This clinical syndrome may result from ineffective pumping of the heart (cardiogenic shock), insufficient volume of circulating blood (hypovolemic shock), or massive vasodilation of the vascular bed causing maldistri-

bution of blood (vasogenic shock). Although the specific definition of shock and strategies for patient management vary according to the underlying pathophysiology, the principle of ineffective or insufficient oxygen delivery to meet the needs of body tissues remains consistent.

Etiology, Risk Factors, and Pathophysiology
The ineffective delivery of oxygen to the tissues leads to cellular dysfunction, rapidly progressing to organ failure and finally to total body system failure. The cause of the initial onset of the shock syndrome may be from any number of underlying problems, including heart problems, fluid loss, and trauma. Because the body responds in the same way, differences between cardiogenic, hypovolemic, and vasogenic shock are obvious to the clinician only after the initial assessment has provided key information about the patient's acute illness. Given the history, the clinician can classify shock into one of three major pathologic groups and proceed to further determine the patient's needs with the help of diagnostic testing. Because interventions for patient management are directed at the cause, it is essential for the underlying pathophysiology to be clearly understood.

Cardiogenic Shock
In cardiogenic shock, the heart is unable to pump enough blood to meet the oxygen and nutrient needs of the body. Pump failure is caused by a variety of factors, the most common being left ventricular failure. A number of other factors may cause pump failure, however, and are typically categorized as coronary or noncoronary causes (Table 9–12).

In all cardiogenic shock cases, the heart ceases to function normally as a pump, resulting in decreases in stroke volume and cardiac output. This leads to a decrease in blood

AT THE BEDSIDE
▶ *Shock Following AMI*

A 49-year-old man was found slumped in his living room chair, cool and clammy but still breathing. His wife phoned emergency medical services, which arranged air transportation to the local emergency room. On arrival, his vital signs were as follows:

BP   68/44
HR   122 beats/min
RR   33 breaths/min
T   36.1°C, orally
SaO$_2$ 91%

Oxygen at 60% by face mask had been initiated in flight, as well as intravenous normal saline running wide open, 450 mL having already infused. Dopamine was started at a rate of 5 mcg/kg/min. A stat ECG showed "tombstone" ST elevation in the anterior leads, with

reciprocal changes in leads II, III, and a VF. The patient was taken for immediate PTCA. In the lab, cardiac catheterization findings were as follows:

LAD   99% proximal lesion
RCA   70% mid lesion
LCX   Normal
LVEF   13%
Wall motion Left ventricular akinesis

On return to the ICU, the nurse obtained hemodynamic parameters as follows:

PA   45/25 mm Hg
RA   15 mm Hg
PCWP 22 mm Hg
CO   4.0 L/min
CI   1.5 L/min/m^2

TABLE 9–12. CAUSES OF CARDIOGENIC SHOCK

Coronary Causes
- MI with resultant cell death in a significant portion of the ventricle
- Rupture of ventricle or papillary muscle secondary to MI
- Dysfunctional ischemic—"shock ventricle"—which occurs as a result of myocardial ischemia, not involving cell death, and is therefore transient

Noncoronary Causes
- Myocardial contusion
- Pericardial tamponade
- Ventricular rupture
- Arrhythmia (PEA—pulseless electrical activity—new name)
- Valvular dysfunction resulting in ventricular congestion
- Cardiomyopathies
- End-stage CHF

pressure and tissue perfusion. The inability of the ventricles, particularly the left ventricle, to empty adequately and maintain adequate forward flow is sometimes referred to as *forward failure* (Figure 9–15). The inadequate emptying of the ventricle increases left atrial pressure, which then increases pulmonary venous pressure. As a result, pulmonary capillary pressure increases, resulting in pulmonary edema. This retrograde congestion is sometimes referred to as *backward failure.*

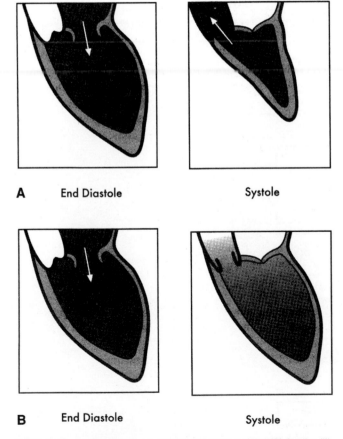

A   End Diastole   Systole

B   End Diastole   Systole

Figure 9–15. Cardiogenic shock. **(A)** Normal cardiac filling. **(B)** Cardiac filling during cardiogenic shock.

Hypovolemic Shock

Hypovolemic shock occurs when there is inadequate volume in the vascular space. This volume depletion may be caused by blood loss, either internal or external, or by the vascular fluid volume shifting out of the vascular space into other body fluid spaces (Table 9–13). The loss of vascular volume results in insufficient circulating blood to maintain tissue perfusion.

The pathophysiology of hypovolemic shock is related directly to decreased circulating blood volume. When an insufficient amount of blood is circulating, the venous blood returning to the heart is insufficient. As a result, right and left ventricular filling pressures are insufficient, decreasing stroke volume and cardiac output. As in cardiogenic shock, when cardiac output is decreased, blood pressure is low and tissue perfusion is poor.

Distributive Shock

Distributive shock is characterized by an abnormal placement or distribution of vascular volume, occurring in three situations: (1) sepsis, (2) neurologic damage, and (3) anaphylaxis. In each of these situations, the pumping function of the heart and the total blood volume are normal, but the blood is not appropriately distributed throughout the vascular bed. Massive vasodilation occurs in each of these situations for various reasons, causing the vascular bed to be much larger than normal. In this enlarged vascular bed, the usual volume of circulating blood (approximately 5 L) is no longer sufficient to fill the vascular space, causing a decrease in blood pressure and inadequate tissue perfusion. For this reason vasogenic shock is also referred to as *relative hypovolemic shock.*

Of the distributive or vasogenic shock syndromes, septic shock is most commonly seen in the critical care setting. In the field or emergency room setting, anaphylaxis and neurogenic shock are also common and typically result from allergic reactions and trauma related spinal cord injury.

Stages of Shock

Regardless of underlying etiology, all three types of shock (cardiogenic, hypovolemic, distributive) activate the sym-

TABLE 9–13. CAUSES OF HYPOVOLEMIC SHOCK

Sources of External Loss of Body Fluid
- Hemorrhage (loss of whole blood)
- Gastrointestinal tract (vomiting, diarrhea, ostomies, fistulas, nasogastric suctioning)
- Renal (diuretic administration, diabetes, insipidus, Addison disease, hyperglycemic osmotic diuresis)

Sources of Internal Loss of Body Fluid
- Internal hemorrhage
- Movement of body fluid into interstitial spaces ("third spacing," often the result of bacterial toxin, thermal injury, or allergic reaction)

pathetic nervous system, which in turn initiates neural, hormonal, and chemical compensatory mechanisms in an attempt to improve tissue perfusion (Figure 9–16). Cellular changes that occur as a result of these compensatory mechanisms are similar in all types of shock. Progression of these cellular changes follows a predictable, four-stage course.

Initial Stage

The initial stage of shock represents the first cellular changes resulting from the decrease in oxygen delivery to the tissue. These changes include decreased aerobic and increased anaerobic metabolism, leading to increases in serum lactic acid. No obvious clinical signs and symptoms are apparent during this stage of shock.

Compensatory Stage

The compensatory stage is composed of a number of physiologic events that represent an attempt to compensate for decreases in cardiac output and restore adequate oxygen and nutrient delivery to the tissues (Figure 9–17). These events can be organized into neural, hormonal, and chemical

responses. Neural responses include pressoreceptors in the aorta and carotid arteries, which detect changes in arterial blood pressure and respond by activating the vasomotor center of the medulla. Hypovolemia and resultant hypotension lead to activation of the sympathetic nervous system. The sympathetic nervous system initiates neural, hormonal, and chemical compensatory mechanisms in an attempt to decrease the vascular space and elevate the blood pressure. The sympathetic nervous system activation produces vasoconstriction of the peripheral circulation, shunting blood to vital organs (autoregulation). As blood is shunted to vital organs, renal blood flow is decreased, stimulating the hormonal response.

Hormonal responses include increased production of catecholamines and adrenocorticotropic hormone (ACTH) and activation of the renin–angiotensin–aldosterone system. As a direct result of decreased renal blood flow, renin is released from the juxtaglomerular cells, combining with angiotensinogen from the liver resulting in the production of angiotensin I. Angiotensin I, circulating in the blood, is converted to angiotensin II in the lungs. As was discussed in

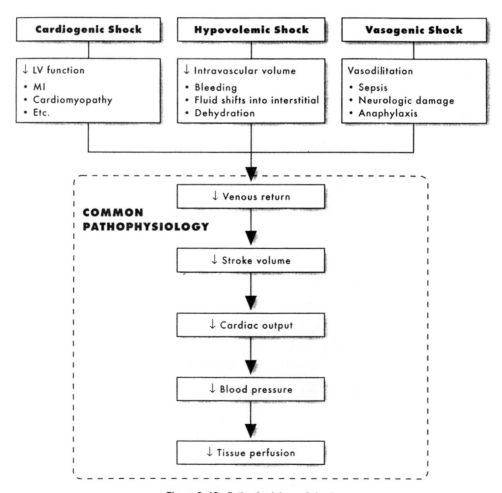

Figure 9–16. Pathophysiology of shock.

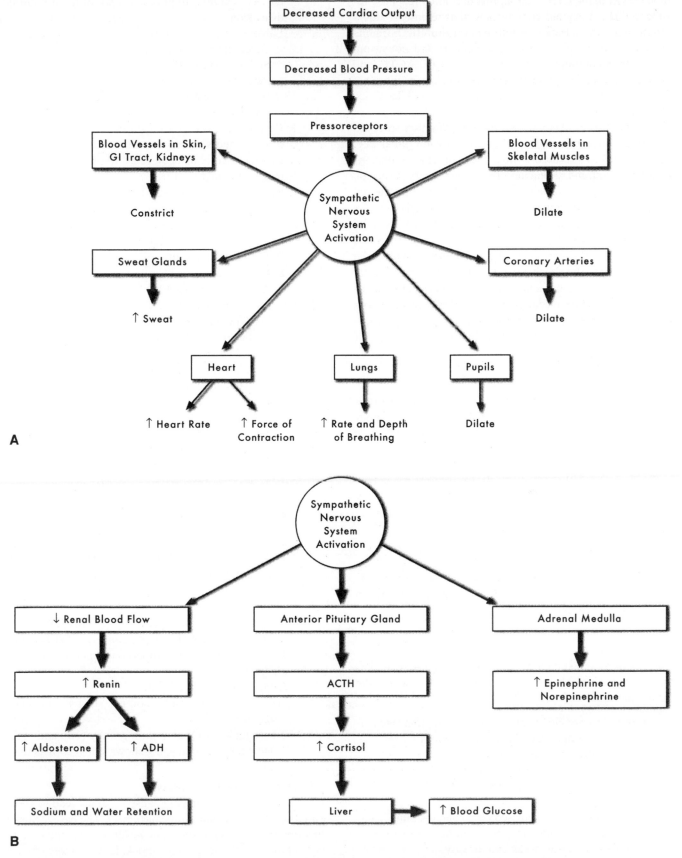

Figure 9–17. Compensatory response to shock. **(A)** Neural compensation. **(B)** Hormonal compensation.

more detail in the CHF section, this hormonal response results in direct vasoconstriction, as well as release of aldosterone from the adrenal cortex and antidiuretic hormone (ADH) from the pituitary gland. Sodium and potassium retention, in conjunction with increased ADH, ACTH, and circulating catecholamines, effectively increases intravascular volume, heart rate, and blood pressure, and decreases urine output.

Chemical responses during the compensatory stage are related to the respiratory ventilation–perfusion imbalance, which occurs as a result of sympathetic stimulation, redistribution of blood, and resultant decreased pulmonary perfusion. A respiratory alkalosis ensues, adversely affecting the patient's level of consciousness, restlessness, and agitation.

These compensatory mechanisms are effective for finite periods of time, which may vary depending on the individual and presence of comorbidities. The younger and healthier the patients prior to the shock episode, the more likely they are to survive a prolonged episode of shock. In the absence of vascular volume replacement, these intrinsic vasopressors eventually fail as a compensatory mechanism, and the patient enters the progressive, and finally refractory, stages of shock, usually resulting in death.

Progressive Stage

The progressive stage is characterized by end organ failure due to cellular damage from prolonged compensatory changes. The compensatory changes, which were effective in supporting blood pressure and therefore tissue perfusion, are no longer effective and severe hypoperfusion ensues. Lack of oxygen and nutrients results in multiple organ failure, typically beginning with gastrointestinal and renal failure, followed by cardiac failure and loss of liver and cerebral function.

Refractory Stage

The refractory stage, as its name implies, is the irreversible stage of shock. At this stage cell death has progressed to such a point as to be irreparable, and death is imminent.

Clinical Presentation

Clinical signs and symptoms vary depending on the underlying cause of shock and the stage of shock in which the patient presents.

- *Initial stage:* No visible signs and symptoms are evident from ongoing cellular changes in this stage.
- *Compensatory stage*
  Consciousness: restless, agitated, confused
  Blood pressure: normal or slightly low
  Heart rate: increased
  Respiratory rate: increased (>20 breaths/min)
  Skin: cool, clammy, may be cyanotic
  Peripheral pulses: weak and thready
  Urine output: concentrated and scant (<30 mL/h)

Bowel sounds: hypoactive, possible abdominal distension
  Labs:
    Glucose: increased
    Sodium: increased
    PaO_2: decreased
    $PaCO_2$: decreased
    pH: increased
- *Progressive stage*
  Consciousness: unresponsive to verbal stimuli
  Blood pressure: inadequate (<90 mm Hg)
  Heart rate: increased
  Respiratory rate: increased, shallow
  Skin: cold, cyanotic, mottled
  Peripheral pulses: weak and thready, may be absent
  Urine output: scant (<20 mL/h)
  Bowel sounds: absent
  Labs:
    Amylase: increased
    Lipase: increased
    SGPT/SGOT: increased
    Lactate dehydrogenase: increased
    CPK: increased
    Creatinine: increased
    Blood urea nitrogen: increased
    PaO_2: increased
    $PaCO_2$: increased
    pH: decreased
    HCO_3: decreased

Diagnostic Tests

- *Cardiogenic*
  ECG: tachycardia
  Pulmonary arterial pressure: PAD/PCWP high (>12 mm Hg), RAP high (>8 mm Hg)
  Echocardiogram: ventricular wall motion abnormalities, cardiac tamponade, ventricular rupture
- *Hypovolemic*
  Pulmonary arterial pressure: PAD/PCWP low (<8 mm Hg), RAP low (<5 mm Hg), RVEDVI low
  Ultrasound: groin or retroperitoneal hemorrhage
- *Distributive*
  Septic: positive blood cultures
  Anaphylactic: arterial blood gas shows inadequate oxygenation
  Neurogenic: computed tomography scan and magnetic resonance imaging shows spinal cord damage

Principles of Management for Shock

Differences in the underlying cause of shock lead to some variation in the principles of management. The basic goals of therapy for all forms of shock, however, include the need to correct the underlying cause of shock, improvement of oxygenation, and restoration of adequate tissue perfusion.

Correction of the Underlying Cause of Shock

- *Cardiogenic:* Remove coronary obstruction, if present, and restore blood flow.
- *Hypovolemic:* Identify source and stop bleeding if possible; correct fluid shunting or third spacing with electrolyte management.
- *Distributive*
  - *Anaphylactic:* Intubate for oxygenation and treat the underlying allergic reaction using antidote or steroid therapy.
  - *Septic:* Antibiotic therapy and removal of infected tissue (e.g., bowel) or device (e.g., central arterial or venous line).
  - *Neurogenic:* Severing of the cord may be irreversible; however, intubation provides respiratory support while the underlying cause is identified.

Improve Oxygenation

- Assess for patent airway and intubate if necessary.
- Administer oxygen at 100% or as necessary until PaO_2 is adequate (>60 to 70 mm Hg).

Restore Adequate Tissue Perfusion

- Administer fluid volume expanders (normal saline, lactated Ringer's solution, or plasmanate) in large rapid boluses. Type and cross-match for blood type and administer blood as necessary for hypovolemic shock.
- Initiate vasoactive drug therapy.

Hypertension

Hypertension is typically a chronic disease of blood pressure elevation that is often masked, especially in the early years of onset, by lack of warning signs or symptoms. Hypertensive crisis is an acute episode or exacerbation, occurring infrequently in a small percentage of hypertensive patients and characterized by the pivotal effect the particular episode and its treatment may have on the patient's long-term outcome. In most cases, the numerical or absolute value of the arterial blood pressure is less important than its impact on the individual's underlying risk of target organ damage, specifically cerebrovascular, coronary, and renal disease.

Etiology, Risk Factors, and Pathophysiology

Although a number of clinical syndromes commonly are associated with hypertension and many underlying etiologies may contribute to the progression of hypertensive disease, the pathophysiology of hypertension is similar regardless of the underlying disease entity.

An acute hypertensive crisis begins with elevation of the systolic or diastolic blood pressure causing a threat, direct or indirect, to an organ or body system. Acute, severe increases in pressure may cause serious, life-threatening cerebrovascular and cardiovascular compromise. Prolonged hypoperfusion of an organ system leads to ischemia, necrosis, and organ system failure.

Classification

Because of the increased risk of such events in all hypertensive patients, morbidity and mortality directly related to hypertension is high, and long-term, consistent therapy in all stages of hypertension is necessary.

- *Benign hypertension:* Benign hypertension is characterized by slightly elevated blood pressure (140 to 150 systolic/90 diastolic, in adults) for long periods of time, with little if any end organ damage. Benign hypertension does not tend to cause acute problems or complications, unless other comorbid conditions, such as atherosclerotic disease, are present. The pressure does not typically exacerbate or precipitate an acute emergent event (generally not greater than 140 to 150 systolic/90 diastolic, in adults).
- *Accelerated hypertension:* Often used interchangeably with malignant hypertension, the stage known as accelerated hypertension is generally considered a precursor to malignant hypertension, and is characterized by an increase in the basal blood pressure.
- *Malignant hypertension:* Hypertension typically is a chronic disease in which elevation in blood pressure occurs slowly, over a period of several years. Because of its gradual onset, the body adapts to increased pressures in the vascular bed and the patient frequently is asymptomatic for years, eventually able to tolerate pressures of up to 200/120 mm Hg without experiencing significant symptoms or clinical events. This type of presentation often is identified "accidentally," secondary to hospitalization for another problem. Generally patients with malignant hypertension are at risk for significant end organ damage because of the severity of high pressure in the vascular bed and inability of the circulatory system to further adapt or compensate in the event of additional stressors.
- *Hypertensive crisis:* Hypertensive crisis is characterized by a severe elevation in blood pressure, relative to the individual's baseline blood pressure, which causes risk of end-organ damage and poor long-term outcome due to permanent organ system damage if the immediate episode is not treated quickly and aggressively.
- *Special populations:* In pregnant women and in children a less severe elevation in blood pressure may result in significant end-organ damage and is therefore considered to be a "hypertensive crisis" at values much lower than would be expected to be problematic in the average adult. The absolute value of the blood pressure varies significantly depending on the

situation and the individual involved. For example, preeclampsia, considered to be a hypertensive crisis in pregnancy, may occur at pressures as low as 130 to 160/100 mm Hg.

Clinical Presentation

Diagnosis of hypertensive crisis is not based on the absolute value of the blood pressure, but rather on the following combined criteria:

- Rapidity of the rise of the blood pressure
- Duration of prior hypertension
- Clinical determination of the immediate threat to vital organ function
- Headache
- Blurred vision
- Nosebleed
- Dizziness or vertigo
- Transient ischemic attack
- Diminished peripheral pulses or bruits
- Carotid or abdominal bruit
- Heart sounds with S_3 and/or S_4
- Systolic and/or diastolic murmurs
- Gastrointestinal bleeding
- Pulmonary edema
- Shortness of breath
- Fatigue
- Malaise
- Weakness
- Nausea and vomiting
- Hematuria
- Dysuria
- Fundoscopic findings: arteriovenous thickening, arteriolar narrowing, hemorrhage, papilledema, or exudates

Diagnostic Tests

- *Chest x-ray:* Myocardial hypertrophy, pulmonary infiltrates
- *Computed tomography:* Arteriolar narrowing and arteriovenous thickening
- Specific tests to target organ damage
  - Renal angiography
  - Coronary angiography
  - Carotid/cerebral angiography
- *Magnetic resonance imaging:* Cerebral vascular malperfusion

Principles of Management for Hypertension

Management of the patient with acute exacerbation of hypertension, or hypertensive crisis, revolves around three primary objectives: reduction of arterial pressure, evaluation and treatment of target organ damage, and preparation and planning for continuous and consistent outpatient follow-up.

Reduction of Arterial Pressure

Ascertain correct arterial blood pressure. Verify arterial blood pressure, being sure to ascertain bilateral measurements with the correct cuff size if using sphygmomanometry, as well as orthostatic pressures if possible (lying and sitting up, if standing is not possible). Each measurement should be 2 minutes apart and both right and left measurements should be documented. If bilateral measurements are greater than 10 mm Hg different, the higher reading should be used to gauge therapy. In most acute situations, priority should be given to establishing a stable arterial access site for direct, invasive monitoring of blood pressure.

Initiate pharmacologic intervention. For acute arterial pressure, pharmacologic intervention is the fastest, most effective means of reducing arterial blood pressure. A number of agents are used in the acute setting for management of hypertensive crisis (Table 9–14). Aggressiveness of pharmacologic intervention should be based on the severity of blood pressure elevation (immediate risk of stroke), the immediate risk of irreversible target organ damage (renal and hepatic function related to drug metabolism and clearance also should be considered), and any confounding conditions or risk factors which are present (for example, the fetus in preeclampsia). In general, acute severe (accelerated malignant/stage 3 and 4) hypertension should be treated as quickly and aggressively as can be tolerated by the patient in order to pre-

TABLE 9–14. COMMON DRUGS USED TO MANAGE ACUTE HYPERTENSIVE EPISODES

Nitroprusside	• Dilates arterioles and veins. • Administer IV at 0.5 to 10.0 mg/kg/min (mix in normal saline only; 100 mg in 500 mL). Cover bottle with foil to avoid light exposure. • Titrate up to desired blood pressure, recognizing that the effect will be evident within 1 minute of change in dose.
Nicardipine	• Calcium channel blocker • Administer 5 mg/h initially, titrate 2.5 mg/h at 5- to 15-min intervals to a maximum dose of 15 mg/h.
Nitroglycerin	• Dilates veins more than arterioles. • Administer IV at a rate of 5 to 100 μg/min. Mix 100 mg in 100 mL NS or D_5 IV.
Diazoxide	• Dilates arteriolar tone only. • No individual titration necessary. • Administer dose of 50 to 150 mg rapidly. Effect noted in 1 to 5 minutes. Repeat same dose in 10 minutes if no effect; total dose not to exceed 600 mg/d. • Do NOT use MI or aortic dissection suspected (diazoxide is a positive inotrope).
Enalapril	• An ACE inhibitor. • Administer IV at a rate of 5 mg/min.
Labetalol	• Beta-receptor agonist (beta-blocker). • Particularly indicated in patients with suspected MI or angina. • Administer 5 mg bolus over 5 minutes and repeat three times. IV drip may then be started.

vent the immediate risk of hypertensive encephalopathy, dissecting aortic aneurysm, MI, or intracranial hemorrhage. Maintenance of cerebral perfusion pressure is imperative during treatment, and overly aggressive pharmacologic management poses the threat of cerebrovascular compromise due to a sudden drop in arterial pressure and inability of the autoregulatory mechanism to adjust. Other organ systems dependent on higher pressure for perfusion include the renal and coronary systems. A sudden, severe drop in systemic arterial pressure may result in ischemic episodes or acute renal failure.

For nonacute arterial pressure, dietary alteration and relaxation or biofeedback techniques may be used in addition to pharmacologic measures to reduce the morbidity and mortality of hypertension. Although these measures are most effective when employed long term as part of a cohesive outpatient follow-up program, initiating these strategies in the acute setting may help to emphasize their importance.

Evaluation and Treatment of Target Organ Disease

Concomitant to initiation of pharmacologic intervention, the assessment and prevention of target organ disease is important to avoid irreversible damage. Target organs typically at risk include the brain, heart, kidneys, and eyes. Strategies to prevent damage to these organ systems during hypertensive crisis include the following.

- *Brain:* Reduce diastolic pressure by one-third (not to go below 95 mm Hg) using aggressive pharmacologic measures (see Table 9–14).
- *Heart:* Reduce diastolic and systolic pressure by one-third; administer combination therapy if possible (vasodilator and beta-blocker) or ACE inhibitor for afterload reduction; monitor for ischemic changes on ECG.
- *Kidneys:* Reduce systolic and diastolic blood pressure using pharmacologic measures; monitor serum creatinine and urine specific gravity as well as proteinuria and hematuria; for patients with severe existing renal impairment, use of ACE inhibitors may exacerbate their renal compromise and is therefore contraindicated in patients with bilateral renal artery stenosis; administer diuretics to maintain serum sodium and adequate diuresis.
- *Eyes:* Reduce systolic and diastolic blood pressure; observe retina for evidence of hemorrhage, exudate, or papilledema; instruct the patient with blurring of vision regarding his or her environment, especially location of the call bell.

Patient Education on Lifestyle Modification and Follow-Up

Following control of hypertension in the acute phase, patient education should be initiated regarding the serious and chronic nature of the disease. Often, the clinician may have an opportunity in the acute stage to make an impact regarding the seriousness of uncontrolled hypertension and its po-

---

AT THE BEDSIDE
▶ *Thinking Critically*

You are taking care of a patient, 4 days post anterior MI, who just transferred into the ICU from an intermediate floor with severe shortness of breath. Your initial assessment reveals the following:

HR	128 beats/min
BP	110/82
RR	36 breaths/min
T	37.6°C, orally
Lung sounds	Coarse, bilateral rales in lower lobes, poor respiratory effort
Heart sounds	S_1, S_2, S_3
Skin	Flushed, diaphoretic, 12 pedal edema (Doppler pulses)
ECG	NSR, with prolonged ventricular repolarization (tall QRS complex)

What is your initial intervention? What is the most likely underlying cause for this patient's respiratory compromise? Management of this condition would most likely include what interventions?

---

tentially debilitating effects. Prior to beginning the educational process, assessment should include:

1. Family history of hypertension, cardiovascular disease, coronary artery disease, stroke, diabetes mellitus, and hyperlipidemia.
2. Lifestyle history including weight gain, exercise, and smoking habits.
3. Dietary patterns including high sodium, alcohol, and dietary fat intake or low potassium intake.
4. Knowledge of hypertension and impact of previous medical therapy for hypertension (compliance, side effects, results, or efficacy).

SELECTED BIBLIOGRAPHY

General Cardiovascular

Andreoli KG, Zipes DP, Wallace AG, et al: *Comprehensive Cardiac Care*, 6th ed. St. Louis, MO: CV Mosby; 1987.

Baas LS: *Essentials of Cardiovascular Nursing*. Gaithersburg, MD: Aspen; 1991.

Wingate S. *Cardiac Nursing: A Clinical Management and Patient Care Resource*. Gaithersburg, MD: Aspen; 1991.

Woods SL, Froelicher ESS, Motzer SA: *Cardiac Nursing*, 4th ed. Philadelphia: Lippincott Williams & Wilkins; 2000.

Coronary Angiography

Tilkian AG, Daily EK: *Cardiovascular Procedures: Diagnostic Techniques and Therapeutic Procedures*. St. Louis, MO: CV Mosby; 1986.

Zorb SL: *Cardiovascular Diagnostic Testing: A Nursing Guide.* Gaithersburg, MD: Aspen; 1991.

Coronary Revascularization

Finkelmeier BA: *Cardiothoracic Surgical Nursing,* 2nd ed. Philadelphia: Lippincott Williams & Wilkins; 2000.

Osguthorpe SG, Tidwell SL, Ryan WJ, et al: Evaluation of the patient having cardiac surgery in the post operative rewarming period. *Heart Lung* 1990;19:570–574.

Seifert, PC: *Cardiac Surgery.* St. Louis, MO: Mosby-Year Book; 1994.

Acute Ischemic Heart Disease

Adams JE, Miracle VA: Cardiac biomarkers: Past, present and future. *Am J Crit Care* 1998;7:418–423.

Califf RM, Mark DB, Wagner GS (eds): *Acute Coronary Care,* 2nd ed. St. Louis, MO: Mosby; 1995, pp. 525–541.

Doering LV: Pathophysiology of acute coronary syndromes leading to acute myocardial infarction. *J Cardiovasc Nurs* 1999;13:1–20.

Fuster V, Dyken ML, Vokonas PS, Hennekens C: Aspirin as a therapeutic agent in cardiovascular disease. *Circulation* 1993;87:659–675.

Murphey MJ, Berding CB: Use of measurements of myoglobin and cardiac troponins in the diagnosis of acute myocardial infarction. *Crit Care Nurse* 1999;19:58–65.

Pasternak R, Braunwald E, Sobel B: Acute myocardial infarction. In Braunwald E (ed): *Heart Disease. A Textbook of Cardiovascular Medicine.* Philadelphia: WB Saunders; 1992, pp. 1200–1291.

Congestive Heart Failure

Albert NM: Cardiac resynchronization therapy through biventricular pacing in patients with heart failure and ventricular dyssynchrony. *Crit Care Nurse* 2003;(suppl):2–16.

English MA: Advanced concepts in heart failure. *Crit Care Nurs Q* 1995;18(1):56–64.

Fara-Erny A. Heart failure: Challenges and outcomes. *J Cardiovasc Nurs* 2000;14(4):v–vii.

Lindpainter K, Ganten D: The cardiac renin-angiotensin system: An appraisal of present experimental and clinical evidence. *Circulation* 1991;68:905–921.

McCullough PA, Joseph K, Mathur VS: Diagnostic and therapeutic utility of B-type natriuretic peptide in patients with renal insufficiency and decompensated heart failure. *Rev Cardiovasc Med* 2003;4(suppl 7):S3–S12.

Packer M: The neurohormonal hypothesis: A theory to explain the mechanism of disease progression in heart failure. *J Am Coll Cardiol* 1992;20:248–254.

Smith T, Braunwald E, Kelly R: The management of heart failure. In Braunwald E (ed): *Heart Disease. A Textbook of Cardiovascular Medicine.* Philadelphia: WB Saunders; 1992, pp. 464–519.

Whitman G (ed): Management of chronic heart failure. *Crit Care Nurs Clin North Am* 1993;5(4).

Shock

Barry WL, Sarembock IJ: Cardiogenic shock: Therapy and prevention. *Clin Cardiol* 1998;21:72–80.

Moscucci M, Bates ER: Cardiogenic shock. *Cardiol Clin* 1995;13:391–406.

Rice V: *Shock, A Clinical Syndrome,* 2nd ed, Parts 1–4. Aliso Viejo, CA: AACN; 1997.

Hypertension

Johannsen JM: Update: Guidelines for treating hypertension. *Am J Nurs* 1993;March:42–49.

Nolan C, Linas S: Accelerated and malignant hypertension. In Schrier R, Gottschalk CW (eds): *Diseases of the Kidney,* 4th ed. Boston: Little Brown; 1988, pp. 1703–1781.

Evidenced-Based Practice Guidelines

Antman EM, Anbe DT, Armstrong PW, et al: ACC/AHA Guidelines for the management of patients with ST-elevation myocardial infarction–Executive summary: A report of the American College of Cardiology/American Heart Association Task Force on Guidelines (Writing Committee to Revise the 1999 Guidelines for the Management of Patients With Acute Myocardial Infarction). ACC/AHA Practice Guideline. *Circulation* 2004;110:588–636.

Braunwald E, Mark D, Jones R, et al: *Unstable Angina: Diagnosis and Management.* Clinical Practice Guideline No. 10. AHCPR Publication number 94-0602. Rockville, MD: Agency for Health Care Policy and Research, Public Health Service, U.S. Department of Health and Human Services; May 1994.

Casey P: Acute coronary syndromes. In Chulay M, Wingate A (eds): *Care of the Cardiovascular Patient Series.* Aliso Viejo, CA: AACN; 2002.

Kirklin JW, Akins CW, Blackstone EH, et al: ACC/AHA guidelines and indications for coronary artery bypass graft surgery. A report of the American College of Cardiology/American Heart Association Task Force on Assessment of Diagnostic and Therapeutic Cardiovascular Procedures (Subcommittee on Coronary Artery Bypass Graft Surgery). *Circulation* 1991;83:1125–1173.

Konstam M, Dracup K, Baker D, et al: *Heart Failure: Evaluation and Care of Patients With Left-Ventricular Systolic Dysfunction.* Clinical Practice Guideline No. 11. AHCPR Publication number 94-0612. Rockville, MD: Agency for Health Care Policy and Research, Public Health Service, U.S. Department of Health and Human Services; June 1994.

National Institutes of Health: *The Fifth Report of the Joint National Committee on Detection, Evaluation, and Treatment of High Blood Pressure* [NIH Publication No. 93-1088]. Bethesda, MD: NIH; January 1993.

Marianne Chulay

▶ Knowledge Competencies

1. Identify various radiologic and pulmonary anatomic
   features relevant to interpretation of chest x-rays.
2. Describe different systems and principles of
   management for chest tubes.
3. Describe the etiology, pathophysiology, clinical
   presentation, patient needs, and principles of
   management of acute respiratory failure (ARF).

4. Compare and contrast the pathophysiology, clinical
   presentation, patient needs, and management
   approaches for common diseases leading to ARF:
   • Acute respiratory distress syndrome (ARDS)
   • ARF in the chronic obstructive pulmonary disease
     patient (asthma, emphysema, bronchitis)
   • Pulmonary embolism

SPECIAL ASSESSMENT TECHNIQUES, DIAGNOSTIC TESTS, AND MONITORING SYSTEMS

Chest X-Rays

Chest radiography is an important tool in respiratory assessment, providing visualization of the heart and lungs. Chest x-rays are a complement to bedside assessment. Critical care nurses need to know basic radiographic concepts and how to optimize portable chest x-ray technique, and need to learn a systematic way for viewing a chest x-ray film.

Chest x-rays are obtained as part of routine screening procedures, when respiratory disease is suspected, to evaluate the status of respiratory abnormalities (e.g., pneumothorax, pleural effusion, tumors), to confirm proper invasive tube placement (i.e., endotracheal, tracheostomy, or chest tubes, and pulmonary artery catheters), or following traumatic chest injury.

Basic Concepts

An x-ray is a form of radiant energy, and a radiographic image is made by x-ray machines. Only a few rays are absorbed by air as beams pass through the atmosphere, whereas all rays are absorbed by metal as the beams attempt to pass through a sheet of metal. When nothing but air lies between the film cassette and the x-ray source, the radiographic image is blackness or radiolucency. If density increases, more beams are absorbed between the film cassette and the x-ray source, and the radiographic image is whiteness or radiopacity. As the x-ray beam passes through the patient, the denser tissues absorb more of the beam, and the less dense tissues absorb less of the beam.

The lungs are primarily sacs of air or gas, so normal lungs look black on chest films. Conversely, the skeletal thorax appears white, because bone is very dense and absorbs the most x-rays (Table 10–1). The heart and mediastinum appear gray because those structures are made up of mostly water. Breast tissue is made up of mostly fat and it appears whitish-gray.

Basic Views of the Chest

The most common method of obtaining a chest x-ray is the posterior-anterior (PA) view. PA chest x-rays are typically done in the radiology department with the machine about 6 feet away from the x-ray film cassette and the patient standing with the anterior chest wall against the x-ray plate and the posterior chest wall toward the x-ray machine. The

TABLE 10–1. BASIC X-RAY DENSITIES

Radiolucent (black)
Gas, air (dark or black)
• Lungs, trachea, bronchi, alveoli
Water (dark or gray)
• Heart, muscle, blood, blood vessels, diaphragm, spleen, liver
Fat (lighter or whitish-gray)
• Breasts, marrow, hilar streaking

Radiopaque (white)
Metal, bone (lightest or white)
• Ribs, scapulae, vertebrae
• Bullets, coins, teeth, ECG electrodes

patient is told to take a deep breath and hold it as the x-ray beam is delivered through the posterior chest wall to the x-ray film cassette. The PA view results in a very accurate, sharp picture of the chest.

Critically ill patients are rarely able to tolerate the positioning requirements of a PA chest x-ray. Most chest x-rays in critical care are obtained with an anterior-posterior (AP) view with the patient supine in bed, with or without back rest elevation. With portable AP chest films, the film cassette is placed behind the patient and the x-ray beam is delivered through the anterior chest to the x-ray film. The x-ray machine is only 3 feet away from the patient, which results in greater distortion of chest images, making the AP chest x-ray less accurate than the PA method. Of particular concern is that the heart size is enlarged on an AP film. When viewing chest x-rays, it is important to know whether a PA or AP view was used to avoid misinterpretation of heart size as cardiomegaly.

Distortions can be minimized by placing the patient in a high Fowler's position, or as erect as possible, with the thorax symmetrically placed on the x-ray film cassette. Explain the procedure to the patient and the need to avoid movement. All unnecessary objects lying on the anterior chest (such as ventilator tubing, safety pins, jewelry, ECG wires, nasogastric tubes, etc.) should be removed if possible. If the patient is unconscious, taping the forehead in a neutral position may be necessary, especially in the high Fowler's position to avoid mispositioning of the head. All caregivers assisting with the chest x-ray need to protect themselves from radiation exposure by positioning themselves behind the x-ray machine or by using lead aprons covering the neck, chest, and abdomen.

Other chest x-ray views include: (1) lateral views to identify normal and abnormal structures behind the heart, along the spine, and at the base of the lung; (2) oblique views to localize lesions without interference from the bony thorax or to get a better picture of the trachea, carina, heart, and great vessels; (3) lordotic views to better visualize the apical and middle regions of the lung and to differentiate anterior from posterior lesions; and (4) lateral decubitus (cross-table) views, done with the patient supine or side-lying, to assess for air–fluid levels or free-flowing pleural fluid.

Systematic Approach to Chest X-Ray Interpretation

A systematic approach should be used when analyzing a chest x-ray film. It is important to first make sure that the film has been properly labeled (correct name and medical record number) and to identify the right and wrong sides before placing the film on the view box. If previous films are available, place them next to the new films for comparison. View the chest x-ray from the lateral borders, moving to the medial aspects of the thorax and asking the series of questions found in Table 10–2.

Begin the chest x-ray analysis by comparing the right side to the left side using the following sequence (Figures 10–1 and 10–2): (1) soft tissues—neck, shoulders, breasts, and subcutaneous fat; (2) trachea—the column of radiolucency readily visible above the clavicles; (3) bony thorax—note size, shape, and symmetry; (4) intercostal spaces (ICS)—note width and angle; (5) diaphragm—dome-shaped with distinct margins, right dome 1 to 3 cm higher than left dome; (6) pleural surfaces—visceral and parietal pleura appear like a thin hairlike line along the apices and lateral chest; (7) mediastinum—size varies with age, gender, and size; (8) hila—large pulmonary arteries and veins; and (9) lung fields—largest area of the chest and most radiolucent (Figure 10–3).

Normal Variants and Common Abnormalities

When the soft tissues are examined, the two sides of the lateral chest should be symmetric. A mastectomy makes one lung look more radiolucent than the other due to the absence of fatty tissue. The trachea should be midline, with the carina visible at the level of the aortic knob or second ICS (see Figure 10–2). The most common cause of tracheal deviation is a pneumothorax, which causes a tracheal and mediastinal shift to the area away from the pneumothorax (Table 10–3).

TABLE 10–2. STEPS FOR INTERPRETATION OF A CHEST X-RAY FILM

Step 1
Look at the different densities (black, gray, and white), and answer the question, *"What is air, fluid, tissue, and bone?"*

Step 2
Look at the shape or form of each density, and answer the question, *"What normal anatomic structure is this?"*

Step 3
Look at both right and left sides, and answer the question, *"Are the findings the same on both sides or are there differences (both physiologic and pathophysiologic)?"*

Step 4
Look at all the structures (bones, mediastinum, diaphragm, pleural space, and lung tissue), and answer the question, *"Are there any abnormalities present?"*

Step 5
Look for all tubes, wires, and lines, and answer the question, *"Are the tubes, wires, and lines in the proper place?"*

From: Thelan L, Davie J, Urden L, Lough M: Critical Care Nursing: Diagnosis and Management, 2nd ed. St. Louis, MO: Mosby-Year Book, 1994.

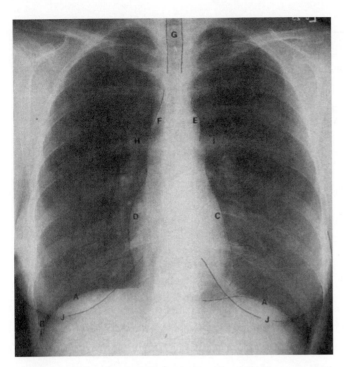

Figure 10–1. Normal chest x-ray. Normal chest x-ray film taken of a 28-year-old woman from a posteroanterior (PA) view. Some anatomic structures can be seen on the x-ray: **(A)** diaphragm; **(B)** costophrenic angle; **(C)** left ventricle; **(D)** right atrium; **(E)** aortic arch (referred to as aortic knob); **(F)** superior vena cava; **(G)** trachea; **(H)** right bronchus (right hilum); **(I)** left bronchus (left hilum); and **(J)** breast shadows.

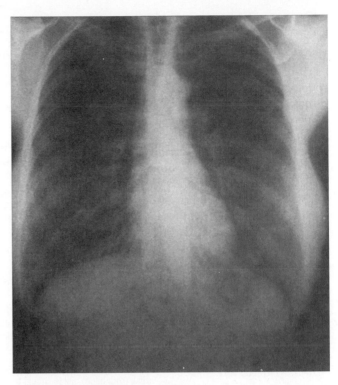

Figure 10–2. Normal chest x-ray. (*From: Sanchez F: Fundamentals of chest x-ray interpretation.* Crit Care Nurse *1986;6:42.*)

Bony thorax inspection reveals general body build. Clavicles should be symmetric and may have an irregular notch or indentation in the inferior medial aspect of the clavicle called a rhomboid fossa, a normal variant. Deformities of the thorax can be detected, such as scoliosis, funnel chest, or pigeon chest. Decreases in the density (less white) of the spine, ribs, and other bones may indicate loss of calcium from the bones due to osteoporosis or long-term steroid dependency. Careful examination of the ICSs and rib angles may indicate pathology. Patients with chronic obstructive pulmonary disease (COPD) have widened ICS and the angle of the ribs to the spine increases to 90° instead of the normal 45° angle because of severe hyperinflation. Conversely, narrowed ICS may be visible in cystic fibrosis patients with severe interstitial fibrosis. Rib fractures, if present, are commonly visible along the lateral borders of the rib cage.

Elevation of the diaphragm can be a result of abdominal distention, phrenic nerve paralysis, or lung collapse. Depression or flattening of the diaphragm can occur when 11 or 12 ribs show on a chest x-ray as a result of COPD. Normal costophrenic angles can be seen where the tapered edges of the diaphragm and the chest wall meet. Because breast tissue can obscure the angles in women, these angles are more distinct in men. Obliteration or "blunting" of the costophrenic angle can occur with pleural effusion or atelectasis.

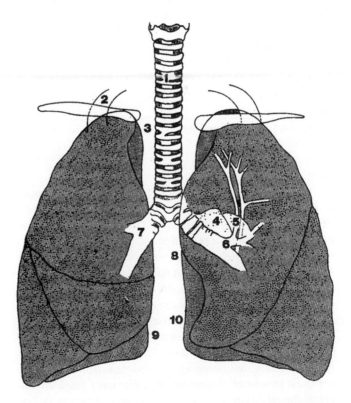

Figure 10–3. Mediastinal structures visible on a chest x-ray. **(1)** Trachea, **(2)** first rib, **(3)** superior vena cava, **(4)** aortic knob, (5) pulmonary artery, **(6)** left main bronchus, **(7)** right main bronchus, **(8)** left atrium, **(9)** right atrium, and **(10)** left ventricle. (*From: Sanchez F: Fundamentals of chest x-ray interpretation.* Crit Care Nurse *1986;6[5]:53.*)

TABLE 10–3. CHEST X-RAY FINDINGS

Assessed Area	Usual Adult Findings	Remarks
Trachea	Midline, translucent, tubelike structure found in the anterior mediastinal cavity	Deviation from the midline suggests tension, pneumothorax, atelectasis, pleural effusion, mass, or collapsed lung
Clavicles	Present in upper thorax and are equally distant from sternum	Malalignment or break indicates fracture
Ribs	Thoracic cavity encasement	Widening of intercostal spaces indicates emphysema; malalignment or break indicates fractured sternum or ribs
Mediastinum	Shadowy-appearing space between the lungs that widens at the hilum	Deviation to either side may indicate pleural effusion, fibrosis, or collapsed lung
Heart	Solid-appearing structure with clear edges visible in the left anterior mediastinal cavity; heart should be less than one-half the width of the chest wall on a posteroanterior film	Shift may indicate atelectasis or tension pneumothorax; if heart is greater than one-half the chest wall width, congestive heart failure or pericardial fluid may be present
Carina	The lowest tracheal cartilage at which the bronchi bifurcate	If the end of the endotracheal tube is seen 3 cm above the carina, it is in the correct position
Main-stem bronchus	The translucent, tubelike structure visible to approximately 2.5 cm from hilum	Densities may indicate bronchogenic cyst
Hilum	Small, white, bilateral densities present where the bronchi join the lungs; left hilum should be 2 to 3 cm higher than the right hilum	A shift to either side indicates atelectasis; accentuated shadows may indicate emphysema or pulmonary abscess
Bronchi (other than main stem)	Not usually visible	If visible, may indicate bronchial pneumonia
Lung fields	Usually not completely visible except as fine white areas from hilum; fields should be clear as normal lung tissue is radiolucent; normal "lung markings" should be present to the periphery	If visible, may indicate atelectasis; patchy densities may be signs of resolving pneumonia, silicosis, or fibrosis; nasogastric tubes, pulmonary artery catheters, and chest tubes will appear as shadows and their positions should be noted
Diaphragm	Rounded structures visible at the bottom of the lung fields; right side is 1 to 2 cm higher than the left; the costophrenic angles should be clear and sharp	An elevated diaphragm may indicate pneumonia, pleurisy, acute bronchitis, or atelectasis; a flattened diaphragm suggests chronic obstructive pulmonary disease; unilateral elevation indicates a pneumothorax or pulmonary infection; the presence of scarring or fluid causes blunting of costophrenic angles; 300 to 500 mL of pleural fluid must be present before blunting is seen

From: Talbot I, Meyers-Marquardt M: Pocket Guide to Critical Assessment. *St. Louis, MO: CV Mosby, 1990.*

Identification of a pleural space on a chest x-ray is an abnormal finding. The pleural space is not visible unless air (pneumothorax) or fluid (pleural effusion) enters it. These findings commonly are seen in the ICU population.

Two terms often heard regarding the mediastinum are *shifting* and *widening*. Mediastinal structures, usually the trachea, bronchi, and heart, can shift with atelectasis, with the shift directed toward the alveolar collapse. Pneumothorax also can shift the mediastinum away from the area of involvement. A widening of the mediastinum can indicate several pathologic conditions, such as cardiomegaly, aneurysms, or aortic disruption. Bleeding into the mediastinum, following chest trauma or cardiac surgery, also may cause widening of the mediastinum.

Heart size can be estimated easily by measuring the cardiothoracic ratio on a PA film. The heart diameter normally is 50% or less of the thoracic diameter to the inside of the ribs on full inspiration. This method for determining normal

heart size cannot be used when viewing AP chest x-rays, the most common type taken of the critically ill.

The lung fields should be assessed for any areas of increased density (whiteness) or increased radiolucency (blackness), which can indicate an abnormality. Density increases when water, pus, or blood accumulates in the lung. Increased radiolucency is caused by increased air in the lungs, as may occur with COPD. A fine line present on the right side of the lung at the sixth rib level (midlung) is a normal finding, representing the horizontal fissure separating the right upper and middle lobes.

Invasive Lines

Chest x-rays are frequently obtained in critical care to confirm proper placement of invasive equipment (endotracheal tubes, central venous and pulmonary artery catheters, intra-aortic balloons, nasogastric tubes, chest tubes). All invasive tubes have radiopaque lines running the length of the tube

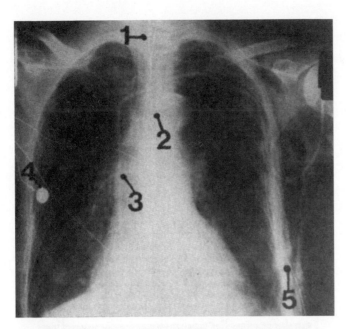

Figure 10–4. Chest x-ray with markers identifying invasive devices. (**1**) Endotracheal tube, (**2**) nasogastric tube, (**3**) pulmonary artery catheter in right pulmonary artery, (**4**) ECG electrode, and (**5**) chest tube. (*From: Sanchez F: Fundamentals of chest x-ray interpretation.* Crit Care Nurse *1986;6[5]:60.*)

that are visible on the x-ray (Figure 10–4). When in the proper position, an endotracheal tube should be 2 to 4 cm above the carina. Look for a thin white line in the trachea and follow it down to the level of the clavicles and measure the space between the end of the tube and the carina. In some patients the tip of the endotracheal tube will be slightly less than 2 cm above the carina to ensure that the inflated balloon is below the vocal cords.

Identify all white lines and follow their paths. The nasogastric tube should run the length of the esophagus with the tip of the tube in the stomach. The stomach can be identified by the radiolucency just under the diaphragm on the left side, which is called the gastric air bubble. Pulmonary artery catheters should be viewed running through the right atrium and right ventricle into the pulmonary artery. These can be difficult to identify at first, but be sure and look at both sides of the hila (right and left pulmonary arteries found on either side of the mediastinum).

Identify all items in the chest, such as temporary or permanent pacing wires, pacing generators, automatic implantable defibrillators, chest tubes, and surgical wires or clips.

Helpful Hints

Chest x-rays should be taken after every attempt to insert central venous catheters to detect the presence of an accidental pneumothorax. A common error is to mistake the scapulae for a pneumothorax, especially on AP views.

Two common abnormal x-ray signs frequently discussed are the silhouette sign and the air bronchogram. For any structure to be visible, the density of its edge must con-

trast with the surrounding density. The loss of contrast is called the silhouette sign. It means that two structures of the same density have come in contact with each other and the borders are lost. For example, the heart is a water density, so if the alveoli near the left heart border fill with fluid, the two densities are the same and there is a loss of contrast and no left heart border. An air bronchogram is air showing through a greater density, such as water. The bronchi are not seen on a normal chest x-ray, except for the main-stem bronchi, because they have thin walls, contain air, and are surrounded by air in the alveoli (two structures of the same density). If water surrounds the bronchi, as in pneumonia and pulmonary edema, then the bronchi filled with air are in contrast to the water density and are visible.

Computed Tomography and Magnetic Resonance Imaging

Computed tomography (CT) and magnetic resonance imaging (MRI) allow for the three-dimensional examination of the chest in situations where two-dimensional chest x-rays are insufficient. CT and MRI are particularly advantageous over chest x-rays to evaluate mediastinal and pleural abnormalities, particularly those with fluid collections. Pleural effusions or empyemas, malpositioned or occluded chest tubes, mediastinal hematomas, and mediastinitis are problems for which CT and MRI are more sensitive than chest x-rays.

The need for transportation to the radiology department and positioning restrictions within the scanning devices pose certain risks to critically ill patients. Of particular concern is the automatic movement of patients during the procedure into and out of the scanning device. Accidental disconnection of invasive devices can easily occur if additional tubing lengths and potential obstructions are not considered. Decreased visualization of patients during the procedures requires vigilant monitoring of cardiovascular and respiratory parameters and devices, as well as establishing a method for conscious patients to alert nearby clinicians in case of difficulties. The strong magnetic field of MRI units may interfere with ventilator performance and necessitate manual ventilation, leading to potential alterations in arterial blood gas values.

MRI testing can be a frightening experience for the patient. Anxiety-related reactions, occurring in up to almost one third of patients, range from mild apprehension to severe anxiety. These reactions can result in cancellation of the test or interference with its results. It is suggested that all patients receive basic information regarding the MRI procedure, including details of the small chamber they will be placed in, the noise and temperature they will experience, and the duration of the procedure. If possible, use of the prone position, some form of relaxation or music tape, and the presence of a family member or friend should be considered. In addition, short-acting anxiolytics should be used for patients who need them.

Pulmonary Angiograms

Pulmonary angiograms are one of the most sensitive tools for diagnosis of pulmonary emboli. Through a catheter advanced into the pulmonary artery, contrast material is injected during rapid filming. Emboli appear as filling defects, or dark circumscribed areas, within the white vascular images of the artery.

The invasive nature of this diagnostic test, coupled with potential reactions to the contrast material, restricts its use to situations where other less invasive tests (e.g., clinical signs or symptoms, ventilation–perfusion scans) are ambiguous.

Chest Tubes

Chest tubes are commonly used in critically ill patients to drain air, blood, or fluid from the pleural spaces (pleural chest tubes) or from the mediastinum (mediastinal tubes). Indications for chest tube insertion are varied (Table 10–4), with no contraindications to chest tube insertion because the need to restore lung function supersedes any potential complications associated with insertion. Pleural tube insertion sites vary based on the type of drainage to be removed (air: second ICS, midclavicular line; fluid: fifth or sixth ICS, midaxillary line). Mediastinal tubes are placed during surgery, exiting from the mediastinum below the xiphoid process.

Following insertion, chest tubes are connected to a closed drainage collection system which uses gravity or suction to restore negative pressure in the pleural space and facilitate drainage of fluids or air (Figure 10–5). Connections to the drainage system must be airtight and secure for proper functioning and to prevent inadvertent entry of air into the pleural space (Figure 10–6). Patency of the system is ensured by avoiding kinking of the drainage tubing, periodic inspection of the tubing for visible clot formation, and gentle squeezing of the tubing between the thumb and index finger.

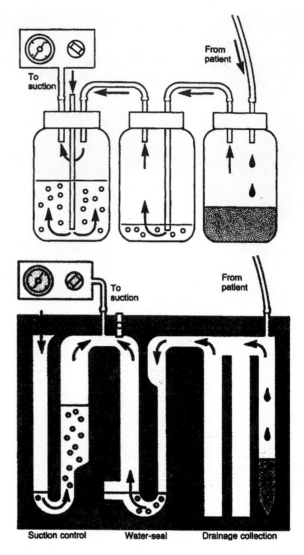

Figure 10–5. Glass bottle (*top*) and disposable drainage systems for chest tubes. (*Reprinted from Luce JM, Tyler ML, Peirson DJ. Intensive Respiratory Care. Philadelphia: WB Saunders; 1984, p. 164, with permission from Elsevier.*)

TABLE 10–4. INDICATIONS FOR CHEST TUBE INSERTION

Pneumothorax
- Open: both chest wall and pleural spaces are penetrated
- Closed: pleural space is penetrated with an intact chest wall, allowing air to enter the pleural space from the lung
- Tension: air leaks into the pleural space through a tear in the lung, with no means to escape the space, leading to lung collapse

Hemothorax

Hemopneumothorax

Thoracostomy

Pyothorax or empyema

Chylothorax

Cholothorax

Hydrothorax

Pleural effusion

Reprinted from: Lawrence D. Performing chest tube placement. In Lynn-McHale DJ, Carlson KK (eds): AACN Procedure Manual for Critical Care, 4th ed. Philadelphia: WB Saunders; 2001, p. 99, with permission from Elsevier.

Removal of the chest tube occurs when restoration of lung expansion and fluid or air removal has been accomplished and the underlying lung abnormality has been resolved or corrected. An occlusive dressing at the chest tube removal site is typically used to prevent introduction of air into the pleural space until the skin has formed a protective seal. Analgesic administration is appropriate prior to removal; discomfort associated with removal is often as much or even greater than during insertion.

PATHOLOGIC CONDITIONS

Acute Respiratory Failure

Each of the case studies below represents a common situation in a critical care unit—respiratory dysfunction. This rapid

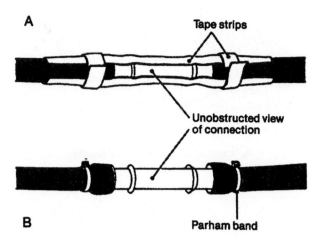

Figure 10–6. Methods for securing connections of chest tube and drainage system. **(A)** Tape. **(B)** Parham bands. (*Reprinted from Kersten LD. Comprehensive Respiratory Nursing: A Decision-Making Approach. Philadelphia: WB Saunders; 1989, p. 783, with permission from Elsevier.*)

onset of respiratory impairment, which is severe enough to cause potential or actual morbidity or mortality if untreated, is termed *acute respiratory failure* (ARF). Although the origin of the respiratory failure may be a medical or surgical problem, the management approaches share similar features.

ARF is a change in respiratory gas exchange (CO_2 and O_2) such that normal cellular function is jeopardized. ARF is defined as a PaO_2 below 60 mm Hg and $PaCO_2$ above 50 mm Hg. Actual PaO_2 and $PaCO_2$ values that define ARF vary, depending on a variety of factors that influence the patient's normal (or baseline) arterial blood gas values. Factors such as age, altitude, chronic cardiopulmonary disease, or metabolic disturbances may alter the "normal" blood gas values for an individual, requiring an adjustment to the classic definition of ARF. For example, if PaO_2 levels in a 75-year-old man living in Denver are normally 56 mm Hg, ARF would not be diagnosed until PaO_2 levels have decreased to 50 mm Hg or less.

Etiology, Risk Factors, and Pathophysiology

Many abnormalities can lead to ARF (Table 10–5). Regardless of the specific underlying cause, the pathophysiology of ARF can be organized into four main components: impaired ventilation, impaired gas exchange, airway obstruction, and ventilation–perfusion abnormalities.

Impaired Ventilation

Conditions that disrupt the muscles of respiration or their neurologic control can impair ventilation and lead to ARF (see Table 10–5). Decreased or absent respiratory muscle movement may be due to fatigue from excessive use, atrophy from disuse, inflammation of nerves, nerve damage (e.g., surgical damage to the vagus nerve during cardiac surgery), neurologic depression, or following administration of neuromuscular blocking agents. Impaired respiratory muscle movement decreases movement of gas into the lungs, result-

ing in alveolar hypoventilation. Inadequate alveolar ventilation causes retention of CO_2 and hypoxemia.

Impaired Gas Exchange

Conditions that damage the alveolar–capillary membrane impair gas exchange. Direct damage to the cells lining the alveoli may be caused by inhalation of toxic substances

---

AT THE BEDSIDE
▶ *Motor Vehicle Accident*

A 22-year-old man was admitted to the surgical ICU following a motor vehicle accident in which he suffered blunt chest trauma, bilateral fractured femurs, and a concussion. During his second day in the unit, his arterial blood gases began deteriorating (decreases in PaO_2, increases in $PaCO_2$), and he required increasing amounts of supplemental oxygen to maintain $PaCO_2$ levels >60 mm Hg. He was dyspneic, restless, and somewhat agitated. He verbalized a fear of impending death.

	Admission	Day 2
Respiration rate	24/min	34/min
Chest x-ray	clear	infiltrates
ABGs	40% FM	100% FM
PaO_2	120 mm Hg	58 mm Hg
$PaCO_2$	33 mm Hg	50 mm Hg
pH	7.42	7.35
HCO_3	24 mEq/L	27 mEq/L

AT THE BEDSIDE
▶ *Postanesthesia*

A woman was admitted to the surgical ICU following thoracic surgery for the removal of a malignant tumor of the right upper lobe. She was intubated and was being manually ventilated by the anesthesiologist with a MRB with 10 L/min of O_2 inflow. A right pleural chest tube was draining minimal amounts of blood, with no evidence of air leaks or obstructions.

The patient was unresponsive to verbal and pain stimulation on admission. No spontaneous respirations were noted after a brief period of disconnection from the MRB. Fifteen minutes after initiation of mechanical ventilation (SIMV of 10 breaths/min, tidal volume of 10 mL/kg, PEEP of 5 cm H_2O, 0.40 FiO_2), ABGs were:

PaO_2	145 mm Hg
$PaCO_2$	41 mm Hg
pH	7.38
HCO_3	24 mEq/L

TABLE 10–5. CAUSES OF ACUTE RESPIRATORY FAILURE IN ADULT

Impaired Ventilation
Spinal cord injury (C4 or higher)
Phrenic nerve damage
Neuromuscular blockade
Guillain–Barré syndrome
CNS depression
   Drug overdoses (narcotics, sedatives, illicit drugs)
   Increased intracranial pressure
   Anesthetic agents
Respiratory muscle fatigue
Impaired Gas Exchange
Pulmonary edema
ARDS
Aspiration pneumonia
Airway Obstruction
Aspiration of foreign body
Thoracic tumors
Asthma
Bronchitis
Pneumonia
Ventilation–Perfusion Abnormalities
Pulmonary embolism
Emphysema

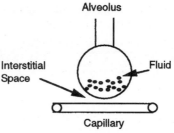

A. Leakage of Fluid into Alveolus

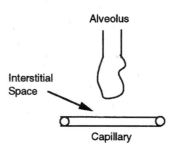

B. Atelectasis

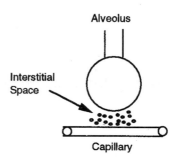

C. Interstitial Edema

Figure 10–7. Pathophysiologic processes in ARF due to impaired gas exchange. **(A)** Increased alveolar membrane permeability. **(B)** Alveolar collapse from decreased surfactant production. **(C)** Increased capillary membrane permeability and interstitial edema.

(gases or gastric contents), leading to two detrimental alveolar changes. The first is an increase in alveolar permeability, increasing the potential for interstitial fluid to leak into the alveoli and cause noncardiac pulmonary edema (Figure 10–7A). The second alveolar change is a decrease in surfactant production by alveolar type II cells, increasing alveolar surface tension, which leads to alveolar collapse (Figure 10–7B).

Another cause of impaired gas exchange occurs when fluid leaks from the intravascular space into the pulmonary interstitial space (Figure 10–7C). The excess fluid increases the distance between the alveolus and the capillary, decreasing the efficiency of the gas exchange process. Interstitial edema also compresses the bronchial airways, which are surrounded by interstitial tissue, causing bronchoconstriction. Capillary leakage may occur when pressures within the cardiovascular system are excessively high (e.g., in heart failure) or when pathologic conditions elsewhere in the body release biochemical substances (e.g., serotonin, endotoxin) that increase capillary permeability.

Airway Obstruction
Conditions that obstruct airways increase resistance to airflow into the lungs, causing alveolar hypoventilation and decreased gas exchange (Figure 10–8). Airway obstructions can be due to conditions that (1) block the inner airway lumen (e.g., excessive secretions or fluid in the airways, inhaled foreign bodies), (2) increase airway wall thickness (e.g., edema or fibrosis) or decrease airway circumference (e.g., bronchoconstriction) as occurs in asthma, or (3) increase peribronchial compression of the airway (e.g., enlarged lymph nodes, interstitial edema, tumors).

Ventilation–Perfusion Abnormalities
Conditions disrupting alveolar ventilation or capillary perfusion lead to an imbalance in ventilation and perfusion. This decreases the efficiency of the respiratory gas exchange

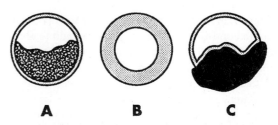

Figure 10–8. Mechanism of airway obstruction. **(A)** Fluid secretions present within airway. **(B)** Intraluminal edema narrowing airway diameter. **(C)** Peribronchial compression of airway.

process. In an effort to keep the ventilation and perfusion ratios balanced, two compensatory changes occur: (1) to avoid wasted alveolar ventilation when capillary perfusion is decreased (e.g., with pulmonary embolism), bronchiolar constriction occurs to limit ventilation to alveoli with poor or absent capillary perfusion (Figure 10–9B); (2) to avoid capillary perfusion of alveoli that are not adequately ventilated (e.g., with atelectasis), arteriole constriction occurs and shunts blood away from hypoventilated alveoli to normally ventilated alveoli (Figure 10–9C). As the number of alveolar–capillary units affected by these compensatory changes increases, gas exchange eventually is affected negatively.

Each of these pathophysiologic changes results in inadequate CO_2 removal, O_2 absorption, or both. The severity of ARF can be further increased when anxiety and fear of

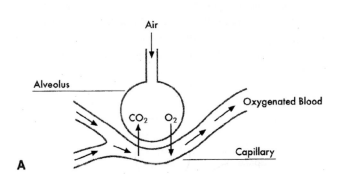

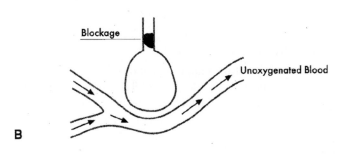

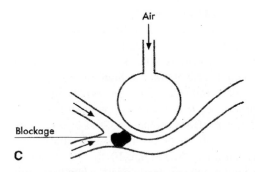

Figure 10–9. Pathophysiologic processes in ARF from ventilation–perfusion abnormalities. **(A)** Normal ventilation and perfusion relationship. **(B)** Decreased ventilation and normal perfusion. **(C)** Normal ventilation and decreased perfusion.

impending death develop, a common consequence of severe dyspnea and hypoxemia. These symptoms increase oxygen demands and the work of breathing, further compromising O_2 availability for crucial organ function and depleting respiratory muscle strength.

Clinical Presentation

Signs and Symptoms

- Hypoxemia (PaO_2 <60 mm Hg)
- Restlessness
- Tachypnea
- Dyspnea
- Tachycardia
- Confusion
- Diaphoresis
- Anxiety
- Hypercarbia ($PaCO_2$ >50 mm Hg)
- Hypertension
- Irritability
- Somnolence (late)
- Cyanosis (late)
- Loss of consciousness (late)
- Pallor or cyanosis of skin
- Use of accessory muscles of respiration
- Abnormal breath sounds (crackles, wheezes)
- Manifestations of primary disease (see description of individual diseases below)

Diagnostic Tests

- Arterial blood gases—PaO_2 <60 mm Hg and $PaCO_2$ >50 mm Hg; or PaO_2 and $PaCO_2$ in abnormal range for that individual
- Tests specific to underlying cause (see description of individual diseases below)

Principles of Management for Acute Respiratory Failure

The management of the patient in ARF revolves around four primary areas: improving oxygenation and ventilation, treating the underlying disease state, reducing anxiety, and preventing and managing complications.

Improving Oxygenation and Ventilation

Most causes of ARF are treatable, with a return of normal respiratory function following resolution of the pathophysiologic condition. Aggressive support of respiratory function is required, though, until there is resolution of the underlying condition.

1. Provide supplemental O_2 to maintain PaO_2 above 60 mm Hg. The use of noninvasive methods for O_2 administration (nasal cannula or face masks) is preferable if acceptable PaO_2 levels can be achieved. Continued hypoxemia despite noninvasive O_2 delivery methods necessitates intubation and mechanical ventilation.

2. Improve ventilation with the administration of bronchodilators, mucolytic agents, and other airway management modalities (chest physiotherapy, suctioning, positioning) as indicated.

3. Intubate and initiate mechanical ventilation if non-invasive methods fail to correct hypoxemia and hypercarbia or if cardiovascular instability develops. The mode of mechanical ventilation, rate, and tidal volume vary depending on the underlying cause of respiratory failure and a variety of clinical factors. Modes of ventilation that decrease the work of breathing (control, assist/control, synchronized intermittent mandatory ventilation [SIMV] with high minute ventilation [MV] rates, pressure support [PS]) are typically used for the first 24 hours because respiratory muscle fatigue is common. Positive end expiratory pressure (PEEP) levels above 5 cm H_2O may be required if Fio_2 levels above 0.6 are needed to eliminate hypoxemia. Closely monitor the cardiovascular status during increases of PEEP, which may decrease venous return and cardiac output. Neuromuscular blockade may be needed initially to prevent ineffective respiratory efforts by the patient and to maximize gas exchange.

4. During suctioning, closely observe for signs and symptoms of hypoxemia (decreases in O_2 saturation; increases in heart rate, respiratory rate, restlessness, diaphoresis, and dysrhythmias). When using a manual resuscitation bag (MRB) for hyperoxygenation, use a MRB that delivers 100% O_2 to prevent cardiopulmonary changes during suctioning, as well as a PEEP valve when ventilator PEEP levels are above 5 cm H_2O. If changes still occur despite these interventions, it may be necessary to keep the patient on the ventilator during hyperoxygenation and suctioning with the use of a closed suction setup or an adaptor for suctioning that is connected to the ventilator tubing. Suctioning should only be performed when clinically indicated, and never on a routine schedule.

5. Prior to intrahospital transport, verify adequacy of ventilatory support equipment to maintain cardiopulmonary stability. Verify that PEEP on the transport equipment is maintained. Some ventilators used for transport do not have the capability to provide more advanced ventilatory modes (e.g., PS, reverse I:E ratio).

Treating the Underlying Disease State

Correction of the underlying cause of the ARF should be done as soon as possible. See specific management approaches later in the chapter for each disease state.

Reducing Anxiety

Maintain a calm, supportive environment to avoid unnecessary escalation of anxiety. Give brief explanations of activities and approaches being done to relieve ARF. Vigilance and presence of health care providers during anxious periods is crucial to avoid panic by patients and visiting family members.

Teach diaphragmatic breathing to slow the rate and increase the depth of respirations. Place one hand on the patient's abdomen. Instruct the patient to inhale deeply, causing the hand on the abdomen to rise. During exhalation, have the patient feel the hand on the belly sink down toward the spine. Explain that the chest should not be moving at all. After a minute or two, ask the patient to place his or her hands on the belly to continue the exercise.

Administer mild doses of anxiolytics (i.e., lorazepam or diazepam) that do not depress respiration.

Preventing and Managing Complications

Ventilator and neuromuscular blockade related; see Chapter 5, Airway and Ventilatory Management, for detailed management strategies.

- *Pulmonary aspiration:* continuous gastric aspiration, ensure proper inflation of endotracheal tube cuff at all times. Refer to additional prevention strategies for ventilator-associated pneumonia listed below.
- *Gastrointestinal (GI) bleeding:* check gastric aspirate for presence of occult blood every 4 to 8 hours. Protect gastric mucosa in high-risk patients with non-alkalinizing gastric protective agents (e.g., sulcralfate).
- *Barotrauma:* avoid unnecessary increases in airway pressures (e.g., "bucking" the ventilator, excessive coughing) and assess for signs and symptoms of pneumothorax, pneumomediastinum, and other barotrauma complications. See Chapter 5, Airway and Ventilatory Management, for additional strategies.

Acute Respiratory Distress Syndrome

The case study of the patient in a motor vehicle accident is typical of a patient who develops ARDS. ARDS is an acute physiologic syndrome characterized by noncardiac pulmonary edema caused by increased alveolar capillary membrane permeability. ARDS is one of the most lethal of the diseases or syndromes that lead to respiratory failure.

Etiology, Risk Factors, and Pathophysiology

Risk factors for the development of ARDS can be categorized into conditions that lead to direct damage to the alveolar–capillary membrane (primary causes) and those that are thought to be mediated by cellular or humoral injury to the capillary endothelial wall (secondary causes) (Table 10–6). Whether primary or secondary causes, the pathologic processes involved in ARDS are characterized by excessive alveolar–capillary membrane permeability, interstitial edema, and diffuse alveolar injury (see Figure 10–8). Direct damage to the alveolar membrane can easily occur when toxic substances are inhaled, such as during fires or chemical spills.

Alveolar and interstitial edema, microatelectasis, and ventilation–perfusion mismatching in ARDS lead to severe

TABLE 10–6. PRIMARY AND SECONDARY CAUSES OF ARDS

Primary Causes (Direct Damage to the Alveolar Membrane)
Aspiration of gastric contents
Pulmonary contusion
Near drowning
Inhalation of smoke or toxic substances
Diffuse pneumonias (viral and bacterial)

Secondary Causes (Mediated by Cellular or Humoral Injury to the Capillary Endothelium)
Systemic sepsis
Hypovolemic shock associated with chest trauma or sepsis
Acute pancreatitis
Fat emboli
Trauma
DIC
Massive blood transfusions

hypoxemia and poor lung compliance ("stiff lungs"). In the setting of trauma and sepsis, this abnormality in microvascular permeability occurs in capillary beds throughout the body. Typically, this multisystem organ dysfunction is not clinically apparent, with clinical manifestations isolated to the respiratory system. When multiple organ dysfunction syndrome does occur, it is seen in ARDS patients who develop bacterial infections and sepsis (see Chapter 11, Multisystem Problems).

The development of a gram-negative pulmonary infection is a frequent sequela of ARDS. The ARDS process disrupts normal macrophage function and increases the risk of infection. Mortality from ARDS is high, frequently occurring several days to weeks after the onset of the syndrome.

Clinical Presentation

Signs and Symptoms

- Dyspnea
- Tachypnea (rates often >40/min)
- Intercostal retractions
- Copious secretions
- Panic, fear of impending death
- Crackles and/or wheezes

Diagnostic Tests

- Chest x-ray shows diffuse, bilateral pulmonary infiltrates without increased cardiac size
- PaO_2/PAO_2 <0.2
- PCWP <18 mm Hg
- Static compliance (tidal volume/[inspiratory plateau pressure PEEP]) <40 mL/cm H_2O

Principles of Management for ARDS

Much of the management of ARDS relies on supportive care and the prevention of complications. To date, interventions to limit the disease progression or reverse the underlying structural defects are not known.

Improving Oxygenation and Ventilation

Interventions specific to ARDS to improve oxygenation and ventilation include the following:

1. Administer high FiO_2 levels with high-flow system or rebreathing mask. A constant positive airway pressure (CPAP) mask may be tolerated in alert, co-operative patients. Continuous, vigilant monitoring for contraindications of noninvasive CPAP (decreased loss of consciousness, nausea/vomiting, increased dyspnea or panic) is imperative.
2. Intubation and mechanical ventilation if cardiovascular instability is present, severe hypoxemia persists, or if fatigue develops.
   - Oxygen support at high FiO_2 levels with PEEP is usually required to achieve an acceptable PaO_2 (>50 mm Hg) without hemodynamic compromise. Decreasing FiO_2 levels to <0.6 once PaO_2 is >50 mm Hg is a primary goal.
   - Decrease work of breathing initially by using ventilator modes and MV rates to decrease respiratory effort by the patient.
   - Adjust tidal volume, inspiratory flow rates and PEEP levels to keep plateau pressures <30 cm H_2O, if possible. Recommended tidal volume is 6 cc/kg.
3. Sedation, and potentially neuromuscular blockade, may be required for the first 24 to 48 hours after intubation to maximize gas exchange. "Fighting the ventilator" is a common complication of ventilatory support in the severely dyspneic, hypoxemic patient.
4. Decrease oxygen consumption by minimizing fever, activity level, and respiratory effort.
5. Improve oxygen-carrying capacity with transfusions for hemoglobin levels below normal.
6. Minimize suctioning the airway to avoid oxygen desaturation. Use of closed system suctioning may be necessary if desaturation is severe during suctioning, particularly in patients on high levels of PEEP and FiO_2.

Reducing Anxiety

Same as previously described for ARF management.

Achieving Effective Communications

Refer to Chapter 6, Pain, Sedation, and Neuromuscular Blockade Management, for detailed discussion of communication techniques for intubated patients.

Maintaining Hemodynamic Stability and Adequate Perfusion

1. Minimize cardiovascular instability by careful hemodynamic monitoring during PEEP therapy; administer fluids to correct hypovolemia.
2. Vasoactive drugs may be required to maintain adequate perfusion.

Preventing Complications
In addition to complications listed for ARF:

1. ARDS patients are at higher risk for development of nosocomial pneumonias. Follow prevention strategies delineated for nosocomial pneumonias below. Prophylactic antibiotics have not been shown to decrease nosocomial pneumonia rates in ARDS patients. Meticulous attention to backrest elevation, hand washing, and removal of invasive devices as soon as possible are key prevention strategies.
2. The incidence of barotrauma, pulmonary embolism, GI bleeding, and electrolyte disorders is particularly high in patients with ARDS.

Acute Respiratory Failure in the Patient With Chronic Obstructive Pulmonary Disease

Individuals with COPD (bronchitis, asthma, emphysema) are at high risk for the development of ARF. Altered host defenses, increased secretion volume and viscosity, impaired secretion clearance and airway changes, and common pathophysiologic changes predispose the patient with COPD to frequent episodes of ARF. The etiology, clinical presentation, and management of ARF in the COPD patient varies somewhat from ARF without chronic underlying pulmonary dysfunction. This section of the chapter highlights differences in ARF management in the patient with underlying COPD.

Etiology, Risk Factors, and Pathophysiology
Any systemic or pulmonary illness can precipitate ARF in patients with COPD. In addition to the etiologies of ARF listed in Table 10–5, diseases or situations that decrease ventilatory drive, muscle strength, chest wall elasticity, or gas exchange capacity, or increase airway resistance or metabolic oxygen requirements can easily lead to ARF in patients with COPD (Table 10–7). The most common precipitating events include:

- *Airway infection* (pneumonia, bronchitis): Frequent antibiotic administration, hospitalization, and impaired cough and host defenses in COPD increase acute airway infections. Infections are commonly caused by gram-negative enteric bacteria or *Legionella,* with *Haemophilus influenzae* and *Streptococcus pneumoniae* causing acute bronchitis.
- *Pulmonary embolus*: The high incidence of right ventricular failure in COPD increases the risk of pulmonary embolus from right ventricular mural thrombi.
- *Congestive heart failure:* In the presence of pulmonary hypertension and right-sided heart failure, treatment of left-sided, congestive heart failure is often delayed due to difficulties in early diagnosis.
- *Noncompliance with medication regime*: The complicated treatment regime for management of COPD,

TABLE 10–7. PRECIPITATING EVENTS OF ACUTE RESPIRATORY FAILURE IN COPD

Decreased Ventilatory Drive
Oversedation
Hypothyroidism
Brain stem lesions
Decreased Muscle Strength
Malnutrition
Shock
Myopathies
Hypophosphatemia
Hypomagnesemia
Hypocalcemia
Decreased Chest Wall Elasticity
Rib fractures
Pleural effusions
Ileus
Ascites
Decreased Lung Capacity for Gas Exchange
Atelectasis
Pulmonary edema
Pneumonia
Pulmonary embolus
Congestive heart failure
Increased Airway Resistance
Bronchospasm
Increased secretions
Upper airway obstructions
Airway edema
Increased Metabolic Oxygen Requirements
Systemic infection
Hyperthyroidism
Fever

which includes frequent administration of both oral and inhaled agents, frequently leads to underuse of medications.

The development of ARF in COPD patients places a tremendous burden on the pulmonary system. The chronic disease process leads to impairment of ventilation, poor gas exchange, and airway obstruction. The additional burden of an acute disease process, even a relatively minor one, further impairs ventilation and gas exchange and increases airway obstruction. Compensatory mechanisms can easily be overwhelmed, with lethal consequences.

Clinical Presentation
Signs and symptoms are similar to ARF, but usually more pronounced.

Diagnostic Tests

- *Chest x-ray:* Evidence of COPD (flat diaphragms, hyperinflation of air fields), in addition to x-ray findings specific to the cause of the ARF.
- *Arterial blood gases:* $PaCO_2$ >45 mm Hg and higher than baseline levels during stable, chronic disease periods.

Principles of Management for ARF in Patients With COPD

The presence of chronic respiratory dysfunction and an acute respiratory problem leads to some changes in the typical management of ARF.

Treating the Underlying Disease State

Treatment is directed at both the acute precipitating event and the chronic airflow obstruction problems associated with COPD.

1. Increase airway diameter with bronchodilators and reduce airway edema with corticosteroids. Beta-adrenergic or anticholinergic agents are more effective bronchodilators than theophylline (Table 10–8). Higher than usual doses may be necessary until the precipitating event is resolved. Bronchospasm that is refractory to bronchodilators in severe asthma cases, also called status asthmaticus, may require subcutaneous epinephrine administration. Epinephrine is only given to young patients with no evidence of cardiac disease.
2. Treat pulmonary infections with appropriate antibiotics.
3. Improve secretion removal. Strategies to improve secretion removal include adequate hydration, corticosteroids, coughing, heated moist aerosolization, and chest physiotherapy. Secretions are particularly thick and tenacious in asthma patients. Monitor response to these therapies and discontinue them if no additional benefits are observed.

Improving Oxygenation and Ventilation

Correction of hypoxemia is done by small increases in FiO_2 levels, preferably with a controlled O_2 delivery device such as a Venturi mask, biphasic intermittent positive airway pressure (BIPAP), or CPAP. Frequent monitoring of arterial blood gases is essential to ensure adequate arterial oxygenation (PaO_2 of 55 to 60 mm Hg or baseline values during nonacute situations) without significantly increasing $PaCO_2$ levels. Higher than necessary FiO_2 levels may increase $PaCO_2$ by suppressing the hypoxic ventilatory drive of some COPD patients or increasing the ventilation–perfusion ratio.

Position the patient to maximize ventilatory efforts and relaxation/rest during spontaneous breathing. A high Fowler's position and leaning on an overbed table is often the position of greatest comfort prior to intubation and mechanical ventilation.

Relaxation techniques and diaphragmatic, pursed lip breathing may be helpful to decrease anxiety and improve ventilatory patterns. Anxiolytics and other sedatives should be used cautiously to avoid decreasing MV.

The decision to intubate and mechanically ventilate the patient is based primarily on the deterioration of mental status, coupled with knowledge of the patient's baseline pulmonary function and functional status, and the reversibility of the underlying cause. Somnolence and inability to cooperate with treatments are other strong indicators for intubation and ventilation. Weaning from mechanical ventilation is frequently more difficult, and in some cases not possible, in the presence of COPD. Informed discussions with the patient and family regarding intubation options should be undertaken. The presence of an advanced directive can help to guide clinician's actions when patients are unable to make treatment decisions themselves.

Ventilatory management of COPD patients differs little from ARF alone. Slow correction of hypercarbia should be done to avoid life-threatening alkalemia from preexisting metabolic compensation. The development of auto-PEEP and barotrauma is increased in patients with COPD, necessitating smaller tidal volumes, higher respiratory rates, and short inspiratory and long expiratory times.

Nutritional Support

Typically, patients with COPD have protein-calorie malnutrition, as well as low levels of phosphate, magnesium, and calcium. These chronic nutritional deficits lead to muscle weakness and may interfere with the weaning process. Early enteral or parenteral feeding of these patients is essential to avoid further deterioration in their nutritional status during acute illness. Parenteral feeding may be best initially because dyspnea in the nonintubated patient makes oral feeding difficult and aerophagia leads to decreased gastrointestinal motility. The administration of lipid calories should account for 50% of the nutritional support during mechanical ventilation. Higher amounts may be needed during weaning attempts to minimize MV requirements related to nutritional CO_2 production.

Preventing and Managing Complications

In addition to the complications associated with ARF, the following complications commonly are observed in COPD patients with ARF:

- *Arrhythmia:* High incidence of both atrial and ventricular arrhythmia in patients with COPD due to hypoxemia, acidosis, heart disease, medications, and electrolyte abnormalities. Cardiac monitoring and correction of the underlying cause is the goal, with pharmacologic treatment of arrhythmia only for life-threatening situations.

TABLE 10–8. BRONCHODILATOR CATEGORIES USED IN STATUS ASTHMATICUS

Category	Examples
Beta-agonists (goal is beta$_2$ specificity)	Albuterol, beta$_2$-specific (often given as a continuous aerosol treatment) Epinephrine (beta$_1$ and beta$_2$)
Anticholinergics	Ipratropium bromide Glycopyrrolate
Methylxanthines	Aminophylline

- *Pulmonary embolus:* High incidence. Observe for signs and symptoms and follow the usual treatment and prevention guidelines.
- *GI distention and ileus:* Aerophagia is common in dyspneic patients, increasing the incidence of this complication.
- *Auto-PEEP and barotrauma:* High incidence, especially in the elderly and in individuals with high ventilation needs.

Pneumonia

Respiratory infection is a common cause of ARF. Infections developed before hospitalization (community acquired) and those acquired during hospitalization (nosocomial) can lead to significant morbidity and mortality, and require critical care management. A variety of respiratory infections occur in critically ill patients, including bronchitis, asthma, and pneumonia. This section focuses on pneumonia, the most common respiratory infection and the most common cause of respiratory failure in critically ill patients.

Etiology, Risk Factors, and Pathophysiology

At high risk for the development of pneumonia are the young, the elderly, those with chronic cardiopulmonary disease, and immunocompromised individuals. In addition, immobility, decreased level of consciousness, and mechanical ventilation place hospitalized patients at high risk for development of nosocomial pneumonias. These latter pneumonias are most commonly referred to as *ventilator-assisted pneumonias.*

The major routes of entry of causative organisms for pneumonia are aspiration of oropharyngeal or gastric contents into the lung (nosocomial), inhalation of aerosols or particles containing the organisms (nosocomial and community acquired), and hematogenous spread of the organism into the lung from another site in the body (nosocomial) (Figure 10–10). Most nosocomial pneumonias are due to aspiration of bacteria colonizing the oropharynx or upper GI tract. Pneumonia develops when the normal bronchomucociliary clearance mechanism or phagocytic cells are overwhelmed by the number or virulence of organisms aspirated or inhaled into the airways. The proliferation of organisms in the pulmonary parenchyma elicits an inflammatory response,

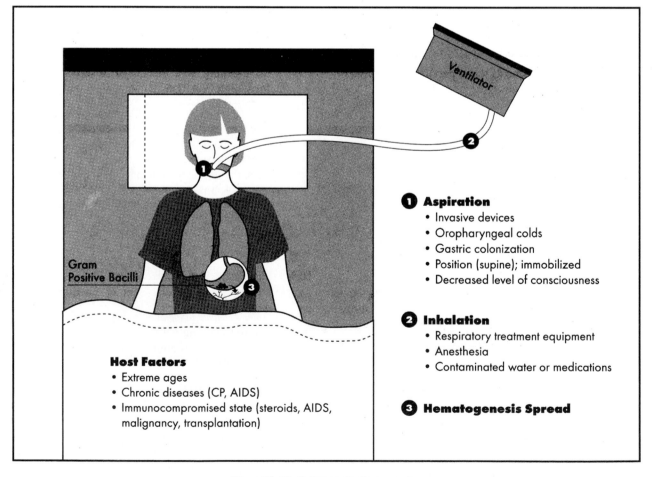

Figure 10–10. Pathogenesis of pneumonia.

with large influxes of phagocytic cells into the alveoli and airways and production of protein-rich exudates. This inflammatory response impairs the distribution of ventilation and decreases lung compliance, resulting in increased work of breathing and the sensation of dyspnea. Hypoxemia results from the shunting of blood through poorly ventilated areas of pulmonary consolidation. The inflammatory response leads to fever and leukocytosis.

Pneumonia also can develop through hematogenous spread, when organisms remote from the lungs gain access to the blood, become lodged in the pulmonary vasculature, and proliferate. Pneumonias with a hematogenous origin usually are distributed diffusely in both lung fields, rather than localized to a single lung or lobe.

Several factors present in critically ill patients increase the risk for the development of nosocomial pneumonia. Aspiration of oropharyngeal and gastric secretions is increased in the presence of endotracheal tubes, nasogastric tubes, poor GI motility, gastric distention, and immobility, all of which are common situations in critically ill patients. Treatments that neutralize the normally acidic gastric contents, such as antacids, H_2 blockers, or tube feeding, allow increased growth of gram-negative bacteria in gastric contents. This increases the potential for aspiration of gram-negative bacteria and/or hematogenous spread.

The high frequency of gastric and pulmonary intubation further increases the risk for pneumonia. Within 24 hours of admission to a critical care unit, there is colonization of the pharynx with gram-negative bacteria. Approximately 25% of colonized patients develop a clinical infection (tracheobronchitis or pneumonia). Critically ill patients at high risk for nosocomial pneumonias are those immunocompromised from malignancy, AIDS, and chronic cardiac or respiratory disease; the elderly; or those with depressed alveolar

macrophage function (oxygen, corticosteroids). Frequent changes in ventilatory equipment also increase the risk for nosocomial pneumonias in patients on ventilators.

Although a variety of similar organisms cause community- and hospital-acquired pneumonias, their frequency distribution is different (Table 10–9). Of particular concern in hospital-acquired infections is the polymicrobial origin of the pneumonia and the potential for causative organisms to be resistant to antimicrobial therapy.

Development of a nosocomial pneumonia is a serious complication in critically ill patients. Increased morbidity and mortality, in addition to increases in critical care and hospital lengths of stay and costs, make nosocomial pneumonias one of the most important sources of negative outcomes for critically ill patients.

Clinical Presentation

Signs and Symptoms

- Fever
- Cough, typically productive
- Purulent sputum or hemoptysis
- Dyspnea
- Pleuritic chest pain
- Tachypnea
- Abnormal breath sounds (crackles, bronchial breath sounds)

Diagnostic Tests

- Gram stain and culture of sputum for causative organisms. May require fiberoptic bronchoscopy with brush specimen or bronchoalveolar lavage specimen retrieval in situations where pneumonia responds poorly to treatment.

TABLE 10–9. INFECTIOUS ETIOLOGIC AGENTS IMPLICATED IN SEVERE COMMUNITY-ACQUIRED PNEUMONIA REQUIRING ICU SUPPORT AND BACTERIAL CAUSES OF NOSOCOMIAL PNEUMONIA IN ICU PATIENTS

Etiologic Agent	Frequency, %	Antibiotic
Community-Acquired Pneumonias		
Streptococcus pneumoniae	40	Penicillin G
Haemophilus influenzae	5	Ampicillin or cefuroxime
Staphylococcus aureus	10	Nafcillin or vancomycin for resistant strains
Enterobacteriaceae	10	Cefotaximine and gentamicin
Legionella pneumophila	10	Erythromycin and rifampin
Mycoplasma pneumoniae	5	Erythromycin
Viral	2	
Lung abscess	10	Penicillin and metronidazole
Nosocomial Pneumonias		
Enterobacteriaceae	30–50	Cefotaximin and gentamicin
Staphylococcus aureus	10–30	Nafcillin or vancomycin for resistant strains
Pseudomonas aeruginosa	10–20	Piperacillin
Streptococci	10–15	Penicillin
Legionella spp.	5–15	Erythromycin and rifampin
Haemophilus influenzae	2–10	Ampicillin or cefuroxime
Anerobes	2–5	Penicillin and metronidazole

Adapted from: Hall JB, Schmidt GA, Woods LD (eds.): Principles of Critical Care. New York: McGraw-Hill, 1992, pp. 1250, 1260, 1261. With permission.

- New or progressive infiltrates on chest x-ray. Infiltrates may be either localized or diffuse in nature.
- Elevated WBC.
- Abnormal arterial blood gases (hypoxemia, hypocapnia).

Principles of Management for Pneumonia

Treating the Underlying Disease

Appropriate antimicrobial therapy should be initiated based on likely causative organisms until definitive culture results are obtained (see Table 10–9). Fluids should be administered to correct hypovolemia and hypotension, if present. Hypotension unresponsive to fluid therapy should alert the clinician to the potential for septic shock.

Improving Oxygenation and Ventilation

Similar to ARF management, with the following additions:

- PEEP and CPAP are unlikely to improve oxygenation in the presence of pneumonia, and may exacerbate the ventilation–perfusion abnormalities associated with pneumonia. These techniques should be used with caution in pneumonia.
- Voluminous, tenacious respiratory secretions may require endotracheal intubation to assist with clearance. Chest physiotherapy may be helpful to increase secretion clearance, particularly when lobar atelectasis is present. Fiberoptic bronchoscopy may also be required to assist with secretion management.

Preventing Nosocomial Pneumonias

In addition to the high morbidity and mortality associated with pneumonia in critically ill patients, high priority must be given to strategies to prevent the development of nosocomial pneumonias. The development of a nosocomial pneumonia in a critically ill patient increases requirements for ventilatory support (mechanical ventilation, oxygen, duration of treatment). It is estimated that a nosocomial pneumonia increases hospitalization 4 to 10 days, and increases costs by $20,000 to $40,000 per episode. Prevention strategies (Table 10–10) include the following:

- Decrease the risk of cross-contamination or colonization via the hands of hospitalized personnel. Hand washing is the most effective strategy.
- Decrease the risk of aspiration. Avoid supine positioning and keep the head of the bed elevated to 30 to 45 degrees at all times, unless medically contraindicated. Use an endotracheal tube with a dorsal lumen above the endotracheal cuff to remove drainage with continuous suction. Suction above the endotracheal tube cuff before removing or repositioning the tube. Assess for, and correct, gastric reflux problems. Ambulate as soon as possible.
- Implement a comprehensive oral hygiene program.

TABLE 10–10. EVIDENCE-BASED PRACTICE GUIDELINES FOR THE PREVENTION OF VENTILATOR-ASSOCIATED PNEUMONIA (VAP)

Preventing Gastric Reflux
1. All mechanically ventilated patients, as well as those at high risk for aspiration (e.g., decreased level of consciousness; enteral tube in place), should have the head of the bed elevated at an angle of 30–45 degrees unless medically contraindicated.[a,b]
2. Routinely verify appropriate placement of the feeding tube.[a]

Airway Management
1. If feasible, use an endotracheal tube with a dorsal lumen above the endotracheal cuff to allow drainage (by continuous or intermittent suctioning) of tracheal secretions that accumulate in the patient's subglottic area.[a,b]
2. Unless contraindicated by the patient's condition, perform orotracheal rather than nasotracheal intubation.[a]
3. ET cuff management: Before deflating the cuff of an endotracheal tube in preparation for tube removal, or before moving the tube, ensure that secretions are cleared from above the tube cuff.[a]
4. Use only sterile fluid to remove secretions from the suction catheter if the catheter is to be used for reentry into the patient's lower respiratory tract.[a]
5. Perform tracheostomy under aseptic conditions.[a]

Oral Care
1. Develop and implement a comprehensive oral hygiene program.[a]
2. Use an oral chlorhexidine gluconate (0.12%) rinse during the perioperative period on patients who undergo cardiac surgery.[a]

Cross-Contamination
1. Hand washing: Decontaminate hands with soap and water or a waterless antiseptic agent after contact with mucous membranes, respiratory secretions, or objects contaminated with respiratory secretions, whether or not gloves are worn.[a]
2. Decontaminate hands with soap and water or a waterless antiseptic agent before and after contact with a patient who has an endotracheal or tracheostomy tube, and before and after contact with any respiratory device that is used on the patient, whether or not gloves are worn.[a]
3. Wear gloves for handling respiratory secretions or objects contaminated with respiratory secretions of any patient.[a]
4. When soiling with respiratory secretions is anticipated, wear a gown and change it after soiling and before providing care to another patient.[a]
5. Room-air humidifiers: Do not use large-volume room-air humidifiers that create aerosols (nebulizers) unless they can be sterilized or subjected to high-level disinfection at least daily and filled only with sterile water.[a]

Mobilization
1. Ambulate as soon as medically indicated in the postoperative period.[a]

Equipment Changes
1. Do not change routinely, on the basis of duration of use, the patient's ventilator circuit. Change the circuit when it is visibly soiled or mechanically malfunctioning. Periodically drain or discard any condensate that collects in the tubing. Do not allow condensate to drain toward the patient.[a,b]
2. Between use on different patients, sterilize or subject to high-level disinfection all MRBs.[a]

Compiled from: [a]Centers for Disease Control and Prevention (2004) and [b]AACN VAP Practice Alert (2004).

- Maintain a closed system on ventilator/humidifier circuits, and avoid pooling of condensation or secretions in the tubing. Do not routinely change the ventilator circuit, except when visibly soiled or malfunctioning.
- Use sterile technique for endotracheal suctioning and suction only when necessary to clear secretions from large airways.
- Provide nutritional support to improve host defenses.

- Eliminate invasive devices and equipment as soon as possible.

Pulmonary Embolism

Etiology, Risk Factors, and Pathophysiology

Pulmonary embolism (PE) is a complication of deep venous thrombosis (DVT), long bone fracture, or air entering the circulatory system. There are many risk factors for pulmonary embolism (Table 10–11), with critically ill patients being especially prone due to the presence of central venous and PA catheters, immobility, use of muscle relaxants, and congestive heart failure.

Thromboemboli

Venous thrombi form at the site of vascular injuries or where venous stasis occurs, primarily in the leg or pelvic veins. Thrombi that dislodge travel through the venous circulation until they become wedged in a branch of the pulmonary circulation. Depending on the size of the thrombi, and the lo-

TABLE 10–11. RISK FACTORS FOR DEVELOPMENT OF PULMONARY EMBOLISM

Thromboemboli
Obesity
Prior history of thromboembolism
Advanced age
Malignancy
Estrogen
Immobility
Paralysis
Congestive heart failure
Postpartum
Postsurgical
Posttrauma
Hypercoagulability states
Central venous and PA catheters

Air Emboli
Neurosurgery
Liver transplant
Harrington rod insertion
Open heart surgery
Arthroscopy
Pacemaker insertion
Cardiopulmonary resuscitation
Gastroscopy
Positive pressure ventilation
Scuba diving
Intravenous infusion
Central venous catheter insertion or removal

Fat Emboli
Long bone fracture
Blunt trauma to liver
Pancreatitis
Lipid infusions
Sickle cell crisis
Burns
Cardiopulmonary bypass
Cyclosporine administration

cation of the occlusion, mild to severe obstruction of blood flow occurs beyond the thrombi.

The primary sequela, and major contributor to mortality, of the pulmonary obstruction is circulatory impairment. The physical obstruction of the pulmonary capillary bed increases right ventricular afterload, dilates the right ventricle, and impedes coronary perfusion. This predisposes the right ventricle to ischemia and right ventricular failure (cor pulmonale).

A secondary consequence of thromboemboli is a mismatching of ventilation to perfusion in gas exchange units beyond the obstruction (see Figure 10–9C), resulting in arterial hypoxemia. This hypoxemia further compromises oxygen delivery to the ischemic right ventricle.

Air Emboli

Air or other nonabsorbable gases entering the venous system also travel to the right heart, pulmonary circulation, arterioles, and capillaries. A variety of surgical and nonsurgical situations predispose patients to the development of air embolization (see Table 10–11). Damage to the pulmonary endothelium occurs from the abnormal air–blood interface, leading to increased capillary permeability and alveolar flooding. Bronchoconstriction also occurs with air embolization. In addition to hypoxemia, P_{CO_2} removal is also impaired.

Arterial embolization may occur if air passes to the left heart through a patent foramen ovale, present in approximately 30% of the population. Peripheral embolization to the brain, extremities, and coronary perfusion leads to ischemic manifestations in these organs.

Fat Emboli

Fat enters the pulmonary circulation most commonly when released from the bone marrow following long bone fractures (see Table 10–11). Nontraumatic origins of fat embolization also occur and are thought to be due to the agglutination of low-density lipoproteins or liposomes from nutritional fat emulsions. The presence of fat in the pulmonary circulation injures the endothelial lining of the capillary, increasing permeability and alveolar flooding.

Clinical Presentation

The diagnosis of PE is based primarily on clinical signs and symptoms. Because many of the signs and symptoms are nonspecific, PE frequently is difficult to diagnosis. In critically ill patients, diagnosis is especially difficult due to alterations in communication and level of consciousness, and the nonspecific nature of other cardiopulmonary alterations.

Signs and Symptoms

- Dyspnea
- Pleuritic pain
- Apprehension
- Diaphoresis
- Evidence of DVT
- Hemoptysis
- Tachypnea

- Fever
- Tachycardia
- Shock symptoms with large PE

Diagnostic Tests

- *Chest x-ray:* Evaluate for basilar atelectasis, elevation of the diaphragm, and pleural effusion, although most patients have nonspecific findings on chest x-ray; diffuse alveolar filling in air embolism.
- *Arterial blood gas analysis:* Hypoxemia with or without hypercarbia.
- *ECG:* Signs of right ventricular strain (right axis deviation, right bundle branch block) or precordial strain; sinus tachycardia.
- *PA pressures:* Elevated with a decreased cardiac output.
- *Ventilation–perfusion scan:* Decreased perfusion to areas with emboli. Scan sensitivity is decreased in intubated patients and in the presence of COPD.
- *Pulmonary angiography:* Slightly higher risk of complications with this procedure, but sensitivity and specificity are high.

Principles of Management for Pulmonary Emboli

The key to preventing morbidity and mortality from pulmonary embolism is early diagnosis and treatment to prevent reembolization. Objectives include the improvement of oxygenation and ventilation, improvement of cardiovascular function, prevention of reembolization, and prevention of pulmonary embolus.

Improving Oxygenation and Ventilation

Oxygen therapy is usually very effective in relieving hypoxemia associated with PE. When cardiopulmonary compromise is severe, mechanical ventilation with neuromuscular blockade may be required to achieve optimal oxygenation.

Improving Cardiovascular Function

Controversy exists as to the benefit of vasoactive drug administration (such as norepinephrine and/or inotropic agents) to improve myocardial perfusion of the right ventricle. In severe embolic events, where cardiac failure is profound, additional therapy to hasten clot resolution, such as use of thrombolytic agents and/or surgical removal of massive emboli may be warranted.

Preventing Reembolization

Several strategies are employed to prevent the likelihood of future embolization and cardiopulmonary compromise:

- Limiting activity to prevent dislodgement of additional clots.
- Use of anticoagulation therapy with heparin to maintain a PTT 1.5 to 2.5 times the control when no contraindication exists.
- Insertion of vena cava filters to prevent emboli from legs, pelvis, and inferior vena cava from migrating to pulmonary circulation if anticoagulation therapy is contraindicated. Filters are placed percutaneously in the inferior vena cava.

Preventing Deep Vein Thrombosis and Pulmonary Embolus

- Subcutaneous, low-dose heparin administration in high-risk patients. Routine use of this prevention strategy in critically ill patients who have no contraindications for heparin therapy has been shown to decrease deep vein thrombosis and resultant PE.
- Sequential compression devices (SCDs) (Table 10–12; Figure 10–11) to prevent venous stasis for high-risk patients (see Table 10–11). In high-risk

---

AT THE BEDSIDE
▶ *Thinking Critically*

You are caring for a patient in ARF with the following interventions:

- Mechanical ventilatory support (assist-control rate 10/min tidal volume 800 mL, PEEP 15 cm H_2O, FiO_2 0.85)
- PaO_2 63 mm Hg
- MAP 68 mm Hg on vasoactive drug support (dopamine 7 mcg/kg/min)
- Neuromuscular blockade (vecuronium)
- Sedation (lorazepam)

How might the level of PEEP this patient is receiving affect his response to suctioning? What precautions could you take to avoid or respond to potential complications?

TABLE 10–12. TIPS FOR SAFE AND EFFECTIVE USE OF SEQUENTIAL COMPRESSION DEVICES

Contraindications for sequential compression device use
- Massive leg edema
- Extreme leg deformities
- Arterial ischemia, severe arteriosclerosis
- Inflammation
- Severe phlebitis
- Trauma
- Pulmonary edema
- Skin disorders in legs (rash, ulcers, new skin grafts)

Follow manufacturer's directions carefully to ensure proper sizing of SCD stockings.

Assess frequently for signs of excessive compression
- Tingling
- Leg pain
- Foot or leg discoloration
- Cool leg extremities
- Change in pulse strength

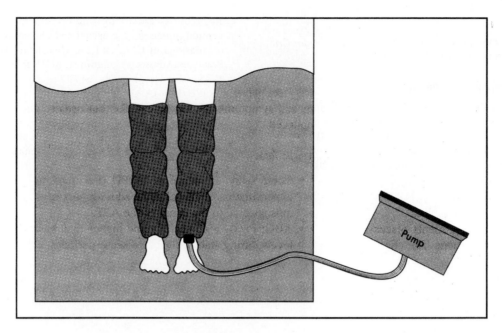

Figure 10–11. Sequential compression device (SCD) for prevention of deep vein thrombosis and pulmonary embolism.

surgical patients, intraoperative application may improve effectiveness.

- Placement of prophylactic vena cava filters in high-risk patients.
- Early fixation of long bone fractures to prevent fat emboli.
- Early mobilization. As soon as hemodynamic stability is achieved, and there are no other contraindications to mobilization, activity level should begin increasing to include sitting in a chair several times per day and short periods of ambulation.

SELECTED BIBLIOGRAPHY

Critical Care Management of Respiratory Problems

Bower R. Mechanical ventilation in acute lung injury and ARDS: Tidal volume reduction. *Crit Care Clin* 2002;18(1):1–13.

Burns S (ed): *Protocols for Practice: Care of the Mechanically Ventilated Patient.* Aliso Viejo, CA: AACN; 1998.

Cardenas VJ: Diagnosis and management of pneumonia in the intensive care unit. *Chest Surg Clin North Am* 2002;12:379–395.

Chastre J, Fagon J: Ventilator-associated pneumonia. In Hall J, Schmidt G, Wood LD (eds): *Principles of Critical Care,* 2nd ed. New York: McGraw-Hill; 1998.

Church V: Staying on guard for DVT and PE. *Nursing* 2000;30–42.

Girou E: Prevention of nosocomial infections in acute respiratory failure patients. *Eur Respir J Suppl* 2003;42:72s–76s.

Hall JB, Schmidt GA, Wood LDH (eds): *Principles of Critical Care,* 2nd ed. New York: McGraw-Hill; 1998.

Kirkwood P: Chest tubes: Ask the experts. *Crit Care Nurse* 2002;22(4):70–72.

Kirkwood P: Chest tubes: Ask the experts. *Crit Care Nurse* 2000; 20(3):97–98.

Lazzara D: Eliminate the air of mystery from chest tubes. *Nursing* 2002,32(6).36–43.

Levy M: Optimal PEEP in ARDS: Changing concepts and current controversies. *Crit Care Clin* 2002;18(1):15–31.

Morrison RJ, Bidani A: Acute respiratory distress syndrome epidemiology and pathophysiology. *Chest Surgery Clin North Am* 2002;12:301–323.

Widemann HP, Arroliga AC, Komara JJ: Emerging systemic pharmacologic approaches in acute respiratory distress syndrome. *Respir Care Clin North Am* 2003;9:419–435.

Chest X-Ray Interpretation

Connolly MA: Black, white, and shades of gray: Common abnormalities in chest radiographs. *AACN Clinical Issues.* 2001; 12(2)259–269.

Detternmeier P: *Radiographic Assessment for Nurses.* St. Louis: Mosby; 1995.

Hall J, Schmidt G, Wood L: *Principles of Critical Care,* 2nd ed. New York: McGraw-Hill; 1998.

Sanchez F: Fundamentals of chest x-ray interpretation. *Crit Care Nurse* 1986;6:41–52.

Siela D: Using chest radiography in the intensive care unit. *Crit Care Nurse* 2002;22(4):18–27.

Talbot I, Meyers-Marquardt M (eds): *Respiratory Assessment. Pocket Guide to Critical Care Assessment,* 3rd ed. St. Louis: Mosby; 1997.

Thelan L, Davie J, Urden L, Lough M: *Critical Care Nursing: Diagnosis and Management,* 4th ed. St. Louis: Mosby; 2002.

Miscellaneous

Lynn-McHale DJ, Carlson KK: *AACN Procedure Manual for Critical Care,* 4th ed. Philadelphia: WB Saunders; 2001.

Evidence-Based Practice Guidelines

Agency for Healthcare Research and Quality: *Prevention of Venous Thromboembolism After Injury* [Evidence Report/Technology Assessment 2001, No 22]. Silver Spring, MD: AHRQ; 2001.

AACN VAP Practice Alert. Aliso Viejo, CA: AACN; 2004. Available: http://www.aacn.org.

Centers for Disease Control and Prevention: Guidelines for prevention of health-care-associated pneumonia, 2003: Recommendations of CDC and the Healthcare Infection Control Practices Advisory Committee. *MMWR* 2004;53(No. RR-3): 1–35.

Gerts WH, Heit JA, Glagett GP, et al: Prevention of venous thromboembolism: 6th ACCP Consensus Conference on Athithrombotic Therapy. *Chest* 2001;119:132S–175S.

Mandell LA, Bartlett JG, Dowell SF, et al: Update of practice guidelines for the management of community-acquired pneumonia in immunocompromised adults: IDSA guidelines. *Clin Infect Diseas* 2003;37:1405–1433.

Multisystem Problems

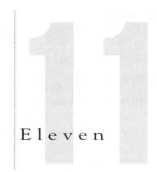

Ruth M. Kleinpell

▶ Knowledge Competencies

1. Identify the relationship between the cellular mediators and clinical manifestations of systemic inflammatory response syndrome (SIRS).

2. Describe the etiology, pathophysiology, clinical manifestations, patient needs, and principles of management of SIRS, sepsis, and associated conditions leading to multisystem problems.

3. Compare and contrast the pathophysiology, clinical manifestations, patient needs, and management approaches for multisystem problems resulting from SIRS, sepsis, multiple organ dysfunction, and overdoses.

PATHOLOGIC CONDITIONS

Sepsis and Multiple Organ Dysfunction Syndrome

Critical illness can predispose patients to several complex conditions including sepsis and multiple organ dysfunction syndrome (MODS) (Table 11–1). Sepsis results from an infectious process and represents a systemic response to infection. Sepsis with acute organ dysfunction (severe sepsis) commonly occurs in critically ill patients. It is estimated that each year there are more than 750,000 cases and approximately 215,000 deaths due to severe sepsis. Severe sepsis is associated with mortality rates of 28% to 50% or more, and is one of the most common causes of death in the intensive care unit (ICU).

The systemic inflammatory response syndrome (SIRS) is a systemic response to a clinical insult, such as an infection or burn (Figure 11–1). In some cases, the syndrome may progress to sepsis and MODS. The stimulus for SIRS can be singular or multifactorial. Examples of situations that can precipitate SIRS are burns, trauma, transfusions, pancreatitis, or infection. Following the insult, an inflammatory response is initiated as a normal physiologic response. The inflammatory response consists of vasodilatation, increased mi-

crovascular permeability, cellular activation and release of mediators, and coagulation (see Figure 11–1). In SIRS, there is an excessive release of these mediators, which may lead to severe tissue damage, with hypoperfusion of organ systems.

SIRS is manifested in a variety of ways: fever, tachycardia, tachypnea, altered level of consciousness, and decreased urine output. These findings may or may not be the result of an infection. If the response progresses unchecked, the result may be the development of sepsis or dysfunction of one or more organ systems, or MODS. The SIRS, sepsis, and MODS may be thought of as progressively severe conditions along a continuum. The key is early identification of the signs and symptoms of SIRS, and prompt development of a treatment plan to avoid further progression. Early intervention is important to ensure good outcomes in these patients.

Etiology, Risk Factors, and Pathophysiology

Systemic Inflammatory Response Syndrome

SIRS consists of a series of systemic events that occur in response to an insult to the body. This response is a cellular reaction that initiates a number of mediator-induced responses, and is both inflammatory and immune in nature (Figure 11–2).

TABLE 11–1. DEFINITIONS

Term	Definition
Bacteremia	The presence of viable bacteria in the blood.
Hypotension	A systolic BP of <90 mm Hg or a reduction of >40 mm Hg from baseline in the absence of other causes for hypotension.
Infection	Microbial phenomenon characterized by an inflammatory response to the presence of microorganisms or the invasion of normally sterile host tissue by those organisms.
MODS	Presence of altered organ function in an acutely ill patient such that homeostasis cannot be maintained without intervention.
Sepsis	The systemic response to infection. This systemic response is manifested by two or more of the following conditions as a result of infection: • Temperature >38.0°C • Heart rate >90/min • Respiratory rate >20 breaths/min or $Paco_2$ <32 mm Hg • WBC >12,000 cells/mm^3, <4000 cells/mm^3, or >10% immature (band) forms
Septic shock	Sepsis with hypotension, despite adequate fluid resuscitation, along with the presence of perfusion abnormalities that may include, but are not limited to, lactic acidosis, oliguria, or an acute alteration in mental status. Patients who are on inotropic or vasopressor agents may not be hypotensive at the time that perfusion abnormalities are measured.
Severe sepsis	Sepsis associated with organ dysfunction, hypoperfusion, or hypotension. Hypoperfusion and perfusion abnormalities may include, but are not limited to, lactic acidosis, oliguria, or an acute alteration in mental status.
SIRS	The systemic inflammatory response to a variety of severe clinical insults. The response is manifested by two or more of the following conditions: • Temperature >38.0°C • Heart rate >90/min • Respiratory rate >20 breaths/min or $Paco_2$ <32 mm Hg • WBC >12,000 cells/mm^3, <4000 cells/mm^3, or >10% immature (band) forms

Data from: ACCP/SCCM Consensus Committee: Crit Care Med *1992;20:866.*

There are essentially four different types of cells that are activated as part of the response to an insult or stimulus: polymorphonuclear cells (neutrophils), macrophages, platelets, and endothelial cells. These cells are activated to become either directly involved in the reaction (i.e., platelet aggregation) or are stimulated to produce and release chemical mediators into the circulation, such as cytokines or plasma enzymes. Once activated, "a checks and balances system" is normally in place to control the inflammatory response. In some situations, however, when the response is large or the injury diffuse, local control of the response is lost, leading to excessive mediator release with consequent organ damage.

AT THE BEDSIDE
▶ Sepsis

A 67-year-old man with a 6-year history of hypertension and a 30-pack per year cigarette history was admitted to the ICU with a diagnosis of cirrhosis secondary to biliary obstruction. He underwent an exploratory laparotomy and cholecystectomy 3 days ago. Postoperatively, he was relatively stable, experiencing an episode of hypotension 12 hours postoperatively, which was corrected by fluid administration. He remains intubated and attempts at weaning have been delayed due to periodic hypoxemia.

He currently has an arterial line, central venous pressure (CVP), pulmonary artery catheter, T-tube drain, and Foley catheter. He is alert and oriented, moving in bed with little assistance. Physical examination reveals that his skin is pale pink, warm to touch, lungs have a few bibasilar rales, 11 pedal edema is present bilaterally. His abdomen is nondistended, no active bowel sounds. His 5-inch midline abdominal wound requires tid dressing changes and is approximated with retention sutures. Current vital signs are:

T	101.0°F core
HR	122

Sinus tachycardia

RR	34
BP	82/60

Current labs are:

ABG:	Ph 7.30, PaO_2 62, $Paco_2$ 46, HCO_3 18, SaO_2 94%
WBC:	22,000, 65 neutrophils, 50 segs, 12 bands, 40,000 platelets
RBC:	4.5, HCT 39, Hgb 13, bili 2.2 mg, LDH 220, NA^1 140, K^1 3.5, CL 100, CO_2 20, BUN 22, creat 1.1

Discussion Questions

1. Why might this patient be at risk for developing sepsis?
2. What clinical signs and symptoms may be evidence of early sepsis?
3. Is he exhibiting SIRS criteria?

Answers

1. Postoperative status, intubated, invasive lines and catheters, abdominal wound requiring dressing changes are risk factors for sepsis in this patient.
2. Elevated temperature, elevated white blood cell count with bandemia, sinus tachycardia, elevated respiratory rate are clinical symptoms of early sepsis.
3. Yes.

A general understanding of the various mediators responsible for the SIRS is important. Mediators can be divided into five groups: cytokines, plasma enzyme cascades, lipid mediators, toxic oxygen-derived metabolites, and unclassified mediators such as nitric oxide and proteases.

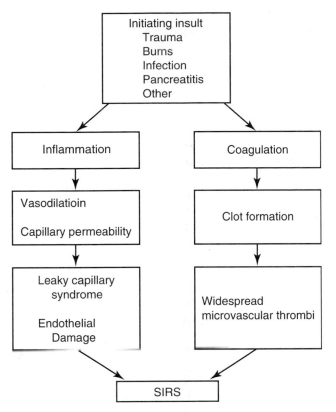

Figure 11–1. The systemic inflammatory response (SIRS) results from activation of interactive cascades of inflammation and coagulation.

cytes or macrophages, they are called *monokines.* Examples of cytokines include tumor necrosis factor, interleukin, interferon, and colony-stimulating factors such as granulocyte colony-stimulating factor.

In addition to cytokines, there is also activation of different enzymatic plasma cascades. Examples of these include the complement cascade and the various coagulation cascades. In addition, there are various lipid mediators that are either stimulated or produced as part of a cellular destructive process. These lipid mediators include arachidonic acid metabolites, leukotrienes, prostaglandins, and platelet activating factor. Oxygen-derived free radicals are another group of mediators that exert a negative effect as part of the SIRS. Examples of these include hydrogen peroxide and hydroxyl radical. Nitric oxide and proteases are other mediators that are not grouped into any of the previous categories, but are mediators that enhance the SIR syndrome.

In addition to the mediators stimulated as part of the inflammatory and immune responses, mediators related to hormonal stimulation and regulation are also produced. The hormonal response component of the SIRS is characterized by the release of stress hormones (catecholamines, glucagon, cortisol, and growth hormone), suppression of thyroid hormone, and hormonal regulation of fluid and electrolyte balance.

These mediators are stimulated after cellular activation in response to a certain stimulus (e.g., infection, trauma, pancreatitis). Cytokines are active chemical substances secreted by cells in response to a stimulus. If secreted by lymphocytes, they are called *lymphokines,* and if secreted by mono-

Sepsis

Sepsis is the manifestation of the SIRS in response to an infectious process (see Table 11–1). The source of infection may be bacterial, viral, fungal, or on rare occasions, rickettsial or protozoal.

The risk factors for development of sepsis are many and include malnutrition, immunosuppression, prolonged antibiotic use, and the presence of invasive devices (Table 11–2).

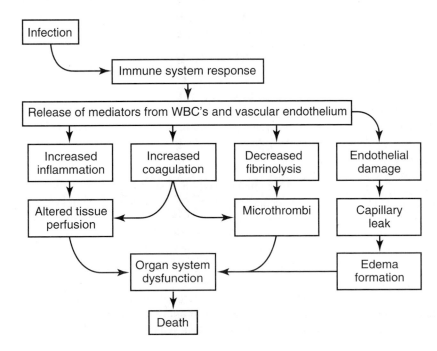

Figure 11–2. Interactive cascade of inflammation and coagulation leading to endothelium damage, diffuse thrombi and organ system dysfunction. (*Reprinted with permission, Kleinpell R:* Nurs Spectrum *2004;17[12]:24–26.*)

It is important to remember that a large number of infections in critically ill patients are hospital acquired and can lead to sepsis. Many of these hospital-acquired infections can be prevented with simple measures. The role of the critical care nurse is instrumental in preventing nosocomial infections. Hand washing remains the single most effective method for preventing nosocomial infections. Recent research suggests that relatively simple measures such as ensuring head-of-bed elevation may prevent ventilator-associated pneumonia, a common source of sepsis in critically ill patients. Therefore, nursing measures to target sepsis prevention as well as early recognition and treatment are important in reducing the high mortality rates associated with severe sepsis (Table 11–3).

TABLE 11–2. RISK FACTORS FOR DEVELOPMENT OF SEPSIS

Host-Related Factors	Treatment-Related Factors
Malnutrition	
Immune deficiency disorders	Invasive diagnostic devices
Immunosuppression	Invasive therapeutic devices
Skin breakdown	Surgical procedures
Fragile skin/mucous membranes	Prolonged hospitalization
Traumatic injuries	Therapeutic immunosuppression
Burns	Chemotherapy
Pressure sores	Radiation therapy
IV drug abuse	Splenectomy
ETOH abuse	Urinary catheters
Chronic illness	Use of H_2 receptor antagonists
Diabetes mellitus	(leading to gastric bacterial
Neoplastic disease	overgrowth and aspiration
Cirrhosis	pneumonia)
Renal failure	Aggressive resuscitation
Cardiac disease	Prolonged TPN
Pulmonary disease	Extensive antibiotic therapy
Pregnancy associated with	Pain/stress
prolonged rupture of membranes	
Immune senescence (elderly)	
Poor mobility	
Bedridden status	
BPH	
Decreased mucociliary transport mechanisms	
Decreased cough and clearance function	
Increased response to influenza vaccine	
UTI	
Vaginal colonization with GBS	
Perineal colonization with Escherichia coli	
Premature rupture of membranes	

Adapted with permission from: Klein DM, Witek-Janusek L: Advances in immunotherapy of sepsis. Dimensions Crit Care Nurs 1992;11(2):75–81.

Severe Sepsis

Sepsis can progress to severe sepsis, with organ dysfunction, hypoperfusion, or severe hypotension. Hypoperfusion and perfusion abnormalities that occur in severe sepsis may include oliguria, lactic acidosis, hypoxemia, and alteration in mental status (Table 11–4). Severe sepsis is associated with three integrated responses: activation of inflammation, activation of coagulation, and impairment of fibrinolysis. The result is systemic inflammation, widespread coagulopathy, and microvascular thrombosis, conditions that often lead to multiple organ dysfunction.

MODS

Multiple organ dysfunction is the worsening progression of the systemic inflammatory response. If SIRS is allowed to persist unchecked, or becomes overwhelming, the patient develops clinical manifestations of organ dysfunction. The mortality rates for MODS vary depending on the underlying cause, with mortality rates ranging from 50% to 100% as the number of involved organs increases.

MODS can be classified as either primary or secondary. In *primary MODS*, organ dysfunction is a direct effect of an insult to an organ that has been compromised. For example, aspiration causes lung dysfunction, or acetaminophen overdose causes liver dysfunction. With primary MODS, the onset occurs relatively soon after the insult. In *secondary MODS*, the organ dysfunction occurs as the result of persistent and prolonged mediator release following an insult such as a thermal burn or pancreatitis. Generally, the time frame for secondary MODS is 7 to 10 days; however, this onset is variable.

Clinical Presentation

SIRS

SIRS is the clinical manifestations of two or more of the following conditions:

- Temperature $>38°C$ or $<36°C$
- Heart rate >90 beats/min
- Respiratory rate >20 breaths/min or $Pa_{CO_2} <32$ mm Hg
- WBC $>12,000$ cells/mm^3, <4000 cells/mm^3, or $>10\%$ immature neutrophils (band) forms.

Close monitoring and assessment are essential for the detection of early signs of SIRS.

Severe Sepsis

The clinical manifestation of severe sepsis is the result of altered perfusion to vital organ systems. Organ system dysfunction develops due to hypoperfusion and microvascular thrombosis. Table 11–4 summarizes the common manifestations of severe sepsis. Signs of organ system dysfunction include cardiovascular alterations (hypotension, tachycardia, dysrhythmias), respiratory system alterations (tachypnea, hypoxemia), renal system alterations (oliguria, elevated creatinine), hematologic system alterations (thrombocytopenia), gastrointestinal alteration (change in bowel sounds, ileus),

TABLE 11–3. NURSING CARE OF PATIENTS WITH SEVERE SEPSIS

Recognition	Early identification of patients at risk for developing sepsis: • Elderly • Immunocompromised • Patients with surgical/invasive procedures • Patients with indwelling catheters • Mechanically ventilated patients
Monitoring physical assessment parameters	Vital signs • Fever/hypothermia • Tachycardia • Tachypnea • Hypotension Hemodynamic parameters • Heart rate/rhythm and presence of ectopy • Hemodynamic monitoring parameter changes (elevated CO and low systemic vascular resistance) Ventilatory parameters • Respiratory rate • Lung sounds • Oxygenation status (pulse oximetry, arterial blood gases, mixed venous oxygen saturation levels) Renal parameters: • Hourly urine output monitoring • Note sudden/gradual decreases in urine output • Monitor laboratory parameters of renal function (creatinine, BUN levels, fractional excretion of sodium levels) Coagulation parameters • Monitor coagulation indices (thrombocytopenia, prothrombin time, activated partial thromboplastin time, INR) • Monitor for bruising, bleeding Metabolic parameters • Provide nutritional support • Recognize role of intact gut barrier in preventing translocation of gram negative bacteria • Maintain nitrogen balance in hypermetabolic state • Provide normalization of hyperglycemia Mental status parameters • Mental status changes (restlessness, confusion) • Changes in GCS
Provide comprehensive sepsis treatment	• Circulatory support with fluids, inotropes, and vasopressors • Supportive treatment with oxygenation and ventilation • Antibiotic administration • Drotrecogin alfa (activated) therapy to appropriate candidates • Monitoring and reporting patient response to treatment
Promote patient and family comfort care	• Promote patient comfort/pain relief/sedation • Turning/skin care • Patient and family teaching • Address needs of families of critically ill patients

Sepsis prevention	• Prevention remains the best treatment
	• Handwashing
	• Universal precautions
	• Measures to prevent hospital acquired infections and iatrogenic complications:
	  – Ventilator-associated pneumonia (see practice guidelines Chapter 10)
	  – DVT and GI prophylaxis
	  – Invasive catheter care
	  – Wound care
	  – Urinary catheter care
	• Astute clinical assessment
	  – Maintain mucosal integrity
	  – Prevent translocation
	• Formulate a sepsis prevention plan
	• Educate members of the health care team on identification and treatment of sepsis
	• Screen patients daily for signs of sepsis
	• Monitor sepsis cases and outcomes
	• Track changes in sepsis incidence rates and outcomes

Adapted from Ely, Kleinpell, and Goyette (2003).

TABLE 11–4. SIGNS OF ACUTE ORGAN SYSTEM DYSFUNCTION

Cardiovascular	• Tachycardia • Dysrhythmias • Hypotension • Elevated central venous and pulmonary artery pressures
Respiratory	• Tachypnea • Hypoxemia
Renal	• Oliguria • Anuria • Elevated creatinine
Hematologic	• Jaundice • Elevated liver enzymes • Decreased albumin • Coagulopathy
Gastrointestinal	• Ileus (absent bowel sounds)
Hepatic	• Thrombocytopenia • Coagulopathy • Decreased protein C levels • Increased D-dimer levels
Neurologic	• Altered consciousness • Confusion • Psychosis

Adapted from Balk R: Pathogenesis and management of multiple organ dysfunction or failure in severe sepsis and septic shock. Crit Care Clin 2000;16(2):337–352.

hepatic alterations (elevated liver enzymes, jaundice, coagulopathies), and neurologic system alterations (confusion, agitation). Early recognition and treatment are extremely important as the prognosis of patients with severe sepsis is related to the number or organs involved and the severity of dysfunction.

MODS

The clinical manifestations of primary and secondary MODS are the same as in SIRS and depend on which organs are affected. In patients with severe sepsis, MODS appears to result from a cascade of inflammatory mediators, endothelial injury, altered perfusion, and microcirculatory failure. Mortality in severe sepsis is directly related to the number of failing organ systems and the severity of dysfunction. MODS is regarded as one of the most common causes of death among patients in the ICU.

Diagnostic Tests

- Complete blood cell count: White blood cell count $>12,000$ cells/mm^3, or <4000 cells/mm^3, or $>10\%$ immature bands
- Arterial blood gas: $PaCO_2$ <32 mm Hg
- Chest x-ray: May be normal or show signs of infiltrates
- Culture and sensitivity: Generally is positive from a normally sterile source
- Computed axial tomography scan: May be negative or show abscess collection

Principles of Management of Sepsis

The treatment of a patient with SIRS or sepsis consists of several objectives: treatment of the underlying cause, maximizing oxygen delivery, and use of evidence-based practice guidelines to ensure that initial resuscitation, organ system support, and targeted interventions are provided. Additional components of the management plan include providing nutrition and providing psychological support for the patient and family.

Treating the Underlying Cause

The management plan begins with recognition and treatment of the source or stimulus of the response. Until this is done, no other therapy may be successfully applied. Examples include the drainage of an abscess or the removal of an infected invasive line, vascular graft, or orthopedic device. Once the source (or presumed source) has been identified, empiric antibiotic therapy is initiated and adjusted when definitive culture results are available.

Maximizing Oxygen Delivery

Parallel to the administration of antibiotics are measures to maximize oxygen delivery. The components of oxygen delivery include cardiac output (CO), oxygen saturation (SaO_2), hemoglobin (Hgb), and to a lesser extent, partial pressure of oxygen (PaO_2).

MAXIMIZE CARDIAC OUTPUT

A significant number of patients with SIRS increase their CO as a compensatory response to meet increased cellular oxygen demands. However, a major pathological problem of SIRS is the increase in the permeability of the capillary bed. As a result, intravascular volume is difficult to maintain. This necessitates the liberal administration of fluids. Typically, a patient requires a combination of both crystalloid and colloid fluid replacement. Pharmacologic support also may be required to maximize CO. Fluid and drug choices are somewhat dependent on clinician preferences as well as the unique requirements of the patient.

MAXIMIZE OXYGENATION

Maintaining SaO_2 above 90% and PaO_2 above 60 mm Hg are acceptable goals.

HEMOGLOBIN

Sufficient hemoglobin is necessary to ensure adequate oxygen-carrying capacity. Disagreement exists as to the appropriate hemoglobin and hematocrit levels for this type of patient; however, as a general rule, 9 g of hemoglobin and 27% hematocrit are acceptable.

DECREASE OXYGEN DEMAND

Decreasing oxygen demand is an important aspect of maximizing oxygen delivery. Methods to reduce oxygen demand include:

1. Reducing tachycardia and tachypnea
2. Reducing hyperthermia
3. Alleviating pain

4. Preventing shivering
5. Providing comfort measures
6. Consolidating activities

By addressing these aspects of supply and demand, unnecessary oxygen consumption may be minimized, thus improving the supply to other tissues in greater need of oxygen.

Notice there has been no mention of maintaining an optimal blood pressure. The reason for this is that although maintenance of blood pressure is critical, adequate blood pressure does not imply adequate perfusion. For this reason, measurements of oxygen delivery and consumption are used to assess adequacy of perfusion, and not blood pressure alone. There is great variability in perfusion among patients with similar mean arterial pressures. A patient with a mean arterial pressure of 100 mm Hg may not have adequate tissue perfusion. In contrast, a patient with a mean arterial pressure of 50 may have sufficient tissue perfusion. The point is that an evaluation of perfusion should not be based on pressure assessment alone.

Supporting Dysfunctional Systems

An important objective in the management of SIRS and MODS is to support dysfunctional organ systems. Renal dysfunction, a common sequela of SIRS, is aggressively managed to prevent fluid and electrolyte imbalances, which contribute to the risk of death. Refer to the chapter in this book specific to each organ system for approaches used to support failing organs.

Evidence-Based Practice Strategies

New evidence-based practice guidelines for managing patients with severe sepsis highlight key recommendations including initial resuscitation to restore perfusion, organ system support, appropriate diagnostic studies, early administration of broad-spectrum antibiotic therapy, vasopressor and inotropic support, lung protective ventilation strategies, use of recombinant activated protein C, glucose control, and goal-directed therapy to improve outcomes for patients with severe sepsis (Table 11–5). Several of the evidence-based practice recommendations have direct implications for nursing care because they require monitoring and oversight. Control of glucose (blood glucose <110 mg/dL) in critically ill patients has been shown to decrease mortality rates and improve outcomes. The use of intravenous insulin to maintain tight glycemic control requires frequent monitoring of glucose (every 1 hour) and is a nurse-driven intervention. Recombinant activated protein C (Xigris) is indicated for patients with three or more SIRS criteria and evidence of early organ system dysfunction. Activated protein C has antithrombotic, anti-inflammatory, and profibrinolytic properties and potentially can correct the pathophysiologic alterations associated with severe sepsis. Identification of patients who are eligible for activated protein C therapy is an essential component of sepsis therapy, and the role of the nurse in monitoring patients receiving the therapy is essential to its optimal and appropriate use.

TABLE 11–5. EVIDENCED-BASED PRACTICE GUIDELINES: SURVIVING SEPSIS CAMPAIGN GUIDELINES FOR THE MANAGEMENT OF SEVERE SEPSIS

Initial resuscitation for sepsis-induced hypoperfusion	Goals: Central venous pressure of 8–12 mm Hg • Mean arterial pressure ≥65 mm Hg • Urine output ≥0.5 mL/kg/h • Central venous (superior vena cava or mixed venous oxygen saturation ≥70% Fluid challenge with crystalloids and/or colloids (e.g., 500–1000 mL of crystalloids or 300–500 mL of colloids over 30 minutes and repeated based on response (increase in blood pressure and urine output) and tolerance (evidence of intravascular volume overload) Administration of vasopressors when appropriate fluid challenge fails to restore adequate blood pressure and organ perfusion (e.g., norepinephrine) Transfusion of packed red blood cells to achieve a hematocrit of ≥30% Administration of inotropic infusion (e.g., dobutamine) to increase CO
Diagnosis	Obtain cultures: At least two blood cultures with one drawn percutaneously and one drawn through each vascular access device; obtain cultures of other sites such as urine, wounds, and respiratory secretions before initiating antibiotic therapy. Diagnostic studies (e.g., ultrasound, imaging studies)
Antibiotic therapy	Empirical antibiotics
Source control	Removal of potentially infected device, drainage of abscess, debridement of infected necrotic tissue
Enhance perfusion	Fluid therapy Vasopressors Inotropic therapy
Steroids	For patients with relative adrenal insufficiency
Recombinant human activated protein C (rhAPC)	For patients with sepsis-induced multiple organ failure with no absolute contra indication related to bleeding risk
Blood product administration	To target hemoglobin of 7.0–9.0 g/dL
Mechanical ventilation	Lung protective ventilation for acute lung injury/acute respiratory distress syndrome (e.g., low tidal volume 6 mL/kg of predicted body weight with the goal of maintaining end inspiratory plateau pressure <30 cm H_2O)
Sedation, analgesia, and neuromuscular blockade	To provide comfort yet avoid prolonged sedation
Glucose control	To maintain blood glucose <150 mg/dL
Renal replacement	For acute renal failure
Prophylaxis measures	Deep vein thrombosis Stress ulcer
Consideration for limitation of support	Discuss end-of-life care for critically ill patients Promote family communication to discuss use of life-sustaining therapies

Adapted from Dellinger, et al: Surviving Sepsis Campaign guidelines for management of severe sepsis and septic shock. Crit Care Med 2004;32:858–873.

Providing Nutritional Support

Nutritional support may be provided by the enteral or parenteral route, although the former is preferred. Most critically ill patients can tolerate a standard type of tube feeding or parenteral formula, with rare situations that require feeding modifications (e.g., volume overload, organ dysfunction, or gastrointestinal abnormalities). General guidelines for nutritional support include 25 to 35 kcal/kg per day for total caloric intake and 1.5 to 2.0 g protein/kg per day. It is helpful to have a nutrition specialist assist with nutritional planning. Refer to Chapter 14, Gastrointestinal System, for more on nutrition.

Providing Psychological Support

Chapter 1, Assessment of Critically Ill Patients and Families, and 2, Planning Care for Critically Ill Patients and Families, discuss many aspects of psychosocial support of critically ill patients and their families. Especially important is the appropriate and timely approach to end-of-life decisions and comfort care for patients with irreversible MODS (refer to Chapter 8, Ethical and Legal Considerations). Table 11–3 outlines important considerations for nursing care of patients with sepsis or MODS.

OVERDOSES

Drug or alcohol overdoses, as well as poisonings, can result in multiple organ dysfunction. Overdoses can be deliberate or accidental. Accidental overdose may involve one or multiple substances, and can be acute (e.g., inaccurate dosing of pediatric medications) or chronic (e.g., inadvertent, unnecessary dosing of asthma medication or over-the-counter medications). The level of intoxication or overdose varies with the element and amount ingested, the time until the patient is treated, and the underlying physical and emotional condition of the patient. The priority of care, as in all emergency situations, is maintenance of the patient's airway, breathing, and circulation.

Etiology, Risk Factors, and Pathophysiology

Alcohol Overdose

Alcohol overdose is most often seen in alcoholics, in young persons who have not yet reached legal drinking age, or in combination with other drugs as a suicidal gesture. There are four types of alcohol intoxication:

- Ethanol (ethyl or grain alcohol)
- Methanol (wood alcohol)
- Ethylene glycol (antifreeze)
- Isopropyl alcohol (rubbing alcohol)

Alcohol dissolves readily in the lipid components of the plasma membranes of the body, and thus enters the brain quickly, resulting in a rapid effect on the central nervous system.

In ethanol intoxication, serum levels range from 200 mg/dL (mild intoxication) to over 500 mg/dL (coma). A serum alcohol level of 100 mg/dL is the legal upper limit for driving a car in most of the United States.

In the case of methanol intoxication, serum levels range from 50 mg/dL (mild intoxication) to 100 mg/dL (severe intoxication). Metabolic acidosis manifests as a decreased bicarbonate level on arterial blood gas analysis, and indicates that the generation of hydrogen ions by the liver exceeds the ability of the kidney to excrete them. This excess of systemic hydrogen ions results in compensatory hyperventilation, as the body attempts to make the pH more alkaline. Refer to Chapter 5, Airway and Ventilatory Management, for further information on acid–base imbalance.

Ethylene glycol intoxication is characterized by neurologic depression, cardiopulmonary complications, pulmonary edema, and renal tubular degeneration. Serum chemistry reveals metabolic acidosis, as described, and renal toxicity. An aggregation of hydrogen ions can result in increased production and accumulation of lactic acid, which tends to impair renal function. Renal toxicity is suspected when the serum pH is below 7.35, serum creatinine is above 2.0 mg/dL, and blood urea nitrogen (BUN) is above 100 mg/dL.

Isopropyl alcohol intoxication is distinguished from other types of alcohol intoxication by the presence of ketoacids in both the urine and serum. Metabolic acidosis is a reflection of excess ketoacids, requiring buffering by the bicarbonate ions.

Clinical Presentation

Excess ingestion of any type of alcohol may cause central nervous system symptoms such as sluggish reflexes, emotional instability, or out-of-character behavior. Amnesia may result for events that occurred during the period of intoxication. Unconsciousness usually occurs before a person can drink enough for fatal consequences to occur, but the rapid consumption of alcohol can cause death by either respiratory depression or aspiration during vomiting. There are signs and symptoms that are specific to each type of alcohol ingested. Descriptions follow.

- *Acute ethanol intoxication:* Muscular incoordination, slurred speech, stupor, hypoglycemia, flushing, seizures, coma, depressed respirations, and hyporeflexia
- *Methanol intoxication:* Neurologic depression, metabolic acidosis, and visual disturbances
- *Ethylene glycol intoxication:* Neurologic depression, cardiopulmonary complications, pulmonary edema, and renal tubular degeneration
- *Isopropyl intoxication:* Neurologic depression, areflexia, respiratory depression, hypothermia, hypotension, and gastrointestinal distress

Diagnostic Tests

A differential diagnosis to rule out other medical conditions, such as hypoglycemia or hyperglycemia, which may mimic

AT THE BEDSIDE
Alcohol Overdose

A 19-year-old man is brought to the ED by his roommates who state that he became unresponsive after drinking at a party. Your initial assessment reveals a depressed level of consciousness, with decreased response to stimuli. While reviewing his initial serum chemistry results, you note that the serum alcohol level is 430 mg/dL. Current vital signs are:

T	97.8°F rectal
HR	120

Sinus tachycardia

RR	16
BP	92/70, pulse oximetry 94%

Discussion Questions

1. What are the priority areas for care for this patient?
2. What information would help to guide the treatment?

Answers

1. Maintenance of airway, stabilization of the patient, establish IV access, provide fluids, and provide detoxification.
2. Amount and type of alcohol ingested, time frame since ingestion (gastric lavage is best considered within 1 hour of ingestion).

Drug Overdose

Drug overdose may involve any type of medication. The majority of overdoses involve analgesics, antidepressants, sedatives, cough and cold drugs, and street drugs (e.g., cocaine, crack cocaine, PCP, LSD). Street drugs are used to induce a relaxed state, elevate mood, or to produce unusual states of consciousness. Psychoactive drugs often are chemically similar to neurotransmitters such as serotonin, dopamine, and norepinephrine, and act by either directly or indirectly altering neurotransmitter–receptor interactions. Medullary inspiratory neurons are highly sensitive to depression by drugs, especially barbiturates and morphine, and death from an overdose of these agents is often secondary to respiratory arrest. Refer to Table 11–6 for presenting signs and symptoms of common agents of drug overdose.

TABLE 11–6. SIGNS AND SYMPTOMS OF OVERDOSE

Opioids	• Change in LOC • Respiratory depression, aspiration • Hypotension • Miosis • Decreased gastric motility
Barbiturates	• Decreased LOC • Hypothermia
Sedatives	• Respiratory depression • Hypnotics • Shock • Cardiac dysrhythmias • Pulmonary edema
Cocaine	• Hyperexcitability • Headache • Hypertension • Tachycardia • Nausea/vomiting, abdominal pain • Fever • Delirium, convulsions, coma
PCP (phenylcyclidine)	• Violent behavior • Hallucinations • Seizures • Rhabdomyolysis • Hypertensive crisis
LSD	• Severe agitation • Dilated pupils • Hallucinations
Tricyclics	• Seizures • Coma • Dysrhythmias, ECG changes • Heart failure • Shock
Salicylates	• Tinnitus • Vertigo • Vomiting • Hyperthermia • Altered mental status
Acetaminophen	• GI distress • Hepatotoxicity • Hepatic necrosis

overdose or intoxication, is an important component of the initial assessment. Because alcohol ingestion interferes with the liver's ability to produce glucose, alcohol-induced hypoglycemia in the intoxicated patient is fairly common.

Prior to obtaining any diagnostic test, it is extremely important to obtain a history either from the patient, family member, friend, or the person who found the patient to determine the probable substance that was ingested. Once the substance is potentially identified there are diagnostic tests helpful in aiding the treatment of patients following alcohol intoxication. These include:

- Ethanol and methanol serum levels. These are elevated if they were ingested. Most labs can run these tests. Isopropyl serum levels are not run as commonly as ethanol and methanol levels.
- Serum creatinine and BUN levels. These may be elevated due to renal dysfunction.
- Liver function studies. The hepatotoxic effects of certain types of alcohol result in abnormal levels.
- Serum glucose and electrolytes. These are often abnormal as described previously.

Clinical Presentation

The specific signs and symptoms of drug overdose depend on the substance ingested. However, there are several signs and symptoms that are commonly seen in most patients. These include changes in mental status (typically, decreased level of consciousness), behavioral changes, and respiratory depression. The signs and symptoms of drug overdose for particular drugs are summarized in Table 11–6.

Diagnostic Tests

Diagnostic studies for patients following drug overdose include the following:

- Toxicology screen, which can be either broad-spectrum tests, including testing for the presence of such substances as amphetamines, barbiturates, benzodiazepines, and narcotics, or specific screens, if the substance is known. Generally these are urine studies.
- Arterial blood gas, to determine the acid–base status.
- Serum glucose and electrolytes, which can be abnormal.

Principles of Management for Overdose

The principles of management of patients following alcohol intoxication or drug overdose are similar. An initial clinical evaluation is conducted with the priority of resuscitating and stabilizing the patient. The principles of management include maintenance of a patent airway, prevention of complications, elimination of ingested substances or toxic metabolites, and maintenance of hemodynamic stability. Specific treatment depends on the agent, route and amount of exposure, and the severity of overdose.

Maintenance of Patent Airway

1. Maintain adequate minute ventilation. Stimulate the patient to breathe. If the patient cannot spontaneously maintain minute ventilation, intubation and mechanical ventilation may be required.
2. Monitor pulse oximetry and blood gas values.
3. Position the patient on their side with the head of the bed elevated >30 degrees if tolerated.
4. Suction the patient's airway as needed.

Circulation and Maintenance of Hemodynamic Stability

1. Ensure venous access (large-bore peripheral or central access).
2. Administer isotonic fluid to maintain intravascular fluid volume. If hypotension is unresponsive to volume expansion, treatment with vasopressors may be necessary.
3. Obtain a 12-lead ECG and maintain on continuous cardiac monitoring.
4. Treatment of arrhythmias: Supraventricular tachycardia with hypertension due to sympathetic nervous system response can be managed with a combination

of beta-blocker and vasodilator therapy (e.g., esmolol and nitroprusside), combined alpha- and beta-blocker (labetalol), or a calcium channel blocker (verapamil or diltiazem). Lidocaine or amiodarone may be used for ventricular tachyarrhythmias.

Neurologic Depression

1. Measure glucose to rule out hypoglycemia and treat with 50% glucose IV if necessary.
2. Evaluate for carbon monoxide poisoning (carboxyhemoglobin), provide oxygen.
3. Administer thiamine (IV for Wernicke's syndrome).
4. Naloxone IV or IM.
5. Flumazenil for benzodiazepine overdose (avoid in those who have potential for seizures).

Catharsis, Clearing Drugs, and Antidotes

1. Ipecac to induce vomiting (in alert patients) can be used for home or prehospital management for ingestants except for caustic acids and alkalis. It is rarely used in the hospital setting and there is little evidence that ipecac prevents drug absorption or systemic toxicity.
2. Gastric lavage decreases ingestant absorption and significant amounts of ingested drug can be recovered the closer that lavage is performed to ingestion. Gastric lavage is contraindicated in corrosive ingestions due to risk of gastroesophageal perforation and with hydrocarbons due to the risk of aspiration-induced hydrocarbon pneumonitis.
3. Activated charcoal: most drugs! Charcoal absorbs ingestants within the gut lumen, allowing the charcoal–toxin complex to be eliminated in the stool. Charcoal is not recommended for patients who have ingested caustic acids and alkalis, alcohols, lithium, or heavy metals.
4. Hemodialysis and hemoperfusion for severe drug intoxication for selected substances. Hemodialysis can be considered for severe poisoning due to methanol, ethylene glycol, salicylates, and lithium. Hemoperfusion, which involves the passage of blood through an absorptive-containing cartridge (usually charcoal), may be indicated for intoxications with carbamazepine, phenobarbital, phenytoin, and theophylline.
5. Renal dialysis: Dialysis may be indicated in cases of severe poisoning due to barbiturates, bromide, chloral hydrate, ethanol, ethylene glycol, isopropyl alcohol, lithium, methanol, procainamide, theophylline, salicylates, and possibly heavy metals. Refer to Chapter 15, Renal System, for more on renal replacement therapies.
6. Methanol: Practice guidelines have been developed by the American Academy of Clinical Toxicology for the treatment of methanol overdose. Folinic acid

(leucovorin) in a dose of 1 mg/kg up to 50 mg every 4 to 6 hours for 24 hours is suggested in methanol poisoning to provide the cofactor for formic acid elimination. Gastric lavage may be considered within 1 hour of ingestion. Activated charcoal does not absorb alcohols, but it may be appropriate to administer if other drugs are suspected. To prevent metabolism of alcohols to toxic metabolites, ethanol can be administered orally or intravenously to maintain a blood concentration of 100 to 150 mg/dL. Hemodialysis is often necessary to remove the alcohol and toxic metabolites and is continued until the acidosis is resolved.

Antidotes

Antidotes help to counteract the effects of poisons by neutralizing them or by antagonizing their effects. Poisons or conditions with specific antidotes include the following:

- Acetaminophen: *N*-acetylcysteine
- Opiates: naloxone
- Benzodiazepines: flumazenil
- Digoxin: digiband
- Cyanide: kelocyanor
- Tricyclic antidepressants: sodium bicarbonate
- Beta-blockers or calcium channel blockers: glucagon and calcium

Preventing Complications

1. Orient the patient to surroundings.
2. Insert a nasogastric tube for stomach decompression and for the delivery of charcoal or other antidotes.
3. Keep the head of the bed elevated to prevent aspiration.
4. Pad bed side rails and restrain the patient as necessary to prevent self-injury.
5. Provide support to the patient and family.

SELECTED BIBLIOGRAPHY

SIRS, Sepsis, and MODS

ACCP/SCCM: ACCP/SCCM consensus conference: Definitions for sepsis and organ failure and guidelines for the use of innovative therapies in sepsis. *Crit Care Med* 1992;20(6):864–874.

Ahrens T, Vollman K: Severe sepsis management are we doing enough? *Crit Care Nurse* 2003;23(5 Suppl):2–1.

Angus DC, Linde-Zwirble WT, Lidicker J, et al: Epidemiology of severe sepsis in the United States: Analysis of incidence, outcome, and associated costs of care. *Crit Care Med* 2001;29:1303–1310.

Balk RA: Pathogenesis and management of multiple organ dysfunction or failure in severe sepsis and septic shock. *Crit Care Clin* 2000;16;337–352.

Balk RA, Goyette RE: The multiple organ dysfunction syndrome in patients with severe sepsis: more than just inflammation. In Balk RA (ed): *Diagnosis and Management of the Patient with Severe Sepsis.* London: Royal Society of Medicine; 2003.

Bernard GR, Vincent JL, Laterre PF, et al: Efficacy and safety of recombinant human activated protein C for severe sepsis. *N Engl J Med* 2001;344:699–709.

Cunneen J, Cartwright M: The puzzle of sepsis. *AACN Clinical Issues* 2004;15:18–44.

Dellinger RP, Carlet JM, Masur H, et al: Surviving Sepsis Campaign guidelines for management of severe sepsis and septic shock. *Crit Care Med* 2004;32:858–872.

Ely EW, Kleinpell RM, Goyette RE: Advances in the understanding of clinical manifestations and therapy of severe sepsis: An update for critical care nurses. *Am J Crit Care* 2003;12(2):120–133.

Hotchkiss RS, Karl IE: The pathophysiology and treatment of sepsis. *N Engl J Med* 2003;348:138–150.

Huddleston VB: *Multisystem Organ Failure. Pathophysiology and Clinical Implications.* St. Louis, MO: Mosby; 1996.

Kleinpell R: Advances in treating patients with severe sepsis: Role of Drotrecogin Alfa (activated). *Crit Care Nurse* 2003;23(3):16–29.

Kleinpell R: The role of the critical care nurse in the assessment and management of the patient with severe sepsis. *Crit Care Nurs Clin North Am* 2003;15(1):27–34.

Levy MM, Fink MP, Marshall JC, et al: 2001 SCCM/ESICM/ACCP/ATS/SIS International Sepsis Definitions Conference. *Crit Care Med* 2003;31(4):1250–1256.

Pronovost P, Berenholtz S: *Improving Sepsis Care in the Intensive Care Unit: An Evidence-Based Approach.* 2004 VHA Research Series. Available: https://www.vha.com/research/public/sepsis_icu.pdf/.

Wheeler AP, Bernard GR: Treating patients with severe sepsis. *N Engl J Med* 1999;340:207–214.

Overdose

American Academy of Clinical Toxicology: American Academy of Clinical Toxicology practice guidelines on the treatment of methanol poisoning. *J Toxicol Clin Toxicol* 2002;40:415–446.

Coughlin C: Poison control: Patient assessment and management. *Emerg Med Services* 2002;31(4):66–71.

Dargan PI, Wallace CI, Jones AL: An evidence based flowchart to guide the management of acute salicylate (aspirin) overdose. *Emerg Med J* 2002;19(3):206–209.

Goldfrank LR, Flomenbaum NE, Lewin NA, et al (eds): *Goldfrank's Toxicologic Emergencies,* 7th ed. New York: McGraw-Hill; 2002.

Hamm J. Acute acetaminophen overdose in adolescents and adults. *Crit Care Nurse* 2000;20(3):69–74.

Harrison's Online 2004. Available: http://harrisons.accessmedicine.com/.

Isbister GK, Downes F, Sibbritt D, et al: Aspiration pneumonitis in an overdose population: frequency, predictors, and outcomes. *Crit Care Med* 2004;32(1):88–93.

Jenkins JL, Braen GR (eds): *Manual of Emergency Medicine.* Philadelphia: Lippincott, Williams & Wilkins; 1999.

Mokhlesi B, Leiken JB, Murray P, Corbridge TC: Adult toxicology in critical care: Part I: General approach to the intoxicated patient. *Chest* 2003;123:577–592.

Mokhlesi B, Leikin JB, Murray P, Corbridge TC: Adult toxicology in critical care: Part II: Specific poisonings. *Chest* 2003;123;897–922.

Newberry L, Sheehy SB (eds): *Sheehy's Emergency Nursing,* 3rd ed. St. Louis, MO: Mosby; 2002.

Nursing 2004 Drug Handbook. Philadelphia: Lippincott; 2004.

Olson KR: *Poisoning and Drug Overdose.* New York: McGraw-Hill; 2003.

Parsons PE: Respiratory failure as a result of drugs, overdoses, and poisonings. *Clin Chest Med* 1994;15(1):93–102.

Soloway RAG: Street-smart advice on treating drug overdoses. *Am J Nurs* 1993;93(4):65–71.

Sue YJ, Shannon M: Pharmacokinetics of drugs in overdose. *Clin Pharm* 1992;23(2):93–105.

Tibbles PM, Perrotta PL: Treatment of carbon monoxide poisoning: A critical review of human outcome studies comparing normobaric oxygen with hyperbaric oxygen. *Ann Emerg Med* 1994; 24(2):269–276.

Verdile VP, Dean BS, Krenzelok EP: Hyperbaric therapy for carbon monoxide poisoning. *Am J Emerg Med* 1994;12(3):389–390.

Weinman SA: Emergency management of drug overdose. *Crit Care Nurse* 1993;13(6):45–51.

Zimmerman JL: Poisonings and overdoses in the intensive care unit: general and specific management issues. *Crit Care Med* 2003;31(12):2794–801.

NEUROLOGIC SYSTEM

Twelve 12

Dea Mahanes

▶ Knowledge Competencies

1. Correlate neurologic assessments to patient problems and diagnostic findings.
2. Identify indications for, complications of, and nursing management of commonly used neurodiagnostic tests.
3. Identify causes of increased intracranial pressure and describe strategies for management.

4. Compare and contrast the etiology, pathophysiology, clinical presentation, patient needs, and nursing management for:
   - Acute ischemic stroke
   - Hemorrhagic stroke
   - Seizure disorders
   - CNS infections
   - Selected neuromuscular diseases

SPECIAL ASSESSMENT TECHNIQUES, DIAGNOSTIC TESTS, AND MONITORING SYSTEMS

Although there is no single method of performing a neurologic evaluation, a systematic, orderly approach offers the best results. Knowledge of neurologic disease processes and neuroanatomy allows the critical care nurse to tailor the assessment to individual patients. Obtaining past medical history and history of present illness or injury is essential and includes preexisting neurologic conditions. The time of symptom onset and mechanism of injury have important implications for diagnostic testing and treatment. The administration of any medications that may potentially alter the neurologic examination, especially sedatives and neuromuscular blockers, is also noted.

Serial assessments, coupled with accurate documentation, allow for detection of subtle changes in neurologic status. Early detection of changes permits rapid intervention and improves patient outcomes. Neurologic assessment in the critical care unit can be broken down into the following components: level of consciousness, mental status, motor examination, sensory examination, and cranial nerve examination. A baseline examination is established and subsequent assessments are compared. At a minimum, serial neurologic assessment includes level of consciousness, orientation, pupillary changes, and motor response.

Level of Consciousness

There are two components to level of consciousness: arousal and awareness. *Arousal* refers to the state of wakefulness; *awareness* reflects the content and quality of interactions with the environment. Arousal reflects function of the reticular activating system and brainstem, and awareness indicates functioning of the cerebral cortex. Level of consciousness is assessed on all patients unless they are pharmacologically sedated and paralyzed. A change in level of consciousness is the most important indicator of neurologic decline and is immediately acted on by the health care team.

Observation of the patient's behavior, appearance, and ability to communicate is the first step in assessing level of consciousness. If the patient responds meaningfully to the examiner without the need for stimulation, then the patient is described as *alert*. If stimulation is required, auditory stimuli are used first. If the patient does not rouse to auditory stimuli, gentle tactile stimuli such as a gentle touch or shake are used, followed by painful stimuli if necessary to elicit a response. Accepted methods of central painful stimulus include squeezing the trapezius or pectoralis major muscle. Supraorbital pressure is also an acceptable pain stimulus, but is not used if there is any suspicion of facial fracture. Use of a sternal rub may result in a motor response that is difficult to interpret (see Glasgow Coma Scale) and often causes bruising. Response to central stimulus is more indicative of cerebral function than peripheral stimulus. Nail bed pressure is a commonly used peripheral pain stimulus. Certain responses to peripheral pain, such as the triple flexion response (flexion of the ankle, knee, and hip), can result from a spinal reflex arc and thus remain present even following death by neurologic criteria (formally called *brain death*).

A variety of terms are used to describe level of consciousness, including *alert, confused, lethargic, obtunded, stuporous,* and *comatose* (Table 12–1). These terms are often misinterpreted, but are included because they are commonly used. It is more useful to describe the patient's response to a particular stimulus such as "no response to verbal stimuli, but opens eyes and localizes with left arm when the right trapezius muscle is squeezed."

Glasgow Coma Scale

The Glasgow Coma Scale (Table 12–2) is used to monitor neurologic status in critically ill patients because it provides a standardized approach to assessing and documenting level of consciousness. Response is determined in three categories: eye opening, verbal response, and motor response. The best response in each category is scored, and the results are added to give a total Glasgow Coma score. Scores range from 3 to 15, with 15 indicating a patient that is alert, fully oriented, and following commands. Coma is generally described as a score of 8 or less.

The eye opening score reflects the amount of stimulation that must be applied for the patient to open his eyes.

TABLE 12–1. DEFINITIONS FOR COMMON TERMS USED TO DESCRIBE LEVEL OF CONSCIOUSNESS

Term	Definition
Alert	Awake and fully conscious: able to demonstrate reliable and responsive behavior.
Confused	Disoriented to time, place, or person; agitation, restlessness, or irritability may be present.
Lethargic	Orientation to time, place, and person, but has a sluggish response time for speech, motor, or cognitive activities.
Obtunded	Arousable with stimulation: responds verbally or follows simple commands with stimulation; else appears sleepy.
Stuporous	Minimal interaction with environment except when maximally stimulated with repeated noxious stimuli; responds with grunts or incomprehensible sounds.
Comatose	Appears to be sleeping; generally has no appropriate interactions with the environment, even with repeated noxious stimuli.

TABLE 12–2. GLASGOW COMA SCALE

Behavior	Score[a]
Eye Opening (E)	
Spontaneous	4
To speech	3
To pain	2
None	1
Motor Response (M)	
Obeys commands	6
Localizes pain	5
Withdraws to pain	4
Abnormal flexion	3
Extensor response	2
None	1
Verbal Response (V)	
Oriented	5
Confused	4
Inappropriate words	3
Incomprehensible sounds	2
None	1

[a]*Coma score = E + M + V (scores range from 3–15).*

Spontaneous eye opening is the best response (4), followed by eye opening to verbal stimulation, then eye opening to painful stimulation. Scoring of the eye opening section of the scale can be complicated by orbital trauma and swelling, and this is documented accordingly.

The motor portion of the Glasgow Coma Scale is the most difficult to assess. Response in each extremity is tested, but only the best motor response is used in calculating a total score. The patient is first asked to follow a command such as "Hold up your thumb" or "Wiggle your toes." A patient who does not follow commands in her or his extremities is asked to look up and down. In certain neurologic disorders (such as basilar artery stroke or high cervical spinal cord injury), the patient may be unable to follow commands with their extremities but still be awake and aware; assessing the ability to look up and down helps to identify these individuals. If the patient does not follow commands, then all four extremities are assessed for response to pain stimuli. Upper extremity response to pain is described as localization, withdrawal, decorticate (flexor) posturing, or decerebrate (extensor) posturing. An attempt by the patient to push the stimulus away is clearly localization, but the response is not always easily apparent. Unfortunately, the interpretation of the response is complicated when a sternal rub is used because with both localization and decorticate posturing, the arms move up toward the stimulus. Reaching across the midline of the body to a stimulus (e.g., if the right arm comes up to the left shoulder when a left trapezius squeeze is applied) is scored as localization. An easy way to remember decorticate and decerebrate posturing is that decorticate is "into the core," or flexion, and decerebrate is away from the body, or extension (Figure 12–1). Decorticate posturing signifies that there is damage in the cerebral hemispheres or

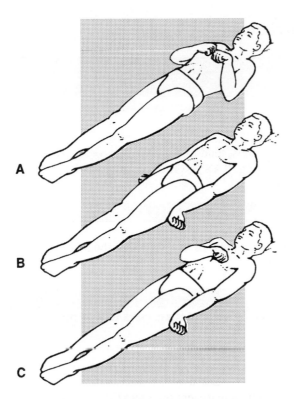

Figure 12–1. Abnormal motor responses. **(A)** Decorticate posturing. **(B)** Decerebrate posturing. **(C)** Decorticate posturing on right side and decerebrate posturing on left side of body. (*Reprinted from Carlson BA: Neurologic clinical assessment. In Urden LD, Stacy KM, Lough ME [eds]: Thelan's Critical Care Nursing: Diagnosis and Management. St. Louis, MO: Mosby; 2002, p. 649.*)

thalamus. Decerebrate posturing indicates damage to the midbrain or pons. The presence of posturing or a change from decorticate to decerebrate posturing should be brought to the attention of the physician immediately. Motor response to pain in the lower extremities is usually graded as withdrawal or triple flexion. In triple flexion, pain stimulus results in stereotypical flexion of the ankle, knee, and hip. This response can be differentiated from withdrawal by applying the pain stimulus to a different area of the lower extremity (e.g., the inside of the knee). If the response is withdrawal, the patient pulls away from the stimulus. If the response is triple flexion, the response is still stereotypical flexion at the ankle, knee, and hip.

The verbal section of the Glasgow Coma Scale assesses a patient's ability to speak coherently and with appropriate content. Orientation to person, place, and time (temporal orientation) is assessed. As mental status declines, temporal orientation is lost first, followed by orientation to place. Orientation to person is seldom lost prior to loss of consciousness. Patients with an endotracheal tube or tracheostomy are commonly assigned a verbal score of *T* and the total GCS is denoted as the sum of the eye opening and motor scores followed by *T*.

Mental Status

Although formal assessments of mental status exist, many critical care patients are unable to complete these assessments because of limited ability to communicate or decreased level of consciousness. Orientation is the component of mental status most often evaluated in the critical care unit. Other components of mental status assessment include attention/concentration, affect, memory, reasoning, and language function. Attention/concentration, affect, and reasoning are typically assessed informally by simply observing the patient throughout daily care. The Confusion Assessment Method for the Intensive Care Unit (described below and in Figure 12–2) includes a more formal assessment of attention. Short-term memory may be evaluated by giving the patient a list of three items and asking him or her to recall them later in the day. However, deficits are often apparent in informal interactions as well. Difficulty with language can be described as *dysarthria* (weakness or lack of coordination of muscles of speech) or *aphasia*. Aphasia can be either expressive (inability to express thoughts), receptive (inability to comprehend), or global (both expressive and receptive). An individual with expressive aphasia may be able to understand everything that is said but be unable to reply, whereas an individual with receptive aphasia may have nonsensical, fluent speech, but cannot comprehend what is said to him. A patient with dysarthria has slurred speech and is difficult to understand, but the content of the speech is appropriate.

Delirium is an alteration in mental status that is of particular importance in general intensive care patients, because the development of delirium is associated with worse clinical outcomes and increased hospitalization costs. Delirium is characterized by acute changes or fluctuations in mental status, inattention, disorganized thinking, and altered level of consciousness. Delirium is usually rapid in onset and reversible. In contrast, *dementia* is a progressive, irreversible loss of intellectual or cognitive abilities like reasoning, math, or abstract thinking and develops more slowly. Delirium and dementia are not mutually exclusive; a patient with mild to moderate dementia may exhibit delirium in the unfamiliar environment of the intensive care unit (ICU). Many tests of delirium are available, but most are difficult to administer in the intensive care setting. The Confusion Assessment Method for the Intensive Care Unit (CAM-ICU) was developed specifically for use in critically ill patients and can be administered to patients receiving mechanical ventilation. The CAM-ICU can be quickly administered and has demonstrated reliability and validity.

Contributing factors to the development of delirium include systemic illness (infection, fever, or metabolic dysfunction), electrolyte abnormalities, the administration of medications including sedative-hypnotics or analgesics, sleep deprivation, and withdrawal from alcohol or other substances. Delirium is more common in elderly patients. The first step in treating delirium is to rule out reversible causes.

CAM-ICU Worksheet

CAM-ICU Features and Descriptions		
1. Acute Onset or Fluctuating Course	**Absent**	**Present**

A. Is there evidence of an acute change in mental status from the baseline?

OR

B. Did the (abnormal) behavior fluctuate during the past 24 hours, that is, tend to come and go, or increase and decrease in severity as evidenced by fluctuation on a sedation scale (e.g. RASS), GCS, or previous delirium assessment?

2. Inattention	**Absent**	**Present**

Did the patient have difficulty focusing attention as evidenced by **scores *less than 8*** on either the auditory or visual component of the **Attention Screening Examination (ASE)**?

3. Disorganized Thinking	**Absent**	**Present**

Is there evidence of disorganized or incoherent thinking as evidenced by **incorrect answers to 2 or more of the 4 questions and/or inability to follow the commands**?

Questions (Alternate Set A and Set B):

Set A	Set B
1. Will a stone float on water?	1. Will a leaf float on water?
2. Are there fish in the sea?	2. Are there elephants in the sea?
3. Does one pound weigh more than two pounds?	3. Do two pounds weigh more than one pound?
4. Can you use a hammer to pound a nail?	4. Can you use a hammer to cut wood?

Other:
1. Are you having any unclear thinking?
2. Hold up this many fingers. (Examiner holds two fingers in front of patient)
3. Now do the same thing with the other hand. (Not repeating the number of fingers)

4. Altered Level of Consciousness	**Absent**	**Present**

Is the patient's level of consciousness anything *other than alert* such as vigilant, lethargic, or stupor? (e.g., RASS other than "0" at time of assessment)

Alert   spontaneously fully aware of environment and interacts appropriately

Vigilant   hyperalert

Lethargic   drowsy but easily aroused, unaware of some elements in the environment, or not spontaneously interacting appropriately with the interviewer; becomes fully aware and appropriately interactive when prodded minimally

Stupor   becomes incompletely aware when prodded strongly; can be aroused only by vigorous and repeated stimuli, and as soon as the stimulus ceases, stuporous subject lapse back into the unresponsive state

Overall CAM-ICU (Features 1 and 2 and either Feature 3 or 4):	**Yes**	**No**

Figure 12–2. Confusion Assessment Method for the Intensive Care Unit (CAM-ICU) Worksheet. Delirium is diagnosed when both I and II are positive, along with either III or IV. (*With permission from E. Wesley Ely, MD, MPH, Vanderbilt University, Nashville, TN, 2002; complete training manual is available at www.ICUdelirium.org*).

Nursing strategies to decrease the effects of delirium include minimizing stimulation in agitated patients, promoting normal sleep–wake cycles, ensuring that assistive devices such as hearing aids and glasses are available, treating pain, and family presence. Family members are educated regarding the condition and provided with guidance in how to interact (speak clearly, provide frequent reorientation, and avoid unnecessary conversation). Attempts are made to avoid the use of restraints unless patient or staff safety is compromised, because this may only add to the patient's confusion and apprehension. In addition to environmental controls, neuroleptic medications such as haloperidol may be useful in the management of delirium.

Patients with organic brain disease, regardless of specific diagnosis, often exhibit challenging behaviors. Examples include agitation, emotional lability, and disinhibition. This can be very disconcerting to family members, especially when the patient has not exhibited these behaviors previously. Dealing with agitated, confused patients can be frustrating for staff as well. Although medicating the patient can be useful, many drugs alter neurologic assessment. Environmental strategies such as decreasing noise and distractions may be very effective and are used when possible.

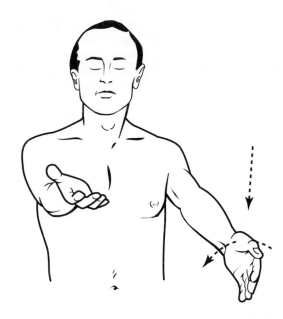

Figure 12–3. Assessment of pronator drift. The patient is asked to hold her or his arms outstretched with the palms supinated and eyes closed. If weakness is present, the weak arm gradually pronates and drifts downward. (*Reprinted from Lindsay KW, Bone I, Callander R:* Neurology and Neurosurgery Illustrated. *New York: Churchill Livingstone; 1997, p. 19.*)

Motor Assessment

Motor assessment includes muscle size, tone, strength, and involuntary movements such as tics or tremors. Motor function is assessed in each extremity. In patients who are able to follow commands, pronator drift is an excellent indicator of upper extremity motor function. Instruct the patient to close his or her eyes and raise his or her arms with the palms facing the ceiling. A normal response is for the patient to maintain this position until told to stop. Patients with focal motor weakness demonstrate varying degrees of pronator drift. Depending on the severity of weakness, the affected side may drift away from its initial position quickly or slowly, or the palm may simply begin to supinate (Figure 12–3). Further assessment of upper extremity strength in cooperative patients involves testing the deltoids, biceps, triceps, and grips. Lower extremity testing includes the hamstrings, quadriceps, dorsiflexion, and plantarflexion. Strength is rated on a 5-point scale (Table 12–3). Motor assessment for patients with spinal cord injury is more complex and is described in Chapter 21, Advanced Neurologic Concepts. In patients who do not follow commands, motor assessment consists of first observing the patient for spontaneous movement. If necessary, a pain stimulus is applied and the patient's response is observed. The response is graded numerically as part of the Glasgow Coma Scale, but may also be described as purposeful, nonpurposeful, or no response.

In an awake, alert patient, complete motor assessment includes testing of coordination, which includes cerebellar function. Common testing mechanisms applicable to the crit-

ical care environment include assessment of rapid alternating movements, finger to nose testing, and the heel slide test. To test rapid alternating movements, ask the patient to supinate and pronate his hands (one extremity at a time) as quickly as possible. In finger to nose testing, the patient is instructed to repeatedly touch his nose, then the examiner's finger. To assess the lower extremities, ask the patient to run the heel of his foot up and down the shin of his opposite leg as quickly as possible. Patients with cerebellar dysfunction display decreased speed and accuracy on these tests.

Sensation

With the exception of patients with suspected spinal cord dysfunction or Guillain-Barré syndrome, nursing assessment of sensation is typically limited in the ICU. There are three sensory pathways: pain/temperature, position/vibration, and light touch. Light touch is the pathway most often assessed

TABLE 12–3. EVALUATION OF MUSCLE STRENGTH

Grade	Definition
0	No movement
1	Muscle contraction only (palpated or visible)
2	Active movement within a single plane (gravity eliminated)
3	Active movement against gravity
4	Active movement against some resistance
5	Active movement against full resistance (normal strength)

in the ICU, but may be preserved even if lesions of the spinal cord exist because of overlapping innervation. Because most patients with intracranial lesions report altered sensation in an entire extremity or one side of the body, assessment of light touch is likely to identify these patients. Ask the patient to close his or her eyes, and lightly touch each extremity working distal to proximal. Facial sensation is also tested and includes all three branches of cranial nerve V (the trigeminal nerve). The three distributions can be tested by touching the forehead, cheek, and mandible.

When a more comprehensive nursing assessment is indicated, testing for pain and position sense provide useful information. A cotton tip applicator with a wooden stem can be broken and used; the end with the cotton is dull and the broken end is sharp. Touch the patient's skin lightly in a random pattern and ask the patient to identify the sensation as sharp or dull. Two seconds should elapse between stimuli and the patient's eyes should remain closed during the assessment. To test position sense, or proprioception, move the patient's index finger or big toe up or down by grasping the digit laterally over the joints. Provide an example of both "up" and "down" positions prior to testing. Repeat these movements in a random order, asking the patient to identify whether the joint is up or down. Always return to the neutral position between movements and carefully grasp the digit to avoid giving the patient clues. Proprioception is tested with the patient's eyes closed. Documentation of comprehensive sensory assessment is best accomplished using a dermatome chart (Figure 12–4). Areas of abnormal sensation can be marked and tracked over time.

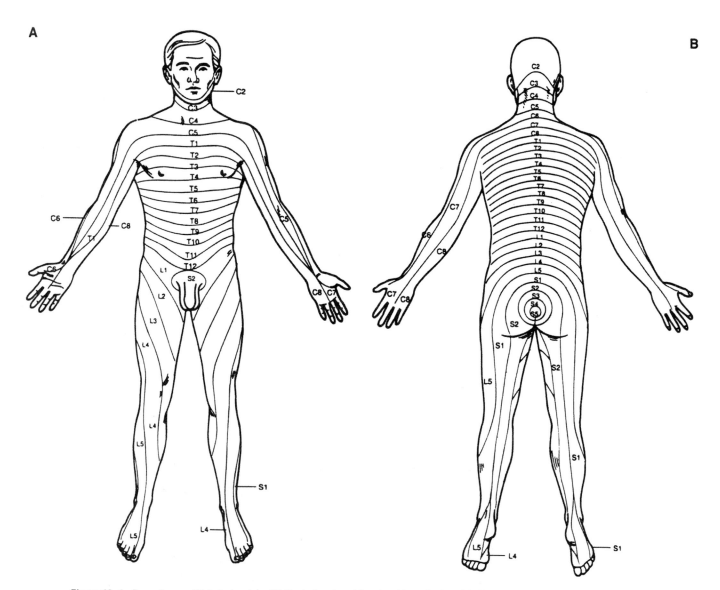

Figure 12–4. Dermatomes. **(A)** Anterior view. **(B)** Posterior view. (*Reprinted from Carlson BA: Neurologic anatomy and physiology. In Urden LD, Stacy KM, Lough ME [eds]: Thelan's Critical Care Nursing: Diagnosis and Management. St. Louis, MO: Mosby; 2002, p. 641.*)

Cranial Nerve Assessment and Assessment of Brainstem Function

Assessment of the cranial nerves provides an indication of the integrity of the nerves themselves and of brainstem function. Cranial nerve assessment can be very complex, but in-depth nursing assessment of each cranial nerve is not realistic or necessary in most critical care patients. A screening examination based on pupillary response and protective reflexes (corneal, gag, cough) is conducted on all patients. Beyond that, the assessment can be customized to the individual based on pathology. Patients with brainstem, cerebellar, or pituitary lesions merit more extensive assessment because of the proximity of the cranial nerves to these structures. The assessments noted below are the most commonly performed tests of cranial nerve function in the critical care unit. Table 12–4 describes the function of all 12 cranial nerves.

Pupil Size and Reaction to Light

Pupillary changes are often seen late in the course of neurologic decline as increased intracranial pressure (ICP) leads to compression of cranial nerve III. Pupils are assessed for size, shape, and reaction to light. Pupils are measured in millimeters, not described by words such as *large, small, pinpoint,* or *blown*. Reaction to light is described as *brisk, sluggish,* or *fixed/nonreactive*. Both eyes are tested for direct and consensual response. To test direct pupillary response, shine a light directly into one eye and observe the response of the pupil in that eye. A normal response is brisk constriction followed by brisk dilation when the light is withdrawn. To test

for consensual pupillary response, shine a light into one eye and observe the pupil of the other eye. It should constrict and dilate similarly. A device (ForSite Pupillometer, Medtronic, Inc) has been developed to objectively quantify pupil size and speed of reaction, but is not in widespread use. Certain medications can affect pupil size and reactivity. For example, atropine can dilate the pupils and narcotics can cause them to become very constricted. Commonly used neuromuscular blockers do not affect pupillary reaction.

Corneal Reflex

The corneal reflex evaluates cranial nerves V (trigeminal) and VII (facial). This test is classically performed with a wisp of cotton lightly drawn across the cornea; a normal response is a blink. A drop of sterile saline can also be used as a stimulus and is less likely to cause corneal abrasions. Patients with cranial nerve VII dysfunction are often unable to completely close their eyes. Strategies to prevent corneal injury include the use of lubricating drops and ointments or taping the lid closed.

Gag and Cough Reflexes

The ability to swallow and the gag reflex are controlled by cranial nerves IX (glossopharyngeal) and X (vagus). To assess the gag reflex in a conscious patient, first explain the procedure and be sure the patient does not have a full stomach. Ask the patient to open his mouth and protrude his tongue (this also provides partial assessment of cranial nerve XII, the hypoglossal nerve). Observe the palate for bilateral elevation when the patient says "ahhh." If the palate rises symmetrically, further assessment is likely unnecessary. If the palate does not elevate symmetrically, lightly touch the back of the throat with a tongue blade and observe the response. Both the left and right sides should be tested. To assess the gag reflex in an unconscious patient use a bite block or rigid suction catheter to keep the patient's teeth separated, then stimulate the back of the throat with a tongue blade. An intact gag reflex is indicated by forward thrusting of the tongue and sometimes the head. The cough reflex is also controlled by cranial nerves IX and X, and can be assessed by noting spontaneous cough or cough in response to suctioning.

Extraocular Eye Movements

Extraocular eye movements are controlled by muscles innervated by cranial nerves III, IV, and VI. To test extraocular movements, the patient is asked to follow an object (usually the examiner's finger) through six positions (Figure 12–5). A normal response consists of the eyes moving in the same direction at the same speed and in constant alignment (conjugate eye movement). Abnormal eye movements include nystagmus (a jerking, rhythmical movement of one or both of the eyes) or an extraocular palsy (eye movement in one or both eyes is inhibited in a certain direction). Mild nystagmus with extreme lateral gaze is normal. Dysconjugate gaze,

TABLE 12–4. CRANIAL NERVE FUNCTION

Nerve	Function
I. Olfactory	Sense of smell
II. Optic	Visual fields, visual acuity
III. Oculomotor	Most extraocular eye movements, ability to elevate eyelid, muscular contraction of the iris in response to light
IV. Abducens	Eye movement down and toward the nose
V. Trigeminal	Facial sensation, including cornea, nasal mucosa, and oral mucosa; muscles of chewing and mastication
VI. Abducens	Lateral eye movement
VII. Facial	Facial muscles, including eyelid closure; taste in anterior two thirds of the tongue; secretion of saliva and tears
VIII. Acoustic	Hearing and equilibrium
IX. Glossopharyngeal	Gag reflex, muscles that control swallowing and phonation; taste in posterior third of tongue
X. Vagus (overlapping innervation)	Salivary gland secretion; vagal control of heart, lungs, and gastrointestinal tract
XI. Spinal accessory	Sternocleidomastoid and trapezius muscle strength
XII. Hypoglossal	Tongue movement

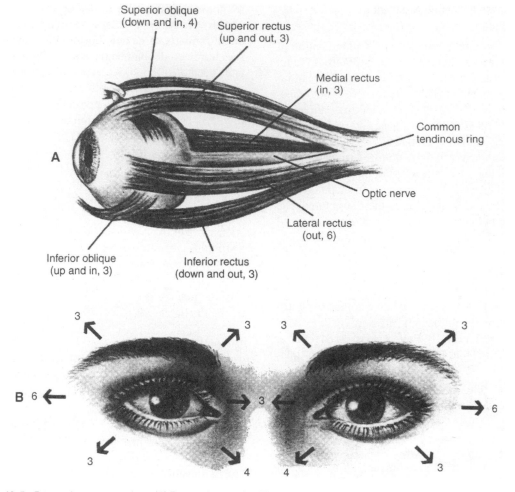

Figure 12–5. Extraocular eye movements. **(A)** Extraocular muscles. The eye movement controlled by the muscle is noted in parentheses, along with the associated cranial nerve supply. **(B)** The six cardinal directions of gaze and associated cranial nerves. (*Reprinted from Carlson BA: Neurologic clinical assessment. In Urden LD, Stacy KM, Lough ME [eds]:* Thelan's Critical Care Nursing: Diagnosis and Management. *St. Louis, MO: Mosby; 2002, p. 652.*)

in which the eyes move independently of each other, is an abnormal finding.

In unconscious patients, the oculocephalic and oculvestibular reflexes are used to test the portion of the brainstem that controls eye movement. Although these reflexes are not included in a typical critical care nursing assessment, it is useful to understand these reflexes and how they are assessed.

To test the oculocephalic reflex (doll's eyes), the patient's eyelids are held open by the examiner and the head is quickly rotated side to side. If the eyes deviate in the opposite direction from which the head is turned, then the pons is intact. If the eyes do not move or movement is asymmetric, this is indicative of pontine dysfunction. The oculocephalic reflex is never evaluated in patients with suspected cervical spine injuries.

Evaluation of the oculovestibular reflex (cold calorics) is also commonly used to determine brainstem function in

unconscious patients. After examination of the external canal for cerumen or perforation of the tympanic membrane, a bolus of 50 to 100 mL of cold water (iced water) is instilled into the ear. In a patient with intact brainstem function, conjugate deviation of the eyes toward the irrigated side occurs. Patients who have interrupted brainstem function either have no response or dysconjugate eye movement.

Vital Sign Alterations in Neurologic Dysfunction

Vital sign changes in neurologic dysfunction occur because of direct brainstem injury or decreased cerebral perfusion. Decreased perfusion causes ischemia and the body's response is to increase the blood pressure in an attempt to provide more nutrients. Hypotension is rarely seen except in the terminal stages of brainstem dysfunction or as the result of loss of sympathetic tone in patients with spinal cord injury. Abnormalities in heart rate and rhythm are common, and can be a cause of neurologic decline due to clot formation or inadequate cardiac output, or be a symptom of neurologic dysfunction (such as ST segment abnormalities following subarachnoid hemorrhage). Respiratory patterns vary widely. Some of the more common patterns are explained in Figure 12–6. It is more important to determine if the patient is ventilating adequately than to determine the specific pattern. Temperature is carefully monitored in patients with neurologic dysfunction, because hyperthermia (regardless of infectious or noninfectious etiology) causes increased cerebral metabolic demand. Hypothermia may result from injury to the brainstem or spinal cord.

Cushing's response refers to a triad of responses seen late in the course of neurologic deterioration. The classic triad is marked by widened pulse pressure, bradycardia, and an irregular respiratory pattern. Cushing's response is of minimal value in identifying early, significant changes in the patient's condition, but it is useful to be alert for components of Cushing's response (e.g., systolic hypertension or change in respiratory pattern).

Death by Neurologic Criteria

Death by neurologic criteria (previously called brain death) indicates an irreversible loss of both cortical and brainstem activity. The procedure that physicians must follow to declare a patient dead by neurologic criteria varies by state law and institutional policy. Conditions that must be ruled out

as causes of coma prior to testing for death by neurologic criteria include the effects of neurologic depressants, hypothermia, and severe metabolic or endocrine disturbance. In addition, the cause of the patient's condition must be established and consistent with irreversible brain injury. Of note, some reflexive motor actions (such as the triple flexion response) are controlled by the spinal cord and may be present even following death by neurologic criteria.

DIAGNOSTIC TESTING

Lumbar Puncture

Lumbar puncture (LP) can be performed for diagnostic or therapeutic purposes. Diagnostic indications for LP include measurement of cerebrospinal fluid (CSF) pressure (an estimation of ICP) and sampling of CSF for analysis when central nervous system (CNS) infection, inflammation, or subarachnoid hemorrhage is suspected. Therapeutic indications for LP include drainage of CSF and the placement of tubes for medication administration or ongoing CSF drainage. Examples of disease processes in which LP is used for diagnostic or therapeutic purposes include meningitis, multiple sclerosis, Guillain-Barré syndrome, hydrocephalus, and subarachnoid hemorrhage. Increased ICP is a theoretical contraindication to LP due to risk of herniation. When increased ICP is suspected, a CT scan (see below) may be performed

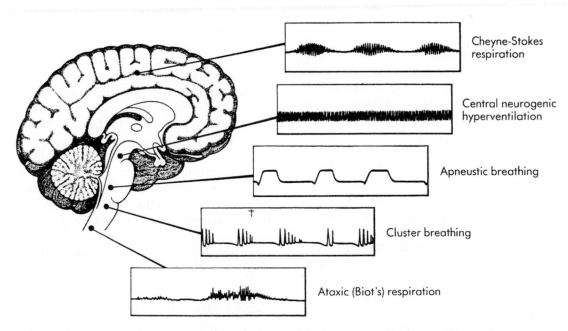

Figure 12–6. Abnormal respiratory patterns. Abnormal respiratory patterns associated with increased intracranial pressure. Cheyne-Stokes respiration, arising from deep inside the cerebral hemispheres and basal ganglia; central neurogenic hyperventilation, from lower midbrain to lower pons; apneustic breathing, from middle to lower pons and brainstem; cluster breathing, from upper medulla; and ataxic (Biot's) respiration, from medulla. (*Reprinted from Barker E: Intracranial pressure and monitoring. In Barker E [ed]: Neuroscience Nursing: A Spectrum of Care. St. Louis, MO: Mosby; 2002, p. 389.*)

prior to proceeding with the LP. Other contraindications include coagulopathy or infection in the area of skin through which the needle will be introduced. Low-molecular-weight heparin is held for 24 hours prior to LP to decrease the risk of formation of a spinal epidural hematoma. Other anticoagulant and antiplatelet medications such as warfarin, aspirin, and clopidogrel are frequently stopped as well, according to physician preference.

When performing a LP, the clinician locates the L3–L4 or L4–L5 intervertebral space and injects a local anesthetic, then inserts a hollow needle with a stylet into the spinal subarachnoid space. The risk of spinal cord injury is minimal because the actual cord ends at L1 and only nerve roots continue below. Proper patient positioning is very important and patients may require sedation if they are unable to remain still. The LP may be performed with the patient sitting up and leaning forward, but a lateral decubitus position is used for most critically ill patients. The patient lies on her or his side with his neck flexed forward and his knees pulled up toward the chest. This position widens the intervertebral space, allowing the needle to pass through more easily. The needle is inserted into the subarachnoid space and the stylet is removed. Flow of cerebral spinal fluid confirms that the needle is in the spinal subarachnoid space. A manometer is attached to the needle and used to measure an opening pressure. Pressures greater than 200 mm H_2O are considered abnormal. The amount of CSF drained varies based on the indication for the procedure, with smaller volumes needed for laboratory analysis than for treatment of hydrocephalus.

Normal CSF is clear and colorless. Infection and blood can change the appearance of CSF. In infection, CSF may be cloudy due to white blood cells and bacteria. Blood causes the CSF to be pink, red, or brown. Although some blood may be present if a small vessel was traumatized during needle insertion, this blood clears as more CSF is drained. Blood due to CNS hemorrhage does not clear. Common tests performed on CSF include analysis of cell counts with differentials, glucose, protein, lactate, gram stain, and culture with sensitivities. Special assays may be requested to look for specific inflammatory or demyelinating disease processes. Once the needle is removed, a small self-adhesive bandage is placed over the insertion site.

Postprocedure care varies with physician preference, hospital protocol, and whether or not the patient complains of headache, but typically involves maintaining the patient on flat bed rest for 1 to 4 hours, encouraging fluids, and monitoring the insertion site for any signs of bleeding, drainage, or development of hematoma. Patients often complain of headaches (due to loss of CSF), local pain at the insertion site, or pain radiating to the thigh if a nerve root was hit during the procedure. Headaches may respond to increased fluid intake, maintaining the head of the bed flat or less than 30°, maintaining a dark quiet room, or administration of analgesics. If the headache persists, an autologous blood patch may be used to stop continued CSF leakage.

Computed Tomography

Computed tomography (CT) is a common diagnostic tool when neurologic dysfunction is suspected. An x-ray beam moves in a 360° arc and a detector measures penetration of the x-ray beam into tissue. Penetration of the x-ray beam varies based on tissue density. The computer translates the collected x-ray beams into images. The result is a series of finely cut pictures showing bony structures, CSF, and brain tissue. Bone is visualized as white because it is most dense. CSF and air are black because of their low density. Brain tissue is seen in varying shades of gray. The appearance of recent intracranial bleeding is white; over time the color darkens as the blood breaks down. CT scans are quick, noninvasive, and easy to perform, and can identify most causes of acute neurologic deterioration, including bleeding, significant edema, and hydrocephalus.

CT scanning can be performed with a contrast medium to allow for better visualization of lesions such as tumors, abscesses, or vascular abnormalities. CT angiography (CTA) uses scanning during intravenous (IV) contrast administration to allow visualization of cerebral blood vessels. CTA is useful in the diagnosis of cerebral vascular anomalies, such as aneurysms or narrowed vessels. A three-dimensional reconstruction of the cerebrovasculature can be created from the images by using a special computer program.

During CT, the patient is placed on a narrow table that is moved up into a donut-shaped gantry. Because the table is very narrow, the patient is positioned carefully and secured with padding or Velcro straps. Patient movement causes blurry images. Sedation may be required for patients that are unable to cooperate. In patients who receive contrast, assessment of renal function (blood urea nitrogen, creatinine) is essential because some of the contrast agents are nephrotoxic. A large-bore IV is required for contrast administration. Due to the increased risk of metformin-induced lactic acidosis following administration of iodinated contrast medium, metformin is discontinued if contrast administration is anticipated and held for at least 48 hours after contrast administration. Renal function is checked prior to resuming metformin.

The primary risks of CT scans result from the use of contrast. Patients with a history of allergic reaction to contrast or iodine require premedication. There are no standard postprocedural interventions associated with this test, with the exception of hydration for patients that received contrast. In patients with preexisting renal compromise, hydration and N-acetylcysteine may be ordered for renal protection, both prior to and following the scan.

Magnetic Resonance Imaging

Magnetic resonance imaging (MRI) offers greater anatomic detail than CT scanning without using ionized radiation. The patient is placed in a strong magnetic field and controlled bursts of radio pulse waves are delivered, causing protons within atomic nuclei to resonate. The radiofrequency signals emitted by the resonating nuclei are measured and used to construct images. Cross-sectional images can be obtained in coronal, sagittal, and oblique planes. Gadolinium, a non–iodine-based contrast agent, is sometimes administered, and highlights areas where the blood–brain barrier is disrupted. MRI scans are most useful in diagnosing disorders of the brainstem, posterior fossa, and spinal cord. MRI scans offer an advantage over CT scans in the identification of demyelinating disorders such as multiple sclerosis or neurodegenerative diseases. MRI can also be used to detect suspected lesions that cannot be seen on CT, such as early cerebral infarction and intramedullary tumors. Magnetic resonance angiography (MRA) uses a specialized computer program to highlight the cerebral vasculature. MRA is useful in the evaluation of suspected arteriovenous malformations, aneurysms, and cavernous angiomas. Acute bleeding and bony abnormalities such as fractures can be better visualized using CT. The time requirement for MRI scans is typically longer than that of CT scans, which can be a disadvantage when needing to make treatment decisions based on diagnostic results. In addition, access to the patient is significantly limited during the scan.

All patients must be screened for the presence of implanted or embedded metal prior to MRI. Metallic objects inside the body may become dislodged or slip in the large magnetic tube and can cause patient injury. Most aneurysm clips are now made of nonferrous material and are safe for MRI; it is important to obtain additional information about the device, including when and where it was placed. Orthopedic hardware may also be safe, depending on the part of the body being imaged and the length of time since the hardware was placed. Patients who are either unable to reliably complete the MRI screening or who have a history of impaled metal fragments or shrapnel must have radiographs taken prior to MRI. The magnet can also damage internally magnetized units, such as cardiac pacemakers, causing them to malfunction or become demagnetized. Devices such as baclofen pumps and spinal cord stimulators are also contraindications to MRI. Most IV pumps and ventilators contain metal and cannot be taken into the room where the MRI machine is located. Long IV tubing and MRI-compatible monitoring equipment are useful in MRI scanning of the critically ill patient. Of note, the same screening precautions apply to the staff member who accompanies the patient to MRI. Any card with a magnetic strip, such as a credit card or even an employee ID, will be damaged by the MRI magnet and is removed. Patient education is important prior to scanning. Patients must be screened closely for any contraindications. In addition, all metal objects, such as jewelry, nonpermanent dentures, prostheses, hairpins, clothing with snaps or zippers, and EKG electrodes with metal snaps must be removed. Patients should be advised of the loud "booming" noise of the scanner. Patients who are claustrophobic may need sedation. Open-sided MRI machines are now available at some institutions and decrease feelings of claustrophobia. Inform the patient that the nurse or technician is in full view of them in the scanner and that they can talk to them if they feel uncomfortable on the table. Ensure the safety and comfort of the patients with safety belts and blankets for positioning. There are no postprocedure interventions associated with this test.

Cerebral Angiography

Cerebral angiography is similar to cardiac catheterization. Angiography can be performed for both diagnostic purposes and therapeutic intervention. Blockages or abnormalities of the cerebral circulation can be visualized, aiding in the diagnosis of vascular malformations (such as aneurysms or arteriovenous malformations) and arterial stenosis. Angioplasty (with or without stent placement) can be performed for narrowed cerebral vessels and medications can be infused directly into the cerebral vasculature. Blood vessels can also be embolized; this is sometimes done to decrease blood supply to a tumor prior to surgical resection. Some aneurysms are treated with embolization.

A catheter is placed in the femoral or brachial artery and threaded up into the carotid or vertebral arteries, and a radiopaque contrast material is injected. The flow of the contrast material is tracked using radiographic films and fluoroscopy. Patients are kept NPO for 6 hours prior to nonemergent angiography, and may need sedation during the procedure. The patient is under a sterile drape during the procedure so it is important to ensure that IV ports are easily accessible for medication administration. Coagulation studies are checked on all patients because coagulopathy is a relative contraindication to cerebral angiography. Many patients require sedation during the procedure. General anesthesia may be needed for uncooperative patients because the risk of vessel injury is increased if the patient moves her or his head during the procedure. Patients may feel a warm or burning sensation in their head when the contrast agent is injected.

Potential complications include neurologic deficit due to injury to an intracranial vessel, allergic reaction to contrast, hematoma formation at the site of catheter insertion, extracranial vessel injury (dissection), retroperitoneal hematoma, and vessel spasm following injection of contrast. All patients undergoing cerebral angiography receive hydration because of the large amount of contrast agent used. *N*-acetylcysteine is sometimes used for renal protection in patients with preexisting renal dysfunction.

Following angiogram, patients are typically kept on bed rest for 6 hours to help prevent hematoma formation at the puncture site. In some cases, a special arterial closure device is used to promote clot formation and allow quicker mobilization; this is reflected in the postangiography orders. The arterial puncture site is monitored frequently for development of a hematoma, and the neurovascular status of the limb is also checked. Careful monitoring of vital signs and neurologic examination aid in the detection of intra- or extracranial emboli or hemorrhage.

Transcranial Doppler Ultrasound

A probe that emits ultrasonic waves is placed on the skin. Structures are differentiated based on how much of the wave is reflected back to the probe. Carotid ultrasound is sometimes used to detect stenosis. A Doppler effect is created when probe detects moving structures, like red blood cells in a blood vessel. Transcranial Doppler ultrasound (TCD) studies allow visualization of the blood flow through major cerebral blood vessels by directing the ultrasonic waves through the thinner parts of the skull bone. The velocity of blood flow can be calculated. TCDs are noninvasive and can be done at the patient's bedside. The use of TCDs varies widely among institutions and can include detection of vasospasm after subarachnoid hemorrhage and monitoring of reperfusion after thrombolytic administration.

Electroencephalography

The electroencephalogram (EEG) is a measurement of the brain's electrical activity. EEG is performed by attaching a number of electrodes to standard locations on the scalp. These electrodes are attached to a recorder, which amplifies the activity and records it on paper. EEG is useful in evaluating causes of coma (structural versus metabolic), identifying seizure disorders, and determining the anatomic origin of seizures.

The EEG usually lasts 40 to 60 minutes with a portable machine for bedside use. The patient is instructed to lie still with their eyes closed. A mild sedative may be prescribed for restless or uncooperative patients, but the interpreter of the EEG must be aware of this because medications may cause changes in the recording. Documentation during the study is done by the technician and may include changes in blood pressure, changes in level of consciousness, medications the patient is currently taking or has taken within 48 hours, movement or posturing of the patient, and any noxious stimuli introduced to the patient. It is best to plan nursing care around the time of the test so that no interventions are done during this examination. When the EEG is complete, the electrode paste is removed with acetone or a special nonflammable solvent. Any medications that were held prior to the study are resumed.

In the setting of status epilepticus, continuous monitoring may be used to guide treatment. Continuous monitoring is also used in the diagnosis and management of intractable or difficult-to-control seizures, usually in conjunction with video monitoring. Continuous monitoring can also be helpful in identifying psychogenic seizures.

Electromyography

Electromyography (EMG) is used in the diagnosis of neuropathies and myopathies. Nerve conduction studies measure the transmission of electrical impulses after stimulation. Conditions in which EMG may aid diagnosis include critical illness myopathy/neuropathy, myasthenia gravis (in which the neuromuscular junction is affected), and Guillain-Barré syndrome. The patient may experience some pain related to insertion of the needle electrodes.

INTRACRANIAL PRESSURE: CONCEPTS AND MONITORING

The skull in adults is a closed, nondistensible compartment that contains three components: brain parenchyma (80%), blood (10%) and CSF (10%). The Monro-Kellie hypothesis states that to maintain a constant intracranial volume, an increase in any of the three components must be accompanied by decrease in one or both of the other components. If this reciprocal decrease does not occur, ICP rises. The body is able to compensate for a limited amount of increased intracranial volume by displacement of intracranial venous blood, decreased production of CSF, or displacement of CSF into the spinal subarachnoid space. ICP rises when these compensatory mechanisms have been exceeded (Figure 12–7). *Compliance* refers to the change in volume needed to result in a given change in pressure and reflects the effectiveness of the compensatory mechanisms. With decreased compliance, a small increase in volume results in a large increase in ICP. Compliance is based on several factors, including the amount of volume increase and the time over which the increase occurs. Smaller increases in volume result in less

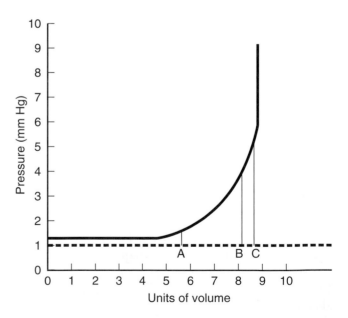

Figure 12–7. Intracranial volume-pressure curve. **(A)** Pressure is normal, and increases in intracranial volume are tolerated due to compensatory mechanisms. **(B)** Increases in volume may cause increases in pressure. **(C)** Small increases in volume may cause large increases in pressure (compensatory mechanisms have been exceeded). (*Reprinted from Mendez KA: Neurologic therapeutic management. In Urden LD, Stacy KM, Lough ME [eds]: Thelan's Critical Care Nursing: Diagnosis and Management. St. Louis, MO: Mosby; 2002, p. 702.*)

increase in pressure. Increases in volume that occur over a long period of time are better tolerated than rapid increases. Older adults typically have increased compliance because of cerebral atrophy. Increased ICP can result in cerebral hypoperfusion, ischemia, herniation, and eventually death.

Cerebral Blood Flow

The brain cannot store oxygen or glucose in significant quantities. Therefore, constant blood flow is required to maintain cerebral metabolism. If cerebral blood flow (CBF) is insufficient, brain cells do not receive sufficient substrate to function and will eventually die. CBF is determined by blood pressure and cerebral vascular resistance.

Autoregulation refers to the ability of cerebral blood vessels to maintain consistent CBF by dilating or constricting in response to changes in blood pressure. Vasodilation occurs in response to decreased blood pressure and an increased blood pressure results in vasoconstriction. In persons without neurologic disease, autoregulation allows consistent cerebral perfusion when mean arterial pressure is 60 to 160 mm Hg. In the injured brain, the autoregulatory response becomes less predictable and CBF becomes dependent on systemic arterial pressure.

Cerebral vascular resistance can also be altered through chemoregulatory processes. An increase in the pressure of arterial carbon dioxide ($PaCO_2$) produces a lower extracellular pH and causes dilation of cerebral vessels. Conversely, a decrease in $PaCO_2$ raises pH and results in cerebral vasoconstriction. Vasodilation also results from PaO_2 levels less than 50 or a buildup of metabolic byproducts such as lactic acid. Other factors can decrease cerebral vascular resistance and thus CBF, including certain anesthetic agents (halothane, nitrous oxide), sodium nitroprusside, and some histamines. Seizures, pain, fever, and agitation increase metabolic demand and produce vasodilation.

Cerebral perfusion pressure (CPP) is a measurement of the pressure at which blood reaches the brain. CPP is an indirect reflection of CBF. It is calculated by subtracting ICP from mean arterial pressure (CPP = MAP − ICP). Decreased CPP occurs as the result of an increase in ICP, a decrease in mean arterial pressure, or both. The normal range for CPP is 70 to 100 mm Hg. A CPP of at least 50 to 60 mm Hg is necessary for adequate cerebral perfusion. CPP below 30 mm Hg results in irreversible neuronal hypoxia. Of note, disagreement exists related to appropriate arterial line leveling. Increasingly, the arterial line transducer is leveled at the foramen of Monro when calculating CPP to reflect the mean arterial pressure in the cerebral vasculature versus systemic mean arterial pressure. Until definitive guidelines emerge, institutional policies are followed.

Causes of Increased Intracranial Pressure

Increased ICP occurs as a result of cerebral edema, mass lesions, increased intracranial blood volume, or increased amounts of CSF. These factors often occur in combination. Pain, emotional distress, suctioning, or an overstimulating environment can also increase ICP.

Cerebral Edema

Cerebral edema is an abnormal accumulation of water or fluid in the intracellular or extracellular space, resulting in increased brain volume. Vasogenic edema results from increased capillary permeability of the vessel walls, which allows plasma and protein to leak into the extracellular space. Cytotoxic edema occurs when fluid collects inside the cells due to failure of cellular metabolism. This causes further breakdown of the cell membrane. Cytotoxic edema can lead to capillary damage, which then results in vasogenic edema.

Mass Lesion

Mass lesions in the brain parenchyma include brain tumor, hematoma, or abscess. In addition to raising ICP, mass lesions contribute to ischemia by compression of cerebral vessels.

Increased Blood Volume

Venous outflow obstruction can result from compression of the jugular veins (neck flexion, hyperextension, rotation). Increased intrathoracic pressure or increased intra-abdominal pressure (Trendelenburg position, prone position, extreme hip flexion, Valsalva maneuver, coughing, PEEP, endotracheal suctioning) also results in venous outflow obstruction. As discussed, cerebral vasodilation occurs as the result of hypoxia, hypercapnia, increased metabolic demands, or drug effects, and causes an overall increase in cerebral blood volume.

Increased CSF Volume

Approximately 500 mL of CSF are produced every day and normally flow through the ventricular system into the subarachnoid space where they are absorbed by the arachnoid granulations (Figure 12–8). Obstruction of CSF flow, decreased reabsorption of CSF, or increased production lead to increased intracranial CSF volume (hydrocephalus). Hydrocephalus is referred to as communicating or noncommunicating (also called obstructive). In meningitis or subarachnoid hemorrhage, the arachnoid granulations become clogged with cellular debris and cannot absorb CSF normally, which leads to communicating hydrocephalus. An example of noncommunicating hydrocephalus is obstruction of CSF flow due to a tumor in the third ventricle of the brain.

Clinical Presentation

Early signs of increased ICP include confusion, restlessness, lethargy, disorientation, headache, and nausea or vomiting. Patients may also report visual abnormalities such as diplopia. Decline in motor function begins with paresis and progresses to plegia, then abnormal posturing. Change in level of consciousness is an important indicator of elevated ICP. Changes in vital signs may occur. Increased systolic

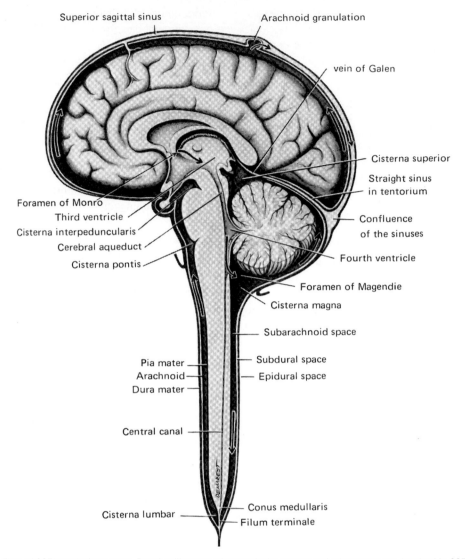

Figure 12–8. Flow of CSF/ventricular system. Drawing illustrates the ventricular system and other structures involved in CSF production, flow, and reabsorption. Arrows indicate the normal direction of flow of CSF. (*Reprinted from Novack CR, Demarest RJ: Meninges, ventricles, and cerebrospinal fluid. In:* The Nervous System: Introduction and Review. *New York: McGraw-Hill; 1986, p. 46.*)

blood pressure is the body's attempt to maintain cerebral perfusion. As ICP worsens, alterations in heart rate or respiratory pattern may also emerge. Pupillary changes are usually late signs of increased ICP, but may occur earlier if the underlying cause is creating pressure on cranial nerve III. Any of these signs and symptoms requires immediate physician notification. Unless the cause of elevated ICP is known, a CT scan is ordered to evaluate for mass lesions (tumor, blood clot) or hydrocephalus.

Monitoring

ICP can be measured in the ventricles, subarachnoid space, epidural space, subdural space, or brain parenchyma (Figure 12–9). Use of an intraventricular catheter remains the gold standard for ICP measurement. Several systems exist, but the basic setup includes a catheter, external transducer, and collection device for CSF. The catheter is placed via a burr hole into the anterior horn of the lateral ventricle and connected to a drainage system and transducer. The transducer is leveled at the external landmark of the foramen of Monro (top of the external auditory canal) and zeroed to atmospheric pressure using manufacturer's specifications. Slightly different anatomic locations are reported in the literature (tragus, outer canthus of the eye, midpoint of an imaginary line drawn between the right and left external auditory canals); the most important factor is consistency among caregivers. The transducer senses the pressure exerted by the CSF in the ventricles and translates it into a

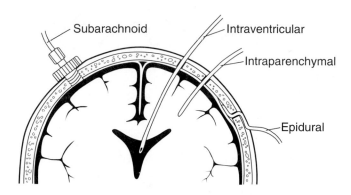

Figure 12–9. Sites for ICP monitoring. Illustration of possible sites for monitoring intracranial pressure: subarachnoid–subdural, intraventricular, intraparenchymal, and epidural. The "gold standard" remains the intraventricular catheter. (*Reprinted from Lee KR, Hoff JT: Intracranial pressure. In Youmans JR [ed]: Neurological Surgery, vol 1. Philadelphia: WB Saunders; 1996, p. 505.*)

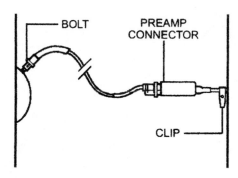

Figure 12–10. ICP monitoring systems. On the right, a ventriculostomy connects to a CSF collection system. A three-way stopcock allows either pressure monitoring or drainage of CSF. On the left, a transducer is inserted into the brain parenchyma and anchored to the skull by a bolt mechanism. The transducer is attached to an external monitoring device. (*Reprinted from Bergsneider M, Becker DP: Intracranial pressure monitoring. In Shoemaker WC, Ayres SM, Grenvik A, Holbrook PR [eds]: Textbook of Critical Care, 3rd ed. Philadelphia: WB Saunders; 1995, p. 313.*)

waveform on the bedside monitor. This system is referred to by several names, including *external ventricle drain, ventriculostomy,* and *intraventricular catheter.* The advantage of using an intraventricular catheter for monitoring is that CSF can be drained, providing a treatment modality for increased ICP. CSF drainage is controlled by adjusting the height of the system relative to the foramen of Monro. The height of the fluid column in the drainage system creates hydrostatic pressure that opposes ICP. If the drainage system is raised, CSF drainage decreases; when the drainage system is lowered, CSF drainage increases. Rapid drainage of CSF can result in ventricular collapse; therefore, CSF is drained in a controlled manner based on a predetermined ICP. This is accomplished by maintaining the drainage system at a specific height, such as 10 cm above the top of the ear. CSF drainage is monitored for amount and color. A physiologic response to elevated ICP is to shunt CSF into the spinal subarachnoid space; this decreases ventricular size and may make intraventricular catheter placement difficult. Risks associated with intraventricular catheter placement include infection and hemorrhage caused by catheter placement. To decrease the risk of infection, preassembled closed drainage systems are available. The catheter may be placed by the physician at the bedside or in the operating room. Sterile technique is essential when the catheter is placed and whenever the system is entered for CSF samples. An occlusive dressing is maintained over the catheter site.

ICP may also be monitored using a fiberoptic transducer or a strain-gauge transducer, either as part of an external ventricular drainage system or alone (Figure 12–10). If placed in the ventricle, these devices have the same risks and benefits as an intraventricular catheter. When placed in the subarachnoid space, epidural space, subdural space, or brain

parenchyma, these monitors are easier to insert and have a lower rate of infection than intraventricular monitors. The transducer is zeroed to atmospheric pressure prior to insertion and cannot be rezeroed. Leveling to the foramen of Monro is not required. Fiberoptic and strain-gauge transducers are connected directly to an independent monitor, which provides an ICP reading. Other technology is available to monitor ICP, including some devices that allow rezeroing after monitor insertion, but these are not commonly used in practice. Normal ICP is 0 to 15 mm Hg in adults. Treatment is typically initiated when ICP is sustained above 20 to 25 mm Hg.

ICP Waveforms

With continuous ICP monitoring, there are fluctuations in waveforms that correlate with specific physiologic events. Examination of these waveforms can be helpful in evaluating changes in the patient's condition.

The ICP pulse waveform is a continuous, real-time pressure display that corresponds to each heartbeat. The normal pulse wave has three or more defined peaks:

- P1 Percussion wave: sharp peak, consistent in amplitude, corresponds to myocardial systole
- P2 Tidal wave: variable in shape and magnitude, corresponds to myocardial diastole
- P3 Dicrotic wave: occurs after dicrotic notch, reflects venous fluctuations

The pulse waveform at low pressures is a descending saw-toothed pattern with a distinct P1 (Figure 12–11). As mean ICP rises, a progressive elevation of P2 occurs, causing the pulse waveform to appear more rounded. When P2 is equal to or higher than P1, decreased compliance exists (Figure 12–12).

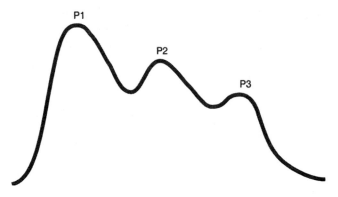

Figure 12–11. Components of a normal ICP waveform.

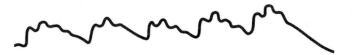

Figure 12–12. ICP waveform demonstrating decreased compliance.

Trend recordings compress continuous ICP recording data into time periods to reflect general trends in ICP over longer time periods (minutes to hours). Three distinct pressure waves have been identified (Figure 12–13). A waves (plateau waves) are sudden increases in pressure lasting 5 to 20 minutes. They begin from a baseline of an already elevated ICP (greater than 20 mm Hg) and reflect cerebral ischemia. B waves are sharp, rhythmic oscillations of pressure (up to 50 mm Hg) occurring every 0.5 to 2 minutes. They are seen in relationship to fluctuations in the respiratory cycle, such as Cheyne-Stokes respirations. They are not clinically significant, but may progress to A waves. C waves are small rhythmic waves with pressures up to 20 mm Hg occurring four to eight times per minute. They relate to normal changes in systemic arterial pressure, and their clinical significance is unknown.

Principles of Management of Increased ICP

Management focuses on avoiding activities known to elevate ICP and on aggressive treatment when increased ICP occurs. The goal is to prevent further neurologic damage.

Treatment is usually initiated when ICP is sustained above 20 to 25 mm Hg for 5 minutes or longer. Principles of management include:

Monitoring Neurologic Status

Assess baseline neurologic signs; then reassess periodically and compare to previous findings. Include level of consciousness, Glasgow Coma Score, pupillary size and reaction to light, eye movement, and motor and sensory function. Assess vital signs and compare with previous findings to identify trends. In patients who are sedated for ICP management, the frequency of neurologic assessment may be decreased by physician order to prevent ICP spikes related to stimulation. Assessment of pupillary size and reaction to light continue, even if the patient is also receiving neuromuscular blockers.

Close monitoring of neurologic status facilitates the identification and treatment of complications, such as the development of an epidural or subdural hematoma. In these cases, surgical evacuation of the hematoma is likely to reduce ICP. In cases of diffuse cerebral edema, a portion of the skull may be removed to increase compliance and allow the brain to swell outside the contained area of the skull. This procedure is referred to as a *craniectomy*.

Adequate Oxygenation and Ventilation

The goal of management is to maintain PaO_2 and $PaCO_2$ at normal levels. For patients with impaired consciousness, intubation and mechanical ventilation may be required. Avoid

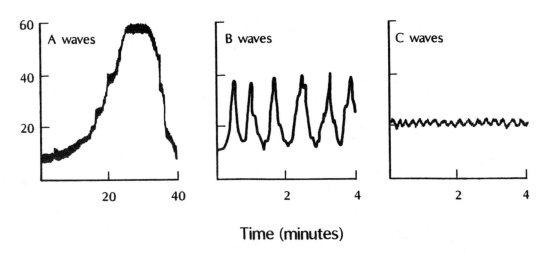

Figure 12–13. ICP trend recordings.

circumferential taping of endotracheal tubes because this may obstruct venous return. Both hypoxemia and hypercarbia can result in cerebral vasodilation and increased ICP. Hyperventilation is no longer routinely used to decrease ICP because the resulting decrease in $Paco_2$ may lead to vasoconstriction and cerebral ischemia. Controlled hyperventilation can be used in the setting of impending herniation to "buy time" for other measures to be implemented and take effect, or when other measures to manage elevated ICP have been unsuccessful. Measures of cerebral oxygenation are useful in determining the impact of $Paco_2$ manipulation on cerebral metabolism (see Chapter 21, Advanced Neurologic Concepts). Suctioning is performed only when necessary. The patient is placed on 100% oxygen and the duration of suctioning is no more than 10 seconds.

Blood Pressure and Fluid Management

Management of blood pressure is determined by the level of ICP and CPP. The goal is to maintain a CPP of at least 60 mm Hg. If the patient is hypotensive, non–glucose-containing fluids are infused to ensure euvolemia. Fluid management is guided by CVP, pulmonary capillary wedge pressure, or both. Vasopressors, such as phenylephrine, may be needed to maintain CPP.

Positioning

Because the venous system of the brain is valveless, increased intrathoracic or intra-abdominal pressure reduces venous return and increases ICP. In general, elevating the head of the bed 30° optimizes ICP and CPP. Hip flexion, especially greater than 90°, is avoided. A bowel regimen is used to avoid constipation.

Neck positioning also effects venous drainage and can raise ICP. The head and neck are maintained in a neutral position, avoiding flexion, hyperextension, or rotation. Cervical collars are carefully applied to avoid decreasing jugular venous return.

Isometric muscle contraction also increases ICP. Examples include pushing up in bed, fighting against restraints, posturing, and shivering.

Minimizing Environmental Stimuli

Maintain a calm, quiet environment. Control the environment for noise, temperature, and other noxious stimuli. Avoid unnecessary conversation at the bedside. The television is turned off. Family members are encouraged to visit and speak quietly to patients and the ICP response is observed. Avoid clustering patient care activities together (suctioning, bathing, turning).

Preventing Increased Metabolic Demand

Seizure activity increases cerebral metabolic demand and ICP. The prophylactic use of anticonvulsants is common in neurologically impaired patients, although this practice is being questioned due to lack of scientific support. Additional information on the management of seizures is included later in this chapter.

Fever increases ICP by increasing metabolic demand. For each elevation of 1°C, cerebral metabolic demand increases by approximately 6%. Methods to normalize temperature include antipyretics, air- or water-filled cooling blankets, and intravascular cooling devices. Shivering also increases metabolic demand and is avoided.

CSF Drainage

Drainage of small amounts of CSF may be used to decrease ICP in patients with an intraventricular catheter. The physician specifies the amount of drainage desired.

Sedation and Analgesia

Sedation and analgesia are used to prevent elevation of ICP due to agitation and pain. Commonly used agents include morphine or fentanyl for analgesia and midazolam or lorazepam for sedation. Propofol (a sedative hypnotic) is commonly used because its short half-life allows for rapid awakening and evaluation of mental status. One of the side effects of propofol is hypotension, especially when given as a bolus; careful use of the drug is required to avoid decreases in CPP.

Neuromuscular Blockade

Neuromuscular blocking agents may be used to prevent increases in intrathoracic and venous pressure that occur with coughing or patient–ventilator asynchrony. Sedation and analgesia are always used in conjunction with neuromuscular blocking agents.

Medications to Decrease Cerebral Edema

Osmotic diuretics reduce cerebral edema by pulling extracellular fluid from brain tissue into the blood vessels. Mannitol is the most commonly used agent and is given as a bolus dose of 0.25 to 1 g/kg body weight. Mannitol is administered using a filter because it crystallizes easily. Euvolemia is maintained and electrolytes are closely monitored. Some also use hypertonic saline to increase serum osmolality and pull water into the vascular space.

Corticosteroids (e.g., dexamethasone) are useful in decreasing cerebral edema associated with intracranial tumors. Steroids are not useful in the management of cerebral edema related to traumatic brain injury or stroke. Potential complications of steroid therapy include gastric irritation or hemorrhage and hyperglycemia.

Barbiturates

Barbiturate coma therapy is sometimes used for the management of uncontrolled intracranial hypertension that does not respond to other therapies. Barbiturates decrease cerebral metabolism, CBF, and ICP. Drugs commonly used are pentobarbital and thiopental. Once the barbiturate coma is induced, the usual parameters of neurologic assessment, such as pupillary, gag, and swallowing reflexes, are lost. However, asymmetrical or dilated pupils may occur in response to brainstem compression, and therefore pupillary assessment is essential to continue. The patient is maintained on a ventilator via an endotracheal tube or tracheostomy tube. Complications associated with barbiturate coma include hypotension and myocardial depression.

Herniation

Folds in the dura mater divide the intracranial cavity into several smaller compartments. Cerebral herniation is the distortion and displacement of the brain from one compartment to another. Herniation is a life-threatening event that occurs with expanding mass lesions or hematomas and rapidly increasing ICP. The classic signs of herniation are:

- Deterioration in the level of consciousness
- Pupillary abnormality—fixed and dilated pupil(s)
- Motor abnormality—hemiplegia, abnormal flexion or decortication, abnormal extension, or decerebration
- Brainstem dysfunction—cranial nerve displacement and compression
- Alteration in vital signs, Cushing's triad, altered respiratory pattern

ACUTE ISCHEMIC STROKE

Etiology, Risk Factors, and Pathophysiology

Stroke is the third leading cause of death in the United States and the leading cause of disability in adults. The brain cannot store oxygen or glucose and therefore requires a constant flow of blood to supply these nutrients. The blood supply to the brain can be altered through several different processes. These include embolism, thrombosis, hemorrhage, and compression or spasm of the vessels. Ischemic stroke due to embolism or thrombus formation accounts for 80% to 85% of all strokes. Edema occurs in the area of ischemic or infracted tissue and contributes to further neuronal cell death.

If ischemia is not reversed, neuronal cell death occurs, leading to infarction of brain tissue. The penumbra is an area of tissue that surrounds the core ischemic area. The penumbra receives some blood flow from adjacent vessels but perfusion is marginal. If CBF is improved, the penumbra may recover.

Risk factors for stroke include hypertension, cardiac disease (atrial fibrillation, patent foramen ovale, carotid artery disease), diabetes, increased age, gender (higher incidence among men), race (African-American), prior stroke, family history, hypercholesterolemia, hypercoagulability (cancer, pregnancy, high RBCs, sickle cell), smoking, diet/obesity, and the use of oral contraceptives. Transient ischemic attack (TIA) is an important warning sign for stroke. With a TIA, stroke symptoms disappear within 24 hours due to resolution of the underlying cause of ischemia. Although most resolve within 10 minutes, an extensive workup to identify treatable causes is warranted with any TIA.

The pathophysiology of stroke varies based on the precipitating event. Thrombosis and embolism formation, described below, result in acute ischemic stroke.

Thrombosis

Thrombosis is the most common cause of ischemic stroke and is usually due to atherosclerosis and the formation of plaque within an artery. Decreased blood flow causes brain tissue ischemia along the course of the affected vessel, which results in infarct if not quickly reversed. Thrombosis due to atherosclerosis of large cerebral vessels results in large areas of infarct. Considerable edema often develops, further increasing ischemia by compressing areas surrounding the infarct. Significant functional deficits are common. If thrombus forms in a smaller branching artery, a lacunar infarct develops. Lacunar infarcts result in smaller areas of neuronal cell death. Deficits are less apparent, unless the infarct is in a crucial area, such as the internal capsule. Patients with a history of atherosclerosis or arteritis are at highest risk for thrombotic strokes. Thrombotic strokes tend to develop during periods of sleep or inactivity, when blood flow is less brisk.

AT THE BEDSIDE
▶ *Acute Ischemic Stroke*

A 64-year-old algebra teacher is admitted to the ICU following thrombolytic therapy for acute ischemic stroke. She has a history of diet-controlled diabetes. For the last 3 weeks, she has complained to her husband about some minor heart palpitations, but has not been to the doctor. She developed left hemiplegia (arm worse than leg), a left facial droop, and slurred speech while eating lunch at her desk. A student found the patient slumped against her desk when he returned to the classroom to retrieve a book. The student called 911. The paramedics established time of symptom onset by discovering that the student last saw her teacher normal about 20 minutes prior. Upon arrival at the ER, she was quickly transported to head CT and the necessary prethrombolytic evaluation was completed by the Stroke Team. No blood was present on CT, and TPA was administered. When JS arrives in the ICU, she continues to have left arm weakness (strength 2/5) but her leg weakness has resolved and her speech is normal. She is monitored in the ICU for 24 hours and diagnosed with atrial fibrillation. After 24 hours in the ICU, she is transferred to a telemetry bed in the stroke unit, where she is started on aspirin and later warfarin. She is discharged home after 7 days in the hospital, with outpatient occupational therapy.

Embolism

Embolism refers to the occlusion of a cerebral vessel, most often by a blood clot but also by infectious particles, fat, air, or tumor fragments. Twenty percent of all strokes are cardioembolic in origin. Embolism is often associated with heart disease that results in bacterial vegetations or blood clots that are easily detached from the wall or valves of the heart. Chronic atrial fibrillation, valvular disease, prosthetic valves, cardiomyopathy, and atherosclerotic lesions of the proximal aorta are common causes of embolism. Less common causes include atrial myxomas, patent foramen ovale, and bacterial endocarditis. The fragmented substance easily lodges at the bifurcation of the middle cerebral artery, sometimes breaking apart and traveling further into the cerebral vascular system. The onset of an embolic occlusion is rapid, with symptoms that develop without warning.

Clinical Presentation

Symptoms range from very mild to significant loss of functional abilities. Common signs and symptoms of stroke include weakness in an extremity or on one side of the body, sensory changes, difficulty speaking or understanding speech, facial droop, and visual changes. Clinical presentation varies based on the area of infarction.

Stroke in a Cerebral Hemisphere

Signs and symptoms occur on the side of the body contralateral to the stroke. Weakness or paralysis occurs in one or both extremities, and sensory loss may also be noted. Visual field deficits are also contralateral to the lesion. The patient often displays an ipsilateral gaze preference, in effect "looking to the lesion." The left hemisphere is dominant in right-handed individuals and in approximately 75% of left-handed patients. As the dominant hemisphere, it controls language functions and language-dependent memory. Dominant hemisphere strokes produce receptive, expressive, or global aphasia. The nondominant hemisphere (usually the right) controls visual-spatial perception and visual memory.

Cerebellar or Brainstem Stroke

Motor and sensory function may be impaired on one or both sides of the body. Loss of equilibrium, decreased fine motor abilities, and nausea/vomiting are typical. Cranial nerve deficits are common and include dysarthria, nystagmus, dysphagia, and decreased cough reflex. Careful evaluation of airway protection and swallowing ability is essential to determine aspiration risk. Patients with severe deficits often require a feeding tube and potentially a tracheostomy. Obstructive hydrocephalus may occur due to occlusion of the ventricular drainage system by edema. Placement of an external ventricular drain may be necessary. Because cortical injury is not present, patients maintain a normal mental status and level of alertness unless pressure in the posterior fossa leads to brainstem compression. Surgical decompression of the posterior fossa may be performed to prevent or relieve brainstem compression.

Diagnostic Tests

The initial diagnostic test in acute ischemic stroke is CT scanning without contrast to rule out intracranial hemorrhage. This is important because treatments for hemorrhagic and ischemic stroke differ significantly. Specialized MRI scans (diffusion-weighted imaging, perfusion-weighted imaging) can detect areas of ischemia before they are apparent on CT, and MRA detects areas of vascular abnormality, as might be seen with clot due to arterial dissection. Other tests that may be done acutely include cerebral angiography, carotid ultrasound, and transcranial Doppler studies. Transthoracic or transesophageal echocardiography is used to assess cardiac causes of stroke. Hypercoagulable states are detected through lab work. All patients who present with stroke require an EKG because of the correlation between cerebrovascular and cardiovascular disease. In addition, conditions that mimic stroke, such as hypoglycemia, must be ruled out.

Principles of Management of Acute Ischemic Stroke

Stroke is a medical emergency and is treated with the same urgency as acute myocardial infarction. Just as "time is muscle" when the heart is ischemic, "time is brain" when cerebral ischemia occurs. The goals of treatment are to restore circulation to the brain when possible, stop the ongoing ischemic process, and prevent secondary complications. Management principles include the following.

Evaluation of Conditions That Mimic Acute Ischemic Stroke

Other conditions may mimic acute ischemic stroke and must be ruled out. Hypoglycemia may cause stroke-like symptoms and is easily detected by using a bedside monitor to check blood glucose. Noncontrast CT scanning is performed on all patients with signs and symptoms of stroke to rule out intracranial bleeding. Other conditions that may mimic acute ischemic stroke include toxic or metabolic disorders, migraines, brain tumors, and seizures.

Thrombolytic Therapy

Thrombolytic therapy is administered in an attempt to restore perfusion to the affected area. IV administration of recombinant tissue plasminogen activator (rtPA) is considered in all patients who meet the inclusion/exclusion criteria (Table 12–5) and can be treated within 3 hours of the onset of symptoms. The recommended dose for rtPA is 0.9 mg/kg, with 10% of the total dose given as a bolus over 1 to 2 minutes followed by the remainder of the dose as an infusion over 1 hour. The maximum dose recommended is 90 mg. In a large-scale study, rtPA administration resulted in improved

TABLE 12–5. CHARACTERISTICS OF PATIENTS WITH ISCHEMIC STROKE WHO COULD BE TREATED WITH rtPA

Diagnosis of ischemic stroke causing measurable neurologic deficit

The neurologic signs should not be clearing spontaneously

The neurologic signs should not be minor and isolated

Caution should be exercised in treating a patient with major deficits

The symptoms of stroke should not be suggestive of subarachnoid hemorrhage

Onset of symptoms <3 h before beginning treatment

No head trauma or prior stroke in previous 3 months

No myocardial infarction in the previous 3 months

No gastrointestinal or urinary tract hemorrhage in previous 21 days

No major surgery in the previous 14 days

No arterial puncture at a noncompressible site in the previous 7 days

No history of previous intracranial hemorrhage

Blood pressure not elevated (systolic <185 mm Hg and diastolic <110 mm Hg)

No evidence of active bleeding or acute trauma (fracture) on examination

Not taking an oral anticoagulant or if anticoagulant being taken, INR ≤1.5

If receiving heparin in previous 48 hours, aPTT must be in normal range

Platelet count ≥100,000 mm^3

Blood glucose concentration ≥50 mg/dL (2.7 mmol/L)

No seizure with postictal residual neurologic impairments

CT does not show a multilobar infarction (hypodensity >⅓ cerebral hemisphere)

The patient or family understand the potential risks and benefits from treatment

outcomes at 3 months post-stroke. There is an increased risk of intracerebral hemorrhage following rtPA administration and for this reason frequent serial neurologic assessments are essential. Vital signs and neurologic checks are done every 15 minutes for the first 2 hours, then every 30 minutes for 6 hours, and then hourly until 24 hours following initial treatment. If neurologic deterioration occurs, notify the physician and prepare for stat head CT. Antiplatelet or anticoagulant meds are avoided for 24 hours following rtPA administration. Placement of nasogastric tubes, bladder catheters, and invasive lines is delayed to decrease the risk of hemorrhage.

Intra-arterial thrombolysis is not FDA approved for the treatment of stroke but is being used at some centers for patients with middle cerebral artery or basilar artery occlusion who do not meet the criteria for IV rtPA. Intra-arterial rtPA is administered by an interventional neuroradiologist (see section on Cerebral Angiography). The time frame for initiation of therapy is 6 hours for middle cerebral artery occlusions. Intra-arterial rtPA for basilar artery occlusion is sometimes administered up to 12 hours (or even longer) after the onset of symptoms under the framework of "compassionate use" because the deficits created by basilar artery occlusion are so devastating that the increased risk of intracerebral hemorrhage (ICH) is tolerated.

Blood Pressure Management

Elevated blood pressure is the body's attempt to maintain perfusion to the ischemic brain and should not be lowered rapidly. Blood pressure management varies based on whether or not the patient is receiving thrombolytics. Recommendations regarding blood pressure management after acute ischemic stroke are summarized in Table 12–6. Induced hypertension is used in some cases in an attempt to increase CBF. This can sometimes be achieved by simply holding the patient's home blood pressure medication. In other cases, IV fluids or vasopressors may be required. The goal blood pressure is determined by the physician.

Management of Increased ICP

Cerebral edema occurs in the area of infarct and leads to increased ICP. For further discussion of treatment options, refer to the section on ICP. Hemicraniectomy may be used to alleviate increased ICP in patients with large infarcts, particularly in the distribution of the middle cerebral artery of the nondominant hemisphere.

Glucose Management

Although hyperglycemia has not been specifically identified as a cause of worse outcomes after stroke, there is a significant correlation. Hyperglycemia is associated with an increased risk of intracranial hemorrhage following tissue plasminogen activator (tPA) administration.

Preventing and Treating Secondary Complications

Patients are at significant risk for decreased airway maintenance and aspiration following stroke. Decreased level of consciousness, facial weakness, and cranial nerve deficits contribute. Intubation may be necessary during the acute phase. Some patients recover enough function to be extubated, but others may need a tracheostomy. Careful assessment of swallowing ability is indicated before any oral intake. Placement of a feeding tube may be indicated.

Deep venous thrombosis is another common complication in stroke patients and may lead to pulmonary embolism. Strategies to decrease risk include elastic compression stockings, pneumatic compression devices, the use of anticoagulants, and early progression in activity. In high-risk cases, an inferior vena cava filter may be placed to decrease the risk of pulmonary embolism.

Preventing Recurrent Stroke

The use of antiplatelet and anticoagulant medications varies depending on the size of the infarct, presumed etiology, and whether or not the patient received thrombolytic therapy. Patients are commonly placed on aspirin soon after the initial event and the decision to use other antiplatelet medications is made on an individual basis. If the stroke is very large, then anticoagulation is typically not used in the acute phase of treatment because it increases the risk of hemor-

TABLE 12–6. APPROACH TO ELEVATED BLOOD PRESSURE IN ACUTE ISCHEMIC STROKE

Blood Pressure Level (mm Hg)	Treatment
Not eligible for thrombolytic therapy	
Systolic <220 *or* diastolic <120	Observe unless other end-organ involvement, e.g., aortic dissection, acute myocardial infarction, pulmonary edema, hypertensive encephalopathy.
	Treat other symptoms of stroke such as headache, pain, agitation, nausea, and vomiting.
	Treat other acute complications of stroke, including hypoxia, increased intracranial pressure, seizures, or hypoglycemia.
Systolic >220 *or* diastolic <121–140	Labetalol 10–20 mg IV over 1–2 min.
	May repeat or double every 10 min (maximum dose 300 mg)
	or
	Nicardipine 5 mg/h IV infusion as initial dose; titrate to desired effect by increasing 2.5 mg/h every 5 min to maximum of 15 mg/h
	Aim for a 10–15% reduction of blood pressure
Diastolic >140	Nitroprusside 0.5 µg/kg/min IV infusion as initial dose with continuous blood pressure monitoring
	Aim for a 10–15% reduction of blood pressure
Eligible for thrombolytic therapy	
Pretreatment	
Systolic >185 *or* diastolic >110	Labetalol 10–20 mg IV over 1–2 min.
	May repeat ×1 *or* Nitropaste 1–2 inches.
	If blood pressure is not reduced and maintained at desired levels (systolic ≤185 and diastolic ≤110), do not administer rtPA.
During and after treatment	
1. Monitor BP	Check BP every 15 min for 2 h, then every 30 min for 6 h, and then every hour for 16 h.
2. Diastolic >140	Sodium nitroprusside 0.5 µg/kg/min IV infusion as initial dose and titrate to desired blood pressure.
3. Systolic >230 *or* diastolic 121–140	Labetalol 10 mg IV over 1–2 min.
	May repeat or double labetalol every 10 min to a maximum dose of 300 mg or give the initial labetalol bolus and then start a labetalol drip at 2 to 8 mg/min
	or
	Nicardipine 5 mg/h IV infusion as initial dose;
	Titrate to desired effect by increasing 2.5 mg/h every 5 min to maximum of 15 mg/h. If BP is not controlled by labetalol, consider sodium nitroprusside.
4. Systolic 180–230 *or* diastolic 105–120	Labetalol 10 mg IV over 1–2 min.
	May repeat or double labetalol every 10–20 min to a maximum dose of 300 mg or give the initial labetalol bolus and then start a labetalol drip at 2–8 mg/min.

rhagic conversion (development of bleeding within the infarcted tissue).

Carotid endarterectomy is the most common surgical procedure to prevent further ischemic strokes, but is not typically performed in the time period immediately following a stroke due to the risk of reperfusion injury and hemorrhage. Carotid endarterectomy is recommended for patients with greater than 70% stenosis. Stenosis may also be treated with angioplasty, with or without stent placement.

The Future of Treatment for Acute Ischemic Stroke
Many clinical trials have investigated the efficacy of neuroprotective agents but to date none have shown significant improvements in outcomes. The use of mild hypothermia (32°C to 34°C) is being tested in several trials and appears promising. In addition, the search for more effective thrombolytics with less risk of hemorrhage is ongoing. Angiographic techniques that permit clot disruption and retrieval are also being investigated.

HEMORRHAGIC STROKE

Etiology, Risk Factors, and Pathophysiology

Approximately 15% of all strokes are hemorrhagic. In subarachnoid hemorrhage, bleeding into the subarachnoid space occurs, usually as the result of a ruptured aneurysm. Although subarachnoid hemorrhage is a type of stroke, management issues vary significantly. Subarachnoid hemorrhage is discussed in Chapter 21, Advanced Neurologic Concepts. Here, *hemorrhagic stroke* refers to intraparenchymal bleeding (also called intracerebral hemorrhage or ICH).

Hypertension is the most common cause of ICH. Other causes include vascular malformations (arteriovenous malformations or cavernous malformations), coagulopathy, amyloid angiopathy, tumor, vasculitis, venous infarction, and illicit drug abuse. Amyloid angiopathy is most common in patients over the age of 70. It is a presumed diagnosis in older patients with repeated ICH, but can only be definitively diagnosed by deposits of beta amyloid protein found in the vessel walls (usually on autopsy). Arteriovenous malformation is a common cause of ICH in younger patients (ages 20 to 40). AVMs are congenital abnormalities in which a tangled mass of blood vessels is present. Within the arteriovenous malformation, the arterial circulation and venous circulation connect without going through a capillary system. Following resolution of the acute ICH, arteriovenous malformations are treated with endovascular embolization, surgical resection, or stereotactic radiosurgery.

In addition to direct tissue injury, the hematoma formed by ICH displaces nearby brain tissue and causes ischemia through compression. Edema occurs around the site of hemorrhage. If the ICH occurs deep within the cerebral hemispheres, it can rupture into the ventricle (intraventricular hemorrhage). The mortality rate is higher in hemorrhagic stroke than ischemic stroke.

Clinical Presentation

ICH presents with a sudden onset of focal neurologic deficits (monoparesis, hemiparesis, monoplegia, or hemiplegia) often associated with a severe headache, nausea/vomiting, decreased consciousness, and sometimes seizures. Neurologic deficits vary based on the area of the brain affected and are similar to the focal deficits experienced by patients with acute ischemic stroke.

Diagnostic Tests

ICH is diagnosed using CT scanning. Tests that may be performed to determine the etiology of the hemorrhage include MRI/MRA and cerebral angiography.

Principles of Management of Intracerebral Hemorrhage

Operative management is based on size and location of hemorrhage. Cerebellar hemorrhage may require a suboccipital craniectomy to evacuate the clot and decrease pressure on vital structures. Blood pressure control and correction of coagulopathy are primary concerns. The blood pressure goal is based on the etiology of the ICH, with lower levels often desired for ICH due to arteriovenous malformation. Intraventricular hemorrhage may cause hydrocephalus, which is treated by placement of an external ventricular drain. The role of intraventricular thrombolytic administration in intraventricular hemorrhage is currently being researched. Antiepileptic medications are typically administered to prevent seizures. Nursing considerations include management of elevated ICP and prevention of secondary complications.

SEIZURES

Etiology, Risk Factors, and Pathophysiology

Seizures are rapid, repeated bursts of abnormal electrical activity within the brain that result from an imbalance of excitatory and inhibitory impulses. Signs and symptoms depend on the location of the abnormal activity. A seizure is often a symptom or consequence of an underlying neurologic problem, such as a tumor, hemorrhage, trauma, or infection. Systemic disturbances such as hypoxia, hypoglycemia, drug overdose, and drug or alcohol withdrawal may also cause seizures. Many seizures are considered idiopathic, but treatable causes must be ruled out.

During a seizure, the metabolic demands of the brain for oxygen and glucose increase dramatically. The body tries to keep up with these increased requirements by increasing CBF. If CBF does not keep up with demand, neurons revert to anaerobic metabolism, which leads to secondary ischemia and brain injury.

Clinical Presentation

Clinical presentation varies based on the origin and extent of the brain's abnormal electrical activity. Seizure types can be identified using the International Classification of Epileptic Seizures.

Partial Seizures

Partial seizures occur when there is a focal discharge in one area of the cerebral cortex. Partial seizures are described as simple or complex. The primary difference is that complex partial seizures cause alterations of consciousness, whereas simple partial seizures do not. Partial seizures may progress to generalized seizures.

Simple Partial Seizures (Also called focal motor or focal sensory seizures) may manifest as

- Motor activity such as twitching or jerking in an extremity or one side of the face
- Sensory symptoms such as an unusual taste or smell
- Autonomic sensations such as sweating or vomiting

Complex Partial Seizures (Also called temporal lobe seizures) may manifest as

- Automatisms (smacking the lips, chewing motions, or fidgeting)
- Purposeless activity such as running or arm jerking
- Change in affect such as elation or fear

Generalized Seizures

Generalized seizures result when the abnormal electrical discharge is bilateral. Patients are more likely to be injured in the course of a generalized seizure than a partial seizure. Following the seizure, the patient may complain of muscle aches related to the violent movements. There are many types of generalized seizures:

- *Absence:* Sudden lapse of consciousness and activity that lasts 3 to 30 seconds. Commonly described as a *staring spell.*

- *Myoclonic:* Sudden, brief muscle jerking of one or more muscle groups. Commonly associated with metabolic, degenerative, and hypoxic causes.
- *Atonic* (also called drop attacks): Sudden loss of muscle tone.
- *Clonic:* Rhythmic muscle jerking.
- *Tonic:* Sustained muscle contraction.
- *Tonic–clonic:* Muscle activity varies between sustained contraction and jerking.

Status Epilepticus

Status epilepticus indicates prolonged or recurring seizures without a return to baseline mental status. A seizure or series of seizures lasting longer than 30 minutes is described as status epilepticus, but treatment is typically instituted much sooner. Status epilepticus is a medical emergency with a significant mortality rate, higher in the elderly or when the seizure is a symptom of an underlying acute process. There are two primary types of status epilepticus—generalized convulsive status epilepticus and nonconvulsive status epilepticus. In generalized convulsive status epilepticus, seizure activity is readily apparent using clinical observation. In nonconvulsive status epilepticus, no outward clinical seizures may be noted but consciousness is impaired and seizure activity is apparent on EEG. Nonconvulsive status epilepticus is believed to be more common than previously thought among patients with decreased level of consciousness of unknown etiology.

AT THE BEDSIDE
► *Status Epilepticus*

A 52-year-old man is admitted to the ICU for management of status epilepticus. He has a long history of seizures following a traumatic brain injury (TBI) 4 years prior. He has returned to work and has no obvious residual deficits of brain injury. He was admitted to the acute care floor yesterday because of increasing seizure frequency. This morning he began having generalized tonic–clonic seizures while eating breakfast. Despite receiving lorazepam, he continues to have seizure activity. His phenytoin level this morning was 25 mcg/mL (normal range 10 to 20 mcg/mL). Upon arrival to the ICU, the patient is intubated for airway management and a midazolam infusion is started. Continuous EEG monitoring is initiated. Both clinical and electrographic evidence of seizure activity stops within 1 hour. The midazolam infusion is weaned over several days with no return of seizure activity and his mental status returns to baseline. He is transferred to the acute care unit for continued adjustments of his antiepileptic medications, and a workup is initiated to evaluate the need for surgical intervention.

Diagnostic Testing

In the critical care environment, management of seizures in a patient without a history of epilepsy is aimed at stopping the seizure and then determining an underlying cause. Diagnostic testing may include:

- *Lab work* to identify electrolyte abnormalities or metabolic etiology.
- *CT* to assess for intracranial processes such as an intracranial hemorrhage or tumor.
- *MRI* to look for structural lesions that may indicate a seizure focus.
- *LP* when an infectious process (e.g., meningitis) is the suspected source of seizure activity.
- One normal *EEG* does not rule out seizure. Patients in status epilepticus may require continuous EEG monitoring. Epileptiform activity may be present on EEG even after the clinical seizure has stopped.
- *Continuous video monitoring* in conjunction with continuous EEG recordings to correlate clinical phenomena with electrical activity in the brain.
- *Intracranial electrodes* in the evaluation of patients with intractable seizures to identify a focus or foci prior to surgical resection. Intracranial electrodes are inserted via burr holes or a craniotomy.

Principles of Management of Seizures

Management of the patient with seizures focuses on controlling the seizure as quickly as possible, preventing recurrence, maintaining patient safety, and identifying the underlying cause. Observation of seizure type, duration, and any precipitating factors is essential. Following a seizure, patients may experience a period of confusion and altered mental status that slowly resolves. They may complain of a headache or muscle aches. Todd's paralysis describes continued focal symptoms that can persist for up to 24 hours after a seizure. Because of the risk of missing underlying intracranial pathology, patients with focal neurologic deficits following a seizure are diagnosed with Todd's paralysis only after other causes have been ruled out.

Maintaining Patient Safety and Airway Management

From a nursing perspective, the first priority is to prevent the patient from further injury. Ensure a safe environment during the seizure by clearing objects out of the area. Padded side rails are indicated for patients at high risk for seizures. During a seizure, attempting to restrain patient movement may result in injury and is avoided.

Airway management assists with maintaining adequate cerebral oxygenation. Maintaining the airway may depend on stopping the seizure. Positioning the patient on his or her side decreases aspiration; supplemental oxygen is provided. Nothing should be placed in the patient's mouth during a seizure. EKG monitoring, continuous pulse oximetry, and blood pressure monitoring are required in patients with prolonged seizures. Hypoglycemia can induce seizure activity, so a glucose level is checked immediately and treated as appropriate.

Medication Administration for Status Epilepticus

The average seizure stops within 2 minutes without requiring medication. Patients with prolonged seizures or status epilepticus receive a benzodiazepine such as lorazepam. Diazepam may be used instead of lorazepam, but is associated with a higher recurrence rate because it has a short duration of action in the brain. The second medication given is typically phenytoin or fosphenytoin. Fosphenytoin is converted to phenytoin in the blood. Fosphenytoin can be administered more quickly than phenytoin and causes less tissue injury should extravasation occur. Both agents can cause cardiovascular side effects, predominately treatment-resistant hypotension, but these side effects are more common with phenytoin. If seizure activity continues, phenobarbital may be used but has significant cardiovascular side effects. Midazolam and propofol are often used as third-line medications in status epilepticus. It is important to remember that neuromuscular blockers, including those used in intubation, stop the motor manifestations of seizure but not the abnormal electrical activity in the brain, and neuronal injury continues.

The prolonged muscle activity that occurs with convulsive status epilepticus may cause tissue breakdown and lead to rhabdomyolysis. Serum creatine phosphokinase is elevated and myoglobin may be present in the urine. Hydration is essential to avoiding renal dysfunction.

Treatment Options for Patients With Seizures

Many patients require ongoing medication for seizure control. Some common medications include phenytoin, phenobarbital, carbamazepine, valproic acid, gabapentin, and levetiracetam. Seventy-five percent of patients treated with medication are able to attain seizure control and live productive lives.

Some patients with seizures uncontrolled by medications may be helped by surgery to remove the seizure focus. These patients most often have complex partial seizures originating from the temporal lobe. Selection criteria include intractable seizures that significantly impact quality of life and are uncontrolled by medication, an identifiable unilateral focus of seizure activity, and seizure focus in an area where removal will cause no major neurologic deficit. A craniotomy is used to access and excise the seizure focus. The primary complications are hemorrhage and infections. The patients are kept on their previous seizure medications during the postoperative period. About 50% of patients become seizure free after surgery and an additional 30% experience a significant improvement in seizure control.

For patients with intractable seizures who do not have an identifiable focus, placement of a vagus nerve stimulator may be considered. Vagal nerve stimulation reduces seizure duration, frequency, or intensity by providing intermittent electrical stimulation of the vagus nerve. The exact mechanism of action has not been determined.

INFECTIONS OF THE CENTRAL NERVOUS SYSTEM

Meningitis

Meningitis is an acute inflammation of the meninges of the brain and spinal cord. Meningitis can be caused by bacteria, viruses, fungi, or parasites. Risk factors include immunocompromise, trauma or surgery that disrupts the meninges, and crowded living conditions. Signs and symptoms include fever, headache, neck stiffness, irritability, vomiting, photophobia, changes in level of consciousness, seizures, weakness, and cranial nerve signs. The classic signs of meningitis include Kernig's sign (severe pain in the hamstring with knee extension when the hip is flexed 90°) and Brudzinski's sign (involuntary flexion of the knees and hips when the neck is flexed). Many patients with meningococcal meningitis have a characteristic rash (petechial rash that progresses to purple blotches). Diagnostic testing includes LP for opening pressure and CSF analysis, blood cultures, sputum cultures, nasopharyngeal cultures, and EEG. CT scanning is performed prior to LP in patients with papilledema or focal neurologic findings. Complications include hydrocephalus, cerebral edema, and vasculitis. Nursing priorities include management of elevated ICP, implementation of seizure precautions, and administration of antimicrobial therapy. Isolation may be required until the causative organism is identified and treated; notify the infection control practitioner and follow institutional guidelines.

Encephalitis

Encephalitis is inflammation of the brain parenchyma. There are many types of encephalitis, including arboviruses such as West Nile, but the most common type seen in most ICUs is encephalitis due to the herpes simplex virus (HSV). HSV encephalitis can result from a new infection, or can represent a reactivation of a preexisting infection. Signs and symptoms include fever, focal or diffuse neurologic changes, headache, seizures, and neck stiffness. HSV encephalitis predominately affects the inferior frontal and temporal lobes. Diagnostic testing includes MRI, EEG, and CSF analysis. The diagnosis is often presumed pending specialized testing of the CSF, and empiric therapy is started with the antiviral agent acyclovir.

Intracranial Abscess

An *intracranial abscess* is a collection of pus in the brain and can be extradural, subdural, or intracerebral. The infective agent enters the brain through the bloodstream, via an opening in the dura (as may occur with a basilar or open skull fracture or following a neurosurgical procedure), or via direct migration from chronic otitis media, poor dentition, frontal sinusitis, or mastoiditis. Signs and symptoms typically develop over a few weeks and may include headache, seizures, fever, neck pain, focal neurologic signs such as hemiparesis, cranial nerve deficits, and change on level of consciousness. Diagnostic testing includes CT with contrast administration, MRI, EEG, and potentially needle aspiration of the lesion for culture. Treatment includes prolonged antibiotic therapy (usually 6 weeks) and in many cases surgical drainage of the abscess.

NEUROMUSCULAR DISEASES

Although there are a number of neuromuscular diseases that may result in hospitalization, only a small number of these patients require admission to the critical care unit. Myasthenia gravis and Guillain-Barré syndrome often cause respiratory muscle weakness requiring mechanical ventilation and are briefly described.

Myasthenia Gravis

In myasthenia gravis, autoimmune-mediated destruction of acetylcholine receptors results in decreased neuromuscular transmission and muscle weakness. Myasthenia gravis is a chronic disease with periodic exacerbations. Diagnostic testing includes laboratory testing for acetylcholine receptor antibodies, EMG, CT scanning of the chest to evaluate for abnormalities of the thymus, and "tensilon testing." Edrophonium chloride (Tensilon) is a short-acting anticholinesterase inhibitor that can be administered intravenously. Improvement in symptoms following edrophonium chloride injection confirms the diagnosis of myasthenic crisis. Adverse effects of edrophonium chloride include bradycardia, asystole, increased oral and bronchial secretions, and bronchoconstriction.

Patients with myasthenia gravis are admitted to the ICU for intubation and mechanical ventilation during acute exacerbation. Treatment includes IV immunoglobulin or plasma exchange in addition to supportive care. Long-term management may include the administration of anticholinesterase medications, thymectomy, or immunosuppression. Priorities of nursing management during an acute exacerbation include close monitoring of respiratory status and prevention of secondary complications.

Guillain-Barré Syndrome

Guillain-Barré syndrome causes progressive muscle weakness, sensory loss, and areflexia due to peripheral nerve demyelination. Symptoms generally start in the lower extremities and ascend. Diagnostic studies include LP and nerve conduction studies. Approximately 25% to 40% of patients require mechanical ventilation. Some patients experience autonomic instability characterized by variations in heart rate and blood pressure. Neuropathic pain related to inflammation and demyelination occurs and requires both pharmacologic and nonpharmacologic treatment. In addition to supportive therapy, patients may receive plasma exchange or IV immune globulin. Most patients recover completely or with minimal deficits, but may require weeks to months of hospitalization. Nursing priorities include close monitoring of respiratory status and prevention of complications related to prolonged immobility.

SELECTED BIBLIOGRAPHY

Assessment and Diagnostic Testing

Bateman DE: Neurological assessment of coma. *J Neurol Neurosurg Psychiatr* 2001;71(suppl 1):113–117.

Bleck TP: Levels of consciousness and attention. In Goetz CG (ed): *Textbook of Clinical Neurology* [electronic version], 2nd ed. Philadelphia: Saunders; 2003.

CAM-ICU web site: www.ICUdelirium.org

Davis AE, Park S, Darwich H, et al: Neurodiagnostic tests. In Bader MK, Littlejohns LR (eds): *AANN Core Curriculum for Neuroscience Nursing,* 4th ed. St. Louis, MO: Saunders; 2004.

Ely EW, Inouye SK, Bernard GR, et al: Delirium in mechanically ventilated patients: Validity and reliability of the Confusion Assessment Method for the Intensive Care Unit (CAM-ICU). *JAMA* 2001;286:2703–2710.

Ely EW, Shintai A, Truman B, et al: Delirium as a predictor of mortality in mechanically ventilated patients in the intensive care unit. *JAMA* 2004;291:1753–1762.

Fischer J, Mathieson C: The history of the Glasgow coma scale: Implications for practice. *Crit Care Nurs Q* 2001;23(4):52–58.

Goldberg S: *The Four Minute Neurologic Exam.* Miami, FL: MedMaster, Inc; 1999.

Hickey JV: *The Clinical Practice of Neurological and Neurosurgical Nursing,* 5th ed. Philadelphia: Lippincott Williams & Wilkins; 2003.

Hobdell EF, Stewart-Amidei C, McNair N, et al: Assessment. In Bader MK, Littlejohns LR (eds): *AANN Core Curriculum for Neuroscience Nursing,* 4th ed. St. Louis, MO: Saunders; 2004.

Lindsay KW, Bone I: *Neurology and Neurosurgery Illustrated.* Edinburgh, UK: Churchill Livingstone; 1997.

McNicoll L, Pisani MA, Zhang Y, et al: Delirium in the intensive care unit: Occurrence and clinical course in older patients. *J Am Geriatr Soc* 2003;51:591–598.

Milbrandt EB, Deppen S, Harrison PL, et al: Costs associated with delirium in mechanically ventilated patients. *Crit Care Med* 2004;32:955–962.

Morcos SK, Thomsen HS: Adverse reactions to iodinated contrast media. *Euro Radiol* 2001;11:1267–1275.

Schuurmans MJ, Deschamps PI, Markham SW, et al: The measurement of delirium: Review of scales. *Res Theory Nurs Pract* 2003;17:207–224.

Thompson EJ, King SL: Acetylcysteine and fenoldopam: Promising new approaches for preventing effects of contrast nephrotoxicity. *Crit Care Nurse* 2003;23(3):39–46.

Intracranial Pressure

Hickey JV: *The Clinical Practice of Neurological and Neurosurgical Nursing,* 5th ed. Philadelphia: Lippincott Williams & Wilkins; 2003.

Kirkness C, March K: Intracranial pressure management. In Bader MK, Littlejohns LR (eds): *AANN Core Curriculum for Neuroscience Nursing,* 4th ed. St. Louis: Saunders; 2004.

Lynn-McHale DJ, Carlson KK: *AACN Procedure Manual for Critical Care,* 4th ed. Philadelphia: WB Saunders; 2001.

March K: Application of technology in the treatment of traumatic brain injury. *Crit Care Nurs Q* 2000;23(3):26–37.

March K, Wellwood J: Intracranial pressure concepts and cerebral blood flow. In Bader MK, Littlejohns LR (eds.): *AANN Core Curriculum for Neuroscience Nursing,* 4th ed. St. Louis: Saunders; 2004.

March K, Wellwood J, Arbour R: Technology. In Bader MK, Littlejohns LR (eds): *AANN Core Curriculum for Neuroscience Nursing,* 4th ed. St. Louis: Saunders; 2004.

Acute Ischemic Stroke and Hemorrhagic Stroke

Adams HP, Adams RJ, Brott T, et al: Guidelines for the early management of patients with ischemic stroke. *Stroke* 2003;34:1056–1083.

Hickey JV. *The Clinical Practice of Neurological and Neurosurgical Nursing,* 5th ed. Philadelphia: Lippincott Williams & Wilkins; 2003.

Hinkle JL, et al: Cerebrovascular events of the nervous system. In Bader MK, Littlejohns LR (eds): *AANN Core Curriculum for Neuroscience Nursing,* 4th ed. St. Louis: Saunders; 2004.

Hinkle JL, Bowman L: Neuroprotection for ischemic stroke. *J Neurosci Nurs* 2003;35(2):114–118.

Lindsay KW, Bone I: *Neurology and Neurosurgery Illustrated,* 3rd ed. Edinburgh, UK: Churchill Livingstone; 1997.

Vance DL: Treating acute ischemic stroke with intravenous alteplase. *Crit Care Nurse* 2001;21(4):25–32.

Seizures

Buelow JM, Long L, Rossi AM, Gilbert KL: Epilepsy. In Bader MK, Littlejohns LR (eds): *AANN Core Curriculum for Neuroscience Nursing,* 4th ed. St. Louis: Saunders; 2004.

Engel J Jr, Weibe S, French J, et al: Practice parameter: Temporal lobe and localized neocortical resections for epilepsy: Report of the Quality Standards Subcommittee of the American Academy of Neurology, in association with the American Epilepsy Society and the AANS. *Neurology* 2003;60:538–47.

Manno EM: New management strategies in the treatment of status epilepticus. *Mayo Clin Proc* 2003;78:508–518.

Varelas PN, Mirski MA: Seizures in the adult intensive care unit. *J Neurosurg Anesthes* 2001;13:163–175.

Infections of the Central Nervous System

Barker E: Central nervous system infections. In Barker E (ed): *Neuroscience Nursing: A Spectrum of Care,* 2nd ed. St. Louis, MO: Saunders; 2002.

Vandemark MV, Lovasik DA, Neatherlin JS, Omert T: Infectious and autoimmune processes. In Bader MK, Littlejohns LR (eds): *AANN Core Curriculum for Neuroscience Nursing,* 4th ed. St. Louis, MO: Saunders; 2004.

Victor M, Ropper AH: Bacterial, spirochetal, fungal, and parasitic infections of the nervous system, and sarcoidosis. In *Adams and Victor's Manual of Neurology,* 7th ed. New York: McGraw-Hill; 2002.

Victor M, Ropper AH: Viral infections of the nervous system. In *Adams and Victor's Manual of Neurology,* 7th ed. New York: McGraw-Hill; 2002.

Neuromuscular Diseases

Chiò A, Cocito D, Leone M, et al, and the Piedmonte and Valle d'Aosta Register for Guillain-Barré Syndrome: Guillain-Barré syndrome: A prospective, population-based incidence and outcome survey. *Neurology* 2003;60(7):1146–1150.

Keesey J: A treatment algorithm for autoimmune myasthenia in adults. *Ann N Y Acad Sci* 1998;841:753–768.

Polak M, Richman J, Lorimer M, et al: Neuromuscular disorders of the nervous system. In Bader MK, Littlejohns LR (eds): *AANN Core Curriculum for Neuroscience Nursing,* 4th ed. St. Louis, MO: Saunders; 2004.

Rees JH, Thompson RD, Smeeton NC, Hughes RA: Epidemiological study of Guillain-Barré syndrome in south east England. *J Neurol Neurosurg Psych* 1998;64:74–77.

Sharshar T, Chevret S, Bourdain F, Raphaël J, for the French Cooperative Group on Plasma Exchange in Guillain-Barré Syndrome: Early predictors of mechanical ventilation in Guillain-Barré syndrome. *Crit Care Med* 2003;31(1):278–283.

Thomas CE, Mayer SA, Gungor Y, et al: Myasthenic crisis: Clinical features, mortality, complications, and risk factors for prolonged intubation. *Neurology* 1997;48(5):1253–1260.

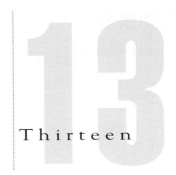

Hematology and Immunology Systems

Thirteen

Diane K. Dressler

▶ Knowledge Competencies

1. Analyze basic laboratory test results used to assess the status of the hematologic and immunologic systems for abnormalities:
   • Complete blood count
   • White blood cell differential
   • Erythrocyte sedimentation rate
   • Prothrombin time/International Normalization Ratio
   • Partial thromboplastin time
   • Fibrinogen
   • Fibrin split products/D-dimer

2. Describe the etiology, pathophysiology, clinical presentation, patient needs, and management

approaches for common hematologic problems in critically ill patients:
   • Anemia
   • Thrombocytopenia
   • Disseminated intravascular coagulation

3. Contrast the clinical presentation, patient needs, and principles of management of the immunocompromised patient with that of a patient with an intact immune response.

SPECIAL ASSESSMENT TECHNIQUES, DIAGNOSTIC TESTS, AND MONITORING SYSTEMS

A complete patient assessment guides the selection of screening tests for hematologic and immunologic problems. Historical data are particularly important and should include family history, occupational exposures, lifestyle behaviors, diet, allergies, past medical problems, surgeries, transfusion of blood or blood products, and current medications. Abnormal physical assessment data from each body system collectively identify risk factors or acute abnormalities pertinent to hematologic and immunologic function. In addition, a variety of laboratory tests assist the clinician to evaluate problems in these systems (Table 13–1).

Complete Blood Count

The complete blood count (CBC) is a primary assessment tool for evaluation of the hematologic and immunologic status. The red blood cell (RBC) count and RBC indices, along

with the hemoglobin and hematocrit levels, provide valuable information regarding the oxygen-carrying capability of the blood. The total white blood cell (WBC) count and the WBC differential reveal the body's ability to muster an immunologic response against foreign substances and to participate in the normal inflammatory process required for tissue restoration. Partial information concerning hemostasis is obtained from the platelet count, with additional studies required to fully evaluate the coagulation process.

Red Blood Cell Count

The RBC count is based on the number of erythrocytes per cubic millimeter of blood. Normal values for men are higher than for women. A decrease in normal RBC count by 10% indicates anemia. Anemia may be caused by decreased production or increased destruction of RBC, or loss of RBC by hemorrhage. An increase in the total number of RBC occurs as a compensatory mechanism in persons with chronic hypoxia or as an adaptation to high altitudes. Further assessment

TABLE 13–1. NORMAL VALUES FOR HEMATOLOGIC AND IMMUNOLOGIC SCREENING TESTS[a]

Laboratory Test	Normal Value
RBC	Males: 4.6–6.2 million/mm^3
	Females: 4.2–5.4 million/mm^3
Hgb	Males: 13–18 g/dL
	Females: 12–16 g/dL
Hct	Males: 45%–54%
	Females: 36%–46%
RBC indices	
MCV	81–98 μm^3
MCH	27–32 pg/cell
MCHC	32%–36%
Total WBC	5000–10,000 mm^3
WBC differential (% of total)	
Neutrophils	60%–70%
Segmented	56%
Bands	3%–6%
Eosinophils	1%–4%
Basophils	0.5%–1.0%
Monocytes	2%–6%
Lymphocytes	20%–40%
Platelet count	150,000–400,000 mm^3
Erythrocyte sedimentation rate	
Westergren method	Males: 0–15 mm/h
	Females: 0–20 mm/h
PT	11–15 sec
Therapeutic anticoagulation	1.5 times normal
INR	1.0–1.2
Therapeutic anticoagulation	2.0–3.0
APTT	<35 sec
Therapeutic anticoagulation	1.5–2.5 times normal
ACT	150–180 sec
Fibrinogen	200–400 mg/dL
FSP	2–10 μg/mL
D-dimer	<200 ng/mL

[a]Normals vary between laboratories. Refer to local laboratory standard values when interpreting test results.

of the ability of the bone marrow to produce RBC is obtained by a reticulocyte count.

Hemoglobin

Hemoglobin is the primary carrier of oxygen to body tissues. As the number of RBC changes, so does the hemoglobin content. The hemoglobin can be estimated by multiplying the total RBC count by 3. A decrease in hemoglobin to a level as low as 7 g/dL can be well tolerated, if the decrease occurs gradually. Patients with underlying cardiac or pulmonary disorders may become symptomatic with even small changes in the hemoglobin content of the blood.

Hematocrit

Hematocrit measures the RBC mass in relationship to a volume of blood. It is usually expressed as the percentage of

cells per 100 milliliter of blood. Multiplying the hemoglobin value by 3 gives an estimate of hematocrit. The hematocrit is particularly sensitive to changes in the volume status of the patient, increasing with fluid losses (hemoconcentration) and decreasing with increased plasma volume (hemodilution). Interpretation of hemoglobin and hematocrit results must also take into account the time the values were obtained in relationship to blood volume loss or fluid administration. For example, values obtained immediately after an acute hemorrhage may appear normal, because compensatory mechanisms have not had time to restore plasma volume. Restoration of plasma volume by compensation or crystalloid resuscitation lowers the hemoglobin and hematocrit.

Red Blood Cell Indices

The RBC indices (mean corpuscular volume, mean corpuscular hemoglobin, mean corpuscular hemoglobin concentration) are mathematical calculations based on the RBC, hemoglobin, and hematocrit and describe the size, weight, and hemoglobin concentration of the individual erythrocyte. These indices are useful in determining the etiology of anemia.

Total White Blood Cell Count

Leukocytes, or WBC circulating in the blood, are measured as an indicator of the total amount of WBC in the body. Most WBCs are not sampled in a CBC because they are marginated along capillary walls, circulating in the lymphatic system, or sequestered in lymph nodes and other body tissues.

Increased WBC, or leukocytosis, usually is caused by an elevation in one type of WBC line. It is most often associated with a normal immune system response to an acute infection, but is also a normal result of the inflammatory process. WBCs are known to have both positive effects (such as phagocytosis of microorganisms) and negative effects. These include the release of toxins and mediators such as oxygen free radicals from neutrophils and cytokines from macrophages. Overproduction of abnormal leukocytes in the bone marrow occurs during leukemia.

Leukopenia refers to a decrease in the total WBC number. This occurs when bone marrow production is inhibited or during infection when rapid consumption of WBC takes place. The life span of a circulating WBC is only hours to days; therefore, a constant replacement process is necessary to prevent leukopenia.

White Blood Cell Differential

Five different categories of leukocytes are measured in the differential and reported as a percentage of the total WBC count. The absolute count is calculated by multiplying the percentage of each type of cell by the total WBC count. Increases or decreases in one cell line help to determine normal immune response or predict impaired immunity.

Neutrophils are the primary responders to infection and inflammation in the body. This type of WBC is released from the bone marrow in an immature form called a band. Bands quickly mature into segmented neutrophils with greater phagocytic properties to respond to infection. Most often leukocytosis is caused by an increased number of segmented neutrophils (neutrophilia). *Left shift* refers to leukocytosis with an increased percentage of bands. Neutropenia, or a decreased number of circulating neutrophils, places the body at increased risk for infection. An absolute neutrophil count of less than $1000/mm^3$ severely compromises immune system function, particularly to bacterial infections.

Monocytes are phagocytic cells that circulate briefly in the blood before leaving the cardiovascular system to mature into macrophages in other body tissues. The circulating monocyte is an important scavenger WBC. As it performs phagocytosis, it sends out chemicals called cytokines, which activate other components of the immune system.

Lymphocytes are the WBCs responsible for the body's specific immune response to infection. Subsets of these lymphocytes exist and are assessed by other laboratory tests. Lack of properly functioning lymphocytes or adequate numbers of these cells places the body at particular risk for viral and fungal infections and certain malignancies. The CD4 cell is a subset of lymphocytes. It is the target of HIV infection leading to the development of acquired immunodeficiency syndrome.

Eosinophils are thought to perform phagocytosis of immune complexes generated during allergic reactions. Therefore, increased percentages of these cells are seen during an allergic response. Basophils are another WBC associated with allergy. They are thought to break down during an allergic reaction, releasing their intracellular contents of heparin and histamine. This destruction causes a lower percentage of basophils following an allergic response.

Platelet Count

Platelets are disc-shaped fragments of megakaryocytes and are not true cells. They are called *thrombocytes* because of their role in the initiation of blood coagulation at the site of damaged blood vessel walls. Two thirds of the body's platelets are circulating in the blood, with the remaining third sequestered within the spleen. Thrombocytopenia (decreased number of platelets) is associated with increased risk of spontaneous bleeding and is caused by decreased production, increased consumption, increased destruction, or increased sequestration of platelets. Hypercoagulability of the blood can result from increased circulating platelets caused by proliferative disorders and inflammation. Qualitative assessment of platelet function is determined by the bleeding time.

Erythrocyte Sedimentation Rate

A nonspecific but useful test in monitoring inflammation and infection in the body is the erythrocyte sedimentation rate (ESR). It measures the rate RBC settle out of unclotted blood. This rate is affected by inflammatory elements in the blood. Women normally have a higher rate than men. Different laboratory techniques have different normal values. Elevated ESR is seen in pregnancy, infection, inflammatory diseases, and cancer. Decreased ESR is seen in sickle cell anemia, polycythemia, or hypofibrinogenemia.

Coagulation Studies

Prothrombin Time and International Normalizing Ratio

The prothrombin time (PT) evaluates the extrinsic pathway of fibrin clot formation stimulated by tissue trauma. Prolonged PT may be caused by abnormalities in coagulation factors V, VII, and X, prothrombin, fibrinogen, and vitamin K, and by liver disease or disseminated intravascular coagulation (DIC). It is a test used to evaluate therapeutic anticoagulation with warfarin. PT results are reported in seconds.

Because of different reagents used in testing, PT values from different facilities are not standardized, so comparing results may lead to discrepancies. The International Normalization Ratio (INR) is a calculation developed to standardize interpretation of PT results. The PT and INR may be reported together, but the INR is now the recommended parameter for establishing the therapeutic range for oral anticoagulant therapy.

Partial Thromboplastin Time and Activated Partial Thromboplastin Time

The partial thromboplastin time (PTT) and activated partial thromboplastin time (APTT) are reported in seconds and are used to evaluate fibrin clot formation stimulated by the intrinsic pathway of coagulation. The APTT is a more sensitive test than the PTT, and is used most often. This test is used to screen for congenital coagulation disorders and for monitoring anticoagulation with unfractionated heparin therapy. Liver disease, vitamin K deficiency, and DIC prolong the APTT.

Activated Coagulation Time

The activated coagulation time is reported in seconds. The test is used most commonly to monitor effects of unfractionated heparin during and following cardiovascular procedures such as cardiopulmonary bypass and percutaneous coronary interventions. It is often performed at the point of care.

Fibrinogen

Fibrinogen, also known as *coagulation factor I*, is the plasma protein that becomes the fibrin clot. Plasma levels may be increased during an inflammatory response, pregnancy, or acute infection. Decreased levels are present with liver disease and DIC. If the fibrinogen level has been elevated, a downward trend, even though within normal range, can indicate a consumptive coagulopathy. Other specific clotting factor assays may be performed if a coagulopathy or hereditary bleeding tendency is suspected.

Fibrin Split Products and Fibrin Degradation Products

The normal breakdown of a fibrin clot releases fragments with mild anticoagulant properties called *fibrin split products* (FSP) or *fibrin degradation products* (FDP). Excessive clot breakdown results in elevated amounts of FSP, contributing to a tendency for bleeding. Increased FSP are observed in DIC, obstetrical complications involving hemorrhage, and thrombotic disorders such as pulmonary embolism. Fibrinolytic drugs such as alteplase and reteplase recombinant, used therapeutically in treating myocardial infarction and other thrombotic events, cause levels of FSP to rise.

D-Dimer

Individual fragments of FSP can be identified. One fragment, the D-dimer, is a very specific indicator of fibrinolysis. Levels of D-dimer are elevated during fibrinolytic drug therapy, in thrombotic conditions, and in DIC.

Additional Tests and Procedures

After obtaining basic laboratory screening tests, additional laboratory and diagnostic testing is necessary to identify specific etiologies for hematologic and immunologic function. For patients with hematologic disorders, a peripheral blood smear, a bone marrow aspiration, or further studies of specific clotting factor assays may be performed.

Microbiological specimens for Gram stain and culture help to identify sources of infection. Molecular diagnostic techniques such as polymerase chain reaction detect infectious agents not readily cultured, such as viruses. Noninvasive studies such as ultrasound may determine liver, spleen, or lymph node abnormalities. Radiologic procedures (radiographs, CT scans, arteriograms) may be needed to identify areas of infection or hemorrhage.

PATHOLOGIC CONDITIONS

Critically ill patients often have combined abnormalities involving the hematologic and immunologic systems. The patient with sepsis and subsequent DIC, as in the case study, typifies this situation. Anemia, immunocompromise, and coagulopathy are three distinct problems faced in the management of this patient. Each of these problems is explored separately.

Anemia

Etiology, Risk Factors, and Pathophysiology

Anemia is the most common condition resulting from hematologic disease. Its etiology may be classified into disorders of RBC production, increased destruction of RBC, or acute blood loss.

A patient history gives important clues to the etiology of anemia. Decreased production may result from nutritional

---

AT THE BEDSIDE
▶ *Sepsis and Disseminated Intravascular Coagulation*

A 72-year-old Caucasian man was admitted to the MICU with hypotension, alteration in mental status, and a fever of 102°F. He has a history of rheumatoid arthritis, right total hip replacement, and gastric ulcers. He is disoriented to place and time. Hemodynamic data revealed values consistent with septic shock. Dressings covering his intravascular lines show evidence of oozing from insertion sites. Nasogastric aspirate is coffee ground in appearance. His initial laboratory data show:

RBC	3.3 million/mm^3
Hemoglobin	10.8 g/dL
Hematocrit	31%
WBC	13,000/mm^3, with 79% segmented neutrophils and 20% bands
Platelets	120,000/mm^3
Fibrinogen	325 mg/dL
INR	2.0
PTT	60 sec
FSP	40 mcg/mL
D-dimer	.250 ng/mL

---

deficiencies in substrates for RBC production—iron, folic acid, or vitamin B_{12}. Those at high risk for iron deficiency anemia include children, adolescents, pregnant women, and patients with malabsorption syndromes. Chronic blood loss from the gastrointestinal (GI) tract or from heavy menstruation is the most common cause. Daily blood testing in hospitalized patients also leads to anemia, because the acutely ill patient's bone marrow cannot keep up with the loss. Folic acid deficiency may be seen in alcoholics. Dietary vitamin B_{12} deficiency may occur in strict vegetarians and from lack of intrinsic factor (postgastrectomy or with pernicious anemia) or Crohn's disease.

Anemia may be associated with chronic illness, such as chronic inflammation, infection, cancer, liver disease, or renal failure. The life span of RBC is decreased in these chronic disease states, and the bone marrow does not compensate adequately with increased production. Cancer specifically involving the bone marrow replaces normal bone marrow and decreases new RBC generation. Anemia associated with chronic renal failure is more severe and involves a decrease in production of erythropoietin, resulting in decreased stimulation of bone marrow production of RBC.

Aplastic anemia (bone marrow suppression) represents a failure of the bone marrow to produce RBCs and other cellular components of blood. A thorough medication history may reveal use of drugs with potential for bone marrow suppressive side effects. Cancer chemotherapeutic agents represent one such category of drugs. Other causes of aplastic anemia include exposure radiation, toxins, and certain infections.

Premature destruction of RBCs leads to hemolytic anemia. This can occur episodically or chronically. Abnormalities intrinsic to the RBC are usually hereditary causes of hemolytic anemia, such as sickle cell disease or G6PD deficiency. Extrinsic sources of hemolysis include immune destruction as in a transfusion reaction, damage by artificial heart valves, cardiopulmonary bypass, or intra-aortic balloon pumping.

Acute hemorrhage also leads to anemia. Trauma, surgical blood loss, DIC, GI bleeding, and bleeding from excessive anticoagulation frequently are encountered as causes of anemia in the critical care patient population. With acute hemorrhage, both cellular components and plasma are lost simultaneously. Until volume replacement from fluid resuscitation or mobilization of fluids from extracellular sources occurs, a drop in hematocrit will not be appreciated.

Regardless of the etiology of anemia, the critical effect of decreased RBC and hemoglobin is a decrease in the oxygen-carrying capacity of the blood. Effects may be well tolerated if anemia develops slowly, but may be life threatening if sudden blood loss occurs. Rapid loss of blood volume results in hypovolemic shock and cardiovascular instability, further reducing delivery of oxygen to body tissues.

Clinical Signs and Symptoms

Clinical manifestations are related to the body's compensatory mechanisms attempting to maintain perfusion of oxygen to vital tissues. As compensatory mechanisms are overwhelmed, more serious signs and symptoms occur. Patients with underlying pathology involving the pulmonary and cardiovascular system do not tolerate the effects of anemia and become symptomatic more quickly.

Cardiovascular

- Tachycardia, palpitations
- Angina
- Increased cardiac output
- Decreased capillary refill
- Orthostatic hypotension
- ECG abnormalities (dysrhythmias, ischemic changes)
- Hypovolemic shock (hypotension, tachycardia, decreased cardiac output, increased systemic vascular resistance)

Respiratory

- Increased respiratory rate
- Dyspnea on exertion, progressing to dyspnea at rest

Skin/Musculoskeletal

- Pallor of skin and mucous membranes
- Dusky nailbeds
- Intermittent claudication

- Muscle cramps
- Decreased skin temperature

Neurologic

- Headache
- Light-headedness
- Faintness
- Irritability
- Restlessness
- Fatigue

Abdominal

- Enlarged liver and/or spleen

Principles of Management of Anemia

The management of the anemic patient must be guided by the severity of symptoms. The level of concern for decreases in hemoglobin and hematocrit is determined by the patient's signs and symptoms and if active bleeding is suspected. Restoration of adequate oxygen delivery to tissues is a priority in the critically ill patient. Identification of the etiology of anemia and resolution of the underlying cause is done simultaneously.

Improving Oxygen Delivery

Oxygen delivery is a product of the amount of hemoglobin in the blood, the saturation of the hemoglobin with oxygen, and the cardiac output. Management strategies focus on optimizing each of those components.

1. Administration of supplemental oxygen can enhance oxygen saturation. Use of oxygen, particularly during activity, may minimize desaturation and dyspnea.
2. Adequate hemoglobin can be replaced in acute situations only by transfusion of RBC. Transfusion of one unit of packed RBC should increase the hemoglobin by 1 g/dL and hematocrit by 2% to 3%.
3. Cardiac output can be optimized with volume replacement, including packed RBC, in situations of bleeding and hypovolemia. Other manipulations of cardiac output must be guided by hemodynamic monitoring and calculations to assess oxygen delivery and oxygen consumption.
4. Monitoring vital signs, oxygen saturation, and subjective patient data before, during, and after a change in therapy or activity identifies the patient's ability to tolerate anemia.
5. Minimizing activity and planning periods of rest are important nursing interventions for the anemic patient.

Identifying and Treating Underlying Disease State

Further diagnostic testing is indicated to determine the etiology of anemia. Radiologic and endoscopic studies to locate sites of bleeding, particularly in the GI tract, may be necessary. Treatment of the underlying cause of anemia may vary from supportive care to the following:

1. Administer recombinant human erythropoietin to restore bone marrow production in chronic anemia. The response may take several weeks so it is not appropriate in situations in which acute correction of anemia is necessary. Chronic renal failure patients and patients receiving chemotherapy may benefit from this treatment.
2. Supplemental oral ferrous sulfate or IV iron sucrose or iron gluconate may be indicated if iron-deficiency anemia is present.
3. Vitamin B_{12} and folic acid–related anemias may also require supplementation.
4. Dietary consultation may be needed prior to discharge to help patients and families plan meals with foods high in iron.

Minimizing Blood Loss and Reducing the Need for Transfusion

1. Use small volume collection tubes and microanalysis techniques.
2. Assess the need for routine and new blood testing daily.
3. Use cell savers and autotransfusion systems in surgical patients.
4. Control hypertension in postoperative patients to avoid stress on vascular suture lines.
5. Use prophylactic agents to reduce the risk of GI bleeding.
6. Screen all patients for anticoagulants and bleeding risk prior to procedures.
7. Accept normovolemic anemia in stable patients.

Immunocompromise

Etiology, Risk Factors, and Pathophysiology

All critically ill patients may be considered compromised hosts because their defense mechanisms are inadequate due to a combination of factors, such as underlying disease, medical therapy, nutritional status, age, or stress. Patients in the critical care unit are much more likely to develop a nosocomial infection than other hospitalized patients. *Immunocompromised* is applied to patients whose immunologic defense mechanisms are defective. Immunocompromised patients may also develop opportunistic infection. Once infection develops in a critically ill patient, it may quickly progress to systemic inflammatory response syndrome or sepsis.

Immune system protection from infection is categorized into three levels: natural defenses, nonspecific responses, and specific responses. Natural defenses include having intact epithelial surfaces (skin and mucous membranes) with normal chemical barriers (pH, secretions) present and all protective reflexes (blink, swallow, cough, gag, sneeze) intact. The invasive catheters and tubes used in critical care bypass these protective barriers.

The nonspecific response to infection is activation of the phagocytic WBC (neutrophils and monocytes) to attack the foreign microorganisms (antigens) that have entered the body by passing or overwhelming the natural defenses. The monocytes play a key role in processing the invading antigen and presenting it to the lymphocytes involved in the specific immune response.

Lymphocytes (B cells and T cells) are responsible for the orchestration of an immune response specific to the antigen. B lymphocytes create antigen-specific antibodies or immunoglobulins to aid in the destruction of the antigen and to protect the body from future encounters with the antigen. This is called *humoral immunity*. T lymphocytes have different subsets of cells created to modulate the immune system response (the T4 or CD4 helper T cells) or cells that have cytotoxic properties (the T8 or cytotoxic CD8 cells) against the antigen. The immune response of the T lymphocytes is called *cell-mediated immunity*. Both types of lymphocytes work closely together in a specific immune response. However, humoral immunity is the primary protection against bacterial invasion and cell-mediated immunity is primarily targeted against infection by intracellular bacteria, viral, and fungal organisms.

Deficiencies in immune system function can be categorized into primary, or congenital, immune system defects and secondary, or acquired, immune system dysfunction. Immune deficiencies may be pinpointed to a specific cell type or may involve abnormalities in multiple components of the immune system. Secondary or acquired immunodeficiencies are the most likely type encountered in the critically ill patient population. Acquired immunodeficiency may be secondary to age, malnutrition, stress, chronic disease states, malignancy, drugs with immunosuppressive effects, or HIV infection.

Today, increased numbers of patients are undergoing organ transplantation and receiving immunosuppressive agents. More aggressive chemotherapeutic treatment of cancer is producing higher numbers of patients with bone marrow suppression. The dramatic growth in the number of people infected with HIV has also increased the number of immunosuppressed patients. All of these patients are at high risk for the development of neutropenia and other manifestations of immunosuppression.

Neutropenia, an absolute neutrophil count below $500/mm^3$, generally increases susceptibility to infection. The cause and duration of neutropenia, the functional capability of the neutrophils, the state of the patient's natural barriers, and the endogenous and exogenous flora also contribute to the susceptibility of the individual patient to infection. The earlier infection can be detected, the more likely therapy is to be effective.

Detection of infection in the immunocompromised patient may be difficult. Due to lack of neutrophils, the patient may not be able to mount a vigorous inflammatory response; therefore, classic signs and symptoms of infection may be diminished or absent. For instance, purulent drainage is largely the result of dying neutrophils at the site of infection. The neutropenic patient may have an infection without evidence of purulent drainage. Pain may be the patient's only complaint. Any complaint of pain in the immunocompromised patient population must be fully investigated. Fever in this patient population is another key sign of infection and warrants aggressive investigation.

Clinical Signs and Symptoms

Local Evidence of Inflammation and Infection

- Redness
- Edema
- Warmth
- Pain
- Purulent drainage

General Evidence of Infection

- Fever or hypothermia
- Rigors or shaking chills
- Fatigue and malaise
- Changes in level of consciousness
- Lymphadenopathy
- Tachycardia
- Tachypnea

System-Specific Evidence

Neurologic

- Headache
- Nuchal rigidity

Respiratory

- Cough
- Change in color, amount of sputum
- Dyspnea, orthopnea

Genitourinary

- Dysuria
- Urgency
- Frequency
- Flank pain
- Abdominal pain
- Cloudy and/or bloody urine

Gastrointestinal

- Nausea
- Vomiting
- Diarrhea
- Cramping abdominal pain
- Enlarged liver or spleen

Principles of Management for Immunompromised Patients

Those patients with high risk for the development of infection must be identified on admission to the critical care unit. Measures to protect and strengthen immune system function should be included in the plan of care. All health care team members must utilize measures to prevent the development of nosocomial infection. Close monitoring for signs and symptoms of a local or systemic inflammatory response to infection is especially important to detect infection early. Identification of the source and likely organisms causing infection allows for initiation of broad-spectrum, empiric antimicrobial coverage. Culture and sensitivity reports guide the choice of drug(s) specific to the organisms isolated from the patient.

Identification of Patients with High Risk of Infection

Risk factors for immunocompromise are as follows.

1. Neonates and the elderly
2. Malnutrition
3. Medications with known immunosuppressive effects such as steroids, cancer chemotherapeutic agents, and transplant immunosuppressive agents
4. Recent radiation therapy
5. Chronic systemic diseases such as renal or hepatic failure or diabetes mellitus
6. Known diseases involving the immune system such as HIV infection
7. Loss of protective epithelial barriers through
   - Oral or nasogastric intubation
   - Presence of decubitus ulcers
   - Burns
   - Surgical wounds
   - Skin and soft tissue trauma
8. Invasive catheters or prosthetic devices in place such as
   - Intravascular catheters
   - Indwelling bladder catheters
   - Heart valve replacements
   - Orthopedic hardware such as artificial joints, pins, plates, or screws
   - Cardiovascular devices such as ventricular assist devices, pacemakers, or implantable defibrillators
   - Synthetic vascular grafts
   - Ventricular shunts

Implementing Measures to Protect and Strengthen Immune System Function

1. Take meticulous care of the skin and mucous membranes to prevent loss of barrier protection.
2. Use the enteral route for feeding when possible to maintain caloric intake and normal gut function.
3. Avoid the use of urinary bladder catheters.
4. Minimize patient stress and the release of endogenous glucocorticoids by relieving pain or using alternative methods such as guided imagery or music

for relaxation, and other comfort measures (positioning, massage).

5. Administer colony stimulating factors (G-CSF or GM-CSF) to stimulate bone marrow production of neutrophils and monocytes.

Implementing Measures to Prevent Nosocomial Infection

1. All personnel and visitors should wash their hands before and after contact with the patient. Hand washing remains the number one method to prevent nosocomial infection.
2. Institute universal blood and body fluid precautions with all patients and appropriate isolation for known or suspected patient infection.
3. Adhere to strict aseptic technique for all care of intravascular catheters and any invasive procedures performed at the patient's bedside.
4. Eliminate environmental sources of infection (e.g., fresh flowers, leftover fluids used for irrigations).
5. Track the time fluids, tubings, and catheters are used in administering IV fluids to the patient and change them at the prescribed intervals.
6. Encourage coughing and deep breathing every 4 hours; ambulate as tolerated.
7. Review facility protocol regarding use of filtered water, restriction of fresh fruits and vegetables, and so on, for immunocompromised patients.

Early Detection of Local or System Inflammatory Response to Infection

1. Monitor the patient closely for signs and symptoms consistent with infection and communicate abnormal findings to the physician.
2. Collect specimens for culture and sensitivity from potential sources of nosocomial infection (e.g., IV catheter tips, urine, sputum, blood, stool, wound drainage).

Coagulopathies

Etiology, Risk Factors, and Pathophysiology

Critically ill patients with coagulopathy may have a problem involving platelets, hemostasis, fibrinolysis, or a combination of these abnormalities. Acquired disorders of coagulation, as opposed to inherited disorders, are seen most frequently in critical care.

Platelets are the first to activate the coagulation process at the site of blood vessel injury. Quantitative platelet disorders can cause traumatic bleeding when the platelet count drops to between 50,000 and 100,000/mm^3. Spontaneous bleeding is possible at counts of 10,000 to 50,000/mm^3. Counts that reach 5000 to 10,000/mm^3 are at high risk for spontaneous hemorrhage. Four general mechanisms are responsible for thrombocytopenia: decreased production of platelets by the bone marrow, shortened survival due to platelet destruction, sequestration of platelets in the spleen, and

intravascular dilution of platelets during massive transfusion.

Thrombocytopenia may also be related to immunologic mechanisms. Drug-induced thrombocytopenia occurs when a drug induces an antigen–antibody reaction that results in the formation of immune complexes that destroy platelets by complement-mediated lysis. There are several types of immune-related thrombocytopenia that are seen in critical care. Heparin-induced thrombocytopenia is an immune reaction to heparin which can result in clinical thrombosis. Immune (idiopathic) thrombocytopenia purpura is another autoimmune disorder characterized by thrombocytopenia, petechiae, and purpura. Thrombotic thrombocytopenia purpura is a complication from infection that can result in widespread vascular occlusion. Hemolytic-uremic syndrome most often results from infectious colitis and the release of bacterial toxins that lead to hemolytic anemia, thrombocytopenia, and acute renal failure.

Patients may have adequate numbers of platelets but still have a bleeding tendency due to qualitative platelet disorders. Drug-induced suppression of platelet function is commonly associated with use of aspirin and nonsteroidal anti-inflammatory agents (NSAIDs). Critically ill patients may be receiving multiple drugs with the potential for impairment of platelet function. Patients with renal failure and uremia also may suffer from platelet dysfunction.

Disorders of hemostasis may be caused by inherited abnormalities of coagulation factors. Hemophilia types A and B are congenital deficiencies in factor VIII and factor IX. Von Willebrand's disease represents a deficiency or dysfunction of the plasma protein of the same name. Replacement of the deficient factor keeps these chronic diseases under control. Patients with these disorders may be monitored in critical care units when undergoing routine surgical procedures or when hospitalized for other medical problems.

Acquired coagulation disorders can be associated with deficient coagulation factor production. This may be caused by a decreased amount of vitamin K, the vitamin essential to the formation of clotting factors II, VII, IX, and X. Critically ill patients are more susceptible to deficiency in vitamin K as a result of dietary deficiency, intestinal malabsorption, liver disease, use of warfarin, or antibiotic therapy. Vitamin K deficiency prolongs the PT/INR. Patients with liver disease have deficiencies of fibrinogen and other factors in addition to the vitamin K–dependent factors.

Many of the drugs used routinely in critical care have anticoagulant and antiplatelet effects (Table 13–2). Therapeutic anticoagulation using heparin, warfarin, and other agents interferes directly with the clotting process. The intrinsic pathway and the final common pathway are affected by the administration of heparin. If bleeding from heparin is minimal, it can be controlled by decreasing the dose or temporarily stopping its administration. If bleeding is severe, the antidote to reverse heparin, protamine sulfate, may be administered intravenously. Low-molecular-weight hep-

TABLE 13–2. ANTICOAGULANTS COMMONLY USED IN CRITICAL CARE

Unfractionated heparin	Heparin sodium
Low-molecular-weight heparins	Dalteparin sodium (Fragmin) Enoxaparin (Lovenox)
Glycoprotein IIb/IIIa inhibitors	Abciximab (Reopro) Eptifibatide (Integrilin) Tirofiban hydrochloride (Aggrastat)
Direct thrombin inhibitors	Argatroban (Acova, Novastan) Bivalirudin (Angiomax) Lepirudin (Refludan)
Thrombolytic agents	Alteplase (Activase) Reteplase recombinant (Retavase) Drotrecogin alfa (Xigris)
Antiplatelet agents	Aspirin Clopidogrel bisulfate (Plavix) Dipyridamole (Persantine) Ticlopidine (Ticlid)

arin is associated with fewer bleeding and immunological complications.

Warfarin acts by inhibiting the production of vitamin K–dependent clotting factors. Effects from warfarin take several days to be observed after initiation of the drug, but may persist for many days following administration. If significant bleeding occurs while on the warfarin, replacement of vitamin K–dependent factors by use of fresh frozen plasma may be necessary. Giving replacement vitamin K may also be helpful, but its effectiveness depends on the time taken by the liver to synthesize new clotting factors.

Use of thrombolytic agents (alteplase, reteplase) to dissolve pathologic fibrin clots may result in patient bleeding from sites where a protective clot has formed. These agents are used in combination with other anticoagulants, and may precipitate obvious or occult bleeding.

DIC is a complex coagulopathy which can develop in patients already critically ill from a wide variety of disorders (Table 13–3). The underlying condition triggers the release of pro-inflammatory cytokines, which activate the coagulation cascade and result in the formation of microclots. The microclots obstruct the capillaries of organs and tissues. This initiates a series of events which result in both bleeding and thrombosis. (Figure 13–1) The acute form of DIC is associated with critical illness. A chronic form of this syndrome is associated with malignancy.

During the process of DIC, stimulation of the clotting cascade rapidly depletes existing platelets and coagulation factors, consuming them at rates faster than the body can replace them. Depletion of substrates of the coagulation process leaves the body at risk for spontaneous bleeding or hemorrhage from surgical sites, or even minimal trauma.

Multiple tiny clots are formed within the blood and flow to the small vessels where they are trapped. Microcirculatory thrombosis then leads to tissue ischemia, infarction, and organ dysfunction. Single or multisystem organ dysfunction may occur.

Simultaneous activation of fibrinolysis releases the enzyme plasmin. Plasmin breaks down some of the fibrin in

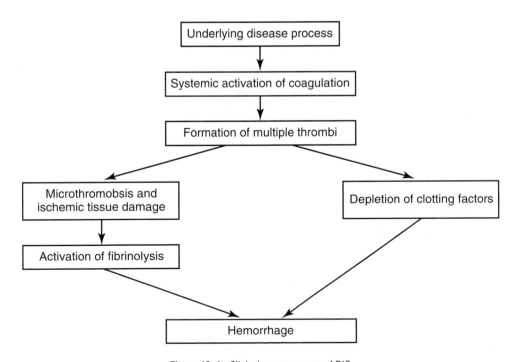

Figure 13–1. Clinical consequences of DIC.

TABLE 13–3. ETIOLOGIES OF DIC

Cardiovascular
Shock
Arterial aneurysm

Tissue Trauma
Burns
Crush injury
Head injury
Extracorporeal circulation
Malignant hyperthermia
Snake venom

Infections
Bacterial
Viral
Fungal

Obstetrical
Eclampsia
Amniotic fluid embolism
Abruptio placentae
Placenta previa
Abortion
Retained dead fetus

Neoplastic Disease
Acute leukemia
Adenocarcinoma

Immunologic Reaction
Incompatible transfusion

a physiologic attempt to open the microcirculation, and this produces FDP. These end products of fibrin breakdown have anticoagulant properties. Overproduction of FDP overwhelms the body's ability to clear them from the circulation, resulting in an increased level of circulating anticoagulants. Clots at new sites of injury are unable to form and existing clots are dissolved, leading to bleeding from both old and new sites.

Laboratory diagnosis of DIC requires careful interpretation of results (Table 13–4). In many cases absolute certainty regarding a diagnosis of DIC may not be possible. With or without a clear diagnosis of DIC, a primary goal of therapy is to treat the underlying condition. In addition, supportive care is provided with volume replacement and support of vital organ systems, including ventilatory assistance. Significant bleeding is managed with blood and component therapy. Heparin may be prescribed for some patients to stop the formation of new thrombi.

TABLE 13–4. LABORATORY RESULTS SUGGESTING DIC

Test	Abnormality
Platelet count	Decreased
PT/INR	Prolonged
PTT/APTT	Prolonged
Fibrinogen	Decreased
FSP/FDP	Increased
D-dimer	Increased

Clinical Signs and Symptoms

Coagulopathy may be a subtle, occult process or a massive, obvious emergency. Assessment must encompass each body system, looking for evidence of abnormality in single or multiple components of the coagulation process.

Abnormal Platelet Numbers or Function

- Petechiae of skin or mucous membranes
- Spontaneous bleeding from gums or nose
- Thrombocytopenia
- Prolonged bleeding time

Abnormal Coagulation Factors

- Hemorrhage into subcutaneous tissue, muscle, or joints
- Ecchymosis, purpura
- Bleeding responds slowly to local pressure
- Prolonged PT/INR, APTT
- Decreased fibrinogen
- Decrease in level of specific coagulation factors

General Assessment for Bleeding or Decreased Organ Perfusion as a Result of Microthrombosis

Skin/Musculoskeletal

- Oozing of blood from multiple sites, including incisions, intravascular catheters
- Petechiae
- Purpura
- Ecchymosis
- Acral cyanosis of toes, fingers, nose, lips, ears
- Pain, swelling, and limited joint mobility
- Increased size of body part, increased girth

Neurologic

- Any change in level of consciousness, pupils, movement or sensation may indicate intracranial bleeding
- Impaired vision with retinal hemorrhage

Gastrointestinal

- Guaiac positive gastric fluids
- Coffee ground emesis or gastric aspirate
- Melena or frank bloody stool
- Abdominal pain
- Enlarged liver or spleen

Genitourinary

- Hematuria
- Decreased urine output
- Vaginal bleeding

Cardiovascular

- Labile blood pressure
- Hypovolemia and/or shock (with rapid loss of large volume of blood)

AT THE BEDSIDE
▶ *Thinking Critically*

As the patient's condition stabilizes, his care plan is revised. His history of rheumatoid arthritis, total hip replacement, and gastric ulcers is taken into consideration. His medications include:

- Prednisone
- Methotrexate
- Omeprazole
- Ferrous sulfate
- Folic acid

What are this patient's risk factors for potential hematologic and immunologic problems while hospitalized?

List interventions that will decrease the risk of anemia, coagulopathy, and nosocomial infection.

Principles of Management of Coagulopathies

The management of coagulopathy varies with the type and severity of the disorder. The overall goal of therapy is to restore normal hemostasis. Supportive care focuses on the control and prevention of further bleeding associated with activities of daily living and therapeutic interventions.

Restoration of Normal Hemostasis

1. Treatment of quantitative platelet disorders may involve transfusion of platelets. One unit of platelets may be expected to increase the platelet count by 5000 to 10,000/mm³. Transfusion is recommended for levels less than 5000/mm³, and prophylactically between 5000 and 33,000/mm³. Increasing the platelet count to higher levels may be necessary for invasive procedures or surgery.
2. Destruction of platelets by immune mechanisms may be treated with steroids or IV immunoglobulin infusion. If related to use of heparin, then heparin should be discontinued. Splenectomy may be performed for severe persistent problems.
3. Dysfunctional platelets may be treated by stopping the offending agent, such as aspirin or NSAIDs. If caused by uremia, short-term improvement may be achieved by administering IV desmopressin. Dialysis improves platelet function in patients with renal failure.
3. Acute replacement of coagulation factors can be accomplished with transfusion of fresh frozen plasma. Cryoprecipitate replaces fibrinogen, factor VIII, and von Willebrand factor. For hemophiliac patients, factor VIII or factor IX concentrates are used to replace the specific factor deficiency.
5. IV vitamin K may be used to treat warfarin-related bleeding or vitamin K deficiency.

6. Heparin therapy may be stopped, or the dosage decreased or reversed with IV protamine sulfate.

Controlling and Preventing Bleeding

1. Modify nursing care measures to minimize trauma and prevent skin and mucous membrane breakdown:
   - Use sponge sticks for oral care.
   - Use electric razor or refrain from shaving.
   - Avoid use of suppositories, tampons, or catheters.
   - Minimize use of automatic blood pressure cuffs.
   - Minimize peripheral blood sampling.
   - Avoid IM injections.
   - Use specialty mattress, pad side rails; avoid restraint use.
   - Handle patients gently when turning or moving.
   - Gently remove adhesive dressings.
   - Avoid nasotracheal suctioning; do not extend suction catheters past end of artificial airways.
2. Modify nursing care procedures to control bleeding:
   - Minimize traumatic procedures; apply direct pressure afterward for at least 5 to 10 minutes or until bleeding has stopped.
   - After removal of intravascular line, elevate arm above level of heart or for central line elevate the head to decrease venous pressure.
   - Use cold saline mouth rinses for oral bleeding.
   - Use ice packs on hematomas or hemarthrosis.
   - Do not dislodge or attempt to remove blood clots.

SELECTED BIBLIOGRAPHY

Anemia

Vernon S, Pfeifer GM: Blood management strategies for critical care patients. *Crit Care Nurse* 2003;23(6):34–41.

Blood Product Administration

Mackersie RC: Transfusion therapy. In Shoemaker WC, Grenvik A, Ayres SM, Holbrook PR (eds): *Textbook of Critical Care Medicine.* Philadelphia: WB Saunders; 2000.

Immunocompromised Patients

Shelton BK: Hematological and immune disorders. In Sole ML, Lamborn ML, Hartshorn JC (eds): *Introduction to Critical Care Nursing,* 3rd ed. Philadelphia: Saunders; 2001.

DIC

Maxson JH. Management of disseminated intravascular coagulation. *Crit Care Nurs Clin North Am* 2000;12(3):341–352.

Evidence-Based Practice Guidelines

Centers for Disease Control and Prevention: *Guidelines for Isolation Precautions in Hospitals, 1997.* Available: www.cdc.gov.

Gastrointestinal System

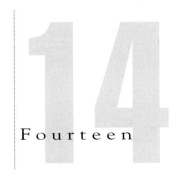

Fourteen

Joanne Krumberger, Carol Rees Parrish, and Joe Krenitsky

▶ Knowledge Competencies

1. Describe the etiology, pathophysiology, clinical presentation, patient needs, and principles of management for
   - Acute upper gastrointestinal bleeding
   - Liver failure
   - Acute pancreatitis
   - Bowel ischemia
   - Bowel obstruction

2. Identify nutritional requirements for enterally fed critically ill patients.

3. List important interventions to decrease the risk for aspiration pneumonia during enteral feeding.

PATHOLOGIC CONDITIONS

Acute Upper Gastrointestinal Bleeding

Life-threatening gastrointestinal (GI) bleeding originates most commonly in the upper GI tract and requires immediate therapy to prevent complications. Although bleeding stops spontaneously in 80% to 90% of cases, patients presenting with sudden blood loss are at risk for decreased tissue perfusion and oxygen-carrying capability, which can affect every organ system in the body. Bleeding that originates distal to the ligament of Treitz is considered to be lower GI bleeding which, different from upper GI bleeding, is not associated with morbidity. Lower GI bleeding is generally a disease of the elderly patient, usually associated with diverticulosis.

Etiology, Risk Factors, and Pathophysiology

A variety of abnormalities within the GI tract can be the source of upper GI bleeding (Table 14–1). The most common cause of upper GI bleeding is peptic ulcer disease. Its pathogenesis is related to hypersecretion of gastric acid, coupled with impaired GI tract mucus secretion. Normally, mucus protects the gastric wall from erosive effects of acid. Peptic ulcers occur in the stomach and the duodenum, and are characterized by a break in the mucosal layer that penetrates the muscularis mucosa (innermost muscular layer), resulting in bleeding. Infection of the mucosa by *Helicobacter pylori,* an organism naturally found in the GI tract, also has been implicated in the pathogenesis of peptic ulcer disease.

Gastroesophageal varices develop when there is increased flow of blood through the portal venous system of the liver. If blood cannot flow easily through the liver because of obstructive disease, it is diverted to collateral channels. These channels are normally low-pressure vessels found in the distal esophagus (esophageal varices), the veins in the proximal stomach (gastric varices), and in the rectal vault (hemorrhoids) (Figure 14–1). Acute upper GI hemorrhage occurs when esophageal and/or gastric varices rupture from increased portal vein pressure (portal hypertension). Portal hypertension is most commonly caused by primary liver disease (see next section), liver trauma, or thrombosis of the splenic or portal veins. Massive upper GI hemorrhage is associated with these variceal bleeds.

Mallory-Weiss syndrome is a linear, nonperforating tear of the gastric mucosa near the gastroesophageal junction. The tear is the result of pressure changes in the stomach that

AT THE BEDSIDE
▶ *Upper GI Bleeding*

A 45-year-old white man is admitted with reports of an 8-hour history of nausea and vomiting of large amounts of "coffee ground secretions" and frequent "maroon-colored" stools. He reports a previous history of peptic ulcer disease diagnosed at age 35 years. He has been hospitalized twice in the past for active GI bleeding. A duodenal ulcer near the pylorus on the posterior wall of the stomach was diagnosed by endoscopy. Significant findings on his admission profile were:

Vital Signs

Blood pressure:	96/60 mm Hg lying; 82/50 mm Hg sitting
Heart rate:	120 beats/min; sinus tachycardia with 2-mm ST-segment elevation
Respiratory rate:	32/min, deep
Temperature:	99.2°F (oral)

Respiratory

Breath sounds clear in all lung fields

Cardiovascular

S_1/S_2 no murmurs
Extremities cool, diaphoretic; pulses present but weak

Abdomen

Distended with hyperactive bowel sounds in all four quadrants

Tender right upper quadrant, no rebound tenderness

Neurologic

Alert, oriented
Anxious

Genitourinary

50 mL of amber cloudy urine following Foley catheter insertion
Stools liquid maroon, guaiac positive

Arterial Blood Gases

pH	7.49
$PaCO_2$	28 mm Hg
HCO_3	19 mEq/L
PaO_2	61 mm Hg on room air
SaO_2	89%
Hematocrit	25%
Hemoglobin	7.0 g/dL
White blood cell count	17,000/mm^3
Prothrombin time	11 sec
Activated partial thromboplastin time	30 sec
Platelet count	110,000/mm^3
Serum potassium	3.5 mEq/L (decreased)
Serum sodium	150 mEq/L
Serum glucose	210 mg/dL
Serum blood urea nitrogen	40
Serum creatinine	0.9
Liver function	Within normal limits

TABLE 14–1. COMMON SOURCES OF UPPER GASTROINTESTINAL BLEEDING

Peptic Ulcer Disease
Gastric ulcer
Duodenal ulcer

Varices
Esophageal
Gastric

Pathologies of the Esophagus
Tumors
Mallory-Weiss syndrome
Inflammation
Ulcers

Pathologies of the Stomach
Cancer
Erosive gastritis
Stress ulcer
Tumors

Pathologies of the Small Intestine
Peptice ulcers
Angiodysplasia

---

occur with vomiting. Alcohol abuse and inflammatory conditions of the stomach and esophagus are also associated with this disorder.

Hemorrhagic gastritis describes gastric lesions that do not penetrate the muscularis mucosa. These are also referred to as stress ulcers. Onset of bleeding is sudden and is often the first symptom. The causes of gastritis are multifactorial (Table 14–2), most commonly associated with nonsteroidal anti-inflammatory drug (NSAID) use, alcohol abuse, and physiologic conditions that cause severe stress (e.g., trauma, surgery, burns, severe medical problems). Alcohol and NSAIDs are known to directly disrupt the mucosal defense mechanisms of the stomach (Figure 14–2). Use of NSAIDs is particularly problematic in the elderly and contributes to increased incidence of symptomatic acute upper GI bleeding in that population.

Regardless of the etiology, upper GI bleeding that results in a sudden loss of blood volume decreases venous return to the heart, with a corresponding decrease in cardiac

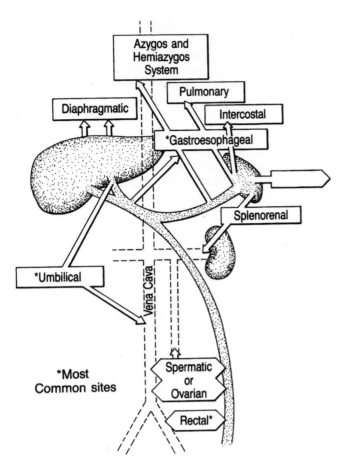

Figure 14–1. The liver with collateral circulation.

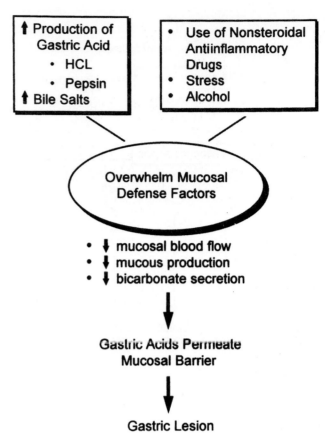

Figure 14–2. Pathogenesis of gastritis.

output (CO). The decrease in CO triggers the release of epinephrine and norepinephrine, causing intense vasoconstriction and tissue ischemia (Figure 14–3). The clinical signs and symptoms of upper GI hemorrhage are directly related to the effects of the decrease in CO and of this vasoconstriction response, typical in hypovolemic shock. In addition, aldosterone and antidiuretic hormones are released, resulting in sodium and water retention.

Clinical Presentation

History
Individuals have a history of peptic ulcer disease, alcohol abuse, severe physiologic stress, NSAID use, or other GI bleeding causes.

Signs and Symptoms
The response of an individual to blood loss depends on the rate and amount of the loss, the patient's age and preexisting physiologic state, and the rapidity of treatment. Specific signs and symptoms include:

- Hematemesis: Bright red blood or coffee ground
- Melena or maroon-colored stools
- Nausea
- Epigastric pain
- Abdominal distension
- Bowel sounds increased or decreased
- If blood loss is greater than 25% of blood volume: hypotension (orthostatic); altered hemodynamic values

TABLE 14–2. CAUSES OF GASTRITIS

Alcohol Abuse
NSAID use
Aspirin
Ascriptin
Ecotrin
Ibuprofen
Naprosyn
Severe Physiologic Stress
Burns (Curling's ulcer)
CNS disease (Cushing's ulcer)
Trauma
Surgery
Medical complications
  Sepsis
  Acute renal failure
  Hepatic failure
Long-term mechanical ventilation

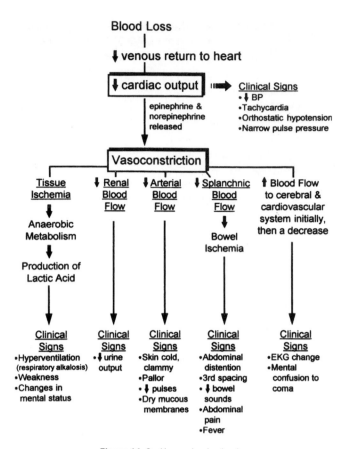

Figure 14–3. Hypovolemic shock.

(decreased central venous pressure [CVP], pulmonary capillary wedge pressure [PCWP], mean arterial pressure [MAP], CO)

- Rapid, deep respirations
- Tachycardia
- Fever
- Cold, clammy skin
- Dry mucous membranes
- Decreased pulses
- Weakness
- Decreased urine output
- Anxiety
- Mental status changes
- Restlessness
- Electrocardiographic (ECG) changes consistent with ischemia (e.g., ST-segment elevation, dysrhythmias)

Diagnostic Tests

- Hematocrit may be normal initially, then decreased with fluid resuscitation and blood loss. It is important to note that the hematocrit may not reflect actual amount of blood loss accurately because equilibrium with extravascular fluid and subsequent hemodilution requires several hours. The hematocrit decreases as extravascular fluid enters the vascular space to restore

volume. This process is not complete for 24 to 72 hours.

- Hemoglobin may be normal initially, then decreased with fluid resuscitation and blood loss.
- White blood cell count is elevated.
- Platelet count is decreased depending on amount of blood loss.
- Serum sodium is usually elevated initially due to hemoconcentration.
- Serum potassium is usually decreased with vomiting.
- Serum blood urea nitrogen (BUN) is mildly elevated.
- Serum creatinine is elevated.
- Serum lactate is elevated with severe bleeding.
- Prothrombin time (PT) is usually decreased.
- Activated thromboplastin time (APTT) is usually decreased.
- Arterial blood gases show respiratory alkalosis (early), metabolic acidosis with severe shock, and hypoxemia.
- Gastric aspirate shows normal or acidotic pH and is guaiac positive.

Principles of Management for Upper GI Bleeding

The management of the patient with acute upper GI bleeding revolves around three major areas: hemodynamic stabilization, identification of the bleeding site, and initiation of definitive medical or surgical therapies to control or stop the bleeding. Measures to decrease anxiety in this patient population are also a focus due to the severity and sudden onset of GI bleeding.

Hemodynamic Stabilization

The initial assessment of GI bleeding focuses on vital signs, which are the most reliable signs of the amount of blood loss. Resuscitation begins immediately in the presence of hemodynamic instability. Risk criteria for patients with acute GI bleed include ongoing bleeding, hemoglobin less than 8 g/dL, systolic blood pressure less than 100 mm on presentation, elevated prothrombin time, erratic mental status, and comorbid disease, such as cardiovascular or liver disease.

1. Monitor and record cardiovascular status (blood pressure, heart rate including orthostatic changes), hemodynamics (CVP, PCWP, CO, MAP), and peripheral pulses.
2. Insert at least two large-bore intravenous (IV) catheters and begin fluid resuscitation with crystalloid solution (e.g., normal saline). Administer fluids to maintain MAP at 60 mm Hg or higher.
3. Obtain blood for hematocrit, hemoglobin, and clotting studies, as well as for typing and cross-matching for packed red blood cells (PRBC). Usually at least 6 units are ordered. The hematocrit taken during the initial resuscitation rarely is useful for transfusion requirements. Estimates for the amount of blood loss are most reliably guided by vital sign values (Table 14–3).

TABLE 14–3. ESTIMATING BLOOD LOSS FROM ACUTE GI BLEEDING

Clinical Signs	Estimated Blood Loss
Systolic BP >90 mm Hg Orthostatic hypotension Heart rate <110 beats/min	20–25% total blood volume (approximately 1000 mL)
Systolic BP 70–90 mm Hg Heart rate 110–130 beats/min	25–40% total blood volume (approximately 1500–2000 mL)

Signs of moderate decreased tissue
  perfusion:
  Anxiety
  Cool, clammy skin
  Decreased urine output
  Hyperventilation
  Diminished pulses	

Systolic blood pressure <70 mm Hg
Mean arterial pressure <60 mm Hg
Signs of severe decreased tissue
  perfusion:
  Impaired mental status
  Cold, clammy, diaphoretic skin
  Thready pulses
  Decreased urine output
  Metabolic acidosis
  ECG changes
  Heart failure
  Respiratory failure
	>40% total blood volume

4. Administer IV colloids, crystalloids, or blood products as prescribed until the patient is stabilized. Blood products may be considered in the initial resuscitation if the hemodynamic response is poor after administering 2 to 3 L of crystalloid fluids. PRBC are used to rapidly increase the hematocrit and with less volume than whole blood. Each unit of PRBC increases the hematocrit by 2% to 3% and improves gas exchange. Up to 24 hours may be required for blood administration to be reflected in the hematocrit values to accurately reflect red blood cell counts, especially if large amounts of crystalloid solutions were administered during the resuscitation.

5. Monitor coagulation studies (e.g., PT/PTT, platelet count).

6. Monitor fluid balance and renal function (intake and output, daily weight, BUN, creatinine, and hourly urine output).

7. Insert a nasogastric tube if bleeding is massive (>40% of blood volume) to assess for the rate of bleeding. Use of gastric lavage in upper GI hemorrhage is controversial. Proponents believe that removing blood clots by gastric lavage is useful in that it allows the stomach to contract and tamponade bleeding vessels. Removal of blood may give some indication of the rate of bleeding and may minimize the chance of pulmonary aspiration. If lavage is ordered, room temperature saline usually is used.

8. Position the patient in the left lateral decubitus position to minimize aspiration associated with hematemesis.

9. Monitor temperature and maintain normothermia. Rapid fluid resuscitation, particularly with blood products, can lead to hypothermia, with interference of normal coagulation. Warming of fluids may be required to prevent hypothermia if traditional measures are insufficient.

10. Prepare for urgent endoscopic therapy if estimated blood loss is greater than 3 units of blood, bright red blood is found in emesis or nasogastric aspirate, or if it is a suspected variceal bleed.

Identify the Bleeding Site

Although the history and physical examination are used to differentiate between upper and lower GI bleeding, endoscopic examination is required to determine the exact site of the bleeding. Endoscopic visualization at the bedside is preferred to allow for early direct visualization of the upper tract during resuscitation measures.

1. Administer sedation (e.g., midazolam [Versed]) as ordered and institute monitoring protocol.

2. Position patient in a left lateral decubitus position to prevent aspiration of GI contents during endoscopy. Have oral-tracheal suction available at the bedside before the procedure begins.

3. Monitor for cardiac ischemia during the exam (e.g., ST-segment changes [see Chapter 18, Advanced ECG Concepts], arrhythmias).

Institute Therapies to Control or Stop Bleeding

Definitive therapies to treat the bleeding differ depending on the cause. A treatment guideline is summarized in Figure 14–4. In nonvariceal upper GI bleeding, endoscopic treatment is widely accepted as the most effective method to control acute ulcer bleeding and has become the standard for prevention of ulcer rebleeding. Although individual studies have been too small to show significant advantage for endoscopic therapy in reducing mortality, a meta-analysis indicates endoscopic therapy prevents not only rebleeding but also death. Several therapeutic interventions are available that commonly include thermal therapy (laser, monopolar electrocoagulation, bipolar electrocoagulation, multipolar electrocoagulation, and heater probe), and injection therapy, also known as *sclerotherapy*. The most frequently used sclerosants are sodium morrhuate, ethanolamine, sodium tetradecyl, and absolute alcohol. Complications of therapeutic endoscopic interventions include further bleeding or perforation. Complications related to the endoscopic procedure are also common, including aspiration or associated sedation protocols. These therapies can also add to the cost of treatment. A number of newer endoscopic therapies are also effective in

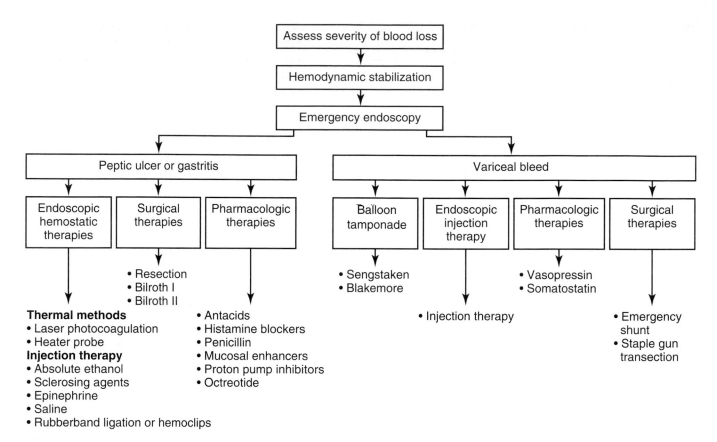

Figure 14–4. Upper GI bleeding treatment guide.

stopping bleeding, but require significant technical expertise to apply. These devices include metal clips, rubber band ligation, endoloops, and sewing devices. As mentioned, their use is limited by technical and practical considerations including the need for multiple bands, clips and loading devices, need for trained assistive personnel, and the inability to reach all lesions. The major complication is rebleeding because the device falls off of the ulcer base. A relatively newer approach is argon plasma coagulation, a device that delivers controlled on contact electrocoagulation by means of high-frequency energy delivered to tissue through nonionized gas (argon plasma). This modality is safe and effective. Pharmacologic treatments may also be used and are summarized in Table 14–4.

Treatment of variceal upper GI bleeding may include endoscopic therapy, banding, tamponade therapy (e.g., Sengstaken-Blakemore tube), pharmacologic therapy to decrease portal hypertension, and surgical therapy to decompress the varices. Sclerotherapy is the treatment of choice for acute variceal bleeding. It is like the procedures and agents described for the treatment of ulcers.

1. Monitor for complications of endoscopic therapy and/or the sclerosing agents used to treat the ulcer or varix. Complications may include fever, pain due to esophageal spasm, motility disturbances of the esophageal sphincter, and perforation. Systemic complications of endoscopic therapy and/or sclerosing agents also may occur and predominantly affect the cardiovascular and respiratory systems. Cardiovascular effects include heart failure, heart block, and pericarditis. Respiratory effects include mediastinitis, aspiration pneumonia, atelectasis, pneumothorax, embolism, and acute respiratory distress syndrome.

2. Institute pharmacologic therapies as prescribed to treat peptic ulcer disease or gastritis (stress ulcers). The most common pharmacologic agents and their actions are reviewed in Table 14–4.

3. Administer pharmacologic therapies as prescribed to treat variceal bleeding (Table 14–5). Pharmacologic agents exert their effect by constricting splanchnic blood flow and thereby reducing portal pressure. Monitor for side effects of systemic vasoconstriction and the cardiac effects of myocardial ischemia and bradycardia (with vasopressin). Administer nitroglycerin titrated to maintain systolic blood pressure between 90 and 100 mm Hg to reduce these side effects and to further reduce portal pressure.

4. Intra-aortic balloon pump therapy may be instituted to achieve temporary vascular control in patients in

TABLE 14–4. PHARMACOLOGIC THERAPIES FOR ULCER DISEASE/GASTRITIS

Agent	Action
Antacids	Acid neutralizers
Histamine blockers Cimetidine Ranitidine Famotidine Nizatidine	Block production of gastric acid (pepsin, HCl) by inhibiting the action of histamine
Cytoprotective agent Sucralfate	Forms protective barrier over ulcer site
Proton pump inhibitors Omeprazole (Prilosec) Lansoprazole (Prevacid) Rabeprazole (Achiphex) Partoprazole (Protonix)-IV	Suppresses secretion of gastric acid
Mucosal barrier enhancers Colloidal bismuth Prostaglandins	Protect mucosa from injurious substances
Penicillins[a] Ampicillin Amoxicillin Mezlocillin	Effective against *Helicobacter pylori*

[a]Several antibiotics must be used in combination; none are effective alone.

shock. This therapy optimizes blood pressure, increases aortic diastolic pressure, increases coronary flow, and allows time for rapid resuscitation.

5. A tamponade tube, most commonly the Sengstaken-Blakemore tube (Figure 14–5) may be used to emergently decrease blood flow through the varix and to control bleeding so that endoscopy can be performed. Rebleeding is common after deflation or removal. Monitor for complications of this tube, including pulmonary aspiration, rupture of the esophagus, asphyxia, and erosion of the esophageal or gastric wall. Maintain esophageal suction to prevent aspiration.

TABLE 14–5. PHARMACOLOGIC THERAPIES FOR VARICEAL UPPER GI BLEEDING

Drug	Action	Administration
Vasopressin	Vasoconstricts splanchnic inflow and reduces portal pressure	Administered by continuous IV infusion at 0.2–0.6 units/min
Somatostatin	Inhibits splanchnic blood flow	Administered by continuous IV infusion at 250 mcg/h
Octreotide	Vasodilates splanchnic vessels to decrease blood flow	IV infusion at 25 mcg/h
Nonselective beta-adrenergic blockers: propranolol, nadolol	Decreases cardiac output and reduces splanic flow (decreases portal hypertension)	Administered orally to reduce resting pulse by 20% or to 55–60 beats/min

Keep a scissors at the bedside to cut and remove the tube if it becomes malpositioned and the tamponade balloon occludes the airway. Endotracheal intubation is usually recommended to prevent most pulmonary complications. Release pressure of the esophageal and or gastric balloons at regular intervals to prevent erosions. Administer frequent mouth care and monitor the skin around the tube to prevent necrosis from traction of the tube.

Surgical Therapies to Stop Bleeding
Surgery is considered for patients who have massive bleeding that is immediately life threatening and for patients who continue to bleed despite aggressive medical therapies. Surgical therapies for peptic ulcer disease or stress ulcers include gastric resections such as antrectomy, gastrectomy, vagotomy, or combination procedures. An antrectomy or gastrectomy may be performed to decrease the acidity of the duodenum or stomach by removing gastric-acid secreting cells. A vagotomy decreases acid secretion in the stomach by dividing the vagus nerve along the esophagus. Combination procedures are common and include Billroth I, which is a vagotomy and antrectomy with anastomosis of the stomach to the duodenum. A Billroth II consists of a vagotomy, a resection of the antrum, and anastomosis of the stomach to the jejunum (Figure 14–6). The latter is preferred over the Billroth I because it prevents dumping syndrome. Gastric perforations can be treated by simple closure.

Surgical decompression of portal hypertension can be accomplished by a procedure called a portacaval shunt. This procedure connects the portal vein to the inferior vena cava, diverting blood from the liver into the vena cava to decrease

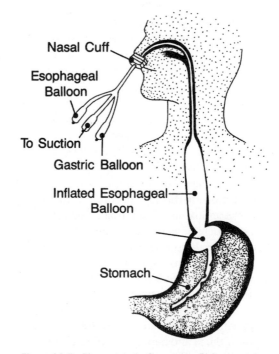

Figure 14–5. Placement of a Sengstaken-Blakemore tube.

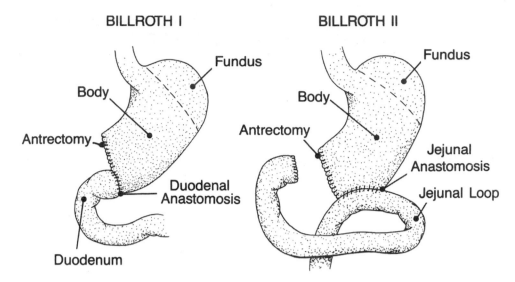

Figure 14–6. Billroth I and II procedures.

portal pressure. Liver transplantation also can relieve portal hypertension, but must be considered by weighing the risks versus the benefits in this patient population.

1. Monitor for fluid and electrolyte imbalances postoperatively due to intraoperative fluid loss and the drains inserted to decompress the stomach or to drain the surgical site.
2. Provide for adequate nutrition to promote wound healing.
3. Monitor the appearance of the incision and surrounding tissue.
4. Document and report all wound drainage (color, amount, odor) and complaints of pain or tenderness.
5. Culture any suspicious drainage.
6. Monitor white blood cell count and temperature trends.

Newer Therapies to Control Bleeding

A newer procedure called the transjugular intrahepatic portosystemic shunt (TIPS) is indicated for control of refractory acute GI bleed from varices or to prevent recurrent bleeding. In the TIPS procedure, a long needle is passed from the right transjugular vein to the hepatic vein into a branch of the portal vein. A stent is placed in the vein. This decreases the pressure in the portal vein (decreases portal pressure) and then pressure on the varices to prevent rupture and bleeding.

The advantage of the TIPS procedure is that it can be performed in the radiology department. Vasopressin, a drug that vasoconstricts GI smooth muscle, lowers venous pressure and decreases venous blood flow, is often administered concurrently. Complications of the TIPS procedures include puncture of the biliary system, bleeding, infection and clotting of the stent. Postprocedural systemic failure (septic shock, renal failure) and hepatic encephalopathy (see next section) are also associated complications.

1. Monitor blood pressure, ECG, and pulse oximetry throughout the procedure.
2. Administer preprocedure antibiotic coverage for gram-negative organisms as prophylaxis for sepsis.
3. Provide moderate IV sedation to treat anxiety.
4. Provide pain medication (e.g., fentanyl). Certain parts of the procedure, such as balloon dilation of the intrahepatic tract, can be painful.
5. Have lidocaine and atropine available to manage potential complications of the procedure. The vasopressin infusion can cause bradyarrhythmias. Due to the proximity of the hepatic vein to the right ventricle of the heart, ventricular ectopy can be induced during the procedure.
6. Have crystalloids, vasopressors, PRBCs, and fresh frozen plasma readily available to manage hypotension from sepsis, bleeding, or sedation.
7. Have continuous and intermittent suction ready to manage bleeding and airway patency.

Reducing Anxiety

1. Encourage communication with a calm, interested, and centered approach; e.g., "Mr. B., you look nervous (worried) to me. Can you tell me what is bothering you?"
2. Assess the patient's previous coping skills that were used in similar difficult situations (e.g., did family presence, watching TV or listening to music, or using relaxation techniques provide support?).
3. Offer appropriate reassurance, facts, and information as requested by the patient. Explain the ICU routine and procedures to the patient. Present information in terms that the patient can understand. Repeat and rephrase the information as necessary.
4. Help the patient to establish a sense of control. Assist the patient to make distinctions among those

things he or she can (and should) control (e.g., bath time, working on reducing anxiety level) and those things that cannot be controlled (e.g., need for vasopressors and monitoring equipment).

5. Guide the patient in discovering that he or she has some control over anxiety and fear. Encourage the patient to participate in breathing and relaxation exercises as a strategy to control the current situation.

Liver Failure

The liver is a complex organ providing numerous metabolic, secretory, and detoxification functions for the body. Disease processes in the liver can affect the liver cells, Kupffer's cells, bile ducts, and blood vessels. If severe, these processes can lead to acute fulminant liver failure. Acute liver failure can be distinguished from chronic liver failure and is characterized by impairment of metabolic and secretory functions in previously healthy livers. In acute failure, there is cellular insult, which overwhelms the normal regenerative response of the liver. Massive cell necrosis results. The liver normally has remarkable regenerative capacity. However, if the necrosis is massive and overwhelms normal liver processes, liver transplantation is usually required. Criteria for transplantation in acute liver failure are summarized in Table 14–6. Liver dysfunction potentially can be reversed. The liver has regenerative capability if the disease process in the liver does not adversely affect the structure of the cells. If the regeneration in liver tissue does not occur in a normal fashion (e.g., with cirrhosis of the liver), fibrous tissue is laid down over time. These fibrotic changes are irreversible, resulting in chronic liver dysfunction and eventual end-stage liver failure.

Etiology, Risk Factors, and Pathogenesis

Causes of liver failure include both inflammatory disease and processes that produce fibrosis of liver tissue (Table 14–7). Hepatitis is the most common form of inflammatory disease of the liver, with at least five different types identified to date. Each type of viral hepatitis has a different mode of transmission and complications (Table 14–8). Hepatitis B is the most serious of these and is vaccine preventable. Health care providers are at risk for contracting this form of hepatitis. The liver is an important site of drug metabolism. Hepatitis D occurs only in combination with hepatitis B. Toxic ingestions of drugs, chemicals, or poisons may also initiate

TABLE 14–6. POSSIBLE CRITERIA FOR LIVER TRANSPLANT IN PATIENTS WITH ALCOHOLIC LIVER DISEASE

Albumin	<3.5 g/dL
Total bilirubin	>2 mg/dL
INR	>1.7
Ascites	Controlled or poorly controlled medically
Encephalopathy	Controlled or poorly controlled medically

TABLE 14–7. COMMON CAUSES OF LIVER FAILURE

Inflammatory Liver Disease
Viruses
  Hepatitis A, B, C, D, and E
  Herpes simplex
  Epstein-Barr
  Cytomegalovirus
  Adenovirus
Parasites
Liver tumors
Toxic ingestion of drugs
  Acetaminophen
  Halothane
  Methyldopa
Toxic ingestion of chemicals and poisons
  Chlorinated hydrocarbons
  Phosphorous
Cirrhosis of the Liver
Alcohol ingestion
Biliary disease
Cardiac disease
Hepatitis

an acute inflammatory process in the liver, causing it to fail. Acetaminophen is a common drug that is associated with liver failure.

Alcohol abuse is the most common cause of cirrhosis of the liver. Alcohol is directly toxic to liver cells, causing them to die. Liver cells are replaced by fibrous tissue which causes the liver progressively to fail.

When the liver fails, the clinical manifestations are directly related to failure of the liver to perform important metabolic processes (Table 14–9). Complications of liver failure include ascites, hepatic encephalopathy, acute respiratory distress syndrome, electrolyte and acid–base imbalances, and hepatorenal syndrome.

TABLE 14–8. VIRAL HEPATITIS

Type of Hepatitis	Mode of Transmission	Potential Complications
A; formerly called infectious hepatitis	Fecal-oral, person-to-person contact; also by uncooked shellfish, fruits, and vegetables, and contaminated water	Acute fulminant hepatitis relapse
B; formerly called serum hepatitis	Blood or body fluids; sexual contact; contaminated needles; and perinatal transmission	Acute fulminant hepatitis, chronic liver disease, cirrhosis, cancer of the liver
C; formerly non-A, non-B hepatitis	Blood	Chronic liver disease, cirrhosis, cancer of the liver
D	Blood and body fluids, sexual contact, and perinatal transmission	Chronic liver disease
E	Fecal-oral	High mortality in pregnant women

TABLE 14–9. SEQUELAE OF LIVER FAILURE

Sequelae	Outcome	Clinical Manifestations
Impaired splanchnic hemodynamics	Portal hypertension	Varices, acute upper GI bleeding
	Hyperdynamic circulation	Increased CO, decreased SVR, decreased perfusion
Reduced liver metabolic processes	Altered fat, protein, and carbohydrate metabolism	Malnutrition, impaired healing
	Decreased phagocytic function of Kupffer cells	Infection
	Decreased synthesis of blood clotting components	Bleeding
	Decreased removal of activated clotting factors	Emboli
	Decreased metabolism of vitamins and iron	Impaired skin integrity
	Impaired detoxification	Increased ammonia, mental status changes, increased drug levels
Impaired bile formation and flow	Impaired bilirubin metabolism	Jaundice

Jaundice

Jaundice (icterus) is caused by the accumulation of bilirubin because the liver cannot conjugate or metabolize it as rapidly as it is formed. *Jaundice* is yellow discoloration of the skin, mucous membranes, and sclera. Pruritis is a common associated symptom that can cause much discomfort for patients.

Ascites

Impaired handling of salt and water by the kidney, as well as alterations in fluid homeostasis, causes the patient to accumulate fluid in the peritoneum. This complication is most problematic because it can impair movement of the diaphragm and cause an ineffective breathing pattern and potentially respiratory failure, as well as serve as a source of infection.

Hepatic Encephalopathy

One of the liver's major functions is detoxification. Normally, the liver detoxifies ammonia, which is produced by bacteria in the bowel and converts it to urea for excretion. When the liver fails, this function of the liver is impaired, allowing ammonia to directly enter the central nervous system. Because ammonia is neurotoxic, as serum ammonia levels rise, the patient often exhibits signs of impaired cerebral functioning or encephalopathy. These signs can range from minor sensory-perceptual changes such as muscle tremors, slurred speech, or slight mental status changes to marked confusion or profound coma. Classifications of deterioration in brain function have been used, from grade I (mild or episodic drowsiness, impaired concentration/intellect, but able to arouse and coherent); grade II (increased drowsiness, confusion, and disorientation, but able to arouse); grade III (very drowsy, agitated, disoriented, but able to respond to simple verbal commands); and grade IV (unresponsive except to painful stimuli). Patients with hepatic encephalopathy need to be carefully assessed for other causes of encephalopathy such as sepsis, uremia, acidosis, alcohol withdrawal, hypoxia, and intracerebral bleed.

Acute Respiratory Distress Syndrome

The major pulmonary complication in liver failure is arterial hypoxemia. The cause has been linked to vascular dilatation in the lung and acute respiratory distress syndrome. Pulmonary edema is also a common finding.

Electrolyte Imbalance

A variety of electrolyte imbalances occur in liver failure. Hypoglycemia develops due to massive hepatic cell necrosis, leading to loss of glycogen stores and diminished glucose release. Hyponatremia is common due to the reduced capacity of the kidneys to excrete free water, leading to a dilutional hyponatremia. Hypokalemia may occur from inadequate oral intake, increased potassium losses from vomiting, or from medical interventions (e.g., nasogastric suction or diuretic therapy). Hypomagnesemia commonly occurs in conjunction with hypokalemia as there is a close relationship between the movement of these electrolytes. Hypocalcemia is a complication of blood transfusions because the citrate used to anticoagulate stored blood causes calcium depletion. Hypophosphatemia also is commonly associated with acute liver failure. The exact mechanisms remain unknown.

Acid–Base Disturbance

Hepatocellular necrosis results in the accumulation of organic acids, primarily lactic acid, causing a metabolic acidosis. Hypoventilation from ascites may complicate this disorder.

Hepatorenal Syndrome

Acute renal failure that occurs with liver failure is called *hepatorenal syndrome.* The pathophysiology of this functional renal failure is not well understood, but presents like acute tubular necrosis (see Chapter 15, Renal System).

Acute Gastrointestinal Bleeding

Bleeding from varices related to portal hypertension is a life-threatening complication (see previous section).

AT THE BEDSIDE
▶ *Liver Failure*

A 54-year-old man is admitted with a 3-day history of shortness of breath, increased confusion, vomiting, and weakness. He was hospitalized in the past year with upper GI bleeding from esophageal and gastric varices. He was diagnosed at that time as having Laînnec's cirrhosis, liver failure due to alcohol abuse. Significant findings on his admission profile were:

History

Complaints of decreased appetite for the past 2 months; also complaints of nausea and weakness.

Vital Signs

Blood pressure: 98/50 lying; 90/54 sitting
Heart rate: Sinus tachycardia with frequent PVCs
Respiratory rate: 28/min; shallow
Temperature: 100°F, orally

Cardiopulmonary

Rales and coarse rhonchi throughout all lung fields
Dyspneic; using accessory muscles
S_3/S_4; no murmurs
Extremities cool, weak pulses
31 edema lower extremities

Neurologic

Alert, but disoriented to time and place
Irritable

Abdomen

Marked ascites, dull to percussion
Hyperactive bowel sounds in all four quadrants

Genitourinary

Urine dark, amber, and cloudy
Large hemorrhoid protruding from rectal vault
Liquid stool; black; guaiac positive

Laboratory Data

Arterial blood gases on 2 L O_2 per nasal cannula

pH	7.49
$PaCO_2$	30 mm Hg
PaO_2	54 mm Hg
SaO_2	87%
HCO_3^2	28
Hematocrit	30%
AST	80 IU/L
ALT	84 IU/L
Bilirubin	Total 10 mg/dl
PT	18 sec
APTT	>45 sec
Fibrinogen	158 mg/dL
Albumin	3.0
Potassium	3.2 mEq/L
Sodium	130 mEq/L
Creatinine	2.8 mg/dL
BUN	40 mg/dL
Glucose	80 mg/dL
Urine electrolytes	
Sodium	5 mEq/L/d
Potassium	10 mEq/L/d

Malnutrition

The liver has many metabolic functions including metabolism of carbohydrates, fats, and proteins. The liver also stores essential minerals such as iron, copper and vitamins A, B_{12}, D, and K. Metabolism and storage function are often seriously impaired in liver failure resulting in profound malnutrition. This affects all cellular functions.

Clinical Presentation

History

- Exposure to contaminated food, water
- Exposure to blood, body fluids
- Alcohol abuse

Signs and Symptoms

Impaired Thought Processes

- Mental status changes (confusion, lethargy)
- Behavioral changes
- Delirium
- Seizures
- Coma

Impaired Gas Exchange

- Hypoxemia
- Pulmonary edema

Fluid Volume Deficit or Excess

- Hypotension
- Skin cool, pale, and dry

- Urine output <30 mL/h
- Tachycardia
- Dry mucous membranes

Hyperdynamic Circulation

- Dysrhythmias
- Fever
- Palmar erythema (flushed palms)
- Jugular vein distension
- Rales
- Murmur
- Increased CO
- Decreased systemic vascular resistance

Altered Nutrition

- Decreased appetite
- Decreased weight
- Nausea and vomiting

Impaired Liver Metabolism

- Jaundice
- Dry skin
- Ascites

Diagnostic Tests

- Total bilirubin >1 mg/dL
- AST >36 IU/L
- ALT >24 IU/L
- PT >13 sec
- APTT >45 sec
- Fibrinogen <200 mg/dL
- Albumin <3.2 g/dL
- Ammonia >45 mg/dL
- Ultrasound, endoscopy, endoscopic retrograde cholangiopancreatography (ERCP), liver angiography/biopsy

Principles of Management for Liver Failure

The management of the patient with liver failure is centered on decreasing the metabolic requirements of the liver, supporting cardiopulmonary status, supporting hematologic and nutritional functions of the liver, and preventing and treating complications.

Decrease Metabolic Requirements of the Liver

1. Place the patient on bed rest to decrease the metabolic needs of the liver. Position the head of the bed at 45 degrees at all times to minimize complications related to ascites. Institute measures to prevent skin breakdown.
2. Monitor drugs that are metabolized or detoxified by the liver, especially narcotics and sedatives.

Support Cardiopulmonary Status

1. Monitor fluid balance. The patient may have a fluid volume deficit related to portal hypertension, third spacing of peritoneal fluid, GI bleeding, or coagulation abnormalities. Fluid overload may be a problem related to sodium excess and hypoalbuminemia.
2. Assist with paracentesis that may be instituted to reduce ascites. Fast removal of fluid via paracentesis requires IV colloid replacement to prevent dehydration. Administer diuretics as prescribed. Weigh patient daily. Monitor abdominal girth when ascites is present.
3. Monitor respiratory status and correlate with arterial blood gas results. Administer oxygen as ordered. Administer sedatives and analgesics cautiously. Assist the patient with maneuvers to improve oxygenation.

Support Hematologic, Nutritional, and Metabolic Functions of the Liver

1. Monitor for signs of bleeding (e.g., gastric contents, stools, urine) and test for occult blood. Observe for petechiae and bruising. Monitor hematologic profile.
2. Administer blood and blood products as ordered.
3. Institute measures for variceal bleeding as needed.
4. Institute measures to provide for safety and to minimize tissue trauma. Provide for frequent mouth care. Avoid use of rectal tubes.
5. Limit protein intake or provide vegetables rich in proteins and branch-chain amino acids; provide calories with carbohydrates and fats. Consider enteral nutrition if oral intake is insufficient.
6. Monitor for signs and symptoms of infection. Maintain sterility of invasive lines and tubes. Maintain aseptic technique when performing procedures.

Preventing and Treating Complications

The most common complications of liver failure are hepatic encephalopathy, fluid and electrolyte imbalances, hepatorenal syndrome, and variceal hemorrhage.

1. Observe for changes in mentation. Institute safety measures during periods of mental status changes. Rule out other causes of encephalopathy. Treat precipitating causes.
2. Administer cleansing enemas and cathartics to keep the bowel empty. Administer oral nonabsorbent antibiotics (neomycin, metronidazole, or vancomycin) to decrease bacteria in the colon. Administer lactulose to decrease intestinal pH and increase ammonia excretion. Monitor patient response to therapy through neurologic assessments and by monitoring serum ammonia levels. Monitor the use of medications metabolized by the liver.
3. Institute protocols for acute upper GI hemorrhage due to variceal rupture (see previous section).

Artificial Liver Support Systems

Efforts to find ways to assist patients with acute liver failure until organ transplantation has led to research in devices that support the liver until an organ is available, or the liver's regenerative systems recover. All artificial liver support system involve extracorporeal circulation of the patient's blood through filters that remove waste products normally filtered by the liver. Several liver support systems are currently in clinical trials in the United States.

Acute Pancreatitis

Acute pancreatitis is inflammation of the pancreas resulting from premature activation of pancreatic exocrine enzymes, such as trypsin, phospholipase A, and elastase within the pancreas. The disease ranges in severity from a mild self-limiting form to a severe process where necrosis of pancreatic cells and release of substrates predominate. The substrates that are released not only cause a local pathology in and around the pancreas, but also can trigger systemic complications when released into the circulation. In the severe acute form, acute pancreatitis results in multisystem failure (see Chapter 11, Multisystem Problems).

Etiologies, Risk Factors, and Pathophysiology

The most common causes of acute pancreatitis are alcohol disease and biliary tract disease (stones). Some drugs also are associated with acute pancreatitis. Those most commonly used in critical care units include acetaminophen, cimetidine, furosemide, procainamide, opiates, and cocaine. Pancreatitis also has been associated with shock states and following organ transplantation

The pathogenesis of acute pancreatitis is not completely clear. The pancreas normally has a protective mechanism, an enzyme called trypsin inhibitor, to prevent activating enzymes before they reach the duodenum, thereby preventing inflammation of pancreatic cells. Regardless of the etiology, the process of premature activation of pancreatic enzymes is characteristic of pancreatitis, leading to local inflammation and potential necrosis of the pancreas. The activated enzymes also can enter the systemic circulation via the portal vein and lymphatics. This is thought to stimulate platelet-activating factor and humoral systems (kinin, complement, fibrinolysis). This results in multisystem failure with a variety of complications (Table 14–10; see also Chapter 11). Septic complications, particularly of the pancreas, also can occur. Pancreatic abscess, pseudocyst, and necrosis are not uncommon with fulminant forms of the disease.

Clinical Presentation

Signs and Symptoms

Pancreatic Inflammation

- Acute pain: Pain rating 6 to 10 on a scale of 1 to 10 (severe, relentless, knifelike; midepigastrium or periumbilical)

TABLE 14–10. COMMON MULTISYSTEM COMPLICATIONS OF ACUTE PANCREATITIS

Pulmonary
Atelectasis
Acute respiratory distress syndrome
Pleural effusions
Cardiovascular
Cardiogenic shock
Neurologic
Pancreatic encephalopathy
Metabolic
Metabolic acidosis
Hypocalcemia
Altered glucose metabolism
Hematologic
Disseminated intravascular coagulation
GI bleeding
Renal
Prerenal failure

- Abdominal guarding
- Nausea
- Rebound tenderness
- Vomiting
- Abdominal distention
- Hypoactive bowel sounds

Fluid Volume Deficit

- Hypotension
- Tachycardia
- Mental status changes
- Cool, clammy skin
- Decreased urine output

Impaired Gas Exchange

- Decreasing PaO_2 (<60 mm Hg) and SaO_2 (<90%)

Diagnostic Tests

- Serum amylase >100 IU/L
- Serum pancreatic isoamylase >50%
- Serum lipase >24 IU/dL
- Serum triglycerides >150 mg/dL
- Urine amylase >14 IU/h
- Serum calcium <8.5 mg/dL
- Serum sodium <135 mEq/L
- Serum potassium <3.5 mEq/L
- Serum magnesium <1.5 mg/dL
- Increased ALT (>120 units/L), in gallstone pancreatitis
- C-reactive protein (>120 mg/L)

Imaging Studies

- Computed tomography
- ERCP
- MRI

Principles of Management of Acute Pancreatitis

The management of the patient with acute pancreatitis centers on disrupting the cycle of enzyme release of the pancreas and treating complications that can occur with multisystem disease. Principles of management include fluid resuscitation, resting the pancreas, pain management, and supporting other organ systems that may fail because of mediators released during the inflammatory process.

Fluid Resuscitation

Patients with acute pancreatitis may have fluid shifts of 4 to 12 L into the retroperitoneal space and peritoneal cavity due to inflammation. In severe acute pancreatitis, blood vessels in and around the pancreas may also become disrupted, resulting in hemorrhage.

1. Replace fluids with colloids, crystalloids, or blood products. High-dose fresh frozen plasma is indicated to replace lost circulating proteins. Monitor outcomes of fluid replacement therapy including blood pressure, heart rate, intake and output, preload indicators (CVP, PCWP), skin turgor, capillary refill, mucous membranes, and urine output.

2. Monitor for signs and symptoms of hemorrhage (low hematocrit and hemoglobin levels). Cullen's sign is a bluish discoloration around the flanks, and Grey Turner's sign is a bluish discoloration around the umbilical area, indicating blood in the peritoneum. Monitor for increasing abdominal girths.

3. Monitor electrolytes for imbalances related to prolonged vomiting or fluid sequestration. Calcium, sodium, magnesium and potassium are most commonly affected. Monitor QT intervals on the electrocardiogram and implement seizure precautions with severe hypocalcemia. Hyperglycemia also may be present due to the stress response and from impaired secretion of insulin by the islet cells in the inflamed pancreas. Administer insulin infusion, then sliding scale insulin to obtain a normoglycemic state.

Pain Management

Acute pain is the only universal sign of acute pancreatitis. It is caused by peritoneal irritation from activated pancreatic exocrine enzymes, edema or distention of the pancreas, or interruption of the blood supply to the pancreas. Treatment of pain is a priority because it causes increased exocrine enzyme release by the pancreas, which may worsen the pathologic process.

1. Assess the degree of pain by having the patient use a pain rating scale.

2. Administer pain analgesics. There is controversy about the use of opiate analgesics (e.g., morphine) because they may cause spasm of the sphincter of Oddi, which may worsen the pain. Use a pain rating scale to assess patient outcomes regardless of what is prescribed. Consider scheduled doses or continuous infusion of pain medication for severe pain. Consider epidural analgesia for unrelieved acute pain.

3. Assess patient anxiety and administer sedatives with analgesics.

4. Assist the patient to a position which promotes comfort. The knee-to-chest position often decreases the intensity of the pain.

Rest the Pancreas

Preventing stimulation of pancreatic exocrine secretion is a priority to interrupt the cycle of pancreatic inflammation.

1. Maintain the patient on NPO status. Avoiding the use of the GI tract is recommended until the patient no longer reports abdominal pain and the serum amylase has returned to normal. Intermittent nasogastric suction also may be used to prevent GI secretions from stimulating the pancreas.

2. Provide nutrition enterally using a jejunal tube to prevent pancreatic enzyme secretion. If parenteral therapy is used, the solution is usually a mixture of hypertonic glucose and amino acids. The use of lipid emulsion is contraindicated during the acute phase because it increases pancreatic exocrine secretion.

3. Encourage bed rest. Bed rest decreases pancreatic exocrine secretion.

4. Administer pharmacologic agents as prescribed to block the secretion of pancreatic enzymes. These include anticholinergic agents, glucagon, cimetidine, calcitonin, and somatostatin.

Treat Local Complications in the Pancreas

Local complications in the pancreas include infected necrosis, pancreatic pseudocyst, and pancreatic abscess. Percutaneous or stent therapies to drain the fluids in and around the pancreas and/or surgical resection or debridement may be required, especially if the pancreas becomes infected. Biliary ERCP and laparoscopic cholecystectomy are indicated for gallstone pancreatitis.

Treat Multisystem Failure

Cardiopulmonary complications are the most common multisystem problems. As mentioned, they are thought to be due to pancreatic enzyme–induced mediators. Pancreatic ischemia is also known to promote the release of myocardial depressant factor. This causes decreased myocardial contractility and CO. Surgical therapies such as a pancreatic resection may be performed to prevent systemic complications of acute necrotizing pancreatitis by removing necrotic or infected tissue. In some cases, a pancreatectomy may be performed, but it is associated with considerable mortality.

1. Administer oxygen therapy to maintain arterial oxygen tension and oxygen saturation. Mechanical ventilation may be used with adjunct therapies to pro-

mote maximal alveolar gas exchange is often used to manage acute respiratory failure (see Chapter 10, Respiratory System).

2. Perform peritoneal lavage. Peritoneal lavage is used to clear activated mediators and enzymes from the peritoneal cavity. The procedure involves placement of a percutaneous peritoneal dialysis catheter and continuous infusion of isotonic solution. Close monitoring of respiratory status during fluid instillation is a priority. Characteristics of pancreatic lavage return should also be monitored.
3. Administer low-dose dopamine to support myocardial contractility. Dobutamine may also be considered if sepsis is not a complication. Avoid alpha constrictors.
4. Institute measures to prevent infection. Monitor for signs and symptoms of sepsis and initiate appropriate treatment if indicated.
5. Manage coagulopathies (see Chapter 13, Hematology and Immune Systems).
6. Treat acute tubular necrosis if a complicating factor (see Chapter 15, Renal System).

Bowel Infarction/Obstruction

Major disorders of the intestine include intestinal ischemia which can lead to infarction, and intestinal obstruction. Both disorders can result in acute abdominal signs with or without peritoneal irritation.

Etiology, Risk Factors, and Pathophysiology

Intestinal ischemia develops from a decrease in blood flow, producing an inadequate oxygen concentration to meet the requirements of the splanchnic bed. Three major arterial trunks—the celiac axis, the superior mesenteric artery, and the inferior mesenteric artery—branch to form the vascular bed referred to as the splanchnic circulation. The splanchnic bed areas receive about 20% of the CO. Factors that can decrease splanchnic blood flow include abdominal distention, alpha-stimulating sympathomimetic amines (epinephrine, norepinephrine), cardiac glycosides, hypovolemia, and decreased CO. The ischemic bowel loses protein, electrolytes, and fluid into the lumen and wall of the bowel. The third-space extracellular fluid loss decreases the circulating blood volume. Bowel ischemia can lead to bowel necrosis and then gangrene of the bowel. Without surgical intervention, this condition usually is fatal.

Intestinal obstructions may be due to mechanical or functional causes. Obstruction of the bowel may cause circulation to the obstructed segment to be impaired. This may progress to gangrene and peritonitis. Mechanical obstruction involves a physical blockage of the bowel lumen. The most common causes are adhesions and strangulated hernias. The ileum is the most common site because it is the narrowest. A mechanical obstruction of the bowel results in the accumulation of intestinal secretions, ingested fluids, and gas proximal to the site of the obstruction. The increased intestinal secretions accumulating in the bowel deplete the extracellular fluid volume. Loss of electrolytes is also common and varies with the site of the obstruction.

A functional obstruction, or paralytic ileus, develops when there is a loss of peristalsis. Conditions that decrease or inhibit intestinal motility are abdominal surgery, intestinal distention, peritonitis, intestinal ischemia, hypokalemia, severe trauma, and severe medical disease.

Clinical Presentation

History

- Ischemia
- Obstruction
- Congestive heart failure
- Abdominal surgery
- Shock
- Hernia
- Atrial fibrillation

Signs and Symptoms

- Crampy umbilical pain
- Abdominal pain (midabdominal)
- Diarrhea
- Cramping
- Abdominal distention
- Weight loss
- Decreased bowel sounds
- GI bleeding
- Muscle guarding and tenderness
- Ileus
- Rebound tenderness
- Vomiting
- Constipation
- Abdominal guarding
- Muscle rigidity
- Fluid volume deficit

Principles of Management for Bowel Obstruction/Infarction

Patient priorities for these disorders revolve around treating the intravascular fluid volume deficit, treating pain related to inflammation and abdominal distension, and measures to decompress the bowel. The major clinical issue for patients with bowel obstruction is to determine if and when surgical intervention is indicated. Patients with high complete small bowel obstruction in particular have a low likelihood of spontaneous resolution and are at high risk for strangulation. Early surgical intervention is usually the treatment course. Medical therapies for treating bowel infarction include relieving the mesenteric vasoconstriction and surgical therapies to resect necrotic bowel. Papaverine is the drug of choice in relieving mesenteric vasoconstriction. It is given intra-arterially after the mesenteric artery is located via radiologic examination. Surgical therapy may also be required to treat bowel obstruction, including lysis of adhesions, reduction of hernias, bypass of obstructions, and excision of obstructions. A colostomy may be performed with left colonic obstructions.

1. Administer colloids and crystalloids to treat the fluid volume deficit. Monitor patient response to fluid resuscitation—hemodynamic parameters (MAP, heart rate), body weight, and intake and output.
2. Administer antimicrobial therapy to treat intra-abdominal infection.
3. Position with head of bed elevated to promote lung expansion to relieve pressure from the distended abdomen. Assist with deep breathing exercises to promote lung expansion, mobilization of secretions, and relaxation.
4. Administer analgesics and sedatives for pain management. Insert a nasogastric tube and apply and maintain suction to drain and decompress the upper GI tract. Avoid excess use of opiates to promote the return of peristalsis.
5. Monitor and report signs and symptoms of ongoing infection.
6. Provide nutrition as prescribed. Total parenteral nutrition may be required early in the course of therapy. Enteral therapy should be begun as early as possible because it promotes the return of peristalsis and may assist in maintaining the gut mucosal barrier function.

NUTRITIONAL SUPPORT FOR CRITICALLY ILL PATIENTS

The negative consequences of malnutrition have been known for centuries, and there is substantial evidence that malnourished hospitalized patients have increased morbidity, compromised surgical outcomes, slower ventilator weaning, and increased mortality rates. However, the science of nutrition support for the critically ill patient is in its infancy. Prospective outcomes research has revealed surprising results in other areas of critical care science, and this has led to the realization that some of the most basic, but important, questions of critical care nutrition remain unanswered. Questions such as the timing of nutrition, nutrient needs, and specific nutrients that best affect outcomes remain active research topics.

There is accumulating evidence that the route of nutrition support can affect morbidity in the critically ill patient. In addition, protocols for the proper initiation and monitoring of patients on nutrition support may reduce complications.

Nutrition Needs

The advent of routine use of total parenteral nutrition in the 1970s allowed the provision of large quantities of calories

TABLE 14–11. POTENTIAL CONSEQUENCES OF OVERFEEDING OF MACRONUTRIENTS[a]

Carbohydrate	Fat
• Hyperglycemia	• Impaired immune response
• Synthesis and storage of fat	• Fat overload syndrome with neurologic, cardiac, pulmonary, hepatic, and renal dysfunction
• Hepatic steatosis	• Thrombocyte adhesiveness
• Increased carbon dioxide production increasing minute ventilation	• Accumulation of lipid in the reticuloendothelial system (RES), leading to RES dysfunction

[a] Remember to look for additional sources of dextrose and fat, such as propofol, intravenous fluid, continuous venovenous hemodialysis, peritoneal dialysis.
Reprinted from: UVAHS Nutrition Services/Morrison Management Specialists. Nutrition Support Traineeship Syllabus. Charlottesville: University of Virginia Health System; 2003, with permission from University of Virginia Health Systems.

and protein in an attempt to improve nutrition status. This ill-advised notion of providing supraphysiologic levels of nutrition, or "hyperalimentation," led to widely published case reports of respiratory failure and hepatic compromise associated with overfeeding. Controlled trials have demonstrated that overfeeding does not provide increased nutritional benefits, and actually has detrimental effects (Table 14–11).

Current recommendations for feeding critically ill patients suggest approximately 25 total calories/kg per day based on the patient's ideal body weight, or 27.5 total calories/kg per day in the presence of systemic inflammatory response syndrome. A total of 1.2 to 1.5 g/kg per day of protein is also recommended.

Total Parenteral Nutrition

Parenteral nutrition is indicated for patients who are malnourished, are at risk for becoming malnourished, and who are unable to receive enteral nutrition (Tables 14–12 and 14–13). Parenteral nutrition can be life saving in some cases, but is not without complications and should be used only when necessary. Prospective trials have demonstrated that the metabolic and infectious complications of total parenteral nutrition outweigh the benefits in patients who do not have significant malnutrition. The need for total parenteral nutrition is evaluated daily in the inpatient setting, and patients who regain GI function are transitioned to enteral feeding.

Enteral Nutrition

Current evidence suggests that enteral nutrition is the preferred method of feeding the critically ill patient. It is associated with less infectious complications, is less expensive and confers some gut protection in terms of immunity, atrophy and attenuation of systemic response (Table 14–14).

Unfortunately, the delivery of enteral nutrition is impeded by various situations that occur in ICUs. For example, enteral feedings may be stopped for diagnostic or therapeutic

TABLE 14–12. INDICATIONS FOR PARENTERAL NUTRITION

Parenteral nutrition is usually indicated in the following situations

- Documented inability to absorb adequate nutrients via the gastrointestinal tract; this may be due to
  - Massive small-bowel resection/short bowel syndrome (at least initially)
  - Radiation enteritis
  - Severe diarrhea
  - Steatorrhea
- Complete bowel obstruction, or intestinal pseudo-obstruction
- Severe catabolism with or without malnutrition when gastrointestinal tract is not usable within 5–7 days
- Inability to obtain enteral access
- Inability to provide sufficient nutrients/fluids enterally
- Pancreatitis accompanied by abdominal pain with jejunal delivery of nutrients
- Persistent GI hemorrhage
- Acute abdomen/ileus
- Lengthy GI workup requiring NPO status
- High output enterocutaneous fistula if feeding ports cannot be distally placed
- Trauma requiring repeat surgical procedures

Parenteral nutrition *may* be indicated in the following situations

- Enterocutaneous fistula
- Inflammatory bowel disease not responding to medical therapy
- Hyperemesis gravidarum when nausea and vomiting persist longer than 5–7 days and enteral nutrition is not possible
- Partial small-bowel obstruction
- Intensive chemotherapy/severe mucositis
- Major surgery/stress when enteral nutrition not expected to resume within 7–10 days
- Intractable vomiting when jejunal feeding is not possible
- Chylous ascites or chylothorax

Reprinted from: UVAHS Nutrition Services/Morrison Management Specialists. Nutrition Support Traineeship Syllabus. Charlottesville: University of Virginia Health System; 2003, with permission from University of Virginia Health Systems.

procedures, in patients who are unstable, or due to clogged or dislodged enteral tubes (Table 14–15).

Successful enteral nutrition is also commonly thwarted by misguided perceptions and beliefs related to the definition of GI "intolerance." Many practices are based on experiential assumptions and practices, as well as beliefs about how the GI tract functions in critical illness. The following sections review these myths and present facts related to GI tolerance or intolerance of enteral feeding.

TABLE 14–13. CONTRAINDICATIONS FOR PARENTERAL NUTRITION

- Functioning gastrointestinal tract
- Treatment anticipated for less than 5 days in patients without severe malnutrition
- Inability to obtain venous access
- A prognosis that does not warrant aggressive nutrition support
- When the risks of parenteral nutrition are judged to exceed the potential benefits

Reprinted from: UVAHS Nutrition Services/Morrison Management Specialists. Nutrition Support Traineeship Syllabus. Charlottesville: University of Virginia Health System; 2003, with permission from University of Virginia Health Systems.

TABLE 14–14. BENEFITS OF ENTERAL FEEDING

- Stimulates immune barrier function
- Physiologic presentation of nutrients
- Maintains gut mucosa
- May prevent bacterial translocation
- Attenuates hypermetabolic response
- Simplifies fluid/electrolyte management
- More "complete" nutrition than total parenteral nutrition
- Fewer infectious complications
- Less expensive (product and septic complications)

Reprinted from: UVAHS Nutrition Services/Morrison Management Specialists. Nutrition Support Traineeship Syllabus. Charlottesville: University of Virginia Health System; 2003, with permission from University of Virginia Health Systems.

Residual Volume

Little evidence exists to support the use of *residual volume,* the volume of fluid in the stomach, as an indicator of GI tolerance and potential clinical outcomes in enterally fed patients. A residual volume is generally expected in the stomach because the physiologic function of the stomach is to act as a reservoir and to control delivery of nutrients into the small bowel. This allows maximal assimilation with bile salts and pancreatic enzymes. A number of factors contribute to the residual volume: endogenous secretions, normal gastric emptying, exogenous fluids, and the cascade effect (Table 14–16).

Endogenous Secretions and Exogenous Additions

Two to four liters per day of saliva and gastric secretions are produced above the pylorus. Conservatively, approximately

TABLE 14–15. COMMON BARRIERS TO OPTIMIZING ENTERAL NUTRITION DELIVERY

- Diagnostic procedures (feedings are stopped)
- Propofol (Diprivan) (calories from the lipid preparation must be calculated as part of the total kcal provided to prevent overfeeding)
- Enteral access issues (clogged/dislodged tubes or obtaining postpyloric access if needed)
- Feedings held due to drug–nutrient interactions
- Hypotensive episodes (patient is often flat in bed necessitating that feedings be turned off)
- Miscalculation of enteral nutrition requirements (orders are hypocaloric, etc.)
- NPO at midnight for tests, surgery, or procedures
- Conditioning regimes and or therapies that require the feedings to be turned off
- Transportation off the unit
- Hemodialysis (enteral nutrition is often stopped during hemodialysis if the patient is deemed unstable by the nurse, often after the patient experiences hypotension)
- Perceived or real "GI intolerance or dysfunction" (gastroparesis, ileus, diarrhea, lack of bowel sounds, residual volumes, aspiration risk, no gag reflex, etc.)

Reprinted from: UVAHS Nutrition Services/Morrison Management Specialists. Nutrition Support Traineeship Syllabus. Charlottesville: University of Virginia Health System; 2003, with permission from University of Virginia Health Systems.

TABLE 14–16. ABSORPTION AND SECRETION OF FLUID IN THE GI TRACT

Additions	mL
Diet	2000
Saliva	1500
Stomach	2500
Pancreas/Bile	2000
Intestine	1000
Subtractions	
Colointestinal	8900
Net stool loss	***100***

3 L of fluid pass the pylorus every 24 hours (an average of 125 mL/h). Once gastric access is obtained, medications, water, and enteral nutrition add to the gastric volume.

The Cascade Effect

The predominant position of ICU patients is supine, preferably with the head of the bed at 30 degrees or higher. In this position, the stomach lies over the spine and is mechanically divided into two parts, the fundus and the antrum. Because the fundus is the noncontractile portion of the stomach, contents fill the fundus until they "cascade over" the spine into the antrum and finally exit through the pylorus. Thus, if the patient's gastric tube feeding port is in the proximal stomach or fundus when the residual volume is checked, the aspirated residual volume may be erroneous. The residual volume in this case is a function of the patient's supine positioning rather than decreased GI motility.

In addition to the effect of positioning on residual volume, another misconception clinicians have is expecting the stomach to be empty. Studies have shown that 40% of healthy volunteers have an average residual volume greater than 100 mL. It is clear that traditional assumptions about what constitutes a significant residual volume during enteral nutrition may be erroneous.

Checking Residual Volume

Finally, the practice of routinely checking residual volume has not been validated. Some of the factors that make the routine assessment of residual volume questionable are listed below.

1. Type of tube (Salem sump versus Dobbhoff-like feeding tube versus percutaneous enteral gastrostomy [PEG]).
2. Location of the feeding port in the patient (fundus, antrum, or PEG).
3. Position of the patient (supine, right or left lateral decubitus, prone).
4. Method of aspiration (20, 35, 50, 60 mL syringe versus gravity drainage versus low constant suction)
5. The volume of the aspirate obtained.

6. Disposition of the aspirate (i.e., reinfused or discarded).
7. The effects of GI stress prophylaxis medications on the production and volume of gastric secretions.
8. Lack of data linking the residual volume to pulmonary aspiration.

A recent consensus statement on aspiration in the critically ill, suggested that the practice of measuring residual volume is poorly standardized. In addition, there are few data demonstrating that residual volume is a valid measure of GI tolerance of enteral feeding or whether the amount of residual volume is linked to the risk for aspiration pneumonia. Until more evidence is available, good clinical judgment is important when evaluating residual volume (Table 14–17).

Aspiration

Aspiration is the passage of materials into the airway below the level of the vocal cords. The aspirated material may be saliva, nasopharyngeal secretions, bacteria, food, beverage,

TABLE 14–17. SUGGESTED APPROACHES TO EVALUATE RESIDUAL VOLUME

1. Determine if it really is a residual (e.g., assess if the volume aspirated is less than the flow rate of enteral nutrition infusing).
2. Assess the appearance of the residual (formula, gastric secretions, bilious looking).
3. Clinically assess the patient for nausea, vomiting, abdominal distension, fullness, bloating, discomfort.
4. Place the patient on his or her right side for 15–20 min before checking a residual volume to avoid the cascade effect.
5. Review all fluids given enterally, including medications and water for flushes and medication delivery.
6. Try a prokinetic agent or antiemetic to decrease residual volume. Typical doses for available prokinetics are:
   - Metoclopramide: 5–20 mg qid (may need to give IV initially)
   - Erythromycin: 50–200 mg qid
   - Domperidone: 10–30 mg qid
7. Consider a transpyloric feeding tube rather than a gastric tube.
8. Switch to a more calorically dense product to decrease the total volume infused.
9. Tighten glucose control to <200 mg% to avoid gastroparesis from hyperglycemia.
10. Consider analgesic alternatives to opiates.
11. Consider a proton pump inhibitor (PPI) to decrease sheer volume of endogenous gastric secretions (e.g., omeprazole, lansoprazole, esomeprazole, pantoprazole, rabeprazole).
12. Raise the threshold for what constitutes a residual volume up to 400–500 mL.
13. Consider stopping the residual volume checks if the patient is clinically stable, has no abdominal complaints, and the residual volume checks have been "acceptable" for 48 hours.

Reprinted from: UVAHS Nutrition Services/Morrison Management Specialists. Nutrition Support Traineeship Syllabus. Charlottesville: University of Virginia Health System; 2003, with permission from University of Virginia Health Systems.

gastric contents, or any other liquid or substance. The incidence of aspiration pneumonia from enteral nutrition is unclear, because it is difficult to identify an aspiration event and definitions of aspiration vary. Commonly quoted aspiration pneumonia rates in enteral nutrition patients, however, are between 5% and 36%.

Detection

Several methods of evaluating patients for aspiration risk have been popularized through "conventional wisdom." These include the routine monitoring of gastric residual volumes (discussed above), evaluation of gag reflex, testing tracheal secretions for the presence of glucose, and the addition of blue food color to feeding formulas.

The gag reflex is the least reliable protective reflex in ensuring that aspiration does not occur. More important to airway protection are reliable cough and swallow reflexes.

The presence of glucose in tracheal secretions is not a specific or sensitive method of detecting aspiration of enteral nutrition. Tracheal glucose can be positive in patients who are not receiving feeding. Finally, some tube feeding formulas have low glucose concentrations and do not result in a positive test when aspirated.

Several studies have demonstrated that adding blue dye to feeding formulas is not a sensitive method for detecting aspiration and should not be used to indicate aspiration of gastric contents. In addition, some food dyes are mitochondrial toxins leading the Food and Drug Administration to release a Public Health Advisory Report noting the toxicity associated with the use of FD&C Blue No. 1 added to enteral feeding solutions.

Reducing Aspiration Risk

Body Position

The position of the patient is one of the primary factors influencing aspiration risk (Table 14–18). Studies have confirmed that aspiration and pneumonia are significantly more likely when patients are supine with the head of the bed elevated at <30 degrees. While the semi-recumbent position with head of the bed elevations of ≥30 degrees cannot guarantee absolute protection against aspiration, it is a method that is inexpensive and relatively easy to accomplish and monitor. Strict use of semi-recumbent position is the most consistent and potent means to reduce the likelihood of aspiration.

Tube Size and Placement Issues

The incidence of aspiration, and subsequently pneumonia, are not affected by the feeding tube size or whether the tube is placed through the nose, mouth, or a gastrostomy stoma. However, regardless of the site, confirmation of accurate placement is essential.

It is commonly believed that placing the tip of the feeding tube beyond the pylorus decreases the incidence of aspiration events. However, despite numerous studies and a meta-analysis on the topic, it remains unclear if a properly positioned jejunal tube can reduce aspiration risk.

The majority of critically ill patients in these studies received gastric tube feedings safely and effectively. In studies that used protocols for the prevention of aspiration, very low rates of aspiration pneumonia were demonstrated. From a purely evidence-based standpoint then, the question of jejunal placement of feeding tubes and aspiration risk remains unanswered.

Considering the time and expense associated with jejunal placement of feeding tubes, it is reasonable to use the gastric route unless intolerance is evident. Exceptions to this approach include patients known to be at increased risk for aspiration due to altered anatomy (e.g., esophagectomy) or motility (e.g., scleroderma, severe gastroparesis). These patients may benefit from jejunally placed tubes.

Feeding Rate

The delivery rate of the feeding formula may influence aspiration and pneumonia. Bolus administration of 350 mL reduces lower esophageal sphincter pressure, which may precipitate reflux. Continuous enteral nutrition (transpyloric-duodenal feeds), have been associated with more rapidly attained feeding tolerance, but no significant change in aspiration incidence. In one study, reduced aspiration events were associated with cyclic infusion feedings (16-hour cycle), compared to continuous feedings. The authors postulated that cyclic enteral feedings resulted in a reduction of gastric pH and subsequently prevented colonization of gastric contents. However, randomized trials have failed to demonstrate associations between gastric pH, gastric colonization, or pneumonia incidence between patients fed with cyclic versus continuous feedings.

Pharmacologic Interventions

Prokinetic medications have been evaluated to determine whether they improve enteral nutrition tolerance. In critically ill patients, metoclopramide and erythromycin improve gastric emptying, but there are few data on these agents reducing the incidence of aspiration pneumonia.

Bowel Sounds

Auscultating the abdomen to determine the presence of bowel sounds, and thus GI tract function, is a well-entrenched practice. Interestingly, no well-designed study exists that correlates bowel sounds to peristalsis or to enteral nutrition tolerance. From a theoretical perspective, if bowel sounds were related to peristalsis, the absence of bowel sounds would mean that a functional ileus existed. If nothing were moving through the GI tract (unlikely because 9 L of secretions are produced daily; see Table 14–16), the patient would require gastric decompression.

In fact, initiating enteral nutrition in patients without bowel sounds may stimulate the bowel to function normally and bowel sounds may emerge in some patients. Furthermore, auscultation of bowel sounds in the clinical setting varies. Clinician assessment practices differ and include how the quadrants are auscultated, the frequency of auscultation, time spent listening for sounds, and the interpretation of the sounds. Bowel sounds are nonspecific and hence are best used in conjunction with the overall clinical assessment of the patient. Suggested approaches to assessment of GI function when bowel sounds are absent can be found in Table 14–19.

Nausea and Vomiting

Many factors contribute to nausea and vomiting in the critical care setting such as medications, the disease process, surgery, procedures, and bedside interventions (e.g., placing a nasogastric tube or suctioning). After careful assessment and treatment of the underlying cause (Table 14–20), antiemetic coverage may allow the continuation of enteral nutrition while making the patient more comfortable. Because PRN orders are often not administered for a variety of reasons (e.g., patient unable or unaware that the medications may be requested), scheduled anti-emetics may be the preferred method. However, it is important that the medications be discontinued when no longer necessary to prevent undesirable side effects.

Osmolality or Hypertonicity of Formula

It is often thought that GI formulas need to be isotonic (300 mOsm) to be tolerated. As a result, many believe that diluting formula is an essential step. Diluting formula prevents nutrient delivery and there is no evidence that it is beneficial.

The GI tract "self-dilutes" all foods and fluids (including fruits, vegetables, grains, natural sugars, sodas, popsicles, and enteral nutrition formulas) by secreting saliva and

TABLE 14–18. EVIDENCE-BASED PRACTICE RECOMMENDATIONS TO REDUCE THE RISK FOR ASPIRATION PNEUMONIA IN CRITICALLY ILL PATIENTS[a,b,c]

- Maintain the head of the bed elevation at ≥30 degrees if no medical contraindication exists.
- Minimize use of opioid narcotics and consider nonopioid analgesics.
- Verify appropriate placement of feeding tube.
- Clinically assess GI tolerance:
  Abdominal distention
  Fullness/discomfort
  Vomiting
  Excessive residual volumes
- Remove nasoenteric or oroenteric feeding tubes as soon as possible.

Data compiled from [a]UVAHS Nutrition Services/Morrison Management Specialists (2003), [b]Centers for Disease Control and Prevention (2003), and [c]AACN VAP Practice Alert (2004).

TABLE 14–19. SUGGESTED APPROACHES FOR ASSESSMENT OF GI FUNCTION WHEN BOWEL SOUNDS ARE ABSENT

- Assess need for, and volume of, gastric decompression (i.e., compare volume aspirated to normal secretions above the pylorus expected over time frame between aspirations).
- Distinguish significance by differentiating those patients requiring:
  Low constant suction versus
  Gravity drainage versus
  An occasional gastric residual check every 4–6 h (small bowel aspirates should not be checked)
- Abdominal exam: firm, distended, tympanic.
- Presence of nausea, bloating, feeling full, vomiting.
- Evaluate whether patient is passing gas or stooling.
- Compare clinical exam with the differential diagnosis, specifically high suspicion for abdominal process.
- Finally, after determining low risk from above, consider a trial of TEN at low rate of 10–20 mL/h and clinically observe for any of the symptoms listed.

Reprinted from: UVAHS Nutrition Services/Morrison Management Specialists. Nutrition Support Traineeship Syllabus. Charlottesville: University of Virginia Health System; 2003, with permission from University of Virginia Health Systems.

gastric and pancreatic juices (including bicarbonate) to ensure isotonicity. In fact, this occurs whether it is delivered gastrically or jejunally. A clear or full liquid diet is far more hypertonic/hyperosmolar than any commercial enteral nutrition product available on the market (Table 14–21), yet these diets are not ordered at quarter or half strength. Some may argue that jejunal feedings circumvent the first step in food processing by bypassing the stomach and as a result should be managed differently than gastric feedings. However, patients who have undergone total gastrectomies, have "functional" jejunostomies as all food is delivered directly from the esophagus into the jejunum. These patients consume a regular diet; there is no evidence that patients fed via the small bowel should be handled any differently.

For patients who require additional frequent water boluses, dilution of the formula may be necessary but the

TABLE 14–20. SUGGESTED APPROACHES TO REDUCE NAUSEA AND VOMITING IN ENTERALLY FED PATIENTS

1. Review medication profile; change suspicious agents to an alternative.
2. Try a prokinetic agent or antiemetic → review orders for PRN versus standing versus elixir versus tablets.
3. Switch to a more calorically dense product to decrease the total volume infused.
4. Seek transpyloric access of feeding tube.
5. Tighten glucose control to <200 mg% to avoid gastroparesis from hyperglycemia.
6. Consider analgesic alternatives to opiates.
7. Consider a proton pump inhibitor to decrease sheer volume of endogenous gastric secretions (e.g., omeprazole, lansoprazole, esomeprazole, pantoprazole, rabeprazole).
8. If bacterial overgrowth is a possibility, treat with enteral antibiotics.

Reprinted from: UVAHS Nutrition Services/Morrison Management Specialists. Nutrition Support Traineeship Syllabus. Charlottesville: University of Virginia Health System; 2003, with permission from University of Virginia Health Systems.

required dose of enteral nutrition should stay the same (the infusion volume increases with the additional water). With this exception, dilution of enteral nutrition is avoided because it delays the attainment of nutrition goals, increases nursing time and potential for error, and increases the chance of introducing nosocomial organisms.

Diarrhea

Diarrhea occurs in patients whether they are eating solid food, are not taking oral nutrition, or are only taking ice chips. The assumption that tube feeding is a major cause of diarrhea is probably a myth. Although definitive evidence is needed to put this notion to rest, work in the area has suggested other compelling reasons for diarrhea such as medications, especially those containing sorbitol, and infectious agents (*Clostridium difficile* in particular). Other commonly cited but unfounded assumptions for the origin of diarrhea include low serum albumin level, strength or osmolality of the formula, formula composition, rate of infusion, fiber-free enteral nutrition, and disuse of the GI tract. After potential reasons for diarrhea are ruled out (Table 14–22), medications to slow GI motility may be warranted.

Flow Rates and Hours of Infusion

Typical infusion rates for the initiation of enteral nutrition range from 10 to 50 mL/h with increases of 10 to 25 mL every 4 to 24 hours. Unfortunately, like other nutrition practices, little science exists to confirm or refute the efficacy of such regimens. Whether enteral nutrition runs continuously, nocturnally, during the day, or is given as a bolus, is often institution specific. However, with the increased use of insulin infusions to ensure "tight glucose control," and thus improve outcomes in critically ill patients, continuous infusions of enteral nutrition may protect the patients from hypoglycemic episodes.

It is clear that it is difficult, in fact rare, to achieve goal enteral nutrition infusion volumes. Frequent interruptions of enteral nutrition are common (see Table 14–15) and feed-

TABLE 14–21. OSMOLALITY OF SELECTED LIQUIDS AND MEDICATIONS

Typical Liquids	mOsm/kg	Drug	mOsm/kg
EN formulas	250–710	Acetaminophen elixir	5400
Milk/eggnog	275/695	Diphenoxylate suspension	8800
Gelatin	535	KCl elixir (sugar-free)	3000
Broth	445	Chloral hydrate syrup	4400
Sodas	695	Furosemide (oral)	3938
Popsicles	720	Metoclopramide	8350
Juices	~990	Multivitamin liquid	5700
Ice cream	1150	Na phosphate	7250
Sherbet	1225	Cimetidine liquid	4035

Reprinted from: UVAHS Nutrition Services/Morrison Management Specialists. Nutrition Support Traineeship Syllabus. Charlottesville: University of Virginia Health System; 2003, with permission from University of Virginia Health Systems.

TABLE 14–22. SYSTEMATIC APPROACH WHEN ADDRESSING DIARRHEA IN ENTERALLY FED PATIENTS

1. Quantify stool volume: determine if it is really diarrhea (>200 mL/d).
2. Review medication list: look for elixirs/suspensions with sorbitol (not always listed on the ingredient list; may need to contact manufacturer).
3. Try to correlate when diarrhea appeared in relation to start of new medication or switch of medications to enteral route once access obtained. Common offenders include:
   - Acetaminophen and theophylline elixir
   - NeutraPhos
   - Lactulose
   - Standing orders for stool softeners/laxatives
4. Check for *C. difficile* or other infectious cause (lactoferrin, leukocytes).
5. Try a fiber-containing formula or add a fiber powder
   - Few clinical studies
   - Supports the health of colonocytes
6. Once infectious causes are ruled out, try an anti-diarrheal agent (may need standing order versus PRN).
7. Check for fecal impaction.
8. Check for excessive hang times of enteral nutrition (appropriate hang times for enteral nutrition range from 8 to 12 hours for open enteral nutrition containers and 24 hours for closed enteral nutrition containers; practices may vary somewhat depending on institutional policy).
9. Consider bolusing protein powders versus adding directly to formulas to decrease contamination risk.
10. Check qualitative fecal fat as last resort, if negative it does not mean patient is not malabsorbing; if positive however, need to look further.
11. Continue to feed.

Reprinted from: UVAHS Nutrition Services/Morrison Management Specialists. Nutrition Support Traineeship Syllabus. Charlottesville: University of Virginia Health System; 2003, with permission from University of Virginia Health Systems.

ings may only be provided for as little as 6 hours during a 24-hour period. As a result, it is reasonable to consider "padding" flow rates by calculating the flow rate on fewer than 24 hours to attain better delivery of the desired dose. Sample tube feeding protocols for enteral nutrition initiation and progression are described in Table 14–23.

Formula Selection

A vast array of tube feeding formulas are available, including specialty formulas marketed for patients with diabetes,

TABLE 14–23. EXAMPLE OF ENTERAL NUTRITION PROGRESSION REGIME

Continuous

Initiation: Full strength at 50 mL/h and increase by 20 mL every 4 hours to goal rate (all products except 2 cal/mL). A 2-cal/mL product is started at 25 mL/h (as few patients need ≥50 mL/h to meet needs). The final goal rate is dependent on the patient's caloric requirements and GI comfort.

Intermittent/Bolus

Initiation: 125 mL, full strength (regardless of product) every 3 hours for two feedings; increase by 125 mL every two feedings to final goal volume per feeding during waking hours.

Reprinted from: UVAHS Nutrition Services/Morrison Management Specialists. Nutrition Support Traineeship Syllabus. Charlottesville: University of Virginia Health System; 2003, with permission from University of Virginia Health Systems.

AT THE BEDSIDE
▶ *Thinking Critically*

You are caring for a patient with acute upper GI hemorrhage with the following patient orders:

- Monitor vital signs q 15 min until stable; then q 1 h
- Stat hemoglobin and hematocrit
- Administer 0.9 NS wide open until MAP is above 60; then call physician

Which of the above interventions gives you the best indication of the amount of blood lost? What do you expect to happen to the serum lab values with the administration of fluid?

---

pulmonary failure, and renal failure. Other formulas contain nutrients that may modulate immune function, or have nutrients in their most basic (elemental) form for patients with pancreatic insufficiency. It is important to remember that medical nutrition products are not required to meet the same level of scientific scrutiny as medications before they are marketed. Many believe that adequate outcome data are not available to warrant the use of these expensive products. Prospective, randomized trials have demonstrated no advantages of specialized "pulmonary" or "glucose control" feeding formulas. The majority of critically ill patients may be fed with "standard" polymeric tube feeding formulas. Most tube feeding formulas provide between 1 and 2 cal/mL.

SELECTED BIBLIOGRAPHY

Upper GI Bleeding

Conrad SA: Acute upper gastrointestinal bleeding in critically ill patients: Causes and modalities. *Crit Care Med* 2002:30(6 suppl): S365–368.

Creed T, Valori T: Can risk stratification improve the management of acute upper bleeding? *Eur J Gastroenterol Hepatol* 2002; 15:475–476.

D'Amico G, Pietrosi G, Tarantino I, et al: Emergency sclerotherapy versus vasoactive drugs for variceal bleeding in cirrhosis: A Cochrane meta-analysis. *Gastroenterology* 2003;124(5):1277–1291.

Funaki B: Endovascular intervention for the treatment of acute arterial gastrointestinal hemorrhage. *Gastroenterol Clin North Am* 2002;31:701–713.

Gosch S, Watts D, Kinnear M: Management of gastrointestinal hemorrhage. *Postgrad Med J* 2002;78:4–14.

Green BT, Rockey DC: Acute gastrointestinal bleeding. *Semin Gastrointest Dis* 2003;14:44–65.

Proctor, DD: Critical issues in digestive diseases. *Clin Chest Med* 2003;24:623–632.

Podila P, Be-Menachem T, Batra SK, et al: Managing patients with acute nonvariceal gastrointestinal hemorrhage: Development and effectiveness of a clinical care pathway. *Am J Gastroenterol* 2001;96:208–219.

Praskash C, Zuckerman GR: Acute small bowel bleeding: A distinct entity with significantly different economic implications compared with GI bleeding from other locations. *Gastrointest Endoscopy* 2003;58:330–335.

Rockey D. Gastrointestinal bleeding. In Feldman M, Friedman L, Sleisenger M (eds): *Gastrointestinal and Liver Disease*, pp. 211–248. Philadelphia: Saunders; 2002.

Rossle M. When endoscopic therapy or pharmacology fails to control variceal bleeding: What should be done? Immediate control of bleeding by TIPS? *Langenbecks Arch Surg* 2003;388: 155–162.

Schuetz A, Jauch KW: Lower gastrointestinal bleeding: Therapeutic strategies, surgical techniques and results. *Curr Concepts Clin Surg* 2001;386:17–15.

Simoens M, Rutgeerts P: Non-variceal upper gastrointestinal bleeding. *Best Prac Res Clin Gastroenterol* 2001;15:121–133.

Sorbi D, Gostout CJ, Peura D, et al: An assessment of the management of acute bleeding varices: A multicenter prospective member-based study. *Am J Gastroenterol* 2003;98:2424–2434.

Targownik L, Gralnek IM: A risk score to predict the need for treatment of upper GI hemorrhage. *Gastrointest Endoscopy* 2001; 54:797–799.

Zuckier L. Acute gastrointestinal bleeding. *Semin Nuclear Med* 2003;33:297–311.

Liver Failure

Boeker K: Treatment of acute liver failure. *Metabolic Brain Dis* 2001;16:103–117.

Campli CD, Gaspari R, Mignani V, et al: MARS treatment in severe cholestatic patients with acute on chronic liver failure. *Artif Organs* 2003;27:565–569.

Kelly DA: Managing liver failure. *Postgrad Med J* 2002;78:660–667.

Krumberger J: Acute liver failure. *RN* 2002;2:46–54.

Maher J: Alcoholic liver disease. In: Feldman M, Friedman L, Sleisenger M, eds: *Gastrointestinal and Liver Disease*, pp 1375–1391. Philadelphia: Saunders; 2002.

Mitzner SR, Stange J, Peszynski P, et al: Extracorporeal support of the failing liver. *Curr Opin Crit Care* 2002;8:171–177.

Starr S, Hand H: Nursing care of chronic and acute liver failure. *Nurs Standard* 2002;16:47–54.

Stockmann HB, Ijzermans JN: Prospects for the temporary treatment of acute liver failure. *Eur J Gastroenterol Hepatol* 2002; 14:195–203.

Acute Pancreatitis

Alsolaiman MM, Green JA, Barkin JS: Should enteral feeding be the standard of care for acute pancreatitis? *Am J Gastroenterol* 2003;98:2565–2567.

Bradley EL: A primer on guidelines in general and pancreatitis in particular. *Pancreatology* 2003;3:139–143.

Hughes E: Understanding the care of patients with acute pancreatitis. *Nurs Standard* 2004;18:45–52.

Isenmann R, Hernne-Bruns D, Adler G: Gastrointestinal disorders of the critically ill. Shock and acute pancreatitis. *Best Prac Res Clin Gastroenterol* 2003;17:345–355.

Kahl S, Zimmerman S, Malfertheiner P: Acute pancreatitis: Treatment strategies. *Dig Dis* 2003;21:30–37.

Krumberger JM: Acute pancreatitis. *Crit Care Nurse* 1998. AACN Self-study. 1–29.

Kusnierz-Cabala B, Kedra B, Sierzega M: Current concepts on diagnosis and treatment of acute pancreatitis. *Adv Clin Chem* 2003;37:47–81.

Mao EQ, Tang YQ, Zhang SD: Formalized therapeutic guideline for hyperlipidemic severe acute pancreatitis. *World J Gastroenterol* 2003;9:2622–2626.

Murphy J, Mehigan BJ, Keane FBV: Acute pancreatitis. *Hosp Med* 2002;63:487–492.

Shi D, Zhang CW, Jiang JS, et al: Enteral nutrition in treatment of severe acute pancreatitis. *Hepatobiliary Pancreatic Dis Int* 2002; 1:146–149.

Nam JH, Murthy S: Acute pancreatitis. The current status in management. *Expert Opin Pharmacother* 2003;4:235–241.

Toouli J, Brooke-Smith M, Bassi C, et al: Guidelines for management of acute pancreatitis. *J Gastroenterol Hepatol* 2002; 17(Suppl):S15–S39.

Varadarajulu S, Noone T, Hawes RH: Pancreatic duct stent insertion for functional smoldering pancreatitis. *Gastrointest Endoscopy* 2003;58:438–441.

Zyromski N, Murr MM: Evolving concepts in the pathophysiology of acute pancreatitis. *Surgery* 2003;133;235–237.

Intestinal Ischemia/Bowel Obstruction

Delgado-Aros S, Camilleri M: Pseudobstruction in the critically ill. *Best Practice Res Clin Gastroenterol* 2003;17:427–444.

Edwards MS, Cherr GS, Craven TE, et al: Acute occlusive mesenteric ischemia: Surgical management and outcomes. *Ann Vasc Surg* 2003;17:72–79.

Kahi CJ, Rex DK: Bowel obstruction and pseudo-obstruction. *Gastroenterol Clin North Am* 2003;32:1229–1247.

Kumar S, Sarr MG, Mamath PS: Current concepts: Mesenteric venous thrombosis. *N Engl J Med* 2001;345:1683–1688.

McConnell EA: What's behind intestinal obstruction? *Nursing* 2001;31(10):58–63.

McNamara I, Tremelling M, Dunkley I, et al: Management of intestinal obstruction in malignant disease. *Clin Med* 2003;3: 311–314.

Potluri V, Zhukovsky DS: Recent advances in malignant bowel obstruction: An interface of old and new. *Curr Pain Headache Rep* 2003;7:270–278.

Sreenarashimhaiah J: Diagnosis and management of intestinal ischaemic disorders. *BMJ* 2003;326:1372–1376.

Von Gunten C, Muir JC: Fast facts and concepts #45: Medical management of bowel obstruction. *J Palliative Med* 2002;5: 739–740.

Nutrition

Bliss D, Guenter PA, Settle RG: Defining and reporting diarrhea in tube-fed patients—What a mess! *Am J Clin Nutr* 1992;55: 753–759.

Booth CM, Heyland DK, Paterson WG: Gastrointestinal promotility drugs in the critical care setting: A systematic review of the evidence. *Crit Care Med* 2002;30:1429–1435.

Braunschweig CL, Levy P, Sheean PM, Wang X: Enteral compared with parenteral nutrition: A meta analysis. *Am J Clin Nutr* 2001; 74:534–542.

Cerra FB, Benitez MR, Blackburn GL, et al: Applied nutrition in ICU patients. A consensus statement of the American College of Chest Physicians. *Chest* 1997;111:769–778.

Dark DS, Pingleton SK, Kerby GR: Hypercapnia during weaning. A complication of nutritional support. *Chest* 1985;88:141–143.

Drover JW, Dhaliwal R, Heyland DK: Small bowel versus gastric feeding in the critically ill patient: Results of a meta-analysis. *Crit Care Med* 2003;30:A44.

FDA Public Health Advisory FDA/Center for Food Safety & Applied Nutrition: *Reports of blue discoloration and death in patients receiving enteral feedings tinted with the dye, FD&C blue NO.* September 29, 2003.

Fisher RL: Hepatobiliary abnormalities associated with total parenteral nutrition. *Gastroenterol Clin North Am* 1989;18:645–666.

Heymsfield SB, Head CA, McManus CB 3rd, Seitz S, Staton GW, Grossman GD: Respiratory, cardiovascular, and metabolic effects of enteral hyperalimentation: Influence of formula dose and composition. *Am J Clin Nutr* 1984;40:116–130.

Marik PE, Zaloga GP: Gastric versus post-pyloric feeding: A systematic review. *Crit Care* 2003;7:R46–R51.

McClave SA, Lukan JK, Stefater JA, et al. Poor validity of residual volumes as a marker for risk of aspiration in critically ill patients. *Crit Care Med* 2005;33:324–330.

McClave SA, Snider HL, Lowen CC, et al: Use of residual volume as a marker for enteral feeding intolerance: Retrospective blinded comparison with physical examination and radiographic findings. *JPEN J Parenter Enteral Nutr* 1992;16:99–105.

McClave SA, DeMeo MT, DeLegge MH, et al: North American Summit on Aspiration in the Critically Ill Patient: Consensus Statement. *J Parenter Enteral Nutr* 2002;26(6 Suppl):S80–S85.

Mentec H, Dupont H, Bocchetti M, Cani P, Ponche F, Bleichner G: Upper digestive intolerance during enteral nutrition in critically ill patients: Frequency, risk factors, and complications. *Crit Care Med* 2001;29:1955–1961.

Metheny NA, Clouse RE: Bedside methods for detecting aspiration in tube fed patients. *Chest* 1997;111:724–731.

Parrish CR, Krenitsky J, Willcutts K: Protocol on nutrition in the mechanically ventilated patient. In Chulay M, Burns S, eds: *AACN Research Based Practice Protocols on Care of the Mechanically Ventilated Patient.* Viejo, CA: AACN; 2004.

Parrish CR: Enteral feeding: The art and the science. *Nutr Clin Pract* 2003;18:76.

Parrish CR, Krenitsky J, McCray S: University of Virginia Health System Nutrition Support Traineeship Syllabus. Charlottesville: University of Virginia Medical Center Nutrition Services Department; 2003.

Sacks G: *Drug–Nutrient Considerations in Patients Receiving Parenteral and Enteral Nutrition Practical Gastroenterology.* Accessed July 2004 from URL: http://www.healthsystem. virginia.edu/internet/digestive-health/nutrition.cfm#ginutlinks.

Spilker CA, Hinthorn DR, Pingleton SK: Intermittent enteral feeding in mechanically ventilated patients. The effect on gastric pH and gastric cultures. *Chest* 1996;110:243–248.

Talpers SS, Romberger DJ, Bunce SB, Pingleton SK: Nutritionally associated increased carbon dioxide production. Excess total calories vs high proportion of carbohydrate calories. *Chest* 1992; 102:551–555.

van den Berghe G, Wouters P, Weekers F, et al: Intensive insulin therapy in critically ill patients. *N Engl J Med* 2001;345:1359–1367.

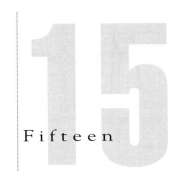

Renal System

Fifteen

Carol Hinkle

► **Knowledge Competencies**

1. Describe the etiology, pathophysiology, clinical presentation, patient needs, and principles of management of acute renal failure (ARF).
2. Differentiate between the three types of ARF:
   • Prerenal
   • Intrarenal
   • Postrenal
3. Compare and contrast the pathophysiology, clinical presentation, patient needs, and management approaches of life-threatening electrolyte imbalances:
   • Sodium (Na^+)

   • Potassium (K^+)
   • Calcium (Ca^{++})
   • Magnesium (Mg^{++})
   • Phosphorous (PO_4)
4. Differentiate between the indications for and the efficacy of the different types of renal replacement therapies.
5. Describe the nursing interventions for patients undergoing renal replacement therapy.

SPECIAL ASSESSMENT TECHNIQUES, DIAGNOSTIC TESTS, AND MONITORING SYSTEMS

There are a wide variety of diagnostic tests available for use in determining the cause and location of renal dysfunction. The creatinine and blood urea nitrogen (BUN) levels are monitored closely, because these levels and their relationship to each other (BUN:creatinine ratio) provide valuable information about the kidney's filtering ability. The BUN level provides valuable information about the state of renal perfusion, whereas the creatinine level is more precise in evaluating actual tubular function. Urine Na^+ values vary as the kidneys attempt to retain or excrete water. Urine volume, specific gravity (SG), and osmolality are useful in identifying the kidney's ability to excrete and concentrate fluid. Comparisons of these test values as found in prerenal and intrarenal failure are shown in Table 15–1. These tests help to establish a firm diagnosis.

PATHOLOGIC CONDITIONS

Acute Renal Failure

The most common renal problem seen in critically ill patients is the development of acute renal failure (ARF). ARF is the abrupt reduction of renal function with progressive retention of metabolic waste products (e.g., creatinine and urea). Oliguria, urine output of less than 400 mL/d, is a common finding in ARF. The development of ARF in the critically ill patient has an estimated mortality of 65%. A history of chronic renal failure (CRF) complicates the clinical course of any critical illness.

Etiology, Risk Factors, and Pathophysiology

ARF is best understood when the condition is considered in terms of the location of damage to the renal system: prerenal, intrarenal, or postrenal causes of failure. Each type of ARF

AT THE BEDSIDE
▶ *Acute Renal Failure*

A 62-year-old woman was initially seen in the emergency department for reports of continued, intense abdominal pain with nausea and vomiting. Following ultrasound, she was taken to the operating room where surgical exploration revealed 5 feet of necrotic bowel, hemorrhagic ascites, and gross peritonitis. The bowel was excised and 460 mL of ascitic fluid was drained.

Upon admission to the critical care unit, the patient was intubated and ventilated, had a pulmonary artery and Foley catheter in situ, and had a nasogastric tube for intermittent suction. Assessment revealed the following:

Skin	Cool and moist
Neurologic	Aroused easily to stimulation, moved all extremities to command
Cardiovascular	Normal heart sounds, no edema or increased neck veins
Respiratory	Diminished breath sounds with crackles bilaterally
Abdomen	Distended, absent bowel sounds, nasogastric drainage minimal (bloody, dark fluid)
Genitourinary	20 mL/h of urine, dark gold in color

Vital Signs

Heart rate	130/min (sinus tachycardia with occasional premature ventricular contractions)
Blood pressure	90/60, labile
Respirations	16/min
Temperature	39.5°C (rectal)

During the first 8 hours postoperatively, she received 5 L of lactated Ringer's solution in an effort to stabilize her blood pressure and increase her urine output.

Aggressive fluid resuscitation was continued throughout her first postoperative day to manage her continued labile blood pressure and poor urine output. Tests at that time revealed the following:

BUN	33 mg/dL
Creatinine	2.8 mg/dL
K^+	6.2 mEq/L

Arterial Blood Gases

pH	7.25
$PaCO_2$	39 mm Hg
HCO_3	14 mEq/L
PaO_2	94 mm Hg

Dobutamine was started at 7.5 mcg/kg per minute. Ventilator changes were made and 88 mEq of $NaHCO_3$ given IV.

On the second postoperative day CVVHD was initiated to correct her increasing renal failure and electrolyte imbalance (BUN 50 mg/dL; creatinine 2.8 mg/dL; K^+ 5.8 mEq/L; arterial pH 7.26). The following day her blood pressure began to stabilize, with decreasing levels of BUN, creatinine, and K^+ and an increase in pH to normal levels.

TABLE 15–1. DIAGNOSTIC TESTS USED IN DIFFERENTIAL DIAGNOSIS OF ARF

Test	Normal Values	Prerenal	Intrarenal
Urine			
Volume	1.0–1.5 L/d	<400 mL/d	<400 mL/d
Specific gravity	1.10–1.20	>1.020	<1.010
Osmolality	500–850 mOsm/kg	>500 mOsm/kg	<350 mOsm/kg
Sodium	40–220 mEq/L/ 24 hours	<20 mEq/L	>30 mEq/L
Serum			
BUN	10–20 mg/dL	>25 mg/dL	>25 mg/dL
Creatinine	0.6–1.2 mg/dL	Normal	>1.2 mg/dL
BUN: creatinine ratio	20:1	>20:1	10:1[a]

[a]Both values elevated but ratio constant.

has different etiologies, pathophysiology, laboratory findings, and clinical presentation.

Prerenal Failure

Physiologic conditions that lead to decreased perfusion of the kidneys, without intrinsic damage to the renal tubules, are identified as prerenal failure (Table 15–2). The decrease in renal arterial perfusion causes a decrease in the rate of filtration of blood through the glomerulus. When perfusion pressure falls below 70 mm Hg, the protection of autoregulation is lost, further decreasing glomerular filtration.

Renal tubular function, at this point, is still completely normal. As a result of the decreased glomerular filtration rate (GFR), the kidneys are unable to filter waste products from the blood. Consequently, more Na^+ and water are reabsorbed, resulting in oliguria. If the decreased perfusion state persists,

TABLE 15–2. CAUSES OF ARF

PRERENAL FAILURE

Hypovolemia
- Burns
- Excessive use of diuretics
- GI losses
- Hemorrhage
- Third spacing
- Shock

Altered Peripheral Vascular Resistance
- Anaphylactic reaction
- Antihypertensive medications
- Neurogenic shock
- Septic shock

Decreased Cardiac Output
- Arrhythmias
- Cardiac tamponade
- Cardiogenic shock
- Congestive heart failure
- Myocardial infarction
- Pulmonary embolism

INTRARENAL FAILURE

Ischemic
- Prolonged decreased renal perfusion
- Septic shock
- Transfusion reaction
- Trauma/crush injury

Nephrotoxic
- Antibiotics
- Fungicides
- Gram negative toxins
- Pesticides
- Radiographic dyes

Inflammatory
- Acute glomerulonephritis
- Acute vasculopathy
- Acute interstitial nephritis

POSTRENAL FAILURE

Mechanical
- Clots
- Stones
- Strictures
- Tumors

Functional
- Medications
- Neurologic disorders

irreversible damage to the renal tubules may occur, resulting in intrarenal failure. Most forms of prerenal failure are easily reversed by treating the cause and increasing renal perfusion.

Intrarenal Failure

Physiologic conditions that damage the renal tubule, nephron, or renal blood vessels are identified as *intrarenal failure* (see Table 15–2). Following prolonged decreases in renal perfusion, the kidneys gradually suffer damage that is not readily reversed with the restoration of renal perfusion. Acute tubular necrosis is the most common form of intrarenal failure.

When the insult to the kidney is nephrotoxic (from drugs or substances that cause direct damage to the kidney), the nephron damage occurs primarily at the epithelial layer. Because this layer has the ability to regenerate, rapid healing often occurs following nephrotoxic insults. When the insult is ischemic or inflammatory, the nephron's basement membrane is also damaged and regeneration is not possible. Ischemic and inflammatory insults are more likely to cause CRF than nephrotoxic insults.

The underlying pathophysiologic abnormality in intrarenal failure is renal cellular damage. In healthy kidneys, the glomerulus normally acts as a filter, preventing the passage of large molecules into the glomerular filtrate. Damage to the glomerulus allows protein and cellular debris to enter the renal tubules, leading to intraluminal obstruction.

Postrenal Failure

Physiologic conditions that partially or completely obstruct urine flow from the kidney to the urethral meatus can cause postrenal failure (see Table 15–2). Partial obstruction increases renal interstitial pressure, which in turn increases Bowman's capsule pressure and opposes glomerular filtration. Complete obstruction leads to urine backup into the kidney, eventually compressing the kidney. With complete obstruction, there is no urine output from the affected kidney. Postrenal failure is an uncommon cause of ARF in critically ill patients. The treatment for postrenal failure is focused on removing the obstruction.

Clinical Phases

There are three clinical phases of ARF, seen primarily in intrarenal failure. The first, the oliguric phase, begins within 48 hours of the insult to the kidney. In intrarenal failure, the oliguric phase is accompanied by a significant rise in BUN and creatinine. The degree of elevation of these waste products is less pronounced in prerenal failure. The most common complications seen in this phase of renal failure are fluid overload and acute hyperkalemia. The oliguric phase may last from a few days to several weeks. The longer the oliguric phase continues, the poorer the patient's prognosis.

The diuretic phase follows the oliguric phase. During this phase, there is a gradual return of renal function. Although the BUN and creatinine continue to rise, there is an increase in urine output. The patient's state of hydration prior to the diuretic phase determines the amount of urine output. A patient who is fluid overloaded may excrete up to 5 L of urine a day and have marked Na^+ wasting. The average time in this phase is 7 to 10 days. Patients must be observed carefully for risk of complications from fluid and electrolyte deficits.

The recovery phase marks the stabilization of laboratory values and can last 3 to 12 months. Some degree of residual renal insufficiency is common following ARF. Some patients never recover renal function and progress to CRF.

Clinical Presentation

The diverse causes of renal failure determine the clinical presentation of the patient. Renal failure can cause multiple organ dysfunction and, therefore, manifests itself in a variety of ways. *Uremia* describes the clinical syndrome that accompanies the detrimental effects of renal dysfunction on the other organ systems. The clinical presentation of the patient in uremia reflects the degree of nephron loss and, correspondingly, the loss of renal function.

Signs and Symptoms

- Oliguria (<400 mL/d) or anuria (<100 mL/d)
- Tachycardia
- Hypotension (prerenal)
- Hypertension (intrarenal)
- Flat neck veins (prerenal)
- Distended neck veins (intrarenal)
- Dry mucous membranes
- Cool, clammy skin
- Lethargy
- Deep, rapid respirations
- Vomiting
- Nausea
- Confusion

Diagnostic Tests

Laboratory tests are extremely important in diagnosing and evaluating the effectiveness of interventions in the ARF patient. Table 15–1 presents the usual laboratory values seen in prerenal and intrarenal failure.

Principles of Management for Renal Failure

A collaborative approach to the treatment of patients in renal failure begins with early recognition of patients at risk for renal failure. The focus is on maintaining adequate renal perfusion and avoiding renal compromise.

Much has changed in the prevention and treatment of ARF over the past several decades. These advances have focused on prompt correction of hypotension and the early use of renal replacement therapies (RRTs) before the development of uremia. Once the patient develops ARF, the goal is to quickly reestablish homeostasis by elimination of the underlying cause. Management of ARF also includes correction of fluid imbalance, prevention and correction of life-threatening electrolyte imbalances, treatment of acidosis, prevention of further renal damage, prevention and treatment of infection, and the improvement of nutritional status.

Correction of Fluid Imbalance

Maintaining fluid balance in the renal failure patient is a challenge. A fine balance must be achieved in providing the fluid necessary for adequate renal perfusion while preventing fluid overload. It is often difficult to assess if the patient is volume depleted or overloaded. A pulmonary artery catheter may be inserted to assist with fluid status evaluation.

1. Calculate daily fluid needs. In prerenal disease, fluid replacement must be matched with fluid loss, both in amount and composition. Insensible fluid losses must be considered in this calculation (Table 15–3). Normal saline volume loading (before a potential insult) of the patient at risk for renal dysfunction is a widely accepted practice. Additionally, volume expansion is certainly beneficial in preventing a volume-depleted patient from progressing from prerenal to intrarenal failure. While oliguric, patients can rarely tolerate more than 1000 mL of fluid per day. It is often necessary to place constraints on other therapies (e.g., IV drug administration, nutritional support) during this phase. During the diuretic phase, the patient may require 1 to 4 L of fluid per day to prevent hypovolemia. The patient is frequently allowed to lose more fluid than is replaced in an effort to facilitate fluid movement from the interstitial and intracellular spaces into the vascular space.

2. Obtain accurate intake and output measurements. All insensible losses should be included in the measurements. Fluid therapy decisions are often based on the patient's output.

3. Obtain daily weights. Body weight should be allowed to decrease by 0.2 to 0.3 kg/d as a result of catabolism. If the patient's weight is stable or increasing, volume expansion is suspected. If weight loss exceeds these recommendations, volume depletion or hypercatabolism is investigated.

4. Administer diuretics to evaluate the patient's response when the patient's fluid status is uncertain. Increasing dosages are used in an attempt to determine the optimal dose. This is often done by doubling the dose (e.g., first dose, 20 mg; second dose, 40 mg; third dose, 80 mg; etc.) every 30 to 60 minutes until diuresis is achieved or a maximum dose is reached. Once renal failure is established, diuretics may be used to avoid fluid overload and to potentiate the effects of antihypertensive medications. Potassium-sparing diuretics are typically avoided because K^+ elimination is diminished in renal failure. Two commonly used diuretics are mannitol and furosemide. Mannitol, an osmotic diuretic, is used in attempts to prevent ARF. It causes vasodilation of the renal

TABLE 15–3. MINIMAL VOLUMES OF FLUID ASSOCIATED WITH INSENSIBLE FLUID LOSSES

Situation/Condition	Volume
Respiratory losses	500–850 mL/d (dependent on minute ventilation rate)
Fever (loss/degree C elevation over 38.0)	200 mL
Diaphoresis	500 mL
Diarrhea	50–200 mL/stool

vessels and expands vascular volume by enhancing movement of fluid from the interstitial space. The beneficial use of mannitol after ARF is established is not clear. Mannitol can contribute to fluid overload without excretory renal function and should be used cautiously. Furosemide, a loop diuretic, is the most common diuretic used in ARF. It works by blocking Na^+ reabsorption in the renal tubules, thereby enhancing excretion of Na^+ and water. It is often used to reduce fluid overload and dialysis frequency in ARF. Furosemide is used cautiously in patients receiving aminoglycoside antibiotics because it potentiates the nephrotoxic effects of these medications.

5. Institute RRT as needed. Until recently, patients in renal failure had either peritoneal dialysis or hemodialysis for assistance in maintaining fluid balance. A number of new continuous filtration devices are now available to increase fluid and metabolic waste product removal during ARF. These newer therapies may be better tolerated in hemodynamically unstable patients than peritoneal dialysis or hemodialysis.

Preventing and Treating Life-Threatening Electrolyte Imbalances

There are a number of electrolyte imbalances that can occur in renal failure, the most common being hyperkalemia, hypocalcemia, hypermagnesemia, and hyperphosphatemia. In ARF, the electrolyte status guides decisions about the type of fluid replacement and RRT. The management of these electrolyte disorders is detailed later in this chapter.

Treating Acidosis

Renal failure patients often develop metabolic acidosis, with a mild respiratory alkalosis compensation.

1. Administer sodium bicarbonate ($NaHCO_3$) as indicated. Treatment is usually not instituted until the serum bicarbonate level drops below 15 mEq/L. Even then, replacement of only half the base deficit is made to avoid overcorrection of the pH. Excessive administration of $NaHCO_3$ can cause metabolic alkalosis, tetany, and pulmonary edema.
2. If a patient is being dialyzed, using a dialysate containing bicarbonate will facilitate buffering of the patient's acidotic state.

Preventing Additional Kidney Damage

In ARF, drugs metabolized or excreted by the kidney require adjustment to avoid excessive blood levels and potential nephrotoxicity. Particular attention must be given to medication scheduling related to RRT schedules. Medications may be eliminated or have their actions potentiated by these therapies. As a result, selected medications, such as antibiotics, are often monitored with peak and trough levels. A clinical pharmacist is a helpful resource on appropriate medication selection, dosing, and monitoring during ARF.

1. Modify medication dosing. Because many medications are eliminated by the kidney, drug administration (dose and schedule) must be altered in the patient with renal failure. Medication dose and schedule decisions are based on the drug and the patient's degree of renal dysfunction. The phase of renal failure and other concomitant treatments help to determine the appropriate dose of medication.
2. Administer antihypertensive agents as needed. Hypertension is a major problem for many renal failure patients, often requiring concomitant use of several antihypertensive agents. Most antihypertensive agents are not removed by RRT. During hemodialysis, it is important to adjust the dosage schedule of antihypertensive agents to avoid hypotensive episodes during dialysis. Some antihypertensive agents, however, are eliminated by the kidney. Therefore, dialysis patients receiving these medications require alterations in their dose or dosing schedule.

Preventing and Treating Infection

Renal failure patients are at high risk for infection and are commonly treated with antimicrobial agents. These antimicrobial agents need to be carefully selected and monitored, and often require dosage adjustment. Careful monitoring of both renal function and drug levels during antimicrobial therapy is imperative to avoid further renal damage.

Improving Nutritional Status

The challenge in the management of the renal failure patient's nutritional status is to provide a balance between sufficient calories and protein to prevent catabolism, yet not create problems, such as fluid and electrolyte imbalances or increase the requirement for RRT. The typical renal failure patient is hypermetabolic, with caloric needs potentially twice normal. Additional stresses, related to being critically ill, can further elevate caloric requirements. Nausea and vomiting, common in uremia, further decrease oral caloric intake. Adequate nutrition is also important in preventing infection by helping to maintain the integrity of the immune system.

1. Restrict the patient's fluid, K^+, Na^+, and protein intake. Because these patients cannot eliminate wastes, fluid, or electrolytes, their dietary intake of these substances is typically restricted. The degree of restriction depends on the cause and severity of their disease. For example, the level of Na^+ restriction is determined by the cause of the renal failure and the serum Na^+ level. Some causes lead to Na^+ wasting and others to Na^+ retention. Phosphorus may need to be restricted and Ca^{++} supplemented if the Ca^{++} level is low in conjunction with normal PO_4^{--} levels.
2. Administer necessary vitamin supplementation. Supplementation of folic acid, pyridoxine, and the water-soluble vitamins is most frequently necessary.

3. Consult a dietitian for a diet plan. Dietary requirements change for patients depending on their renal status and the severity of their underlying condition. Although the precise role of nutrition in ARF is controversial, malnutrition is thought to increase morbidity and mortality. Nutrition, enteral or parenteral, used in conjunction with daily RRT, is thought to improve survival and promote healing of renal tubular cells.

The usual approach to hypercatabolic states is to provide adequate proteins and carbohydrates to provide for resynthesis of damaged or lost tissue elements. Protein requirements may range initially from 0.5 to 1 g/kg per day and increase with RRT to 1 to 1.5 g/kg per day. Nonprotein calories, usually in the form of fat, are given for nonanabolic metabolic needs.

Life-Threatening Electrolyte Imbalances

The kidneys play a major role in the regulation of fluid and electrolyte balance in the body. Regulation of body fluids and electrolytes helps to ensure a stable internal environment, resulting in maximal intracellular function. Any renal dysfunction results in abnormalities in both fluid and electrolyte balance.

For all of the electrolyte disorders, the indications for treatment vary from patient to patient. The signs and symptoms of any electrolyte imbalance are not necessarily determined by the degree of abnormality. Rather, the signs and symptoms are determined by the cause of the condition, as well as the magnitude and rapidity of onset. For many of the electrolyte imbalances, it is difficult to determine at precisely what level signs or symptoms may occur.

Sodium Imbalance: Hyperosmolar Disorders
Etiologies, Risk Factors, and Pathophysiology
Serum osmolality, a measure of the number of particles in a unit of blood volume, is an important indicator of fluid status. Because serum osmolality is determined primarily by the serum Na^+ level, evaluation of Na^+ levels provides valuable information on serum osmolality and potential excesses or deficits of total body water. A quick estimate of serum osmolality can be calculated by simply doubling the serum Na^+ value. Normal serum osmolality values are 285 to 295 mOsm/kg. Abnormal serum Na^+ levels are classified as disorders of osmolality, with hyperosmolality referring to high Na^+ levels, which may be indicative of water deficit, or hypoosmolality referring to low sodium levels, which may be indicative of water excess.

Critically ill patients often are at risk for disorders of osmolality, with children and the elderly at highest risk. As a person ages, the hypothalamus becomes less sensitive to changes in osmolality and is, therefore, less able to alert the body to abnormalities through normal mechanisms. Additionally, the neurologic signs indicative of osmolality dis-

orders are often ignored or assessed as being related to age rather than to a physiologic abnormality.

Hyperosmolar disorders are the result of a deficit of water. The causes of hyperosmolality include inadequate intake of water, excessive loss of water, or conditions that cause an inhibition of antidiuretic hormone (ADH). In the critically ill patient, hyperosmolar disorders develop because of inadequate intake, usually related to loss of consciousness or endotracheal intubation, and ADH inhibition, as manifested by diabetes insipidus in a patient with a head injury. The signs and symptoms seen are the result of the ensuing cerebral dehydration. Water is pulled from the intracellular space to enhance intravascular volume, leaving the cells dehydrated.

Clinical Presentation

Signs and Symptoms

- Lethargy
- Restlessness
- Disorientation
- Delusions
- Seizures
- Oliguria
- Hypotension
- Thirst
- Tachycardia
- Dry mucous membranes
- Coma

Diagnostic Tests

- Serum Na^+ >145 mEq/L
- Serum osmolality >295 mOsm/kg
- Urine SG >1.030

Sodium Imbalance: Hypoosmolar Disorders
Hypoosmolality disorders are the result of an excess of water. The causes of hypoosmolality include excess intake or impaired secretion of water, excess ADH as in the syndrome of inappropriate ADH, replacement of volume loss with pure water, and salt wasting disorders. Hypoosmolar disorders are extremely common in critically ill patients, most often related to the use of D_5W IV solutions. Because these patients have often lost some volume, balanced fluid replacement is extremely important. The signs and symptoms seen with hypoosmolar disorders are related to cerebral intracellular swelling, as water moves from the intravascular to the intracellular spaces.

Clinical Presentation

Signs and Symptoms

- Confusion
- Delirium
- Seizures
- Muscle twitching

- Nausea
- Weight gain
- Headache
- Personality changes
- Coma
- Anorexia
- Vomiting

Diagnostic Tests

- Serum Na^+ <136 mEq/L
- Serum osmolality <280 mOsm/kg
- Urine SG <1.010

Potassium Imbalance: Hyperkalemia
Etiologies, Risk Factors, and Pathophysiology

There are three primary causes of hyperkalemia: increased intake, decreased excretion, and redistribution of K^+ from intracellular to extracellular fluid. Rarely is increased intake a sole cause of hyperkalemia, but it is commonly found in combination with decreased K^+ excretion. The most common causes of hyperkalemia in the critically ill are ARF, cellular destruction (e.g., from crush injuries), and excess supplementation. Because cardiac tissue is sensitive to K^+ levels, hyperkalemia often manifests first as changes in the electrical conduction, demonstrated by changes on ECG tracings. Elevated serum K^+ levels alter the conduction of electrical impulses, particularly in cardiac and muscle tissue. These conduction abnormalities can lead to serious cardiac arrhythmias and death.

Clinical Presentation

Because K^+ impacts normal neuromuscular and cardiac function, these systems are carefully evaluated when hyperkalemia is suspected. It is important to note that a patient may be experiencing hyperkalemia and have no ECG or rhythm changes.

Signs and Symptoms

- Vague muscle weakness
- Decreased deep tendon reflexes
- Flaccid paralysis
- Mental confusion
- Nausea
- Diarrhea
- Cramping

ECG Changes

- Tall, tented T waves
- QT interval may shorten
- Intraventricular conduction is slowed
- Widened QRS
- Wide P waves
- Bradycardia
- First-degree atrioventricular (AV) block

- Advanced AV block with ventricular escape rhythms, ventricular fibrillation, or asystole

Diagnostic Tests

- Serum K^+ >5.5 mEq/L

Potassium Imbalance: Hypokalemia
Etiologies, Risk Factors, and Pathophysiology

The causes of hypokalemia include decreased intake, increased excretion or impaired conservation of potassium, excess or abnormal loss, and increased movement of K^+ into the cells. In the critically ill patient, hypokalemia is often related to the use of diuretics and excess losses through the gastrointestinal tract. Muscle weakness, including cardiac muscle, is the hallmark sign of hypokalemia. Asystole can result from severe hypokalemia. Depressed levels of serum K^+ lead to increased irritability of cardiac muscle and neuromuscular cells. Serious cardiac arrhythmias, and death, may result from hypokalemia.

Clinical Presentation

Signs and Symptoms

- Weakness
- Respiratory muscle weakness, hypoventilation
- Paralytic ileus
- Abdominal distention
- Cramping
- Confusion, irritability
- Lethargy

ECG Changes

- Ventricular ectopy and flat, inverted T waves
- QT interval prolongation
- U-wave development
- ST segment shortening and depression

Diagnostic Tests

- Serum K^+ <3.5 mEq/L

Calcium Imbalance: Hypercalcemia
Etiologies, Risk Factors, and Pathophysiology

The causes of hypercalcemia are threefold: increased Ca^{++} release from the bone, increased Ca^{++} absorption from the gastrointestinal tract, and decreased Ca^{++} excretion.

Clinical Presentation

Signs and Symptoms

- Somnolence
- Stupor
- Nausea
- Anorexia
- Polyuria
- Lethargy
- Coma

- Vomiting
- Constipation
- Renal calculi

ECG Changes

- Arrhythmias
- Prolonged QT interval
- Prolonged ST segment
- Flat, inverted T waves

Diagnostic Tests

- Serum Ca^{++} >10.5 mg/dL

Calcium Imbalance: Hypocalcemia

Etiologies, Risk Factors, and Pathophysiology

True hypocalcemia is rare. The causes of hypocalcemia are classified into three categories: decreased absorption of Ca^{++}, increased loss of Ca^{++}, and decreased amounts of physiologically active Ca^{++}. Critically ill patients develop hypocalcemia infrequently, most often related to either gastrointestinal losses or malabsorption. The low Ca^{++} levels result in muscle contraction, seen as tetany, and bronchospasm.

Clinical Presentation

Signs and Symptoms

- Positive Chvostek's sign (twitching of the upper lip in response to tapping of the facial nerve)
- Positive Trousseau's sign (carpopedal spasm in response to occlusion of circulation to the extremity for 3 minutes)
- Tetany
- Seizures
- Respiratory arrest
- Bronchospasms
- Stridor
- Wheezing
- Paralytic ileus
- Diarrhea

ECG Changes

- Arrhythmias
- Shortened QT interval
- ST-segment sagging and shortening
- T-wave inversion

Diagnostic Tests

- Serum Ca^{++} <8.5 mg/dL

Magnesium Imbalance: Hypermagnesemia

Etiologies, Risk Factors, and Pathophysiology

Hypermagnesemia is most commonly seen in renal failure patients with an inability to excrete Mg^{++} or with increased intake of Mg^{++} from antacid. ARF is the most common etiology of hypermagnesemia in critically ill patients. Both neuromuscular and cardiac depression are observed. Hypermagnesemia may also develop in non–renal failure situations when Mg^{++} intake is increased, excretion is decreased, or adrenal insufficiency or hyperparathyroidism causes increased Mg^{++}.

Clinical Presentation

Signs and Symptoms

- Respiratory depression
- Diminished deep tendon reflexes
- Flaccid paralysis
- Drowsiness
- Lethargy

ECG Changes

- Cardiac arrest
- Prolonged PR and QT intervals
- Widened QRS
- Increased T-wave amplitude
- Bradycardia

Diagnostic Tests

- Serum Mg^{++} >2.5 mEq/L

Magnesium Imbalance: Hypomagnesemia

Etiologies, Risk Factors, and Pathophysiology

Hypomagnesemia frequently occurs in alcoholic and critically ill patients and is often associated with hypocalcemia and hypokalemia. Hypomagnesemia can be caused by decreased intake; increased excretion, such as with diuretic therapy; and excessive loss of body fluids. The hypomagnesemia seen in the critically ill is most often the manifestation of a compromised nutritional status, secondary to starvation and malabsorption.

Clinical Presentation

Signs and Symptoms

- Hyperreflexia
- Positive Chvostek's and Trousseau's signs
- Nystagmus
- Seizures
- Tetany

ECG Changes

- Prolonged PR and QT intervals
- Broad, flat T waves
- Ventricular arrhythmias

Diagnostic Tests

- Serum Mg^{++} <1.5 mEq/L

Phosphate Imbalance: Hyperphosphatemia

Etiologies, Risk Factors, and Pathophysiology

The most common cause of hyperphosphatemia in all patients, including the critically ill, is renal failure; the regulation of phosphate in the body is regulated by the kidneys. Hyperphosphatemia is also seen in hypoparathyroidism, excessive intake of alkali or vitamin D, Addison's disease, and with bone tumors or fractures. Hyperphosphatemia is often associated with hypocalcemia.

Clinical Presentation

Signs and Symptoms

- Muscle cramps
- Joint pain
- Seizures

Diagnostic Tests

- Serum phosphate >4.5 mg/dL

Phosphate Imbalance: Hypophosphatemia
Etiologies, Risk Factors, and Pathophysiology
Hypophosphatemia is caused by hyperparathyroidism, hyperinsulinism, administration of IV glucose, and conditions that cause bone deterioration, such as osteomalacia. This condition is not often seen in critically ill patients. When seen, it is frequently in conjunction with hypercalcemia.

Clinical Presentation

Signs and Symptoms

- Muscle weakness and wasting
- Fatigue
- Confusion
- Oliguria
- Tachycardia
- Anorexia
- Dyspnea
- Cool skin

Diagnostic Tests

- Serum phosphate <3.0 mg/dL

Principles of Management for Electrolyte Imbalances
Hyperosmolar Disorders

1. Administer free water. Fluid replacement can be given orally, if feasible, or with intravenous administration of D_5W. The goal is to normalize the serum Na^+ level over a 48- to 72-hour period. A gradual return to normal avoids cellular overhydration.
2. Monitor Na^+ and serum osmolality level frequently. Care must be taken to correct the Na^+ and osmolality level gradually. Correcting these levels too quickly may precipitate hypoosmolar conditions and seizures.
4. Administer desmopressin (nasally) or vasopressin (IV, IM, subcutaneously) in diabetes insipidus. These medications inhibit the action of ADH.

Hypoosmolar Disorders

1. Restrict water intake. Mild, asymptomatic hyponatremia often is not treated or is treated only with a water restriction.
2. Institute RRT. RRT is indicated for severe fluid overload in the presence of renal failure.
3. Administer hypertonic saline. Hypertonic saline may be needed to correct Na^+ levels below 115 mEq/L when the patient is symptomatic. Careful, slow administration of hypertonic saline is important to avoid sudden shifts in serum osmolality and subsequent hyperosmolality.
4. Monitor Na^+ and serum osmolality levels frequently. Care must be taken to correct these levels gradually. Rapid correction can precipitate hyperosmolar conditions and seizures.

Hyperkalemia
Of all the potential electrolyte disorders, hyperkalemia is considered the most life threatening because of potassium's profound impact on the electrophysiology of the heart. Hyperkalemia is also the most common reason for initiation of dialysis in the ARF patient.

1. Initiate cardiac monitoring. Because hyperkalemia does affect cardiac tissue, continuous ECG monitoring assists in recognizing cardiac manifestations of altered K^+ levels.
2. Restrict dietary intake of K^+ to 40 mEq/d. A dietary restriction is considered conservative management and is usually instituted in conjunction with other therapies aimed at removing K^+ from the body.
3. Administer cation-exchange resins. Sodium polystyrene sulfonate (Kayexalate) is used to increase K^+ excretion and is administered by mouth or enema with sorbitol. Sorbitol acts to draw fluid into the bowel where the polystyrene causes an exchange between Na^+ and K^+ ions. The K^+ is then eliminated from the body through feces.
4. Administer hypertonic (50%) glucose and regular insulin. Insulin acts to drive K^+ into the cells on a temporary basis, thereby protecting the heart from the effect of the elevated serum (extracellular) K^+ level.
5. Administer $NaHCO_3$. The administration of sodium bicarbonate causes movement of K^+ into the cell, encouraging the exchange of hydrogen (H^+) ion inside the cells with the excess K^+ ion outside the cell.
6. Administer calcium salts, such as calcium gluconate. Calcium elevates the stimulation threshold, protecting the patient from the negative myocardial effects of hyperkalemia. The administration of calcium does not change the level of K^+ in the extracellular fluid.
7. Institute RRT. Hemodialysis may be necessary for rapidly removing K^+ when the patient's K^+ level cannot be controlled by other methods.

Hypokalemia

1. Administer K^+ supplementation. Depending on the severity of the deficit, oral or IV replacements can be utilized. Ideally, supplementation of K^+ is given through a central line due to the irritating nature of K^+ to the tissues. Potassium replacement is given in at least 50 mL of fluid with no more than 20 mEq replaced per hour. It is common for patients to be unable to tolerate more than 10 mEq/h if the supplementation is given peripherally. Because K^+ is primarily an intracellular cation, allow at least 1 hour after administration for the movement of the K^+ into the cells before evaluating the serum K^+ level. A level obtained too quickly after supplementation is completed may reflect an artificially high serum value.
2. Evaluate the patient's diuretic therapy.

Hypercalcemia

1. Administer normal saline IV and diuretics. In the presence of normal renal function, normal saline infusions given with diuretics increase the GFR and enhance Ca^{++} excretion from the kidneys.
2. Administer corticosteroids. Corticosteroids decrease absorption of Ca^{++} from the gastrointestinal tract.
3. Administer plicamycin. Plicamycin increases the bone uptake and storage of Ca^{++}.
4. Administer oral phosphate (PO_4^{--}) supplementation. PO_4^{--} binds Ca^{++} so that it is excreted in stool.

Hypocalcemia

1. Administer Ca^{++} supplementation. Calcium-containing antacids may be used. Often Ca^{++} supplementation is done concurrently with the administration of PO_4^{--} binders, such as aluminum hydroxide. There is a reciprocal relationship between Ca^{++} and PO_4^{--} levels in the body. Calcium may be given orally in the form of antacids or intravenously as calcium gluconate or calcium chloride when symptoms are serious.
2. Administer vitamin D supplementation. Vitamin D is necessary for Ca^{++} to be absorbed from the gastrointestinal tract.
3. Institute seizure precautions. Patients with hypocalcemia are at risk for developing tetany and seizures.

Hypermagnesemia

1. Institute RRT. See below.
2. Discontinue use of Mg^{++}-containing antacids.
3. Administer normal saline and diuretics. If the patient has normal renal function, the administration of saline and diuretics increases GFR and enhances excretion of Mg^{++}.

Hypomagnesemia

1. Administer Mg^{++} supplementation. Oral administration or Mg^{++} sulfate IM or IV may be used. IV Mg^{++} should not be given faster than 150 mg/min. Total daily replacement should not exceed 30 to 40 g.
2. Reduce auditory, pressure, and visual stimuli.

Hyperphosphatemia

1. Administer aluminum hydroxide binding gels. These gels bind with phosphate in the intestine, limiting the absorption, promoting excretion, and decreasing the serum level.
2. Institute RRT. If the patient is symptomatic, hemodialysis is the most effective choice to rapidly decrease the serum levels.
3. Administer acetazolamide. Acetazolamide increases the urinary excretion of phosphate.

Hypophosphatemia

1. Administer phosphate supplementation. Supplementation can be administered by mouth or IV.
2. Discontinue use of phosphate binding gels.

RENAL REPLACEMENT THERAPY

For many years hemodialysis and peritoneal dialysis were the only therapies available to manage renal failure or situations in which the patient becomes volume overloaded. Many critically ill patients cannot tolerate the rapid fluid and electrolyte shifts associated with traditional hemodialysis because of hemodynamic instability and cardiac arrhythmias. Peritoneal dialysis, an option for patients who cannot tolerate the hemodynamic changes associated with hemodialysis, is limited to patients without recent abdominal incisions, respiratory distress, or bowel perforations.

Several alternative therapies to manage acute fluid and electrolyte problems have been introduced during the past 25 years, beginning with continuous arteriovenous hemofiltration (CAVH). A number of additional continuous renal replacement therapies (CRRTs) have been introduced, offering more treatment options for the critically ill patient with renal failure or fluid overload. These therapies include using a double-lumen venous access and a pump for continuous venovenous hemofiltration (CVVH) and the addition of dialysate for continuous venovenous hemodialysis (CVVHD). Continuous venovenous hemodiafiltration (CVVHDF) combines the principles of CVVH and CVVHD. Some patients may benefit from high-volume hemofiltration to promote even higher clearances of substances from the bloodstream. Using CRRT, many of the desirable outcomes of hemodialysis can be accomplished without the associated hemodynamic instability.

The goal of any type of RRT is the removal of excess fluid and uremic toxins and correction of electrolyte imbalances. Each of the RRT methods are able to accomplish that goal, with varying levels of success. These homeostatic corrections are accomplished through the processes of diffusion, osmosis, filtration, or convection. *Diffusion,* the process by which substrates move from an area of high concentration to one of a lesser concentration, provides for movement of fluids and electrolytes from the body into the filtrate. Through *osmosis,* water from an area of lesser solute concentration moves to an area of greater solute concentration, becoming part of the filtrate. *Filtration* also occurs, allowing for movement of water and solute as a result of a difference in hydrostatic pressure. *Convection* involves the movement of fluids and solutes being pushed through a membrane by pressure and creating a drag, which pulls larger particles along with the fluid.

RRTs are grouped into three general categories: those requiring arteriovenous access, those requiring venous access only, or those requiring a peritoneal access (Table 15–4). RRT is applied for periods of 4 hours or more, with some requiring continuous use. Except for peritoneal dialysis, all of the RRT devices require extracorporeal blood flow. This flow is accomplished through the use of two catheters, one arterial and one venous, or through a single venous catheter with two lumens. Filtration and dialysis occur as the blood moves through a dialyzer or hemofilter.

Access

Before any type of RRT can be performed, access to the bloodstream or peritoneum is necessary. The type of access is determined by the reason for initiation and method of renal replacement. It can be either temporary or permanent.

Permanent Vascular Access

Permanent access is achieved by placement of either an arteriovenous fistula or graft. A *fistula* is a surgically created anastomosis between an artery, usually the radial, brachial, or femoral, and an adjacent vein. This anastomosis allows arterial blood to flow through the vein, causing venous enlargement and engorgement. Permanent access is necessary for patients requiring chronic dialysis.

Arteriovenous grafts are placed in patients who do not have adequate vessels to create a fistula. A prosthetic graft is implanted subcutaneously and used to anastomose an artery to a vein. A period of maturation, usually 2 to 3 weeks, is necessary before the access can be used. This maturation time allows for the venous side to dilate and the vessel wall to thicken, permitting repeated insertion of dialysis needles.

Temporary Vascular Access

Temporary access to the bloodstream is obtained through cannulation of an artery and/or a large-diameter vein, with a large-bore, double- or single-lumen catheter specifically designed for dialysis. These catheters are inserted and maintained similarly to other arterial and central venous devices, but are used primarily for dialysis treatments. A single double-lumen catheter is more commonly used than a single-lumen, single-vessel catheter to maximize the filtration and dialysis capabilities of the renal replacement devices. These catheters can be used for extended periods of time with meticulous attention to sterile technique. The location for catheter placement is chosen to maximize blood flow and prevent kinking of the catheter with patient movement. To initiate CVVH, hemodialysis (CVVHD), or hemodiafiltration (CVVHDF), a single 14- to 16-gauge double-lumen catheter is placed in the subclavian, jugular, or femoral vein.

TABLE 15–4. SUMMARY OF RENAL REPLACEMENT THERAPIES

Type	Indications	Contraindications	Complications
Hemodialysis	Life-threatening fluid/electrolyte imbalances Renal failure Poisoning/drug overdose	Hemodynamic instability Hypovolemia Coagulation disorders	Blood loss
Peritoneal dialysis	Fluid/electrolyte imbalances Renal failure	Recent abdominal surgery Abdominal adhesions Peritonitis Respiratory distress Pregnancy	Peritonitis
Continuous renal replacement therapy SCUF CAVH CAVHD CAVHDF CVVH CVVHD CVVHDF	Fluid/electrolyte imbalances Renal failure Fluid overload	Inadequate blood pressure for CAVH, CAVHD, or CAVHDF	Filter clotting Worsening uremia for SCUF

Abbreviations: CAVH, continuous arteriovenous hemofiltration; CAVHD, continuous arteriovenous hemodialysis; CAVHDF, continuous arteriovenous hemodiafiltration; CVVH, continuous venovenous hemofiltration; CVVHD, continuous venovenous hemodialysis; CVVHDF, continuous venovenous hemodiafiltration; SCUF, slow continuous ultrafiltration.

Peritoneal Access

Peritoneal catheters are made of silastic tubing, with multiple perforations to allow for fluid exchange, and an attached cuff, soft disk, or balloon to anchor the catheter. When peritoneal dialysis needs to be initiated immediately, a rigid stylet, designed for single acute use only, is inserted. Both types of catheters are inserted through small incisions in the abdomen and threaded into the peritoneal space.

Dialyzer/Hemofilters/Dialysate

There are a variety of dialyzers and hemofilters available for use. The type of dialyzer or hemofilter chosen is determined by the patient's condition and desired outcomes of the RRT. All dialyzers have a blood and dialysate compartment, separated by a semipermeable membrane. The dialyzer has two inlet ports and two outlet ports, one each for blood and dialysate. During dialysis, blood and dialysate are pumped through the dialyzer in opposite directions.

Hemofilters are made of highly permeable hollow fibers or plates. These fibers or plates are surrounded by an ultrafiltrate space and have arterial and venous blood ports. Plasma water and certain solutes are separated from the blood by the hemofilter and drain into a collection device.

Dialysate solution, used in any therapy that has dialysis as a component, is specifically designed to create concentration gradients so that optimal removal of wastes, acid–base and electrolyte balance, and maintenance of extracellular fluid balance can be achieved. The specific solution is determined by the patient's condition and desired outcomes. Although standard solutions may initially be used, they can be tailored to meet the individual patient's needs and contain varying concentrations of Na^+, K^+, Mg^+, Ca^{++}, Cl^-, glucose, and buffers.

Procedures

Hemodialysis

Initiation of hemodialysis through a temporary access is accomplished using a procedure called *coupling*. During coupling, the dialysis catheter and the dialysis circuitry are connected, using sterile technique. To initiate dialysis through a permanent access, two 14- or 16-gauge needles are inserted into the dilated vein of the fistula or the graft portion of the synthetic graft. One needle is considered arterial, used for blood outflow, and the other is considered venous, used for blood return.

The basic components of a hemodialysis system are shown in Figure 15–1. Blood, leaving the patient through the arterial needle, is pumped through the circuitry and returned to the patient through the venous needle. A blood pump moves the blood through the dialysis circuitry and dialyzer, allowing for different flow rates. Both arterial and venous pressures are monitored in the circuitry.

Peritoneal Dialysis

Peritoneal dialysis is accomplished through a series of cycles or exchanges. The dialysate, administered into the peritoneal cavity, remains in the cavity for a preset amount of time (dwell time) and then is drained. Each set of these activities is called a *cycle* or *exchange*. Dialysate flows into the peritoneal cavity by gravity, taking approximately 10 minutes for 2 L of fluid to infuse. During the dwell time, diffusion, osmosis, and ultrafiltration occur. Typically, dwell times range from 10 to 30 minutes. With an optimally functioning catheter, it takes 2 L of fluid 10 minutes to drain from the abdomen.

Continuous Renal Replacement Therapy

In CRRT, the blood lines are primed with a saline solution with or without heparin as an anticoagulant and then attached to the appropriate vascular access catheter arm (arterial or venous outflow and venous inflow). Blood flow is pumped from the outflow side and passes through the hemofilter. The blood returns to the body via the inflow tubing after fluid and electrolytes are moved into the ultrafiltrate. The ultrafiltrate is collected in a bag after removal. In CVVHD, blood leaves the patient through the outflow catheter and is pumped through a dialyzer rather than a hemofilter. Wastes and fluid are removed and drained into an ultrafiltrate bag. The blood is then returned to the body through the inflow catheter. The dialysate is pumped through the dialyzer countercurrent to blood flow. Figure 15–2 shows the basic setup of CVVHD. In CVVHDF, both dialysis fluid and replacement fluids are used to make the system more efficient.

Indications for and Efficacy of Renal Replacement Therapy Modes

Each type of RRT is indicated for different clinical situations and achieves different goals. The goals of therapy are clearly delineated before selection of the type of therapy.

Hemodialysis

Hemodialysis is implemented when aggressive therapy is indicated in acute situations. Hemodialysis is contraindicated in patients with hemodynamic instability (although hypotension may be a relative contraindication), hypovolemia, coagulation disorders, or vascular access problems.

Considered the gold standard for the treatment of ARF and CRF, hemodialysis is considered the most effective of all of the RRTs. Fluid and uremic wastes can be eliminated from the body during a 4- to 6-hour treatment. Approximately 200 mL of blood is utilized in the circuit, which can add to a patient's unstable condition.

Peritoneal Dialysis

Most often, peritoneal dialysis is indicated for critically ill patients who need dialysis but are unable to tolerate the

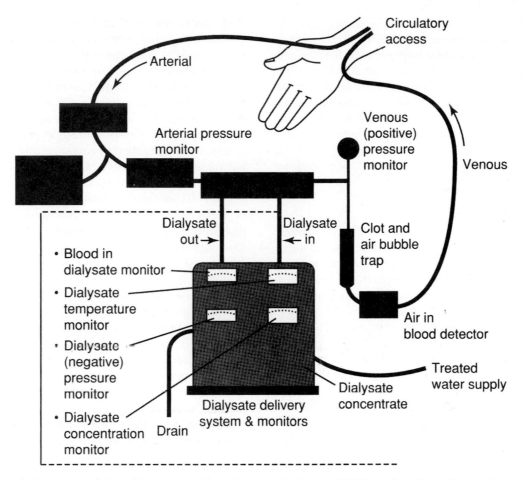

Figure 15–1. Components of a hemodialysis system. (*From: Thompson JM, McFarland GK, Hirsch JE, et al [eds]: Mosby's Manual of Clinical Nursing, p. 592. St. Louis, MO: Mosby, 1990.*)

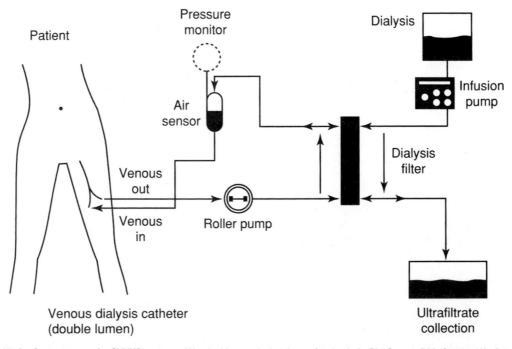

Figure 15–2. Components of a CVVHD system. (*Used with permission from: Strohschein BL, Caruso DM, Greene KA: Continuous venovenous hemodialysis. Am J Crit Care 1994;3:95.*)

hemodynamic changes associated with hemodialysis. Peritoneal dialysis may also be performed in a critical care unit for a patient who is on chronic peritoneal dialysis and presently hospitalized with an acute illness. Utilizing the peritoneal membrane as the dialyzer, effective elimination of fluid and waste products can be achieved. Peritoneal dialysis is slower and less effective than hemodialysis.

Peritoneal dialysis is contraindicated in patients who have had recent or extensive abdominal surgery; who have abdominal adhesions, peritonitis, or respiratory distress; or who are pregnant.

Continuous Renal Replacement Therapy

Patients appropriate for CRRT are chosen after evaluating their clinical diagnosis, hemodynamic parameters, and metabolic status. The specific type of CRRT is selected after considering the patient's fluid and electrolyte status, metabolic needs, and severity of uremia. The most commonly used forms of CRRT are CVVHD and CVVHDF.

Slow Continuous Ultrafiltration

When slow continuous ultrafiltration is desired, slow continuous ultrafiltration (SCUF) is the therapy of choice. This therapy is primarily for use in patients with a fluid volume excess and some degree of renal function. Because fluid removal is the primary goal, this procedure is performed without simultaneous fluid replacement. There is a minimal impact on the urea and creatinine levels.

Continuous Venovenous Hemofiltration

The main objective of CVVH is fluid removal. Although large changes in blood chemistries are not expected, it is possible for a patient to achieve and maintain a stable volume and composition of electrolytes in his or her extracellular fluid. Because large volumes of fluid can be removed, the health care team has more flexibility in treating patients. Nutrition, a problem in many critically ill patients, can often be enhanced in these patients because nutrition (even total parenteral nutrition when enteral cannot be tolerated) can be provided without fear of fluid overload.

CVVH, in some institutions, has become the treatment of choice when patients have contraindications to hemodialysis or peritoneal dialysis. Fluid shifts in CVVH are less rapid than with hemodialysis, making the therapy attractive when persistent hemodynamic instability, especially hypotension, is present. Other patients who may benefit from CVVH are patients with uncontrolled congestive heart failure, pulmonary edema, or hepatorenal syndrome. Patients can be maintained on CVVH for several weeks until either long-term hemodialysis can be initiated or there is return of renal function. There are no absolute contraindications for CVVH. A major advantage of CVVH over CAVH is a decrease in access-related complications because there is no need for an arterial access. Unfortunately, the therapy has to be discontinued for transportation off the unit such as for selected diagnostic tests (e.g., computed tomographic scans) and the continuous nature of the therapy limits mo-

---

AT THE BEDSIDE
Thinking Critically

A 60-year-old gentleman was admitted through the emergency department following the onset of severe abdominal and back pain. On arrival, his blood pressure was 80/60, and pulse was 120 and regular. He was slightly dyspneic. His abdomen was large and rigid, and bowel tones were absent. Within an hour, he received 1200 mL of albumin and 1500 mL of normal saline. When his blood pressure did not respond to the fluid challenge, he was placed on a dopamine drip at 5 mcg/kg per min. A Foley catheter was placed with only 35 mL of urine output. After a CAT scan, he was taken to the OR for repair of a ruptured aortic aneurysm. Estimated blood loss was 12,000 mL, with replacement of 11,000 mL of whole blood, 600 mL of fresh frozen plasma, and 1250 mL of albumin. He was admitted to the critical care unit following surgery with no urine output.

- What therapies would you consider at this time?
- Would initiation of a diuretic be appropriate?

His BP continued to be low (80/60). A pulmonary artery catheter was placed to assist in evaluation of his fluid status. Pulmonary artery pressures were 20/7 mm Hg, with a PAOP of 8 mm Hg.

- What type of fluid therapy should this patient be given?

While his BP was gradually increased using fluids and dopamine, he continued to have a rocky course. By his third postoperative day, he still had a low urine output. His creatinine had climbed quickly to 7.5 mg/dL and BUN to 90 mg/dL. His potassium was 5.8 mEq/L. Hemodialysis was instituted.

- What special considerations should be made for his medication therapy while he is being treated with dialysis?
- What should the team consider to meet his increased caloric demands?

After 2 weeks on dialysis, the patient's urine output began to gradually increase. His wound bleeding stopped, and he became hemodynamically more stable. He had been started on total parenteral nutrition, which was stopped as soon as he started eating an adequate diet. Seven weeks after the rupture, he was ready for discharge. His urine output was averaging 1200 mL/d; BUN and creatinine were 28 and 1.9 mg/dL, respectively.

bility, particularly if a femoral access is used (e.g., out of bed to chair).

Continuous Venovenous Hemodialysis

CVVHD combines the principles of hemofiltration with a slow form of dialysis (see Figure 15–2). More aggressive removal of fluid and solute is possible than with CVVH. Dialysate is infused through a dialyzer, countercurrent to the patient's blood flow.

The indications for CVVHD are similar to those for hemodialysis. Selection of CVVHD is generally made because a patient is unstable and not able to tolerate the rapid fluid and electrolyte shifts that occur with hemodialysis. CVVHD provides an avenue for these hemodynamically unstable patients to achieve a stable fluid and electrolyte balance without further compromise of their status. There are no absolute contraindications for CVVHD. Maintaining patency of the dialyzer is key to successful CVVHD. Patients with coagulopathies require special monitoring.

General Renal Replacement Therapy Interventions

The frequency of RRT as a therapy in critical care units is on the rise. Some practitioners feel CRRT will replace hemodialysis as the therapy of choice for ARF in the critically ill patient.

Although each therapy has unique characteristics, all require similar interventions. Careful observations and interventions are essential, as is accurate fluid management. Close monitoring of mean arterial pressure, urine output, cardiac output, central venous pressure, pulmonary artery occlusion pressure, daily weights, and state of anticoagulation are critical. Careful monitoring of acid–base and serum chemistries is mandatory. The critical care nurse assumes a primary responsibility for early recognition and initial interventions for patient and system problems.

SELECTED BIBLIOGRAPHY

General Renal

Carlson KK: Acute renal failure. In Urban N, Greenlee K, Krumberger J, Winkleman C, eds: *Guidelines for Critical Care Nursing.* St. Louis: Mosby, 1995.

Stark JL: The renal system. In Alspach G, ed: *Core Curriculum for Critical Care Nursing,* 5th ed, pp. 464–563. Philadelphia: WB Saunders, 1998.

Urden LD, Stacy KM, Lough, ME, et al: Renal alterations. In: *Critical Care Nursing: Diagnosis and Management,* 4th ed. St. Louis, MO: Mosby, 2002.

Nutrition in the Acute Renal Failure Patient

Wolfson M, Kopple JD: Nutritional management of acute renal failure. In Lazarus L, Brenner J, eds: *Acute Renal Failure,* 3rd ed, pp. 467–485. New York: Churchill Livingston, 1993.

Hemodialysis

Carlson KK: Hemodialysis. In Urban N, Greenlee K, Krumberger J, Winkleman C, eds: *Guidelines for Critical Care Nursing.* St. Louis, MO: Mosby, 1995.

Giuliano KK: Hemodialysis. In Lynn-McHale DJ, Carlson KK, eds: *AACN Procedure Manual for Critical Care,* 4th ed, pp. 733–745. Philadelphia: WB Saunders, 2001.

Peritoneal Dialysis

Carlson KK: Peritoneal dialysis. In Urban N, Greenlee K, Krumberger J, Winkleman C, eds: *Guidelines for Critical Care Nursing.* St. Louis, MO: Mosby, 1995.

Giuliano KK: Peritoneal Dialysis. In Lynn-McHale DJ, Carlson KK, eds: *AACN Procedure Manual for Critical Care,* 4th ed, pp. 746–752. Philadelphia: WB Saunders, 2001.

Stark JL: The renal system. In Alspach G, ed: *Core Curriculum for Critical Care Nursing,* 5th ed, pp 511–513. Philadelphia: Saunders, 1998.

Continuous Renal Replacement Therapies

Carlson KK: Continuous renal replacement therapies. In Urban N, Greenlee K, Krumberger J, Winkleman C, eds: *Guidelines for Critical Care Nursing.* St. Louis, MO: Mosby, 1995.

Dirkes SM: Continuous renal replacement therapy: Dialytic therapy for acute renal failure in intensive care. *Nephrol Nurs J* 2000; 27:581–592.

Giuliano KK: Continuous renal replacement therapies. In Lynn-McHale DJ, Carlson KK, eds: *AACN Procedure Manual for Critical Care,* 4th ed, pp. 717–732. Philadelphia: Saunders, 2001.

Mehta RL: Continuous renal replacement therapies in the acute renal failure setting: Current concepts. *Adv Renal Replace Ther* 1997;4(Suppl 1):81–92.

Ronco C, Bellomo R, Kellum JA: Continuous renal replacement therapy: Opinions and evidence. *Adv Renal Replace Ther* 2002; 9:229–244.

Stark JL: The renal system. In Alspach G, ed: *Core Curriculum for Critical Care Nursing,* 5th ed, pp. 513–515. Philadelphia: WB Saunders, 1998.

Strohschein BL, Caruso DM, Greene KA: Continuous venovenous hemodialysis. *Am J Crit Care* 1994;3:92–101.

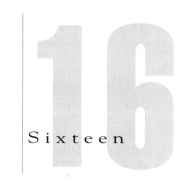

Endocrine System

Sixteen 16

Joanne Krumberger

▶ Knowledge Competencies

1. Outline the nursing management of patients receiving blood glucose monitoring.
2. Describe the etiology, pathophysiology, clinical presentation, patient needs, and principles of management for
   - Diabetic ketoacidosis
   - Hyperosmolar hyperglycemic states
   - Acute hypoglycemia
   - Syndrome of inappropriate antidiuretic hormone secretion
   - Diabetes insipidus

SPECIAL ASSESSMENT TECHNIQUES, DIAGNOSTIC TESTS, AND MONITORING SYSTEMS

Blood Glucose Monitoring

Frequent assessments of blood glucose levels in the critically ill patient commonly are performed at the bedside by placing a drop of blood on a chemical reagent strip and observing color changes to estimate glucose levels by simple visual observation or with a glucometer (Figure 16–1). Bedside glucose monitoring allows more rapid treatments of glucose abnormalities than laboratory analysis. New strip technology and meters eliminate the common problem of not getting enough blood on the strip, resulting in more accurate readings. The newer reagent strips are designed to pull blood into the strip by capillary action.

Large discrepancies between laboratory serum blood glucose and capillary blood glucose monitoring (BGM) results should be investigated. Most authors recommend that BGM readings be within a 20% to 30% variance of the laboratory values to be acceptable. Clinical signs and symptoms of the patient always need to be considered when interpreting results.

Equipment-Related Discrepancies

Some older models of BGM measure the glucose level of whole blood, whereas newer meters measures the glucose level of plasma. When using a meter that gives whole blood glucose levels, the fasting target goal is between 80 and 120 mg/dL. When using a meter that gives plasma glucose levels, the fasting target goal is between 90 and 130 mg/dL. There also may be variations between the laboratory and BGM results depending on the source of blood (capillary, venous, or arterial). Other sources of error include use of expired strip reagents and errors in following the procedure for proper use of the device. Obtaining a simultaneous laboratory sample and bedside BGM reading periodically identifies discrepancies and allows for more accurate interpretation of the bedside BGM reading. In general, a capillary BGM result of greater than 500 mg/dL should always be checked with a laboratory specimen, because BGM meters are not considered reliable for serum glucose levels above 500 mg/dL.

Patient-Related Discrepancies

Several clinical conditions may also influence bedside BGM measurements (Table 16–1). The presence of hypovolemia

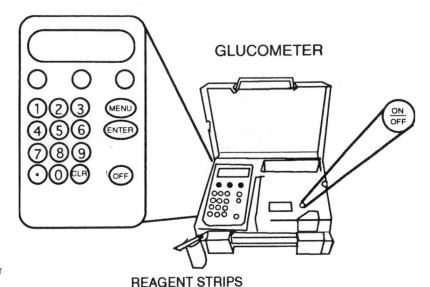

Figure 16–1. Reagent strip and glucometer for bedside testing of blood glucose levels.

REAGENT STRIPS

or abnormal hematocrit values (<30% or >55%) fall outside the BGM instrument's hematocrit range and may cause inaccurate results. Higher than normal hematocrit levels result in underestimation of the blood glucose. Lower than normal hematocrit levels result in overestimating blood glucose. In addition, conditions that lead to inadequate tissue perfusion in the fingers, such as hypotensive shock or edema, make unreliable any capillary BGM done by fingerstick (underestimation of the blood glucose). Finally, patients receiving large doses of acetaminophen may cause a chemical reaction on some BGM strips which also may introduce error into the result. Tips for BGM are reviewed in Table 16–2.

Patient Teaching

The specific procedure for BGM needs to be taught to the patient. The goal of treatment is to maintain a fasting glucose less than 140 mg/dL. Higher serum glucose target values for older patients may be more appropriate because they are more vulnerable to hypoglycemia. Patients on insulin should be encouraged to test their glucose before each meal and at bedtime to evaluate the effectiveness of their insulin dose. If this is not feasible, patients should be encouraged to test at least two times a day at alternating times so they can track glucose patterns at all four times of day. For non–insulin-dependent diabetics, BGM is recommended before breakfast and 2 hours before, during, and after exercise and whenever they experience signs and symptoms of hyperglycemia. They should also check more frequently during any illness or major changes in eating patterns. Patients should also be instructed to test their meter control at least once per week.

Continuous glucose monitoring with glucose sensors are now available, and although relatively expensive, they can supply the patient with all of the information needed to optimize insulin therapy and metabolic control. Clinical trials are needed to clearly demonstrate the long-term benefits of this new therapy.

TABLE 16–1. CLINICAL SITUATIONS THAT MAY AFFECT THE ACCURACY OF BEDSIDE BGM

Blood glucose levels >500 mg/dL

Hct <30% or >55%

Inadequate tissue perfusion
  Hypovolemia

High blood levels of acetaminophen

Use of vasoactive drugs

Patients requiring control of hypoglycemic or hyperglycemic states

Neonates

TABLE 16–2. TIPS FOR BGM USE

- Review the manufacturer's guidelines for specific procedures related to the use of your BGM device. User error is the most common reason for inaccurate readings.
- Ensure that the BGM device is calibrated and clean before using.
- Do not use alcohol to clean the machine.
- For patients with cold hands, let the hand hang down below the level of the heart so that blood can flow to the fingertips.
- Obtain a large drop of blood and let it drop down onto the reagent pad. Distribute evenly over the entire pad, but do not smear the blood.
- Use the side of the finger rather than the underside as it has fewer nerve endings (therefore is less painful) and more capillaries (will get larger drop of blood).
- Correlate the BGM device reading with the clinical assessment of the patient.
- Use universal precautions during the entire procedure.

PATHOLOGIC CONDITIONS

Hyperglycemic Emergencies

The two most common endocrine crises which require critical care admission are diabetic ketoacidosis (DKA) and hyperosmolar hyperglycemic states (HHS). DKA is defined as acute hyperglycemia with acidosis, and HHS is classified as acute hyperglycemia without acidosis (nonketotic). Diabetes is the fourth most common comorbid condition complicating all hospital discharges. Evidence suggests in-hospital morbidity and mortality are increased by hyperglycemia for many conditions, particularly in the critically ill.

The common feature of these hyperglycemic emergencies is diabetes mellitus (DM). There are four clinical classifications of DM: type I diabetes mellitus; type II diabetes mellitus; other specific types; and gestational diabetes mellitus. Critically ill patients with DM typically present with type 1 or type 2 diabetes.

DM is a metabolic disease that is caused by ineffective uptake of glucose by cells. There are several types of diabetes, the two most common being insulin-dependent DM (type I DM) and non–insulin-dependent DM (type II DM). Type I DM usually has a juvenile or early adult onset and is characterized by little or no insulin being produced by pancreatic beta cells. Type II DM usually occurs in older adults and is associated with below normal, normal, or above normal insulin production. Although hyperglycemia is the common feature, the etiology, risk factors, pathophysiology, and management priorities vary considerably for each of these disorders.

Etiology, Risk Factors, and Pathophysiology

Insulin is normally released from the pancreas by beta cells of the islets of Langerhans in response to increases in blood glucose. Insulin is necessary for cellular uptake of glucose by most cells in the body (except brain and liver cells). Without insulin, the glucose fails to enter cells and accumulates in the blood, resulting in hyperglycemia. Cells without glucose begin to starve and begin to use existing stores of fat and protein to provide energy for body processes (gluconeogenesis). This triggers a complex series of physiologic processes, which account for the major signs and symptoms associated with DKA and HHS.

Diabetic Ketoacidosis

The most common causes of DKA include previously undiagnosed type I DM, infections, and omission of insulin (Table 16–3). Other acute illness such as myocardial infarction, stroke, trauma, or pancreatitis are also commonly associated with DKA. DKA is described by three clinical features: hyperglycemia, ketoruia/ketonemia, and acidosis. By definition, the following lab values are present with DKA: serum glucose greater than 250 mg/dL, moderate or large ketonuria/ketonemia, and arterial pH less than 7.30 or serum bicarbonate less than 15 mEq/L.

AT THE BEDSIDE
▶ *Diabetic Ketoacidosis*

An 18-year-old woman was admitted to the MICU with a diagnosis of DKA. She was diagnosed with insulin-dependent diabetes mellitus (IDDM) 9 months earlier. Her roommate reported that she had consumed approximately six or seven beers at a school party when she "passed out" and was difficult to arouse. Her friend also reported that the patient had been complaining of flulike symptoms (vomiting, diarrhea) for 2 or 3 days prior to admission. On arrival in the ED, the patient was alert, but confused. Significant findings on her admission profile were:

Respiratory rate	38/min, deep ("fruity" breath)
Blood pressure	98/50 mm Hg
Heart rate	110 beats/min; sinus tachycardia
Skin	Warm and flushed
Arterial blood gases	pH 7.20
	$PaCO_2$ 24 mm Hg
	PaO_2 60 mm Hg
	HCO_3^- 11 mEq/L
	SaO_2 91%
Serum glucose	440 mg/dL
Serum acetone	3
Serum ketones	3+
Serum osmolality	310 mOsm/kg
Anion gap	22 mEq/L
Serum potassium	5.8 mEq/L
Serum BUN	28 mg/dL
Serum creatinine	1.5 mg/dL
Serum sodium	130 mEq/L
Serum magnesium	1.1 mg/dL
Serum phosphate	2.2 mg/dL
Serum chloride	94 mEq/L
White blood cell count	14,000/mm^3
Urine glucose	2+ (large)
Urine ketone	3+ (large)

The initiating event in DKA is an insufficient or absent level of circulating insulin. This insulin deficiency results in increased fatty acid metabolism, increased liver gluconeogenesis (formation of glucose from amino acids and proteins), and increased secretion of counterregulatory hormones, including glucagon and the stress hormones (catecholamines, cortisol, and growth hormone). These hormones counteract the glucose-lowering effects of insulin and are released in response to stress and other stimuli. The pathophysiology of DKA can be organized into two main components: fluid volume deficit and acid–base imbalance (Figure 16–2).

Fluid Volume Deficit With Associated Electrolyte Imbalance

Because of the insulin deficiency, there is both hyperglycemia and increased amino acid release from cells. The

AT THE BEDSIDE
▶ *Hyperosmolar Hyperglycemic State*

A 72-year-old man was admitted to the MICU with a diagnosis of hyperglycemic crisis. He lives with his small dog. His daughter dialed 911 after finding her father nonarousable at his home. She reported that he had complained of flulike symptoms 3 weeks earlier. His history is significant for congestive heart failure and adult-onset type II DM. His daily medications include: digoxin 0.25 mg/d orally, Lasix 10 mg orally twice a day, KCl 20 mEq/d orally, and glyburide 10 mg orally twice a day. On arrival in the ED the patient was comatose. Significant findings on his admission profile were:

Blood pressure	82/44 mm Hg; MAP 56 mm Hg
Heart rate	121 beats/min
Respiratory rate	14/min, shallow
Skin	Dry, poor turgor; dry mucous membranes
Arterial blood gases on cannula	pH 7.35
	2 L/min O_2 per nasal
	$PaCO_2$ 49 mm Hg
	PaO_2 56 mm Hg
	HCO_3^- 22 mEq/L
	SaO_2 88%
Serum glucose	1100 mg/dL
Serum osmolality	362 mOsm/kg
Serum potassium	2.8 mEq/L
Serum BUN	41 mg/dL
Serum creatinine	2.2 mg/dL
Serum sodium	152 mEq/L
Serum phosphate	2.0 mg/dL
Serum chloride	121 mEq/L

stress response in the body leads to metabolic decompensation, and stress hormones further trigger a rise in plasma glucose and ketones. The hyperglycemia causes an osmotic diuresis and hypotonic losses leading to fluid volume deficits (intracellular and extracellular) and electrolyte losses. As serum glucose exceeds the renal threshold, glycosuria results. In the absence of insulin, protein stores are also broken down by the liver into amino acids and then into glucose for energy. This further increases serum blood glucose, increases urine glucose, and worsens the osmotic diuresis and ketonemia. Urinary losses of water, sodium, magnesium, calcium, and phosphorous cause an increase in serum osmolality and decreased electrolyte levels. Potassium levels may be increased or decreased, depending on the amount of nausea and vomiting, acid–base balance, and fluid status of the patient. This hyperosmolality causes additional fluid shifts from the intracellular to the extracellular space, increasing dehydration. Hypovolemic shock can result from severe fluid losses in DKA (see Chapter 11, Multisystem Problems). Volume depletion decreases glomerular filtration

TABLE 16–3. CAUSES OF DKA

Initial presentation of previously undiagnosed patients with DM.

Type I IDDM who omits insulin dose, decreases dose, does not adhere to diet, or experiences severe stress or increased exercise without adequate insulin adjustment.

Type II NIDDM with severe medical problems or stress

Stressors
    Infections
    Trauma
    Surgery
    Pregnancy
    Acute illness
    Renal failure
    Myocardial ischemia

Impairment of glucose metabolism by drugs
    Thiazide diuretics
    Phenytoin
    Beta blockers
    Calcium channel blockers
    Steroids
    Epinephrine
    Analgesics
    Psychotropics

Intoxication
    Alcohol
    Salicylate

of glucose and creates a cycle of progressive hyperglycemia. The increase in serum osmolarity also is thought to further impair insulin secretion and promote insulin resistance. The altered neurologic status frequently seen in these patients is due primarily to cellular dehydration and serum hyperosmolarity.

Acid–Base Imbalance

Cells without glucose starve and begin to use existing stores of fat and protein to provide energy for body processes (gluconeogenesis). Fats are broken down faster than they can be metabolized in the liver, which results in an accumulation of ketone acids. Ketone acids accumulate in the blood stream where hydrogen ions (H^+) dissociate, causing a metabolic acidosis. Acetone also is formed during this process and is responsible for the "fruity breath" found in these patients.

This acidosis may be worsened with severe fluid volume deficits because hypovolemia results in hypoperfusion and production of lactic acids from anaerobic metabolism. Excess lactic acid results in what is called *increased anion gap* (increased body acids). Sodium, potassium, chloride, and bicarbonate are responsible for maintaining a normal anion gap in the body which is normally less than 12 to 14 mEq/L (Table 16–4). Ketone accumulation, a byproduct of gluconeogenesis, causes an increase in the anion gap above 14 mEq/L.

The normal physiologic response to metabolic acidosis is to produce bicarbonate to buffer the ketones and H^+ ions.

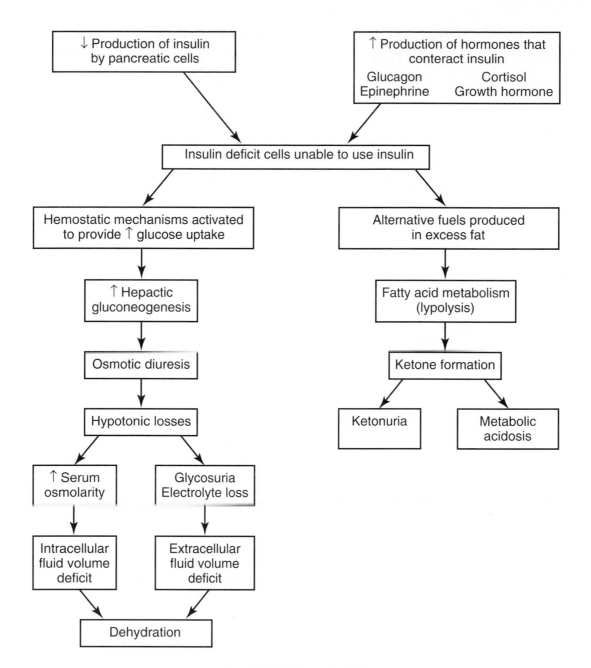

Figure 16–2. Pathogenesis of DKA.

The patient with DKA often has diminished bicarbonate levels because of the osmotic diuresis. The respiratory system attempts to compensate by eliminating acids by blowing off carbon dioxide to restore normal blood pH. This ex-

plains the deep rapid breathing, called Kussmaul's respirations, seen in these patients.

Metabolic acidosis also results in potentially life-threatening electrolyte imbalances. Serum potassium is elevated initially in DKA probably due to potassium shifts from the intracellular to the extracellular space because of the acidosis. Later, hypokalemia is common due to increased urinary excretion of potassium with the osmotic diuresis.

Hyperosmolar Hyperglycemic States

The pathogenesis of HHS is similar to the pathogenesis of DKA with the following differences. HHS is classified as

TABLE 16–4. CALCULATION OF ANION GAP (NORMAL <12 mEq/L)

$Na^+ - (Cl^- + HCO_3^-)$ = anion gap

Example from DKA case study:

   128 − (94 + 12) = 22 mEq/L (anion gap acidosis)

Example from HHNK case study:

   152 − (121 + 22) = 10 mEq/L (no anion gap)

hyperglycemia with profound dehydration without ketosis. The onset of hyperglycemia in HHS is progressive because many patients have a history of type II DM with some circulating insulin levels. The extremely severe hyperglycemia in HHS results in profound extracellular fluid volume contraction, marked intracellular dehydration, and excessive loss of electrolytes. In addition, because there is some insulin, lipolysis is suppressed; therefore, there is no production of ketones and no specific physical signs and symptoms of ketosis (no Kussmaul's respiration, renal excretion of ketones, abdominal pain, nausea, vomiting, or anorexia). Because of the lack of these emergent signs and symptoms, many of these patients do not seek early treatment. Sustained osmotic diuresis results, leading to massive volume losses, electrolyte imbalance, and central nervous system (CNS) dysfunction. Mortality rates, therefore, are higher with HHS, both because of the severe volume loss and because it occurs more frequently in a more elderly population. Death results from CNS depression of vital body functions (cardiac and respiratory centers in the brain are depressed), cerebral edema, cardiovascular collapse, renal shutdown, and vascular embolism.

Clinical Presentation

DKA	HHS
History	
Younger with history of type I IDDM or previously undiagnosed; preexisting infection common	Elderly with history of type II IDDM, and preexisting chronic illnesses which are associated with decreased renal glucose excretion, concurrent illness frequently precipitates viral infections or pneumonia
Signs and Symptoms	
Nonspecific: polyuria, polydipsia, weakness	Nonspecific: polyuria, polydipsia, weakness
Specific: nausea, vomiting, anorexia, Kussmaul's respiration, fruity breath	Specific: none
Diagnostic Tests	
Serum glucose 250 to 800 mg/dL	Serum glucose At least 600 mg/dL, often >1000 mg/dL
Serum osmolality <330 mOSm/Kg/H$_2$O	Serum osmolality >350 mOsm/kg/H$_2$O
Ketoacidosis Marked pH <7.30 HCO$_3$ <15 mEq/L Serum ketones >2+	Ketoacidosis Not a feature pH >7.30 HCO$_3^-$ >15 mEq/L
Positive urine ketones Kussmaul's respirations Acetone breath Positive anion gap	Serum ketones below 2+ Minimal urine ketones
Dehydration Volume depletion (intracellular and extracellular)	Dehydration Severe volume depletion (intracellular and extracellular)
Renal function Increased BUN/creatinine ratio Urine ketones +2	Renal function Marked increase in BUN: creatinine ratio
Neurologic impairment Common	Neurologic impairment Common due to serum osmolality
Electrolyte depletion Potassium, magnesium, phosphate	Electrolyte depletion Potassium, magnesium, phosphate, sodium

Principles of Management for Hyperglycemic Emergencies

The management of the patient in acute DKA and HHS revolves around six primary areas: fluid replacement, treatment of hyperglycemia, electrolyte replacement, treatment of any underlying disorders, prevention and management of complications, and patient/family teaching.

Fluid Replacement

Treatment of intracellular and extracellular fluid volume deficits is a priority for both DKA and HHS to restore intravascular volume and prevent cardiovascular collapse. Initial volume replacement is based on assessment of vascular status.

1. Administer normal saline (0.9%). The choice of intravenous (IV) fluid depends on the initial blood pressure readings and the serum sodium level. The presence of hyperglycemia and dehydration masks the true serum sodium level, requiring a correction of serum sodium levels prior to IV fluid selection (Table 16–5). IV fluids are generally infused at rapid rates (1000 to 2000 mL in the first hour, 1000 mL in the second hour, and then at 500 mL/h) until fluid volume is restored or initially around 15 to 20 mL/kg per hour.

2. Titrate the rate of infusion based on urine output, mean arterial blood pressure, and central venous

TABLE 16–5. CORRECTION OF SERUM SODIUM LEVELS IN THE PRESENCE OF HYPERGLYCEMIA

$$\text{Corrected sodium} = (\text{serum sodium}) + 1.6 \times \left[\frac{\text{glucose (mg/dL)} - 100}{100} \right]$$

pressure measurements. Typically, the patient with HHS has more profound fluid volume deficits, but because the patient is older and often has other underlying medical problems, the rate of fluid replacement needs to be carefully titrated. Serum glucose falls with initiation of fluids alone. It is critical that insulin therapy not be started without simultaneously correcting the fluid deficit. Otherwise, the result is an acute loss of vascular volume, worsening of the hypernatremia, shock, and increased risk of mortality.

3. Change IV fluid to 5% dextrose with 0.45 NaCl at 150 to 200 mL/h when serum glucose reaches 250 mg/dL. Maintain insulin therapy (see next section).

Treating Hyperglycemia

In both DKA and HHS some insulin replacement is needed, although the requirements in HHS are typically low.

1. Regular insulin 0.15 units/kg as IV bolus.
2. Initiate low-dose IV regular insulin at a rate of 0.1 units/kg per hour. If serum glucose does not fall by 50 to 70 mg/dL in the first hour, double insulin infusion on an hourly basis until glucose falls by 50 to 70 mg/dL.
3. Monitor serum glucose levels closely and titrate insulin infusion accordingly. Once the serum glucose reaches 250 mg/dL, the insulin infusion should be decreased to a rate of 2 to 4 units/h and the IV fluids changed to half normal saline with glucose (D5-1/2NS). This ensures that hypoglycemia does not occur during ongoing treatment of the acute condition. It is essential that insulin therapy continues in the patient with DKA until the serum pH is corrected to avoid intracellular hypokalemia. Additional glucose may be needed to keep the insulin drip infusing to achieve this outcome. Glucose-containing solution should also be started in the patient with HHS when serum glucose reaches 250 to 300 mg/dL to protect against cerebral edema.

Electrolyte Replacement

Electrolyte deficits are usually present in both DKA and HHS due to the osmotic diuresis.

1. Administer potassium supplements according to serum levels:
   - If serum K^+ is less than 3.3 mEq/L, hold insulin and give 40 mEq K^+/h (2/3 KCl and 1/3 KPO_4^-) until K^+ is greater than 3.3 mEq/L.
   - If serum K^+ is >5.0, hold K^+ and check K^+ every 2 hours.
   - If serum K^+ is >3.3 mEq/L <5.0 mEq/L give 20 to 30 mEq K^+ in each liter of volume replacement.

Replacement of potassium is a priority during the correction of hyperglycemia to avoid hypokalemia during rehydration, when potassium moves into the cell along with glucose. To avoid cardiac dysrhythmias associated with hypokalemia, delay insulin administration until serum potassium levels are greater than 3.3 mEq/L. The rate of potassium chloride infusion should be adjusted according to frequently monitored serum potassium levels and the urine output.

2. Monitor magnesium, calcium, and phosphate levels every 2 hours during rehydration. Hemodilution may further decrease serum levels of these electrolytes. Magnesium and calcium replacements are given based on serum levels. Total body phosphorous levels are depleted due to osmotic diuresis. This may result in impaired cardiac and respiratory functions. The administration of potassium phosphate 20 mEq/L is the best method of phosphate replacement as it replaces both potassium and phosphate simultaneously. Phosphate replacements should not be administered in patients with renal failure. If hypokalemia is refractory to potassium replacement, magnesium replacement should be considered.

3. Assess need for bicarbonate:
   - If pH is less than 6.9, dilute $NaHCO_3^-$ (100 mmol) in 400 mL H_2O. Infuse at 200 mL/h.
   - If pH is 6.9 to 7.0, dilute $NaHCO_3^-$ (50 mmol) in 200 mL H_2O. Infuse at 200 mL/h.
   - If pH is greater than 7.0, hold $NaHCO_3^-$.

   Repeat HCO_3 administration every 2 hours until pH is greater than 7.0. Monitor serum K^+ closely.

Treating Underlying Disorders

The precipitating cause for the hyperglycemic emergency needs to be determined. Underlying infection is a common precipitating factor in both DKA and HHS.

1. Investigate precipitating factors through the following tests: urinalysis, complete blood count, ECG, chest x-ray, and appropriate cultures. Administer antibiotics as appropriate if infection is suspected.
2. Obtain history from patient and family about the possibility of missed insulin doses.

Preventing and Managing Complications

1. Monitor serum glucose, electrolytes (sodium and potassium), and arterial blood gases (DKA only) every 1 to 2 hours until normal levels are approached.
2. Measure serum phosphate and magnesium initially and repeat as necessary.
3. Monitor temperature, blood pressure, pulse, respiratory rate, pulse oximetry, urinary output, and central venous pressure at frequent intervals.
4. Evaluate neurologic status at frequent intervals. Institute seizure precautions if cerebral edema is suspected. Institute measures to avoid aspiration in pa-

tients with altered mental status. Administer dexamethasone and mannitol if appropriate.

5. Titrate fluid replacement carefully to prevent congestive heart failure. Auscultate lung sounds frequently during fluid replacement.
6. Administer anticoagulants as ordered. Hyperosmolar patients are at great risk of thrombosis.

Patient and Family Education

Particularly in type I DM, the key to prevention of recurrent DKA is adequate patient education regarding diabetes management. Teach the skills needed to manage diabetes. Table 16–6 outlines the required skills for diabetic management. Return demonstrations by the patient or designated caregiver are essential. Instruction regarding the need for routine medical follow-up and the availability of hospital and community resources is also an important component of the diabetes management plan.

Acute Hypoglycemia

Hypoglycemia is a blood glucose level less than 60 mg/dL and is a common endocrine emergency. Hypoglycemia results from the imbalance between glucose production and glucose utilization. Of the acute complications, hypoglycemia is most common in insulin-dependent diabetics, but it also can occur with type II diabetics who are treated with insulin or oral hypoglycemic agents, such as chlorpropamide (Diabinese).

Etiology, Risk Factors, and Pathophysiology

Hypoglycemia can be divided into two categories: fasting hypoglycemia (more than 5 hours after a meal) and postprandial hypoglycemia (1 to 2 hours after a meal) (Table 16–7). *Fasting hypoglycemia* occurs when the normal physiologic response to a falling glucose level is altered and there is an imbalance in glucose production and use. Hypoglycemia in a diabetic person is most commonly caused by excessive insulin or oral hypoglycemic agent, too much exercise, or not enough food. Excessive insulin doses usually result from errors in administration technique, especially in diabetics with decreased visual acuity. The most common cause of postprandial hypoglycemia is gastric surgery because after this surgery, food passes more rapidly through the small intestine, causing glucose levels to fall.

Glucose is the obligate fuel for the brain and CNS. The brain is unable to synthesize or store glucose and must rely on circulating plasma blood glucose levels for survival. As blood glucose declines rapidly, epinephrine, glucagon, glucocorticoids, and growth hormones are released. Patients exhibit adrenergic symptoms—tachycardia, anxiety, sweating, trembling, and hunger. These symptoms can occur even if the blood glucose is normal but there is a sudden acute decline (i.e., blood glucose level decrease from 180 to 90 mg/dL). In moderate to severe hypoglycemic reactions, the CNS is affected, signifying that the brain is being deprived of the glucose it needs.

Hypoglycemic unawareness is used for diabetics whose first initial manifestation of hypoglycemia is CNS symptoms, at which time it may be too late for self-treatment. Hypoglycemic unawareness is defined as the loss of adrenergic symptoms of hypoglycemia that prompt a patient to act to prevent the progression of severe hypoglycemia. It results from altered counterregulation systems described. Type I diabetics are known to have deficiencies in counterregulation systems. It is not known whether this is true for type II diabetics.

Clinical Presentation

Signs and Symptoms

- Mild hypoglycemic symptoms (adrenergic response)
  - Tremors
  - Shakiness

TABLE 16–6. SKILLS FOR DIABETIC MANAGEMENT

Blood glucose monitoring
Insulin administration
Diet therapy
Meal planning
Exercise therapy
Urine ketone testing
Sick day management
Recognition of signs and symptoms of hypoglycemia and hyperglycemia
Proper treatments for hypoglycemia and hyperglycemia

Expected Outcomes

1. The patient or caregiver will be able to verbalize essential aspects of diet therapy, meal planning, exercise therapy, sick day management, signs and symptoms of hypoglycemia and hyperglycemia, and proper treatments for hypoglycemia and hyperglycemia.
2. The patient or caregiver will be able to demonstrate blood glucose monitoring, insulin administration, and urine ketone testing.

TABLE 16–7. CAUSES OF HYPOGLYCEMIA (PARTIAL LISTING)

Fasting Hypoglycemia
Excessive insulin dosage
Decreased need for insulin
   Decreased food intake
   Increased exercise
   Renal failure
   Liver failure
   Congestive heart failure
Drugs
   Oral hypoglycemic agents
   Alcohol
   Salicylates
   Beta-adrenergic blockers
Postprandial Hypoglycemia
Excessive insulin effect
Postgastric surgery

– Tachycardia
– Paresthesias
– Pallor
– Excessive hunger
– Anxiety
– Diaphoresis

• Moderate to severe hypoglycemic symptoms (CNS or neuroglycopenic symptoms)
  – Headache
  – Inability to concentrate
  – Mood changes
  – Drowsiness
  – Irritability
  – Confusion
  – Impaired judgment
  – Slurred speech
  – Staggering gait
  – Double or blurred vision
  – Morning headaches
  – Nightmares
  – Psychosis (late)
  – Seizures
  – Coma

Diagnostic Tests

• Serum blood glucose level for fingerstick glucose less than 60 mg/dL

Principles of Management for Acute Hypoglycemia

The management of the patient with acute hypoglycemia depends on the severity of the reaction. Principles of management include normalization of blood glucose concentrations and patient teaching.

Normalization of Blood Glucose Concentrations

Treatment of the hypoglycemia depends on its severity.

Mild Reaction

1. Administer 10 to 15 g carbohydrate (Table 16–8). Follow in 10 minutes with another 10 to 15 g if the

TABLE 16–8. EXAMPLES OF FOODS WITH 10 TO 15 GRAMS OF CARBOHYDRATE EQUIVALENTS FOR TREATMENT OF MILD HYPOGLYCEMIC REACTIONS

4 oz orange juice
6 oz regular (nondiet) cola
3 glucose tablets
6 to 8 oz 2% fat or skim milk
3 graham cracker squares
6 to 8 Lifesavers
6 jelly beans
2 tbsp raisins
1 small (2-oz) tube of cake icing

condition does not improve.
2. Obtain a blood glucose measurement.
3. If the next meal is more than 2 hours away, provide the patient with a complex carbohydrate (i.e., 4 oz milk).
4. If patient is not alert enough to swallow or unable to do so, inject 1 mg glucagon. If the patient cannot swallow and has a feeding tube, administer a liquid source of glucose (soda).

Moderate and Severe Reactions

1. Administer IV glucose. The initial bolus is 50% dextrose (equivalent of 25 g glucose) followed by a continuous IV infusion until oral replacement is possible.
2. Provide for patient rest.
3. Monitor glucose levels frequently for several hours.

Patient Teaching

The best treatment for hypoglycemia is prevention.

1. Teach the early signs and symptoms of hypoglycemia. Instruct the patient to always carry a source of fast-acting carbohydrate (see Table 16–8).
2. Advise the patient not to skip or delay meals and snacks more than 30 minutes; to limit alcohol to no more than 2 oz hard liquor, 8 oz wine, or 24 oz beer per week; and to never drink on an empty stomach.
3. Evaluate the patient's pattern of blood glucose self-monitoring.
4. Teach the patient and family or friends how to give glucagon for severe reactions.
5. Stress the importance of wearing visible health identification.
6. Assess the patient's exercise pattern.

Syndrome of Inappropriate Antidiuretic Hormone Secretion

Antidiuretic hormone (ADH), also known as arginine vasopressin, is produced by the hypothalamus and is stored in the posterior pituitary gland. In response to changes that occur in the blood osmolality and blood volume, ADH exerts its effect on the kidney, causing concentration of the urine and body water conservation. Syndrome of inappropriate antidiuretic hormone (SIADH) and diabetes insipidus (DI) are the most common disorders that affect ADH secretion in the critically ill.

Etiology, Risk Factors, and Pathophysiology

The SIADH is characterized by excessive release of ADH unrelated to the plasma osmolality, or the concentration of electrolytes and other osmotically active particles. Normal mechanisms that control ADH secretion fail, causing impaired water excretion and profound hyponatremia. SIADH is a syndrome of water intoxication.

There are many causes of SIADH (Table 16–9). Vasopressin can be produced by a variety of malignancies, most commonly oat cell carcinoma of the lung. Therefore, patients who develop "idiopathic" SIADH are screened for malignant tumors. SIADH is also commonly associated with pulmonary diseases or conditions, disorders of the CNS, and drugs, particularly chlorpropamide, thiazide diuretics, narcotics, and barbiturates.

Surgical patients are also at risk because many operative procedures are followed by increased vasopressin secretion, usually during the first 3 to 4 days postoperatively.

Clinically, SIADH is distinguished by hyponatremia and water retention that progresses to water intoxication. The seriousness of the patient's signs and symptoms depends on how low the serum sodium falls and how rapidly the fluid accumulates. As water intoxication progresses and the serum becomes more hypotonic, brain cells swell, causing neurologic problems. Without treatment, irreversible brain damage and death can occur.

Clinical Presentation

Signs and Symptoms

Early

- Urine volume decreased and concentrated
- Nausea
- Vomiting
- Headache
- Impaired taste

TABLE 16–9. ETIOLOGIES OF SIADH (PARTIAL LISTING)

Malignancies
Lung
Lymphoma
Gastrointestinal

Pulmonary Diseases/Conditions
Positive pressure ventilation
Asthma
Pneumonia
Chronic obstructive pulmonary disease
Acute respiratory failure
Tuberculosis

CNS Disorders
Head trauma
Meningitis, encephalitis
Cerebrovascular accidents
Brain tumors
Guillian-Barré syndrome

Drugs
Vasopressin
Desmopressin
Thiazide diuretics
Narcotics
Barbiturates
Nicotine
Antineoplastic drugs
Tricyclic antidepressants

- Dulled sensorium
- Muscle weakness and cramps
- Anorexia
- Weight gain
- Adventitious breath
- Dyspnea sounds
- Increased CVP, PCWP
- Weakness/fatigue

Late

- Confusion
- Hostility
- Aberrant respirations
- Hypothermia
- Coma
- Convulsions

Diagnostic Tests

- Serum Na^+ <130 mEq/L
- Serum osmolality <280 mOsm/kg
- Increased urine osmolality >500 mOsm/kg
- Urine sodium >20 mEq/L
- Blood urea nitrogen and creatinine decreased (hemodilution)

Principles of Management for SIADH

Principles of management depend on the severity and duration of the hyponatremia. Recognition of early clinical manifestations of SIADH is key to prevent life-threatening complications. Continued assessment of neuromuscular, cardiac, gastrointestinal, and renal systems is important. Generally, treatment focuses on restricting fluids, replenishing sodium deficits, and in severe cases of hyponatremia, inhibiting antidiuretic actions. Treatment of the underlying disorder is also a priority.

Fluid Restriction and Treating Hyponatremia

Fluid restriction is the mainstay of treatment and, to be effective, a negative water balance must be achieved.

1. Treatment of mild hyponatremia (sodium level >125 mEq/L) includes fluid restriction of 800 to 1000 mL/d. This allows sodium level to correct over 3 to 10 days. If fluid restriction alone is not effective, demeclocycline (Declomycin) can be administered. Democlocycline allows excretion of water because it inhibits the effect of ADH on the renal tubules.

2. If severe neurologic symptoms of SIADH are present along with severe hyponatremia (<105 mEq/L, administer 3% saline infusion over 2 to 3 hours). Furosemide is also given to increase urinary water excretion.

3. Assess cardiovascular and respiratory functions closely to evaluate the effects of the excess volume on these systems. Right and left ventricular volumes may

increase, causing heart failure. Tachypnea, reports of shortness of breath, and fine crackles are indicators of fluid overload and impending heart failure.

4. Provide for patient comfort with limited fluid intake. Provide for frequent mouth care. Explain why fluid is being restricted and allow the patient to develop the schedule for allotted fluid intake. If the patient complains of nausea, administer an antiemetic prior to meals.

Replenish Sodium Deficits

1. In severe symptomatic hyponatremia, infuse 3% saline at a rate of 0.1 mL/kg per minute for 2 hours to raise plasma sodium. Monitor closely for signs of hypernatremia, fluid overload, and heart failure because this treatment causes a transient increase in the serum sodium.
2. Monitor neurologic status closely and protect the patient from harm. Institute seizure precautions as necessary. Monitor respiratory status closely.

Inhibit Antidiuretic Hormone Actions

In cases where SIADH does not resolve within 1 to 2 weeks, drugs that interfere with the renal effect of vasopressin, such as demeclocycline, may be ordered. The full effect of these drugs are unsuitable for acute management of the syndrome.

Diabetes Insipidus

Etiology, Risk Factors, and Pathophysiology

Diabetes insipidus results from a group of disorders in which there is an absolute or relative deficiency of ADH (called *central DI*) or an insensitivity to its effects on the renal tubules (called *nephrogenic DI*) (Figure 16–3). Diabetes insipidus may complicate the course of the critically ill patient and can result in acute fluid and electrolyte disturbances.

There are many causes of DI (Table 16–10). Neurogenic DI results from damage to the hypothalamic system. An absolute deficiency of ADH results in impaired urine-concentrating ability, polyuria, and a subsequent tendency to dehydration. Patients with head trauma or those who have had neurosurgery must be watched closely for at least 7 to 10 days after the injury for evidence of DI. Nephrogenic DI is characterized by renal tubule insensitivity to ADH and develops because of structural or functional changes in the kidney. This results in an impairment in urine-concentrating ability and free water conservation.

Regardless of the etiology, in DI the ability of the body to increase ADH secretion or respond to ADH is impaired. A persistent output of dilute urine despite increasing hemoconcentration is the hallmark of DI. Signs and symptoms of dehydration are present in those patients in whom the thirst mechanism has been impaired (neurogenic DI) or in whom there is inadequate fluid replacement. In addition, if a hyperosmolar state exists, intracellular brain volume depletion occurs as water moves from within the brain cells to the plasma.

Clinical Presentation

Signs and Symptoms

ADH Deficiency

- Polydipsia (if alert)
- Polyuria (5 to 20 L in 24 hours)

Fluid Volume Deficit

- Orthostatic hypotension
- Weight loss
- Tachycardia
- Decreased CVP, PCWP
- Poor skin turgor

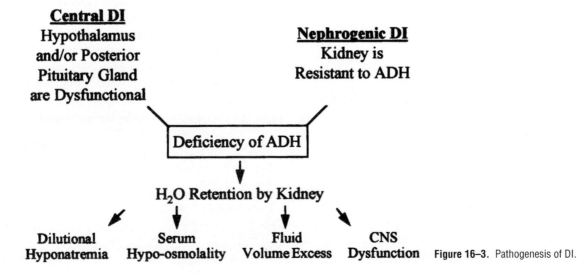

Figure 16–3. Pathogenesis of DI.

TABLE 16–10. CAUSES OF DI

ADH Insufficiency (Neurogenic DI)
Familial (hereditary)
Trauma
Neoplasms
Infections
   Tuberculosis
   Cryptococcosis
   Syphilis
   CNS infections
Vascular
   Cerebrovascular hemorrhage
   Aneurysm (circle of Willis)
   Cerebral thrombosis
ADH Insensitivity (Nephrogenic DI)
Familial (hereditary)
Drug induced
   Lithium
   Demeclocycline
   Glyburide
   Colchicine
   Amphotericin B
   Gentamicin
   Furosemide
Electrolyte disorders
   Hypokalemia
   Hypercalcemia
Renal disease
Excessive Water Intake (Secondary DI)
Excessive IV fluid administration
Psychogenic polydipsia (lesion in thirst center)

- Dry mucous membranes

Intracellular Brain Volume Depletion

- Confusion
- Restlessness
- Lethargy
- Irritability
- Seizures
- Coma

Diagnostic Tests

- Serum sodium >145 mEq/L
- Serum osmolality >295 mOsm/kg/H_2O
- Urine osmolality inappropriately low with high serum osmolality
- Urine specific gravity decreased
- BUN and creatinine increased (hemoconcentration)

Principles of Management for Diabetes Insipidus

The management of the patient in DI is directed at correcting the profound fluid volume deficit and electrolyte imbalances associated with this condition. If fluid losses are not replaced, hypovolemic shock can rapidly develop (see Chapter 9, Cardiovascular System). In some cases of DI, vaso-pressin or agents that simulate ADH release and renal response to ADH are prescribed to treat the disorder. As with other disorders, location and treatment of the cause of DI are priorities.

Fluid Volume Replacement

If the patient is alert and the thirst mechanism is not impaired, allow the patient to drink water to maintain normal serum osmolality. In many critically ill patients, this is not possible.

1. Administer dextrose in water IV as prescribed to restore fluid volume. The administration of normal saline to replace volume is usually contraindicated because it presents an added renal load, promoting osmotic diuresis and worsening dehydration. In severe DI, where large amounts of fluid replacement are required, the IV intake is usually titrated to urine output. For example, 400 mL of urine output for 1 hour is replaced with 400 mL IV fluid the next hour. Hypotonic saline solutions are usually used (quarter-strength or half-strength saline) because the solutions are hypotonic.
2. Monitor fluid status: intake and output, daily weight, and urine specific gravity. Monitor for signs of continuing fluid volume deficit. Expected outcomes for the patient with DI are listed in Table 16–11.
3. Monitor neurologic status continuously. An altered level of consciousness indicates intracellular dehydration and hypovolemia.

Vasopressin Administration

Exogenous vasopressin (Pitressin), which replaces the absent or reduced ADH may be used to restore normal serum ADH levels. Carbamazepine or chlorpropamide may be used to enhance the release of ADH and increase the renal response to ADH.

1. Administer 5 to 10 units Pitressin subcutaneously or IM. Major side effects to watch for include headache, abdominal cramps, vasoconstrictive effects, or allergic reactions. Monitor for overmedication, which may precipitate hypervolemia. Signs and symptoms of fluid volume excess include dyspnea, hypertension, weight gain, and angina.
2. For central DI, administer vasopressin and carba-

TABLE 16–11. EXPECTED OUTCOMES FOR THE PATIENT WITH DI

Adequate fluid balance is maintained/restored as evidenced by:
   Blood pressure within 10 mm Hg of patient baseline
   Heart rate 60–100 beats/min
   Normal skin turgor
   Peripheral pulses return to baseline
   CVP and PCWP within patient norms
   Serum osmolality 275–295 mOsm/kg
   Serum sodium 135–145 mEq/L
   Urine osmolality appropriate for serum osmolality

AT THE BEDSIDE
► *Thinking Critically*

You are caring for a patient in acute DKA with the following interventions and laboratory results:

- 0.9 NS with 20 mEq KCl at 150 mL/h
- Insulin (regular) drip at 20 units/h
- Oxygen 6 L/min by nasal cannula
- Arterial blood gases

pH	7.16
PaCO$_2$	24 mm Hg
PaO$_2$	59 mm Hg
SaO$_2$	89%
HCO$_3$$^-$	14 mEq/L

Which intervention is most important in correcting the acidosis in this case? Why isn't sodium bicarbonate ordered to correct the acidosis?

mazepine as prescribed and monitor for fluid overload.
3. For nephrogenic DI, administer chlorpropamide. Because of this agent's antidiabetic properties, monitor for hypoglycemia.

SELECTED BIBLIOGRAPHY

Blood Glucose Monitoring

American College of Endocrinology. Position Statement on Inpatient Diabetes and Metabolic Control. *Endocrine Prac* 2004; 10:78–82.

Cefalu W, Weir G. New technologies in diabetes care. *Patient Care Nurse Practition* 2003:1–11.

Heinemann L, Koschinsky T. Continuous glucose monitoring: an overview of today's technologies and their clinical applications. *Int J Clin Pract Suppl* 2002;129:75–79.

Meldrum M. Home blood glucose monitoring: A guide for nurses and pharmacists. *J Diabetes Nurs* 2003;7(4):125–7.

Vineze G, Barner J, Lopez D. Factors associated with adherence to self-monitoring of blood glucose among persons with diabetes. *Diabetes Ed* 2004;30(1):112–125.

DKA and HHS

Chiasson JL, Aris-Jilwan N, Belanger, R et al. Diagnosis and treatment of diabetic ketoacidosis and the hyperglycemic hyperosmolar states. *CMAJ Can Med Assoc J* 2003;168:859–866.

Deepak PJ, Sunitha K, Nagarj J, et al. Inpatient management of diabetes: Survey in a tertiary care centre. *Postgrad Med J* 2003: 79:585–587.

Fillbin MR, Brown DF, Nadel ES. Hyperglycemic hyperosmolar nonketotic coma. *J Emerg Med* 2001;20:285–290.

Freeland B. Diabetic ketoacidosis. *Today's Educator* 2003;29:385–395.

Magee MF, Bhatt BA. Management of decompensated diabetes. Diabetic ketoacidosis and hyperglycemic hyperosmolar syndrome. *Crit Care Clin* 2001;17:75–106.

Quinn L. Diabetic emergencies in patient with type 2 diabetes. *Nurs Clin North Am* 2001;36:341–360.

Quinn L. Pharmacologic treatment of the critically ill patient with diabetes. *Crit Care Nurs Clin North Am* 2002;14:81–98.

Hypoglycemia

Cryer PE, Davis SN, Shamoon H. Hypoglycemia in diabetes. *Diabetes Care* 2003;26:1902–1912.

Kerr D, Everett JD. Assessment of reduced awareness of hypoglycaemia. *J Diabetes Nurs* 2003;7:130–133.

Sammer CE. How should you respond to hypoglycemia. *Nursing* 2001;31(7):48–50.

Watts SA, Anselmo JM, Smith MA. Combating hypoglycemia in the hospital and at home: Learn how to handle the crisis and what to teach your patient to manage the problem after discharge. *Nursing* 2003;33(3):1–5.

Disorders of Antidiuretic Hormone Secretion (SIADH and DI)

Flounders J. Syndrome of inappropriate antidiuretic hormone. *Online exclusive: Cont Ed* 2003;30(3):E63–68.

Holcomb SS. Diabetes insipidus. *Dimen Crit Care Nurs* 2002; 21(3):94–97.

Miller M. Syndromes of excess antidiuretic hormone release. *Crit Care Clin* 2001;17:11–21.

Moore K, Thompson C, Trainer P. Disorders of water balance. *Clin Med* 2003;3:28–33.

Seventeen

Trauma

17

Carol A. Rauen and Jamie B. Sinks

▶ Knowledge Competencies

1. Describe the mechanisms of traumatic injury and relate them to accurate assessment of obvious and subtle injuries.

2. Discuss the common physiologic and psychosocial effects on the patient and family because of major traumatic injury.

3. Identify the unique needs of the trauma patient in the critical care unit.

4. Apply selected management principles to treat trauma patients with thoracic, abdominal, and musculoskeletal injuries.

SPECIALIZED ASSESSMENT TECHNIQUES, DIAGNOSTIC TESTS, AND MONITORING SYSTEMS

Trauma is an increasing health care problem in the United States. The cost of treating trauma exceeds $400 billion annually. For Americans between the ages of 1 and 44, trauma is the leading cause of death, surpassing cancer and atherosclerosis. Although the death rate is high for this patient population, the disability rate is even greater. This chapter focuses on thoracic, abdominal, musculoskeletal, and pelvic trauma. Although traumatic brain injury and spinal cord injury account for approximately 50% of all trauma deaths, these topics are covered in Chapter 21, Advanced Neurologic Concepts.

Critically ill trauma patients are unlike other hospitalized patients and require specialized assessment and monitoring. For the trauma victim, admission to the critical care setting is sudden and unplanned, with no time for psychological preparation or the stabilization of chronic conditions. Trauma patients are often young; however, trauma among the elderly is an increasing problem because of the population's longer life span. Traumatic injuries may be subtle, and complications are common (Table 17–1). Alcohol or drug abuse plays a major role in the cause of the trauma and subsequent treatment. Rehabilitation is often needed after injury, and a trauma victim's quality of life may never return to preinjury status. This is especially true for traumatic brain and spinal cord injuries; however, even in lower extremity trauma, it may take a full year for an individual to return to work. Trauma takes a significant emotional and financial toll on the patient, family, and society.

Management of traumatic injury in the initial phases of care occurs in tandem with assessment. For example, the control and insertion of an airway, the administration of fluids, and pain medication may all be provided before the site of bleeding is identified and controlled. One of the most important aspects of assessing the traumatically injured patient is to determine the mechanism of injury, whether blunt or penetrating trauma. Based on this information, an "index of suspicion" regarding specific injuries is developed to ensure that no injuries are overlooked and a trauma patient plan of care is developed.

Primary and Secondary Trauma Survey Assessment

The life-threatening nature of trauma requires a reorganization of the traditional assessment priorities (Tables 17–2 and 17–3). The primary and secondary surveys reveal immediate

TABLE 17–1. MAJOR COMPLICATIONS IN TRAUMA

Complication	Associated Conditions	What to Look for	Nursing Interventions
Hypovolemia	Internal hemorrhage Multiple-system injuries Fractures of major bones Coagulopathies	Decreased blood pressure Tachycardia, tachypnea Cool, clammy skin Pallor Decreased urine output Frank hemorrhage Anxiety Obtunded sensorium	Notify physician immediately Type and cross-match patient's blood Check amount of blood on hand in blood bank Administer transfusion as ordered Elevate patient's legs while patient is supine, with head elevated as necessary to facilitate respiration Administer medications as ordered Monitor vital signs every 15 min
Sepsis	Systemic infection Peritonitis	Increased WBCs Increased or decreased temperature Tachycardia Sudden hypotension Increased serum glucose Decreased platelets, decreased Pao_2 Confusion/disorientation Diaphoresis/flushed face	Monitor ABGs Notify physician Monitor vital signs every 15 min Administer fluid replacement and medications as ordered Monitor ABGs, electrolytes, and CBC Maintain normothermia
Neurogenic shock	Spinal cord injury	Hypotension Hypothermia with absence of sweating below injury level Flaccid paralysis below injury level Bradycardia	Notify physician Administer medications and IV fluids as ordered Monitor vital signs every 15 min Insert Foley catheter and nasogastric tube as ordered
Pulmonary embolism	Immobility Fracture of the long bones, pelvis, or ribs Improper handling of fractures before and during admission	Chest pain Shortness of breath Sudden disorientation Petechiae over axillae and chest (fat) Decreased Pao_2 Tachycardia	Notify physician Assist with transport to lung scan Monitor ECG Administer O_2 Draw ABGs STAT and serially Assist ventilation as ordered
ARDS	Chest trauma Sepsis Multiple transfusions Brain injuries Multiple-system injuries	Decreased $Paco_2$, decreased Pao_2 Decreased lung compliance Decreased tidal volume Increased airway pressures Increased WBC	Assess chest, monitor lung volumes and compliance Draw serial ABGs Administer O_2 or ventilator therapy as ordered Suction as needed Administer medications as ordered Monitor ECG
Pneumonia	Blunt chest trauma Immobility Atelectasis Endotracheal intubation	Increased temperature Increased WBC Decreased breath sounds Rales, some bronchi on auscultation Radiologic changes Positive sputum cultures	Assess chest Use sterile suction technique and chest physiotherapy for pulmonary hygiene as needed Supplemental O_2 as needed Serial chest x-rays as ordered
Wound dehiscence	Abdominal surgery Wound infection Poor nutritional status	Pink serous wound exudate Poor wound edge approximation	Notify physician Have sterile saline and dressings on hand Prevent/correct abdominal distention
Gastrointestinal fistula	Penetrating abdominal trauma Sepsis	Bile, fecal, or pancreatic drainage from wounds or drain sites	Monitor amount, odor, and color of drainage Meticulous skin care around drainage sites Perform dressing changes as necessary
Stress ulcers	Multiple-system trauma Patient kept NPO for prolonged periods Head injury Sepsis Continuous mechanical ventilation Prolonged ICU stay	NG aspirate hemopositive Decreased pH of NG aspirate Stools hemopositive Decreased hematocrit Malena	Administer medications as ordered Chilled saline lavage until clear Administer transfusions, medications, and fluid replacement as ordered
Pneumothorax (simple)	Mechanical ventilation	Decreased or absent breath sounds Radiologic evidence Decreased Pao_2, cyanosis Unequal chest expansion Hyperresonance over affected area	Notify physician Administer supplemental O_2 Assist with chest tube insertion or thoracentesis

Complication	Etiology	Signs and Symptoms	Interventions
Pneumothorax (tension)	PEEP; Improper CVP line placement	Decreased Pao₂, cyanosis; Decreased tidal volume, unequal chest expansion; Decreased lung compliance; Breath sounds absent; Tracheal deviation; Increased airway pressures; Restlessness; Hyperresonance over affected area; Hemodynamic instability	Notify physician STAT; Insert 18-gauge needle into 2nd intercostal space laterally if certified; Assist with chest tube insertion; If chest tubes in place, check for patency and suction; Monitor vital signs every 15 min
Renal failure	Prolonged hypotension; Sepsis; Ruptured aorta; Toxic drug reaction; ARDS	Increased serum BUN and creatinine; Decreased urine output, decreased specific gravity; Increased serum potassium; Increased confusion; Uremic frost	Record hourly intake and output; Foley catheter care daily; Monitor tab values; Administer hemodialysis or peritoneal dialysis as ordered; Daily weights
Bronchoesophageal fistula	Prolonged tracheostomy; Overinflation of cuff balloon; Prolonged need for NG tube	Gastric contents suctioned through tracheostomy; Radiologic confirmation; Respiratory distress	Maintain NPO; Maintain proper positioning of endotracheal tube to maintain ventilation; Administer feedings as ordered via gastrostomy or jejunostomy
Diabetes insipidus	Brain injuries	Increased urine output; Decreased urine specific gravity; Decreased urine osmolality; Severe thirst	Record hourly intake and output, check urine specific gravity every 4 hours; Maintain fluid balance; Replace urine output as ordered; Administer Pitressin as ordered
Ruptured innominate artery	Tracheostomy; Tracheal tube too long; Inadvertent traction on tracheal tube when moving patient; Prolonged overinflation of tracheal tube cuff	Visible pulsation of trachea; Frank bleeding from trachea	Elevate tracheal flange with 4 × 4's if arterial pulsations present; If rupture occurs, slide finger down outside of outer cannula and attempt to tamponade innominate artery against clavicle
Atelectasis	Immobility; Prolonged anesthesia; Blunt chest trauma; Pain; Endotracheal intubation	Radiologic changes; Decreased Pao₂; Inability to cough; Decreased breath sounds	Provide pulmonary hygiene and chest physiotherapy; Turn and position every 1-2 hours; Kinetic therapy; Encourage coughing and deep breathing; Draw serial ABGs; Administer O₂ as needed; Incentive spirometer
Empyema	Blunt chest trauma; Pneumonia; Prolonged atelectasis; Pleural effusion; Open chest wound	Purulent chest drainage; Increased temperature; Increased WBC; Generalized malaise; Radiologic confirmation; Sepsis	Monitor amount and consistency of chest tube drainage as ordered; Culture chest tube drainage as ordered; Maintain chest tube patency; Provide pulmonary hygiene and chest physiotherapy
Aspiration	Unconscious patients; Spinal cord injury; Sudden vomiting; Malfunctioning NG tube; Decreased gag reflex; Prolonged endotracheal intubation	Suctioning of gastric contents from tracheal tube or ET tube; Radiologic confirmation; Increased temperature and WBCs; Decreased Pao₂	Notify physician immediately; Take chest x-ray STAT; Turn patient to side or suction if vomits; Elevate head of bed when giving tube feedings
Meningitis	Brain injury; Skull fracture; Maxillofacial trauma; Intraventricular catheter placement	Increased temperature; Increased WBC; Positive spinal fluid cultures; Changes in neurological status	Administer medications as ordered; Monitor every hour; Do neurologic checks every hour; Assist with spinal tap; Draw serial WBCs
Sensory deprivation/ICU psychosis	Prolonged stay in ICU; Sleep deprivation	Confusion; Disorientation; Hallucinations; Restlessness; Combativeness	Arrange for psychiatric consult if necessary; Provide quiet environment; Plan nursing care in blocks of time to promote sleep; Administer medications as ordered; Use consistent approach to orient to reality

From: Cardona VD, Hurn PD, Mason PJB, Scanlon AM, Veise-Berry SW (eds): Trauma nursing from resuscitation through rehabilitation, pp. 840–841, Philadelphia: WB Saunders; 1994.

TABLE 17–2. PRIMARY SURVEY AND RESUSCITATION

Airway with cervical spinal protection	Assessment • Ascertain patency • Rapidly assess for airway obstruction Management—Establish a patent airway • Perform a chin lift or jaw thrust maneuver • Clear the airway of foreign bodies • Insert an oropharyngeal or nasopharyngeal airway • Establish a definitive airway Maintain the cervical spine in a neutral position with manual immobilization as necessary when establishing an airway Reinstate immobilization of the C-spine with appropriate devices after establishing an airway
Breathing: Ventilation and oxygenation	Assessment • Expose the neck and chest: Ensure immobilization of the head and neck • Determine the rate and depth of respirations • Inspect and palpate the neck and chest for tracheal deviation, unilateral and bilateral chest movement, use of accessory muscles, and any signs of injury • Percuss the chest for presence of dullness or hyperresonance • Auscultate the chest bilaterally Management • Administer high concentrations of oxygen • Ventilate with a bag–valve–mask device • Alleviate tension pneumothorax • Seal open pneumothorax • Attach a CO_2 monitoring device to the endotracheal tube • Attach the patient to a pulse oximeter
Circulation and hemorrhage control	Assessment • Identify source of external, exsanguinating hemorrhage • Identify potential source(s) of internal hemorrhage • Pulse: Quality, rate, regularity, paradox • Skin color • Blood pressure, time permitting Management • Apply direct pressure to external bleeding site • Consider presence of internal hemorrhage and potential need for operative intervention, and obtain surgical consult • Insert two large-caliber IV catheters • Simultaneously obtain blood for hematologic and chemical analyses, pregnancy test, type and cross-match, and arterial blood gases • Initiate IV fluid therapy with warmed Ringer's lactate solution and blood replacement • Apply the pneumatic antishock garment or pneumatic splints as indicated to control hemorrhage • Prevent hypothermia
Disability: brief neurologic examination	• Determine the level of consciousness • Assess the pupils for size, equality, and reaction
Exposure/environment	• Completely undress the patient, but prevent hypothermia

Modified with permission from American College of Surgeons' Committee on Trauma: Advanced Trauma Life Support® for Doctors (ATLS®) Student Manual, 6th ed, pp. 51–53. Chicago: American College of Surgeons; 1997.

life-threatening injuries and direct the trauma team toward an individualized resuscitation. This approach ensures that common causes of tissue injury are rapidly identified so appropriate therapeutic interventions can begin. If the patient's status changes at any time during the secondary survey the practitioner must return to the primary survey to again review airway, breathing, circulation, disability, and environment/exposure to determine if there has been any decompensation.

Diagnostic Studies

Diagnostic Peritoneal Lavage, Ultrasound, and Computed Axial Tomography

Hemorrhage is of major concern during the primary survey of the trauma patient. Both external and occult bleeding must be considered. Secondary survey diagnostic studies may include diagnostic peritoneal lavage (DPL), ultrasound, and computed axial tomography to diagnose occult hemorrhage.

TABLE 17–3. SECONDARY SURVEY

Item to Assess	Establishes/Identifies	Assess	Finding	Confirm By
Level of consciousness	• Severity of head injury	• GCS score	• ≤8, severe head injury • 9–12, moderate head injury • 13–15, minor head injury	• CT scan • Repeat without paralyzing agents
Pupils	• Type of head injury • Presence of eye injury	• Size • Shape • Reactivity	• Mass effect • Diffuse axonal injury • Ophthalmic injury	• CT scan
Head	• Scalp injury • Skull injury	• Inspect for lacerations and skull fractures • Palpable defects	• Scalp laceration • Depressed skull fracture • Basilar skull fracture	• CT scan
Maxillofacial	• Soft-tissue injury • Bone injury • Nerve injury • Teeth/mouth injury	• Visual deformity • Malocclusion • Palpation for crepitus	• Facial fracture • Soft-tissue injury bones	• Facial bone x-ray • CT scan or facial bones
Neck	• Laryngeal injury • C-spine injury • Vascular injury • Esophageal injury • Neurologic deficit	• Visual inspection • Palpation • Auscultation	• Laryngeal deformity • Subq emphysema • Hematoma • Bruit • Platysmal penetration • Pain, tenderness of C-spine	• C-spine x-ray • Angiography/duplex exam • Esophagoscopy • Laryngoscopy
Thorax	• Thoracic wall injury • Subq emphysema • Pneumo/hemothorax • Bronchial injury • Pulmonary contusion • Thoracic aortic disruption	• Visual inspection • Palpation • Auscultation	• Bruising, deformity, or paradoxical motion • Chest wall tenderness, crepitus • Diminished breath sounds • Muffled heart tones • Mediastinal crepitus • Severe back pain	• Chest x-ray • CT scan • Angiography • Bronchoscopy • Tube thoracostomy • Pericardiocentesis • TE ultrasound

Abdomen/flank	• Abdominal wall injury
	• Intraperitoneal injury
	• Retroperitoneal injury
		• Visual inspection
		• Palpation
		• Auscultation
		• Determine path of penetration
			• Abdominal wall pain/tenderness
			• Peritoneal irritation
			  • Visceral injury
			  • Retroperitoneal organ injury
				• DPL/ultrasound
				• CT scan
				• Celiotomy
				• Contrast GI x-ray studies
				• Angiography

Pelvis	• GU tract injuries
	• Pelvic fracture(s)
		• Palpate symphysis pubis for widening
		• Palpate bony pelvis for tenderness
		• Determine pelvic stability only once
		• Inspect perineum
		• Rectal/vaginal exam
			• GU tract injury (hematuria)
			• Pelvic fracture
			• Rectal, vaginal, perineal injury
				• Pelvic x-ray
				• GU contrast studies
				  • Urethrogram
				  • Cystogram
				  • IVP
				  • Contrast-enhanced CT

Spinal cord	• Cranial injury • Cord injury • Peripheral nerve(s) injury	• Motor response • Pain response	• Unilateral cranial mass effect • Quadriplegia • Paraplegia • Nerve root injury	• Plain spine x-rays • MRI
Vertebral column	• Column injury • Vertebral instability • Nerve injury	• Verbal response to pain, lateralizing signs • Palpate for tenderness • Deformity	• Fracture vs. dislocation	• Plain x-rays • CT scan
Extremities	• Soft-tissue injury • Bony deformities • Joint abnormalities • Neurovascular deficits	• Visual inspection • Palpation	• Swelling, bruising, pallor • Malalignment • Pain, tenderness, crepitus • Absence/diminished pulses • Tense muscular compartments • Neurologic deficits	• Specific x-rays • Doppler examination • Compartment pressures • Angiography

DPL is performed to detect free blood in the peritoneal cavity. The physician instills and then removes sterile fluid into the patient's peritoneal cavity. If the fluid is blood tinged on removal, the test is considered to be positive and may indicate the need for emergency exploratory surgery. The test is especially important in the blunt, multiple trauma patient who is unconscious or unable to verbalize abdominal pain on palpation.

Under local anesthetic, a lavage catheter is percutaneously placed into the abdomen. If no blood or fluid is aspirated, a liter of normal saline solution is instilled and then drained. Bloody return or drainage with red blood cells greater than 100,000 cells/mm^3 demonstrates a positive DPL. However, retroperitoneal injuries, such as pancreatic injury, do show up as positive with a lavage, so vigilant observation of abdominal expansion is required by the nurse.

Ultrasound is used increasingly to diagnose hemorrhage in the trauma patient. This noninvasive technique may quickly show injury in the hemodynamically unstable patient. However, the usefulness of ultrasound depends on the experience of the person performing the study; a DPL may have to be performed for confirmation of hemoperitoneum that was observed by ultrasound.

Computed axial tomography (CAT) is a good alternative to DPL in the stable trauma patient. CAT scanning continues to be the gold standard for diagnosis of injury if the patient is hemodynamically stable. For a comparison of DPL, ultrasound, and CAT, refer to Table 17–4.

Cervical Spine Radiograph

A cervical spine (C-spine) x-ray is one of the first priorities of assessment after the primary survey. All trauma patients are presumed to have a C-spine injury until all seven cervical vertebrae have been cleared or visualized as intact on x-ray. A cervical collar to immobilize the neck is applied until the C-spine has been visualized and no injuries are found.

Radiographic Studies

Radiographic studies are performed after the primary survey. These studies should not delay resuscitation, but may be essential in determining the extent of injury. Depending on the mechanism of injury, common x-rays may include chest, pelvis, and musculoskeletal studies.

Serial Examinations

Trauma patients require frequent reexamination to ensure that all injuries are identified and that the patient's status is not deteriorating. Missed injuries may lead to pain, disability, and increased mortality for the patient. Examples of trauma where repeated assessments by the same provider are recommended include traumatic brain injury and abdominal injuries. Intercranial or occult abdominal bleeding may not be evident initially. Having a high degree of suspicion for traumatic injuries comes from knowledge of mechanism of injury and the specific injuries created by destructive blunt or penetrating forces.

Mechanism of Injury

The principles of mechanism of injury help the trauma team to "make sense" of the injuries sustained by the patient. How an injury occurred, the nature of the forces involved, and suspected tissue and organ damage are all important aspects of mechanism of injury. This knowledge is required when assessing a trauma patient at the scene and in the emergency department, as well as in the critical care unit. Knowing this information helps anticipate potential complications.

Injuries result when a body is exposed to an uncontrolled outside source of energy that disrupts the body's integrity or functional ability. This energy can come from a variety of sources, and can be kinetic, penetrating, chemical, thermal, electrical, or radiating energy. The severity of the resultant injury is determined by several factors: the force or speed of impact, the length of the impact or exposure, the total surface area exposed, and related risk factors such as age, gender, preinjury health, and alcohol/drug ingestion.

Mechanisms of injury are typically divided into two major categories: blunt and penetrating. *Blunt trauma* is defined as injuries without communication with the environment and *penetrating* as injuries where the tissue has been pierced. Blunt trauma usually results from motor vehicle or motorcycle collisions, assaults, falls, contact sports injuries, pedestrian/vehicle collisions, or blast injuries. Assessment strategies useful in diagnosing blunt traumatic injuries include physical assessment, ultrasound, DPL, CT scanning, radiographic studies angiography, and blood count, and blood chemistry analysis. Penetrating trauma is commonly caused

TABLE 17–4. DPL VERSUS ULTRASOUND VERSUS COMPUTED TOMOGRAPHY IN BLUNT ABDOMINAL TRAUMA

	DPL	Ultrasound	CT Scan
Indication	Document bleeding if decreased BP	Document fluid if decreased BP	Document organ injury if BP normal
Advantages	Early diagnosis and sensitive; 98% accurate	Early diagnosis; noninvasive and repeatable; 86–97% accurate	Most specific for injury, 92–98% accurate
Disadvantages	Invasive; misses injury to diaphragm or retroperitoneum	Operator dependent; bowel gas and subcutaneous air distortion, misses diaphragm, bowel, and some pancreatic injuries	Cost and time; misses diaphragm, bowel tract, and some pancreatic injuries

Reproduced with permission from American College of Surgeons' Committee on Trauma: Advanced Trauma Life Support ® for Doctors (ATLS ®) Student Manual, *6th ed, p. 166. Chicago: American College of Surgeons; 1997.*

by bullets or knives in urban areas and by farm or industrial equipment in rural areas.

Knowledge of mechanism of injury provides clinicians with information to determine patterns of injury. These common patterns are helpful when assessing trauma patients who cannot speak to indicate areas of pain. Patterns of injury offer the trauma team an index of suspicion and direction to focus the primary and secondary surveys. Such injury patterns help determine which tests and the sequence of the diagnostic tests needed to identify each of the patient's injuries. For example, in motor vehicle crashes, the common pattern of injury for the unrestrained driver include head, pelvis, chest, and musculoskeletal areas (e.g., hip, ankle, and foot trauma) (Figure 17–1A). Thoracic trauma is often due to impact with a steering wheel. Other patterns of injuries to unrestrained passengers demonstrate an increased incidence of craniofacial trauma resulting from hitting the head on the windshield (Figure 17–1B). Fractures of the clavicle and humerus are more frequent among passengers, possibly due to the defensive reflex action of raising the arms prior to impact. Similar patterns of injury have been identified for victims of falls and pedestrians struck by motor vehicles (Figure 17–2). Knowledge of these patterns of injuries also helps to prevent further damage or complications during the resuscitation efforts. For example, if a patient has sustained a head injury with a high suspicion of basilar skull fracture, a nasogastric tube should not be inserted because it could be passed through the fracture directly into the brain. A Foley catheter should not be inserted if the mechanism of injury suggests bladder rupture or trauma.

Physiologic Consequences of Trauma

Traumatic injury unleashes a cascade of vasoactive mediators, such as various hormones, prostaglandins, and cytokines that serve a protective function through the stress response. However, in severe multisystem trauma, these same mediators that help the trauma patient survive the initial injury may prolong the stress response and contribute to complications and even death. This response is best limited by enhancing the patient's healing ability through attention to physiologic and psychosocial care. Priorities include supporting tissue oxygenation through hemodynamic monitoring and ventilatory support. The trauma patient undergoes continuous vital sign monitoring, including pulse oximetry. Pain and anxiety are treated at the same time as injuries are assessed.

Traumatic injury creates fractures, wounds, and crushed tissues that may not be readily visible. Once the ABCs or primary trauma survey has been completed and management begins, the head-to-toe in-depth assessment, known as the *secondary survey,* is initiated. In secondary survey, evidence is accumulated for the detailed diagnosis of multiple trauma and definitive care is planned. A high index of suspicion is needed to link patterns of trauma, mechanism of

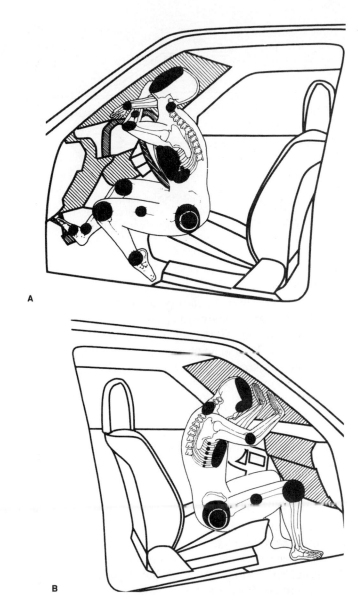

A

B

Figure 17–1. Major areas of impact injuries (solid dark areas). The "hostile" contact areas are striped (windshield, steering column, dashboard, and foot pedals). **(A)** Unrestrained drivers. **(B)** Unrestrained front seat passengers. (*From: Daffner R, Deeb Z, Lupetin A, Rothfus W: Patterns of high speed impact injuries in motor vehicle occupants.* J Trauma *1988;28:499–500.*)

injury, and physiologic consequences to the traumatic injuries. The critical care nurse assists in stabilizing the patient with fluids, ventilatory and circulatory support, while also providing emotional support during diagnostic tests. Many times the nurse is responsible for addressing pain control for the patient and the psychosocial needs of the patient and family.

Consequences of traumatic injury include blood loss, tissue destruction, intense pain due to damaged tissues, and altered oxygenation and ventilation. Fluid balance, airway management, aggressive pain control, and wound care are priorities. Stabilization of fractures and surgical repair of in-

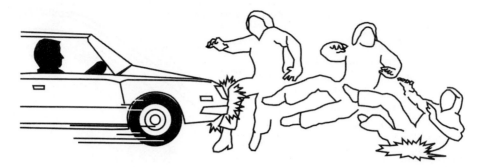

Figure 17–2. Waddell's triad in adult pedestrians. Impact (1) with the bumper or hood and lateral rotation (2) produce injury to the upper and/or lower leg (3). (*Reprinted with permission from Weigelt J, Klein J: Mechanism of injury. In McQuillan K, VonReuden K, Hartsock, et al.* [*eds.*]: Trauma Nursing from Resuscitation Through Rehabilitation, *3rd ed., p. 94. St. Louis, MO: Mosby; 2002.*)

jured organs are accomplished in the early operative period. The priority for care in the early phases of trauma is to optimize tissue oxygenation (see Chapter 19, Advanced Cardiovascular Concepts). Although patients in critical care settings frequently have more than one injured system, a focus on one body system at a time assists in providing an organized management plan.

COMMON INJURIES IN THE CRITICALLY ILL TRAUMA PATIENT

Thoracic Trauma

Etiology and Pathophysiology

Thoracic trauma accounts for approximately 25% of all trauma-related deaths and may include injuries created by fractured ribs, blunt cardiac injury, vascular injury, and contused or punctured lung tissue. Common mechanisms of injury include a motor vehicle crash where the torso is crushed between the steering wheel and the front seat, especially in the unbelted driver, or a gun shot or stabbing wound to the chest. Common injuries associated with thoracic trauma include tension pneumothorax, hemothorax, open pneumothorax, pulmonary contusion, rib fractures/flail chest, cardiac tamponade, or aortic disruption (Figure 17–3).

Injury to the lung parenchyma may cause a tension pneumothorax, which may result in hemodynamic collapse and is therefore a medical emergency. Air collects under positive pressure in the pleural space, collapses the lung, and shifts the heart and great vessels to the opposite side of the chest from the injury causing hemodynamic collapse. Management consists of early detection of the tension pneumothorax and insertion of a chest tube. In emergent situations, if a chest tube insertion is not an option, a needle can be inserted to the chest wall at the midclavicular line, second intercostal space to relieve the pressure and tension.

A *hemothorax* is defined as blood in the pleural space. Fractures to the first and second ribs are considered most serious. If these ribs are broken, one can assume significant force was sustained in the traumatic event, therefore damage to the underlying vessels is possible. An initial chest x-ray demonstrating a widened mediastinum often confirms this suspicion of hemothorax. If the hemothorax is large enough and the patient is experiencing respiratory difficulty, a chest tube is placed to drain the hemothorax. If the patient is hemodynamically unstable, the physician may need to perform an open thoracotomy to control the bleeding.

An *open pneumothorax* is present when there is passage of air in and out of the pleural space. This usually occurs when there is a penetrating injury to the chest wall by either a gunshot or stab wound. A dressing may be applied to the open sucking chest wound with careful attention to taping only three sides of the dressing. If the dressing is made occlusive, a tension pneumothorax may occur. The patient needs a chest tube placed in the affected side.

Pulmonary contusion is injury to the lung parenchyma, which commonly occurs after blunt injury to the chest. A pulmonary contusion may lead to alveolar capillary membrane disruption. Depending on the severity of the contusion, hypoxemia occurs, which may worsen several days after the injury, progressing to respiratory failure and acute respiratory distress syndrome (ARDS). Pulmonary contusions can easily be missed during the initial trauma resuscitation because clinical findings may not occur until several hours after the injury. This injury is an example of when an index of suspicion and knowing the mechanism of injury assists the critical care nurse to anticipate pulmonary complications such as hypoxemia progressing to respiratory failure and ARDS.

Fractured ribs are also common in blunt trauma. Fractured lower ribs can damage the liver or spleen, and upper rib fractures may puncture lung tissue. All patients with rib fractures are suspected of having a pulmonary contusion. A *flail chest* may occur when three or more adjacent ribs are fractured in two segments, creating a "floating segment" that

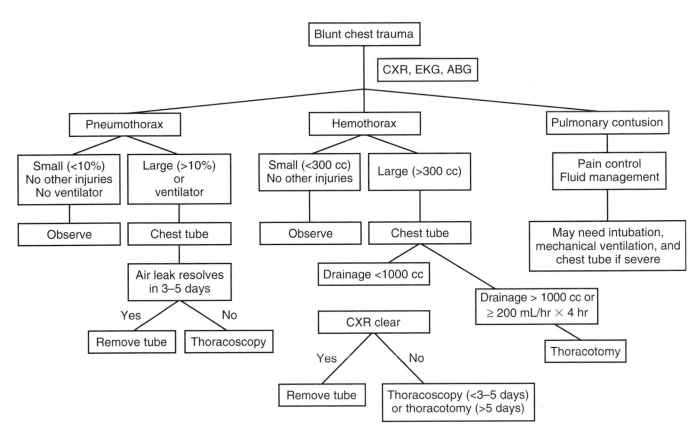

Figure 17–3. Algorithm: therapeutic approach to the patient with blunt chest trauma. (*From Mattox K, Feliciano D, Moore F [eds.]*: Trauma, *4th ed, p. 525. New York: McGraw Hill; 2000.*)

may puncture the lung and compromise effective ventilation efforts. Diagnosis of a flail chest is made by observing inward movement of the chest during inspiration and outward movement during expiration. This injury is best assessed when the patient is breathing spontaneously. The paradoxical motion of the chest wall creates hypoxemia from a decreased tidal volume and atelectasis. Because patients are unable to take a deep breath without pain, pneumonia and respiratory failure may ensue.

Blunt cardiac injury results from damage to the myocardium without involving the coronary arteries and may occur with blunt chest trauma. Diagnosis is based on ECG changes suggestive of ischemia, elevation of troponin levels, and by the use of echocardiography. These tests do not always demonstrate changes, but blunt cardiac injury should be anticipated in major trauma to the chest. Arrhythmias such as sinus tachycardia, atrial fibrillation, and premature ventricular contractions are the chief concern in blunt cardiac injury in the first 12 hours after injury.

Cardiac tamponade is a life-threatening complication of penetrating chest injury but may also occur with blunt chest trauma. Bleeding into the pericardial sac causes compression on the heart, which then compromises cardiac function. The pericardial sac is stiff and noncompliant. The rate at which fluid accumulates around the heart in the pericardial

one determines if the patient is able to compensate for the increase in pressure around the heart. A rapid accumulation of blood does not allow the pericardial sac to stretch and the tamponade may lead to cardiogenic shock.

Traumatic aortic disruption is a surgical emergency and a common cause of death in the thoracic trauma patient. A clinician with a high index of suspicion and knowledge of mechanism of injury, such as a high-speed motor vehicle crash, can help these patients survive. A widened mediastinum may be seen on chest x-ray but angiography is considered the gold standard for detecting this injury.

Principles of Management for Thoracic Trauma
Management of the patient with trauma to the chest must be individualized to the patient and includes four basic principles: ventilatory support to prevent hypoxemia, monitoring chest tubes for drainage, providing optimal pain control, and positioning to promote adequate oxygenation and decrease complications of immobility.

Ventilatory Support
The goals for ventilatory support of the trauma patient are the same as the ventilatory goals for any patient in the critical care unit. Management focuses on improving oxygenation, correcting acidosis, and easing the work of breathing.

Ventilatory therapy may be definitive or supportive, depending on the patient's injury and requirements. Definitive care for a flail chest may include the use of the ventilatory support to stabilize the chest wall. Supportive ventilatory care is imperative in the patient with a pulmonary contusion who exhibits signs of ARDS. The nurse caring for the trauma patient must be comfortable with the modes of conventional mechanical ventilation and have an awareness of some of the nonconventional ventilatory techniques (see Chapter 5, Airway and Ventilation Management, and Chapter 20, Advanced Respiratory Concepts).

Monitoring Chest Tubes

Chest tubes are inserted for patients with chest wall injuries and punctured lung tissue. Care of the patient with chest tubes includes observing for drainage characteristics, signs of a resolving air leak, and prevention of infection with meticulous attention to sterile technique. Trauma patients may have draining wounds adjacent to the chest tube site, which can make dressing changes more complicated.

Pain Control

Pain control, both systemic and local, is needed and may even preempt the need for mechanical ventilation in patients with milder degrees of thoracic trauma. For example, when patients are able to breathe deeply and cough effectively, smaller airways remain open, atelectasis is avoided, and healing can occur. Patient-controlled analgesia (PCA), epidural narcotic infusions, or local anesthetics can be used for aggressive pain control in the trauma patient to allow for enhanced pulmonary function exercises and avoid the need for mechanical ventilation.

Patients report that chest tubes, suctioning, and turning are all extremely painful. Attacking a patient's pain aggressively is not only a humane concern, but it also allows the patient to focus energy on healing. Pain can be controlled through narcotics that act centrally, locally, or regionally, and through drugs that act at the periphery to interrupt the painful stimulus (see Chapter 7, Pharmacology). Nonpharmacologic approaches can also operate at the central level through cognitive distraction or relaxation, and peripherally by using positioning or application of heat and cold.

PCA gives the patient control to request pain medication at a preset time interval. Epidural PCA is used with success in patients with rib fractures and may eliminate the need for mechanical ventilation, an important benefit in older trauma patients. Vigilant nursing is essential because the epidural catheter may migrate and not provide adequate pain relief. A patient's report of pain relief needs to be requested by the nurse at hourly intervals initially; it is the only reliable measurement for pain.

A variety of nonpharmacologic pain-reducing strategies are useful in patients with trauma, and the nurse needs to combine these with drug therapy for maximal gain. Because narcotics have side effects, combining them with a non-steroidal anti-inflammatory agent and a cognitive intervention may offer the patient the best pain reduction possible. Cognitive interventions for pain includes relaxation, guided imagery, music therapy, and hypnosis. Clear documentation of what strategies or combinations work best for the individual is needed. This approach requires an established communication system between patient and nurse. Anxiety and sleeplessness contribute to the pain response and should be addressed by asking the patients how they typically try to relax and by eliminating as much environmental noise as possible. Encouraging rest and sleep and limiting patient interruptions provides better pain management.

Positioning

Early mobilization of the trauma patient assists in promoting oxygenation and other complications of immobility. This includes positioning the patient in and out of bed. Information obtained from daily chest x-ray results is essential for accurate positioning of the patient. Positions to be considered include: sitting, prone, and lateral decubitus. The lateral decubitus position with the good lung down is especially important to maximize oxygenation if there is unilateral lung disease or injury to one side of the chest. An example of how the concept of therapeutic positioning can be used by the nurse is to position the patient and observe chest excursion, respiratory rate, pulse oximetry, peak inspiratory pressures, and if applicable, hemodynamic data for improvement. A continuous lateral rotation bed may be helpful for certain patients.

Abdominal Trauma

Etiology and Pathophysiology

Trauma to the abdomen may occur to organs in three distinct abdominal regions: peritoneal cavity, retroperitoneum, and pelvis. Pain and physical examination in the awake patient assist in diagnosing trauma to the spleen, liver, or peritoneal organs. If the patient is hemodynamically unstable, a DPL is necessary to diagnose abdominal injury. Another useful diagnostic tool to diagnose hemoperitoneum is focused abdominal sonography for trauma (FAST). Although FAST is being used more frequently by trauma specialists, a negative or indeterminate FAST requires performance of a DPL. Retroperitoneal trauma occurs when the pancreas or kidneys are injured. A DPL typically cannot discover a retroperitoneal bleed and the patient requires a CT scan. Bladder trauma is an example of pelvic area injury and can accompany fractures of the pelvis. Depending on the mechanism of injury, identification of the injured organs is accomplished through a history of the traumatic event, performing serial physical examinations, and interpretation of CT scans and DPL where appropriate. Trauma to the spleen is one of the most frequently encountered abdominal injuries after a motor vehicle crash. Depending on severity of splenic injury, interventions range from nonoperative observation and bedrest for mild lacerations to removal of a massively ruptured spleen. Liver trauma runs the spectrum from minor injury to severe laceration requiring operative repair and packing.

Typically, presenting signs and symptoms in abdominal trauma include pain and hypovolemia. Complications from abdominal trauma are directly linked to the function of the gastrointestinal tract and include metabolic/nutritional alterations, infections such as peritonitis, and pancreatitis. Patients may require extensive dressing changes if the wound is open or requires frequent trips to the operating suite for staged repair of the abdominal organs.

Principles of Management for Abdominal Trauma

Selected principles of caring for the patient with abdominal trauma include monitoring for bleeding, providing optimum wound care, and initiating early (within 24 to 48 hours) nutritional support.

Monitoring for Bleeding

Acute hemorrhage is commonly addressed during the primary survey. However, occult bleeding may not be initially evident and later discovered by the critical care nurse. Common abdominal injuries that may not initially exhibit signs and symptoms of bleeding include liver laceration, splenic fractures, and slow retroperitoneal bleeds.

Salvage of the spleen by performing a splenorrhaphy, repair of the spleen, or watchful waiting is increasing in popularity. The goal is to allow the spleen to heal and preserve the valuable immunoprotective function. Overwhelming postsplenectomy sepsis can occur as a serious complication years after removal of the spleen and efforts to optimally care for the damaged spleen, especially in children, are warranted. If splenectomy is indicated due to massive injury, patients are given polyvalent pneumococcal vaccine within 72 hours after surgery to prevent infection with pneumococci. Management also includes monitoring for rebleeding during 3 days of bedrest and preventing the complications of immobility.

Wound Care

The major goal in traumatic wound care is prevention of infection. Traumatic wounds can be simple lacerations or abrasions from a motor vehicle crash. With abdominal trauma, the patient may have a major abdominal surgical incision and drains. Wound care for the patient with a large abdominal wound is directed by the type of wound (open or closed) and the degree of intracompartment contamination due to the injury. Open abdominal wounds may require packing with dressing changes by the nurse and frequent trips to the operating room. Careful consideration of antimicrobial therapy must also be considered with contaminated wounds. The dressing changes are frequently performed by the critical care nursing staff so assessment for signs of infection as well as wound healing is essential during these dressing changes. Premedicating the patient or timing dressing changes around pain medication administration is another important role of the nurse providing holistic care.

Nutritional Support

Nutritional support in the trauma patient is multifactorial and an integral part of trauma care. Management focuses on the route and timing of nutritional support. Other considerations include composition of nutrient formulation, assessment of laboratory tests that measure nutrition and enteral verses parenteral feedings. Trauma patients have increased metabolic needs due to a hypermetabolic stress response caused by severe injuries, wound healing and sepsis.

Enteral nutrition is encouraged whenever possible at the earliest time after injury. Even a small amount of nutrition delivered via tube feeding to the gut is believed to be beneficial. A variety of metabolic derangements in the hypermetabolic trauma patient make nutritional support an early imperative. Insertion and maintenance of a small-bowel feeding tube, percutaneous gastrostomy tube, or jejunostomy tube is often required after injury until the patient can be orally fed. Total parenteral nutrition is recommended only if the gastrointestinal tract is unable to tolerate adequate nutrients. Accurate nutritional assessment conducted in collaboration with the nutritionist is essential, as trauma patients are at risk of complications from overfeeding as well as underfeeding. Diarrhea, inappropriate withholding of tube feedings, and the potential for increased aspiration are issues that need to be addressed for trauma patients (see Chapter 14, Gastrointestinal System).

Musculoskeletal Trauma

Etiology and Pathophysiology

Trauma to the musculoskeletal system accounts for approximately 70% to 85% of polytrauma injuries. Patients in the critical care setting with extremity or pelvic fractures often have other injuries due to the significant physical impact to the body. Motor vehicle trauma, falls, sports injuries, and industrial trauma are all frequent causes of musculoskeletal trauma. Victims of motorcycle accidents frequently have severe fractures with extensive soft tissue damage. Massive blood loss, edema of tissues, tissue destruction, and pain accompany musculoskeletal injuries.

Compartment syndrome is a serious complication of extremity trauma as a result of contused tissue swelling in a specific muscle compartment (Figure 17–4). This may lead to lack of perfusion and nerve compression in the area. Muscle compartments are located in the forearm, leg, hand, foot, thigh, abdomen, and chest. The nurse should assess for signs of compartment syndrome and should perform early and consistent neurovascular checks. However, neurovascular assessment and pain may not provide accurate early assessment of rising compartment pressures. Optimal assessment for compartment pressures is with a specialized needle that is inserted directly into the tissue compartment by a physician. Even open fractures may have significantly increased compartment pressures (normal pressure 0 to 8 mm Hg). If compartment pressures are found to be high, a physician relieves pressure with a fas-

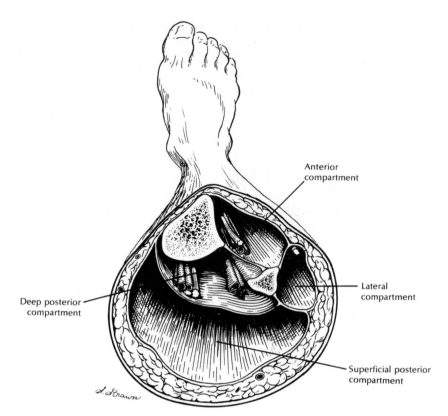

Figure 17–4. Compartments of the lower leg. (*From Bess R: Fasciotomy. In Moore E, Elsman B, Van Way C* [*eds.*]: *Critical Decisions in Trauma, p. 530. St. Louis: CV Mosby; 1984.*)

ciotomy. A fasciotomy entails surgically opening the skin and fascia to relieve the pressure in a muscle compartment and is the treatment of choice to treat compartment syndrome.

Principles of Management for Musculoskeletal Trauma

Management of extremity trauma focuses on early stabilization of fractures to prevent further tissue damage, infection, bleeding, and disability. Complications from musculoskeletal trauma include immobility, which can lead to increased incidence of pulmonary emboli, fat emboli, deep venous thrombosis, and decubitus ulcers. Pain control to promote mobility, and assessment of neurovascular status are key components to managing these patients (Table 17–5).

The risk of pulmonary embolism and deep vein thrombosis are extremely high in the trauma population. Guidelines for the management of venous thromboembolism for trauma patients include thromboprophylaxis and mechanical prophylactic devices, such as sequential compression devices (Table 17–6).

Stabilizing Fractures

Fractures are repaired early after a traumatic injury to decrease further bleeding and to limit pulmonary embolism complications. External fixation is used for pelvic fractures and lower limb fractures. Frequent sensation, movement, and vascular checks on affected extremities are essential. If the presence of pulses is in doubt, Doppler ultrasound should be used at the bedside.

Pain Control

Pain control is best achieved with an individualized strategy of medications and nonpharmacologic therapies. Patients respond best when strict attention is paid to pain control and their own unique coping style is used. Patients are expected to move in bed and get out of bed as soon as possible after an injury. Titrated pain medication is required to achieve this goal using PCA or continuous infusion. Nurses need to determine patient anxieties regarding the trauma and promote adequate sleep and rest. Sleep deprivation from a noisy environment, constant worry, and needless pain only makes the patient perceive a more intense pain.

COMPLICATIONS OF TRAUMATIC INJURY IN SEVERE MULTISYSTEM TRAUMA

The key to survival for patients with multiple trauma is to limit the extent of complications experienced and increase the delivery of oxygen to the tissues during the initial phase of trauma. In the history of trauma as a clinical specialty this has been called the "golden hour." The resuscitation goal is

TABLE 17–5. PHYSICAL COMPLICATIONS RELATED TO IMMOBILITY COMMONLY SEEN IN TRAUMA PATIENTS

Body System	Complications	Pathophysiology	Prevention
Neurologic	Potentially affects all body systems	Caused by decreased level of consciousness; injury to cortex, motor, or sensory systems	• Neurologic assessment • Specific focus on the effects seen in other body systems • Understand neurologic basis of complication
Respiratory	Fatigue, decreased productivity; infection, pneumonia, respiratory acidosis	Decreased respiratory movement, unable to mobilize secretions, alterations in blood gases	• Assessment of respiratory status and changes in level of consciousness • Mobilization of secretions by turning, coughing, and deep breathing; postural drainage, percussion, vibration, early ambulation, humidification
Cardiovascular	Osthostatic hypotension, fatigue, increased cardiac workload, thrombosis, embolus	Increased heart rate, cardiac output, stroke volume in supine position; loss of supporting muscle tone resulting in venous stasis; orthostatic neurovascular receptors cannot adjust to position changes; hypercoagulability and external pressure to vessels	• Cardiovascular assessment • Encourage mobilization, exercise, range of motion, positioning • Antiembolic stockings • Provide adequate hydration • Avoid Valsalva maneuver
Gastrointestinal	Anorexia, fatigue, malnutrition, constipation, impaction, bowel obstruction, diarrhea, dehydration	Negative nitrogen balance and protein deficiency; stress; decreased appetite creates bowel intolerance; muscle weakness; diminished ability to apply abdominal pressure needed for evacuation; psychologic factors and position for defecation may increase difficulty	• Assessment of GI functioning, including baseline history of nutrition, exercise, and bowel habits • Coordinate bowel plan with nutrition specialist • Adequate hydration • Positioning and privacy • Gastrocolic reflex timing factors; use of digital stimulation • Stool softeners and suppositories for stimulation • Adjust tube feedings to avoid constipation or diarrhea • Small, frequent feedings to increase tolerance and decrease anorexia • Encourage intake of protein, fluids, bulk foods
Urinary	Urinary reflux, incontinence, urinary stasis, renal calculi, urinary tract infection	Loss of effect of gravity, urinary stasis in renal pelvis; increased calculi formation from urine sediment in renal pelvis; diminished coordination of sphincters and muscles in supine position; bladder distention, overflow incontinence	• Assess urinary tract function • Promote movement and exercise • Maintain fluid intake • Decrease calcium intake • Monitor distention and voiding patterns • Prevent incontinence • Use upright or sitting position for voiding if possible • Intermittent catheters preferred to indwelling
Musculoskeletal	Muscle atrophy, contractures	Muscles shorten and atrophy; loss of ROM as supporting ligaments, tendons, and capsule lose mobility; loss of ROM becomes permanent; spasticity of antagonistic muscle with weakness of opposing muscle creates contracture	• Ongoing assessment • Passive, active, and active-assisted ROM exercises • Appropriate positioning and body alignment in both bed and chair
	Osteoporosis, stress fractures, heterotrophic ossification	Normal bone-building activities depend on weight bearing and movement; increased destruction of bone, release of calcium; bone becomes porous and fragile; abnormal calcification over large joints may also occur	• Calcium supplement to diet is not recommended • Promote weight bearing
Integumentary	Skin breakdown; stage I–IV skin ulcers; secondary infection of skin ulcers, sepsis	Prolonged pressure to skin diminishes capillary blood supply and stops flow of nutrients to cells; necrosis of cells results in skin breakdown, allowing infection to enter body	• Assessment of skin integrity, nutritional status, and risk factors for breakdown • Reposition; shift pressure and patient weight frequently; "every 2 hours" rule may not be adequate • Check for changes in blanching, sustained redness • Keep off all red areas • Massage at-risk areas to promote circulation • Teach patient to inspect own skin and shift weight • Increase protein in diet • Take immediate, consistent action on any areas of breakdown

TABLE 17–6. EVIDENCE-BASED PRACTICE: MANAGEMENT OF VENOUS THROMBOEMBOLISM IN TRAUMA PATIENTS[a,b]

Risk Factors
- Patients with major trauma, spinal cord or spinal fractures are at high risk for venous thromboembolism (VTE) following trauma.
- Older age is an increased factor for venous thromboembolism but it is not clear at which exact age the risk increases substantially.

The Role of Low-Molecular-Weight Heparin (LMWH)
- There are insufficient data to make recommendations for general use of LMWH as VTE prophylaxis in trauma patients.
- LMWH could be used for VTE prophylaxis in trauma patients with the following patterns: (1) pelvic fracture requiring operative fixation or prolonged bed rest (>5 days); (2) complex lower extremity fractures (defined as open fractures or multiple fractures in one extremity) requiring operative fixation or prolonged bed rest (>5 days); (3) spinal cord injury with complete or incomplete motor paralysis. The use of LMWH is predicted on the fact that these patients do not have other injuries that put them at high risk for bleeding.
- The use of LMWH or oral anticoagulants for several weeks postinjury should be considered in patients who remain at high risk for VTE (i.e., elderly pelvic fracture patients, spinal cord injury patients, patients who remain at prolonged bed rest (>5 days), and patients who require prolonged hospitalization or rehabilitation).

The Use of Low-Dose Heparin
- There is little evidence to support a benefit of low-dose heparin as a sole agent for prophylaxis in the trauma patient at high risk for VTE.
- For patients in whom bleeding could exacerbate their injuries, the safety of low-dose heparin has not been established and an individual decision should be made when considering anticoagulant prophylaxis.

The Use of Sequential Compression Devices (SCD)
- There are insufficient data to support a standard on this topic.
- In the subset of spine-injured, head-injured patients, SCD may have some benefit.
- For patients in whom the lower extremity is inaccessible to place SCDs at the calf level, foot pumps may act as an effective alternative to lower the rate of DVT formation.

The Role of A-V Foot Pumps
- There are insufficient data to suggest recommendations for this topic.
- Foot pumps are less effective than SCD for prevention of DVT.
- A-V foot pumps may be used as a substitute for sequential compression devices (SCDs) in those high-risk trauma patients who cannot wear SCDs due to external fixators or casts.

The Role of the Vena Cava Filter
A vena cava filter should be inserted in patients with
- Recurrent PE despite full anticoagulation,
- Proximal DVT and contraindications to full anticoagulation,
- Proximal DVT and major bleeding while on full anticoagulation, or
- Progression of iliofemoral clot despite anticoagulation (rare).

Extended indications for prophylactic vena cava filter placement in a patient with established DVT or PE include
- Large free-floating thrombus in the iliac vein or IVC,
- Following massive PE in which recurrent emboli may prove fatal, or
- During and after surgical embolectomy.

Data compiled from: [a]Eastern Association for the Surgery of Trauma: *Practice Management Guidelines for Venous Thromboembolism in Trauma Patients.* Available: www.east.org or www.guidelines.gov; Retrieved June 29, 2004; and [b]Gerts et al (2001).

to stop the deprivation of oxygen (hypoperfusion) and identify and eliminate what caused the problem. Shock, by definition, occurs when cellular oxygen delivery does not meet oxygen demands, which leads to cellular hypoxia. When adequate oxygen and blood flow are provided during the initial phase of trauma, the frequency of shock and complications decrease. Heart rate and blood pressure are not considered adequate parameters to judge the effectiveness of resuscitation, because they indicate only the body's compensation for the stress of trauma and not real-time tissue oxygenation. Appropriate measures to evaluate resuscitation should focus on assessing tissue oxygen delivery, including oxygen transport, delivery, and utilization (see Chapter 19, Advanced Cardiovascular Concepts). Serum lactate rises with inadequate oxygenation and is an additional diagnostic indicator of the adequacy of reperfusion and oxygen delivery.

Common complications of trauma are infection/sepsis, ARDS, and systemic inflammatory response syndrome (SIRS) (see Chapter 10, Respiratory System, and Chapter 11, Multisystem Problems). Patients with sepsis and SIRS experience a persistent inflammatory response which can lead to acute lung injury and multiple organ dysfunction syndrome (MODS). Oxygen debt occurs when resuscitation is delayed or inadequate and refers to the body's unmet and continuous need for oxygen. Delivering oxygen to the tissues by maintaining increased blood flow during resuscitation and early critical care phases is believed to decrease the incidence of oxygen debt and these often lethal complications.

Achieving adequate oxygen delivery to the tissues requires oxygen, hemoglobin, and sufficient cardiac output to deliver them to the organs and cells. This is typically accomplished with massive fluid and or blood resuscitation. Massive transfusion is defined as the administration of more than 10 units of blood (whole blood or packed red blood cells) within 24 hours, replacing the patient's total blood volume. Trauma patients are at risk of experiencing significant complications after massive fluid/blood administration. This same treatment, believed to prevent the complications of decreased oxygen delivery, has specific consequences the clinician needs to monitor. Coagulopathy, acidosis, electrolyte imbalances, pulmonary dysfunction, and altered membrane permeability (edema) are potential complications associated with massive fluid/blood replacement. Monitoring for and treating these complications are essential during the critical care phase of trauma patient care.

Acute Respiratory Distress Syndrome

The complications of ARDS, infections, and SIRS are interrelated in the trauma patient but require specific monitoring and treatment. Patients with trauma have an increased incidence of the severe respiratory dysfunction known as ARDS (see Chapter 10, Respiratory System). Precipitating factors for ARDS in the trauma patient include a prolonged shock state, massive fluid resuscitation, a direct lung injury, and sepsis. Patients with rib fractures and large pulmonary contusions may also develop respiratory failure and ARDS.

Standard treatment for ARDS includes mechanical ventilation, oxygen titrated to maintain PaO_2 above 60 mm Hg, positive end-expiratory pressure and/or pressure ventilatory modes to recruit closed alveoli and decrease lung injury. In addition to mechanical ventilation, another common treatment to improve oxygenation is positioning for optimal ventilation and perfusion. This is a unique challenge for the critically ill trauma patient because their traumatic injuries may preclude many positions. For example, the patient with an unstable pelvic fracture, a spinal cord injury, or lower extremity fractures may be difficult or impossible to turn.

Infection/Sepsis

Trauma patients are at high risk of developing an infection and possibly sepsis. This is because of the nature of the injury, the environment in which the injury occurred, the non-sterile conditions in which invasive devices may have been initially placed, and the multiple invasive procedures, including surgery, necessary for trauma resuscitation and management. The procedures preformed during resuscitation are best preformed under clean conditions. The trauma resuscitation areas do not have the same level of sterility focus and attention as is used in the operating room. All invasive devices placed in the field and the emergency department should be replaced within the first 24 hours of admission.

The classic signs and symptoms of infection are sometimes difficult to isolate in a recovering critically ill trauma patient. Fever, tachycardia, elevated white blood cell count, inflammation, pain, and a hyperdynamic state are classic indicators of infection and sepsis. These assessment parameters are also common after injury, resuscitation, and during the healing process. Due to the high probability that a trauma patient has an infection, clinicians should always focus their assessment looking for this common complication. The classic rule in trauma critical care is that there is an infection—it just needs to be found and treated. Meticulous attention to sterile technique and hand washing is essential.

Systemic Inflammatory Response Syndrome

Identification and management of SIRS requires knowledge of the underlying inflammatory process (see Chapter 11, Multisystem Problems). Assessment criteria for SIRS includes two or more of the following: temperature greater than 38°C or less than 36°C, heart rate greater than 90 beats/min, respiratory rate greater than 20/min, $PaCO_2$ less than 32 mm Hg, and white blood cell count greater than 12,000/mm^3 or less than 4000/mm^3. The systemic inflammatory response has occurred because of direct injury to tissues/organs and lack of oxygen delivery (hypoperfusion) during the shock state.

These circumstances lead to the release of biological mediators from injured tissue/cells, which cause an intense systemic inflammation, vasodilatation, and increased membrane permeability (edema, leaky tissue). The cardiopulmonary changes typical in SIRS include high cardiac output, decreased systemic vascular resistance, and elevated oxygen requirements and consumption.

Goals for managing the patient with SIRS are to provide the essentials such as oxygenation and nutrition, limit known stressors such as pain and fever, and support organ system function. The delivery of oxygen and nutrients requires a strong cardiac output, oxygen saturated hemoglobin, and an environment (pH) in which the cells can extract and utilize the delivered oxygen. Inotropic drug support to maximize the heart's ability to generate the work needed to sustain the patient through SIRS is often required.

The individual's response to SIRS may be prolonged and destructive, leading to MODS. As organs begin to dysfunction and fail, treatments such as maximal ventilatory support and hemodialysis may be necessary. Mortality remains high for MODS, requiring increased attention to prevention of early oxygen debts. Limiting the initial shock (hypoperfusion) state decreases the likelihood of SIRS and therefore MODS. In trauma care, the critical care team's interventions in the first 24 hours of injury often determines survival.

PSYCHOLOGICAL CONSEQUENCES OF TRAUMA

Critical illness places many stresses on patients and families. Critical illness as a result of trauma has unique psychosocial implications. Trauma injury is by nature unexpected. It typically affects young healthy individuals and can launch both the patient and family into a cycle of chaos and crisis. Common responses to trauma include anxiety, fear, grief, loss, guilt, depression, denial, hopelessness, and sleeplessness.

Fear begins immediately as the awake trauma patient is transported from the scene. Fear is related to the unknown, the specifics of the injuries, and impact on the patient's future, including body image, family, and career. Loss typifies the experience of trauma and can be characterized as loss of physical functioning, loss of quality of life, or even loss of significant others due to the traumatic event. Guilt may ensue as the patient may perceive responsibility for the event (directly or indirectly), and this can be overwhelming. Depression and denial are common coping mechanisms used during personal crises and may be exhibited in a variety of ways by trauma victims. It should be noted that although the injuries were sustained by the patient, the family members and family structure frequently are also traumatized.

Monitoring the patient's response to injury is as much the responsibility of the nurse as monitoring the patient's blood pressure. As there are long-term physiologic effects of a low blood pressure (shock), so are there long-term psychological effects of unmet or unidentified emotional needs. There are also psychoneuroimmunology responses that can impact the physical recovery. The emotional response to injury should be assessed. Talk to the patient and really listen to their responses and perceptions. Help them to identify and articulate their concerns and fears.

Fear creates anxiety in the trauma patient, and unrelieved pain may worsen anxiety. With the intense monitoring and frequent care interruptions in the critical care environment, sleep may be impossible. A vicious cycle is thus initiated whereby sleeplessness leads to an increased perception of pain, which in turn creates needles anxiety and inhibits sleep. The importance of viewing these responses as cyclical emphasizes that the critical care nurse may intervene anywhere in the cycle of responses and make a major impact on all three. For example, providing pain-relieving strategies that permit sleep automatically decreases anxiety. A focus on information sharing may ease the patient's mind so that sleep can occur and pain perception decreases. The nurse has a significant role in intervening to stop this vicious cycle through a variety of holistic strategies.

All families of trauma patients experience a crisis. Families may have no idea of how to act or what the health care team expects of them. Clinicians have a key role in providing the right amount of support and information to meet family needs, and in identifying family coping mechanisms. Knowing the phases of family emotional response and suggested interventions is useful (Table 17–7). Early assessment of

family system structure, relationship process, and family functioning are keys to effective management of the psychosocial needs of the patient and family. Getting to know and work with family members in trauma care is essential and can be best facilitated with flexible visiting policies, family presence during rounds, procedures, and codes when appropriate, and where family members are wanted and expected by the patient, the nurse, and the entire team.

SELECTED BIBLIOGRAPHY

General Trauma

Abou-Khalil B, Scalea TM, Trooskin SZ, Henry SM, Hitchcock R: Hemodynamic responses to shock in young trauma patients: Need for invasive monitoring. *Crit Care Med* 1994;22:633–639.

ACCP-SCCM Consensus Conference Committee: Definitions for sepsis and organ failure and guidelines for the use of innovative therapies in sepsis. *Chest* 1992;101:1644–1655.

American College of Surgeons Committee on Trauma: *Advanced Trauma Life Support for Doctors,* 6th ed. Chicago: ACS; 1997.

Cunnenn J, Cartwright M: The puzzle of sepsis: Fitting the pieces of inflammatory response with treatment. *AACN Clin Iss* 2004:15:18–44.

DeKeyser F: Psychoneuroimmunology in critical ill patients. *AACN Clin Iss* 2003;14:25–32.

DePalma J, Redorka P, Simkko L: Quality of life experienced by severely injured trauma survivors. *AACN Clin Iss* 2003;14:42–53.

Emergency Nurses Association: *Trauma Nursing Core Course-Provider Manual,* 5th ed. Chicago, IL: Emergency Nursing Association; 2000.

Farrar JA: Trauma. In Kinney M, Dunbar S, Brooks-Brunn, JA, et al (eds): *AACN's Clinical Reference for Critical-Care Nursing,* 4th ed, pp. 1091–1123. St. Louis, MO: Mosby; 1998.

Freeman B, Parrillo J, Natanson C: Septic shock and multiple organ failure. In Parrillo J, Dellinger R, eds: *Critical Care Medicine,* 2nd ed, pp. 437–452. St. Louis, MO: Mosby; 2001.

Kinney M, Dunbar S, Brooks-Brunn J, Vitello-Cicciu J: *AACN Clinical Reference for Critical Care Nursing,* 4th ed. St. Louis, MO: Mosby; 1998.

Kleinpell R: The role of the critical care nurse in the assessment and management of the patient with severe sepsis. *Crit Care Clin North Am* 2003;5:27–34.

Makic-Flynn M, Mclesky S: Shock, systemic inflammatory response syndrome and multiple organ dysfunction syndrome. In Morton P, Fontaine D, eds: *Critical Care Nursing: A Holistic Approach,* 8th ed. Philadelphia: Lippincott, Williams & Wilkins; 2004.

Mattox K, Feliciano D, Moore E, eds: *Trauma,* 4th ed. New York: McGraw Hill; 2000.

McQuillan K, Von Rueden K, Hartsock R, Flynn MB, Whalen E (eds): *Trauma Nursing from Resuscitation Through Rehabilitation,* 3rd ed. Philadelphia: WB Saunders; 2002.

Montonye JM: Abdominal injuries. In McQuillan K, Von Rueden K, Hartsock R, Flynn MB, Whalen E (eds): *Trauma Nursing from Resuscitation Through Rehabilitation,* 3rd ed, pp. 591–616. Philadelphia: WB Saunders; 2002.

Romito RA: Early administration of enteral nutrients in critically ill patients. *AACN Clin Iss* 1995;6:242–256.

TABLE 17–7. PHASES AND MANIFESTATIONS OF STRESS AND NURSING INTERVENTIONS FOR FAMILIES OF TRAUMA PATIENTS

Phase	Manifestations	Interventions
High anxiety	Restlessness Fainting Nausea High-pitched voice	Encourage ventilation of feelings Provide accurate information
Denial	Families commonly state, "Everything will be all right"	Reiterate the facts of the situation
Anger	Verbal abuse directed toward health care staff	Active listening Allow ventilation of angry feelings Help to refocus on the real cause of anger
Remorse	Elements of guilt and sorrow "If only" stage	Listen to family's expressions of remorse Interject reality
Grief	Intense period of sadness Crying	Encourage flow of tears Provide empathetic gestures such as silent physical closeness, holding a trembling hand, embracing limp shoulders

From: Hopkins AG: The trauma nurse's role with families in crisis. Critical Care Nurse. 1994;14(2):37; and Epperson M: Families in sudden crisis: Process and intervention in a critical care center. Social Work in Health Care. 1977;2:265–273.

Scalea T, Boswell S: Initial management of trauma shock. In McQuillan K, Von Rueden K, Hartsock R, Flynn MB, Whalen E (eds): *Trauma Nursing from Resuscitation Through Rehabilitation,* 3rd ed. Philadelphia: WB Saunders; 2002.

Sherwood SF, Hartsock RL: Thoracic injuries. In McQuillan KA, Von Rueden KT, Hartsock RL, Flynn MB, Whalen E (eds): *Trauma Nursing from Resuscitation Through Rehabilitation,* 3rd ed, pp. 543–588. Philadelphia: WB Saunders; 2002.

Shapiro M. Traumatic shock: Nonsurgical management. In Parrillo J, Dellinger R: *Critical Care Medicine,* 2nd ed, pp. 501–512, St. Louis, MO: Mosby; 2001.

Vary T, McLean B, VonRueden K: Shock and multiple organ dysfunction syndrome. In McQuillan K, Von Rueden K, Hartsock R, Flynn MB, Whalen E (eds): *Trauma Nursing from Resuscitation Through Rehabilitation,* 3rd ed. Philadelphia: Saunders; 2002.

Wachtel TL: Critical care concepts in the management of abdominal trauma. *Crit Care Nurs Q* 1994;17(2):34–50.

Selected Web-Sites

http//:www.aacn.org
http//:www.east.org
http//:www.trauma.org
http//:www.facs.org

http//:www.sccm.org
http//:www.ena.org

Evidence-Based Practice

Dellinger P, Carlet J, Masur H, et al: Surviving sepsis campaign guidelines for management of severe sepsis and septic shock. *Crit Care Med* 2004;32:858–873.

Gerts W, Heit J, Clagett G, et al: Prevention of venous thromboembolism. *Chest* 2001;119:132S–175S.

Eastern Association for the Surgery of Trauma (EAST): *Practice Management Guidelines for the Management of Venous Thromboembolism in Trauma Patients.* Available: www.east.org

Eastern Association for the Surgery of Trauma (EAST): *Practice Management Guidelines for the Evaluation of Blunt Abdominal Trauma.* Available: www.east.org

Eastern Association for the Surgery of Trauma (EAST): *Practice Management Guidelines for the Screening of Blunt Cardiac Trauma.* Available: www.east.org

Eastern Association for the Surgery of Trauma (EAST): *Practice Management Guidelines for Nutritional Support of the Trauma Patient.* Available: www.east.org

Rivers E, Nguyen B, Havstad S, et al: Early goal-directed therapy in the treatment of severe sepsis and septic shock. *N Engl J Med* 2001;345:1368–1377.

Advanced Concepts in Caring for the Critically Ill Patient

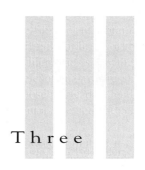

Three

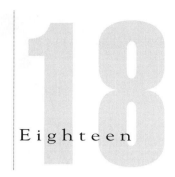

Carol Jacobson

▶ Knowledge Competencies

1. Identify electrocardiogram (ECG) characteristics and treatment approaches for each of the following advanced arrhythmias:
   • Supraventricular tachycardias
   • Wide QRS beats and rhythms
2. Using the 12-lead ECG, determine the following:
   • Bundle branch blocks

• Axis of the heart
• Patterns of myocardial ischemia, injury, and infarct
3. Identify ECG characteristics of single- and dual-chamber pacemakers during normal and abnormal functioning.

THE 12-LEAD ELECTROCARDIOGRAM

The 12-lead ECG records electrical activity as it spreads through the heart from 12 different leads, which are in turn recorded by electrodes placed on the arms and legs and in specific spots on the chest. Each lead represents a different "view" of the heart and consists of two electrodes. A bipolar lead has two poles—one positive and one negative. A unipolar lead has one positive pole and a reference pole that is a point in the center of the chest that is mathematically determined by the ECG machine. The standard 12-lead ECG consists of six frontal plane limb leads that record electrical activity traveling up/down and right/left in the heart, and six precordial leads that record electrical activity in the horizontal plane traveling anterior/posterior and right/left. Limb leads are recorded by electrodes placed on the arms and legs, and precordial leads are recorded by electrodes placed on the chest (Figure 18–1).

A camera analogy makes the 12-lead ECG easier to understand. Each lead of the ECG represents a picture of the electrical activity in the heart taken by the camera. In any lead, the positive electrode is the recording electrode or the camera lens. The negative electrode tells the camera which way to "shoot" its picture and determines the direction in which the positive electrode records. When the positive electrode sees electrical activity traveling toward it, it records an upright deflection on the ECG. When the positive electrode sees electrical activity traveling away from it, it records a negative deflection (Figure 18–2). If the electrical activity travels perpendicular to a positive electrode, either a diphasic deflection or no activity is recorded. The ECG records three bipolar frontal plane leads (lead I, lead II, and lead III) and three unipolar frontal plane leads (aVR, aVL, and aVF). In addition, there are six unipolar precordial leads: V_1, V_2, V_3, V_4, V_5, and V_6.

The three bipolar frontal plane leads are illustrated in Figure 18–3A. In each lead, the camera represents the positive pole of the lead. In lead I, the positive electrode is on the left arm and the negative electrode is on the right arm. Any electrical activity in the heart that travels toward the positive electrode (camera lens) on the left arm is recorded as an upright deflection and any traveling away from it is recorded as a negative deflection. In lead II, the positive electrode is on the left leg and the negative electrode is on the right arm. Any electrical activity traveling toward the left leg electrode (camera lens) is recorded as an upright deflection and any traveling away from it toward the right arm electrode is recorded as a negative deflection. In lead III, the positive

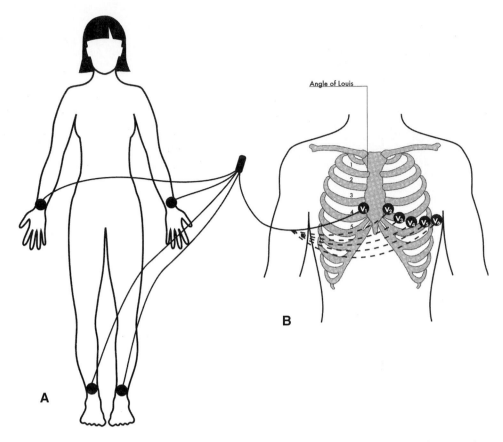

Figure 18–1. (A) Limb electrodes can be placed anywhere on arms and legs. Standard placement is shown here on wrists and ankles. **(B)** Chest electrode placement. V_1 = fourth intercostal space to right of sternum; V_2 = fourth intercostal space to left of sternum; V_3 = halfway between V_2 and V_4 in a straight line; V_4 = fifth intercostal space at midclavicular line; V_5 = same level as V_4 at anterior axillary line; V_6 = same level as V_4 at midaxillary line.

electrode is on the left leg and the negative electrode is on the left arm. Any electrical activity coming toward the left leg electrode (camera lens) is recorded upright and any traveling away from it toward the left arm is recorded negative.

The view of the heart by the bipolar leads can be compared to a wide-angle camera lens.

The three unipolar frontal plane leads, aVR, aVL, and aVF, are illustrated in Figure 18–3B. The camera represents

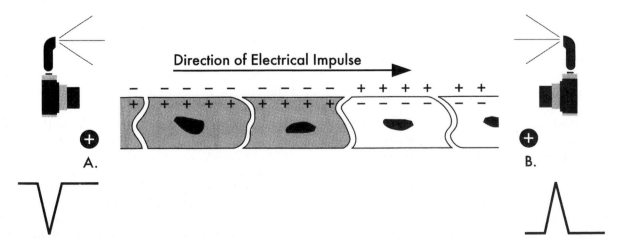

Figure 18–2. A strip of cardiac muscle depolarizing in the direction of the arrow. A positive electrode at *B* sees depolarization coming toward it and records an upright deflection. A positive electrode at *A* sees depolarization going away from it and records a negative deflection.

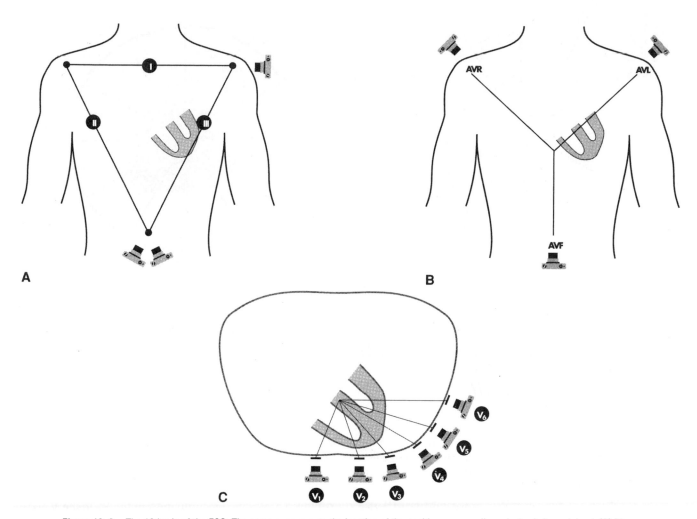

Figure 18–3. The 12 leads of the ECG. The camera represents the location of the positive, or recording, electrode in each lead. **(A)** Bipolar frontal plane leads I, II, and III. **(B)** Unipolar frontal plane leads aVR, aVL, and aVF. **(C)** Unipolar precordial leads V₁ to V₆.

the location of the positive electrode: on the right shoulder for aVR, on the left shoulder for aVL, and at the foot for aVF. The "negative end" of the unipolar lead is a reference spot in the center of the chest that is mathematically determined by the ECG machine. The same principles apply to unipolar leads: any electrical activity traveling toward the positive electrode is recorded as an upright deflection and any traveling away from it is recorded as a negative deflection. The six unipolar precordial leads are recorded from their locations on the chest as shown in Figure 18–3C. The view of the heart by unipolar leads can be compared to a telephoto lens on the camera, "zooming in" on the electrical activity in the heart.

The hexaxial reference system (or axis wheel) is formed when the six frontal plane leads are moved together in such a way that they bisect each other in the center (Figure 18–4A). Each lead is labeled at its positive end to make it easy to remember where the positive electrode is. In Figure 18–4B, the hexaxial reference system is superimposed over a drawing of the heart to illustrate how each lead views the heart.

The normal sequence of depolarization through the heart begins with an electrical impulse originating in the sinus node, high in the right atrium, and spreading leftward through the left atrium and downward toward the AV node low in the right atrium (Figure 18–5A). Leads I and aVL, with their positive electrodes (camera lens) on the left side of the body, record this leftward electrical activity as an upright P wave, and leads II, III, and aVF, with their positive electrodes at the bottom of the heart, record the downward spread of activity as upright P waves. Lead aVR, with its positive electrode on the right shoulder, sees the electrical activity moving away from it and records a negative P wave.

As the impulse spreads through the AV node, no electrical activity is recorded because the AV node is too small to be recorded by surface leads. As the impulse exits the AV node, it moves through the bundle of His and enters the right and left bundle branches. The left bundle branch sprouts some Purkinje fibers high on the left side of the septum that carry the impulse into the septum and cause it to depolarize

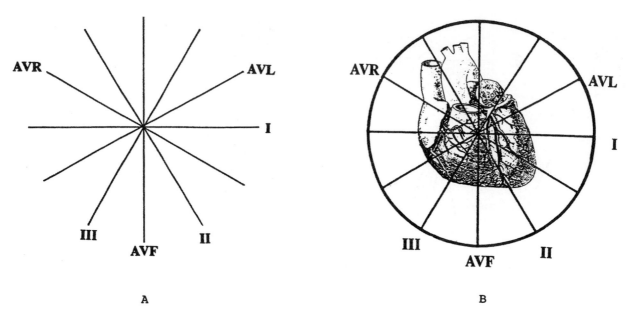

Figure 18–4. Hexaxial reference system (or axis wheel). **(A)** All six frontal plane leads bisecting each other. Each lead is labeled at its positive end. **(B)** The axis wheel superimposed on the heart to demonstrate each lead's view of the heart. Leads I and aVL face the left lateral wall; leads II, III, and aVF face the inferior wall.

first in a left-to-right direction. The electrical impulse then enters the Purkinje system of both ventricular free walls simultaneously and depolarizes them from endocardium to epicardium, as shown by the small arrows through the ventricular wall in Figure 18–5A. The millions of electrical forces travel through the heart in three dimensions simultaneously, but if averaged together they move downward, leftward, and posteriorly toward the large left ventricle, as indicated by the large arrow in the same figure. This large arrow represents the mean axis, which is the net direction of electrical depolarization through the ventricles when all the smaller arrows are averaged together.

The QRS complex is recorded as the ventricles depolarize. Leads I and aVL, with their positive electrodes on the left side of the body, see the septum depolarizing away from them and record a small negative deflection (Q wave). These leads then see the large left ventricular free wall depolarizing toward them and record an upright deflection (R wave). Leads II, III, and aVF, with their positive electrodes at the bottom of the heart, may not see septal activity at all and record no deflections. However, if these leads see septal electrical activity coming slightly toward them, they record a positive deflection. As the forces continue moving downward toward leads II, III, and aVF, an upright deflection (R wave) is recorded. Lead aVR, positive on the right shoulder, sees all activity moving away from it and records a negative deflection (QS complex). Figure 18–5B illustrates how the six precordial leads record normal electrical activity as it spreads through the ventricles.

The six precordial leads record electrical activity traveling in the horizontal plane. Figure 18–5B illustrates the po-

sition of the precordial leads and how they record electrical activity as it spreads through the ventricles. Lead V_1 is located on the front of the chest and records a small R wave as the septum depolarizes toward it from left to right. It then records a deep S wave as depolarization spreads away from it through the thick left ventricle. As the positive electrode is moved across the precordium from the V_1 to the V_6 position, it records progressively more left ventricular forces and the R wave gets progressively larger. Lead V_6 is located on the left side of the chest and usually records a small Q wave as the septum depolarizes from left to right away from the positive electrode, and it records a large R wave as electrical activity spreads toward the positive electrode through the thick left ventricle.

In addition to P waves and QRS complexes, the ECG records T waves as the ventricles repolarize. Normal T waves are slightly asymmetrical with an ascending limb that is more gradual than the descending limb. T waves are usually upright in leads I, II, and $V_{3–6}$, and negative in lead aVR. T waves can vary in other leads. A normal T wave is not taller than 5 mm in a limb lead or 10 mm in a chest lead. Tall T waves can indicate hyperkalemia or myocardial ischemia or infarction.

The ST segment begins at the end of the QRS complex (the J point) and ends at the beginning of the T wave. It is normally at the baseline (the isoelectric segment between the T wave and the next P wave), and should not stay on the baseline for longer than 0.12 second (Figure 18–6). The ST segment should gently curve upward into the T wave without forming a sharp angle. Normal ST-segment elevation and depression is discussed under "ST-Segment Monitoring" later in this chapter.

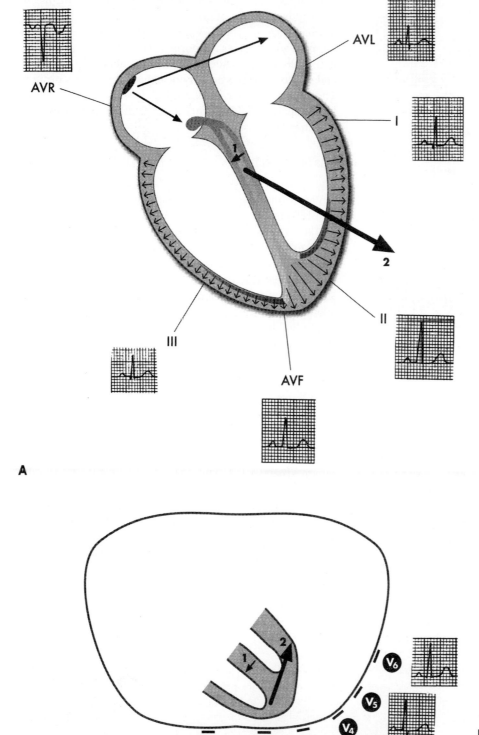

Figure 18–5. **(A)** Normal sequence of depolarization through the heart as recorded by each of the frontal plane leads. **(B)** Cross-section of the thorax illustrating how the six precordial leads record normal electrical activity in the ventricles. The small arrow (*1*) shows the initial direction of depolarization through the septum, followed by the direction of ventricular depolarization, indicated by the larger arrow (*2*).

Lead II   Lead V₁

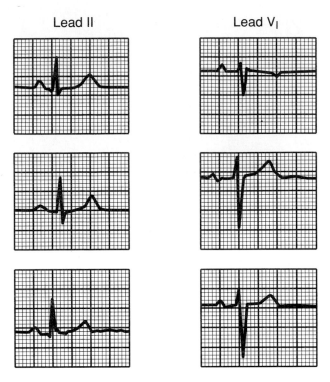

Figure 18–6. Normal ST segment and T waves.

The U wave is sometimes seen following the T wave, and when present it should be smaller than the T wave and point in the same direction as the T wave. U waves are thought to represent either repolarization of the terminal portion of the Purkinje system or of the papillary muscles. Large U waves can be seen in hypokalemia and with certain drugs, like quinidine. Inverted U waves can indicate myocardial ischemia.

Figure 18–7 shows a normal 12-lead ECG. Normal sinus rhythm is present, and the axis is +45°. P waves are normal (they are flat in V₂, but this is not necessarily abnormal), and T waves are normal. The QRS complex is normal (0.08-second wide), there are no abnormal Q waves, and R-wave progression is normal across the precordium. The ST segment is at baseline in all leads. This ECG is used for comparison as abnormalities are discussed throughout this chapter.

Axis Determination

The *hexaxial reference system* (axis wheel) forms a 360° circle surrounding the heart that by convention is divided into 180 positive degrees (+180°) and 180 negative degrees (−180°) (Figure 18–8). The normal QRS axis is defined as −30° to +110° because most of the electrical forces in a normal heart are directed downward and leftward toward the large left ventricle. Left axis deviation is defined as an axis of −30° to −90° and occurs when most of the forces move in a leftward and superior direction, as can happen in a variety of conditions, such as left ventricular hypertrophy, left anterior fascicular block, inferior myocardial infarction (MI), or left bundle branch block (LBBB) (Table 18–1). Right axis deviation is defined as +110° to +180° and occurs when most of the forces move rightward, as can happen in conditions such as right ventricular hypertrophy, left posterior fascicular block, and right bundle branch block (RBBB) (see Table 18–1). When most of the forces are directed superior and rightward between −90° and −180°, the term *indeterminate axis* is used. This axis can occur with ventricular tachycardia and occasionally with bifasicular block.

The mean frontal plane QRS axis can be determined in a number of ways. The most accurate method is to average the forces moving right and left with those moving up and down. Because this represents the frontal plane, lead I is the

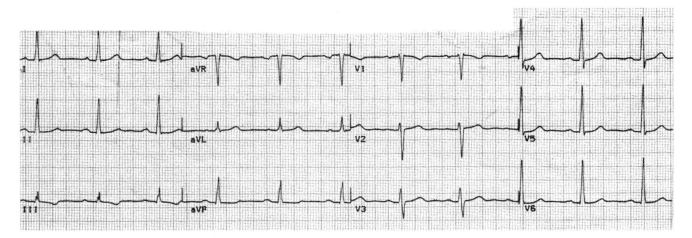

Figure 18–7. Normal 12-lead ECG.

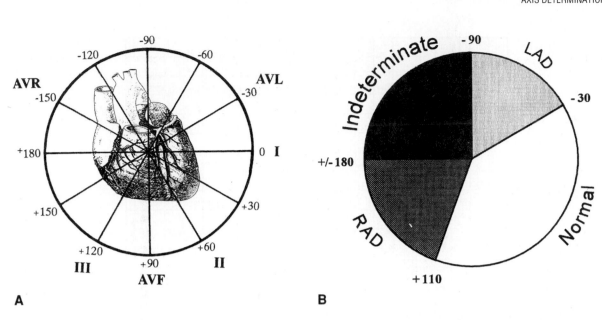

Figure 18–8. (A) Degrees of the axis wheel. **(B)** Normal axis = −30° to 110°; Left axis deviation = −30° to −90°; right axis deviation = +110° to +180°; indeterminate axis = −90° to −180°.

"pure" right/left lead and lead aVF is the "pure" up/down lead; it is easiest to use these two perpendicular leads to calculate the mean axis. Figure 18–9A shows the frontal plane leads of a 12-lead ECG. Leads I and aVF are shown enlarged along with the axis wheel with small hash marks along the axes of lead I and lead aVF (Figure 18–9B). These hash marks represent the small, 1-mV boxes on the ECG paper. To determine the mean QRS axis, follow these steps:

1. Look at the QRS complex in lead I and count the number of positive and negative boxes. Mark the net

TABLE 18–1. SUMMARY OF CAUSES OF AXIS DEVIATIONS

Axis: −30° to +110°
• Normal

Left Axis Deviation: −31° to −90°
• Left ventricular hypertrophy
• Left anterior fascicular block
• Inferior myocardial infarction
• Left bundle branch block (LBBB)
• Congenital defects
• Ventricular tachycardia
• Wolff-Parkinson-White syndrome

Right Axis Deviation: +110° to +180°
• Right ventricular hypertrophy
• Left posterior fascicular block
• Right bundle branch block (RBBB)
• Dextrocardia
• Ventricular tachycardia
• Wolff-Parkinson-White syndrome

Intermediate Axis: −90° to −180°
• Ventricular tachycardia
• Bifascicular block

vector along the appropriate end of lead I on the axis wheel. In Figure 18–9B, the QRS complex in lead I is 5 boxes positive and 2 boxes negative, resulting in a net 3 boxes positive, or +3. Count 3 hash marks toward the positive end of lead I and put a mark on the axis wheel at that spot.

2. Look at the QRS complex in aVF and follow the same procedure as above. In this example, the QRS complex in aVF is 8 boxes positive and has two very small negative deflections that equal approximately 1 box when combined, resulting in a net +7. Count 7 hash marks along the positive end of aVF's axis and place a mark at that spot.

3. Draw a perpendicular line down from the mark on lead I's axis and a perpendicular line across from the mark on aVF's axis.

4. Draw a line from the center of the axis wheel to the spot where the two perpendicular lines meet. This line represents the mean QRS axis. In the example in Figure 18–9B, the axis is about +65°.

A quick but less accurate method of axis determination is to place the axis in its proper quadrant of the axis wheel by looking at leads I and aVF, because these leads divide the wheel into four quadrants. As illustrated in Figure 18–10, if both of these leads are positive, the axis falls in the normal quadrant, 0° to +90°. If lead I is positive and aVF is negative, the axis falls in the left quadrant, 0° to −90°. If lead I is negative and aVF is positive, the axis falls in the right quadrant, +90° to +180°. If both leads are negative, the axis falls in the indeterminate quadrant or "no-mans-land," −90° to −180°. Locating the correct quadrant is sometimes adequate, but because 30° of the left quadrant is considered normal, it is

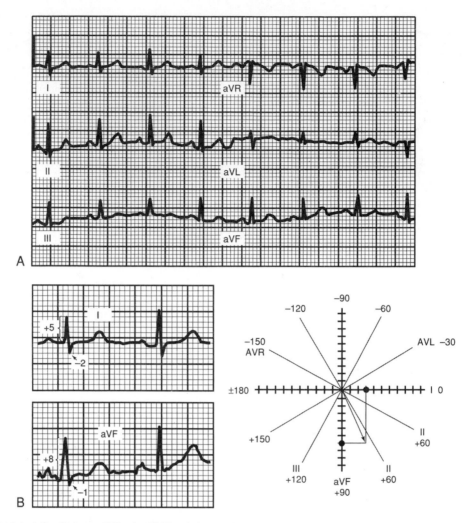

Figure 18–9. Calculating the mean QRS axis. **(A)** The six frontal plane leads of an ECG. **(B)** Leads I and aVF enlarged. See the text for instructions on calculating the axis using leads I and aVF on the axis wheel.

necessary to be more precise in describing the axis when it falls in the left quadrant. To "fine-tune" the axis quickly, find the limb lead with the smallest or most biphasic QRS complex. This lead must not be seeing much electrical force if it is the smallest; therefore, its perpendicular lead must be seeing most of the forces. Locate the perpendicular lead (leads I and aVF, leads II and aVL, leads III and aVR) and see if the QRS is positive or negative in that lead. If it is positive, the axis is directed toward the positive end of the lead; if it is negative, the axis is directed toward the negative end of the lead. Using the ECG in Figure 18–9A do the following:

1. Place the axis in its correct quadrant by looking at leads I and aVF. Because both leads are positive, the axis is in the normal quadrant.
2. Find the smallest or most diphasic limb lead. Lead aVL is the most diphasic lead in this example.
3. Find the lead that is perpendicular to the diphasic lead and note if it is positive or negative. Lead II is

perpendicular to aVL and lead II is positive in this example. Therefore, the axis is directed toward the positive end of lead II, which is +60°.

Using the ECG in Figure 18–11A, first place the axis in the appropriate quadrant by using leads I and aVF. Lead I is upright and aVF is negative, placing the axis in the left quadrant. However, because 30° of the left quadrant is considered normal, we need to fine-tune the axis to determine where within the left quadrant it actually falls. Lead aVR is the most biphasic lead in this ECG, which means that most of the electrical force is moving perpendicular to aVR. Lead III is perpendicular to aVR, and lead III is negative in this ECG, indicating that the axis is directed toward the negative pole of lead III. The axis is −60°. The axis wheel shows how to count boxes in this example.

Using the ECG in Figure 18–11B, place the axis in the appropriate quadrant. Because lead I is negative and aVF is positive, the axis is in the right quadrant. The most diphasic

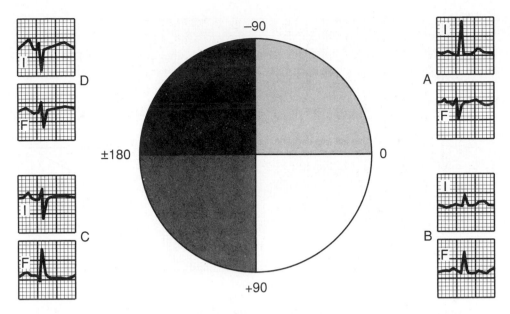

Figure 18–10. The four quadrants of the axis wheel. **(A)** Left axis deviation quadrant; lead I is positive and lead aVF is negative. **(B)** Normal axis quadrant; leads I and aVF are both positive. **(C)** Right axis deviation quadrant; lead I is negative and lead aVF is positive. **(D)** Indeterminate axis quadrant; leads I and aVF are both negative. (*With permission from: Marriott HJL. Practical Electrocardiography, 8th ed, p. 35. Baltimore: Williams & Wilkins; 1988.*)

lead is aVR, and lead III is perpendicular to aVR. Because lead III is positive, the axis is directed toward the positive pole of lead III, or $+150°$. The axis wheel shows how boxes are counted in this example.

Bundle Branch Block

When one of the bundle branches is blocked, the ventricles depolarize asynchronously. Bundle branch block is characterized by a delay of excitation to one ventricle and an abnormal spread of electrical activity through the ventricle whose bundle is blocked. This delayed conduction results in widening of the QRS complex to 0.12 second or more and a characteristic pattern best recognized in precordial leads V_1 and V_6 and limb leads I and aVL.

Normal ventricular depolarization as recorded by leads V_1 and V_6 is illustrated in Figure 18–12. The positive electrode for V_1 is located on the front of the chest at the fourth intercostal space to the right of the sternum, close to the right ventricle. The positive electrode for V_6 is located in the left midaxillary line at the fifth intercostal space, close to the left ventricle. Lead V_1 records a small R wave as the septum depolarizes from left to right toward the positive electrode. It then records a negative deflection (S wave) as the main forces travel away from the positive electrode toward the left ventricle, resulting in the normal rS complex in V_1. Lead V_6 records a small Q wave as the septum depolarizes left to right away from the positive electrode. It then records a tall R wave as the main forces travel toward the left ventricle, resulting in

the normal qR complex in V_6. When both ventricles depolarize together, the QRS width is less than 0.12 second.

Right Bundle Branch Block

The presence of a block in the right bundle branch causes a different spread of electrical forces in the ventricles and thus a different pattern to the QRS complex. Three separate forces occur, as seen in Figure 18–13A.

1. Septal activation occurs first from left to right (*arrow 1*), resulting in the normal small R wave in V_1 and small Q wave in V_6.
2. The left ventricle is activated next through the normally functioning left bundle branch. Depolarization spreads normally through the Purkinje fibers in the left ventricle (*arrow 2*), causing an S wave in V_1 as the impulse travels away from its positive electrode and an R wave in V_6 as the impulse travels toward the positive electrode in V_6.
3. The right ventricle depolarizes late and abnormally as the impulse spreads via cell-to-cell conduction through the right ventricle (*arrow 3*). This abnormal activation causes a wide second R wave (called R prime [R′]) in V_1 as it travels toward the positive electrode in V_1 and a wide S wave in V_6 as it travels away from the positive electrode in V_6. Because muscle cell-to-cell conduction is much slower than conduction through the Purkinje system, the QRS complex widens to 0.12 second or greater.

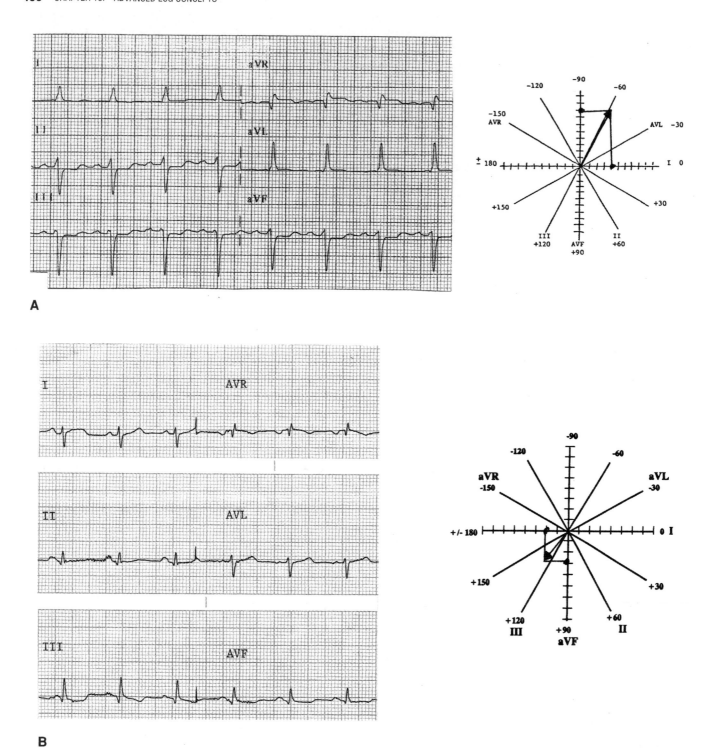

Figure 18–11. (A) Frontal plane leads demonstrating left axis deviation. Lead I is 5 boxes positive; aVF is 2 boxes positive and 10 boxes negative for a net of −8. The axis is −60°. **(B)** Frontal plane leads demonstrating right axis deviation. Lead I is 2 boxes positive and 5 boxes negative for a net of −3; lead aVF is 2 boxes positive. The axis is +150°.

RBBB can be recognized by a wide rSR′ pattern in V_1 and a wide qRs pattern in V_6, I, and aVL, because the positive electrode in these two limb leads is located on the left side of the body. The ECG in Figure 18–13B illustrates RBBB.

Left Bundle Branch Block

Figure 18–14 illustrates the spread of electrical forces through the ventricles when the left bundle branch is blocked. In LBBB, the septum does not depolarize in its normal left-to-right direction because the block occurs above the Pur-

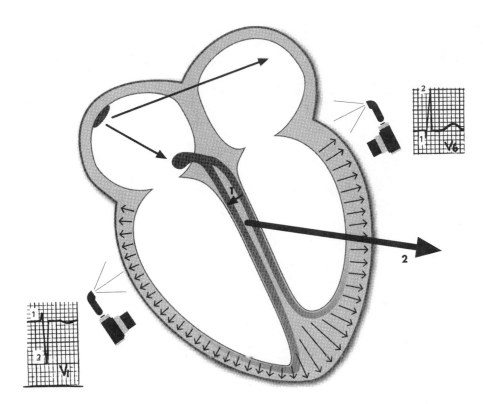

Figure 18-12. Normal ventricular activation as recorded by leads V_1 and V_6. See the text for discussion.

kinje fibers that normally activate the left side of the septum. This results in the loss of the normal small R wave in V_1 and loss of the Q wave in V_6, I, and aVL. Two main forces occur in LBBB:

1. The right ventricle is activated first through the Purkinje fibers (*arrow 1*). Because the right ventricular free wall is so much thinner than that of the left ventricle, forces traveling through it are often not recorded in V_1. Sometimes a small, narrow R wave is recorded in V_1 during LBBB, and this is most likely the result of forces traveling through the right ventricular free wall.

2. The left ventricle depolarizes late and abnormally as the impulse spreads via cell-to-cell conduction through the thick left ventricle (*arrow 2*). This causes V_1 to record a wide negative QS complex as the impulse travels away from its positive electrode. The lateral leads V_6, I, and aVL record a wide R wave as the impulse travels through the large left ventricle toward their positive electrodes. The QRS widens to 0.12 second or greater due to the slow cell-to-cell conduction in the left ventricle.

LBBB can be recognized by a wide QS complex in V_1 and wide R waves with no Q waves in V_6, I, and aVL. The ECG in Figure 18–14B illustrates LBBB.

Myocardial Ischemia, Injury, and Infarction

Myocardial ischemia is the result of an imbalance between myocardial O_2 supply and demand and is a reversible process if blood flow is restored before cellular damage occurs. If ischemia is severe and blood flow is not restored relatively soon, cellular injury and eventually necrosis (infarction) results. When infarction does occur, there are three "zones" of tissue involvement, each of which produces characteristic changes on the ECG (Figure 18–15).

Myocardial ischemia can result in several changes on the ECG (Figure 18–16). The most familiar patterns of ischemia are ST-segment depression of 0.5 mm or more and T-wave inversion. Other indicators of ischemia include an ST segment that remains on the baseline longer than 0.12 second, an ST segment that forms a sharp angle with the T wave, tall, wide-based T waves, and inverted U waves.

Myocardial injury is most often indicated by ST-segment elevation of 1 mm or more above the baseline (Figure 18–17). Other signs of acute injury include an ST segment that slopes up to the peak of the T wave without spending any time on the baseline, tall, peaked T waves, and symmetrical T-wave inversion.

Necrosis or death of myocardial tissue is indicated on the ECG by development of Q waves that are greater than 0.03-second wide. Infarction Q waves are also deeper than normal, with criteria ranging from 2 mm deep to 25% of the R-wave amplitude (see Figures 18–5A and 18–9 for normal Q waves and Figures 18–18 and 18–19 for abnormal Q waves). Traditionally, it was taught that the presence of Q waves indicates transmural MI extending through the entire thickness of the muscle, and that subendocardial infarction involving less than the entire thickness of the muscle does not produce Q waves. Now it is thought that Q waves

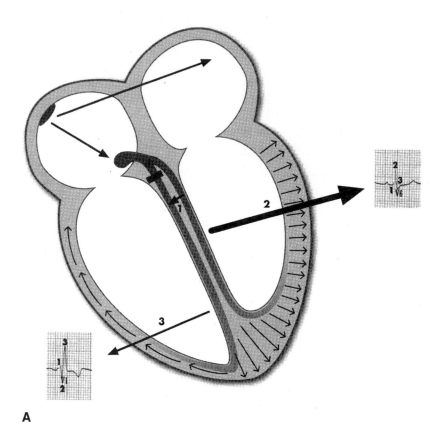

A

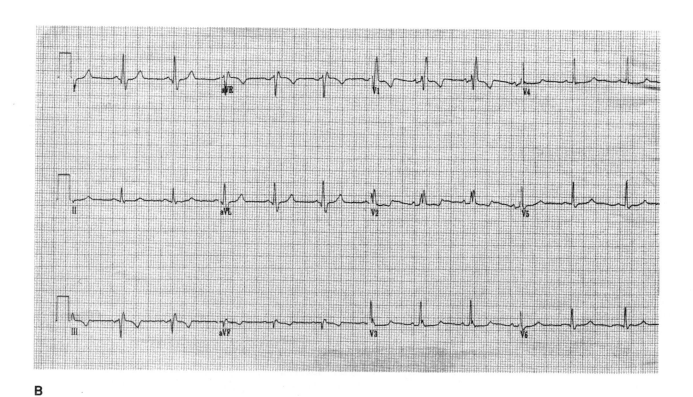

B

Figure 18–13. (A) Ventricular depolarization with RBBB as recorded by leads V_1 and V_6. See the text for details. **(B)** 12-lead ECG illustrating RBBB.

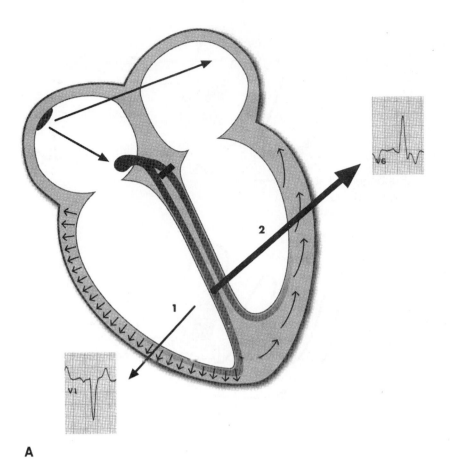

A

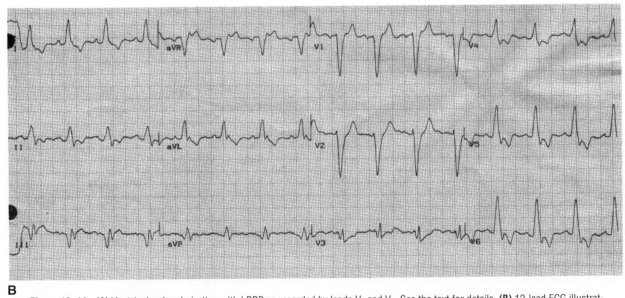

B

Figure 18–14. (A) Ventricular depolarization with LBBB as recorded by leads V_1 and V_6. See the text for details. **(B)** 12-lead ECG illustrating LBBB.

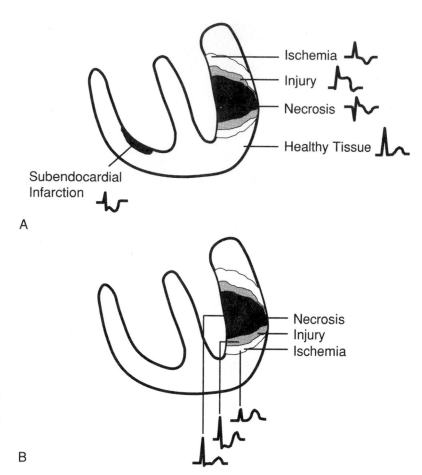

Figure 18–15. Zones of myocardial ischemia, injury, and infarction with associated ECG changes. **(A)** Indicative changes of ischemia, injury, and necrosis seen in leads facing the injured area. **(B)** Reciprocal changes often seen in leads not directly facing the involved area.

can develop transiently with severe ischemia and that infarction can occur without the development of Q waves. Subendocardial infarction is recognized by decreased amplitude of R waves, ST depression, and T-wave inversion. The newer terms *Q-wave* and *non–Q-wave MI* are replacing the older terms of *transmural* and *subendocardial infarction,* respectively. In any case, the presence of Q waves is still considered indicative of myocardial necrosis.

The ECG reflects the evolution of the infarction from the acute stage through the fully evolved stage. Very early MI often causes peaking and widening of the T waves, followed within minutes by ST-segment elevation. ST elevation can persist for hours to several days, but resolves more quickly with successful reperfusion. Once the ST segment has returned to baseline, ECG evidence of the acute infarction stage is lost. Q waves appear within hours of pain onset and usually remain forever, although sometimes Q waves disappear over the years following infarction. T-wave inversion occurs within hours after infarction and can last for months. T waves often return to their previous upright position within a few months after acute MI. Thus an "evolving" infarct is one in which the ECG shows ST segments returning toward baseline, the development of Q waves, and T-wave inversion. The terms *old infarction* or *infarct of in-*

determinate age are used when the first ECG recorded shows Q waves, ST segment at baseline, and T waves either inverted or upright, indicating that an MI occurred at some point in the past.

Locating the Infarction From the ECG

ST-segment elevation, Q waves, and T-wave inversion are recorded in leads facing the damaged myocardium and are called the *indicative changes of infarction.* Leads not facing the involved tissue often show changes related to the loss of electrical forces (depolarization and repolarization) in the damaged tissue. These leads record mirror-image changes that are called *reciprocal changes.* Figure 18–15 illustrates indicative and reciprocal changes associated with MI, and Table 18–2 lists leads in which indicative and reciprocal changes are found in each of the major types of MI.

Anterior wall MI is recognized by indicative changes in leads facing the anterior wall precordial leads V_1 to V_4 (see Figure 18–18). Reciprocal changes are often recorded in the lateral leads I and aVL, as well as in the inferior leads II, III, and aVF. Inferior wall MI is diagnosed by indicative changes in leads II, III, and aVF (see Figure 18–19). Reciprocal changes are often seen in leads I and aVL and/or the V leads. Lateral wall MI presents with indicative changes in leads I,

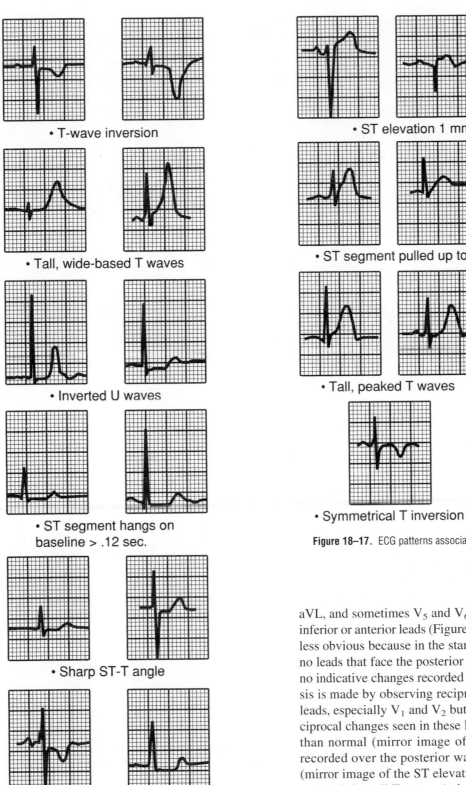

- T-wave inversion

- Tall, wide-based T waves

- Inverted U waves

- ST segment hangs on
baseline > .12 sec.

- Sharp ST-T angle

- ST depression
(horizontal or downsloping)

Figure 18–16. ECG patterns associated with myocardial ischemia.

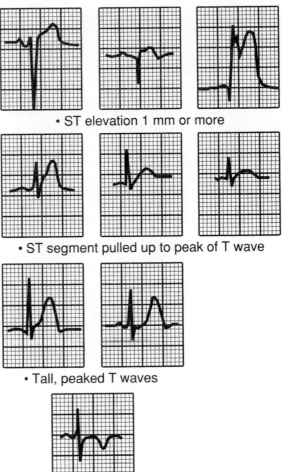

- ST elevation 1 mm or more

- ST segment pulled up to peak of T wave

- Tall, peaked T waves

- Symmetrical T inversion

Figure 18–17. ECG patterns associated with acute myocardial injury.

aVL, and sometimes V_5 and V_6, with reciprocal changes in inferior or anterior leads (Figure 18–20). Posterior wall MI is less obvious because in the standard 12-lead ECG there are no leads that face the posterior wall, and therefore there are no indicative changes recorded (Figure 18–21). The diagnosis is made by observing reciprocal changes in the anterior leads, especially V_1 and V_2 but often all the way to V_4. Reciprocal changes seen in these leads include a taller R wave than normal (mirror image of the Q wave that would be recorded over the posterior wall), ST-segment depression (mirror image of the ST elevation from the posterior wall), and upright, tall T waves (mirror image of the T-wave inversion from the posterior wall).

Right ventricular MI occurs in up to 45% of inferior MIs; therefore, it usually is associated with indicative changes in the inferior leads II, III, and aVF (Figure 18–22). In addition, it is not uncommon to see ST elevation in V_1 as well, because V_1 is the chest lead that is closest to the right

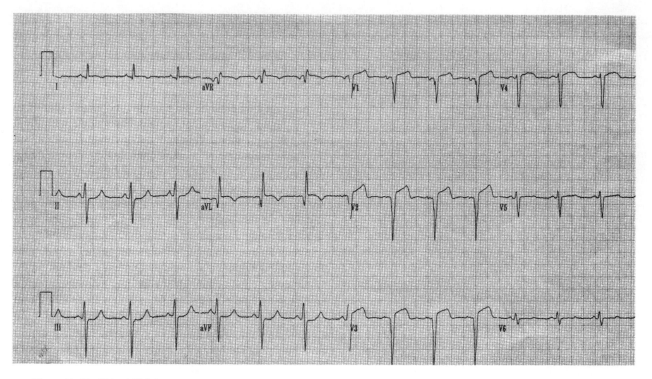

Figure 18–18. 12-lead ECG demonstrating acute anterior wall MI. Q waves are present in V_1 to V_3 and ST-segment elevation is present in V_1 to V_4. An abnormal Q wave is also present in aVL.

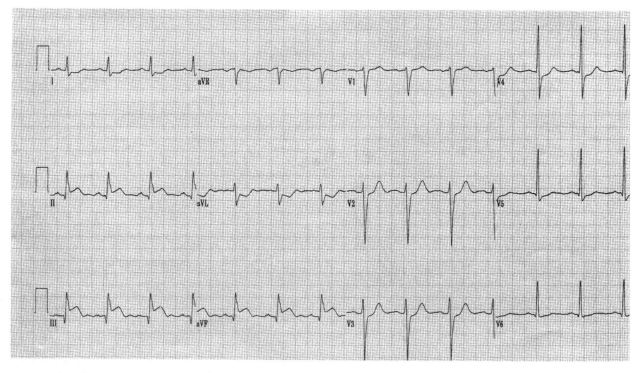

Figure 18–19. 12-lead ECG demonstrating acute inferior wall MI. ST elevation is present in II, III, and aVF; reciprocal ST depression is present in I, aVL, and V_2 to V_4. Q waves can be seen in III and aVF.

TABLE 18–2. ECG CHANGES ASSOCIATED WITH MYOCARDIAL INFARCTION

Location of MI	Indicative Changes	Reciprocal Changes
Anterior	V_1 to V_4	I, aVL, II, III, aVF
Septal	V_1, V_2	I, aVL
Inferior	II, III, aVF	I, aVL, V_1 to V_4
Posterior	None	V_1 to V_4
Lateral	I, aVL, V_5, V_6	II, III, aVF, V_1, V_2
Right ventricle	V_3R to V_6R	

ventricle. ST elevation in V_1, together with ST elevation in the inferior leads, is suspicious for right ventricular MI. Another clue is discordance between the ST segment in V_1 and the ST segment in V_2. Normally, when the ST segment in V_1 is elevated, it is related to anterior or septal MI, in which case the ST in V_2 is also elevated. *Discordance* means that the ST segments do not point in the same direction—V_1 shows ST elevation while V_2 is either normal or shows ST depression. This finding is suspicious of right ventricular MI. When right ventricular MI is suspected, right-sided chest leads should be obtained (Figure 18–23). Leads V_3R through V_6R develop ST elevation when acute right ventricular MI is present. Lead V_4R is the most sensitive and specific lead for recognition of right ventricular MI.

Preexcitation Syndromes

Preexcitation means early activation of the ventricle by supraventricular impulses that reach the ventricle through an accessory conduction pathway faster than they travel through the AV node. Many people have tracts of tissue, often referred to as "bypass tracts" or "accessory pathways," that can carry electrical impulses directly from atria to ventricles, bypassing the delay in the AV node and causing early and abnormal depolarization of the ventricles. These accessory pathways can be found anywhere around the tricuspid or mitral valve rings. The most common type of preexcitation syndrome is the Wolff-Parkinson-White syndrome, in which the impulse travels down the accessory pathway from the atria directly into the ventricles, completely bypassing AV node delay. Other anatomic connections exist that can bypass the normal AV node delay or create connections between different parts of the conduction system and the ventricles and cause variations of the preexcitation pattern. Fibers originating in the atria and inserting into the His bundle have been demonstrated anatomically and can result in a short PR interval and normal QRS complex (formerly called Lown-Ganong-Levine syndrome).

Wolff-Parkinson-White Syndrome

In Wolff-Parkinson-White syndrome, the ventricle is stimulated prematurely by an electrical impulse traveling through the accessory pathway while the impulse simultaneously

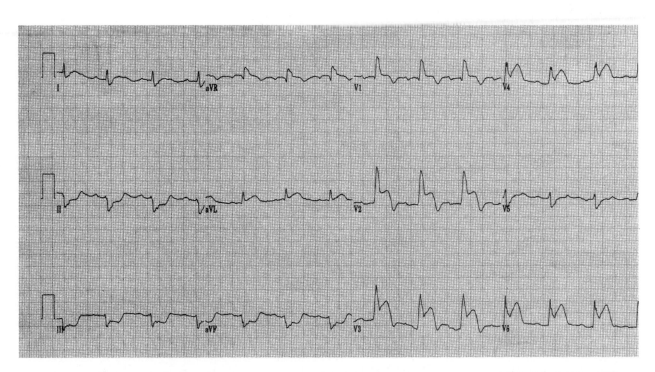

Figure 18–20. 12-lead ECG demonstrating acute anterolateral wall MI. ST elevation is present in I, aVL, V_2 to V_4, and V_6. Reciprocal ST depression is present in III, aVF, and aVR.

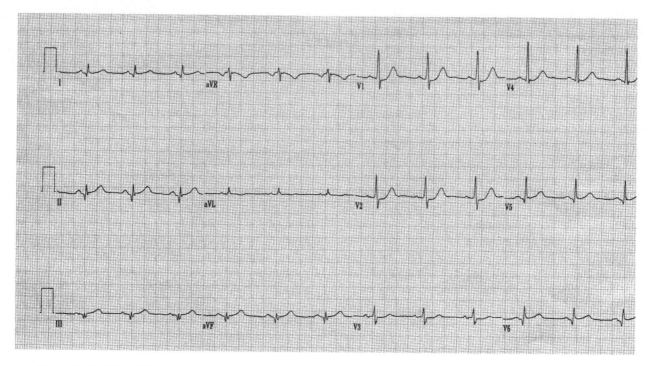

Figure 18–21. 12-lead ECG demonstrating posterior wall MI. Large R waves and ST depression are present in V_1 and V_2. Q waves and wide-based T waves in II, III, and aVF probably indicate inferior infarction as well.

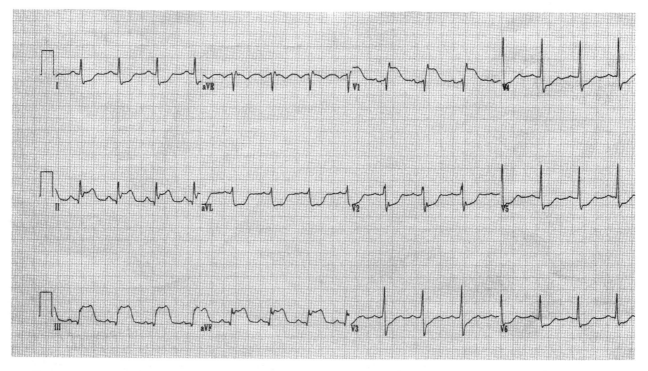

Figure 18–22. 12-lead ECG demonstrating acute right ventricular MI. ST elevation is present in II, III, aVF, and V_1; reciprocal ST depression is present in all other leads. Note the discordant ST elevation in V_1 and ST depression in V_2.

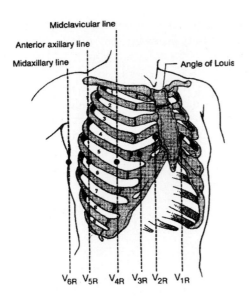

Figure 18–23. Right side chest lead placement. (*From Drew BJ, Ide B: Right ventricular infarction.* Prog Cardiovasc Nurs *1995;10:54–46.*)

descends normally through the AV node (Figure 18–24A). Impulses travel faster through the accessory pathway because they bypass the normal AV node delay. Part of the ventricle receives the impulse early via the accessory pathway and begins to depolarize before the rest of the ventricle is activated through the His–Purkinje system. Early stimulation of the ventricle results in a short PR interval and a widened QRS complex as the impulse begins to depolarize the ventricle via muscle cell-to-cell conduction. Premature stimulation of the ventricle causes a characteristic slurring of the initial part of the QRS complex, called a delta wave. The remainder of the QRS complex is normal because the rest of the ventricle is depolarized normally through the Purkinje system. This preexcitation results in ventricular fusion beats as the ventricles are depolarized simultaneously by the impulse coming through the accessory pathway and through the normal AV node. The degree of preexcitation varies, depending on the relative rates of conduction down the accessory pathway and through the AV node, and it determines the length of the PR interval and size of the delta wave (Figures 18–24A to 18–24C).

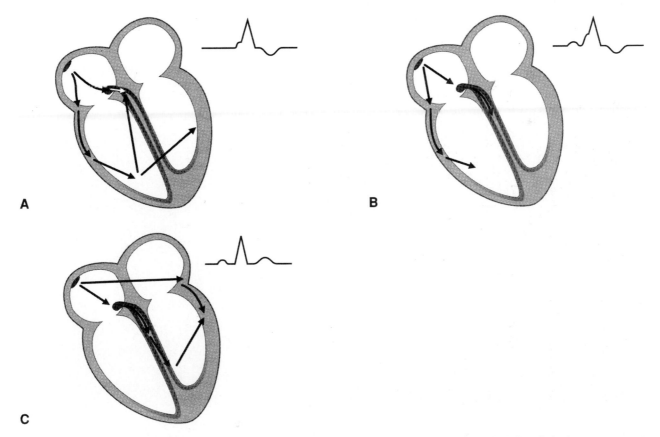

Figure 18–24. Varying degrees of preexcitation. **(A)** Maximal preexcitation when the ventricles are activated totally by the accessory pathway. **(B)** Less-than-maximal preexcitation when the ventricles are activated by the impulse traveling through both the accessory pathway and the normal AV conduction system. **(C)** Concealed accessory pathway. The ventricles are activated through the normal AV conduction system with no participation of the accessory pathway, resulting in a normal PR interval and normal QRS complex.

Wolff-Parkinson-White syndrome is recognized on the ECG by the presence of a short PR interval (<0.12 second) and delta waves in many leads. Figures 18–25 and 18–26 show two examples of this type of pattern. Preexcitation syndromes are clinically significant because the presence of two pathways into the ventricle is a setup for reentrant tachycardias, which occur frequently in people with accessory pathways and are a part of the "syndrome" of Wolff-Parkinson-White. See the section on supraventricular tachycardias later in this chapter for more information on arrhythmias associated with accessory pathways.

Treatment

Wolff-Parkinson-White syndrome does not require treatment unless it is associated with symptomatic tachycardias. Specific therapy depends on the mechanism of the tachyarrhythmia, the effect of drugs on conduction through the AV node and the accessory pathway, and on the patient's tolerance of

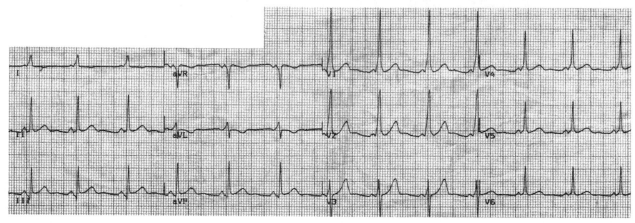

A

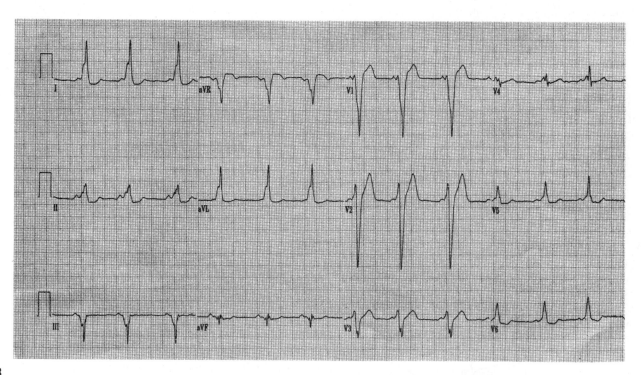

B

Figure 18–25. (A) 12-lead ECG demonstrating Wolff-Parkinson-White syndrome with short PR interval and delta waves. Lead V₁ is positive, sometimes called type A Wolff-Parkinson-White syndrome, indicating a posterior accessory pathway. (*From: Jacobson C: Arrhythmias and conduction disturbances. In Woods SL, et al [eds]: Cardiac Nursing, 3rd ed, p. 338. Philadelphia: JB Lippincott; 1995.*) **(B)** Wolff-Parkinson-White syndrome with short PR and delta waves with a negative V₁, sometimes called type B Wolff-Parkinson-White syndrome, indicating an anterior or right-sided accessory pathway.

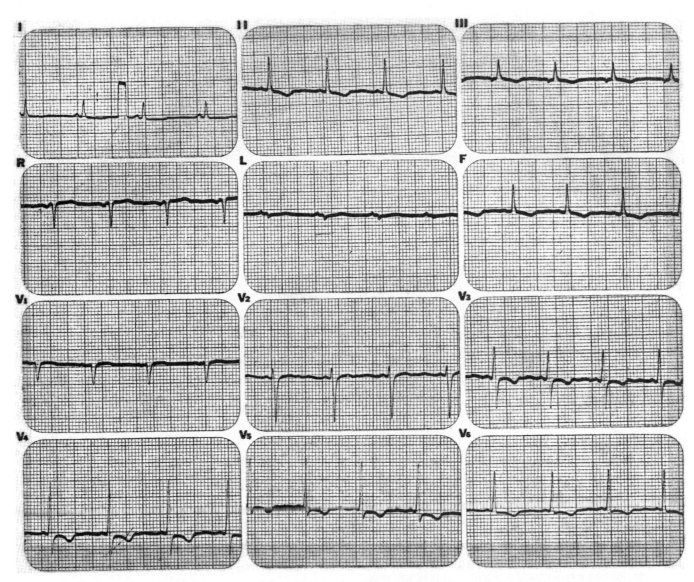

Figure 18–26. ECG demonstrating a short PR interval and normal QRS (formerly called Lown-Ganong-Levine pattern). (*From Jacobson C: Arrhythmias and conduction disturbances. In Woods SL, et al [eds]: Cardiac Nursing, 3rd ed, p. 339. Philadelphia: JB Lippincott; 1995.*)

the arrhythmia. The section on supraventricular tachycardias later in this chapter discusses drug treatment of tachycardias associated with accessory pathways.

Radio-frequency (RF) catheter ablation of the bypass tract provides a cure for the tachyarrhythmias associated with accessory pathways in many patients. RF ablation is an invasive procedure that requires the introduction of several catheters into the heart through the venous and sometimes arterial systems. An electrophysiology study is done first to record intracardiac signals and determine the mechanism of the tachycardia. The electrophysiology study confirms the presence and location of the accessory pathway, participation of the pathway in maintaining the tachycardia, and conduction characteristics of the accessory pathway. A special ablation catheter is then positioned next to the bypass tract

and RF energy is delivered through the catheter to the tract, destroying the tissue and preventing it from being able to conduct. Permanent tissue damage in the accessory pathway is the goal of RF ablation, and when successful, it prevents further episodes of tachycardia.

ADVANCED ARRHYTHMIA INTERPRETATION

The study of cardiac rhythms provides a never-ending challenge to those interested in learning about arrhythmias. In most basic ECG classes the content presented is limited to basic rhythms originating in the sinus node, atria, AV junction, and ventricles, and to basic AV conduction abnormalities. Rarely does time permit the inclusion of more advanced concepts. This section discusses some of these more advanced concepts of arrhythmia interpretation and provides clues to aid in recognition of selected arrhythmias not usually covered in a basic course.

Supraventricular Tachycardias

Supraventricular tachycardia (SVT) describes a rapid rhythm that arises above the level of the ventricles (atria or AV junction) but whose exact origin is not known. Usually, *SVT* is used to describe a narrow QRS tachycardia where atrial activity (P waves) cannot be identified, and therefore the origin of the tachycardia cannot be determined from the surface ECG. The presence of the narrow QRS indicates the supraventricular origin of the rhythm and conduction through the normal His–Purkinje system into the ventricles. Sometimes SVT conducts with bundle branch block, which results in a wide QRS but does not change the fact that the rhythm is supraventricular in origin. Thus, *SVT* can be used for narrow QRS tachycardias whose mechanism is uncertain or for wide QRS tachycardias that are known to be coming from above the ventricles.

SVTs can be classified into those that are AV nodal passive and those that are AV nodal active. *AV nodal passive SVTs* are those in which the AV node is not required for the maintenance of the tachycardia but serves only to passively conduct supraventricular impulses into the ventricles. Examples of AV nodal passive arrhythmias include atrial tachycardia, atrial flutter, and atrial fibrillation, all of which originate within the atria and do not need the AV node to sustain the atrial arrhythmia. In these rhythms, the AV node passively conducts the atrial impulses into the ventricles but does not participate in the maintenance of the arrhythmia itself. *AV nodal active tachycardias* require participation of the AV node in the maintenance of the tachycardia. The two most common causes of a regular, narrow QRS tachycardia are AV nodal reentry tachycardia and circus movement tachycardia using an accessory pathway, both of which require the active participation of the AV node in maintaining the tachycardia.

Atrial fibrillation is a supraventricular rhythm that is usually easily recognized because of its irregularity, but atrial tachycardia, atrial flutter, junctional tachycardia, AV nodal reentry tachycardia, and circus movement tachycardia can all present as regular narrow QRS tachycardias whose mechanism often cannot be determined from the ECG. Because AV nodal reentry tachycardia and circus movement tachycardia are the most common causes of a regular narrow QRS tachycardia, they are discussed in detail here.

Atrioventricular Nodal Reentry Tachycardia

In people with AV nodal reentry tachycardia (AVNRT), the AV node has two pathways that are capable of conducting the impulse into the ventricles. One pathway conducts more rapidly and has a longer refractory period than the other

pathway (Figure 18–27A). In AVNRT, a reentry circuit is set up within the AV node, usually using the slow pathway as the antegrade limb into the ventricle and the fast pathway as the retrograde limb back into the atria (Figure 18–27C).

The sinus impulse normally conducts down the fast pathway into the ventricles, resulting in a normal PR interval of 0.12 to 0.20 second. If a PAC occurs and enters the AV node before the fast pathway with its longer refractory period has recovered its ability to conduct, the impulse conducts down the slow pathway into the ventricle because of its shorter refractory period (Figure 18–27B). This slow conduction causes the PR interval of the PAC to be longer than the PR interval of sinus beats. The long conduction time through the slow pathway allows the fast pathway time to recover, making it possible for the impulse to conduct backward through the fast pathway into the atria. This returning impulse may then reenter the slow pathway, which is again ready to conduct antegrade because of its short refractory period, thus setting up a reentry circuit within the AV node and resulting in AVNRT. Figure 18–27C illustrates the mechanism of the most common type of AVNRT in which antegrade conduction occurs over the slow pathway and retrograde conduction over the fast pathway. The resulting rhythm is usually a narrow QRS tachycardia because the ventricles are activated through the normal His–Purkinje system. P waves are either not seen at all or are barely visible peeking out at the tail end of the QRS complex because the atria and ventricles depolarize almost simultaneously (Figure 18–28). In the presence of preexisting bundle branch block or rate-dependent bundle branch block, the QRS in AVNRT is wide.

In about 4% of cases of AVNRT, the impulse conducts antegrade into the ventricle through the fast pathway and retrograde into the atria through the slow pathway, reversing the circuit within the AV node. This reversal of the circuit in the AV node results in P waves that appear immediately in front of the QRS because atrial activation is delayed because of slow conduction backward through the slow pathway. These P waves are inverted in inferior leads because the atria depolarize in a retrograde direction.

Treatment

AVNRT is an AV nodal active SVT because the AV node is required for the maintenance of the tachycardia. Therefore, anything that causes block in the AV node, such as vagal stimulation or drugs like adenosine, beta-blockers, or calcium channel blockers, can terminate the rhythm. AVNRT is usually well tolerated unless the rate is extremely rapid. Episodes can become frequent and, if not controlled with drugs, can interfere with lifestyle. Many people learn to stop the rhythm by coughing or breath holding, which stimulates the vagus nerve. Acute medical treatment involves administering any drug that blocks AV node conduction, but adenosine is usually used first because of its rapid effect, short duration of action, and lack of significant side effects. RF ablation can destroy the slow pathway and prevent recurrence of the arrhythmia.

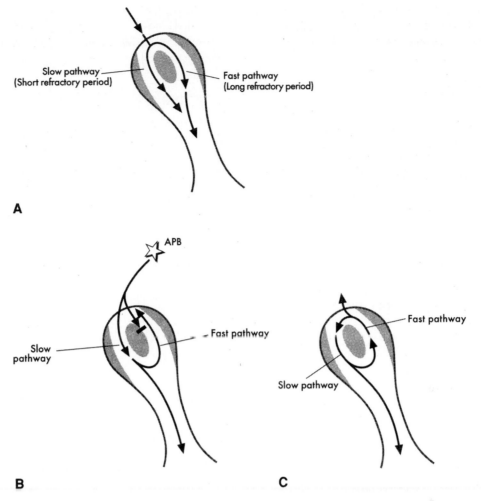

Figure 18–27. **(A)** Illustration of two conduction pathways within the AV node. The fast conducting pathway has a longer refractory period than the slow conducting pathway. Normal conduction occurs through the fast pathway. **(B)** A PAC finds the fast pathway still refractory so it conducts to the ventricle through the slow pathway, resulting in a long PR interval. Slow conduction through the slow pathway allows the fast pathway to recover and allows retrograde conduction. **(C)** Reentry within the AV node using the slow pathway as the antegrade limb and the fast pathway as the retrograde limb of the circuit, resulting in AVNRT. Atrial and ventricular depolarization occur simultaneously. (*From Marriott HJL, Conover M:* Advanced Concepts in Arrhythmias, *2nd ed, pp. 121–123. St. Louis, MO: Mosby; 1989.*)

Circus Movement Tachycardia

Circus movement tachycardia is an SVT that occurs in people who have accessory pathways (see the section on preexcitation syndromes above). *AV reentrant tachycardia* (AVRT) is also used to describe this arrhythmia, but to avoid confusion between AVRT and AVNRT, *circus movement tachycardia* is used here.

In circus movement tachycardia, an impulse travels a reentry circuit that involves the atria, AV node, ventricles, and accessory pathway. *Orthodromic* is used to describe the most common type of circus movement tachycardia, in which the impulse travels antegrade through the AV node into the ventricles and retrograde back into the atria through the accessory pathway (Figure 18–29A). The result is a regular narrow QRS tachycardia because the ventricles are activated through the normal His–Purkinje system. In the presence of bundle branch block a wide QRS pattern is present. Because the atria and ventricles depolarize separately, P waves, if visible at all, are seen following the QRS complex in the ST segment or between two QRS complexes, usually closest to the first QRS.

Antidromic describes the rare form of circus movement tachycardia in which the accessory pathway conducts the impulse from atria to ventricles and the AV node conducts it retrograde back to the atria (see Figure 18–28B). Antidromic circus movement tachycardia is a regular wide QRS tachycardia because the ventricles depolarize abnormally through the accessory pathway. This form of SVT is often indistinguishable from ventricular tachycardia on the ECG.

Treatment

Circus movement tachycardia is an AV nodal active tachycardia because the AV node is necessary for maintenance of

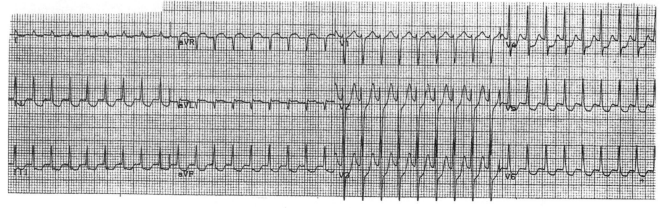

A

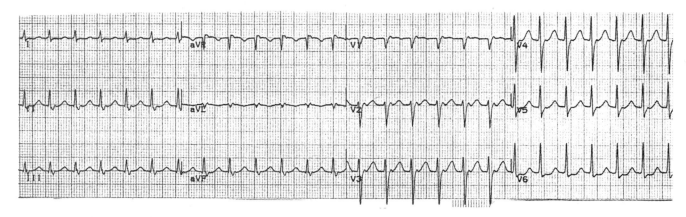

Figure 18–28. (A) AVNRT, rate 214. No P waves are visible. **(B)** AVNRT, rate 150. P waves distort the end of the QRS complex in leads II, III, aVF, and V₁ to V₃. (*From Jacobson C: Arrhythmias and conduction disturbances. In Woods SL, et al [eds]: Cardiac Nursing, 3rd ed, p. 341. Philadelphia: JB Lippincott; 1995.*)

the arrhythmia. Vagal maneuvers and drugs that block AV conduction can be used to terminate an episode of tachycardia. Acute treatment is aimed at slowing conduction through the AV node with adenosine, beta-blockers, or calcium channel blockers, or at slowing accessory pathway conduction with drugs like procainamide or amiodarone. Chronic therapy with class IC drugs (moricizine, flecainide, propafenone), or amiodarone can be used to slow conduction through the accessory pathway and the AV node, and may also suppress PACs and PVCs that initiate the tachycardia RF ablation of the accessory pathway has become the first line treatment for circus movement tachycardia.

Atrial Fibrillation in Wolff-Parkinson-White Syndrome

Atrial fibrillation occurs more frequently in people with accessory pathways than in the general population and can be life threatening. Atrial flutter and fibrillation are especially dangerous in the presence of an accessory pathway because the pathway can conduct impulses rapidly and without delay into the ventricles, resulting in dangerously fast ventricular rates (Figure 18–30). These rapid ventricular rates can degenerate into ventricular fibrillation and result in sudden

death. When atrial fibrillation is the mechanism of the tachycardia in Wolff-Parkinson-White syndrome, the QRS complex is wide and bizarre due to conduction of the impulses into the ventricle through the bypass tract. The ventricular response to the atrial fibrillation is irregular and very rapid, often approaching rates of 300 beats/min or more due to lack of delay in conduction through the accessory pathway. Atrial fibrillation with accessory pathway conduction must be recognized and differentiated from atrial fibrillation conducting through the AV node because treatment is different for the two situations. When accessory pathway conduction is known or suspected, the drug of choice is procainamide because it prolongs the refractory period of the accessory pathway and slows ventricular rate. Verapamil often is used to slow AV conduction in atrial fibrillation conducting into the ventricles through the AV node, but can be very dangerous and even lethal when used in the presence of an accessory pathway. Digitalis, verapamil, diltiazem, and similar calcium channel blocking agents can shorten the refractory period in the accessory pathway, resulting in even faster ventricular rates and degeneration into ventricular fibrillation. In addition, the hypotensive effects of these agents may inten-

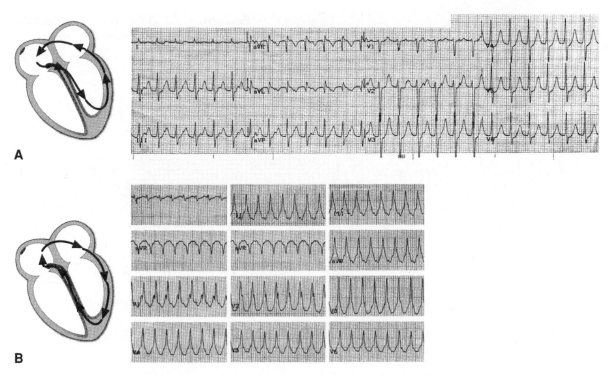

Figure 18–29. **(A)** Orthodromic circus movement tachycardia. P waves are visible on the upstroke of the T wave in leads II, III, aVF, and V₁ to V₃. (*From Jacobson C: Arrhythmias and conduction disturbances. In Woods SL, et al [eds]*: Cardiac Nursing, *3rd ed, p. 342. Philadelphia: JB Lippincott; 1995.*) **(B)** Antidromic circus movement tachycardia.

sify the hypotension related to the arrhythmia's rapid ventricular rate.

Differentiating Wide QRS Beats and Rhythms

Determining the origin of a wide QRS beat or a wide QRS tachycardia is one of the most common problems encountered when caring for monitored patients. A supraventricular beat with abnormal, or aberrant, conduction through the ventricles, can look almost identical to a beat that originates in the ventricle. The problem with aberration is that it can mimic ventricular arrhythmias, which require different therapy and carry a different prognosis than aberrancy. Aberrancy is always secondary to some other primary disturbance and does not itself require treatment. Nurses must be able to identify accurately which mechanism is responsible for the wide QRS rhythm be-

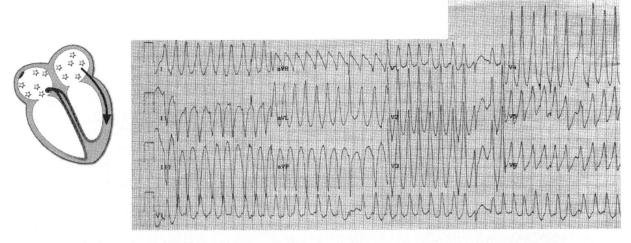

Figure 18–30. Atrial fibrillation conducting into the ventricle through an accessory pathway. Note the extremely short RR intervals in the V leads. QRS is fast, wide, and irregular.

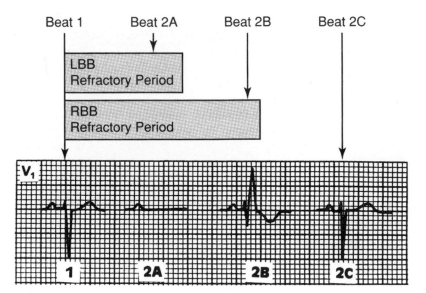

Figure 18–31. Diagram of refractory periods in the bundle branches and the effect of cycle length on conduction. The right bundle has a longer refractory period than the left. Beat 2A occurs so early that it cannot conduct through either bundle branch. Beat 2B encounters a refractory right bundle and conducts with RBBB. Beat 2C falls outside the refractory period of both bundles and is able to conduct normally.

ing observed whenever possible, initiate appropriate treatment when needed, and avoid inappropriate treatment.

Mechanisms of Aberration

Aberrancy is the temporary abnormal intraventricular conduction of supraventricular impulses. Aberration occurs whenever the His–Purkinje system or ventricle is still partly refractory when a supraventricular impulse attempts to travel through it. The refractory period of the conduction system is directly proportional to preceding cycle length. Long cycles are followed by long refractory periods, and short cycles are followed by short refractory periods. An early supraventricular beat, such as a PAC, may enter the conduction system during a portion of its refractory period, forcing conduction through the ventricles to occur in an abnormal manner. Beats that follow a sudden lengthening of the cycle may conduct aberrantly because of the increased length of the refractory period that occurs when the cycle lengthens (Figure 18–31). The right bundle branch has a longer refractory period than the left; therefore, aberrant beats tend to conduct most often with a RBBB pattern, although LBBB aberration is common in people with cardiac disease.

Electrocardiographic Clues to the Origin of Wide QRS Beats and Rhythms

P Waves

If P waves can be seen during a wide QRS tachycardia, they are very helpful in making the differential diagnosis of aberration versus ventricular ectopy. Atrial activity, represented by the P wave on the ECG and preceding a wide QRS beat or run of tachycardia, strongly favors a supraventricular origin of the arrhythmia. Figure 18–32 shows three wide QRS beats that could easily be mistaken for PVCs if not for the obvious presence of the early P wave initiating the run.

An exception to the preceding P-wave rule occurs with end-diastolic PVCs. *End-diastolic PVCs* occur at the end of diastole, after the sinus P wave has been recorded but before it has a chance to conduct through the AV node into the ventricle. Figure 18–33 shows sinus rhythm with an end-

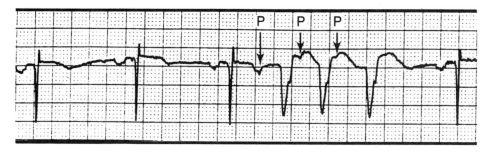

Figure 18–32. Sinus rhythm with PACs and three wide QRS beats that could be mistaken for ventricular tachycardia. The second beat in the strip is a PAC that conducts normally. Note the P waves preceding the wide QRS complexes, indicating aberrant conduction. (*From: Jacobson C: Arrhythmias and conduction disturbances. In Woods SL, et al [eds]: Cardiac Nursing, 3rd ed, p. 346. Philadelphia: JB Lippincott; 1995.*)

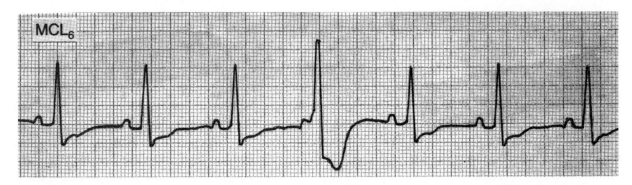

Figure 18–33. Sinus rhythm with an end-diastolic PVC. The P wave preceding the PVC is the sinus P wave that coincidentally occurs just before the PVC. (*From Jacobson C: Arrhythmias and conduction disturbances. In Woods SL, et al [eds]*: Cardiac Nursing, *3rd ed, p. 347. Philadelphia: JB Lippincott; 1995.*)

diastolic PVC occurring immediately after the sinus P wave. Here, the P wave preceding the wide QRS is merely a coincidence and does not indicate aberrant conduction. The PR interval is much too short to have conducted that QRS complex. In addition, the P wave preceding the wide QRS is not early; it is the regularly scheduled sinus beat coming on time. Thus, early P waves that precede early wide QRS complexes are usually "married to" those QRSs and indicate aberrant conduction, while "on-time" P waves in front of end-diastolic PVCs are not early and do not cause the wide QRS.

P waves seen during a wide QRS tachycardia also can be very helpful in making the differential diagnosis between SVTs with aberration and ventricular tachycardia. If P waves are seen associated with every QRS, the rhythm is supraven-

tricular in origin (Figure 18–34A). P waves that occur independently of the QRS and have no consistent relationship to QRS complexes indicate the presence of AV dissociation, which means that the atria and the ventricles are under the control of separate pacemakers and strongly favors ventricular tachycardia (Figure 18–34B).

QRS Morphology

The shape of the QRS complex is very helpful in determining the origin of a wide QRS rhythm. When using QRS morphology clues, it is extremely important to examine the correct leads and apply the criteria only to leads that have been proven helpful. Many practitioners prefer to monitor with lead II because usually it shows an upright QRS

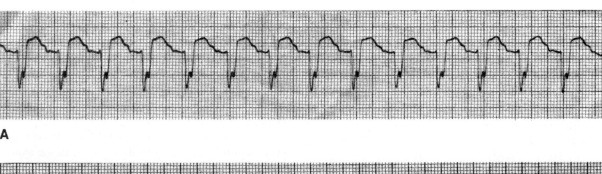

A

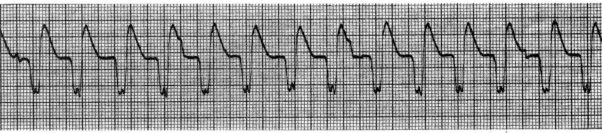

B

Figure 18–34. Two very similar wide QRS tachycardias. **(A)** Sinus tachycardia, rate 115. P waves can be seen on the downslope of the T wave preceding each QRS, indicating a supraventricular origin of the tachycardia. **(B)** P waves are independent of QRS complexes, indicating AV dissociation, which favors ventricular tachycardia. (*From Jacobson C: Arrhythmias and conduction disturbances. In Woods SL, et al [eds]*: Cardiac Nursing, *3rd ed, p. 347. Philadelphia: JB Lippincott; 1995.*)

complex and clear P wave. Lead II, however, has no value in determining the origin of a wide QRS rhythm. The single best arrhythmia monitoring lead is V_1, followed by V_6 and V_2 in certain situations.

When applying QRS morphology criteria for wide QRS rhythms, it is helpful to first decide whether the QRS complexes have a RBBB morphology or a LBBB morphology (Figure 18–35). RBBB morphology rhythms have an upright QRS in lead V_1, while LBBB morphology rhythms have a negative QRS complex in V_1.

When dealing with a wide QRS rhythm of RBBB morphology (upright in V_1), follow these steps to evaluate QRS morphology (Figures 18–35 and 18–36A):

1. Look at V_1 and determine if the upright QRS complex is monophasic (R wave), diphasic (qR), or triphasic

RBBB MORPHOLOGY

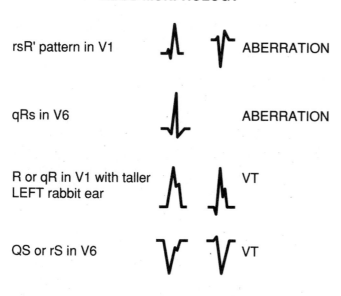

rsR' pattern in V1   ABERRATION

qRs in V6   ABERRATION

R or qR in V1 with taller LEFT rabbit ear   VT

QS or rS in V6   VT

LBBB MORPHOLOGY

In Leads V1 or V2:

Wide R (>.03 sec) Slurred downstroke >.06 sec to nadir of S   VT

Any Q (qR or QS) in V6   VT

Figure 18–35. Morphology clues for wide QRS beats and rhythms with RBBB and LBBB patterns. (*From Jacobson, C: Arrhythmias and conduction disturbances. In Woods SL, et al [eds]: Cardiac Nursing, 3rd ed, p. 348. Philadelphia: JB Lippincott; 1995.*)

(rsR'). Monophasic and diphasic complexes favor a ventricular origin, whereas the triphasic rsR' is typical of RBBB aberration in V_1.

2. Look at V_6 and determine if the QRS is monophasic (all negative QS), diphasic (rS), or triphasic (qRs). A monophasic or diphasic complex in V_6 favors a ventricular origin, and the triphasic qRs complex is typical of RBBB aberration in V_6.

3. If the QRS in V_1 has "rabbit ears" (two peaks), determine if the left or the right rabbit ear is taller. A taller left rabbit ear favors a ventricular origin, whereas a taller right rabbit ear does not favor either diagnosis.

If the QRS has a LBBB morphology (negative in V_1), follow these steps to evaluate morphology (Figures 18–35 and 18–36B):

1. Look at V_1 or V_2 (both are helpful in this case) and determine if the R wave (if present) is wide or narrow. A wide R wave of more than 0.03 second favors a ventricular rhythm, and a narrow R wave favors a supraventricular origin with LBBB aberration.

2. Next look at the downstroke of the S wave in V_1 or V_2. Slurring or notching on the downstroke favors a ventricular origin. LBBB aberration typically slurs on the upstroke if it slurs at all.

3. Measure from the onset of the QRS complex to the deepest part of the S wave in V_1 or V_2. A measurement of more than 0.06 second favors a ventricular rhythm and a narrower measurement favors LBBB aberration. Note that this measurement can be prolonged due to either a wide R wave or slurring on the downstroke of the S wave, either one of which favors the ventricular origin of the rhythm.

4. Look at V_6 and determine if a Q wave is present. Any Q wave (either a QS or qR complex) favors a ventricular origin.

Concordance

Concordance means that all the QRS complexes across the precordium from V_1 through V_6 point in the same direction; positive concordance means they are all upright, and negative concordance means they are all negative (Figure 18–37A). Negative concordance favors a diagnosis of ventricular tachycardia when it occurs in a wide QRS tachycardia, and positive concordance favors ventricular tachycardia as long as Wolff-Parkinson-White syndrome can be ruled out.

FUSION AND CAPTURE BEATS

Ventricular fusion beats occur when the ventricles are depolarized by two different wavefronts of electrical activity at the same time. Fusion often results when a supraventricular impulse travels through the AV node and begins to depolarize the ventricles at the same time that an impulse from a

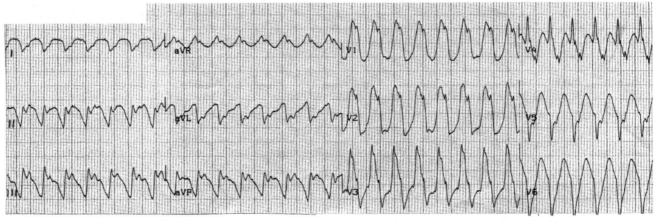

A

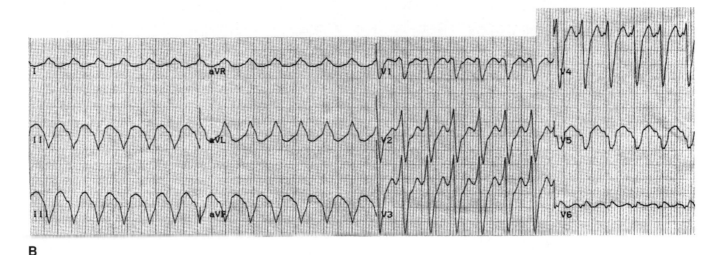

B

Figure 18–36. 12-lead ECG of ventricular tachycardia. **(A)** With RBBB morphology. Note monophasic R wave with taller left rabbit ear in V_1 and QS complex in V_6. **(B)** With LBBB morphology. Note wide R wave in V_1 and V_2, and qR pattern in V_6.

ventricular focus depolarizes the ventricles. When two different impulses contribute to ventricular depolarization, the resulting QRS shape and width are determined by the relative contributions of both the supraventricular and the ventricular impulses. In the presence of a wide QRS tachycardia, the presence of fusion beats indicates AV dissociation, which means that the atria and ventricles are under the control of separate pacemakers. Capture beats occur when the supraventricular impulse manages to conduct all the way into and through the ventricle, depolarizing ("capturing") the ventricle and resulting in a normal QRS in the midst of the wide QRS tachycardia. The presence of fusion and capture beats in a wide QRS tachycardia is strong evidence supporting the diagnosis of ventricular tachycardia, but they occur rarely and cannot be counted on to make the diagnosis. Figure 18–37B shows fusion beats in a wide QRS tachycardia. Helpful ECG clues for differentiating aberrancy from ventricular ectopy are summarized in Table 18–3.

ST-SEGMENT MONITORING

Many bedside monitors have software programs that allow for continuous monitoring of the ST segment in addition to routine arrhythmia monitoring. Continuous ST-segment monitoring can detect ischemia related to reocclusion of the involved artery in patients with acute MI who have received thrombolytic therapy, angioplasty, or other interventional cardiologic procedures aimed at opening occluded coronary arteries. ST-segment monitoring is also useful in detecting silent ischemia (ischemic episodes that occur in the absence of chest pain or other symptoms) that would otherwise go unnoticed with symptom and arrhythmia monitoring alone. Early detection of ischemic changes is critical in identifying patients who need interventions to reestablish blood flow to myocardium before permanent damage occurs.

ST elevation in leads facing damaged myocardium is the ECG sign of myocardial injury. ST depression is often

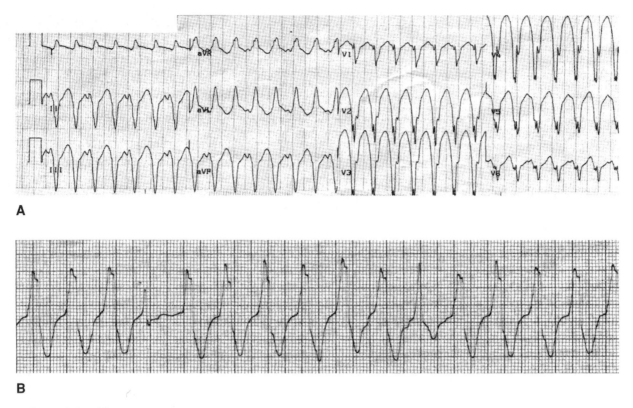

Figure 18–37. (A) 12-lead ECG of ventricular tachycardia with negative concordance. **(B)** Rhythm strips of ventricular tachycardia with fusion beats.

recorded as a reciprocal change in leads that do not directly face involved myocardium. In addition, ST depression can be recorded in leads facing ischemic tissue. Therefore, either ST elevation or ST depression indicates myocardium at risk for infarction and a patient potentially at risk for complications related to infarction. The sooner the artery is opened and blood flow reestablished to ischemic or injured tissue, the more myocardium is salvaged and the fewer complications and deaths occur.

Measuring the ST Segment

Clinically significant ST-segment deviation is defined as ST elevation or depression 1 mm or more from the baseline, or isoelectric line, measured 80 msec (0.08 sec) after the J point. The J point is the point at which the QRS ends and the ST segment begins. Some sources recommend measuring the ST segment 60 msec (0.06 sec) after the J point, but this may lead to more false-positive ST changes when there is no myo-

TABLE 18–3. ECG CLUES FOR DIFFERENTIATING ABERRATION FROM VENTRICULAR ECTOPY

	Aberrancy	Ventricular Ectopy
P Waves	Precede QRS complexes	Dissociated from QRS or occur at rate slower than QRS; if 1:1 V-A conduction is present, retrograde P waves follow every QRS
Precordial QRS concordance	Positive concordance may occur with WPW	Negative concordance favors VT; positive concordance favors VT if WPW ruled out
Fusion or capture beats		Strong evidence in favor of VT
QRS axis	Often normal; may be deviated to right or left	Intermediate axis favors VT; often deviated to left or right
RBBB QRS morphology	Triphasic rsR′ in V_1: triphasic qRs in V_6	Monophasic R wave or diphasic qR complex in V_1: left "rabbit ear" taller in V_1: monophasic QS or diphasic rS in V_6
LBBB QRS morphology	Narrow R wave (<0.04 sec) in V_1; straight downstroke of S wave in V_1 (often slurs or notches on upstroke); usually no Q wave in V_6	Wide R wave (>0.03 sec) in V_1 or V_2; slurring or notching on downstroke of S wave in V_1; delay of greater than 0.06 second to nadir of S wave in V_1 or V_2; any Q wave in V_6

cardial ischemia. Figure 18–38 illustrates a normal ST segment, and ST-segment elevation and depression.

ST-segment monitoring software in newer bedside monitors defines the baseline and the ST-segment measuring point. It also sets default alarm parameters so the equipment can audibly notify the nurse when the patient's ST segment falls outside the defined parameters. Most monitors allow the user to redefine the baseline, reset the J point, choose where the ST segment is measured, and change the alarm parameters to account for individual patient variations. The monitor then displays the ST-segment measurement in millimeters on the screen, and most monitors also allow for trending of the ST segment over specified time intervals.

Choosing the Best Leads for ST-Segment Monitoring

Some monitoring systems offer continuous 12-lead ECG monitoring, which eliminates the need to select the "best" leads to monitor for a given clinical situation. Most newer generation bedside monitors offer at least two leads for simultaneous ECG monitoring and some offer three leads. The single best lead for arrhythmia monitoring is V_1, with V_6 being next best. Using two or three leads for ST-segment monitoring is optimal because a single lead may miss significant ST-segment deviations. Because current bedside monitors allow for the use of only one V lead at a time, using V_1 as the arrhythmia monitoring lead (or V_6 if V_1 is not available because of dressings, etc.) means that limb leads must be used for ST-segment monitoring. The best limb leads are discussed below.

The best way to choose leads for ST-segment monitoring is to know the patient's "ischemic fingerprint." To determine the patient's ischemic fingerprint, obtain a 12-lead ECG during a pain episode or with inflation of the balloon during angioplasty and note which leads show the most ST-segment displacement (either elevation or depression) during the acute ischemic event. Choose the lead or leads with the most ST-segment displacement as the bedside ST-segment monitoring leads.

If no ischemic fingerprint is available, use a lead or leads that have been determined through research to be best for the artery involved (Table 18–4). The limb leads that have been shown to best detect ischemia related to all three major coronary arteries (right coronary, left anterior descending, and circumflex) are leads III and aVF. In the case of the right coronary artery (RCA), leads III and aVF directly face the inferior wall supplied by this artery and record ST elevation with inferior wall injury. The left anterior descending and circumflex artery supply the anterior and lateral walls, respectively. Because these walls are not directly

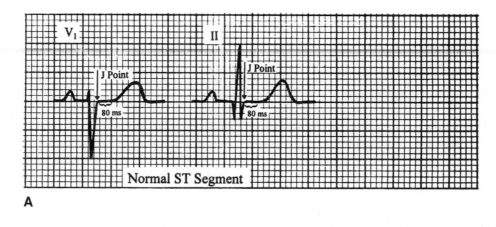

A

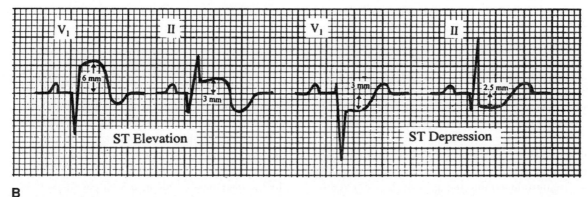

B

Figure 18–38. **(A)** Normal ST segment on the baseline in leads V_1 and II. **(B)** ST-segment elevation and ST-segment depression.

TABLE 18–4. RECOMMENDED LEADS FOR CONTINUOUS ECG MONITORING

Purpose	Best Leads
Arrhythmia detection	V_1 or MCL_1 (V_6 or MCL_6 next best)
RCA ischemia, inferior MI	III, AVF
LAD ischemia, anterior MI	V_2, V_3 V_4 (III, aVF best limb leads)
Circumflex ischemia, lateral MI	III, aVF, V_2
RV infarction	V_4R
Wellens warming	V_2 or V_3
Axis shifts	I and aVF together

faced by leads III and aVF, ST-segment depression is recorded as a reciprocal change when anterior or lateral wall injury occurs. Table 18–5 summarizes critical elements of ST segment monitoring.

CARDIAC PACEMAKERS

Chapter 3, Interpretation and Management of Basic Cardiac Rhythms, describes the components of a temporary pacing system and basic pacemaker operation. This section discusses single-chamber and dual-chamber pacemaker function and evaluation of pacemaker rhythm strips for appropriate capture and sensing.

Cardiac pacemakers are classified by a standardized five-letter pacemaker code that describes the location of the pacing wire(s) and the expected function of the pacemaker. Table 18–6 illustrates the five-letter code. The first letter in the pacemaker code describes the chamber that is paced (A = atrium, V = ventricle, D = dual [atrium and ventricle], 0 = none). The letter in the second position describes the chamber where intrinsic electrical activity is sensed (A = atrium, V = ventricle, D = dual, 0 = none). The letter in the third position describes the pacemaker's response to sensing of intrinsic electrical activity (I = inhibited, T = triggered, D = dual [inhibited or triggered], 0 = none). The fourth letter describes programmable functions of the pacemaker or the presence of rate modulation, and the fifth letter describes antitachycardia pacing functions. To know how a pacemaker should function, it is necessary to know at a minimum the first three letters of the code, which describe where the pacemaker is supposed to pace, where it is supposed to sense, and what it should do when it senses. The last two codes, representing advanced pacemaker function, are not covered in this text; see the recommended references at the end of the chapter.

Three types of temporary pacing are commonly used in the critical care setting. The first is transvenous pacing through a wire introduced into the apex of the right ventricle via a peripheral or central vein and set in the demand mode (sensitive to intrinsic ventricular activity). Ventricular

TABLE 18–5. EVIDENCED-BASED PRACTICE: ST SEGMENT MONITORING

Patient Selection

Class I: ST segment monitoring recommended for the following types of patients:
- Patients in the early phase of acute coronary syndromes (unstable angina, "rule-out MI, ST elevation MI, non–ST-elevation MI).[a,c]
- Patients presenting to emergency department with chest pain or anginal equivalent symptoms.[a,c]
- Patients who have undergone nonurgent percutaneous coronary intervention who have suboptimal angiographic results.[a,c]
- Patients with possible variant angina due to coronary vasospasm.[a,c]

Class II: ST segment monitoring may be of benefit in some patients but is not considered essential for all:
- Patients with post-acute MI (after 24–48 h).[a]
- Patients who have undergone nonurgent, uncomplicated percutaneous coronary intervention 1.
- Patients at high risk for ischemia after cardiac or noncardiac surgery.[a]
- Pediatric patients at risk of ischemia or infarction due to congenital or acquired conditions.[a]

Electrode Application
- Make sure skin is clean and dry before applying monitoring electrodes.[a,b,c]
- Place electrodes according to manufacturer recommendations when using a derived 12-lead ECG system.[a]
- When using a 3- or 5-wire monitoring system, place electrodes as follows:
  - Place arm electrodes in infraclavicular fossa close to shoulder[a] or on top or back of shoulder as close to where arm joins torso as possible.
  - Place leg electrodes at lowest point on rib cage or on hips.[a,b]
  - Place V_1 electrode at the fourth intercostal space at right sternal border.[b]
  - Place V_6 electrode at the fifth intercostal space at left midaxillary line.[b]
- Mark electrode placement with indelible ink.[a,c]
- Replace electrodes every 48 hours or more often if skin irritation occurs.[b]

Lead Selection
- Monitor all 12 leads continuously if using a 12-lead monitoring system.[b]
- Use V_1 (or V_6 if V_1 is not possible due to dressings, etc.) for arrhythmia monitoring in all multilead combinations.[b]
- Choose the ST-segment monitoring lead according to the patient's "ischemic fingerprint" obtained during an ischemic event whenever possible.[b,c] Use the lead with the largest ST-segment deviation (elevation or depression).[b]
- If no ischemic fingerprint is available, use either lead III[b,c] or aVF (whichever has tallest QRS complex)[b] for ST-segment monitoring.
- Lead V_3 is the best lead for detecting anterior wall ST-segment deviation,[c] but can only be used if the chest lead is not being used for arrhythmia monitoring in lead V_1.

Alarm Limits
- Establish baseline ST level with patient in the supine position.[a,c]
- Set ST alarm parameters at 1 mm above and below the patient's baseline ST level in patients at high risk for ischemia.[a]
- Set ST alarm parameters at 2 mm above and below the patient's baseline ST level in more stable patients.[a]

Data compiled from [a]Drew et al (in press), [b]Jacobson (2004), and [c]AACN (2004).

pacing is always done in the demand mode to avoid the delivery of pacing stimuli into the vulnerable period of the cardiac cycle, which could induce ventricular tachycardia or fibrillation (see Chapter 3, Interpretation and Management of Basic Cardiac Rhythms). This type of pacing is described by the pacemaker code as a VVI pacemaker—it paces the ventricle, senses intrinsic ventricular electrical activity, and inhibits its output when sensing occurs.

TABLE 18–6. PACEMAKER CODES

First Letter: Chamber Paced	Second Letter: Chamber Sensed	Third Letter: Response to Sensing	Fourth Letter: Programmability, Rate Modulation	Fifth Letter: Antitachycardia Pacing Functions
0 = None	0 = None	0 = None	0 = None	0 = None
A = Atrium	A = Atrium	I = Inhibited	P = Simple programmable	P = Pacing (Antitachycardia)
V = Ventricle	V = Ventricle	T = Triggered	M = Multiprogrammable	S = Shock
D = Dual (A&V)	D = Dual (A&V)	D = Dual (I&T)	C = Communicating	D = Dual (P&S)
			R = Rate modulation	

The second type of pacing done in critical care is temporary epicardial pacing (either atrial, ventricular, or dual chamber) via pacing wires attached to the atria and/or ventricles during cardiac surgery. If atrial pacing is done with no sensing of atrial electrical activity, also called asynchronous mode, the pacemaker operates as an A00 pacemaker—it paces the atria, does not sense, and therefore does not respond to sensing. If atrial pacing is done with sensing of atrial electrical activity, also called the demand mode, the pacemaker operates as an AAI pacemaker—it paces the atria, senses atrial activity, and inhibits its output when it senses. Dual-chamber pacing can be done in several modes involving pacing and sensing functions in one or both chambers and described by the pacemaker code according to the mode chosen. The two most common dual-chamber modes used with temporary epicardial pacing (and occasionally with temporary transvenous pacing) are DVI (paces atria and ventricles, senses only in the ventricle, and inhibits pacing output when sensing occurs) and DDD (paces both chambers, senses both chambers, and either triggers or inhibits pacing output in response to sensing). The common dual-chamber pacing modes are listed in Table 18–7.

The third type of temporary pacing is external (transcutaneous) pacing. External pacing is done in emergency situations requiring immediate pacing when placement of a temporary transvenous pacing wire is not feasible. External pacing is not as reliable as transvenous or epicardial pacing and is used as a temporary measure until transvenous pacing can be instituted. External pacing is briefly described in Chapter 3, Interpretation and Management of Basic Cardiac Rhythms.

Evaluating Pacemaker Function

Evaluating pacemaker function requires knowledge of the mode of pacing expected (VVI, AAI, etc.); the minimum rate of the pacemaker, or pacing interval; and any other programmed parameters in the pacemaker. The basic functions of a pacemaker include stimulus release, capture, and sensing. *Stimulus release* refers to pacemaker output, or the ability of the pacemaker to generate and release a pacing impulse. *Capture* is the ability of the pacing stimulus to result in depolarization of the chamber being paced. *Sensing* is the ability of the pacemaker to recognize and respond to intrinsic electrical activity in the heart. Pacemaker operation is evaluated according to these three functions. Single-chamber pacemaker evaluation is much less complicated than dual-chamber evaluation. Because single-chamber ventricular pacing is a very common type of temporary pacing in critical care and telemetry units, VVI pacemaker evaluation is discussed here.

VVI Pacemaker Evaluation

Stimulus release, capture, and sensing must all be assessed when evaluating VVI pacemakers. A VVI pacemaker is expected to pace the ventricle at the set rate unless spontaneous ventricular activity occurs to inhibit pacing. The set rate of the pacemaker, or *pacing interval,* is measured from one pacing stimulus to the next consecutive stimulus. Pacemakers have a *refractory period,* which is a period following either pacing or sensing in the chamber, during which the pacemaker is unable to respond to intrinsic activity. During the refractory period, the pacemaker in effect has its eyes closed and is not able to see spontaneous activity. In a normally

TABLE 18–7. DUAL-CHAMBER PACING MODES

Mode	Chamber(s) Paced	Chamber(s) Sensed	Response to Sensing
DVI	Atrium and ventricle	Ventricle	Inhibited
VDD	Ventricle	Atrium and ventricle	Atrial sensing triggers ventricular pacing Ventricular sensing inhibits ventricular pacing
DDI	Atrium and ventricle	Atrium and ventricle	Inhibited
DDD	Atrium and ventricle	Atrium and ventricle	Atrial sensing inhibits atrial pacing, triggers ventricular pacing Ventricular sensing inhibits atrial and ventricular pacing

functioning VVI pacemaker, pacing spikes occur at the set pacing interval and each spike results in a ventricular depolarization (capture). If spontaneous ventricular activity occurs (either a normally conducted QRS or a PVC), that activity is sensed and the next pacing stimulus is inhibited. Figure 18–39 shows normal VVI pacemaker function.

Stimulus Release

Stimulus release depends on a pacemaker with enough battery power to generate the electrical impulse, and on an intact pacemaker lead system to deliver the electrical stimulus to the heart. The presence of a pacer spike on the rhythm strip or monitor indicates that the stimulus was released from the generator and entered the body. The presence of the spike does not indicate where the stimulus was delivered (e.g., atria or ventricles), only that it entered the body somewhere. Total absence of pacing stimuli, when they should be present, can indicate a faulty pulse generator or battery, or a break or disconnection in the lead system. Pacing stimuli also can be absent when pacing is inhibited by the sensing of intrinsic electrical activity. Figure 18–40 illustrates total

loss of stimulus release in a patient whose pacemaker battery was dead.

Capture

Capture is indicated by a wide QRS complex immediately following the pacemaker spike and represents the ability of the pacing stimulus to depolarize the ventricle. Loss of capture is recognized by the presence of pacer spikes that are not followed by paced ventricular complexes (Figure 18–41). Causes of loss of capture include:

- Inadequate stimulus strength, which can be corrected by increasing the electrical output of the pacemaker (turning up the milliampere level).
- Pacing wire out of position and not in contact with myocardium, which can be corrected by repositioning the wire and sometimes by repositioning the patient.
- Pacing lead positioned in infarcted tissue, which can be corrected by repositioning the wire to a place where the myocardium is not injured and is capable of responding to the stimulus.

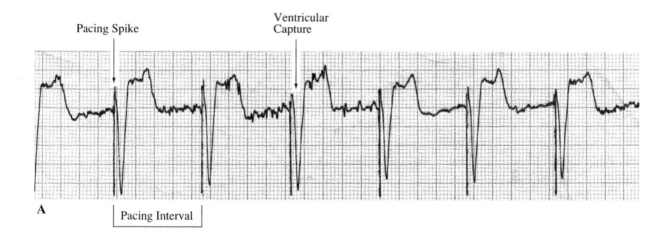

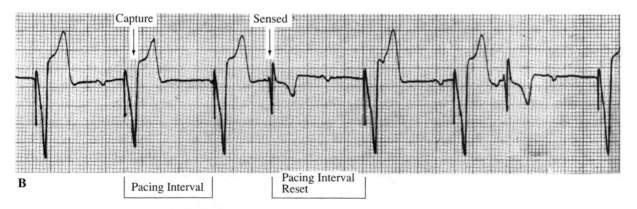

Figure 18–39. Normal VVI pacemaker function. **(A)** Pacing electrical activity ("pacer spike") followed by a wide QRS complex indicating ventricular capture. Pacemaker sensing cannot be evaluated because no intrinsic QRS complexes are present. **(B)** Pacemaker capture and sensing both normal. Intrinsic QRS complexes are sensed, inhibiting ventricular pacing output, and resetting the pacing interval. Absence of intrinsic ventricular electrical activity causes pacing to occur with capture.

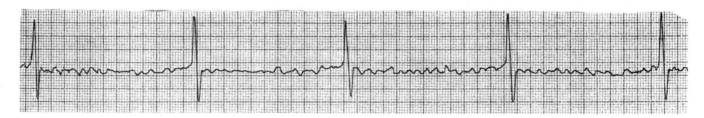

Figure 18–40. Absence of stimulus release in a patient with a permanent pacemaker. Underlying rhythm is atrial fibrillation with complete AV block and a very slow ventricular rate. The battery in the pacemaker generator was dead.

- Electrolyte imbalances or drugs that alter the ability of the heart to respond to the pacing stimulus.
- Delivery of a pacing stimulus during the ventricles refractory period when the heart is physiologically unable to respond to the stimulus. This problem occurs with loss of sensing (undersensing) and can be corrected by correcting the sensing problem (Figure 18–42A).

Sensing

Sensing of intrinsic ventricular electrical activity inhibits the next pacing stimulus and resets the pacing interval. Sensing cannot occur unless the pacemaker is given the opportunity to sense. It must be in the demand mode and there must be intrinsic ventricular activity that occurs for the pacemaker to have an opportunity to sense. In Figure 18–39A, sensing cannot be evaluated because there is no intrinsic ventricular activity that occurs, and therefore the pacemaker is not given an opportunity to sense. In Figure 18–39B, the occurrence of

two spontaneous QRS complexes provides the pacemaker with an opportunity to sense. In this example, sensing occurred normally, as indicated by the absence of the next expected pacing stimulus and resetting of the pacing interval by the intrinsic QRS complex.

Two sensing problems can occur: undersensing and oversensing. Undersensing, also called "failure to sense" or "loss of sensing," can be caused by:

- Asynchronous (fixed rate) mode in which the sensing circuit is off. This problem can be corrected by turning the sensitivity control to the demand mode.
- Pacing catheter out of position or lying in infarcted tissue, which can be corrected by repositioning the wire. Pacing wire repositioning must be done by a physician; however, turning the patient onto his or her side sometimes temporarily works when the pacing wire loses contact with the ventricle.
- Intrinsic QRS voltage too low to be sensed by the pacemaker. Turning the sensitivity control clockwise

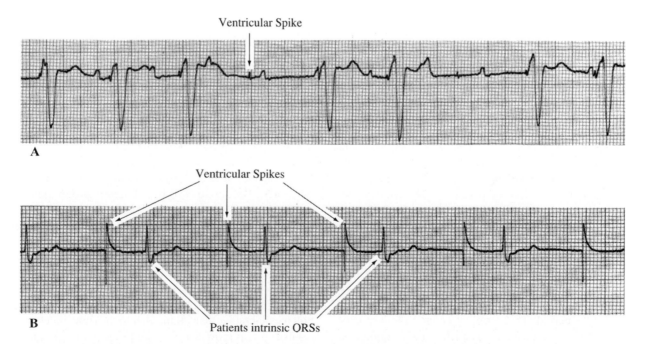

Figure 18–41. **(A)** VVI pacemaker with intermittent loss of capture. **(B)** VVI pacemaker with total loss of capture.

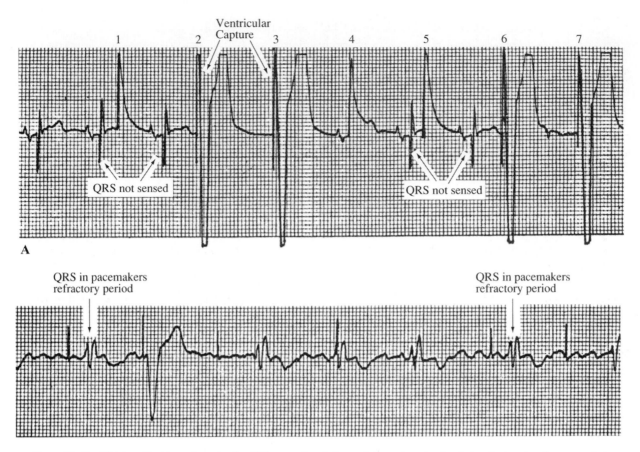

Figure 18–42. (A) Intermittent loss of sensing in a VVI pacemaker. Delivery of the pacing stimulus during the heart's refractory period makes it appear that capture is lost as well. Because the heart is physiologically unable to respond to the pacing stimulus when it falls in the refractory period, this is not a capture problem. Pacer spikes 1, 2, 5, and 6 should not have occurred; their presence is due to loss of sensing. Pacer spike 4 occurred coincident with the normal QRS complex, resulting in a "pseudofusion" beat, and does not represent loss of sensing. **(B)** Loss of capture in a VVI pacemaker. Only one pacer spike captures the ventricle. Two QRS complexes occur during the pacemaker's refractory period and thus are not sensed. This does not represent loss of sensing because the pacemaker has its "eyes closed" during the time intrinsic ventricular activity occurred.

or decreasing the sensitivity number increases the sensitivity of the pacemaker and makes it able to "see" smaller intrinsic electrical signals. Repositioning the wire sometimes helps.

- Break in connections, battery failure, or faulty pulse generator. Check and tighten all connections along the pacing system, and replace the battery if it is low. A chest x-ray may detect wire fracture. Change the pulse generator if problems cannot be corrected any other way.

- Intrinsic ventricular activity falling in the pacemaker's refractory period. If a spontaneous QRS complex occurs during the time the pacemaker has its eyes closed, the pacemaker cannot see it. This event occurs when the pacemaker fails to capture, which can allow an intrinsic QRS to occur during the pacemaker's refractory period. This problem is due to loss of capture and does not reflect a sensing malfunction (see Figure 18–42).

Oversensing means that the pacemaker is so sensitive that it inappropriately senses internal or outside signals as QRS complexes and inhibits its output. Common sources of outside signals that can interfere with pacemaker function include electromagnetic or RF signals, or electronic equipment in use near the pacemaker. Internal sources of interference can include large P waves, large T-wave voltage, local myopotentials in the heart, or skeletal muscle potentials (Figure 18–43B). Because a VVI pacemaker is programmed to inhibit its output when it senses, oversensing can be a dangerous situation in a pacemaker-dependent patient, resulting in ventricular asystole. Oversensing is usually due to the sensitivity control being set too high, which can be corrected by turning the sensitivity dial counterclockwise and reducing the pacemaker's sensitivity. It is recommended that the sensitivity control be set between the 1 and 3 o'clock positions on the dial rather than all the way to the right, unless a higher sensitivity is required to make the pacemaker sense QRS complexes.

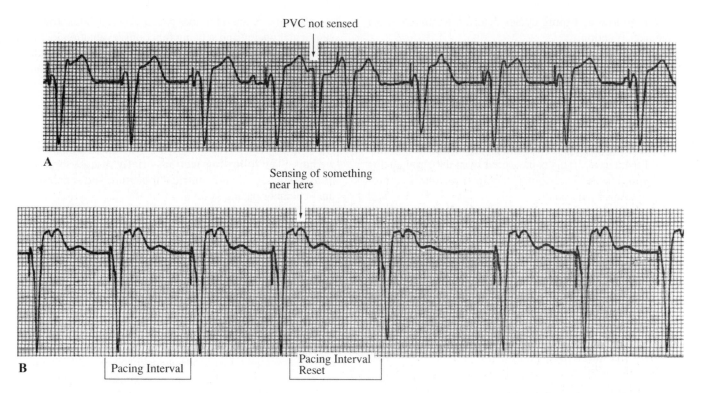

Figure 18–43. **(A)** Undersensing in a VVI pacemaker. The PVC is not sensed and pacing occurs at the programmed pacing interval, resulting in a pacemaker spike on the T wave of the PVC without capture. **(B)** Oversensing in a VVI pacemaker. The pacing rate slows for two intervals, presumably due to sensing of something near the T wave, which resets the pacing interval from the point where sensing occurred.

Stimulation Threshold Testing

The stimulation threshold is the minimum output of the pacemaker necessary to capture the heart consistently. The stimulation threshold changes over time; when the pacing lead is first placed, the stimulation threshold is usually very low. Over time, the threshold increases and it takes more output to result in capture. When caring for a patient with a temporary pacemaker, stimulation threshold testing should be done every shift until a stable threshold is reached. Once the threshold has been determined, set the output two to three times higher than threshold to ensure an adequate safety margin for capture. To determine the stimulation threshold, follow these steps:

- Verify that the patient is in a paced rhythm. The pacing rate may need to be temporarily increased to override an intrinsic rhythm.
- Watch the monitor continuously while slowly decreasing output by turning the output control counterclockwise.
- Note when the pacing stimulus no longer captures the heart (a pacing spike not followed by a paced beat).
- Slowly increase the output until 1:1 capture resumes. This is the stimulation threshold.
- Set the output two to three times higher than threshold (i.e., if threshold is 2 mA, set output between 4 and 6 mA).

DDD Pacemaker Evaluation

Dual-chamber pacemakers have become very complicated, with multiple programmable parameters and varying functions depending on the manufacturer. It is impossible to present dual-chamber pacemaker function in detail in a single chapter. To understand dual-chamber pacemaker function, it is necessary to understand the timing cycles involved in dual-chamber pacing. This information is best obtained in a class sponsored by a pacemaker manufacturer or from a pacemaker technical manual. In this section, the major timing cycles are defined and basic DDD pacemaker evaluation is covered in a very generic manner, because each pacemaker is different depending on the manufacturer. Dual-chamber pacemakers can function in a variety of modes (see Table 18–6). Because the DDD mode is most commonly used, basic DDD function is described here.

According to the pacemaker code, DDD means that both chambers (atria and ventricles) are paced, both chambers are sensed, and the mode of response to sensed events is either inhibited or triggered, depending on which chamber is sensed. When atrial activity is sensed, pacing is triggered in the ventricle after the programmed AV delay. When ventricular activity is sensed, all pacemaker output is inhibited.

The following timing cycles determine dual-chamber pacemaker function:

- *Pacing interval* (or lower rate limit): the base rate of the pacemaker, measured between two consecutive atrial pacing stimuli. The pacing interval is a programmed parameter.
- *AV delay* (or AV interval): the amount of time between atrial and ventricular pacing, or the "electronic PR interval." This is measured from the atrial pacing spike to the ventricular pacing spike and is a programmed parameter.
- *Atrial escape interval* (or VA interval): the interval from a sensed or paced ventricular event to the next atrial pacing output. The VA interval represents the amount of time the pacemaker waits after it paces in the ventricle or senses ventricular activity before pacing the atrium. The atrial escape interval is not a programmed parameter, but is derived by subtracting the AV delay from the pacing interval. Its length can be estimated by measuring from a ventricular spike to the next atrial pacing spike.
- *Total atrial refractory period* (TARP): the period of time following a sensed P wave or a paced atrial event during which the atrial channel will not respond to sensed events (i.e., "has its eyes closed"). The TARP consists of the AV delay and the PVARP (see below).
- *Postventricular atrial refractory period* (PVARP): the period of time following an intrinsic QRS or a paced ventricular beat during which the atrial channel is refractory and will not respond to sensed atrial activity. PVARP is a programmable parameter but is not evident on a rhythm strip.
- *Blanking period:* the very short ventricular refractory period (VRP) that occurs with every atrial pacemaker output. The ventricular channel "blinks its eyes" so it does not sense the atrial output and inappropriately inhibit ventricular pacing. The blanking period is a programmable parameter but is not evident on a rhythm strip.
- *Ventricular refractory period*: the period of time following a paced ventricular beat or a sensed QRS during which the ventricular channel ignores intrinsic ventricular activity (i.e., "has its eyes closed"). VRP is a programmable parameter but is not evident on a rhythm strip.
- *Maximum tracking interval* (or upper rate limit): the maximum rate at which the ventricular channel will track atrial activity. The upper rate limit prevents rapid ventricular pacing in response to very rapid atrial activity, such as atrial tachycardia or atrial flutter. The maximum tracking interval is a programmable parameter and usually is set according to how active a patient is expected to be and how fast a ventricular rate is likely to be tolerated.

Because a dual-chamber pacemaker has both atrial and ventricular pacing and sensing functions, evaluation includes assessing atrial capture, atrial sensing, ventricular capture, and ventricular sensing. To evaluate dual-chamber pacemaker function accurately, it is necessary to know the following information: mode of function (DDD, DVI, etc.), minimum rate, upper rate limit, AV delay, and atrial and VRPs. In the real world of bedside nursing, this information is not always available, so we do the best we can with what we have. The following sections briefly discuss the issues of assessing atrial and ventricular capture and sensing in a dual-chamber pacing system.

Atrial Capture

Atrial capture, unlike ventricular capture, is not always easy to see. Often, the atrial response to pacing is so small that it cannot be seen in many monitoring leads, so we cannot rely on the presence of a P wave following every atrial pacer spike as evidence of atrial capture. If a clear P wave is present after every atrial pacemaker spike, atrial capture can be assumed. In the absence of a clear P wave, atrial capture can only be assumed when an atrial pacer spike is followed by a normally conducted QRS complex within the programmed AV delay. If the atrial spike captures the atrium and there is intact AV conduction, the presence of the normal QRS indicates that the atrium must have been captured for conduction to have occurred into the ventricles before the ventricular pacing stimulus was delivered. Because a DDD pacemaker paces the ventricle at a preset AV interval following atrial pacing, the presence of a ventricular paced beat following an atrial paced beat does not verify capture, because the ventricle paces at the end of the AV delay whether atrial capture occurs or not. Therefore, atrial capture can only be assumed when there is an obvious P wave after every atrial pacing spike or when an atrial pacing spike is followed by a normal QRS within the programmed AV delay.

Atrial Sensing

Atrial sensing is verified by the presence of a spontaneous P wave that is followed by a paced ventricular beat at the end of the programmed AV delay. If a P wave is sensed, it starts the AV delay and ventricular pacing is triggered at the end of the AV delay unless AV conduction is intact and results in a normal QRS. The presence of a normal P wave followed by a normal QRS only proves that AV conduction is intact, not that the P wave was sensed by the pacemaker. Therefore, atrial sensing is verified by a spontaneous P wave followed by a paced QRS.

Ventricular Capture

Ventricular capture is recognized by a wide QRS immediately following a ventricular pacing spike. Ventricular capture is much easier to recognize than atrial capture and is no different than with single-chamber ventricular pacing.

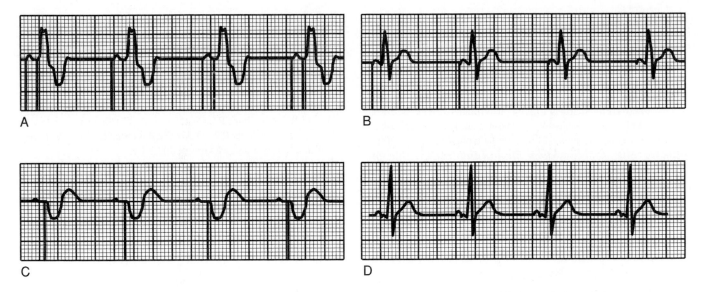

Figure 18–44. Four states of DDD pacing. **(A)** Atrial and ventricular pacing (AV sequential pacing state). **(B)** Atrial pacing, ventricular sensing. **(C)** Atrial sensing, ventricular pacing (atrial tracking state). **(D)** Atrial and ventricular sensing (inhibited pacing state).

Ventricular Sensing

Ventricular sensing can only be verified if there is spontaneous ventricular activity present for the pacemaker to sense. Ventricular sensing is verified by an atrial pacer spike followed by a normal QRS that inhibits the ventricular pacing spike, which is the same event that proves atrial capture. If a QRS is sensed before the next atrial pacing spike is due, both the atrial and ventricular pacing stimuli are inhibited and the VA interval (atrial escape interval) is reset.

Dual-chamber pacemakers are capable of operating in four states of pacing: atrial and ventricular pacing, atrial pacing with ventricular sensing, atrial sensing with ventricular pacing, and atrial and ventricular sensing. All four states of pacing can occur within a short period of time, and the timing cycles determine which state of pacing is done. Figure 18–44 shows the four states of dual-chamber pacing, and Figure 18–45 illustrates the basic principles of dual-chamber pacemaker evaluation.

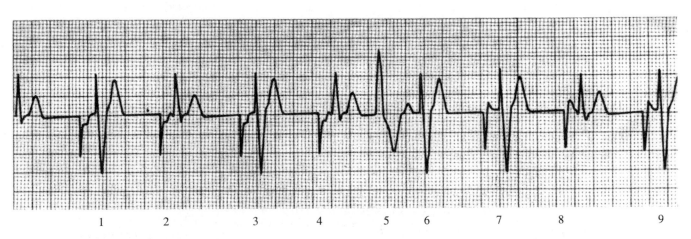

Figure 18–45. DDD pacemaker operating in all four states of pacing. Beat 1 = AV sequential pacing; beat 2 = atrial pacing, ventricular sensing; beat 3 = AV sequential pacing; beat 4 = atrial pacing, ventricular sensing; beat 5 = PVC; beat 6 = atrial sensing, ventricular pacing; beat 7 = AV sequential pacing; beat 8 = atrial pacing, ventricular sensing; beat 9 = AV sequential pacing. Atrial capture is proven by beats 2, 4, and 8 (atrial spike followed by normal QRS within the programmed AV delay). Atrial sensing is proven by beat 6 (normal P followed by paced V at end of AV delay). Ventricular capture is verified by beats 1, 3, 6, 7, and 9 (wide paced QRS following ventricular pacing spike). Ventricular sensing is proven by beats 2, 4, and 8 (atrial spike followed by normal QRS which inhibited ventricular cardiac spike).

SELECTED BIBLIOGRAPHY

General Electrocardiography

Bharucha B, Podrid PJ. Use of the electrocardiogram in the diagnosis of arrhythmia. In Podrid PJ, Kowey PR (eds): *Cardiac Arrhythmia: Mechanisms, Diagnosis & Management,* 2nd ed, pp. 127–164. Philadelphia: Lippincott Williams & Wilkins; 2001.

Braunwald E, Zipes DP, Libby P: *Heart Disease: A Textbook of Cardiovascular Medicine,* 6th ed. Philadelphia: Saunders; 2001.

Conover MB: *Understanding Electrocardiography,* 7th ed. St. Louis, MO: Mosby; 1996.

Fuster V, Alexander RW, O'Rourke RA (eds): *Hurst's The Heart,* 10th ed. New York: McGraw-Hill; 2001.

Jacobson C: Electrocardiography. In Woods SL, Froelicher ES, Motzer SU, Bridges EJ (eds): *Cardiac Nursing,* 5th ed. Philadelphia: JB Lippincott; 2005.

Marriott HJL: *Practical Electrocardiography,* 8th ed. Baltimore: Williams & Wilkins; 1988.

Wagoner GS: *Marriott's Practical Electrocardiography,* 9th ed. Baltimore: Williams & Wilkins; 1994.

Wellens HJJ, Conover MB: *The ECG in Emergency Decision Making.* Philadelphia: WB Saunders; 1992.

ST-Segment Monitoring

Drew B, Tisdale LA: ST segment monitoring for coronary artery reocclusion following thrombolytic therapy and coronary angioplasty: Identification of optimal bedside monitoring leads. *Am J Crit Care* 1993;2:280–292.

Drew BJ, Califf RM, Funk M, et al: Practice standards for electrocardiographic monitoring in hospital settings: A report for healthcare professionals by a task force of American Heart Association Councils on Cardiovascular Nursing, Clinical Cardiology, and Cardiovascular Disease in the Young, and the International Society of Computerized *Circulation* 2004;110:2721–2746.

Tisdale LA, Drew B: ST segment monitoring for myocardial ischemia. *AACN Clinical Issues.* 1993;4:34–43.

Cardiac Pacing

Barold SS, Stroobandt RX, Sinnaeve AF: *Cardiac Pacemakers Step by Step.* Malden, MA: Blackwell Futura; 2004.

Barold SS, Mugica J: *Recent Advances in Cardiac Pacing.* Armonk, NY: Futura; 1998.

Furman S, Hayes D, Holmes D: *A Practice of Cardiac Pacing,* 3rd ed. New York: Futura; 1993.

Hayes DL, Zipes DP: Cardiac pacemakers and cardioverter-defibrillators. In Braunwald E, Zipes DP, Libby P (eds): *Heart Disease, vol. 1,* 6th ed. Philadelphia: WB Saunders; 2001.

Mitrani RD, Myerburg RJ, Castellanos A: Cardiac pacemakers. In Fuster V, Alexander RW, O'Rourke RA (eds): *Hurst's The Heart,* 10th ed. New York: McGraw-Hill; 2001.

Shanker A, Saksena S: Cardiac pacemakers. In Podrid PJ, Kowey PR (eds): *Cardiac Arrhythmia: Mechanisms, Diagnosis, and Management,* 2nd ed, pp. 323–356. Philadelphia: Lippincott Williams & Wilkins; 2001.

Siemens Pacesetter: Pacemaker technology for nurses and allied health professionals. Norcross, GA: Siemens Pacesetter Education Department.

Advanced Arrhythmia Interpretation

Jacobson C: Arrhythmias and conduction disturbances. In Woods SL, Froelicher ES, Motzer SU, Bridges EJ (eds): *Cardiac Nursing,* 5th ed. Philadelphia: JB Lippincott; 2005.

Marriott HJL, Conover M: *Advanced Concepts in Arrhythmias,* 3rd ed. St. Louis, MO: Mosby; 1998.

Olgin JE, Zipes DP: Specific arrhythmias: diagnosis and treatment. In Braunwald E, Zipes DP, Libby P (eds): *Heart Disease,* 6th ed, pp. 659–699. Philadelphia: WB Saunders; 2001.

Podrid PJ, Kowey PR (eds): *Cardiac Arrhythmia: Mechanisms, Diagnosis & Management,* 2nd ed. Philadelphia: Lippincott Williams & Wilkins; 2001.

Zipes DP, Jalife J (eds): *Cardiac Electrophysiology: From Cell to Bedside,* 3rd ed. Philadelphia: WB Saunders; 2000.

Evidence-Based Medicine

American Association of Critical Care Nurses (AACN): *Practice Alert: ST Segment Monitoring.* Aliso Viejo, CA: AACN; 2004.

Jacobson C: Bedside cardiac monitoring. In Chulay M, Burns S (eds): *AACN's Protocols for Practice: Technology Series,* 2nd ed. Aliso Viejo, CA: AACN; 2004.

Advanced Cardiovascular Concepts

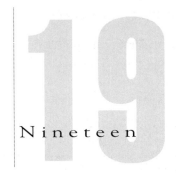

Nineteen

19

Barbara Leeper

▶ **Knowledge Competencies**

1. Describe the etiology, pathophysiology, clinical presentation, patient needs, and principles of management of
   - Cardiomyopathy
   - Valvular disease
   - Pericarditis
   - Aortic aneurysm
   - Cardiac transplantation
2. Compare and contrast the pathophysiology, clinical presentation, patient needs, and management approaches of
   - Cardiomyopathy

- Valvular disease
- Pericarditis
- Aortic aneurysm
- Cardiac transplantation

3. Identify indications for, complications of, and nursing management of patients receiving intraaortic balloon pump and ventricular assist device therapy.

PATHOLOGIC CONDITIONS

Cardiomyopathy

Cardiomyopathy is a disease that involves destruction of the cardiac muscle fibers, leading to impaired cardiac function. The cause of cardiomyopathy is often unknown. Cardiomyopathy commonly is classified into three types: dilated, hypertrophic, and restrictive (Figure 19–1).

The two case studies involve patients with dilated cardiomyopathy. As is typical with this type of cardiomyopathy, myocardial contractility is impaired and ventricular filling pressures are increased. Dilated cardiomyopathy is the most common type of cardiomyopathy, frequently affecting men during midlife.

Hypertrophic cardiomyopathy may occur in both the young and the elderly. Hypertrophic cardiomyopathy often is categorized as obstructive or nonobstructive. Ventricular hypertrophy occurs in both types. The diagnosis of obstructive

hypertrophic cardiomyopathy is made if hypertrophy of the intraventricular septum is also present. The hypertrophied septum obstructs left ventricular ejection.

Restrictive cardiomyopathy is the least common type. A classic finding for this type of cardiomyopathy is ventricular fibrosis. The fibrosis causes the ventricles to become rigid, thus limiting their compliance or ability to distend.

Etiology and Pathophysiology

The etiology of cardiomyopathy is unclear. It is postulated that a variety of conditions may cause or contribute to the development of cardiomyopathy (Table 19–1).

Pathophysiology of Dilated Cardiomyopathy

Dilated cardiomyopathy begins with gradual destruction of the myocardial fibers, limiting the ability of cardiac muscle to forcefully contract. As the disease progresses, left ventricular dilatation occurs, with increases of blood volume in the

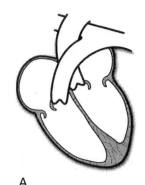 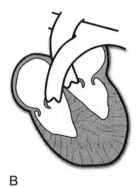 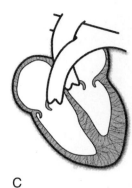

Figure 19–1. Types of cardiomyopathies. **(A)** Dilated (cardiac dilatation and impaired contractility). **(B)** Hypertrophic (decreased size of ventricular chambers and increased ventricular muscle mass). **(C)** Restrictive (decreased ventricular compliance).

A   B   C

left ventricle. This causes increased filling pressures and a decrease in cardiac output (CO). Left atrial volume and pressure eventually increase as the atrium struggles to eject blood into a fluid-overloaded left ventricle. Increased left atrial pressure may lead to increased pulmonary vascular pressure as blood backs up into the pulmonary system. Right-sided heart failure may result from increased pulmonary vascular pressure or destruction of right atrial and ventricular myocardial fibers. Last, the atrioventricular valves (mitral and tricuspid) may develop insufficiency due to the increased ventricular pressures.

Pathophysiology of Hypertrophic Cardiomyopathy
Patients with hypertrophic cardiomyopathy have a greatly enlarged ventricular wall (see Figure 19–1). It is not uncommon for the ventricular chamber size to be dramatically reduced from the hypertrophy. In obstructive cardiomyopathy the intraventricular septum is also involved in the hypertrophic process, whereas in nonobstructive cardiomyopathy the septum is relatively normal. This excessive myocardial muscle development causes the ventricle to become rigid,

leading to decreased ventricular compliance and distensibility. This causes a decrease in the force of each myocardial contraction. As the strength of myocardial contractions decrease, left ventricular ejection into the aorta and cardiac output also decrease. Left ventricular systolic ejection may be further compromised by obstruction of the outflow tract as the anterior leaflet of the mitral valve presses against an enlarged intraventricular septum (obstructive cardiomyopathy).

Stress is placed on the left atrium as it attempts to propel blood forward into the stiff left ventricle. It is not uncommon for left atrial enlargement to develop as the left atrium is forced to contract against high left ventricular resistance. In addition, mitral insufficiency may occur as elevated left ventricular end-diastolic pressure places added stress and pressure on the closed mitral valve.

AT THE BEDSIDE
▶ *Cardiomyopathy*

A 56-year-old man was admitted to the emergency room with shortness of breath. His chest x-ray revealed an enlarged heart and pulmonary congestion. His 12-lead ECG was consistent with left ventricular hypertrophy. His rhythm was AF with a ventricular rate of 102. Clinical findings included bilateral rales auscultated one-third up from the bases, bilateral lower extremity 41 pitting edema to the midcalf, JVD, an S₃, and a systolic murmur heard best at the apex. An emergency echocardiogram showed limited contractility of a dilated left ventricle.

AT THE BEDSIDE
▶ *Cardiomyopathy*

A 32-year-old woman was admitted to the high-risk perinatal unit at 31 weeks' gestation with dyspnea and fatigue. She had bilateral, basilar rales and her oxygen saturation via pulse oximetry was 88%. An echocardiogram showed a markedly dilated left ventricle with diffuse hypokinesis and an ejection fraction of 20% to 25%.

A pulmonary artery catheter was placed with the following parameters obtained:

RA	12 mm Hg
PA	48/26 mm Hg
PCW	24 mm Hg
CO	3.7 L/min
CI	1.8 L/min/m²

A dobutamine infusion was initiated at 5 mcg/kg/min and oxygen was applied at 6 L/min via nasal cannula.

TABLE 19–1. ETIOLOGY OF CARDIOMYOPATHY

Dilated Cardiomyopathy
Idiopathic
Toxins, such as lead, alcohol, cocaine
Muscle dystrophy
Myotonic dystrophy
Hypophosphatemia
Hypocalcemia
Hypokalemia
Viral, bacterial, or fungal infections
Lupus erythematosus
Peripartum or postpartum status
Rheumatoid disease
Scleroderma
Hypertension
Thiamine deficiency
Microvascular spasm

Hypertrophic Cardiomyopathy
Idiopathic
Genetic transmission
Friedreich's ataxia
Hypoparathyroidism

Restrictive Cardiomyopathy
Idiopathic
Myocardial fibrosis
Infiltration
Hypertrophy
Amyloidosis
Hemochromatosis
Glycogen deposition
Scleroderma

Similar changes may occur on the right side of the heart. These may produce changes in the right atrium, right ventricle, and tricuspid valve.

Pathophysiology of Restrictive Cardiomyopathy
The ventricles of patients with restrictive cardiomyopathy become rigid as fibrotic tissue infiltrates the myocardium. This stiffness of the ventricles decreases the compliance, or distensibility, of the ventricles, thus decreasing ventricular filling and increasing end-diastolic pressures. The strength of the myocardial contraction is diminished, leading to decreases in cardiac output. As with the other types of cardiomyopathy, atrial workload is increased as the atria attempt to propel blood forward into stiff ventricles. It is not uncommon for atrioventricular valve insufficiency to develop, and for fluid to back up into the pulmonary and venous systems.

Clinical Presentation
Patients may be asymptomatic for lengthy periods of time (months to years) prior to being diagnosed with cardiomyopathy. By the time patients develop symptoms, significant cardiac dysfunction already may have occurred.

An increase in heart rate may occur initially as the heart attempts to maintain an adequate cardiac output. As the disease progresses and/or during physical exertion, the dysfunctional myocardium is usually unable to maintain an increase in heart rate and cardiac output begins to decrease.

Dilated Cardiomyopathy

1. Inability to maintain adequate cardiac output
   - Fatigue
   - Weakness
   - Sinus tachycardia
   - Pulses alternans
   - Narrowed pulse pressure
   - Decreased CO
2. Increased left ventricular filling pressures
   - Dyspnea
   - Orthopnea
   - Paroxysmal nocturnal dyspnea
   - Rales
   - S_3/S_4
   - Arrhythmias
   - Systolic murmur with mitral valve insufficiency
   - Abnormal hemodynamic profile:
     – Increased pulmonary artery systolic (PAS) and diastolic (PAD) pressures
     – Elevated pulmonary capillary wedge (PCW) pressures
     – Increased systemic vascular resistance (SVR)
     – Elevated V wave on PCW waveform with mitral valve insufficiency
3. Increased right ventricular filling pressures
   - Peripheral edema
   - Jugular vein distention (JVD)
   - Hepatomegaly
   - Elevated V wave on the right atrial (RA) waveform and systolic murmur with tricuspid valve insufficiency
4. Increased atrial pressure
   - Palpitations
   - S_4 may develop as the atria attempt to eject blood into rigid ventricles
   - Atrial arrhythmias may occur, such as premature atrial complexes (PACs) or atrial fibrillation (AF), due to the increase in atrial pressure
   - Elevated A wave on PCW waveform
   - Elevated RA pressures
   - Elevated A wave on the RA waveform

Hypertrophic Cardiomyopathy

1. Inability to maintain adequate cardiac output
   - Angina
   - Syncope
   - Fatigue
   - Sinus tachycardia

- Ventricular fibrillation
- Cardiac output is initially normal, then decreases
2. Increased ventricular filling pressures
   - Dyspnea
   - Orthopnea
   - Arrhythmias, such as premature ventricular contractions or ventricular tachycardia
   - Abnormal hemodynamic profile:
     – Elevated PAS and PAD pressures
     – Elevated PCW pressure
     – Increased SVR
3. Increased atrial pressure
   - S_4 may develop as the atria attempt to eject blood into rigid ventricles
   - Atrial arrhythmias may occur (e.g., PAC, AF) due to the increase in atrial pressure
   - Palpitations
   - Elevated A wave on PCW waveform
   - Elevated RA pressure
4. Left outflow tract obstruction
   - Systolic murmur as blood flows through a narrowed outflow tract due to septal hypertrophy; heard at apex

Restrictive Cardiomyopathy

Signs and symptoms of restrictive cardiomyopathy and pericarditis are similar. Diagnosis can usually be made after an echocardiogram.

1. Inability to maintain adequate cardiac output
   - Activity intolerance
   - Weakness
   - Sinus tachycardia
   - Arrhythmias
   - Decreased CO/cardiac index (CI)
2. Increased left ventricular filling pressures
   - Dyspnea
   - JVD
   - S_3
   - Narrowed pulse pressure
   - Systolic murmur with mitral valve insufficiency
   - Abnormal hemodynamic profile:
     – Elevated PAS, PAD, and PCW pressures
     – Elevated SVR
     – Elevated V wave on PCW waveform with mitral valve insufficiency
3. Increased right ventricular pressures
   - Peripheral edema
   - Hepatomegaly
   - Jaundice
   - JVD
   - Systolic murmur with tricuspid valve insufficiency
   - Kussmaul's sign (increased neck vein distention with inspiration)

- Elevated V wave on the RA waveform if tricuspid valve insufficient
4. Increased atrial pressures
   - Palpitations
   - S_4 may develop as the atria attempt to eject blood into rigid ventricles
   - Atrial arrhythmias may occur (e.g., PAC, AF) due to the increase in atrial pressure
   - Elevated A wave on PCW waveform
   - Elevated RA pressure
   - Elevated A wave on the RA waveform

Diagnostic Tests

Dilated Cardiomyopathy

- *Chest x-ray:* Left ventricular dilation with potential enlargement and dilatation of all four cardiac chambers.
- *12-Lead ECG:* ST-segment and T-wave changes; left axis deviation; left bundle branch block and left ventricular hypertrophy.
- *Echocardiography:* Dilated left ventricle with an increase in chamber size (other chambers may be enlarged also); diminished ventricular contractility; decreased septal movement; elevated ventricular volumes and decreased ejection fraction.
- *Endomyocardial biopsy:* Not usually done.

Hypertrophic Cardiomyopathy

- *Chest x-ray:* Normal or left atrial and ventricular dilatation (potential enlargement of right heart chambers).
- *12-Lead ECG:* ST-segment and T-wave changes; septal Q waves due to septal hypertrophy; left ventricular hypertrophy.
- *Echocardiography:* Thickened ventricular walls with a decrease in chamber size; left ventricular obstruction created by thickened ventricular septum and motion of mitral valve leaflet.
- *Endomyocardial biopsy:* Abnormal myocardial fibers that are in disarray.

Restrictive Cardiomyopathy

- *Chest x-ray:* Normal or slight enlargement of left atria and ventricle.
- *12-Lead ECG:* ST-segment and T-wave changes; low QRS amplitude.
- *Echocardiography:* Thickened ventricular walls; enlarged atria; diminished ventricular contractility; decreased ventricular volumes; elevated ventricular end-diastolic pressures.
- *Endomyocardial biopsy:* Not usually done.

Principles of Management for Cardiomyopathy

The primary objectives in the management of cardiomyopathy are to treat the underlying cause (if known); maximize cardiac function; assist the patient and family members to cope with a debilitating, chronic disease; and prevent complications associated with cardiomyopathy.

Improvement of Cardiac Function
Dilated Cardiomyopathy

1. *Improve myocardial oxygenation.* As ventricular dilatation occurs, ventricular wall tension increases, increasing the myocardial workload and oxygen consumption. Oxygen therapy should be initiated as necessary to increase oxygenation saturation. Pulse oximetry, mixed venous oxygenation saturation (SvO_2), and arterial blood gases are helpful in guiding sufficient oxygen therapy.
2. *Increase myocardial contractility.* Inotropic agents (e.g., digoxin, dobutamine) strengthen myocardial contractions; phosphodiesterase inhibitors (e.g., amrinone, milrinone) cause vasodilation and produce a positive inotropic effect, decreasing the workload of the failing ventricle.
3. *Decrease preload and afterload.* Diuretics decrease excess fluid and ventricular end-diastolic volumes; fluid and sodium restrictions also may be necessary. Vasodilators (e.g., nitroprusside, hydralazine) dilate arterial and venous vessels, decreasing venous return and resistance to ventricular systolic ejection.
4. *Mechanical cardiac assist devices* (e.g., intraaortic balloon therapy, hemopump therapy, ventricular assist device therapy) may be instituted to assist with the augmentation of adequate CO/CI.
5. *Dynamic cardiomyoplasty.* This is a relatively new surgical procedure that has grown in popularity since 1985. During surgery the latissimus dorsi muscle is dissected and wrapped around the cardiac muscle. The muscle is electrically stimulated to contract in harmony with ventricular systole to strengthen myocardial contraction and improve CO.
6. *Cardiac transplantation* may be necessary if medical therapy does not relieve patient symptoms.

Hypertrophic Cardiomyopathy

The management of the patient with hypertrophic cardiomyopathy focuses on promoting myocardial relaxation and decreasing left ventricular obstruction.

1. *Decrease myocardial contractility.* Use beta-blockers and/or calcium channel blockers to decrease heart rate, contractility, and myocardial oxygen consumption. One or both types of medications may be given in an effort to increase ventricular compliance, decrease ventricular outflow obstruction, and improve left ventricular function.
2. The following *medications* are usually contraindicated in patients with hypertrophic cardiomyopathy:
   - *Diuretics,* because a decrease in fluid volume decreases ventricle filling pressures and decreases CO.
   - *Inotropes* (e.g., digoxin, dobutamine), because an increase in contractility contributes to an increase in the left ventricular outflow obstruction.
   - *Vasodilators* (e.g., nitroglycerin, nitroprusside), because they decrease end-diastolic volume, leading to an increase in left ventricular outflow obstruction.
3. *Reduce physical and psychological stress.* Patients with hypertrophic cardiomyopathy are at an increased risk for sudden cardiac death, which may occur during stressful periods. It is important that strenuous physical activity be limited. In addition, sudden changes in position should be avoided, because the heart cannot respond to fluid shifts created by sudden position changes. Valsalva's maneuver should also be avoided. Psychological stress should also be decreased. Teach patients strategies to use to enhance self-relaxation. Relaxation therapy may include rhythmic breathing, biofeedback, and imagery.
4. *Cardiac surgery.* Myectomy may be indicated for individuals who do not respond to medical management and have severe left ventricular outflow obstruction. Myectomy involves removal of a portion of the enlarged intraventricular septum in an attempt to decrease left ventricular outflow obstruction and improve myocardial functioning.
5. *Ethanol ablation.* In recent years a new therapy for hypertrophic obstructive cardiomyopathy has emerged. Absolute alcohol (98% ethanol) is instilled into selected septal perforator branches of the left anterior descending coronary artery resulting in a therapeutic myocardial infarction (MI). The resultant outcome is reduction of left ventricular outflow obstruction and improved CO. The procedure is performed in the cardiac catheterization laboratory by the interventional cardiologists. It has been found to be associated with less risk than myectomy because it is less invasive. Long-term outcomes of this procedure have yet to be determined.

Restrictive Cardiomyopathy

1. *Decrease preload.* Diuretics, sodium and fluid restrictions, and vasodilators decrease ventricular end-diastolic volumes. The rigid ventricle is very sensitive to small fluid changes, significantly increasing ventricular end-diastolic pressure.

Facilitate Coping

For most patients, cardiomyopathy is a chronic, potentially life-threatening disease. Patients and their families often face an uncertain long-term prognosis. Emotions may vacillate as the family struggles to cope with the implications of the disease and its effect on lifestyle. Emphasis is placed on assisting the patient to remain active and to cope with a progressive disease. Involvement of the family unit in symptom management is also important. Relaxation therapy can benefit not only the patient, but also the family.

Preventing and Managing Complications

1. *Arrhythmias.* Continuous ECG monitoring; observe for potential side effects of cardiac medications; encourage family to learn cardiopulmonary resuscitation (CPR).
2. *Hemodynamic instability.* Pulmonary artery pressure monitoring; manage patient based on trends in hemodynamic parameters (i.e., RA, PAS, PAD, and PCW pressures; CO; CI; SVR; and PVR).
3. *Thromboembolic event.* Anticoagulation is necessary for patients with severely compromised left ventricular function and for patients experiencing AF. In both circumstances, thrombi may develop due to increased fluid volume and stasis.
4. *Endocarditis.* Antibiotic prophylaxis is recommended for patients with valve involvement. Prophylaxis should be given prior to dental work, surgery, or other invasive procedures.

Valvular Disease

Valvular disorders result from both congenital and acquired causes. Valves on the left side of the heart are more commonly affected because they are constantly exposed to higher pressures. Normally, when a valve opens, there are no pressure gradients, or differences, between the structures (chamber or vessel) above and below the valve. As valve disease progresses, pressure gradients between the two structures develop.

Valvular disorders are commonly classified as valve stenosis or valve insufficiency. A *stenotic valve* has a narrowed opening, permitting less blood to flow forward through it. An *insufficient valve* does not close properly, thus permitting some blood to flow backward instead of forward. Valve insufficiency is also referred to as valve regurgitation. Valve dysfunction may affect one or more valves.

The development of valve disease is usually a gradual process. As the case study illustrates, the patient's valvular problems began with a bacterial endocarditis 15 years prior to the onset of her symptoms of mitral valve insufficiency.

Etiology and Pathophysiology

Valve disorders are caused by either congenital or acquired diseases (Table 19–2). Congenital valve disorders may affect any of the four valves and result in valve stenosis or insufficiency. An example of a congenital valve disorder is an aortic valve with only one, instead of three, cusps. The unicusp valve causes an increase in turbulence as blood flows through the narrowed orifice. The individual may be asymp-

---

AT THE BEDSIDE
▶ *Valvular Disorder*

A 48-year-old woman was admitted to the coronary care unit with increasing shortness of breath and fatigue. She had bacterial endocarditis 15 years ago, which resulted in mitral valve insufficiency. On admission, she was in normal sinus rhythm with frequent premature atrial contractions, with a blood pressure of 150/94. Chest auscultation revealed rales in the left lower area. Hemodynamic parameters included:

RAP	12 mm Hg
PAP	35/25 mm Hg
PCWP	24 mm Hg
CO	4.8 L/min
CI	1.9 L/min/m^2
SVR	2100 dynes/sec/cm^5

---

tomatic until later in life when fibrotic tissue and calcium deposits form on the abnormal valve, leading to stenosis.

There are three types of acquired valve disorders: degenerative disease, rheumatic disease, or infective endocarditis. Degenerative disease may occur as the valve is damaged over time due to constant mechanical stress. This may occur with aging, or may be aggravated by conditions such as hypertension. Hypertension places significant pressure on the aortic valve, often causing insufficiency.

Individuals who develop rheumatic fever often experience valvular disease years later. Rheumatic disease contributes to gradual fibrotic changes of the valve, in addition to calcification of the valve cusps. Shortening of the chordae tendineae also may occur. Rheumatic fever commonly affects the mitral valve.

Infective endocarditis may occur as a primary or secondary infection. The valve tissue is destroyed by the infectious organism. Table 19–2 lists other conditions that cause valve disease.

Pathophysiology of Mitral Stenosis

Several processes occur that together cause stenosis or narrowing of the mitral valve orifice (Figure 19–2). Gradual fusion of the commissures (the valve leaflet edges) and fibrosis of the valve leaflets are common. In addition, calcium deposits may invade the valve leaflets, further impeding their movement. As the mitral valve becomes increasingly stenotic, the left atrium has to generate significant amounts of pressure to propel blood forward through the mitral valve and into the left ventricle. Left atrial pressures are commonly increased, with left atrial dilatation occurring as the stenosis worsens. Increased left atrial pressures may lead to increased pulmonary vascular pressures as fluid backs up into the pulmonary system, resulting in right-sided heart failure.

TABLE 19–2. ETIOLOGY OF VALVULAR DISORDERS

Mitral Stenosis
Rheumatic disease
Endocarditis
Degenerative process

Mitral Insufficiency
Rheumatic disease
Congenital
Endocarditis
Mitral valve prolapse
Papillary muscle dysfunction
Chordae tendineae dysfunction

Aortic Stenosis
Rheumatic disease
Congenital
Degenerative process

Aortic Insufficiency
Rheumatic disease
Congenital
Hypertension
Endocarditis
Marfan syndrome

Tricuspid Stenosis
Rheumatic disease
Congenital
Endocarditis

Tricuspid Insufficiency
Rheumatic disease
Marfan syndrome
Endocarditis
Ebstein's anomaly
Congenital
Secondary to left-sided valve disease
IV drug use

Pulmonic Stenosis
Rheumatic disease
Congenital
Endocarditis

Pulmonic Insufficiency
Primary pulmonary artery hypertension
Secondary to left-sided valve disease
Marfan syndrome
Endocarditis

Pathophysiology of Mitral Insufficiency

Adequate closure of the mitral valve is important so that blood is ejected forward, not backward, during ventricular systole. Damage to the mitral valve can affect the valve's ability to close properly (Figure 19–3). During ventricular systole, as blood is ejected forward into the aorta, blood is also ejected backward through the insufficient mitral valve. This abnormal blood flow contributes to an increase in left atrial volume, pressure, and eventually dilatation. Increased left atrial pressures may lead to increased pulmonary vascular pressures and right-sided heart failure. The left ventricle usually dilates and hypertrophies over time as end-diastolic volumes increase and cardiac output decreases.

Acute mitral insufficiency may occur due to dysfunction of the papillary muscles. Papillary muscle contraction is an important component of adequate mitral valve leaflet closure. Papillary muscles may rupture during an acute MI if blood supply is diminished or eliminated by coronary artery disease. Loss of a papillary muscle causes sudden, severe insufficiency of the mitral valve, resulting in rapid increase in both left ventricular and atrial volumes and pressures. The pulmonary vascular system is quickly affected by the high left-sided pressures, with pulmonary edema developing acutely. In acute mitral insufficiency, there is no time for the heart to compensate for the sudden increases in volume and pressure, as there is with long-standing mitral insufficiency.

Pathophysiology of Aortic Stenosis

A similar process occurs in aortic stenosis as occurs in mitral stenosis (Figure 19–4). Fusion of the commissures, fibrosis of the valve leaflets, and calcium deposits may occur on the aortic valve leaflets, impeding their movement. In aortic stenosis, the left ventricle has to generate a significant amount of pressure to propel blood forward through the aortic valve into the aorta. Left ventricular pressure increases lead to left ventricular dilatation and hypertrophy, as well as decreases in cardiac output. Left atrial volume and pressure may increase as pressure backs up from the left ventricle. Left atrial dilatation may eventually occur, and fluid may continue to back up into the pulmonary vascular system and to the right side of the heart, eventually causing right-sided heart failure.

Pathophysiology of Aortic Insufficiency

A similar process also occurs in aortic insufficiency as occurs with mitral insufficiency (Figure 19–5). Adequate closure of the aortic valve is even more important than adequate closure of the mitral valve. If the aortic valve is not closed properly, blood flows backward from the aorta into the left ventricle during diastole. This can seriously affect forward blood flow into the aorta, and thus cardiac output. This causes significant increases in the volumes and pressures of the left ventricle, with the gradual development of left ventricular dilatation and hypertrophy. As with other left-sided valve dysfunctions, pulmonary vascular system dysfunction and right-sided failure can also occur.

Pathophysiology of Tricuspid Stenosis

Fused commissures or fibrosis of the valve leaflets may also narrow the tricuspid valve orifice. Right atrial pressures increase as the right atrium attempts to propel blood forward into the right ventricle. Eventually, right atrial dilatation occurs and fluid may back up into the venous system.

Pathophysiology of Tricuspid Insufficiency

Damage to the tricuspid valve that prevents complete closure during ventricular systole causes the abnormal ejection of blood through the tricuspid valve into the right atrium. Right atrial volumes and pressures increase, leading eventually to dilatation and possible decreases in cardiac output.

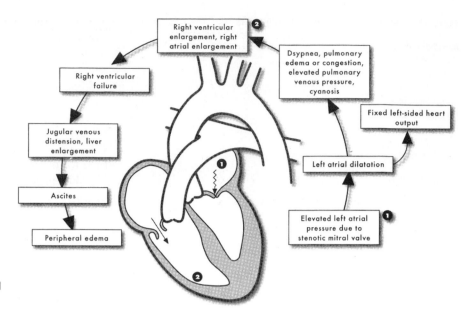

Figure 19–2. Cardiovascular effects of mitral stenosis.

Pathophysiology of Pulmonic Stenosis
Pulmonic stenosis develops as the pulmonic valve orifice becomes narrowed. Right ventricular pressures increase as the right ventricle attempts to eject blood forward into the pulmonary artery. Over time, right ventricular dilatation may occur, with decreases in right-sided cardiac output. The increased pressure may back up into the right atrium, causing an increase in volume and pressure, and eventually leading to dilatation. This can lead to volume and pressure increases in the venous system.

Pathophysiology of Pulmonic Insufficiency
Closure of the pulmonic valve prevents blood from backing up from the pulmonary artery into the right ventricle during

diastole. An insufficient pulmonic valve permits blood to flow backward into the right ventricle during diastole. Right-sided cardiac output decreases as blood flows backward instead of forward. An increase in right ventricular volume and pressure occurs, which may eventually lead to dilatation. The backflow of pressure may continue to the right atrium and then to the venous system.

Clinical Presentation

Mitral and Aortic Disease
The following signs and symptoms are found in all of the valvular disorders of the left side of the heart:

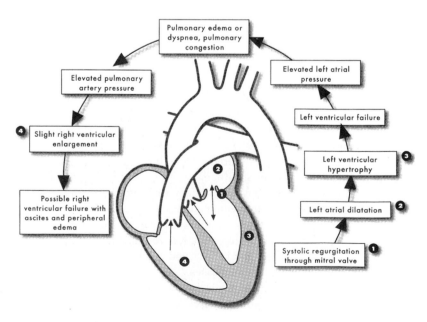

Figure 19–3. Cardiovascular effects of mitral insufficiency.

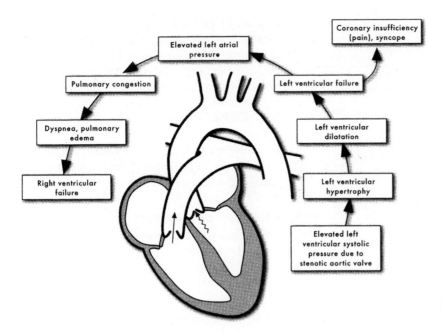

Figure 19–4. Cardiovascular effects of aortic stenosis.

- Dyspnea
- Fatigue
- Increased pulmonary artery pressures (PAS, PAD, PCW)
- Decreased CO

Mitral Stenosis

- Palpitations
- Hemoptysis
- Hoarseness
- Dysphagia

- JVD
- Orthopnea
- Cough
- Diastolic murmur
- Atrial arrhythmias (PAC, AF)
- Elevated A wave on PCW pressure waveform

Mitral Insufficiency

- Paroxysmal nocturnal dyspnea
- Orthopnea
- Palpitations

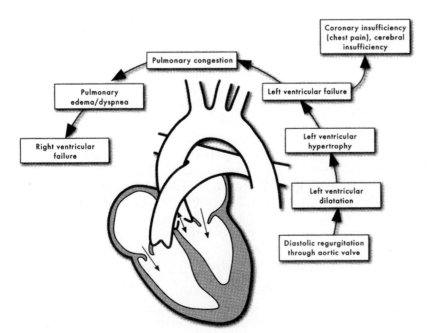

Figure 19–5. Cardiovascular effects of aortic insufficiency.

- S_3 and/or S_4
- Rales
- Systolic murmur
- Atrial arrhythmias
- Elevated V wave on PCW pressure waveform

Aortic Stenosis

- Angina
- Syncope
- Decreased SVR
- S_3 and/or S_4
- Systolic murmur
- Narrowed pulse pressure

Aortic Insufficiency

- Angina
- S_3
- Diastolic murmur
- Widened pulse pressure
- de Musset's sign (nodding of the head)

Tricuspid and Pulmonary Valve Disease
The following signs and symptoms are found in all of the valvular disorders of the right side of the heart:

- Dyspnea
- Fatigue
- Increased RA pressures
- Peripheral edema
- Hepatomegaly
- JVD

Tricuspid Stenosis

- Atrial arrhythmias
- Diastolic murmur
- Decreased CO
- Elevated A wave on RA pressure waveform

Tricuspid Insufficiency

- Conduction delays
- Supraventricular tachycardia
- Systolic murmur
- Elevated V wave on RA pressure waveform

Pulmonic Stenosis

- Cyanosis
- Systolic murmur
- Elevated A wave on RA pressure waveform

Pulmonic Insufficiency

- Diastolic murmur
- Elevated A wave on RA pressure waveform

Diagnostic Tests
- *Chest x-ray:* Shows specific cardiac chamber enlargement, pulmonary congestion, presence of valve calcification.

- *12-Lead ECG:* Useful in the diagnosis of right ventricular, left ventricular, and left atrial hypertrophy.
- *Echocardiogram:* Demonstrates the size of the four cardiac chambers, presence of hypertrophy, specific valve dysfunction, ejection fraction, and amount of regurgitant flow, if present.
- *Radionuclide studies:* Identify abnormal ejection fraction during inactivity and activity.
- *Cardiac catheterization:* Determines cardiac chamber pressures, ejection fraction, regurgitation, and pressure gradients, if present.

Principles of Management for Valvular Disorders
The primary objectives in the management of valvular disorders are to maximize cardiac function, reduce anxiety, and prevent complications associated with valve disease.

Maximize Cardiac Function

Medical Management

1. *Improve myocardial oxygenation.* As ventricular dilatation occurs, there is an increase in ventricular wall tension, myocardial workload, and oxygen consumption. Oxygen therapy should be initiated, as necessary, to increase oxygen saturation. Pulse oximetry, mixed venous oxygenation saturation (Svo_2), and arterial blood gases are helpful in guiding sufficient oxygen therapy.
2. *Decrease preload.* Diuretics decrease excess fluid and ventricular end-diastolic volumes. Fluid and sodium restrictions also may be necessary. (*Exception:* Preload usually is not decreased in patients with aortic insufficiency, because decreased left ventricular end-diastolic volumes may accentuate decreases in CO.)
3. *Decrease afterload.* Afterload reduction may be indicated for patients with increased SVR and impaired left ventricular function (e.g., aortic stenosis or mitral insufficiency).
4. *Improve contractility.* Inotropic agents (e.g., digoxin, dobutamine) strengthen myocardial contractions and improve CO.
5. *Modify activity.* Activity limitation helps to decrease myocardial oxygen consumption. Teach patients the importance of rest between activities.
6. *Balloon valvuloplasty* may be an option for stenotic mitral or aortic valves. A percutaneous catheter is inserted via the femoral artery under fluoroscopy and the balloon is inflated at the stenotic lesion in an effort to force open the fused commissures and improve valve leaflet mobility.

Surgical Management
Cardiac surgery is indicated when medical management does not alleviate patient symptoms. Patients may have better sur-

gical outcomes if surgery is done prior to left ventricular dysfunction.

1. *Valve repair.* An increasing trend today is to have dysfunctional valves repaired instead of replaced. The hemodynamic function of the inherent valve is superior to any prosthetic valve. In addition, the risks associated with valve replacement are avoided. An open commissurotomy may be performed to relieve stenosis of any of the four heart valves. During open commissurotomy, the fused commissures are incised, thus mobilizing the valve leaflets. Valve leaflet reconstruction also may be done to patch tears in valve leaflets using pericardial patches for the repair. Chordae tendineae reconstruction may be performed to elongate fibrotic tendineae or to shorten excessively stretched tendineae. An annuloplasty ring may also be inserted to correct dilatation of the valve annulus.

2. *Prosthetic valve replacement.* Replacement of the native valve with a prosthetic, or artificial, valve is done for severely damaged valves or when repair is not possible. The entire native valve is removed and replaced with a mechanical or biological (porcine, bovine, or allograft) prosthetic valve.

3. *Postoperative management* after cardiac surgery is similar to coronary artery bypass surgery management (see Chapter 9, Cardiovascular System). Special considerations for patients having valve repair or replacement include the following:

   - *Maintain adequate preload.* Patients with valvular disease usually are accustomed to increased end-diastolic volumes. Although the valve is repaired, the heart needs time to adjust to the hemodynamic changes. Most patients do better in the postoperative phase if fluids are adjusted based on presurgical RA and PCW pressures.

   - *Monitor for conduction disturbances.* The mitral, tricuspid, and aortic valves lie in close proximity to conduction pathways. Conduction disorders may be treated by temporary or permanent cardiac pacing.

   - *Initiate anticoagulation therapy.* Anticoagulation therapy is usually initiated for patients having valve replacement after the epicardial pacing wires are removed. This may be as early as the first postoperative day.

Reducing Anxiety

1. *Teach the patient relaxation techniques.* Deep breathing or imagery may help alleviate anxiety especially when symptoms of valve dysfunction occur.

Preventing and Managing Complications

1. *Arrhythmias:* Continuous ECG monitoring; daily 12-lead ECG; observe for side effects of specific cardiac medications.

2. *Hemodynamic instability:* Pulmonary artery pressure (PAP) monitoring, manage patient based on trends in hemodynamic monitoring.

3. *Thromboembolic event:* Anticoagulation is necessary for patients with severely compromised left ventricular function or AF, and after valve surgery. Lifelong anticoagulation therapy is indicated for patients after mechanical valve replacement. Short-term anticoagulation therapy is usually initiated for patients having a biological valve replacement.

3. *Endocarditis:* Antibiotic prophylaxis is recommended for patients with valve disorders and for patients with prosthetic valves. Prophylaxis should be given prior to dental work, surgery, or other invasive procedures. Prior to discharge, teach the patient and family the importance of prophylaxis.

4. *Prosthetic valve dysfunction:* Biological valve dysfunction usually develops slowly with gradual signs and symptoms (e.g., presence of a new murmur, dyspnea, syncope). Mechanical valve dysfunction may occur slowly or suddenly. Rapid valve dysfunction requires emergency intervention as the patient presents with signs and symptoms of acute cardiac failure (hypotension, tachycardia, low CO/CI, congestive heart failure, cardiac arrest).

Pericarditis

Pericarditis is a chronic or acute inflammation of the pericardial lining of the heart. Acute pericarditis usually occurs secondary to another disease process and usually resolves within 6 weeks. Chronic pericarditis, however, may last for months.

Pericarditis may lead to pericardial effusion or cardiac tamponade. Pericardial effusion occurs as fluid builds up within the pericardial sac. Cardiac tamponade can occur as the pericardial fluid compresses the heart, restricts ventricular end-diastolic filling, and compromises cardiac function.

AT THE BEDSIDE
▶ *Pericarditis*

A woman had an acute anterior myocardial infarction 5 days ago. She was readmitted to the CCU with dull, substernal chest pain, shortness of breath, and ST-segment elevations in the precordial leads and in leads I and II. The chest pain was unrelieved with nitroglycerin. Her pain was decreased after receiving 4 mg of morphine IV. Her pain was completely relieved when her nurse had her sit up and lean forward so that he could auscultate posterior breath sounds.

The case study is an example of the importance of accurate diagnosis of patients with chest pain. The pain of pericarditis may be similar to anginal pain, but the treatment is very different.

Etiology and Pathophysiology

A number of different conditions and situations can cause pericarditis (Table 19–3). Common causes include MI, infections, neoplasm, radiation therapy, and uremia.

Normally, the pericardial sac contains a small amount of clear serous fluid, typically less than 50 mL. This fluid lies between the visceral and parietal pleura and contributes to the ease with which the heart expands and contracts. An inflammation of the pericardium causes friction between the visceral and parietal pleura.

Inflammation of the pericardium causes an increase in pericardial fluid production, with increases of up to 1 L or more. A gradual buildup of fluid may have little compromising effect on the heart as the pericardium expands and hemodynamic functioning is not altered. A sudden increase in pericardial fluid, however, has dramatic effects on hemodynamic functioning.

Chronic pericarditis causes fibrotic changes within the pericardial lining. The visceral and parietal pleura eventually adhere to each other, restricting the filling of the heart. This condition may be referred to as *constrictive pericarditis*. The pressure created by the constricted pericardium affects the heart's ability to distend properly, causing decreases in end-diastolic volume and cardiac output. These changes may contribute to increases in atrial pressures, leading to increases in pulmonary vascular and venous system pressures.

Clinical Presentation

Acute Pericarditis

- Sharp, stabbing, burning, dull, or aching pain in the substernal or precordial area, which increases with movement, inspiration, or coughing, or when the patient is in a recumbent position
- Pericardial friction rub
- Fever
- Sinus tachycardia

TABLE 19–3. ETIOLOGY OF PERICARDITIS

Idiopathic
Infections (viral/bacterial)
Myocardial infarction
Cardiac surgery
Neoplasm
Radiation therapy
Rheumatic disease
Lupus erythematosus
Scleroderma
Uremia
Medication induced

- Dyspnea, orthopnea
- Cough
- Fatigue
- Narrowed pulse pressure
- Hypotension
- Arrhythmias
- Elevated cardiac pressures (PA, PCW, RA)
- Decreased CO
- Peripheral edema
- JVD

Chronic Pericarditis

- Dyspnea
- Anorexia
- Fatigue
- Abdominal discomfort
- Weight gain
- Activity intolerance
- JVD
- Peripheral edema
- Hepatomegaly
- Kussmaul's sign (increase in RA pressure during inspiration)

Diagnostic Tests

- *Chest x-ray:* Normal or enlarged heart; chronic pericarditis may reveal a decrease in heart size.
- *ECG:* ST-segment elevation in precordial leads (V leads) and leads I, II, or III; T-wave inversion after ST-segment returns to isoelectric line; decrease in QRS voltage.
- *Echocardiogram:* Presence of increased fluid in pericardial sac; chronic, constrictive pericarditis may demonstrate a thickened pericardium and diminished ventricular contractility.
- *Laboratory:* Elevated sedimentation rate and elevated WBC; causative organisms may be identified from blood cultures.
- *CT/MRI Scan:* Detects a thickened pericardium for patients with chronic pericarditis.

Principles of Management for Pericarditis

The primary principles of management of pericarditis are to correct the underlying cause, relieve pain and promote comfort, relieve pericardial effusion, and prevent and manage complications associated with pericarditis.

Promoting Comfort and Relieving Pain

1. *Decrease pain.* Teach the patient that chest pain may be decreased or relieved by sitting up and/or leaning forward. Analgesics (e.g., aspirin) and narcotics (e.g., morphine) administered around the clock assist in pain relief.
2. *Promote relaxation.* Teach the patient relaxation techniques such as progressive muscle relaxation

and visualization. This may assist the patient to cope. Relaxation techniques that include deep breathing should be avoided because pericardial pain usually increases with deep inspiration.

3. *Limit activity.* This is especially important during the acute period of inflammation. Activity can be gradually increased as fever and chest pain decrease. Assist patients to find a position of comfort. Patients often are more comfortable sitting up and leaning slightly forward.

Correcting the Underlying Cause

1. *Decrease pericardial inflammation.* Nonsteroidal anti-inflammatory agents (e.g., indomethacin, ibuprofen) assist to decrease inflammation of the pericardium and the associated pain. Chronic, recurrent pericarditis may require corticosteroid therapy.
2. *Eliminate infection.* If the cause of the pericarditis is an infectious process, appropriate medications, including antibiotic therapy, are necessary.

Relieving Pericardial Effusion

1. *Pericardiocentesis.* A needle is placed within the pericardial sac and fluid is withdrawn via the needle or is attached to a catheter and drained into a bottle. This procedure is performed to decrease fluid in the pericardium, in an effort to improve myocardial function. Culture specimens of the drained fluid should be obtained and sent to the laboratory for analysis. The drain may be left in for several days until the volume of drainage is minimal.
2. *Pericardiotomy/pericardial window.* This is a surgical procedure in which a section of the pericardium is removed in an effort to decrease pericardial pressure on the heart and to allow pericardial fluid to drain more readily. It may be performed for recurrent pericardial effusions.
3. *Pericardiectomy.* This involves surgically removing the entire pericardium. This may be necessary for chronic pericarditis that is refractory to other interventions.

Preventing and Managing Complications

1. *Monitor for signs and symptoms of acute heart failure.* These include hypotension, tachycardia, increased respiration, extreme dyspnea, pink frothy sputum, decreased oxygen saturation, decreased peripheral pulses, and decreased urinary output. Oxygen therapy and inotropic agents assist in improvement of myocardial contractility. Assessment of the need for surgical intervention for pericarditis may be indicated.
2. *Cardiac tamponade.* Monitor for signs and symptoms of cardiac tamponade. These include hypotension, tachycardia, tachypnea, dyspnea, pulsus paradoxus, narrowed pulse pressure, muffled heart sounds, and distended neck veins. Emergency pericardiocentesis is necessary to prevent further hemodynamic compromise.

Aortic Aneurysm

An *aortic aneurysm* is an area of aortic wall dilatation. Aneurysms are most prevalent in men, commonly occurring during their early 50s to late 60s. Without treatment, mortality from aneurysms is high.

Aneurysms frequently are classified by types (Figure 19–6). A *fusiform aneurysm* is characterized by distention of the entire circumference of the affected portion of the aorta. A *saccular aneurysm* is characterized by distention of one side of the aorta. The distention of a saccular aneurysm resembles a bulging sac. Aneurysms may also be classified according to their location (Figure 19–7):

- *Ascending:* between the aortic valve and the innominate artery
- *Transverse:* between the innominate artery and the left subclavian artery
- *Descending:* from the left subclavian artery to the diaphragm
- *Thoracoabdominal:* from the diaphragm to the aortic bifurcation

Aneurysms have the potential to dissect or rupture. *Dissection* occurs when the intimal aortic wall is disrupted and blood extends into the aortic vessel layers (Figure 19–6C and 19–6D). *Rupture* occurs when all three layers of the aorta are disrupted and massive hemorrhage occurs. Both dissection and rupture are life-threatening events. The case study demonstrates the sudden onset of signs and symptoms associated with aortic rupture and the emergent need for lifesaving interventions.

Etiology and Pathophysiology

Aortic aneurysms are caused by a variety of conditions, including atherosclerosis, cystic medial necrosis, genetic link, congenital abnormality, hypertension, Marfan syndrome, and trauma to the chest.

The aorta is composed of three layers: the intima, media, and tunica adventitia. Aneurysm development is initiated by degeneration of smooth muscle cells and elastic tissue in the medial layer of the aorta. This weakens the vessel wall, potentially leading to dilatation of all layers of the aorta. The aortic wall may be further weakened with age, as well as from hypertension.

As the aortic aneurysm gradually expands, there is an increase in the risk for aortic dissection. Dissection is caused by a tear in the intima. Blood leaves the central aorta via the intimal tear and flows through the medial layer of the aorta (Figure 19–6C and 19–6D). This creates a false lumen. As the amount of blood increases in the medial layer, the pres-

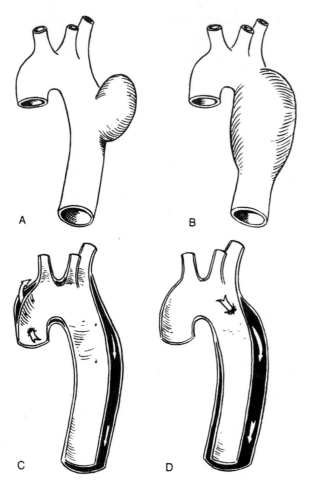

Figure 19–6. Diagram of different types of aortic aneurysms. **(A)** Fusiform aneurysm. **(B)** Saccular aneurysm. **(C, D)** Two aortic dissections. (*From Underhill SL, Woods SL, Sivarajan ES, Halpenny CJ:* Cardiac Nursing, *p. 680. Philadelphia: JB Lippincott; 1982.*)

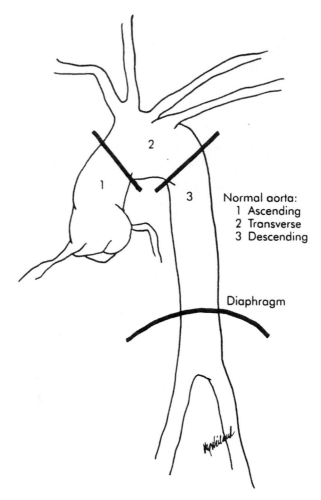

Figure 19–7. Classification of aortic aneurysms according to location. (*From: Seifert PC:* Cardiac Surgery, *p. 321. St. Louis, MO: Mosby Yearbook; 1994.*)

sure in the false lumen increases, compressing the central aorta (Figure 19–6D). This compression may decrease or totally obstruct blood flow through the aorta and/or its arterial branches. Dissections are classified as acute if they have occurred less than 2 weeks since the onset of symptoms. They are classified as chronic if they occurred more than 2 weeks since the onset of symptoms.

Two additional classifications exist for identifying the location of aortic dissections (Figure 19–8). The first classifies the dissection as type A, involving the ascending aorta, or type B, involving the descending aorta (distal to the left subclavian artery). Another classification system for aortic dissection has three categories for the dissection: Type I, the original intimal tear begins in the ascending aorta and the dissection extends to the descending aorta; type II, the original intimal tear begins and is contained in the ascending aorta; and type III: the original intimal tear begins and is contained in the descending aorta.

Clinical Presentation

Patients rarely demonstrate early signs of an aortic aneurysm. Diagnosis is commonly made during a routine physical examination or chest x-ray. Signs and symptoms of an aortic aneurysm occur as the aneurysm enlarges and compresses adjacent organs, structures, and/or nerve pathways.

Thoracic Aneurysm

- Ripping, tearing, or splitting pain, located at the anterior chest or posterior chest between the scapula, of an intense or excruciating nature
- Dysphagia
- Hoarseness, cough
- Dyspnea
- Different blood pressures when comparing right and left arms
- Different pulses when comparing right and left peripheral pulses

AT THE BEDSIDE
▶ *Aortic Aneurysm*

A 62-year-old man was admitted to the ICU with substernal chest pain. The chest pain was unrelieved by nitroglycerin. The pain decreased in intensity after 8 mg of morphine sulfate. His admitting ECG was normal. His chest x-ray revealed a widened mediastinum, and an aortogram demonstrated a thoracic aneurysm. He has nitroprusside infusing at 1.0 mcg/kg/min to maintain his systolic blood pressure below 100 mm Hg. Suddenly, the patient yells out, "The pain, the pain . . . it's back . . . it's even worse than before." A rapid assessment reveals the following:

BP	190/100 mm Hg
HR	110 beats/min
RR	30 breaths/min
Color	Gray
Skin	Moist and cool
Pain	Rated 10 on a 0 to 10 scale, described as tearing in the middle of his chest and between his shoulder blades

Abdominal Aneurysm

- Dull, constant abdominal or low back or lumbar pain
- Abdominal mass
- Pulsations in the abdomen
- Reduced lower extremity pulses

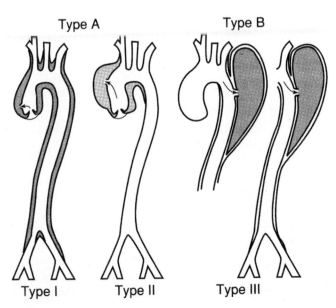

Figure 19–8. Classification for the location of aortic dissections. The Stanford system classifies aortic dissections based on involvement (type A) of the ascending aorta or noninvolvement (type B). The DeBakey system classifies dissections into types I, II, or III. (*From DeBakey ME, et al: Surgical management of dissecting aneurysms of the aorta.* J Thorac Cardiovasc Surg *1965;49:131; adapted by Seifert PC:* Cardiac Surgery, *p. 321. St. Louis, MO: Mosby Yearbook; 1994.*)

- Nausea and/or vomiting

Aortic Dissection

- Sudden intense pain in chest or back (or sudden increase in the intensity of pain)
- Dyspnea
- Syncope
- Abdominal discomfort or bloating
- Extremity weakness
- Oliguria or hematuria
- Hemiparesis, hemiplegia, or paraplegia
- Speech or visual disturbances
- Decreased hemoglobin and hematocrit

Aortic Rupture

- Sudden cessation of pain
- Reoccurrence of pain
- Signs and symptoms of shock, with the exception of blood pressure (high in rupture), including tachycardia, increased respiratory rate, pallor, moist skin, and restlessness

Diagnostic Tests

- *Chest x-ray:* Shows the dilated aorta, widening of the mediastinum, and mediastinal mass.
- *Aortography:* Determines the origin, size, and location of the aneurysm and involvement of additional arterial branches.
- *CT/MRI Scan:* Determines the size of the aorta, size of the aneurysm, extent of a dissection, involvement of additional arterial branches, lumen diameter, and wall thickness.

Principles of Management for Aortic Aneurysm

The primary objectives in the management of aortic aneurysm are relieving pain and anxiety, decreasing stress on the aneurysm, surgical repair, patient teaching, and prevention of complications.

Relieving Pain and Anxiety

Administer narcotics (e.g., morphine) as necessary. Unrelieved pain is likely to increase anxiety, tachycardia, and hypertension, all of which may aggravate the condition. Relaxation therapy, with deep breathing exercises or imagery, may be extremely helpful.

Decreasing Stress on Aneurysm Wall

1. *Decrease afterload.* Vasodilators (e.g., nitroprusside, nicardipine) may be prescribed to lower blood pressure and thus pressure on the aneurysm. Blood pressures should be maintained as low as possible (systolic blood pressure 90 to 120 mm Hg), without compromising perfusion to vital organs.

2. *Decrease preload.* Limit oral and IV fluids, decrease sodium intake, and administer diuretics as indicated. A decrease in preload decreases the circulating blood volume, thus decreasing pressure on the aneurysm.
3. *Decrease myocardial contractility* with beta-blockers (e.g., esmolol, labetalol). A decrease in the strength of each cardiac contraction decreases the pulsatile pressure on the aneurysm.

Patient Teaching

1. *Follow-up.* If the patient is to be medically managed, follow-up chest x-rays, CT scans, MRI scans, and/or ultrasounds will be needed at 6-month intervals to assess the status of the aneurysm. The importance of these studies should be stressed.
2. *Diet modification.* Teach the patient and family the importance of following a low-sodium diet. Consult a nutritionist for recipes and tips for food preparation.
3. *Smoking cessation.* Assist patient with programs available to assist with smoking cessation.
4. *Physical/psychological stress modification.* Teach the patient and family the hazardous effects of stress and the importance for modification. Discuss activity limitations and relaxation therapy.
5. *Medications.* Teach the patient and family the importance of compliance with the medication regimen. Stress that the medications are essential even though the patient may be asymptomatic.

Surgical Management
Surgery is indicated for acute aneurysm rupture, aortic dissection in the ascending aorta, aortic dissection refractory to medical therapy, and asymptomatic patients with a fusiform aneurysm 6 or more cm in diameter (normal diameter is 2.5 to 3 cm).

1. During surgery the aortic aneurysm is resected and a prosthetic graft is sutured in place. The original aortic wall may be wrapped around the prosthetic graft for additional support.
2. If an acute dissection or rupture occurs and the patient is waiting for the operating room team to arrive,
   • Administer narcotics for pain.
   • Titrate vasodilators to maintain the patient's blood pressure as low as possible (90 to 120 mm Hg if tolerated). This decreases the pressure on the aneurysm.
   • Administer fluids to prevent hypovolemia.
   • Administer blood replacement products to maintain adequate hemoglobin and hematocrit levels.
3. Postoperative management:
   • Same interventions as described to relieve pain and anxiety and decrease stress on the aorta wall.

It is important to decrease pressure on the repaired aorta so that suture lines can heal and bleeding is kept to a minimum.
   • Continuous ECG and hemodynamic monitoring.
   • Continuous spinal pressure monitoring (for surgical repair of descending thoracic aortic dissection) draining spinal fluid as necessary to maintain pressure at 10 mm Hg or less.
   • Complete assessment every 1 to 2 hours.
   • Gradual rewarming of the patient is important. Prevent postoperative shivering, which increases blood pressure and places additional stress on suture lines.
   • Ventilator management to maximize oxygenation.
   • Keep the head of the bed less than 45° the first 2 postoperative days to avoid additional tension on the prosthetic graft. Activity may be progressed more rapidly depending on institution standards and surgeon preference.
   • Monitor renal function [urine output, blood urea nitrogen (BUN)], and creatinine, especially if the aorta was cross-clamped above the renal arteries.
   • Initiate anticoagulation. Anticoagulation therapy is initiated for patients receiving prosthetic valves.

Preventing and Managing Complications

1. *Hemorrhage.* Hourly assessment of vital signs and hemodynamic parameters. Daily hemoglobin and hematocrit.
2. *Arrhythmias.* Continuous ECG monitoring; daily 12-lead ECGs.
3. *Hemodynamic instability.* Arterial and pulmonary artery pressure monitoring; manage hemodynamic parameters based on trends.
4. *Altered perfusion.* Arteries originating from the aorta may be compromised, leading to MI, cerebral insufficiency/cerebrovascular accident, bowel necrosis, renal failure, paraplegia, and limb ischemia. Assess and monitor the patient for these conditions.
5. *Aortic insufficiency.* Aortic insufficiency may develop if the aneurysm is located in the ascending aorta. Enlargement or dissection of the aneurysm may dilate or damage the aortic valve, causing signs of acute congestive heart failure and pulmonary edema.

Cardiac Transplantation

From the early work of Dr. Christian Barnard in 1967, cardiac transplantation has evolved over nearly four decades to a standard modality for the treatment of end-stage cardiac disease. When medical, surgical, or pharmacologic interventions have failed to improve quality of life and functional capacity, cardiac transplantation offers patients improved survival. The international survival rate is 80% to 90% at 1 year and 72% at 10 years. The primary indications for cardiac transplantation include cardiomyopathies or ischemic heart disease. Other indications include cardiac valvular disease, congenital heart disease, and myocarditis.

Candidate Selection

Patients usually have a less than 1-year survival without cardiac transplant and are in New York Heart Association (NYHA) functional class III or IV. Because of the shortage of available organs, the patient must pass an extensive screening process to ascertain that he or she is appropriate for the candidate list (Table 19–4). Patients must be emotionally stable and free of alcohol or drug addictions. They must demonstrate a commitment to the rigors of being a candidate and eventual recipient through compliance with their medical regimens.

The period of waiting for an available donor can be extremely stressful for the patients and their families. It is important to explore their perceptions of the transplant process, what outcomes they are anticipating, and what methods they have utilized to cope in the past. Support group participation or meetings with a psychiatric clinical nurse specialist or nurse practitioner may be beneficial. Fear of death and critical illness may heighten the patient's anxiety. Family members may need proximity to the patient, and this may assist in alleviating anxiety. Incorporating their involvement in direct patient care may enhance their coping abilities.

Pretransplant Process

The greatest delay for cardiac transplantation occurs because of the shortage of donors. When a brain-dead donor is identified, he or she must be carefully managed to maintain cardiovascular stability and avoid electrolyte and renal complications. The United Network for Organ Sharing (UNOS) coordinates the allocation of organs based on a nationwide waiting list. The donor must be of a compatible ABO blood type to the recipient and of similar body size and weight. The recipient is tested for relative immunologic compatibility with the donor to avoid hyperacute rejection. Panel-reactive antibody screening is performed using the recipient's serum with a random pool of lymphocytes. If no lymphocyte destruction occurs, the cross-match is negative and the transplant may proceed. The donor's cardiac function must be normal as assessed by an echocardiogram, nuclear studies, or cardiac catheterization. The donor should have stable hemodynamic profiles on minimal inotropic support.

This process may take several hours, and it is imperative that the patient and family be frequently updated and made aware of the clinical plan of care. Pretransplant teaching should be reviewed to clarify misconceptions and correct knowledge deficits. If cardiac output is compromised, decreased cerebral perfusion may compromise the attention

---

TABLE 19–4. RECIPIENT SELECTION CRITERIA FOR CARDIAC TRANSPLANTATION

End-stage cardiac disease
Condition that can no longer be managed by conventional medical or
    surgical therapy
Placement in NYHA functional class III or IV
Life expectancy <1 year
Age <65 years
Absence of other conditions that limit survival:
    Fixed pulmonary vascular resistance >6–8 Wood units
    Systemic infection
    Irreversible renal insufficiency
    Irreversible pulmonary insufficiency
    Recent pulmonary embolus
    Active peptic ulcer
    Malignancy
Absence of smoking or alcohol and drug abuse
Compliant, well-motivated patient

From: Dressler DK: The patient undergoing cardiac transplant surgery. In Guzzetta CE, Dossey BM [eds.]: Cardiovascular Nursing Holistic Practice. St. Louis, MO: Mosby-Year Book, 1992.

AT THE BEDSIDE
▶ *Cardiac Transplant*

A 54-year-old, white, married, unemployed man is admitted to the surgical ICU for idiopathic cardiomyopathy after an orthotopic heart transplant (OHT). He is orally intubated with a mediastinal chest tube draining 60 mL of sanguinous fluid per hour. Atrial and ventricular epicardial wires, a left radial arterial line, and a right subclavian Swan-Ganz catheter are in place.

Temperature	35.88°C
BP	140/82 mm Hg
HR	90/min NSR without ectopy; remnant P wave present
RR	18/min
Ventilator settings	0.50 FiO_2
	TV of 700 mL
	Assist control mode, rate of 14/min
	PEEP 5 cm H_2O
CO	3.80 L/min
Urine	60 mL/h
CI	2.0 L/min/m^2
Mediastinal tube	60 mL/h
SVR	1800 dyne/sec/cm^5
SvO_2	58%
SPO_2	96%
Neurology	Moves all extremities on command; neurologically intact

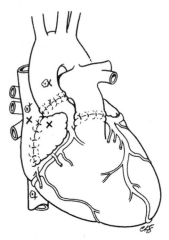

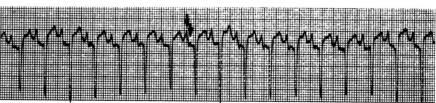

Figure 19–9. Orthotopic method of transplantation. Both the donor and the recipient SA nodes are intact (x). This results in an ECG tracing as shown. Note the double P wave, at independent rates. (*From: Weber BL: Cardiac surgery and heart transplantation. In Hudak CM, Gallo BM [eds]: Critical Care Nursing: A Holistic Approach. Philadelphia: JB Lippincott; 1994.*)

span. During this time, the recipient needs close monitoring to maintain cardiovascular stability. The recipient may require antidysrhythmic therapy, inotropes, diuretics, or afterload reduction agents to achieve major organ perfusion adequate for cellular function. Anticoagulation therapy may be instituted to decrease risk of embolization secondary to AF, reduced left ventricular function, or peripheral venous stasis.

The most unstable patient may be maintained on a cardiac assist device such as the intra-aortic balloon pump (IABP) or ventricular assist device (VAD) to promote stabilization or to "bridge" him or her to transplantation.

Transplant Surgical Techniques

In the past, there were two surgical options for cardiac transplantation. Today, almost all are orthotopic transplants in which the recipient's heart is removed and replaced by the donor heart in the normal anatomic position (Figure 19–9). The surgical approach is a median sternotomy; the recipient's heart is incised at the superior and inferior vena cavae, pulmonary artery, and aorta. The donor and recipient's vena cavae, aortas, and pulmonary arteries are aligned and anastomosed. The fact that the donor's heart is denervated results in no sympathetic or parasympathetic influence, so the donor heart must rely on noncardiac mediators to increase cardiac output.

The other surgical option was a heterotopic approach, which is interesting from a historical perspective. It was used in about 5% of cardiac transplants at one point and was also known as a "piggyback" approach. The donor heart was placed to the right side of the pleural cavity and performed as an auxiliary pump for the native heart (Figure 19–10). This was used as an option in a size mismatch between donor and recipient or for severe pulmonary hypertension. This approach is rarely performed any more.

Principles of Management for Cardiac Transplantation

The postsurgical care is similar to care following conventional open heart surgery (see Chapter 9, Cardiovascular System). The primary objectives in the early postoperative period include stabilizing cardiovascular function, monitoring altered immune response and graft protection, and providing posttransplant psychological adjustment.

Stabilizing Cardiovascular Function

1. *Cardiac denervation.* Postoperatively there is loss of vagal influence, and the patient usually has a higher resting heart rate than normal.
   - The posttransplant patient requires more stabilization prior to exercise or position changes to avoid orthostasis due to these effects from denervation. With loss of vagal tone, should the sinus rate decrease, there is a stronger potential for junctional rhythms to result.
   - *Surgical manipulation and postoperative edema* may decrease donor SA node automaticity, and therefore the patient may require temporary pacing or isoproterenol (Isuprel) to increase the heart rate.
   - Should *arrhythmias* such as SVT occur, the denervated heart does not respond to digitalis, Valsalva's maneuver, or carotid sinus pressure. Beta-blockers or calcium channel blockers are used to decrease heart rate in these circumstances. It is important to assess the patient for response to iso-

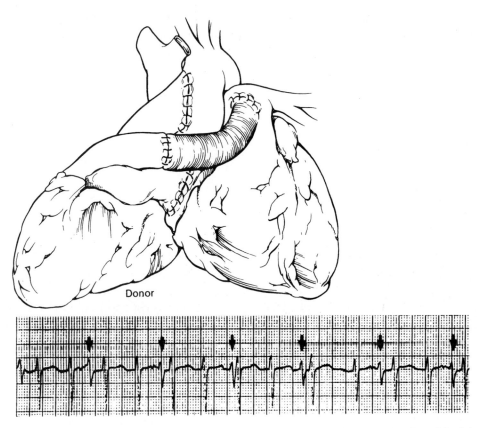

Donor

Figure 19–10. Heterotopic method of transplantation. The donor heart is anastomosed with a Dacron graft to the recipient's heart. This results in an ECG tracing as shown. Note the "extra" QRS at an independent rate. (*From: Weber BL: Cardiac surgery and heart transplantation. In Hudak CM, Gallo BM [eds]: Critical Care Nursing: A Holistic Approach. Philadelphia: JB Lippincott; 1994.*)

proterenol, because the drug can increase myocardial oxygen consumption.

- *Denervation* creates a more long-term concern in these patients because the patient no longer experiences angina if the myocardium becomes ischemic. Pain impulses are not transmitted to the brain, so patients must be taught to report other signs of declining cardiac function (i.e., decreased exercise tolerance). This is seen in chronic rejection where even with diffuse coronary artery disease, the patient does not experience angina. The patient transplanted for ischemic cardiac disease may find this difficult to comprehend.

2. *Ventricular failure.* Any element of pulmonary hypertension can result in right ventricular dysfunction and eventually compromise left ventricular function also. Inotropic and vasodilating agents may be required to enhance cardiac function. It is essential to rule out any cardiac injury during harvesting and implantation that may have an impact on cardiac function. In reviewing the operative procedure, rule out reperfusion injuries or postbypass problems.

3. *Bleeding.* Risk factors include cardiopulmonary bypass (CPB), altered coagulation factors if right ventricular failure compromised hepatic function, and preoperative anticoagulation therapy. The recipient's pericardium may be enlarged from pretransplant cardiomegaly. With a smaller donor heart there is more room for blood accumulation without early detection. If there is greater than 100 to 200 mL/h of bleeding for 2 hours, the patient may need to be reexplored. All medications should be reviewed for potential effect on platelet function and coagulation factors.

Monitoring Altered Immune Response and Graft Protection

After cardiac transplantation, the patient is pharmacologically managed with immunosuppressive treatment for graft protection, with titrating for the best graft function with the least adverse effects. By virtue of these agents, patient survival has been tremendously enhanced, with a decrease in the need for retransplantation.

1. *Immunosuppression.* Most patients are maintained on triple-therapy immunosuppression: cyclosporine, mycophenolate mofetil (Cellcept), and corticosteroids.
   - Cyclosporine creates a "selective immunosuppression" by selectively inhibiting T cells. T cells dependent on humoral immunity continue intact and no bone marrow suppression occurs. T-cell lym-

phocytes become unresponsive to interleukin (IL)-1, ultimately preventing maturation of helper and cytotoxic T cells. Adverse effects include hypertension, nephrotoxicity, hepatotoxicity, hirsutism, tremors, and gum hyperplasia. When the first intravenous (IV) dose is administered, it is important to assess the patient closely for potential histamine-type reactions with cardiovascular collapse. This is related to the IV solution preparation and is not seen with the oral preparation. A daily trough level is measured to assess therapeutic dosage and avoid toxicity.

- Basilixmab (Simulect) is an immunosuppressive agent that is an IL-2 antagonist. It is indicated for patients with renal insufficiency related to their chronic low CO because it is renal sparing. This drug is given preoperatively and then 2 to 4 days postoperatively.

- Mycophenolate mofetil has potent cytotoxic effects on lymphocytes. It inhibits the proliferative responses of T and B lymphocytes to both mytogenic and allospecific stimulation. It also suppresses antibody formation against B lymphocytes. It is given in 1.5-g dose twice a day. The side effects include gastrointestinal tract ulceration, nausea, vomiting, and diarrhea. It has severe neutropenic effects and can cause anemia, leukopenia, and thrombocytopenia.

- Corticosteroids are administered to both prevent and treat rejection. They are able to decrease antibody production and inhibit antigen-antibody production, as well as interfere with production of mediators IL-1 and IL-2. Both their anti-inflammatory and immunosuppressive properties offer the patient benefits. Immediately postoperatively, they are administered in high doses, and then tapered over the next 6 months. However, if the patient experiences two or more episodes of acute rejection, the patient remains on a maintenance dose. In situations of acute or chronic rejection the patient may be "pulsed" with steroids. These doses are 500 to 1000 mg IV every day for 3 days, during which other steroids are discontinued. The patient then resumes another tapering wean to maintenance dose steroids. Complications from steroid treatment are numerous and include infection, hyperlipidemia, diabetes, hypertension, osteoporosis, sodium and water retention, metabolic alkalosis, peptic ulceration, pancreatitis, increased appetite, adrenopituitary suppression, lymphocytopenia, opportunistic infections, and aseptic necrosis of femoral and humoral heads. The patient often receives ulcer prophylaxis with a histamine blocker or antacids. Strict fluid and electrolyte balance must be maintained, and close assessment must

be maintained for glucose intolerance. The anti-inflammatory response may mask an infection; therefore, identification of malaise, anorexia, myalgias, change in wound appearance, cough, or sore throat must be reported. With all these immunosuppressive agents, the patient has an intrinsic risk for malignancies and needs comprehensive teaching regarding this and all preventive therapies to follow.

- Newer therapies offer further improvement in transplant outcomes. OKT3 (Orthoclone), a monoclonal antibody, may be given to reverse acute rejection although rarely is used. Antibodies that react with T_3 cells' surface antigens are produced, interfering with T-cell antigen recognition and making it more difficult for active T cells to recognize the target organ. OKT3 is administered for a 10- to 14-day course of therapy as a daily bolus dose of 5 to 10 mg IV. There is a danger of flash pulmonary edema; therefore the patient is premedicated with steroids, acetaminophen, and diphenhydramine. Vital signs are monitored every 15 minutes for 1 hour after the dose is given with emergency intubation and resuscitative equipment available. While receiving the treatment of OKT3, cyclosporine is usually held and then titrated back up during the last 3 days of treatment. CD3 levels are monitored in the laboratory on the 4th and 10th days of therapy to assess effectiveness. Some centers utilize a monoclonal or polyclonal antibody for induction therapy in the immediate postoperative period. Others reserve medications such as OKT3 for rescue therapy.

2. *Infection risk.* The immunosuppressive drugs decrease the normal immune response, increasing the risk for nosocomial or suprainfections (Table 19–5). In the immediate posttransplant period, when steroid doses are highest, the patient is more vulnerable to these infections. Infections are a major cause of morbidity and mortality, and prevention and early detection are crucial.

- The most challenging aspect of determining an infection is the clinical presentation, which is often masked by immunosuppressive therapy. The patient's temperature may not elevate as high as in nonimmunosuppressed patients and the WBC may not elevate as rapidly. It is imperative to assess the individual trend in each patient and have a strong suspicion if patients appear more fatigued, complain of sore throats, develop a new cough, or run low-grade temperatures. Bacterial, fungal, viral, and protozoal infections may compromise the posttransplant recipient.

- Aggressive skin care to decrease dermal injuries, adequate nutrition and hydration, removing all in-

TABLE 19–5. COMMON INFECTIONS IN CARDIAC RECIPIENTS

Bacterial Infections

Early
  Escherichia coli
  Enterococci
  Klebsiella organisms
  Pseudomonas organisms
  Serratia organisms
  Staphylococcus organisms
  Streptococcus organisms

Late
  Legionella organisms
  Listeria organisms
  Mycobacterium organisms
  Nocardia organisms
  Salmonella organisms

Viral Infections
CMV
Herpes simplex
Epstein-Barr virus
Varicella-zoster virus

Fungal Infections
Aspergillus organisms
Cryptococcus organisms
Histoplasmosis
Coccidiodomycosis
Blastomycosis
Candida organisms

Parasitic Infections
Pneumocystis organisms
Toxoplasmosis

From: Dressler DK: The patient undergoing cardiac transplant surgery. In Guzzetta CE, Dossey BM [eds.]: Cardiovascular Nursing Holistic Practice, St. Louis, MO: Mosby-Year Book, 1992.

and chest x-ray every 6 months may be performed. Cyclosporine levels are measured monthly. These data provide further guidance for earlier detection of rejection.

Providing Posttransplant Psychological Adjustment
Many emotions impact on the posttransplant patient. Often the patient and family have altered their roles and responsibilities during the illness. The posttransplant goal is to encourage role readjustment and resumption of pre-illness activities of daily living. The return to independence may frighten them after the "security" of the hospital environment.

1. They must be supported and assisted toward their return to home and with the plan of care.
2. Involvement in a transplant support group may benefit the patient and family, reduce anxieties, and clarify misconceptions. Meeting other recipients may validate their feelings and enhance the patient's adjustments.
3. Some recipients experience body image concerns related to hirsutism and increased weight. Reviewing cosmetic methods for dealing with these changes may decrease their concerns.
4. Weight loss may be enhanced through dietary counseling and participation in cardiac rehabilitation activities.
5. Quality-of-life issues should be explored with patients to heighten the positive side of transplantation and the future that awaits them.

vasive devices as soon as possible, and limiting unnecessary procedures may assist in reducing risks for sepsis. Patients and families should receive thorough education regarding transmission of infections. Antimicrobial therapy is instituted postoperatively while invasive devices are in place but should be utilized appropriately to avoid growth of antibiotic-resistant organisms. Thorough skin and oral assessments should be incorporated into daily assessment to rule out viral or fungal infections.

3. *Assessing for rejection.* Routinely, the patient undergoes a posttransplant endomyocardial biopsy to rule out rejection (Figure 19–11). Under fluoroscopy, utilizing a cardiac bioptome via the right internal jugular vein into the right ventricle, multiple (three to five) samples are taken of the myocardium to rule out rejection. The patient is then treated with the appropriate protocol (pulsed steroids or monoclonal antibodies). These biopsies are performed serially posttransplant during clinic visits to monitor for rejection. Other diagnostic procedures such as transesophageal echocardiogram

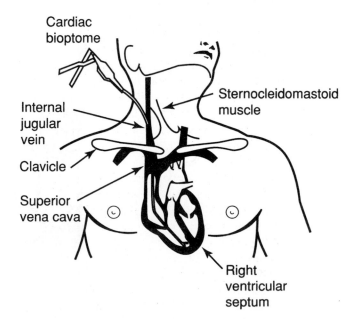

Figure 19–11. Endomyocardial biopsy technique. (*From Macdonald SN: Heart transplantation. In Smith SL:* Tissue and Organ Transplantation: Implications for Professional Nursing Practice. *St. Louis, MO: Mosby-Year Book; 1990, used with permission from AACN.*)

6. Steroids may cause periods of mood swings from episodes of depression to euphoria. Counseling with the patient and family may reduce confusion over the cause of personality changes. During pulsed steroid therapy it is very important to assess for steroid psychosis. Closer monitoring and reassurance during this therapy may assist in diminishing this side effect.

Intra-Aortic Balloon Pump Therapy

The IABP provides cardiac assistance by improving myocardial oxygen supply and reducing cardiac workload. The IABP catheter is inserted percutaneously or via a surgical incision into the femoral artery. It is advanced into the aorta and, when correctly positioned, lies below the subclavian artery and above the renal arteries.

The IABP works on the principle of counterpulsation. Gas (helium or CO_2) moves back and forth from the IABP console to the IABP catheter, causing the balloon to inflate and deflate (Figure 19–12). The balloon inflates during ventricular diastole, increasing intra-aortic pressure and blood flow to the coronary arteries. The balloon deflates just prior to ventricular systole, decreasing intra-aortic pressure. This pressure decrease reduces the resistance to left ventricular ejection, or afterload.

Indications and Contraindications

Common indications for IABP therapy include angina refractory to medical therapy, left ventricular failure, cardiogenic shock, and failure to wean from CPB after cardiac surgery. Patient symptoms necessitating the need for IABP therapy include symptoms of cardiogenic shock (tachycardia,

systolic BP <90 mm Hg, mean arterial pressure <70 mm Hg, CI <2.2–2.5 L/min/m^2, PCW pressure <18 mm Hg), decreased oxygenation, unstable angina, inadequate peripheral perfusion, and decreased urine output. The Thrombolysis and Counterpulsation to Improve Cardiogenic Shock Survival Trial demonstrated that augmentation of diastolic arterial pressure by IABP counterpulsation enhances thrombolysis and leads to faster reperfusion. Contraindications to IABP therapy include moderate to severe aortic insufficiency and aortic aneurysms.

IABP Timing

Balloon inflation and deflation are synchronized to left ventricular systole and diastole from the ECG signal and arterial pressure waveform. Accurate timing of the IABP is essential to avoid obstructing left ventricular ejection and severely compromising cardiac function. An ECG lead should be selected that optimizes the R wave. This is important because the IABP is usually set to deflate when it sees the R wave, which represents the beginning of ventricular depolarization just prior to ventricular systole. Inflation of the balloon is timed by observing the arterial pressure waveform for the dicrotic notch, an indicator of aortic valve closure at the beginning of diastole. Proper timing of IABP requires extensive knowledge and skill development, which is beyond the scope of this book. Refer to specific IABP manufacturers' recommendations for timing guidelines. A general overview of the process, however, is described in the following section.

Prior to assessing IABP timing, set the IABP frequency to 1:2 (Figure 19–13). In this mode the IABP will assist every other beat.

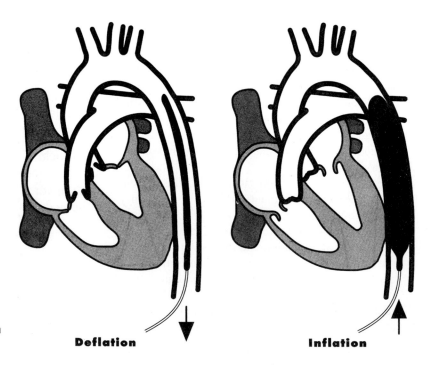

Figure 19–12. Counterpulsation. IABP inflation and deflation within the aorta.

Deflation

Inflation

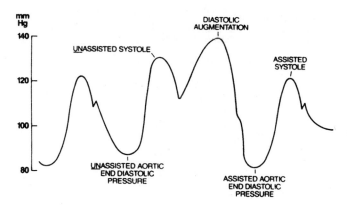

Figure 19–13. IABP frequency of 1:2. (*Datascope Corporation: Mechanics of intraaortic balloon counterpulsation. Montvale, NJ: Datascope, 1989.*)

Inflation

- Identify the dicrotic notch of the assisted systolic waveform.
- Adjust inflation slightly after the dicrotic notch of the unassisted systolic waveform.
- Adjust inflation to occur just before the dicrotic notch and a sharp V wave is formed. The dicrotic notch will no longer be visible.
- The diastolic augmentation should be equal to or greater than the unassisted systole.

Deflation

- Set the balloon to deflate so that the balloon-assisted aortic end-diastolic pressure is as low as possible, while maintaining optimal diastolic augmentation and not impeding on the next systole.
- Resume 1:1 pumping and observe the arterial waveform for characteristics of proper timing (Figure 19–14). Many of the IABP consoles perform automatic timing. Even if this mode is used, hourly assessment of the accuracy of timing is essential.

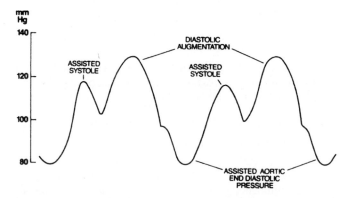

Figure 19–14. IABP frequency of 1:1. (*Datascope Corporation: Mechanics of intraaortic balloon counterpulsation. Montvale, NJ: Datascope, 1989.*)

Inaccurate IABP Timing

Inaccurate timing of the IABP decreases, instead of increases, myocardial performance. Common IABP timing errors include early and late inflation, as well as early and late deflation.

Early Inflation

Early inflation occurs when the IABP inflates too soon, thus impeding systolic ejection or the unassisted systolic pressure (Figure 19–15A). This timing error can lead to aortic regurgitation, premature closure of the aortic valve, and an increase in left ventricular end-diastolic volume.

Late Inflation

If the IABP inflates too late, the diastolic augmentation effect of the IABP is diminished (Figure 19–15B). This decreases the amount of perfusion to the coronary arteries.

Early Deflation

Early deflation occurs when the IABP does not remain inflated long enough, resulting in reduced diastolic augmentation (Figure 19–15C). This may result in an increase, instead of a decrease, in the assisted systolic pressure. Early deflation also decreases coronary artery perfusion and inhibits optimal afterload reduction.

Late Deflation

Late deflation occurs when the IABP remains inflated too long, thus impeding the patient's next systolic ejection or the assisted systolic pressure (Figure 19–15D). This results in a decrease in left ventricular ejection and an increase in afterload.

IABP Weaning

Weaning can be done by gradually decreasing the frequency of the IABP ratio (1:1 to 1:8, depending on the balloon console) or by decreasing the IABP volume. Patients are ready to wean from the IABP when:

- Heart rate and rhythm are normal.
- Mean arterial pressure is greater than 70 mm Hg with minimal vasopressor support.
- CI is greater than 2.2 to 2.5 L/min/m^2.
- Pulmonary wedge pressure is less than 18 mm Hg.
- Oxygenation saturation is adequate.
- Urine output is adequate.

Principles of Management for IABP Therapy

IABP Maintenance

1. Monitor hemodynamic parameters to evaluate the effectiveness of IABP therapy and to identify the need to adjust prescribed vasoactive agents.

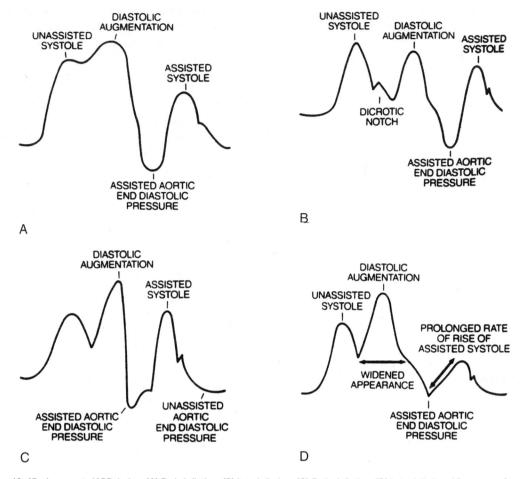

Figure 19–15. Inaccurate IABP timing. **(A)** Early inflation. **(B)** Late inflation. **(C)** Early deflation. **(D)** Late deflation. (*Datascope Corporation: Mechanics of intraaortic balloon counterpulsation. Montvale, NJ: Datascope, 1989.*)

2. Frequently (every hour) monitor neurologic status and circulation to the extremity distal to the balloon catheter.
3. Limit activity to maintain proper catheter position.
   • Maintain bed rest.
   • Immobilize the affected leg so that the IABP catheter does not become dislodged or kinked.
   • Maintain head of bed less than 45° to avoid catheter kinking.
   • Log roll every 2 hours and perform range of motion for the affected extremity.
4. Check the insertion site every 2 hours for bleeding or hematoma formation.
5. Change the insertion site dressing daily using aseptic technique.

IABP Removal

1. Discontinue anticoagulant therapy 4 to 6 hours prior to IABP removal.
2. Turn the IABP off just prior to removal.
3. Assist the physician with removal of the balloon.

4. Ensure that hemostasis is obtained after pressure is maintained on the insertion site for 30 to 45 minutes after balloon catheter removal.
5. Apply a pressure dressing to the insertion site for 2 to 4 hours.
6. Monitor vital signs and hemodynamic parameters every 15 minutes for 1 hour, every 30 minutes for 1 hour, and then every hour.
7. Assess peripheral perfusion to the affected extremity after catheter removal every hour for 2 hours, and then every 2 hours.
8. Restrict activity of the decannulated extremity and maintain bed rest with the patient's head of bed no greater than 45° for 24 hours.

Preventing and Managing Complications

1. *IABP catheter misalignment.* If the IABP catheter is advanced too far, the brachial artery may become occluded; thus left arm (brachial, radial) pulses are diminished or absent and signs of limb ischemia are present. If the catheter is not in far enough, the mesenteric and/or renal arteries may be occluded.

Signs of this include decreased or absent bowel sounds, increased abdominal girth or firmness, and decreased urine output.

2. *Thromboemboli.* Anticoagulation is recommended to decrease the development of thromboemboli related to the indwelling IABP catheter. Fast flushing and withdrawing blood samples should be avoided from the central aortic lumen of the IAB catheter. If this must be done, ensure that the IABP is on standby and that extreme care is taken to ensure that air bubbles are not introduced into the system. If the patient experiences asystole, turn the IABP console to the internal mode. In this mode, the catheter will flutter within the aorta so that thrombi formation is prevented. Refer to specific IABP manufacturer recommendations.

3. *Hemorrhage.* Monitor the central aortic pressure via the IABP catheter. This should be connected to a transducer, a pressured flush system, and an alarm system. Accidental disconnection of the central aortic lumen could cause rapid exsanguination.

4. *Intraaortic balloon rupture.* Signs of rupture include:
   - Loss of balloon augmentation.
   - Obvious blood or brown particles in the IAB catheter tubing.
   - Depending on the model of the IABP console, "a catheter problem" alarm may be activated.
   - Sudden hemodynamic instability.

If the intra-aortic balloon ruptures, turn the IABP console off, clamp the IABP catheter, notify the physician, and prepare for IABP removal or replacement. Observe your patient's hemodynamic status and adjust vasoactive medications accordingly.

Ventricular Assist Devices

Patients with cardiogenic shock following a MI, coming off CPB, or with cardiomyopathies may require additional assistance when cardiac output remains low despite maximal medical therapy. IABP support offers 8% to 12% augmentation to the patient's cardiac output, but this may be inadequate, requiring placement of a VAD. Greater support for the failing ventricle(s) can be provided with a VAD. The goals of utilizing a VAD are to reduce myocardial ischemia and workload, limit permanent cardiac damage, and restore adequate organ perfusion.

Indications

Appropriate candidates for VAD include those patients with end-stage cardiac disease, cardiomyopathies, post-CPB, and acute MI with cardiogenic shock. Another indication for insertion is to "bridge" the patient prior to cardiac transplantation until a suitable donor is located. Post-MI, a patient may be "bridged" in the hope of myocardial recovery and

eventual weaning from the device. More recently, VADs (left ventricular) have been approved for "destination therapy"; for example, once the VAD is inserted and the patient recovers, the patient is discharged home. The patient is also taken off the transplant list or moved to a lower priority of need. Recently, there have been reports of myocardial recovery allowing for surgical explantation of the VAD.

The appropriate selection of a candidate for these devices is based on hemodynamic criteria. If preload has been maximized, afterload reduced, and drug therapy instituted to maximal levels, and yet the patient is still cardiovascularly compromised, a VAD may be critical to achieve survival. Appropriate parameters to consider for VAD placement are:

- CI <2 L/min/m^2
- SVR >2100 dyne/sec/cm^5
- Mean arterial pressure <60 mm Hg
- Left or right atrial pressure >20 mm Hg
- Urine output <30 mL/h
- Pulmonary wedge pressure $>15–20$ mm Hg

The exclusion criteria for use of a VAD include the following:

- Shock $>12–18$ hours where reversibility is unlikely
- Acute cerebral vascular damage
- Cancer with metastasis
- Renal failure (unrelated to cardiac failure)
- Severe hepatic disease
- Coagulopathy
- Severe systemic sepsis, resistant to therapy
- Severe pulmonary disease
- Severe peripheral vascular disease
- Psychological instability
- Alcohol or drug addiction

General Description of VAD Principles

The VAD "unloads" the native ventricle or ventricles by way of artificial ventricles or a blood pump. Cardiac output is enhanced by blood circulating at a physiologic rate and by augmenting systemic and coronary circulation.

VAD support is predominately utilized for the left ventricle. However, if the right ventricle is compromised, support can be provided to both ventricles. This would necessitate separate VADs, yet the systems would function in tandem.

VADs are composed of nonpulsatile pumps (roller and centrifugal) or pulsatile pumps (pneumatically driven or implantable electromagnetically driven). Nonpulsatile pumps are inserted in the operating room (Figure 19–16). Atrial cannulation is via the right superior pulmonary vein or into the upper portion of the left atria at the junction with the right superior pulmonary vein. Aortic cannulation is placed low in the ascending aorta. Blood flow is diverted via the atrial cannulation and is returned via the aortic cannulation.

Roller pumps deliver blood flow by compressing blood and moving it forward. Flow is continuous, but nonpulsatile.

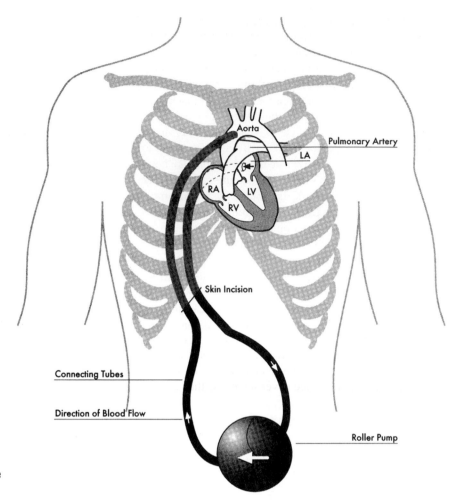

Figure 19–16. Left VAD cannula inserted into the left atria and the aorta.

Generally this is chosen for resuscitative purposes. Centrifugal pumps are vortex pumps with two magnetic cones rotating to create a "tornado effect." Blood flow is adjusted by liter per minute based on revolutions per minute. These pumps are nonthrombogenic acrylic cones and flow is designed to reduce turbulence, thereby reducing hemolysis.

Pulsatile pumps include internal or external pneumatic pumps and electric pumps. Pulsatile flow is believed to reduce microcirculatory shunting and edema formation and yield more physiologically acceptable assistance. There is superior flow assistance with pulsatile systems because they can assume flow for the assisted ventricle even during ventricular tachycardia or fibrillation.

The external pneumatic pump contains inflow and outflow valves that keep blood moving forward. The pumping chambers rest close to the thorax and are connected by transcutaneous cannula to the inflow and outflow sites. The inflow cannula is surgically placed in either the left atrium or left ventricle. Atrial cannulation is associated with less bleeding and less trauma to the ventricle. However, if the patient is a transplant candidate, it is more important to use left ventricle cannulation. This affords left atrium protection,

which will be anastomosed to the donor heart. The outflow exits the chest below the costal margin and connects to the pneumatic pump, returning to the aorta.

The inflow conduit of the internal pneumatic pump is inserted into the left ventricular cavity after excising a core of the left ventricular apex. The outflow conduit is anastomosed to the ascending aorta. Blood flows from the left ventricle into the inflow to the pump and is ejected into the ascending aorta.

The electric pump consists of an abdominally placed, battery-powered titanium blood pump. The inflow conduit is inserted into the left ventricular cavity and the outflow conduit is placed into the aorta. A percutaneous electric line connects the blood pump to the portable system controller, which clips to a belt or waistband. The pump can generate a cardiac output up to 10 L/min. The patients can wear either a shoulder holster or a belt bag with 5 to 8 hours battery life to increase mobility, even permitting them to go home and await transplantation.

The hemopump is a temporary cardiac assist device that employs an axial flow pump to augment left ventricular output. The catheter is inserted through the femoral artery, advanced into the aorta, through the aortic valve, and is placed into the left ventricle. Power is transmitted to the pump via a flexible drive shaft from an external motor and rotating magnet, which connects to an external power source. The hemopump does not require left ventricular synchronization and can generate 3.5 L/min of nonpulsatile blood flow.

Weaning and Recovery

The plan for weaning should revolve around hemodynamic stability and the patient's other physiologic systems' response. Neurologic, pulmonary, renal, and hematologic systems must be recovered from multiorgan insults. Assessment of cardiac output, CI, SVR, PCW pressure, mean arterial pressure, and SvO_2 guides decisions for initiating weaning. Pharmacologic support should be at a stable level with good major organ perfusion.

The arterial line waveform is assessed for the dicrotic notch appearance, evidence that there is adequate left ventricular pressure for aortic opening. A MUGA scan may be done with the VAD off for 4 minutes and if the ejection fraction is >30% with the VAD off, then weaning can start. The VAD is turned down at small increments to assess tolerance throughout the weaning process. Heparin must be initiated before weaning and the device never set at less than 2 L/min flow to avoid clot formation. At completion of weaning, the patient returns to the operating room for surgical removal.

Principles of Management for VAD

The primary objectives in managing the patient with a VAD are to optimize cardiac output, maximize coping, and prevent complications.

Optimizing Cardiac Output

1. Initially, the risk of biventricular failure still is paramount after the device's insertion and the patient must be closely evaluated. Cardiovascular profiles should be measured every 2 to 4 hours and changes in CO and CI reported to the physician. Pharmacologic support should be titrated to achieve the most stable mean arterial pressure and adequate SvO_2.
2. The VAD should be assessed for proper function to achieve an improved cardiovascular profile. The amount the VAD is delivering should be considered when measuring CO to assess for the natural heart's intrinsic CO. As myocardial recovery occurs, more support occurs from the heart and less from the VAD. The patient can then support CO without as much mechanical support.

Maximizing Coping

The patient and family may be overwhelmed by the suddenness of the disease, the ICU environment, the equipment related to the VAD, and the threat of loss of life. Transplantation, if discussed, may significantly increase their stress. They may require intense information sharing and clarification of misconceptions.

1. Promote emotional and psychological adaptation and assess for nonverbal clues of fear or anxiety. Frequent updates regarding goals for the day and present plan of care need to be provided in an interdisciplinary manner. The advanced practice nurse and the patient's primary nurse may coordinate this process.
2. Realistic information related to prognosis needs to be addressed with the patient and family. Often, 20% to 40% of patients on VAD die awaiting a donor heart, and families need support to cope with this possibility. Early involvement with social work and chaplains also may assist patients and families. Closely assess for other situational stressors and review prior coping strategies the patient or family found helpful.

Preventing Complications

1. *Thromboembolism.* Anticoagulation therapy may include heparin, dextran, or aspirin to reduce the risk for thromboembolism. Peripheral vascular impairment may occur secondary to vascular catheters. Frequent neurovascular checks should be performed and any change reported immediately. Assess for the 5 Ps of vascular complications:
   * Pallor
   * Pain
   * Parasthesia
   * Paralysis
   * Pulselessness
2. *Bleeding.* Monitor hemoglobin, hematocrit, and coagulation factors frequently. Assess all catheter sites and wounds for oozing. The patient needs to be evaluated for spontaneous oozing or occult bleeding. The patient needs close monitoring of therapy so he or she is safely anticoagulated but not in a dangerous range should a sudden match for a transplantation heart occur. Ideally the partial thromboplastin time (PTT) should be 1.5 times normal. The anticoagulation therapy may increase the propensity for cardiac tamponade to occur. This is a surgical emergency and may require reoperation for stabilization. Clues to this complication include the following:
   * Elevated atrial pressures
   * Reduced CO as pump cannot fill properly
   * Elevated pulmonary pressures
   * Diastolic equalization
   * Reduced mean arterial pressure
   * Declining MvO_2
3. *Arrhythmias.* Possible treatment with medications or electrical cardioversion may be required. Biventricular support may maintain nearly normal hemodynamics during arrhythmias. Assess the effect of arrhythmias on CO and augment the VAD accordingly. Treat all electrolyte abnormalities aggressively

to enhance contractility. Validate with physicians whether CPR may be performed for asystole, depending on the specific VAD.

4. *Decreased renal function.* Possible etiologies in the VAD patient for reduced renal function include hypoperfusion before VAD insertion, prolonged CPB time, massive transfusions, and hemolysis with release of hemoglobin. Assess daily BUN and creatinine values for further decline in renal function. It is imperative that all medications be assessed for nephrotoxicity and doses be based on creatinine clearance. Adequate vasopressor therapy in the dopaminergic range is beneficial to enhance renal perfusion. Maintain adequate fluid balance so preload is within normal limits. Monitor urinalysis for potential abnormalities, and avoid any period of hypotension which could further insult the kidneys.

5. *Infection.* The large cannulas exiting the skin create great portals of entry for pathologic organisms. Patients on VAD support are so metabolically stressed that they are more prone to infections, and strict precautions need to be followed. It is imperative they not become colonized, especially if they are pretransplant, because sepsis could preclude their receiving a heart. The best plan of action is prevention and includes:
   • Strict hand washing before and after all patient care activities.
   • Strict aseptic technique.
   • Pan-culture for temperature >101°F.
   • Monitor wounds for erythema, exudate, or edema.
   • Assess for shift to the left on differential count.

6. *Immobility.* Dermal injury may arise from the degree of immobility during the patient's critical phase of illness. Meticulous skin care and frequent position changes assist in reducing problems. Aggressive nutritional support assists in decreasing the degree of catabolism. Immobility may result in significant muscle mass loss and negative nitrogen balance. Bedside physical therapy is crucial until the patient is more stable and can begin ambulating. Foot splints may be applied to diminish the risk of foot drop.

7. *Poor device performance.* Dangers related to VAD mechanical problems include thrombus formation, in-flow obstructions, or device failures. Frequent device evaluation is needed, particularly with any change in the patient's clinical status. Device failure may result in inadequate or no systemic perfusion, so emergency measures must be implemented rapidly (Table 19–6).

TABLE 19–6. EMERGENCY MEASURES FOR VAD FAILURE OR CARDIAC ARREST

• Back-up VAD in place and ready for operation if mechanical failure occurs.
• Discuss with surgeons if CPR can be performed.
• Assess availability of blood products should emergency transfusions be necessary.
• Have vascular clamps available for cannula disconnections.
• Educate all team members regarding emergency measures if problem with VAD occurs.
• Patients can be safely cardioverted and defibrillated with VAD in place.
• Connect to emergency power outlets in case of an electrical outage.

AT THE BEDSIDE
Thinking Critically

You are caring for a patient who just returned to the SICU from cardiac surgery. He was admitted to the hospital with mitral insufficiency and today he had a St. Jude mechanical valve inserted into the mitral position. Your assessment includes:

Temperature	36.28°C
HR	Temporarily atrial paced at 80 beats/min
BP	86/60 mm Hg
RR	Assist control of 12 via the Bear ventilator
PAS	15 mm Hg
PAD	8 mm Hg
PCW	4 mm Hg
RA	3 mm Hg
CO	4.9 L/min
CI	1.9 L/min/m^2
SVR	2200 dynes/sec/cm^5

What is the probable reason for his hypotension and low CO/CI? What interventions should be immediately initiated to improve his cardiac status?

SELECTED BIBLIOGRAPHY

Cardiomyopathy

Albert NM: Surgical management of heart failure. *Crit Care Nurs Clin North Am* 2003;15:477–486.

Barkman A, Pooler C: Carvedilol: A countermeasure to heart failure. *DCCN* 2001;20(5):11–16.

Bristow MR: Management of heart failure. In Braunwald E, Zipes DP, Libby P (eds): *Heart Disease,* 6th ed, pp. 635–651. Philadelphia: WB Saunders; 2001.

Brown DL: *Cardiac Intensive Care.* Philadelphia: WB Saunders; 1998.

Cheever KH, Kitzes B, Genthner D: Epoprostenol therapy for primary pulmonary hypertension. *Crit Care Nurse* 1999;19(4):20–27.

Colucci WS, Braunwald E: Pathophysiology of heart failure. In Braunwald E, Zipes DP, Libby P (eds): *Heart Disease,* 6th ed, pp. 503–533. Philadelphia: WB Saunders; 2001.

Dimengo JM: Surgical alternatives in the treatment of heart failure. *AACN Clin Iss Crit Care* 1998;9(2):192–207.

Goran SF, Johantgen M: Heart failure. In Kinney MR, Dunbar SB, Brooks-Braun JA, Molter N, Vitello-Cicciu JM (eds): *AACN Clinical Reference for Critical Care Nursing,* 4th ed, pp. 429–460. St. Louis, MO: Mosby; 1998.

Leeper B, Legge D: Resynchronization therapy for management of heart failure. *Crit Care Nurs Clin North Am* 2003; 15:467–476.

Lewis PS, Boyd CM, Hubert NE, Steele MC: Ethanol-induced therapeutic myocardial infarction to treat hypertrophic obstructive cardiomyopathy. *Crit Care Nurse* 2001;21(2):20–34.

MacKlin M: Managing heart failure: A case study approach. *Crit Care Nurse* 2001;21(2):36–48.

Mann DL: *Heart Failure: A Companion to Braunwald's Heart Disease.* Philadelphia: Elsevier; 2004.

Michael KA, Parnell KJ: Innovations in the pharmacologic management of heart failure. *AACN Clin Iss Crit Care* 1998;9(2): 172–191.

Moser DK: Pathophysiology of heart failure update: The role of neurohumoral activation in the progression of heart failure. *AACN Clin Iss* 1998;9(2):157–171.

Moser DK, Frazier SK: Care of the patient with heart failure. In Chulay M, Wingate S: *Care of the Cardiovascular Patient Series.* Aliso Viejo, CA: AACN; 2001.

Paul S: Diastolic dysfunction. *Crit Care Nurs Clin North Am* 2003;15:495–500.

Paul S: Ventricular remodeling. *Crit Care Nurs Clin North Am* 2003;15:407–412.

Pettrey LJ, Leflar-DiLeva KM: Preventing complications in the dynamic cardiomyoplasty patient. *Dimens Crit Care Nurs* 1994; 13(5):238–240.

Pettrey LJ, Leflar-DiLeva KM: Preparing for cardiomyoplasty: A new horizon in cardiac surgery. *Dimens Crit Care Nurs* 1994; 13(5):226–237.

Piano MR, Prasun M: Neuorhormone activation. *Crit Care Nurs Clin North Am* 2003;15:413–422.

Rogers JM, Reeder SJ: Current therapies in the management of systolic and diastolic dysfunction. *DCCN* 2001;20(6):2–10.

Rudisill PT, Kennedy C, Paul S: The use of β-blockers in the treatment of chronic heart failure. *Crit Care Nurs Clin North Am* 2003;15:439–446.

Starling RC, McCarthy PM, Yamani MH: Surgical treatment of chronic CHF. In Mann DL (ed): *Heart Failure: A Companion to Braunwald's Heat Disease,* pp. 717–736. Philadelphia: Elsevier; 2004.

Tarolli KA: Left ventricular systolic dysfunction and nonischemic cardiomyopathy. *Crit Care Nurs Q* 2003;26(1):16–21.

Wynn J, Braunwald E: The cardiomyopathies and myocarditides. In Braunwald E, Zipes DP, Libby P (eds): *Heart Disease,* 6th ed, pp. 1751–1806. Philadelphia: WB Saunders; 2001.

Young J. Congestive heart failure. In Fuster V, Alexander RW, O'Rourke RA (eds): *Hurst's The Heart,* 10th ed, pp. 663–665. New York: McGraw-Hill; 2001.

Heart Transplantation

Augustine SM: Heart transplantation: Long term management related to immunosuppression, complications, and psychosocial adjustments. *Crit Care Nurs Clin North Am* 2000;12:69–78.

Bush WW: Overview of transplantation immunology and the pharmacotherapy of adult solid organ transplant recipients: Focus on immunosuppression. *AACN Clin Iss Crit Care* 1998;9:253–269.

Collins EG, White-Williams C, Jalowiec A: Spouse quality of life before and 1 year after heart transplantation. *Crit Care Nurs Clin North Am* 2000;12:103–110.

Cupples SA, Sprull LC: Evaluation criteria for the pretransplant patient. *Crit Care Nurs Clin North Am* 2000;12:35–48.

Guido GW: Heart transplantation from an ethical perspective. *Crit Care Nurs Clin North Am* 2000;12:111–121.

Krau SD: The evolution of heart transplantation. *Crit Care Nurs Clin North Am* 2000;12:1–10.

Miniati DN, Robbins RC, Reitz BA: Heart and heart lung transplant. In Braunwald E, Zipes DP, Libby P (eds): *Heart Disease,* 6th ed. Philadelphia: WB Saunders; 2001.

Rourke TK, Droogan MT, Ohler L: Heart transplantation: State of the art. *AACN Clin Iss Crit Care* 1998;9:185–201.

Smith L, Farroni J, Baillie BR, Haynes H: Heart transplantation: An answer for end-stage heat failure. *Crit Care Nurs Clin North Am* 2003;15:489–494.

Tokarczyk TR: Cardiac transplantation as a treatment option for the heart failure patient. *Crit Care Nurs Q* 2003;26:61–68.

Torre-Amiobe G, Koerner MM, Lisman KA, Thohan V: Cardiac transplantation. In Mann DL (ed): *Heart Failure: A Companion to Braunwald's Heat Disease,* pp. 706–736. Philadelphia: Elsevier; 2004.

Trupp RJ, Abraham WT, Lamba S: Future therapies for heart failure. *Crit Care Nurs Clin North Am* 2003;15:525–530.

Walton J, St. Clair K: "A Beacon of Light": Spirituality in the heart transplant patient. *Crit Care Nurs Clin North Am* 2000;12:87–102.

Valvular Disorders

Blaisdell MW, Good L, Gentzler RD: Percutaneous transluminal valvuloplasty. *Crit Care Nurse* 1989;9(3):62–68.

Braunwald E: Valvular heart disease. In Braunwald E, Zipes DP, Libby P (eds): *Heart Disease,* 6th ed, pp. 1643–1713. Philadelphia: WB Saunders; 2001.

Brown MM, Fitzgerald C, Morse K, Doyle JE: Cardiovascular surgery. In Kinney MR, Dunbar SB, Brooks-Braun JA, Molter N, Vitello-Cicciu JM (eds): *AACN Clinical Reference for Critical Care Nursing,* 4th ed, pp. 383–428. St. Louis: Mosby; 1998.

Holloway S, Feldman T. An alternative to valvular surgery in the treatment of mitral stenosis: Balloon mitral valvotomy. *Crit Care Nurse* 1997;17(3):27–36.

Finkelmeier BA (ed): *Cardiothoracic Surgical Nursing,* 3rd ed. Philadelphia: JB Lippincott; 2004.

Nauer KA, Schouchoff B, Demitras K: Minimally invasive aortic valve surgery. *Crit Care Q* 2000;23(1):66–71.

Weigand DL, Pruess T: Care of the patient undergoing cardiovascular surgery. In Chulay M, Wingate S (eds): *Care of the Cardiovascular Patient Series.* Aliso Viejo, CA: AACN; 2002.

Woods SL, Froelicher ESS, Motzer SU (eds): *Cardiac Nursing,* 4th ed. Philadelphia: JB Lippincott; 2000.

Pericarditis

Dziadulewicz L, Shannon-Stone M: Postpericardiectomy syndrome: A complication of cardiac surgery. *AACN Clin Iss Crit Care* 1998;9:464–470.

Hamel W: Care of patients with an indwelling pericardial catheter. *Crit Care Nurse* 1998;18(5):40–45.

Finkelmeier BA (ed): *Cardiothoracic Surgical Nursing,* 3rd ed. Philadelphia: JB Lippincott; 2004.

Spodick DH: Pericardial diseases. In Braunwald E, Zipes DP, Libby P (eds): *Heart Disease,* 6th ed, pp. 1823–1876. Philadelphia: WB Saunders; 2001.

Woods SL, Froelicher ESS, Motzer SU (eds): *Cardiac Nursing,* 4th ed. Philadelphia: JB Lippincott; 2000.

Thoracoabdominal Aneurysms

Anderson LA: Abdominal aortic aneurysm. *J Cardiovasc Nurs* 2001;15(4):1–14.

Cronewett JL (ed): Arterial aneurysms. In Rutherford RB (ed): *Vascular Surgery,* 5th ed, pp. 1241–1344. Philadelphia: WB Saunders; 2000.

Finkelmeier BA, Marolda D. Aortic dissection. *J Cardiovasc Nurs* 2001;15(1):15–24.

Iacono LA: Naloxone infusion and drainage of cerebrospinal fluid as adjuncts to postoperative care after repair of thoracoabdominal aneurysms. *Crit Care Nurse* 1999;19(5):37–47.

House-Fanchier MA: Aortic dissection: pathophysiology, diagnosis, and acute care management. *AACN Clin Iss Crit Care* 1995; 6:602–613.

Fahey V: *Vascular Nursing,* 3rd ed. Philadelphia: WB Saunders; 2003.

Finkelmeier BA (ed): *Cardiothoracic Surgical Nursing,* 3rd ed. Philadelphia: JB Lippincott; 2004.

Isselbacher EM: Diseases of the aorta. In Braunwald E, Zipes DP, Libby P (eds): *Heart Disease,* 6th ed. Philadelphia: WB Saunders; 2001.

McClarren-Curry C, Shaughnessy K: Acute thoracic aortic dissection: How to diffuse a time bomb. *DCCN* 1999;18(4):26–29.

Morresey NJ, Hamilton IN, Holier LH: Thoracoabdominal aortic aneurysms. In Moore WS (ed): *Vascular Surgery: A Comprehensive Review,* 6th ed, pp. 437–456. Philadelphia: WB Saunders; 2002.

IABP Therapy

Ardire L, Boswell J: Intraaortic balloon pump timing in the patient with hypotension. *Focus Crit Care* 1992;19(2):146–149.

Quaal SJ: Care of the patient with an intra-aortic balloon pump. In Chulay M, Wingate S (eds): *Care of the Cardiovascular Patient Series.* Aliso Viejo, CA: AACN; 2002.

Goran S: Vascular complications of the patient undergoing intraaortic balloon pumping. *Crit Care Nurs Clin North Am* 1989; 1:459–467.

Lynn-McHale DJ, McGrory J: Intraaortic balloon pump management. In Boggs RL, Wooldridge-King M (eds): *AACN Procedure Manual,* 3rd ed. Philadelphia: WB Saunders; 1993.

Quall SJ: *Comprehensive Intraaortic Balloon Pumping.* St. Louis, MO: CV Mosby; 1984.

Shinn AE, Joseph D: Concepts of intraaortic balloon counterpulsation. *J Cardiovasc Nurs* 1994;8(2):45–60.

Shoulders-Odom B: Managing the challenge of IABP therapy. *Crit Care Nurse* 1991;11(2):60–62.

Whitman G: Intraaortic balloon pumping and cardiac mechanics: A programmed lesson. *Heart Lung* 1978;7:1034–1050.

Wojner AW: Assessing the five points of the intra-aortic balloon pump waveform. *Crit Care Nurse* 1994;14(3):48–52.

Ventricular Assist Devices

Abou-Awadi NL, Joseph KA: Hemopump left ventricular support in the peripartum cardiomyopathy patient. *J Cardiovasc Nurs* 1994;8(2):36–44.

Bond AE, Nelson K, Germany CL, et al: The left ventricular assist device. *Am J Nurs* 2003;103(1):32–41.

Bond AE, Bolton B, Nelson K: Nursing education and implications for left ventricular assist device destination therapy. *Prog Cardiovasc Nurs* 2004;29(3):95–101.

Camp D: The left ventricular assist device (LVAD): A bridge to heart transplantation. *Crit Care Nurs Clin North Am* 2000;12(1): 61–68.

Cianci P, Lonergan-Thomas H, Slaughter M, Silver MA: Current and potential applications of left ventricular assist devices. *J Cardiovasc Nurs* 2003;18(1):17–22.

Couper GS, Dekkers RJ, Adams DH: The logistics and cost-effectives of circulatory support: Advantages of the Abiomed BVS 5000. *Ann Thoracic Surg* 1999;68:646–649.

Curtis JJ, Wells JT, Wagner-Moore CA, et al: Centrifugal pumps: Description of devices and surgical techniques. *Ann Thoracic Surg* 1999;68:666–671.

DeBakey ME: A miniature implantable axial flow ventricular assist device. *Ann Thoracic Surg* 1999;68:637–640.

Delgado RM, Frazier OH, Razeghi P, Taegtmeyer H: Mechanical circulatory support in patients with heart failure. In Mann DL (ed): *Heart Failure: A Companion to Braunwald's Heart Disease.* Philadelphia: Elsevier; 2004.

Duke T, Perna J: The ventricular assist device as a bridge to cardiac transplantation. *AACN Clin Iss Crit Care* 1998;9:217–228.

Finkelmeier BA: Mechanical assist devices. In: *Cardiothoracic Surgical Nursing.* Philadelphia: JB Lippincott; 1995.

Frazier OH, Myers TJ: Left ventricular assist system as a bridge to myocardial recovery. *Ann Thoracic Surg* 1999;68:734–741.

Holmes EC: AbioCor totally implantable replacement heart. *J Cardiovasc Nurs* 2003;18(1):23–29.

Lewandowski AV: The bridge to cardiac transplantation: Ventricular assist device. *Dimens Crit Care Nurs* 1995; 14(1):17–25.

McCauley MF: Pulmonary artery balloon counterpulsation as a treatment for right ventricular failure. *J Cardiovasc Nurs* 1994; 8(2):61–68.

Moroney DA, Reedy JE: Understanding ventricular assist devices: A self-study guide. *J Cardiovasc Nurs* 1994;8(2):1–15.

Richenbreler WE, Pierce WS: Treatment of heart failure: Assisted circulation. In Braunwald E, Zipes DP, Libby P (eds): *Heart Disease,* 6th ed. Philadelphia: WB Saunders; 2001.

Rose EA, Moskowitz AJ, Packer M, et al: The REMATCH trial: Rationale, design and end points. *Ann Thorac Surg* 1999;67:723–730.

Rose EA, Gelijns AC, Moskowitz AJ: Long term mechanical therapy left ventricular assistance for end-stage heart failure. *N Engl J Med* 2001;345:1435–1443.

Savage L: Quality of life among patients with a left ventricular assist device: What is new? *AACN Clin Iss* 2003;14:64–72.

Evidenced-Based Practice and Guidelines

Lee TH: Guidelines: Management of valvular heart disease. In Braunwald E, Zipes DP, Libby P (eds): *Heart Disease,* 6th ed, pp. 1714–1722. Philadelphia: WB Saunders; 2001.

Hunt SA, Baker, DW, Chin MH, et al: ACC/AHA Guidelines for the evaluation and management of chronic heart failure in the adult. Available: http://www.acc.org/clinical/guidelines/failure/hf_index.htm. 2001.

Moser DK, Frazier SK: Care of the patient with heart failure. In Chulay M, Wingate S (eds): *Care of the Cardiovascular Patient Series.* Aliso Viejo, CA: AACN; 2001.

Quaal SJ: Care of the patient with an intra-aortic balloon pump. In Chulay M, Wingate S (eds): *Care of the Cardiovascular Patient Series.* Aliso Viejo, CA: AACN; 2002.

Schakenbach L: Care of the patient with a ventricular assist device. In Chulay M, Wingate S (eds): *Care of the Cardiovascular Patient Series.* Aliso Viejo, CA: AACN; 2001.

ADVANCED RESPIRATORY CONCEPTS

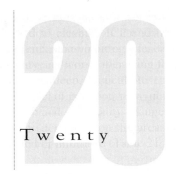

Twenty

Suzanne M. Burns

▶ **Knowledge Competencies**

1. Discuss the definition, patient selection process, application, assessment, and complications of pressure support ventilation, bi-level positive airway pressure, pressure-controlled/Inverse ratio, volume-guaranteed pressure modes, airway pressure release ventilation, bi-phasic ventilation, and high-frequency ventilation in critically ill patients

2. Describe the use of minimum minute volume and flow-by as ventilator options for critically ill patients.

3. Identify pulmonary and nonpulmonary factors important to the promotion of positive weaning outcomes in long-term mechanically ventilated patients.

4. Describe the concepts of respiratory muscle fatigue, rest, and conditioning as they relate to the mechanically ventilated weaning patient.

5. Identify essential components for the successful design of weaning predictors, protocols for weaning trials, and multidisciplinary institutional approaches to the care of long-term mechanically ventilated patients.

ADVANCED MODES OF MECHANICAL VENTILATION

New Concepts: Mechanical Ventilation

For years, volume ventilation was the dominant form of ventilation. Recently, numerous pressure modes emerged and are commonly used in critical care units to ventilate patients from the acute to weaning stages of illness. Although selected characteristics of the pressure modes are attractive, some of the modes are not well understood and outcomes associated with their use are not yet determined. Results of recent studies of acute respiratory distress syndrome (ARDS) suggest that traditional ventilatory methods are injurious to the lung. Thus, clinical applications of ventilation and the use of specific modes during the acute stage of illness focus on "protecting the lung" and improving patient outcomes.

Mechanical Ventilation of Acute Lung Injury and Acute Respiratory Distress Syndrome

Acute respiratory distress syndrome, the most severe presentation of acute lung injury (ALI), results from an acute insult to the body that may be direct (i.e., specific lung condition such as pneumonia) or indirect (i.e., condition outside the lung such as sepsis). The release of mediators and a host of other toxic substances affect the alveolar–capillary permeability adversely and result in a noncardiac pulmonary edema. Pathology includes decreased compliance, shunting, and refractory hypoxemia. Mortality rates are as high as 50%. To date, there is no definitive treatment for ARDS. Therapy focuses on managing the underlying condition and on supportive mechanical ventilation. Recently, however, the understanding of which ventilatory strategies are helpful (or harmful) has been challenged.

Study results of animals and patients with ARDS show that large tidal volume delivery results in greater lung damage and higher mortality rates than low lung volume ventilation. Although low volume ventilation leads to hypoventilation in the ARDS patient and hypercarbia, or permissive hypercarbia, mortality rates are lower with this approach. In addition, studies show that the use of positive end expiratory pressure (PEEP) decreases mortality in ARDS by opening collapsed lung units. This effect is called lung recruitment.

463

Results of recent studies changed the way patients with ARDS are managed during the acute stage, however, questions about whether pressure targeted ventilation is the equivalent of low volume ventilation and how to best determine the optimal PEEP level remain. It is clear that to "protect the lung," high tidal volumes and high plateau pressures should no longer be used for ventilating the ARDS patient. Acute respiratory distress syndrome patients should be ventilated with low volume ventilation, which may result in permissive hypercarbia, to prevent volutrauma and death. Traditional therapeutic clinical end points, such as the attainment of normal arterial blood gases, are no longer sufficient for guiding ventilatory management strategies.

Volume versus Pressure Ventilation

Volume ventilation delivers a prescribed volume at a set flow rate regardless of the pressure required (see Chapter 5, Air-

way and Ventilatory Management). In contrast, with pressure ventilation, pressure is stable and tidal volume varies with the selected pressure level, changing airway resistance, and lung and chest wall compliance. The characteristic decelerating flow pattern associated with pressure support ventilation (PSV) (Figure 20–1A) is one of the positive characteristics of pressure support ventilation: improved gas distribution. In contrast, volume ventilation provides a steady gas flow throughout inspiration. This is referred to as a square flow pattern (Figure 20–1B).

Flow patterns are important because they affect lung filling. Gas moving down the airways takes the path of least resistance and tends to preferentially fill alveoli that are open and compliant. Closed or partially open alveoli are less compliant and do not fill easily. With volume ventilation, gas flow can be quite turbulent (especially when short inspiratory times are used) and the distribution of gas is uneven; closed alveoli stay closed, while compliant alveoli receive the bulk of the fresh gases. With pressure ventilation, flow is high initially but slows toward the end of the breath; gas distributes more evenly. It is thought that this is because the slower end-inspiratory flow rate results in less turbulent gas flow

---

AT THE BEDSIDE
▶ *Complex Ventilator Modes: PC/IRV*

A patient was admitted to the RICU in respiratory distress. Her history included a flulike illness that progressively got worse, necessitating a trip to the ER. Her chest radiograph showed bilateral diffuse infiltrates in a honeycomb pattern consistent with ARDS. Once intubated, she was placed on assist-control at a rate of 20/min. Her plateau pressure was very high (60 cm H_2O) and she required an FiO_2 of 1.0 and 10 cm H_2O of PEEP. ABGs on these settings were pH 7.23, $PaCO_2$ 38 mm Hg, and PaO_2 52 mm Hg. She was agitated, thrashing, and asynchronous with the ventilator, despite a sensitivity setting of 21 cm H_2O, a short inspiratory time, and a high ventilator rate.

The decision was made to sedate and paralyze this patient and place her on the PC/IRV mode. Settings were:

PC level	30 cm H_2O
V_t	6 mL/kg
Rate	20/min
I:E ratio	2:1
FiO_2	0.6
PEEP	10 cm H_2O (auto-PEEP on these settings was 5 cm H_2O, providing a total PEEP level of 15 cm H_2O)

ABGs after 30 minutes were

pH	7.34
$PaCO_2$	55 mm Hg
PaO_2	66 mm Hg

The team felt that the positive results were reflective of the improved gas distribution associated with the pressure ventilation and the use of sedation and paralytics. Further, by decreasing or controlling the plateau pressure, which resulted in lower tidal volumes, the risk of volutrauma was lessened.

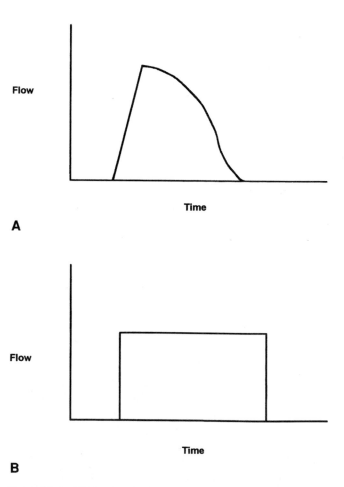

Figure 20–1. (A) Decelerating flow pattern seen with pressure support ventilation. **(B)** Square flow pattern seen with volume ventilation.

(called laminar flow). A wide variety of pressure modes are available for application during the acute stage of illness and for weaning.

Pressure Support Ventilation

Pressure support ventilation (PSV), first described in the early 1980s as a form of ventilation for the stable, spontaneously breathing patient during weaning, is now a popular mode of ventilation in most critical care units. The clinical success of pressure support resulted in the use of many other pressure modes.

Pressure support ventilation is designed for the spontaneously breathing patient but requires that a pressure level be selected by the clinician. Then, when the patient initiates a breath, the ventilator senses the negative pressure (the sensitivity "trigger" is usually set at -1 to 2 cm H$_2$O) and delivers a high flow of gas to the patient until the selected pressure level is reached early in inspiration. This pressure level is then maintained throughout the inspiratory phase. The ventilator cycles off and exhalation begins when flow decreases to approximately one-quarter of the original flow (the cycle-off mechanism varies with different ventilators). This occurs as the lungs fill toward the end of the inspiration. An important characteristic of PSV is that it enables the patient to determine inspiratory time, volume, and respiratory rate. This characteristic is thought to explain why pressure support is a "comfortable" mode for spontaneously breathing patients. In addition, PSV decreases the work of breathing associated with circuits, high breathing rates, and small endotracheal tubes. Because the level of support can be gradually reduced, the mode is especially helpful for weaning. This method may be used in less stable patients as well, provided that the tidal volume is closely monitored. Patient selection, application, assessment, and potential complications are delineated in Table 20–1.

Bi-Level Positive Airway Pressure

Bi-level positive airway pressure (BIPAP) is a noninvasive mode of ventilation that combines two levels of positive pressure (PSV and PEEP) by means of a full face mask, nasal mask (most common), or nasal pillows. The ventilator is designed to compensate for leaks in the set-up, but sometimes a chin strap is used to prevent excessive leaks around the mouth. This form of therapy can be very labor intensive, especially when used to prevent reintubation following extubation. Full face mask ventilation is cautiously used because the potential for aspiration is high. If full face mask ventilation is chosen, the patient should be able to remove the mask quickly if nausea occurs or vomiting is imminent. Obtunded patients and those with excessive secretions are not good choices for BIPAP ventilation.

A number of options are available with BIPAP and include a spontaneous mode where the patient initiates all the pressure supported breaths; a spontaneous-timed option,

TABLE 20–1. PRESSURE SUPPORT VENTILATION (PSV)

Definition
Pressure support ventilation (PSV) is a form of ventilation used to augment spontaneous respirations with a selected amount of positive airway pressure. There are two applications of PSV: (1) stand-alone mode and (2) mixed mode where a back-up rate is set. As with any pressure mode of ventilation, changes in compliance or resistance can result in changes in tidal volume.

Patient Selection
1. Patients who are stable, ready to wean, and with a dependable ventilatory drive.
2. PSV helps overcome resistance associated with circuits and airways.
3. In less stable patients, close monitoring of tidal volume and respiratory rate is necessary.

Application
1. *Rest* (called PSV max): Adjust PSV level to obtain a respiratory rate of less than 20 breaths per minute, a tidal volume of 8–12 mL/kg and an eupneic respiratory pattern.
2. *Work:* Decrease PSV level as tolerated. The speed of PSV decrease varies between patients (from hours to days) and may be defined by protocol. Respiratory rate may be higher and tidal volumes lower during work intervals. Monitor both parameters hourly and stop if the predetermined thresholds are exceeded.

Assessment
1. *Comfort:* The patient controls inspiratory and expiratory time, rate, and volume. The patient should be comfortable and without dyspnea.
2. *Secretions* can increase resistance and decrease tidal volume. Ensure airway patency with adequate humidification and suctioning as needed. If secretions are copious, pressure support may be contraindicated.
3. *Compliance changes:* Any change in lung status (i.e., pulmonary edema) results in a decreased tidal volume.
4. *Conditioning:* PSV is good for promoting endurance of the respiratory muscles by gradually increasing workload over time. For example, when the PSV level is set at a higher level, little effort (work) is required. The work is increased as the PSV level is gradually lowered. It is important to remember that when other activities are taking place (i.e., sitting up in a chair, physical therapies) or when there are physical impediments to breathing (i.e., ascites, obesity, distention), the PSV level may need to be increased. Use respiratory rate and tidal volume to determine optimal level of support.

Complications
1. Use caution when chest tube leaks and cuff leaks are present: Patients with large air leaks from chest tubes and/or endotracheal tube cuffs should not be placed on PSV. When a leak is present, the patient may not be able to control the parameters of inspiratory time, rate, or volume.
2. PSV should be used very cautiously in patients with asthma or in patients with rapidly changing physical status (i.e., with acute bronchospasm, airway resistance increases and tidal volume will decrease).

similar to PSV with a backup rate (some vendors call this A/C); and a control mode. The control mode requires the selection of a control rate and inspiratory time. High Fio$_2$ requirements are a relative contraindication for the use of BIPAP because generally, oxygen is bled into the system.

BIPAP is used successfully in critically ill ICU patients to prevent intubation, and also to prevent reintubation following extubation. It may be especially helpful in patients with chronic obstructive pulmonary disease and with congestive heart failure, particularly because these patients are often difficult to wean from conventional ventilation given their underlying disease processes. Study results also demonstrate that outcomes in immunocompromised patients may be better with noninvasive ventilation. Patient selection, application, assessment, and potential complications are delineated in Table 20–2.

Pressure Control and Pressure Controlled/Inverse Ratio Ventilation

Pressure controlled/inverse ratio ventilation (PC/IRV) is actually two modes of ventilation used in combination and designed to ventilate patients with ARDS. The pressure control option allows the clinician to control (or limit) the pressure during inspiration to a level that is less likely to result in barotrauma (less than 35 cm H_2O). Because the tendency of the stiff ARDS lung is to collapse, a prolonged inspiratory time may be used to prevent alveolar closing (derecruitment) Inspiratory to expiratory ratios (I/E), which are normally 1:2

or 1:3, are increased to 1:1, 2:1, 3:1, or 4:1. The short expiratory time is generally sufficient for complete exhalation, however, in some cases, auto-PEEP may be an expected and even desirable outcome.

The options of controlling pressure and prolonging inspiration, in conjunction with the decelerating flow pattern (see Figure 20–1A) are beneficial aspects of this pressure mode. Use of PC/IRV frequently requires that the patient be heavily sedated and/or chemically paralyzed to assure patient/ventilator synchrony. Guidelines for patient selection, application, assessment, and potential complications of PC/IRV are summarized in Table 20–3.

Volume-Guaranteed Pressure Modes of Ventilation

As noted earlier, a major drawback to the use of pressure ventilation is the inability to ensure consistent volume delivery. Delivered volume is dependent on compliance, resistance, and pressure level. In severely ill patients, such as the patient with ARDS, changes in compliance can result in changes in volume delivery and ultimately acid–base disturbances. Ventilator manufacturers responded to this concern by designing mode options that guarantee a prescribed tidal

---

TABLE 20–2. BI-LEVEL POSITIVE AIRWAY PRESSURE (BIPAP)

Definition

BIPAP is pressure support with PEEP provided through a face mask, nasal pillows or nasal mask (although it may also be provided through a tracheostomy tube, that application is rarely used in the critical care environment).

Patient Selection

Patients in whom invasive ventilation is not desired, for sleep apnea or hypoventilation syndrome, to prevent intubation or reintubation, and to treat congestive heart failure. The mode should not be used in those who cannot protect their airway or in those with very high Fio_2 requirements.

Application

1. *Select mode* (names vary with the manufacturer): spontaneous, spontaneous-timed (assist-controlled), or controlled.
2. *Spontaneous mode:* select the level of pressure support (inspiratory pressure level) and the PEEP level (generally there must be at least 5 cm H_2O pressure difference between these).
3. *Spontaneous timed:* pressure support level; PEEP and backup rate are selected.
4. *Controlled:* pressure support level, PEEP, rate and inspiratory time are selected.
5. Fio_2 is adjusted by means of a flow meter and "bled" into the circuit to attain appropriate Sao_2 or Pao_2. The ventilator function is adversely affected if the flow rate is too high. Refer to manufacturers limits as this varies with the ventilator make and model.

Assessment

1. *Rate and pattern of breathing:* The patient should look comfortable with no evidence of accessory muscle use and a reasonable respiratory rate.
2. Although ABGs are often obtained, Sao_2, in conjunction with assessment of rate and pattern of breathing, mental status and vital signs, tells us much about how the patient is tolerating the mode.
3. This method of ventilation is labor intensive and requires that the nurse and respiratory therapist work together to determine the best settings for the patient.

Complications

1. Decreased mental status is a relative contraindication for BiPAP because the patient may not be able to protect the airway. Any acute change in mental status should be promptly reported and continued use of BiPAP carefully evaluated. Intubation may be necessary.
2. If the patient becomes nauseated, aspiration risk is increased. Make sure the patient can quickly remove the face or nasal mask if necessary.

TABLE 20–3. PRESSURE CONTROLLED/INVERSE RATIO VENTILATION (PC/IRV)

Definition

PC/IRV is actually two modes of ventilation used in combination to lower peak airway pressure and improve gas distribution (and oxygenation).

Patient Selection

Patients with ARDS with Pao_2 ≤60 mm Hg and peak inspiratory pressures ≥60 mm H_2O in whom the risk of barotrauma is present.

Application

1. Select the pressure level: Generally this is around 30–35 cm H_2O initially. This can be lowered over time to ensure lower tidal volumes or plateau pressures.
2. Select inspiratory/expiratory ratio (1:1, 2:1, 3:1, and 4:1).
3. Select respiratory rate (this is usually high—in most cases >20).
4. Set PEEP (the amount dialed in) may stay the same initially. However, with the prolonged inspiratory time secondary to inverse ratios, auto-PEEP may occur. Auto-PEEP may be a desirable outcome.
5. Fio_2 is initially high but can be decreased as oxygenation improves.
6. Patients placed on PC/IRV require sedation, and often, paralytic agents. This is because the inverse ratio is not physiologic and patient/ventilator asynchrony results in inadequate ventilation.

Assessment

1. Arterial blood gases, end-tidal CO_2, and pulse oximetry to monitor adequacy of oxygenation and ventilation.
2. With changing compliance or resistance (agitation, secretions, pneumothorax, bronchospasm, abdominal distention, fluid overload, etc.), tidal volume is affected. Monitor tidal volume hourly and with any position change.
3. Patient comfort/synchrony: If paralytic agents are used, the appropriate use of sedatives and analgesics should be ensured.

Complications

1. A high index of suspicion for barotrauma: Acute changes in oxygenation, ventilation, tidal volume, and vital signs may herald a pneumothorax.
2. Acute changes in lung compliance and resistance affect tidal volume.

volume while delivering the volume as a pressure breath (decelerating flow pattern, etc.). The technology associated with these new mode options is sophisticated and characteristics vary between manufacturers. However, the inherent concepts are similar and can be applied in the clinical setting. Two different examples of volume-guaranteed pressure modes of ventilation are described as follows.

Volume-Assured Pressure Support Ventilation (VAPS), Pressure Augmentation (Bear 1000, Bear Medical Systems, Riverside, CA)
This mode option allows the clinician to select the desired tidal volume with a pressure option (called pressure augmentation). This option provides for all the delivered ventilator breaths to be pressure breaths unless it is determined (i.e., by internal calculations of compliance and flow during breath delivery) that the prescribed tidal volume goal will not be reached. If this occurs, the ventilator automatically delivers the rest of the inspiration as a volume breath (Figure 20–2C). The pressure waveforms vary and will change as the clinician adjusts the pressure level. In nonspontaneously breathing patients, a rate is also set.

Volume Support (VS) and Pressure-Regulated Volume Control (PRVC) (Siemens Medical, Iselin, NJ)
These mode options are similar to VAPS in that the breaths are delivered as pressure breaths and volume is ensured. The difference between them, however, is in the manner that the breaths are delivered. With VS, the pressure level for the breaths is adjusted on a breath-to-breath basis to maintain the desired volume. The pressure waveforms (Figure 20–3) show step-wise changes in pressure levels as needed in the spontaneously breathing patient. In the nonspontaneously breathing patient, the same mechanism is in place to ensure that the desired tidal volume is maintained. A mandatory rate and inspiratory time also are selected for the breaths. This mode option is called PRVC. Table 20–4 summarizes the selection criteria, application, assessment, and potential complications associated with volume-guaranteed pressure modes (VAPS, VS, PRVC, etc.) of ventilation.

Airway Pressure Release Ventilation (APRV) and Bi-Phasic Ventilation (BiLevel Puritan Bennett Pleasanton, CA)

APRV and bi-phasic ventilation are relatively new options and are only available on some ventilators. Both options are used for patients with ARDS. The APRV option employs a high level of CPAP to recruit the lung (i.e., open alveoli and restore FRC) and uses brief expiratory "releases" (no longer than 1.5 sec), provided at set intervals, to enhance CO_2 clearance. In contrast, the bi-phasic mode uses two different levels of CPAP called high-PEEP and low-PEEP. A rate and inspiratory time are set as in PC/IRV. A major difference between PC/IRV and bi-phasic ventilation is that flow is available to the patient for spontaneous breathing at both pressure levels. Pressure support may also be added to decrease the work associated with spontaneous breathing. This

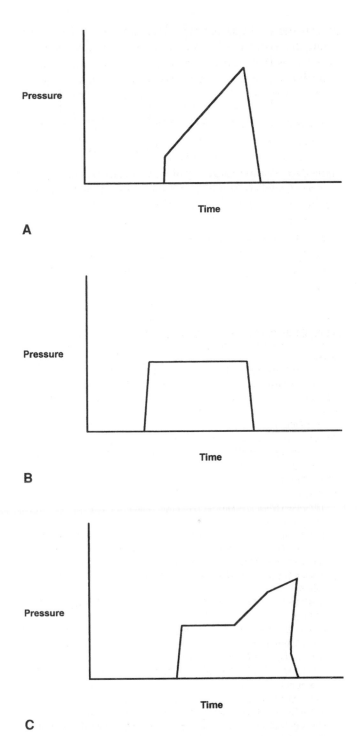

Figure 20–2. **(A)** Accelerating pressure waveform seen with volume ventilation. **(B)** Square pressure waveform associated with pressure ventilation. **(C)** Pressure augmentation breath begins as pressure breath (square waveform), but when the ventilator senses that desired volume will not be reached, the rest of the breath is delivered as a volume breath (accelerating waveform).

feature of unrestricted breathing, allowed at high levels of pressure, make the mode desirable because the use of heavy sedation and paralytics may not be necessary. Table 20–5 summarizes the selection, application, assessment, and potential complications of these mode options.

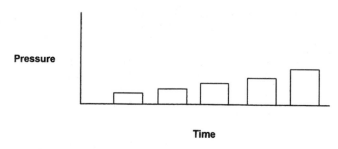

Figure 20–3. Volume support (VS) pressure waveforms (square) adjusted on breath-to-breath basis. Note how the level of pressure support changes to deliver the desired tidal volume. These changes are made in a gradual, step-wise fashion.

TABLE 20–4. VOLUME-GUARANTEED PRESSURE MODES (VAPS, VS, PRVC)

Definition

Volume-guaranteed pressure modes provide spontaneous and controlled pressure ventilation mode options while ensuring that a predetermined tidal volume is delivered. The volume-guarantee characteristic is provided in one of two ways. Either the pressure level is automatically adjusted by the ventilator to attain the predetermined volume, or the breath starts as a pressure breath but is completed as a volume breath. The decelerating flow pattern characterized by pressure ventilation is a desired outcome of these modes.

Patient Selection

1. *Acutely ill patients:* This mode can be selected so that volume is guaranteed while providing pressure ventilation.
2. *Chronically ill patients:* This option may be used as a "safety" in spontaneously breathing patients in whom pressure ventilation is desired. May be especially helpful for night use (when respiratory rates and volumes normally decrease) and in patients in whom secretions are a problem. (For example, as secretions build, resistance increases and tidal volume goes down. This mode option prevents the decreased tidal volume and potential atelectasis.)

Application

Application varies with specific ventilators.

1. Volume desired is selected and mode selection (pressure augmentation, volume support, etc.) is activated.
2. Pressure level is adjusted (i.e., in VAPS) to attain acceptable tidal volume while delivering it as a pressure breath (this is automatically done with VS).
3. Respiratory rate is selected for controlled modes and as a backup.
4. Airway pressure monitoring is necessary with these modes to accurately apply and assess the mode options.

Assessment

1. Arterial blood gases, end-tidal CO_2, and pulse oximetry.
2. Monitor pressure waveforms to determine the need for pressure/volume adjustment (alarms also indicate when pressure limits are exceeded, indicating compliance changes).

Complications

1. Barotrauma is a potential complication of all mechanical ventilation.
2. These modes, if not understood, are hard to assess. An understanding of the specific ventilator mode characteristics and the ability to interpret airway pressure waveforms are essential to prevent errors in mode application.

TABLE 20–5. AIRWAY PRESSURE RELEASE VENTILATION (APRV) AND BI-PHASIC VENTILATION[a]

Definitions

APRV: High level of CPAP provided with short releases at regular intervals.
Bi-Phasic: Two levels of PEEP (high and low levels) with spontaneous breathing allowed at both pressure levels.

Patient Selection

Patients with ARDS or with decreased lung compliance in whom lung recruitment is desired.

Application

1. *APRV:* CPAP level, Fio_2 and pressure release interval (similar to frequency or rate) and duration (no more than 1.5 seconds; longer releases result in lung "de-recruitment" and are to be avoided).
2. *BiPhasic:* This is similar to setting PC ventilation. Select a high PEEP level (this is like setting the inspiratory pressure level) and a low PEEP level (this is PEEP). A rate is set for the releases to the low PEEP level and the inspiratory time is also set.
3. Heavy sedation and paralytics should not be necessary because the patient can breathe at both levels of support. PSV may be set to assist with the patient's spontaneous breaths at the levels of support.

Assessment

Although comfort is a goal for the application of all mechanical ventilation, patients on these modes may be very tachypneic yet comfortable.

Complications

As per all modes of ventilation used in the acutely ill ventilated patient with noncompliant lungs.

[a]Bilevel, Puritan Bennett, Pleasanton, CA.

High-Frequency Ventilation and High-Frequency Oscillation

High-frequency ventilation (HFV), once considered an extreme but promising mode of ventilation for adults, only gained true widespread acceptance in neonatal critical care. High-frequency jet ventilation and high-frequency oscillation (HFO) are two types of HFV used in adults. These forms of ventilation are not easily categorized as either volume or pressure modes. Instead they demonstrate the characteristics of both.

HFV is defined as mechanical ventilation using higher than normal breathing rates. Generally, this means greater than 100 breaths per minute in the adult. The volumes delivered with HFV are very small (dead-space ventilation), with higher mean airway pressures, but lower peak airway pressures, than those found with conventional ventilation. How gases actually move through the lungs with HFV is not clear but is sometimes referred to as augmented dispersion. This mechanism is quite different than with conventional ventilation, where gases are delivered by bulk flow and include phenomena such as Taylor dispersion (how the gases in front of the bulk flow move through the lungs), molecular diffusion (the traditional concept of how gases mix in the alveoli secondary to diffusion), and the Pendelluft phenomenon (intra-unit gas mixing).

Recently, HFO was proposed for use in ARDS patients. With HFO, a bias flow of gases is provided via an oscillator, which disperses the gases throughout the lung at very high frequencies. The bias flow, combined with the oscillatory activity (extremely rapid pulses in a back and forth motion), result in the constant infusion of fresh gases and evacuation of old gases. The method provides oscillation around a constant mean airway pressure, the lung is recruited and a chest vibration ("wiggle") results. Some practitioners believe that this mode of ventilation may recruit alveoli and prevent tidal stress (since very small volumes result), to date, only one randomized controlled trial was done. The Multicenter Oscillatory Ventilation for Acute Respiratory Distress Syndrome Trial (MOAT) demonstrated that no substantial benefit in mortality rates was achieved with HFO over conventional ventilation. Additional concern about HFO rests with the fact that heavy sedation and often paralytics are necessary to assure compliance with the mode. These aspects, in addition to the fact that it is somewhat difficult to become proficient in the use of the mode, are limitations to its widespread applicability. Indications for, uses of, and complications associated with HFV are summarized in Table 20–6.

Alternative Ventilator Options

It is clear that pressure modes of ventilation appear especially promising and will continue to be popular choices for ventilating critical care and progressive care patients. However, other mode options continue to emerge for use in selected clinical situations. Two commonly used examples include the minimum minute volume option and flow-by.

Minimum Minute Volume

The minimum minute volume (MMV) mode option is only available on a few ventilators. MMV ensures that spontaneously breathing patients on CPAP, SIMV, PSV, or other spontaneous ventilatory modes receive a minimum minute volume. To do this, tidal volume, rate, and minimum minute volume are set by the clinician. As long as the patient meets the minimum minute volume requirement, the ventilator does not provide additional support. However, should the minimum minute volume not be attained, additional "back-up" breaths are delivered to achieve the MMV level. Because minute volume is determined by respiratory rate and tidal volume, a negative aspect of this mode option is that the patient may potentially meet the minute volume requirement by breathing rapidly and shallowly. To prevent this, safeguards, such as high rate alarms, are activated to alert the clinician to undesirable respiratory rates and patterns.

Flow-By

Also available only on some ventilators, this option provides for a high flow of gas past the patient's airway opening (patient wye) during spontaneous breathing intervals (e.g., SIMV). Spontaneous inspirations are "flow triggered." With this option, flow is always present in the system and triggering occurs when the ventilator senses a flow difference (between flow entering and exiting the system) indicating the

TABLE 20–6. HIGH-FREQUENCY VENTILATION (HFV) AND HIGH-FREQUENCY OSCILLATION (HFO)

Definition
Adult HFV is mechanical ventilation using respiratory rates higher than 100 breaths/min. The rationale for using HFV is to reduce airway pressure swings associated with barotrauma and to improve the efficiency of ventilation. Two systems commonly are employed to deliver gas at high frequencies: jets and oscillators.

Patient Selection
1. Patients with large pulmonary air leaks (i.e., bronchopleural fistulas) in whom a decreased pressure and improved gas distribution are desired (and in whom conventional modes have failed).
2. In lithotripsy when a quiet thoraco-abdominal wall is indicated.
3. Airway surgical procedures.

Jets
With high-frequency jet ventilation (HFJV) a small tube is placed in the circuit or airway (generally as far down the airway as possible), and a high-velocity "jet" of gas is injected at desired frequencies. Exhalation is passive and additional fresh gases are entrained from a bias (or cross) flow of source gas. Tidal volume is difficult to assess and is the product of rate, frequency, and the entrained gases. Jet ventilation is associated with frequencies between 100 to 600 breaths/min.

Application
Rate, inspiratory time, jet pressure, and PEEP are all set by monitoring pressure, chest movement, and arterial blood gases.

Oscillators
High-frequency oscillators (HFO) move in a back-and-forth motion (piston generated) and so have "inspiratory" and "expiratory" phases. Fresh gas is supplied by a bias flow. Tidal volume is dependent on the oscillator displacement volume and the magnitude and location of the bias flow.

Application
- *Bias flow:* In liters per minute (LPM; somewhere around 40–50 LPM).
- *Oscillatory frequency (fx):* In Hz.
- *Mean airway pressure:* Generally a bit above conventional ventilation to begin.
- *ΔP:* The change in pressure or pressure amplitude (generally adjusted to achieve chest wall vibration).
- *Fio_2 level and PEEP level:* As in conventional (generally PEEP is >10).
- *% inspiratory time:* Controls the percentage of time the oscillator spends in the inspiratory phase.

Assessment
1. Arterial blood gases, pulse oximetry, and end-tidal CO_2 monitoring.
2. Chest movement: Generally the chest is seen to "vibrate." With adequate gas exchange, the patient may not initiate spontaneous breaths. Return of spontaneous effort may be indicative of increased $Paco_2$.
3. Auto-PEEP is a common and often desirable outcome of these modes, but may be excessive and result in barotrauma and decreased cardiac output.

Complications
1. Adequate humidification is often difficult to attain, and airway obstruction is possible.
2. Tracheobronchitis (especially with jet ventilation).
3. Barotrauma.

beginning of inspiration. The flow-triggering sensitivity is adjusted by the clinician. This method differs from traditional pressure-triggered systems, which require that a negative pressure be sensed within the ventilator before a breath is delivered. Research demonstrated that the flow-by method of gas flow delivery can result in decreased work of breathing for the patient.

WEANING PATIENTS FROM LONG-TERM MECHANICAL VENTILATION

Weaning refers to the process of liberating patients from mechanical ventilation. In patients ventilated over the short-term (less than 3 days), weaning is rarely a problem because ventilatory support may be rapidly withdrawn. In other patients, the process takes longer than 3 days, sometimes requiring weeks or even months to accomplish. In these long-term mechanically ventilated (LTMV) patients, the weaning process varies and consists of four stages. The first stage is marked by instability and high ventilatory support requirements. During the second stage, called the prewean stage, many physiologic factors continue to require attention, and the patient's overall status may fluctuate. Ventilatory requirements are less and adjustments are made to maintain oxygenation and acid–base status as well as provide ventilatory muscle conditioning. The third, or weaning stage, is evident when the patient is stable, and rapid progress with weaning trials is possible. Finally, the last stage is called the outcome stage, which consists of extubation or partial or full ventilatory support.

Long-term mechanical ventilation is associated with high morbidity and mortality rates, and institutions lose money on patients ventilated long-term because reimbursement rarely covers the associated costs. As a result clinicians, scientists, and institutions are interested in testing methods of care delivery that improve the clinical and financial outcomes of the patients. Research in the area of weaning offers guidance to clinicians working with these patients. The following discussions of weaning addresses wean assessment, wean planning, and weaning modes and methods, including comprehensive institutional approaches.

Wean Assessment

Traditionally, the decision about when to begin the weaning process is determined once the condition that necessitates mechanical ventilation is improved or resolved. During this prewean stage, other factors that contribute to wean ability are considered prior to attempting weaning trials. In the past, "traditional" weaning predictors were used in an attempt to determine the optimal timing for extubation. More recently, investigators combined pulmonary elements to improve predictive ability. An example is the index of rapid shallow breathing, also known as the frequency (fx)/tidal volume (V_t) index, which integrates rate and tidal volume. Unfortunately, predictors have not predicted wean-ability. This is in part because they focus exclusively on pulmonary specific components to the exclusion of other important nonpulmonary factors (Table 20–7). Although the standard weaning criteria are not predictive, the components are helpful for assessing the patient's overall condition and readiness for weaning.

As noted, assessment of weaning potential starts with an evaluation of the underlying reason for mechanical ventilation (sepsis, pneumonia, trauma, etc.). Resolution of the underlying cause is necessary before gains in the weaning process can be expected. However, it is important to remember that resolution alone is frequently not sufficient to ensure successful weaning. Patients who require prolonged ventilation, sometimes referred to as the "chronically, critically ill,"

AT THE BEDSIDE
▶ *Weaning*

A 75-year-old man was admitted to the ER in respiratory distress. He was intubated and placed on the ventilator secondary to profound hypercarbia and acidosis and then transferred to the MICU for management of respiratory failure and right upper lobe pneumonia.

After 2 days of treatment with mechanical ventilation (AC of 14/min), antibiotics, fluid and nutritional replacement, and bronchodilators, the care team reassessed the patient's wean potential. Major impediments to weaning included factors such as:

• Poor nutritional status (albumin <1.8 g/dL)
• Anxiety and agitation
• Immobility
• Persistent upper lobe infiltrate
• Copious secretions
• NIP <15 cm H_2O
• Minute ventilation >15 L/min with a $PaCO_2$ of 50 mm Hg

The team recognized that these factors contributed to his high work of breathing (secretions, respiratory rate, minute ventilation) and his overall weak and debilitated state (nutrition, immobility, NIP). They acknowledged that these factors must be addressed before active weaning could successfully occur. It was likely that prolonged ventilation would be necessary. After 2 days of "complete rest," a ventilatory mode was selected that would allow for gradual respiratory muscle conditioning while overall improvement in physical status occurred. PSV was selected at PSV max (which in this case was 20 cm H_2O). This setting resulted in a respiratory rate of 16 breaths/min, a tidal volume of 8 mL/kg, and an eupneic respiratory pattern. PSV max was used for rest during the day and at night. For gradual conditioning trials, the PSV level was decreased in increments of 5 cm HO as defined by the PSV protocol.

Three days later, the patient was sitting in a chair at the bedside and beginning to ambulate with the help of the nurse and physical therapist. Enteral nutrition was provided via an oral gastric tube. Serial BWAP assessments demonstrated improvement (47–55%) but it was recognized that his recovery would likely take weeks. A tracheostomy was placed for comfort, to enhance mobility, and so that he could eat and talk. It took him 2 more weeks to finally reach a PSV of 5 (the lowest level of the plan), and it was at that time that the team initiated tracheostomy collar trials. Night rest was continued until the patient could tolerate 12 hours without signs of intolerance. He was decannulated and sent home with his family 1 week later.

TABLE 20-7. PULMONARY SPECIFIC WEAN CRITERIA THRESHOLDS

Traditional Weaning Criteria
- Negative inspiratory pressure (NIP) $\leq$20 cm H_2O
- Positive expiratory pressure (PEP) $\geq$30 cm H_2O
- Spontaneous tidal volume (SV_t) $\geq$5 mL/kg
- Vital capacity (VC) $\geq$15 mL/kg
- Fraction of inspired oxygen (Fio_2) $\leq$50%
- Minute ventilation (MV) $\leq$10 L/min

Integrated Weaning Criteria
- Index of rapid shallow breathing or frequency tidal volume ratio (fx/V_t) $\leq$105

---

often suffer from a myriad of symptoms that impede weaning. Even with resolution of the disease or condition that necessitated mechanical ventilation, the patient's overall status is often below baseline (weak, malnourished, etc.). Therefore, a systematic, comprehensive approach to weaning assessment is important. One example of a tool that encourages such an approach is the Burns Wean Assessment Program (BWAP) (Table 20–8). The BWAP score is used to track the progress of the patient and keep care planning on target. Factors important to weaning are listed in the BWAP bedside checklist.

Wean Planning

Once impediments to weaning are identified, plans that focus on improving the impediments are made in collaboration with a multidisciplinary team. A collaborative approach to assessment and planning greatly enhances positive outcomes in the LTMV patient. However, for care planning to be successful, it must also be systematic. The wean process is dynamic and regular reassessment and adjustment of plans are necessary. Tools like the BWAP can be used to systematically assess and track weaning progress. Other methods that have demonstrated efficacy in assuring consistency in care management and good outcomes for the patients include care delivery models using clinical pathways, protocols for weaning, and institution-wide approaches to managing and monitoring the patients.

Weaning Trials, Modes, and Methods

A wide variety of weaning modes and methods are available. To date, no data support the superiority of any one mode for weaning, however, methods using protocols and other systematic, multidisciplinary approaches do appear to make a difference and are to be encouraged. These methods are described following a discussion of respiratory muscle fatigue, rest, and conditioning because the concepts are integrated into the section on protocols.

Respiratory Fatigue, Rest, and Conditioning

Respiratory muscle fatigue is common in ventilated weaning patients and occurs when the respiratory workload is excessive. When the workload exceeds metabolic stores, fatigue and

---

TABLE 20–8. BURNS' WEAN ASSESSMENT PROGRAM (BWAP)[a]

I. General Assessment

Yes	No	Not Assessed	
___	___	___	1. Hemodynamically stable (pulse rate, cardiac output)?
___	___	___	2. Free from factors that increase or decrease metabolic rate (seizures, temperature, sepsis, bacteremia, hypo/hyperthyroid)?
___	___	___	3. Hematocrit >25% (or baseline)?
___	___	___	4. Systemically hydrated (weight at or near baseline, balanced intake and output)?
___	___	___	5. Nourished (albumin >2.5, parenteral/enteral feedings maximized)? *If albumin is low and anasarca or third spacing is present, score for hydration should be "no."
___	___	___	6. Electrolytes within normal limits (including Ca^{++}, Mg^+, PO_4)? *Correct Ca^{++} for albumin level.
___	___	___	7. Pain controlled (subjective determination)?
___	___	___	8. Adequate sleep/rest (subjective determination)?
___	___	___	9. Appropriate level of anxiety and nervousness (subjective determination)?
___	___	___	10. Absence of bowel problems (diarrhea, constipation, ileus)?
___	___	___	11. Improved general body strength/endurance (i.e., out of bed in chair, progressive activity program)?
___	___	___	12. Chest x-ray improving?

II. Respiratory Assessment

Yes	No	Not Assessed	
Gas Flow and Work of Breathing			
___	___	___	13. Eupneic respiratory rate and pattern (spontaneous RR <25, without dyspnea, absence of accessory muscle use)? *This is assessed off the ventilator while measuring #20–23.
___	___	___	14. Absence of adventitious breath sounds (rhonchi, rales, wheezing)?
___	___	___	15. Secretions thin and minimal?
___	___	___	16. Absence of neuromuscular disease/deformity?
___	___	___	17. Absence of abdominal distention/obesity/ascites?
___	___	___	18. Oral ETT > #7.5 or trach > #6.5?
Airway Clearance			
___	___	___	19. Cough and swallow reflexes adequate?
Strength			
___	___	___	20. NIP <20 (negative inspiratory pressure)?
___	___	___	21. PEP >30 (positive expiratory pressure)?
Endurance			
___	___	___	22. STV >5 mL/kg (spontaneous tidal volume)?
___	___	___	23. VC >10–15 mL/kg (vital capacity)?
ABGs			
___	___	___	24. pH 7.30–7.45?
___	___	___	25. $Paco_2$, 40 mm Hg (or baseline) with mV <10 L/min? *This is evaluated while on ventilator.
___	___	___	26. Pao_2 >60 on Fio_2 <40%?

[a]The BWAP score is obtained by dividing the total number of BWAP factors scored as "yes" by 26. ©Burns 1990.

hypercarbic respiratory failure ensue. Examples of those at risk include patients who are hypermetabolic, weak, or malnourished. Signs of fatigue include dyspnea, tachypnea, chest-abdominal asynchrony, and elevated $PaCO_2$ (a late sign). These signs and symptoms indicate a need for increased ventilatory support. Once fatigued, the muscles require 12 to 24 hours of rest to recover, and careful application of selected modes of ventilation is required.

For the respiratory muscles to recover from fatigue, the inspiratory workload must be decreased. In the case of volume ventilation (e.g., assist-control, intermittent mandatory ventilation), this means complete cessation of spontaneous effort, but in the case of pressure ventilation, a high level of PSV may accomplish the necessary "unloading." Generally, this means increasing the PSV level to attain a spontaneous respiratory rate of 20 breaths per minute or less and the absence of accessory muscle activity.

Respiratory muscle conditioning employs concepts borrowed from exercise physiology. To condition muscles and attain an optimal training effect from exercise, the concepts of endurance and strength conditioning must be considered. With strength training, a large force is moved a short distance. The muscles are worked to fatigue (short duration intervals) and rested for long periods of time. Spontaneous breathing trials on t-piece or continuous positive airway pressure (CPAP) both mimic this type of training because they employ high pressure and low-volume work. Endurance conditioning, which requires that the workload be increased gradually, is easily accomplished with PSV because the level of support can be decreased over time. This kind of endurance training employs low pressure and high-volume work. Central to the application of both conditioning methods is the provision of adequate respiratory muscle rest between trials. Prolonging trials once the patient is fatigued serves no useful purpose and may be extremely detrimental physiologically and psychologically.

Wean Trial Protocols

Recent study results suggest that no mode of ventilation is superior for weaning, however, the method of weaning, specifically the use of protocols, decreases variations in care and improves outcomes. Protocols direct caregivers by clearly delineating the protocol components. The protocol components consist of weaning readiness criteria ("wean screens"), weaning trial method and duration (i.e., CPAP, t-piece, or PSV), and definitions of intolerance and respiratory muscle rest. An example of a weaning protocol containing these components is found in Table 20-9.

In most cases, the choice between PSV (an endurance mode) and t-piece or CPAP (strengthening modes) is somewhat arbitrary if the protocol is appropriately aggressive, and easily understood and applied by the caregivers. There are some conditions that require more selective decision making. One example is that of patients with congestive heart fail-

TABLE 20–9. EXAMPLE OF WEANING PROTOCOL COMPONENTS

Weaning Trial Screen
1. Hemodynamic stability
2. $FiO_2 \leq 50\%$
3. PEEP ≤ 8 cm H_2O
4. BWAP $\geq 50\%$ (within the last 48 h)

Signs of Intolerance of Wean Trials
1. RR ≥ 35/min
2. O_2 Sat $\leq 90\%$ (or a decrease of 4%)
3. HR ≥ 140
4. Sustained change in HR of 20% (in either direction)
5. Systolic BP ≥ 180 or ≤ 90 mm Hg
6. Excessive anxiety or agitation
7. Diaphoresis

Wean Trial: CPAP
1. One trial of CPAP attempted daily. Each trial may last *no more than* 2 hours total.
2. If any signs of intolerance emerge (defined above), the trial is discontinued and the patient is rested.
3. Once the trial is sustained without signs of intolerance, the team is approached and extubation potential is discussed.
4. Full respiratory muscle rest is provided between trials and at night (definition below).

OR,

Wean Trial: PSV
1. Start at PSV max level (level to attain RR ≤ 20 with eupneic pattern).
2. Decrease PSV by 5 cm H_2O.
3. If no signs of intolerance are evident during the first 4-hour trial, the PSV is decreased by another 5 cm H_2O for the second trial.
4. With any signs of intolerance during trials, patient is returned to previous level for the second 4-hour trial.
5. If unable to tolerate, the patient is fully rested until the next day when the process begins again.
6. Once the patient is able to sustain the lowest level of PSV (as determined by the team) for 4 hours, extubation potential is discussed.

Definition of Rest (Both Protocols)
1. PSV max: PSV max is that pressure level required to attain a RR of 20 or less with V_t between 8 and 10 mL/kg and synchronous respiratory pattern without respiratory muscle use.
2. With volume modes of ventilation (i.e., A/C or IMV), respiratory muscle rest is not assured unless there is cessation of respiratory muscle activity. Therefore, rest is considered that level of support required to prevent patient-initiated breaths. When IMV is used, PSV may be added for protection (i.e., as a "safety"). Regardless, the goal is cessation of spontaneous effort.

ure. In these patients, the use of t-piece or CPAP can result in an increased venous return during the wean trial that may overwhelm the heart's ability to compensate. While appropriate preload and after-load reduction is addressed, PSV may be a gentler method of weaning. Another example is that of patients with profound myopathies or extremely debilitated states that may benefit from more gradual increases in work such as provided by PSV.

A popular and common sense approach to wean trial progression is to attempt weaning trials during the daytime, allowing the patient to rest at night until the protocol threshold for extubation is reached. In the case of the patient with a tracheostomy, progressively longer episodes of spontaneous breathing, usually on tracheostomy collar or t-piece, are accomplished until tolerated for a specified amount of time. Then, decisions about discontinuation of ventilation and tracheostomy downsizing or decannulation may be made (see Chapter 5, Airway and Ventilatory Management). Wean plans need to be communicated clearly to all members of the health care team (especially the patient) so that the plan is sufficiently aggressive but safe and effective. It is important that the philosophy of weaning is accepted by the health care team so that care planning is consistent and effective. Table 20-10 describes some general wean philosophy concepts.

Other Protocols for Use

Patients who require LTMV often are affected by a variety of clinical conditions that prolong ventilator duration and other clinical outcomes such as length of stay and death. Recent studies demonstrated that outcomes of critically ill patients are improved with protocol-directed sedation management and glucose control as compared to "traditional" or "standard" methods

---

TABLE 20–10. GENERAL WEANING GUIDELINES FOR LTMV PATIENTS

Active Weaning Should Occur
1. When patient is stable and reason for mechanical ventilation is resolved or improving.
2. When the wean score indices (BWAP, etc.) are improving and or when the "wean screen protocol criteria" are attained. A temporary hold and even an increase in support may be necessary when setbacks occur.
3. During the daytime, not at night (to allow respiratory muscle rest).

Considerations for Temporary Hold
1. When wean score drops (investigate factors and intervene as necessary).
2. During procedures that require that the patient be flat or in the Trendelenburg position (i.e., during line insertion).
3. During "road trips" (increased ventilatory support will protect the patient while off the unit).
4. If suctioning is excessive (every half hour).
5. When febrile, bacteremic, septic, or with *Clostridium difficile* disease.
6. During acute events (bronchospasm, hypotension).

Rest and Sleep
Rest is important for psychological and physiologic reasons. Complete rest in the mechanically ventilated patient is defined as that level of ventilatory support that offsets the work of breathing and decreases fatigue (refer to detailed description in text). Decisions about when rest is important include the following:
1. When an acute event has occurred (i.e., hypercarbic respiratory failure, pulmonary embolus, pulmonary edema).
2. A reasonable approach for the chronic or nonacute patient is to work on active weaning trials during the day with rest at night until most of the daytime wean is accomplished ($\geq$10 hours). Then, nighttime wean trials can be accomplished fairly rapidly. At night, the patient is allowed to sleep—if work of breathing is high, sleep is not possible. Ventilator rate should be high enough to allow for relaxation and optimal resting. If night sleeping aids are used, administer them early in the night to enhance sleep and ventilatory synchronization and so that the drugs can be metabolized before the daytime trials begin.

Critical Pathways

Critical pathways are used to assure that evidence-based care is provided and that variation in care delivery is reduced. The pathways may be very directive in selected categories of patients, such as those patients with hip replacements, where progression can be anticipated by hours or days, such specificity is not possible in the ventilated patient. Instead, pathways for the LTMV patient combine elements of care by specific time intervals (i.e., begin deep vein thrombosis prophylaxis by day 1) with those that are designated by the stage of illness (i.e., patient up to the chair during the prewean stage). In addition to providing an evidence-based blueprint for a wide variety of care elements, the pathways encourage multidisciplinary input and collaboration. In general, they are incorporated into systematic institutional approaches to care of the LTMV patient population.

Systematic Institutional Initiatives for the Management of the LTMV Patient Population

Given the importance of systematic assessment and care planning, it is not surprising that many institutions have taken a very comprehensive approach to the care for the LTMV patient. Solutions to reduce variation and promote standardization of care are implemented to ensure that best practices are adhered to and good outcomes result.

Smyrinos used an algorithmic approach to weaning in three adult ICUs. The investigator used nurses to manage the process and focused on the outcomes of ventilator duration, ICU and hospital lengths of stay (LOS), mortality rate, and cost savings to determine efficacy. Burns and colleagues demonstrated that care managed and monitored by advanced practice nurses (called Outcomes Managers) using a multidisciplinary clinical pathway and protocols for the management of sedation and weaning trials was both clinically and cost effective. The two studies demonstrated that statistically significant positive differences in most variables of interest were attainable with the approaches.

The health care environment is often chaotic. Short lengths of stay and decreased staffing levels affect the continuity of care and contribute to gaps in practice and care planning. Given the complexity of the care of the ventilated patient, it is clear that approaches to care that decrease variation may improve patient outcomes and are to be encouraged.

SELECTED BIBLIOGRAPHY

Acute Respiratory Distress Syndrome

The Acute Respiratory Distress Syndrome Network: Ventilation with lower tidal volumes as compared with traditional tidal volumes for acute lung injury and the acute respiratory distress syndrome. *N Eng J Med* 2000;342:1301–1307.

Amato MBP, Barbas CSV, Medeiros DM, et al: Effect of protective ventilation strategies on mortality in the acute respiratory distress syndrome. *N Engl J Med* 1998;338:347–354.

Bidani A, Tzouanakis AE, Cardenas VJ Jr, Zwischenberger JB: Permissive hypercapnia in acute respiratory failure. *JAMA* 1994; 272:957–962.

Dreyfuss D, Saumon G: The role of V_T, FRC, and end-inspiratory volume in the development of pulmonary edema following mechanical ventilation. *Am Rev Respir Dis* 1993;148:1194–1203.

Fu Z, Costell ML, Tsukimoto K, et al: High lung volume increases stress failure in pulmonary capillaries. *J Appl Physiol* 1992;73: 123–133.

Hickling KG, Walsh J, Henderson S, Jackson R: Low mortality rate in acute respiratory distress syndrome using low volume, pressure limited ventilation with permissive hypercapnia: A prospective study. *Crit Care Med* 1994;22:1568–1578.

Parker JC, Hernandez LA, Peevy KJ: Mechanisms of ventilator-induced lung injury. *Crit Care Med* 1993;21:131–143.

Slutsky AS: Consensus conference on mechanical ventilation, January 28–30, 1993 at Northbrook, Il, USA. Parts 1 & 2. *Intensive Care Med* 1994;20:64–79, 150–162.

West JB, Tsukimoto K, Mathieu-Costello O, et al: Stress fracture in pulmonary capillaries. *J Appl Physiol* 1991;70:1731–1742.

Mechanical Ventilation: Modes

Amato MBP, Barbas CSV, Bonassa J, Saldiva PHN, Zin WA, de-Carvalho CRR: Volume-assured, pressure support ventilation (VAPSV): A new approach for reducing muscle workload during acute respiratory failure. *Chest* 1992;102:1225–1234.

Brochard L, Harf A, Lorino H, Lemaire F: Inspiratory pressure support prevents diaphragmatic fatigue during weaning from mechanical ventilation. *Am Rev Respir Dis* 1989;139:513–521.

Brochard L, Pluskwa F, Lemaire R: Improved efficacy of spontaneous breathing with inspiratory pressure support. *Am Rev Respir Dis* 1987;136:411–415.

Derak S, Mehta S, Stewart TE, et al: High-frequency oscillatory ventilation for acute respiratory distress syndrome in adults: A randomized controlled trial. *Am J Respir Crit Care Med* 2002; 166:801–808.

Fiastro JF, Habib MP, Quan SF: Pressure support compensation for respiratory work due to endotracheal tubes and demand continuous positive airway pressure. *Chest* 1998;93:499–505.

Frawley PM, Habashi N: Airway pressure release ventilation: Theory and practice. *AACN Clinical Issues* 2001;12:234–246.

Hilbert G, Gruson D, Vargas F, et al: Noninvasive ventilation in immunosuppressed patients with pulmonary infiltrates, fever and acute respiratory failure. *N Engl J Med* 2001;344:481–487.

MacIntyre NR: Respiratory function during pressure support ventilation. *Chest* 1986;89:677–683.

Marini JJ, Rodriguez M, Lamb V: The inspiratory workload of patient-initiated mechanical ventilation. *Am Rev Respir Dis* 1986; 134:902–909.

Peter JV, Moran JL, Phillips-Hughes J, Warn D: Noninvasive ventilation in acute respiratory failure—A meta analysis update. *Crit Care Med* 2002;30:555–562.

Stock M, Downs JB: Airway pressure release ventilation: A new approach to ventilatory support during acute lung injury. *Respir Care* 1987;32:517–524.

Weaning From Long-Term Mechanical Ventilation

Bellemare F, Grassino A: Evaluation of human diaphragm fatigue. *J Appl Physiol* 1982;53:1196–1206.

Brochard L, Harf A, Lorino H, Lemarie F: Inspiratory pressure support prevents diaphragmatic fatigue during weaning from mechanical ventilation. *Am Rev Respir Dis* 1989;139:513–521.

Brochard L, Pluskwa F, Lemaire F: Improved efficacy of spontaneous breathing with inspiratory pressure support. *Am Rev Respir Dis* 1987;136:411–415.

Brook AD, Ahrens TS, Schaiff R, et al: Effect of a nursing-implemented sedation protocol on the duration of mechanical ventilation. *Crit Care Med* 1999;27:2609–2615.

Burns SM, Ryan B, Burns JE: The weaning continuum: Use of APACHE III, BWAP, TISS, and WI scores to establish stages of weaning. *Crit Care Med* 2000;28:2259–2267.

Burns SM, Earven D, Fisher C, et al: Implementation of an institutional program to improve clinical and financial outcomes of patients requiring mechanical ventilation: One year outcomes and lessons learned. *Crit Care Med* 2003;31:2752–2763.

Burns SM, Burns JE, Truwit JD: Comparison of five clinical weaning indices. *Am J Crit Care* 1994;3:342–352.

Cohen CA, Zagelbaum G, Gross D, Roussos CH, Macklem PT: Clinical manifestations of inspiratory muscle fatigue. *Am J Med* 1982;73:308–316.

Cook D, Meade M, Guyatt G, Griffith L, Booker L: Evidence report on criteria for weaning from mechanical ventilation. Contract No. 290-97-0017. Rockville, MD: Agency for Health Care Policy and Research; November 1999.

Ely EW, Baker AM, Dunagan DP, et al: Effect on the duration of mechanical ventilation of identifying patients capable of breathing spontaneously. *N Engl J Med* 1998;335:1864–1869.

Kollef MH, Shapiro SD, Silver P, et al: A randomized, controlled trial of protocol-directed versus physician-directed weaning from mechanical ventilation. *Crit Care Med* 1997;25:557–574.

Knebel A, Shekleton MD, Burns S, et al: Weaning from mechanical ventilatory support: Refinement of a model. *Am J Crit Care* 1998;7:149–152.

Kress JP, Pohlman AS, O'Connor MF, Hall JB: Daily interruption of sedative infusions in critically ill patients undergoing mechanical ventilation. *N Engl J Med* 2000;342:1471–1477.

MacIntyre NR, Cook DJ, Ely EW Jr, et al: Evidence-based guidelines for weaning and discontinuing ventilatory support: A collective task force facilitated by the American College of Chest Physicians; the American Association for Respiratory Care; and the American College of Critical Care Medicine. *Chest* 2001; 120(6 Suppl):375S–395S.

Marini JJ, Smith TC, Lamb VJ: External work output and force generation during synchronized intermittent mechanical ventilation: Effect of machine assistance on breath effort. *Am Rev Respir Dis* 1998;138:1169–1179.

Smyrnios NA, Connolly A, Wilson MM, et al: Effects of a multifaceted, multidisciplinary, hospital-wide quality improvement program on weaning from mechanical ventilation. *Crit Care Med* 2002;30:1224–1230.

Tobin MJ, Geunther S, Perez W, et al: Konno-Mead analysis of ribcage-abdominal motion during successful and unsuccessful trials of weaning from mechanical ventilation. *Am Rev Respir Dis* 1987;135:1320–1328.

Van DE, Berge G, Wouters PJ, et al: Outcome benefit of intensive insulin therapy in the critically ill: Insulin dose versus glycemic control. *Crit Care Med* 2003;31:359–366.

Yang KL, Tobin MJ: A prospective study of indexes predicting the outcome of trials of weaning from mechanical ventilation. *N Engl J Med* 1991;324:1445–1450.

Evidence-Based Practice

Pierce LNB: Traditional and non-traditional modes of mechanical ventilation. In: Chulay M (exec ed), Burns SM (series ed): *Protocols for Practice: Care of the Mechanically Ventilated Patient. AACN Critical Care.* Aliso Viejo, CA: AACN; 1998.

Burns SM: AACN protocol for practice: Weaning from long-term mechanical ventilation. In: Chulay M, Burns SM (eds): *Protocols for Practice: Care of the Mechanically Ventilated Patient. AACN Critical Care.* Aliso Viejo, CA: AACN; 1998.

Additional Reading

Burns SM: Mechanical ventilation and weaning. In: Kinney MR, Dunbar SB, Brooks-Brunn J, Molter N, Vitello-Cicciu JM (eds): *AACN Clinical Reference for Critical Care Nursing,* 4th ed. St. Louis, MO: Mosby–Year Book; 1998:607–633.

Hess D, Kacmarack R: *Essentials of Mechanical Ventilation.* New York: McGraw-Hill/Appleton & Lange; 2002.

ADVANCED NEUROLOGIC CONCEPTS

Dea Mahanes

▶ **Knowledge Competencies**

1. Compare and contrast the pathophysiology, clinical presentation, patient needs, and management approaches for the following conditions:
   • Subarachnoid hemorrhage
   • Traumatic brain injury

   • Acute spinal cord injury
   • Brain tumor
2. Describe the concept of cerebral oxygenation and monitoring modalities.

SUBARACHNOID HEMORRHAGE

Etiology, Risk Factors, and Pathophysiology

Subarachnoid hemorrhage (SAH) can result from trauma, aneurysm, or other vascular malformations. This discussion focuses on SAH due to the rupture of an intracranial aneurysm. Intracranial aneurysms usually occur in the circle of Willis at arterial bifurcations or trifurcations (Figure 21–1). Aneurysms vary in size and shape (Figure 21–2); saccular (also called berry) aneurysms are the most common and most amenable to treatment. When an intracranial aneurysm ruptures, blood is forcibly expelled into the subarachnoid space and coats the brain surfaces. Clot may form in the ventricular system or in the brain parenchyma. Blood in the subarachnoid space causes obstruction of cerebrospinal fluid (CSF) flow through the ventricles or clogs the arachnoid granulations that absorb CSF, resulting in hydrocephalus. Although the mechanism is not well understood, arterial spasm occurs in a significant number of patients and correlates temporally with the breakdown of the subarachnoid blood. There are several scales used to grade the severity of a SAH. The Hunt and Hess scale (Table 21–1) is most commonly used in the published nursing research.

Significant risk factors associated with SAH include smoking, hypertension, heredity (higher incidence in first degree relatives), and autosomal dominant polycystic kidney disease. Twenty percent of patients have multiple aneurysms. Other factors that have been associated with aneurysm rupture include heavy alcohol intake (more than 2 to 3 drinks per day), illicit drug use, low body mass index, and size of the aneurysm. SAH is most common in men until age 50 years; the incidence is higher in women after age 50 years and in the overall population. Predictors of outcome include neurologic condition on admission, age, and the amount of blood on the initial CT scan.

Clinical Presentation

Most patients are asymptomatic until the time of aneurysm rupture, but some have prodromal signs such as headache and visual changes. Upon aneurysm rupture, most patients experience a sudden, severe headache, sometimes described as "explosive" or "the worst headache of my life." Transient or prolonged loss of consciousness can occur. Bystanders may describe seizure activity; it is unclear whether this is an actual seizure or abnormal posturing related to a sudden increase in intracranial pressure (ICP). Other common signs and symptoms include nausea and vomiting, stiff neck, blurred vision, mental status changes, and photophobia. Focal deficits, such as hemiparesis, hemiplegia, or aphasia, may also occur.

477

AT THE BEDSIDE
▶ *Subarachnoid Hemorrhage*

A 54-year-old loan officer at a bank experienced the sudden onset of a severe headache while at work. She was taken to the emergency department of a local hospital where she described her headache as the "worst headache of my life." The diagnosis of subarachnoid hemorrhage was made by CT scan. Angiography revealed an aneurysm of the left internal carotid artery. The aneurysm was successfully clipped and she returned to the ICU following surgery. On the fifth day postbleed, the nurse noted that this patient was difficult to rouse and once awake had right upper extremity weakness and difficulty speaking. She was taken to CT scan, which revealed normal postoperative changes, and then to neuroradiology. Cerebral angiography revealed severe vasospasm of the left middle cerebral artery. Balloon angioplasty was performed with improvement in vasospasm.

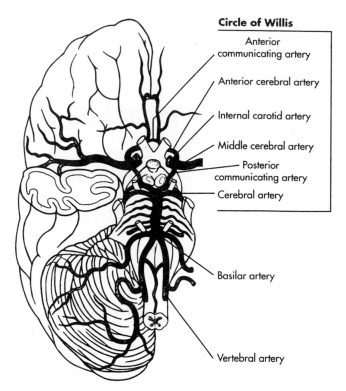

Figure 21–1. The circle of Willis as seen from below the brain. (*Reprinted from: Perry L, Sands JK: Vascular and degenerative problems of the brain. In: Phipps WJ, Marek JF, Monahan FD, Neighbors M, Sands JK [eds]: Medical-Surgical Nursing: Health and Illness Perspectives, p. 1365. St. Louis, MO: Mosby, 2003.*)

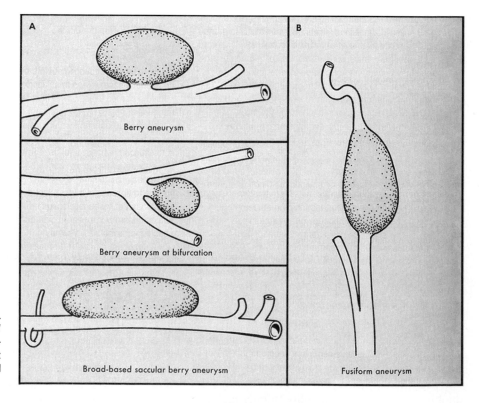

Figure 21–2. Types of cerebral aneurysms. (*Reprinted from Boss BJ, Heath J, Sunderland PM: Alterations of neurologic function. In: McCance KL, Huether SE [eds.]: Pathophysiology: The Biological Basis for Disease in Adults and Children, p. 496. St. Louis, MO: Mosby; 1990.*)

TABLE 21–1. HUNT AND HESS SCALE FOR THE CLASSIFICATION OF PATIENTS WITH INTRACRANIAL ANEURYSMS

Category	Criteria
Grade I	Asymptomatic, or minimal headache and slight nuchal rigidity.
Grade II	Moderate to severe headache, nuchal rigidity, no neurological deficit other than cranial nerve palsy.
Grade III	Drowsiness, confusion, or mild focal deficit.
Grade IV	Stupor, moderate to severe hemiparesis, possible early decerebrate rigidity and vegetative disturbances.
Grade V	Deep coma, decerebrate rigidity, moribund appearance.

Reprinted from Hunt WE, Hess RM: Surgical risk as related to time of intervention in the repair of intracranial aneurysms. J Neurosurg *1968;28:14.*

Diagnostic Tests

CT Scan
A CT scan is used to determine if subarachnoid hemorrhage has occurred and to assess for hydrocephalus. CT angiography can be performed quickly at the time of the initial scan and is increasingly used to detect aneurysm location, but catheter angiography remains the gold standard. The amount of blood present on the CT scan is predictive of vasospasm risk. Recently, the use of CT angiography or CT perfusion was proposed as a method for evaluation of vasospasm, but conclusive research is not yet available.

Lumbar Puncture
A lumbar puncture (LP) is performed when CT fails to demonstrate SAH in a patient with a history highly suspicious for SAH. LP is avoided in patients with signs or symptoms of increased intracranial pressure due to the risk of herniation. LP is performed at least 6 to 12 hours after the onset of symptoms to allow red blood cells (RBCs) in the CSF to start to break down. This breakdown in RBCs gives a yellow tinge to the CSF after centrifugation. This pigmentation is called xanthochromia and will not be present if blood in the CSF is due to a traumatic LP.

Cerebral Angiography
Cerebral angiography is performed to identify the location, size, and shape of the aneurysm or other vascular anomalies, and to determine the presence of vasospasm. The initial angiogram will not reveal an aneurysm in approximately 10% to 20% of patients with SAH. Repeat angiogram after several days will reveal an aneurysm in a small number of these patients. Negative angiogram and a distinct pattern of bleeding on CT scan may also indicate a nonaneurysmal perimesencephalic SAH; patients with this diagnosis have an excellent prognosis and do not develop the typical complications of SAH, such as vasospasm.

MRI and MRA
Used to identify aneurysm location and look for other vascular abnormalities, MRI and MRA is especially useful in patients with a negative angiogram.

Principles of Management of Aneurysmal Subarachnoid Hemorrhage
Patients who survive the initial rupture of a cerebral aneurysm are at risk to develop complications that increase their chances for morbidity and death. Primary CNS complications include rebleeding, hydrocephalus, and delayed ischemic neurologic deficit due to vasospasm.

Rebleeding
Prior to the aneurysm being secured, the biggest risk to the patient is that the aneurysm will bleed again. This risk is highest within the first 24 hours. The probability of death is markedly increased by rebleed. Signs and symptoms of rebleeding include a sudden increase in headache, nausea, and vomiting, decrease in the level of consciousness, and new focal neurologic deficits. The most definitive method to prevent rebleeding is to secure the aneurysm using surgical clipping or endovascular embolization.

In the interim between admission and definitive treatment, strategies such as blood pressure management and prevention of activities that increase intracranial pressure are used to decrease the risk of rebleeding. The goal for blood pressure management varies by patient history, examination findings, and physician preference. The goal is to treat hypertension without dropping the blood pressure to a level that decreases cerebral perfusion. Systolic BP goals with an upper range of 150 to 160 mm Hg are common. Two frequently used antihypertensive medications used in patients with SAH are intravenous labetalol and nicardipine infusion.

Bed rest is typically ordered but may be adapted with physician approval to meet patient needs (for example, a patient who becomes anxious and hypertensive when using a bedpan may be allowed to use a bedside commode). Prophylaxis for deep vein thrombosis, including elastic compression stockings and sequential compression devices, is implemented. Stool softeners are used to prevent straining due to constipation, which will increase ICP. Pain is treated with analgesics, usually short-acting narcotics. A calm, quiet environment is maintained. Anxiety is reduced through explanations of care and psychological support. Neurologic assessment is performed hourly (or more frequently if indicated) to promptly identify changes related to rebleeding or hydrocephalus. An external ventricular drain may be placed for assessment and management of elevated intracranial pressure, especially in patients with poor-grade SAH (Hunt and Hess IV or V), or if hydrocephalus is apparent on CT scan. Careful management of external ventricular drains is essential to prevent over-drainage of CSF, which can result in rebleeding due to a change in mural pressure.

Two management options exist to secure the aneurysm and prevent another rupture: surgical clipping of the aneurysm via craniotomy and endovascular embolization of the aneurysm via catheter angiography. The decision to use surgery versus an endovascular procedure is made on the basis of aneurysm location, comorbidities, and the severity of neurologic deficits on admission. Endovascular treatment is limited to centers with physicians trained in the procedure.

Current practice is to secure the aneurysm as soon as possible, prior to the period of time when patients are most at risk for vasospasm. With the aneurysm secured, standard management strategies for vasospasm can be implemented without the risk of causing additional hemorrhage. Aneurysm surgery is performed via a craniotomy incision. The surgeon carefully dissects tissue away from the aneurysm and places a titanium or titanium alloy clip across the base (Figure 21–3). Different sizes and shapes of clips are available. Following surgery, the patient returns to the ICU for continued management. Follow-up radiologic studies may be done, including CT scanning to look for bleeding at the operative site and angiography to evaluate clip position. Postoperative care includes frequent neurologic assessment (every 15 minutes initially), pain management, and prevention of complications. The postoperative neurologic assessment is compared to the preoperative assessment and any changes are reported to the neurosurgeon.

Endovascular embolization is increasingly used in the management of aneurysmal SAH, especially when the aneurysm is difficult to access or the patient has multiple medical problems that would make surgery inadvisable. Using cerebral angiography, the interventional radiologist threads a wire with a helical platinum coil at the end into the cerebral vasculature. The coil is manipulated into the body of the aneurysm and detached from the wire using a small electrical current. The neck of the aneurysm must be narrow enough for the coils to be retained in the aneurysm instead

of floating back out into the vessel lumen. Multiple coils may be needed to completely fill the aneurysm. The coils cause the aneurysm to clot, preventing blood flow into the aneurysm and decreasing the likelihood of rebleed. The primary risks associated with coil embolization are aneurysmal rupture during the procedure and ischemia related to clot formation in other vessels. Postprocedure care for the patient who has received embolization is similar to that of a patient postsurgical clipping, with the addition of the postangiography care as described in Chapter 12, Neurologic System.

In some instances, the aneurysm cannot be treated via either surgery or embolization, and the decision is made to occlude the parent vessel that leads to the aneurysm. This occurs most often with large aneurysms in the internal carotid artery and is possible because of collateral circulation permitted by the circle of Willis. A catheter with a temporary balloon attached is threaded into the parent artery and inflated. The patient is monitored closely for neurologic changes, usually for 30 minutes. If no neurologic changes occur, a permanent balloon is placed.

Hydrocephalus

SAH disrupts normal CSF flow through two mechanisms. Intraventricular blood may create a blockage in the ventricular drainage system and cause CSF to build up (obstructive or noncommunicating hydrocephalus). In addition, the arachnoid granulations that absorb CSF may become blocked with cellular debris. This results in decreased reabsorption of CSF and communicating hydrocephalus. Signs and symptoms relate to increased intracranial pressure. Acute hydrocephalus after SAH is managed by external ventricular drainage or, less commonly, serial lumbar punctures. Some SAH patients later require placement of a ventricular shunt due to continued hydrocephalus.

Vasospasm

Cerebral vasospasm is the narrowing of cerebral arteries, which cause decreased perfusion, ischemia, and infarction of cerebral tissue. Vasospasm develops 4 to 14 days after initial hemorrhage, with peak incidence around day 7, and is the biggest contributor to morbidity and mortality rates in patients with SAH who survive to hospital admission. Approximately one third of patients with aneurysmal SAH will develop delayed ischemic neurologic deficits due to vasospasm, and another third will have angiographic evidence of vasospasm without neurologic decline. At many institutions, transcranial Doppler studies (TCDs, see Chapter 12, Neurologic System) are used to monitor the development of vasospasm, but angiography is the gold standard for diagnosis. Vasospasm is suspected in any patient who develops neurologic decline, especially a decrease in level of consciousness, paresis or paralysis of a limb or side of the body, or aphasia. Early identification of neurologic deficits allows rapid intervention to improve cerebral perfusion.

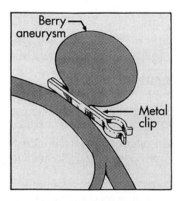

Figure 21–3. Aneurysm clipping. A titanium or titanium alloy clip is placed across the neck of the aneurysm. Flow through the parent artery is maintained, but blood can no longer flow into the aneurysm. (*From: Chipps EM, Clanin NJ, Cambell VG: Central nervous system disorders. In: Chipps EM [eds.]: Neurologic Disorders, p. 85. St. Louis, MO: Mosby; 1992.*)

Maintenance of euvolemia is essential to decrease the risk of vasospasm. Dehydration increases blood viscosity and decreases cerebral perfusion. SAH patients are at risk for dehydration because of cerebral salt wasting, in which excessive sodium is excreted, leading to increased water loss and hypovolemia. If serum sodium falls, volume restriction is contraindicated because of increased risk of cerebral ischemic deficits. Infusion of hypertonic saline (either 1.8% or 3% saline) is often used for treatment of hyponatremia. The calcium channel blocker, nimodipine, does not significantly decrease angiographic vasospasm but a large trial showed improved outcomes at 3 months after aneurysmal SAH. This medication should never be given sublingually as a precipitous drop in blood pressure may occur, resulting in decreased cerebral perfusion. If blood pressure drops with the standard dosing regimen of 60 mg orally or via gastric tube every 4 hours, the dose can be divided and 30 mg can be given every 2 hours.

Hypervolemic, hypertensive, hemodilution (triple-H) therapy is used to increase cerebral perfusion in patients with vasospasm. In most patients, a pulmonary artery catheter is used to guide treatment. Intravascular volume is increased (hypervolemia) through the infusion of crystalloids or colloids, although recent study results suggest that hypervolemia is less important than avoiding hypovolemia. At least 3 L of fluid a day are typically administered, but some patients may require more. Careful attention to fluid balance is essential, and must include recognition of insensible fluid loss. Hypertension is induced using intravenous fluids and vasopressors. Blood pressure goals vary based on the patient response but are typically in the range of 160 to 200 mm Hg. The rationale for induced hypertension is that the loss of cerebral autoregulation makes the brain more dependent on systemic blood pressure for adequate perfusion. Hemodilution occurs as the result of operative blood loss, laboratory work, and the administration of intravenous fluids. A hematocrit of 30% to 35% is considered optimal. Recent evidence suggests benefit from increasing cardiac output through the use of hydration and inotropic medications (e.g., dobutamine). Goals of vasospasm treatment are primarily based on improvement in neurologic examination instead of a strict range of hemodynamic values.

Vasospasm can be definitively treated by transluminal balloon angioplasty, provided that the vessel in spasm is proximal enough to be reached by the angiography catheter. When vasospasm occurs in a distal vessel, intra-arterial infusion of a calcium channel antagonist, such as verapamil, is sometimes used. Intra-arterial infusion of papaverine, a vasodilator, provides transient relief of vasospasm but may cause side effects including elevated ICP. As the use of other agents becomes more common, the use of papaverine is decreasing. Other strategies that may be of benefit in the prevention or treatment of vasospasm include intraoperative removal of clot, intrathecal administration of thrombolytics, lumbar drainage, and intraventric-

ular administration of a number of vasoactive agents (e.g., sodium nitroprusside, nicardipine); multiple clinical trials are ongoing.

Additional Management Strategies and Prevention of Complications
The use of anticonvulsants and steroids in the management of SAH is not well-supported in published research results but continues to be common practice at some institutions. Systemic complications of SAH include myocardial dysfunction, cardiac arrhythmias, and neurogenic pulmonary edema. Cardiac complications are believed to be due to massive catecholamine release at the time of initial hemorrhage. Left ventricular dysfunction occurs, but typically returns to baseline over days to weeks. The most common ECG changes associated with SAH are ST-segment abnormalities, T wave inversion, and prolonged QTc interval. Neurogenic pulmonary edema is believed to result from a CNS-mediated increase in intravascular permeability or massive sympathetic discharge, or a combination of these factors. Neurogenic pulmonary edema occurs rapidly and presents with signs and symptoms similar to those of cardiogenic pulmonary edema; however, pulmonary artery occlusion pressure is normal or only mildly elevated. Treatment is supportive and often includes mechanical ventilation. Diuresis is done gently (if at all) to avoid increasing vasospasm risk. Neurogenic pulmonary edema typically resolves within 72 hours.

TRAUMATIC BRAIN INJURY

Etiology, Risk Factors, and Pathophysiology
Major causes of traumatic brain injury (TBI) are motor vehicle accidents (MVAs), falls, and acts of violence. Falls are more common in the elderly, and acts of violence are more prevalent in urban areas. The incidence of TBI is higher in males than females and higher in people 15 to 24 years of age or older than 75 years. TBI can be classified by severity using the Glasgow Coma Scale score (GCS, see Chapter 12). Mild brain injury refers to patients with a GCS score of 13 to 15, moderate indicates a GCS score of 9 to 12, and patients with a score of 8 or less are categorized as having severe brain injury. Mild TBI can cause significant functional deficits that become apparent in the weeks and months following injury; however, these patients are not admitted to the ICU unless they have other injuries. Patients with moderate TBI are typically admitted to the ICU for close monitoring and may require aggressive intervention. Patients with severe TBI are among the sickest patients admitted to the intensive care unit and require frequent interventions to prevent secondary brain injury. The majority of this discussion is limited to moderate and severe TBI.

The damage that occurs following TBI is described as primary or secondary. Primary injury occurs due to the bio-

AT THE BEDSIDE
▶ *Traumatic Brain Injury*

A 30-year-old construction worker was involved in a single-vehicle, high-speed, rollover accident. On EMS arrival, the patient did not open his eyes, displayed decorticate posturing, and did not verbalize (GCS score 5). He was intubated and transported by helicopter to the nearest Level 1 trauma center, where a CT scan revealed diffuse cerebral edema and some small (punctate) hemorrhages. The rest of his trauma evaluation was negative except for a broken right clavicle. An ICP monitor was placed with an initial reading of 18 mm Hg. The patient was admitted to the ICU, where he remained on sedation and analgesics for several days. He also received several doses of mannitol and meticulous attention to prevention of complications. On the seventh day postinjury, he opened his eyes to painful stimulation and attempted to push the stimulus away with his right hand (localization). Tracheostomy and gastric tubes were placed the next day. About 3 weeks after his injury, the patient was opening his eyes spontaneously and followed very simple commands. He was transferred to a rehabilitation hospital. About 2 months after his accident, he was discharged into the care of his parents. He was able to perform ADLs, but remained unable to work because of decreased judgment and cognitive skills.

mechanical effects of trauma on the brain and skull as a result of the initial insult. Prevention is the only way to avoid primary injury. Secondary injury refers to the complications that result in additional pathophysiologic changes and dysfunction of the brain tissue. There are many causes of secondary brain injury, including hypoxemia, hypotension, increased ICP, infection, and electrolyte imbalances. These problems compromise the oxygen and nutrient supply necessary for adequate cerebral cell metabolism, result in the build-up of waste products, and contribute to cerebral ischemia and poor patient outcomes. TBI can be further classified on the basis of mechanism of injury and the type of injury.

Mechanism of Injury
TBI occurs as the result of blunt trauma (a direct blow to the head) or penetrating trauma (missile or impaled object). Blunt injury occurs as the result of:

- *Deceleration:* The head is moving and strikes a stationary object (e.g., pavement).
- *Acceleration:* A moving object (e.g., baseball bat) strikes the head.
- *Acceleration–deceleration:* The brain moves rapidly within the skull, resulting in a combination of injury-causing forces.
- *Rotation:* Twisting motion of the brain occurs within the skull, usually due to side impact.

- *Deformation/compression:* Direct injury to the head changes the shape of the skull, resulting in compression of brain tissue.

In the United States, gunshot wound (GSW) is the most common type of penetrating brain trauma. The degree of injury caused by a GSW varies based on the type of firearm, bullet type, and trajectory of the bullet. Tissue is destroyed by the bullet, and shock waves and cavity formation occur along the bullet's path. Some bullets will ricochet once inside the skull, creating more tissue destruction. Other causes of penetrating brain injury include nail guns and stab wounds. Surgical management of penetrating trauma to the brain differs from the management of closed injury, but many of the issues relevant to critical care nurses remain the same.

Skull Fractures
Skull fractures can result in injury to the underlying brain tissue, but can occur in isolation. Skull fractures are classified as linear, depressed, or basilar.

- Linear skull fractures resemble a line or single crack in the skull. Generally, they are not displaced and require no treatment.
- Depressed skull fractures are characterized by an inward depression of bone fragments. Depressed skull fractures require surgery to elevate the depressed bone. In the case of an open fracture, the wound is also washed out to decontaminate the area and decrease the risk of infection. If the fractured portion of skull cannot be replaced due to contamination or the presence of multiple fragments, a plate made of acrylic or metal may be placed.
- Basilar skull fractures involve the base of the skull, including the anterior, middle, or posterior fossa. Clinical manifestations of a basilar skull fracture include periorbital ecchymosis (raccoon's eyes), mastoid ecchymosis (Battle's sign), rhinorrhea (CSF or blood leaking from the nose), otorrhea (CSF or blood leaking from the ears), hemotympanum (CSF or blood behind the tympanic membrane), conjunctival hemorrhage, and cranial nerve dysfunction. The presence of otorrhea or rhinorrhea indicates a dural tear with increased risk of meningitis. Although most CSF leaks stop spontaneously, those that persist after 7 to 14 days may require dural repair. Management includes elevating the head of bed, antibiotics, and, occasionally, lumbar drainage of CSF to decrease pressure on the healing dura.

Primary Brain Injury
Primary injury occurs at the time of initial impact and causes focal or diffuse anatomic changes to the cerebral tissue or cerebral vasculature. Focal injuries are produced by an object striking the head or acceleration-deceleration forces. Focal lesions result in local damage at the site of injury,

which takes up space, increases ICP, and may cause brain shift and herniation. Examples of focal injury include cerebral contusions and hematomas. Diffuse brain injuries involve microscopic damage to cells deep in the white matter. They occur as lateral head motion produces angular movement of the brain within the skull causing shearing or stretching of axonal nerve fibers. Damage is variable and dependent on the amount of accelerative force transmitted to the brain. Examples of primary injury follow.

- *Cerebral contusion, laceration, and intracerebral hematoma.* Contusions are cortical bruises caused by the brain impacting the inside of the skull. They may be described as coup (occurring at the site of impact) or contrecoup (occurring opposite the site of impact). The frontal and temporal lobes are common sites of contusions. Lacerations are actual tears in the brain surface and often occur in conjunction with contusions. Clinical presentation depends on the site and extent of brain injury. Progressive focal edema and mass effect may result in neurologic deterioration. The severity of injury may not be apparent on the initial CT scan, because bleeding into the contused or lacerated tissue often occurs and results in intracerebral hematoma. Repeat CT scanning may be performed to evaluate for injury progression.
- *Epidural hematoma* (EDH, Figure 21–4). EDH is a blood clot located between the dura and the skull, most often associated with skull fractures that lacerate an underlying artery. EDH is most common in the temporal region due to tearing of the middle meningeal artery. The clot expands rapidly, displacing brain structures and causing increased ICP. Symptoms include a decrease in consciousness, headache, seizures,

vomiting, hemiparesis, and pupillary dilation. Management includes emergency surgery to evacuate the hematoma.
- *Subdural hematoma* (SDH, Figure 21–5). Bleeding occurs within the subdural space between the dura and arachnoid layer, creating direct pressure on the brain. Bleeding results from rupture of the bridging veins between the brain and dura, bleeding from contused or lacerated brain tissue, or extension from an intracerebral hematoma. SDH is described as acute if symptoms begin within the first 48 hours after injury. Many patients experience significant symptoms immediately following the injury or much sooner than 48 hours. Patients with acute SDH present with progressive decline in level of consciousness, headache, agitation, and confusion. Motor deficits, pupillary changes, and cranial nerve dysfunction may be seen, reflecting the primary brain injury and compressive effects. Treatment of acute SDH consists of evacuation of the hematoma via craniotomy. Blood may also collect in the subdural space more slowly, over days to weeks (subacute SDH) or weeks to months (chronic SDH). The onset of symptoms is insidious because the brain can better compensate for this slow increase in mass. Symptoms include an increasingly severe headache, confusion, drowsiness, and, possibly, seizures, pupillary abnormalities, or motor dysfunction. Predisposing conditions include advanced age, alcoholism, and disorders or treatments that result in prolonged coagulation times. Treatment of subacute or chronic SDH includes evacuation via burr holes or craniotomy.
- *Traumatic subarachnoid hemorrhage.* Traumatic SAH can occur alone or in combination with other types

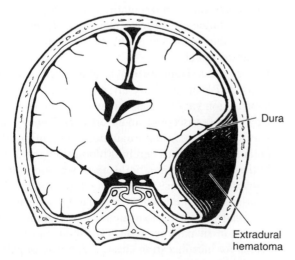

Figure 21–4. Schematic illustration of an epidural hemorrhage. (*Reprinted from Waxman SG: Vascular supply. In:* Clinical Neuroanatomy, *p. 187. New York: Lange Medical Books/McGraw-Hill; 2003.*)

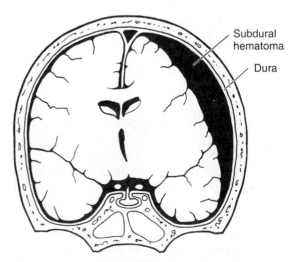

Figure 21–5. Schematic illustration of a subdural hemorrhage. (*Reprinted from Waxman SG: Vascular supply. In:* Clinical Neuroanatomy, *p. 187. New York: Lange Medical Books/McGraw-Hill; 2003.*)

of primary brain injury. The risk of vasospasm is markedly less than that associated with aneurysmal SAH. In patients who present with traumatic SAH, the possibility that the patient experienced an aneurysmal SAH (which then caused the traumatic event) should be investigated.

- *Diffuse injury.* Diffuse traumatic brain injury exists on a continuum from cerebral concussion to severe diffuse axonal injury (DAI). Cerebral concussion is a transient, temporary neurologic dysfunction caused by rapid acceleration–deceleration or by a sudden blow to the head. Symptoms include headache, confusion, disorientation, and amnesia. The decision to admit a patient with concussion is made on a case-by-case basis, but these patients will not be admitted to the critical care unit unless required by other multisystem injuries. In patients with DAI, also called "shearing" injury, the initial CT scan may appear normal, show signs of diffuse cerebral edema (decreased ventricle size, loss of differentiation between gray and white matter, and loss of sulci), or show very small areas of hemorrhage (punctate hemorrhage). The clinical course and outcome are dependent upon the severity of axonal injury. Patients with DAI typically experience an immediate and prolonged loss of consciousness and display abnormal posturing.

Secondary Brain Injury

Secondary brain injury refers the ongoing neuronal damage that occurs following a TBI as the result of multiple systemic and neurologic complications. These factors do not occur in isolation. The management of severe TBI focuses on minimizing secondary injury by improving the supply of oxygenated blood to the brain and decreasing cerebral metabolic demands. Major contributors to secondary injury include the following:

- *Hypoxemia.* The brain needs a constant supply of oxygen to function, and is very sensitive to systemic insults that create hypoxemia. Causes of hypoxemia in patients with TBI include pneumonia, atelectasis, chest trauma, neurogenic pulmonary edema, airway obstruction, and pulmonary embolus. Hypoxemia results in cerebral tissue hypoxia and anaerobic metabolism. Anaerobic metabolism produces less energy than aerobic metabolism and results in a number of metabolic byproducts. These metabolic byproducts cause further cell damage. Airway management and maintaining adequate oxygenation are essential to avoid secondary injury due to hypoxemia.
- *Anemia.* Anemia causes secondary injury by decreasing oxygen delivery to the brain. Controversy exists regarding the optimal hematocrit in patients with cerebral insults. Transfusion to maintain a hematocrit of 30% or greater is common.

- *Hypoglycemia or hyperglycemia.* The brain cannot store glucose and is dependent on a constant supply to maintain metabolic function. Hypoglycemia disrupts this supply and leads to cellular dysfunction. Significant hypoglycemia is uncommon following TBI but can occur in patients with diabetes who have taken antihyperglycemic medication prior to injury. Hyperglycemia is more common and is associated with increased mortality; it is unclear whether elevated blood glucose is a marker of severity of injury or contributes to pathologic changes that increase mortality. Hyperglycemia may increase secondary injury by causing intracellular acidosis. Blood glucose monitoring and management is essential to the care of all ICU patients.
- *Increased metabolic demands.* Fever, agitation, and seizures increase metabolic demand. Fever increases intracranial pressure and can be due to an infectious process or injury to the hypothalamus. In nonintubated patients who experience seizures, hypoxemia due to loss of airway may result and also contributes to secondary injury.
- *Loss of autoregulatory mechanisms.* As discussed in Chapter 12, Neurologic System, in the section on ICP, autoregulatory mechanisms in the uninjured brain maintain constant cerebral blood flow over a wide range of cerebral perfusion pressure (CPP) (between 50 and 150 mm Hg) and within a wide range of blood pressures and ICP. When CPP decreases, cerebral vasodilation occurs to maintain CBF by increasing cerebral blood volume. When CPP increases, cerebral vasoconstriction occurs, maintaining CBF with a lower cerebral blood volume. The ability to autoregulate blood flow can be lost in the injured brain. Cerebral blood flow becomes dependent on changes in blood pressure and CPP. The extent of this autoregulatory loss varies in traumatic brain injury patients. Because of the loss of cerebral autoregulation, the injured brain is more susceptible to ischemia caused by decreased blood flow.
- *Hypotension.* Hypotension is associated with increased risk of mortality after TBI. Definitions of hypotension vary between studies. The injured brain may be more susceptible to the effects of hypotension due to changes in autoregulatory capability. Hypotension decreases cerebral blood flow, resulting in tissue ischemia and build-up of waste products. Causes of hypotension following TBI include other injuries, the administration of sedating medications, and hypovolemia due to mannitol administration. Hypotension in patients with TBI should prompt a search for bleeding from chest, abdominal, or pelvic injuries.
- *Increased intracranial pressure.* Increased ICP negatively effects cerebral perfusion and the viability

of neurons. When cerebral perfusion pressure is sustained at a low level, irreversible neuronal changes occur. The major sources of increased ICP in head injuries are cerebral edema and expanding lesions, such as hematomas. Compression of blood vessels can result in ischemia and infarction of specific areas. Cerebral edema commonly contributes to elevations in ICP after severe TBI. Edema may be localized to the site of the injury or diffuse, with maximal edema occurring 2 to 5 days after injury. ICP increases when the normal compensatory mechanisms are exhausted.

- *Hypocapnia or hypercapnia.* Hypocapnia decreases cerebral blood flow by increasing pH and causing cerebral vasoconstriction. Hypercapnia results in cerebral vasodilation and may increase cerebral blood flow, but can also increase ICP. In the absence of signs of herniation, the goal is to maintain eucapnia ($Paco_2$ between 35 and 45). Measurements of cerebral oxygenation (see section at the end of this chapter) can assist practitioners in balancing $Paco_2$ levels to maintain cerebral oxygenation without causing unacceptable increases in ICP.
- *Biochemical changes.* A number of biochemical changes occur following TBI, including the release of excitatory amino acids, free radical production, inflammation, and abnormal calcium shifts. A complete explanation of the processes underlying these changes is beyond the scope of this text. All factors contribute to changes in cellular function and eventually can cause cell death. Much research has been completed in an attempt to stop these biochemical changes and confer neuroprotection; to date, none of these trials demonstrated significant improvement in outcomes. Biochemical substances, such as lactate, excitatory amino acids, and free radicals, are present following severe TBI and cause cytotoxic edema. With focal injuries, loss of autoregulation results in a local increase in CBF. These changes increase the pressure in the capillaries and venules and alter the blood–brain barrier, resulting in the movement of fluid, plasma proteins, and electrolytes into the cerebral extracellular space, which causes vasogenic edema.

Clinical Presentation

- *External signs of injury including lacerations or signs of basilar skull fracture.* Signs of basilar skull fracture include bruising of the mastoid (Battle's sign), periorbital ecchymosis (raccoon's eyes), drainage from the nose or ears, subconjunctival hemorrhage, and cranial nerve dysfunction.

- *Level of consciousness.* A Glasgow Coma Scale (GCS) score of 13 to 15 indicates mild traumatic brain injury; 9 to 12 indicates moderate TBI; and a score of 8 or less indicates severe TBI. A decreasing GCS score indicates neurologic deterioration and warrants notification of the physician.
- *Pupillary response and shape.* Changes in pupil size, shape, or reactivity indicate neurologic deterioration and warrant physician notification. Pupillary asymmetry of 1 mm or greater, an irregularly shaped or oval pupil, and sluggishly reacting pupils are all significant signs.
- *Vital signs.* Vital signs are assessed frequently to ensure adequate perfusion to the brain. ICP and CPP are monitored for changes. As ICP rises and CBF falls, the systemic arterial blood pressure rises to maintain adequate cerebral perfusion. A change in blood pressure and heart rate without an accompanying change in the level of consciousness should prompt a search for nonneurologic causes (such as abdominal bleeding).
- *Motor function.* Hemiparesis, hemiplegia, flexor posturing, or extensor posturing can all be noted in TBI. However, a patient may be strong and purposeful with all extremities and still have a severe injury.

Diagnostic Tests

CT scanning is used to rapidly identify hematomas in need of evacuation. Other bleeding (such as into the subarachnoid space), contusions, skull fractures, and cerebral edema can be detected on CT. MRI is useful in the detection of DAI, brain stem injury, and traumatic aneurysms. The diagnostic work-up of the TBI patient includes a search for other injuries as appropriate to the mechanism of injury.

Principles of Management of Traumatic Brain Injury

The management of patients with severe TBI is focused on optimizing functional recovery by minimizing secondary brain injury. Supporting cerebral perfusion and preventing cerebral ischemia are the principal goals of treatment. Guidelines for the management of severe traumatic brain injury were developed by the Brain Trauma Foundation and the American Association of Neurological Surgeons in 1995 and 2000, and an update on CPP management was released in 2003. In addition, much research related to traumatic brain injury has been published over the last decade. General principles of management relevant to critical care nurses include the following topics.

Airway Management

Patients with a GCS score of 8 or less require intubation and mechanical ventilation. Oral intubation is recommended instead of nasal intubation. This is recommended because of the possibility of skull fractures and to decrease secondary complications such as sinusitis. Patients with TBI are treated with spine precautions until fracture can be ruled out, and require manual in-line stabilization during intubation. Endotracheal tubes and tracheostomies should be secured without causing pressure on the jugular veins; pressure decreases venous return and potentially increases ICP.

Oxygenation
Hypoxemia ($Paco_2$ less than 60 mm Hg or oxygen saturation less than 90%) is associated with a poor outcome. The $Paco_2$ levels required to maintain adequate oxygenation to the injured brain can be higher due to increased metabolic demand. Cerebral oxygenation is compromised by systemic hypoxia due to pulmonary contusion, atelectasis, pneumonia, pneumothorax and hemothorax, neurogenic pulmonary edema, and other respiratory complications.

The use of PEEP can increase ICP in some patients, but the improvement in oxygenation seen with PEEP typically outweighs any minor effect on ICP. Endotracheal suctioning is performed only when clinically indicated. Patients are preoxygenated prior to suctioning.

Ventilation
Prolonged or prophylactic hyperventilation ($Paco_2$ less than or equal to 25 mm Hg) is not recommended and contributes to cerebral ischemia by decreasing carbon dioxide levels in the blood, leading to a rise in pH and cerebral vasoconstriction. Controlled hyperventilation is used as a temporary measure to lower ICP in the setting of impending herniation while other more definitive measures are implemented. The use of devices that monitor cerebral oxygenation assists the practitioner in ventilatory management by providing information about the effects of $Paco_2$ on tissue oxygenation. For further information about cerebral oxygenation monitoring, refer to the section at the end of this chapter.

Fluid and Volume Management
The goal of fluid management is to maintain euvolemia. A central venous catheter or pulmonary artery catheter is useful in managing volume status. Hypotonic solutions are avoided because they increase cerebral edema. Glucose-containing solutions are also avoided. Historically, blood glucose was treated to maintain a level of 150 mg/dL or below. After a large-scale trial that demonstrated improved outcomes in ICU patients with strict blood glucose control, most practitioners now recommend that glucose levels be maintained in the range of 80 to 110 mg/dL.

There is no research that definitively identifies the role of colloids and blood products in the management of traumatic brain injury. Blood transfusion is often used to maintain the hematocrit at or above 30%, but this varies among practitioners. Normal saline is used initially in volume resuscitation because it is isotonic. Lactated Ringer's solution is also frequently used. Hypertonic saline (as a bolus or continuous infusion) is under investigation for use as both a resuscitation fluid and a treatment for elevated ICP. Hypertonic saline increases the serum sodium and osmolality by drawing fluid from the tissue into the intravascular space.

Managing Increased Intracranial Pressure
Treatment to decrease ICP is initiated when ICP is sustained above 20 to 25 mm Hg. Nursing measures to prevent and manage elevations in ICP are discussed in Chapter 12, Neurologic System. In addition to surgical evacuation of hematomas, operative strategies to decrease ICP include resection of severely contused tissue and craniectomy (removal of a portion of the skull to decrease ICP and allow swelling to occur). An external ventricular drain can be placed both for ICP monitoring and to permit drainage of CSF. Drainage of even small amounts (2–5 mL) of CSF may decrease ICP. Steroids do not improve the outcome following severe traumatic brain injury and are associated with secondary complications such as gastrointestinal hemorrhage and hyperglycemia.

In the Brain Trauma Foundation guidelines, the use of mannitol to decrease ICP is recommended as an option in patients with progressive deterioration in neurologic status or signs of herniation, even prior to the initiation of ICP monitoring. Mannitol is given as a bolus of 0.25 to 1 g/kg. Mannitol crystallizes easily, especially at lower temperatures, and is given through a filter. At most institutions, mannitol is held if serum osmolality exceeds 320 mOsm.

Managing Cerebral Perfusion
Hypotension (systolic BP <90 mm Hg) is associated with a poor outcome in TBI patients. Hypertension is a normal response by the body to maintain cerebral blood flow, and modest elevations in blood pressure do not increase and may even decrease ICP. Hypotension does not occur until late in the progression of herniation syndromes and prompts a search for other causes, such as blood loss from injuries to the abdomen, chest, or pelvis.

Cerebral perfusion pressure (CPP; see Chapter 12, Neurologic System) is maintained at levels of at least 60 mm Hg. Values greater than 70 mm Hg are not found to improve outcomes and may be associated with a higher incidence of acute respiratory distress syndrome. To maintain a CPP of 60, most patients will require a mean arterial pressure of at least 70 to 80 mm Hg. Brain tissue oxygen monitoring (see section at the end of this chapter) is useful in determining critical CPP values for individual patients. Once euvolemia is established, vasopressors, such as phenylephrine, norepinephrine, and dopamine, can be used to increase MAP and thus CPP. The other component of CPP is ICP, and effective management of elevated ICP will also improve cerebral perfusion.

Preventing Increased Cerebral Oxygen Demand
An anticonvulsant, usually phenytoin, is used to prevent early post-traumatic seizures during the first 7 days after injury. Continued seizure prophylaxis does not impact the development of late post-traumatic seizures and is not recom-

mended. Patients with penetrating injuries are at a higher risk for seizures than those with blunt injuries.

The results of several studies showed no benefit from the use of induced hypothermia after TBI, although additional studies are ongoing. Fever is known to be detrimental to the injured brain. Brain temperature is typically 0.5°C to 2.0° C higher than core temperature. For every 1°C increase in fever, cerebral metabolism increases by approximately 6%. Normothermia can be attained using antipyretics, cooling blankets, and intravascular cooling systems. Preventing fever decreases the demands on the brain, but increased vigilance is required to identify infectious causes. Shivering markedly increases cerebral metabolic demands and is avoided. Focal hand warming and the use of sedative medications can decrease shivering.

Agitation also increases cerebral oxygen demand and can worsen secondary injury. Strategies to avoid agitation include maintaining a calm, quiet environment and the use of sedating medications. Both analgesics (e.g., morphine or fentanyl) and sedatives (e.g., midazolam or lorazepam) are typically used. Propofol (a sedative hypnotic) is commonly used in the care of neurology patients due to its short half-life, but care must be taken to avoid hypotension and decreased CPP. Neuromuscular blocking agents can be used if sedation alone does not control ICP or in patients who are difficult to ventilate. Methods of monitoring sedation and neuromuscular blockade are discussed in Chapter 6, Pain, Sedation, and Neuromuscular Blockade.

High-Dose Barbiturates

The use of high-dose barbiturates is effective for lowering ICP, but is not proven to improve outcomes. Complications of barbiturate coma include hypotension, myocardial suppression, and pupil dilation. Patients receiving high-dose barbiturates are monitored using continuous EEG or bispectral index monitoring.

Preventing Secondary Complications

Common secondary complications include pneumonia and other infections, deep venous thrombosis (DVT), pulmonary embolism, gastric ulcers, and skin breakdown. Nutrition is started within the first 3 days after injury. Patients who are not paralyzed receive 140% of their estimated nutritional needs, while patients who are paralyzed receive 100%. DVT prophylaxis is initiated on admission with graduated compression stockings and sequential compression devices. Pharmacologic prophylaxis varies by practitioner but may include low-molecular-weight heparin or low-dose subcutaneous unfractionated heparin. Some institutions regularly screen for DVT by using Doppler ultrasound. Inferior vena cava filters are often placed in patients who develop DVT and cannot be anticoagulated.

Complications of immobility are common in patients with TBI. Progression of activity is optimized with early spine clearance. Institutional protocols vary, but typically include a series of spine x-rays, CT scanning, and potentially MRI to rule out injury to the bones and ligaments of the spine.

Coagulopathy is also a common problem following severe TBI. Coagulopathy occurs when injury to the brain tissue leads to release of tissue stores of thromboplastin, which creates a fibrinolytic state. Treatment is based on laboratory normals and physician orders.

Family Education and Support

Traumatic brain injury alters the life of the injured individual and his or her family forever. The unpredictable nature of brain injury recovery is difficult to comprehend. Family members may feel that information provided by different caregivers is inconsistent, or that insufficient information is being provided. Family members of patients with TBI also express the need to be involved in care—to be "part of the team." Critical care nurses can best support families of patients with TBI by providing direct, honest communication (including recognition of the difficulty of predicting prognosis) and by recognizing the need for their presence and involvement in care.

TRAUMATIC SPINAL CORD INJURY

Etiology, Risk Factors, and Pathophysiology

Common causes of spinal cord injury (SCI) include motor vehicle accidents, falls, acts of violence, and sports-related injuries. Over 80% of individuals with SCI are male. Two thirds of all injuries occur in people under the age of 30 years, and over 50% involve the cervical region of the spinal cord. SCI causes varying degrees of paralysis and loss of sensation below the level of injury, and impacts physical, emotional, and social function. Similar to brain injury, deficits are due to both the initial impact (primary injury) and ongoing physiologic changes (secondary injury).

The spinal column consists of stacked vertebrae joined by bony facet joints and intervertebral disks. Ligaments provide structure and support to prevent the vertebrae from moving. The ring-like structure of the stacked vertebrae creates a hollow canal through which the spinal cord runs. SCI occurs when something (e.g., bone, disk material, or foreign object) enters the spinal canal and disrupts the spinal cord or its blood supply. Mechanisms of injury include hyperflexion, hyperextension, axial loading and vertical compression, rotation, and penetrating trauma (Figure 21–6). Damage to the spinal cord can be characterized as concussion, contusion, laceration, transection, hemorrhage, or damage to the blood vessels that supply the spinal cord. Concussion causes temporary loss of function. Contusion is bruising of the spinal cord that includes bleeding into the spinal cord, subsequent edema, and possible neuronal death from compression by the edema or damage to the tissue. The extent of neurologic deficits depends on the severity of the contu-

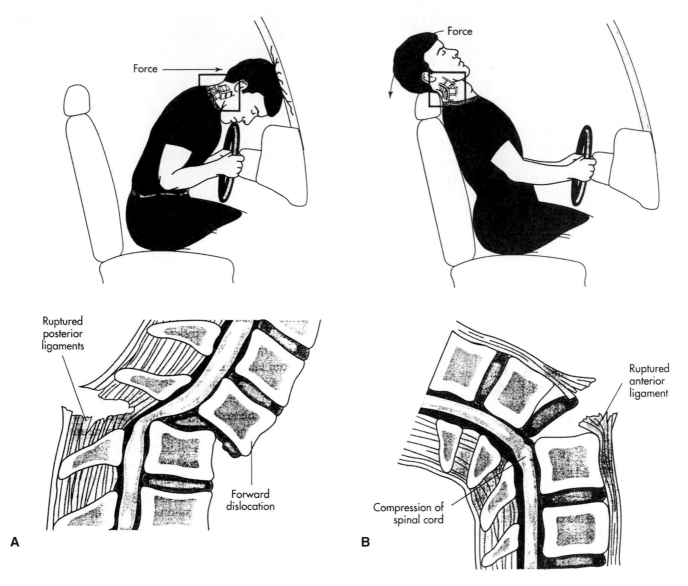

Figure 21–6. Mechanisms of spinal cord injury. **(A)** Hyperflexion. **(B)** Hyperextension. (*Reprinted from Sands JK: Spinal cord and peripheral nerve problems. In: Phipps WJ, Marek JF, Monahan FD, Neighbors M, Sands JK [eds]: Medical-Surgical Nursing: Health and Illness Perspectives, pp. 1405–1406. St. Louis, MO: Mosby; 2003*).

sion. Laceration is an actual tear in the spinal cord that results in permanent injury. Contusion, edema, and cord compression are seen with a laceration. Transection is a severing of the spinal cord resulting in complete loss of function below the level of the injury. Hemorrhage is bleeding that occurs in and around the spinal cord, resulting in edema and cord compression. Damage to the blood vessels that supply the spinal cord can result in ischemia and infarction. Regardless of the type of primary injury, secondary insults occur from cellular damage to the spinal cord, hemorrhage, vascular damage, structural changes in the gray and white matter, and subsequent biochemical responses. Blood flow to the spinal cord

is decreased significantly during the acute phase of injury, resulting in changes in metabolic function, destruction of cell membranes, and the release of free radicals. Neurogenic shock occurs following cervical and upper thoracic cord injury (at or above T6). Neurogenic shock results from the loss of sympathetic nervous system influences from the T1 to L2 area of the spinal cord, which normally increase heart rate and constricts the blood vessel walls. Loss of sympathetic outflow results in bradycardia and decreased vascular resistance. Blood pools in the peripheral vasculature, resulting in hypotension and decreased cardiac output. Neurogenic shock contributes to hypoperfusion and secondary injury.

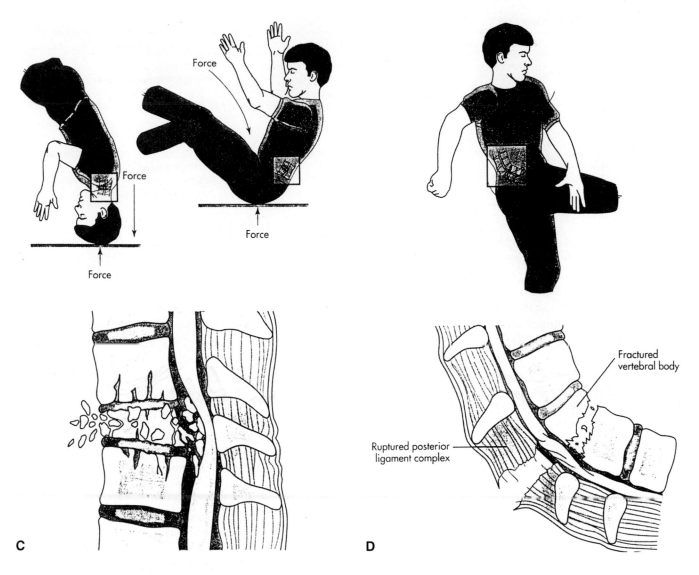

Figure 21–6. (Continued) Mechanisms of spinal cord injury. **(C)** Axial loading/vertical compression. **(D)** Rotation. (*Reprinted from Sands JK: Spinal cord and peripheral nerve problems. In: Phipps WJ, Marek JF, Monahan FD, Neighbors M, Sands JK [eds]:* Medical-Surgical Nursing: Health and Illness Perspectives, *pp. 1405–1406. St. Louis, MO: Mosby; 2003*).

Clinical Presentation

Assessment of the patient with SCI begins with evaluation of airway, breathing, and circulation, with attention to immobilization of the spine to prevent further injury. The focus then shifts to obtaining a baseline assessment of motor and sensory function. Assessment of motor function is performed at least every 4 hours during the acute postinjury period. Decreased motor function may be seen with swelling at the injury site, loss of vertebral alignment, or intrathecal hematoma formation. Changes in function warrant physician notification.

The severity of deficits caused by spinal cord injury is determined by whether the injury is complete or incomplete and the level of the spinal cord affected. Acute spinal cord injury can result in the temporary suppression of reflexes controlled by segments below the level of injury, a phenomenon referred to as "spinal shock." The completeness of SCI cannot be formally determined until spinal shock is resolved. Complete SCI results in total loss of sensory and motor function below the level of injury due to complete interruption of motor and sensory pathways. Incomplete SCI results in mixed loss of motor and sensory function because some spinal tracts remain intact. Incomplete SCI is divided into five syndromes (Table 21–2). Deficits caused by SCI relate to the level at which the injury occurs (cervical, thoracic, or lumbar). Cervical and lumbar injuries are more

TABLE 21–2. INCOMPLETE SCI SYNDROMES

Type	Mechanism of Injury	Motor Deficits	Sensory Deficits
Central cord syndrome	Hyperextension	Weakness/paralysis of upper extremities greater than lower extremities	Same as motor distribution Varying bowel and bladder dysfunction
Anterior cord syndrome	Hyperflexion	Paralysis below injury level	Loss of temperature and pain sensation below injury level
Posterior cord syndrome	Blunt or penetrating trauma	None	Loss of touch, position, and vibration sensation below injury level
Brown-Séquard's syndrome (lateral cord syndrome)	Penetrating trauma	Ipsilateral motor paralysis below injury level	Contralateral loss of pain and temperature sensation below injury level Ipsilateral loss of touch, pressure, and vibration sensation below injury level

common because these areas have the greatest flexibility and movement. A cervical injury can result in paralysis of all four extremities, or tetraplegia (previously called quadriplegia). Injuries to the thoracic and lumbar areas can result in paraplegia. The ASIA scale (Figure 21–7) frequently is used to assess and document motor and sensory function. Specific functional losses from SCI are summarized in Table 21–3.

Diagnostic Tests

- *X-rays.* Cervical, thoracic, and lumbar spine x-rays identify presence of injury. Immobilization of the spinal column must be maintained to prevent additional trauma.
- *CT scanning.* Identifies bone injury and cord compression.
- *MRI.* Detects soft tissue involvement. Useful in diagnosing ligamentous injury, which can be present without bony abnormality.

Future Spinal Cord Injury Treatment

Currently, much research is focused on SCI. The major areas of investigations include limiting the neuronal damage caused by secondary injury (neuroprotection), enhancing regrowth of neurons (nerve regeneration), and encouraging increased activity of functioning neurons (synaptic plasticity). One resource for patients and families who request information about clinical trials is a website sponsored by the National Institutes of Health, www.clinicaltrials.gov.

Principles of Management of Acute Spinal Cord Injury

As with brain injury, critical care management is based on decreasing secondary injury and preventing complications. Patients with cervical SCI are typically admitted to the intensive care unit due to the risk of neuromuscular respiratory failure.

Immobilization and Prevention of Further Injury

All trauma patients are treated as if they have a SCI until proven otherwise. This includes spinal immobilization with a hard cervical collar and backboard in the prehospital environment and a cervical collar and bed rest in the ICU until injury is ruled out or confirmed clinically and radiographically. Some mattresses (such as air mattresses) do not provide adequate stability to the spinal column; follow manufacturer and institutional guidelines. Specialty beds designed to maintain spine immobilization and provide kinetic therapy are available.

Establishing an Airway

Loss of airway protection may be related to poor cough effort, concomitant brain injury, or facial trauma. Patients can develop neuromuscular respiratory failure and require an endotracheal tube for mechanical ventilation. Intubation is performed with careful attention to maintaining spine immobilization. Techniques include the use of manual in-line stabilization with direct laryngoscopy or fiber-optic awake intubation. The neuromuscular blocking agent succinylcholine is not used if more than 24 hours have elapsed since the time of injury. Succinylcholine administration can cause massive release of skeletal muscle potassium, resulting in serum hyperkalemia and potentially cardiac arrest.

Maintaining Adequate Oxygenation and Ventilation

Altered respiratory function is a major problem for patients with high thoracic or cervical SCI. Impaired oxygenation contributes to secondary injury. Patients with complete injuries at or above the C2 level require mechanical ventilation due to the loss of diaphragmatic innervation. The diaphragm is controlled by the phrenic nerve, which exits the spinal cord at the C3 to C5 level. Patients with injuries below the level of diaphragmatic innervation will initiate breaths but still experience respiratory compromise due to paralysis of the intercostal and abdominal muscles. Paralysis of the intercostal muscles causes the chest wall to be flaccid. Contraction of the diaphragm creates a negative pressure in the thoracic cavity and the intercostal muscles retract, decreasing lung capacity. Upright positioning creates further downward displacement of the diaphragm and increases intercostal retraction; flat positioning actually can improve respiratory function in pa-

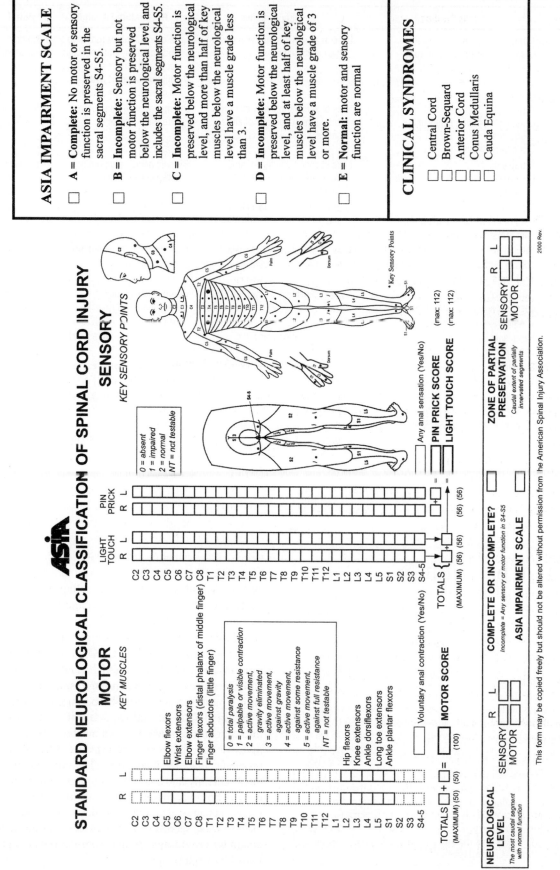

Figure 21–7. ASIA scale for the evaluation of patients with SCI. (Copyright American Spinal Injury Association, 2000, reprinted with permission.)

491

TABLE 21–3. FUNCTIONAL LOSSES FROM SCI

Level of Injury	Motor Function	Sensory Function	Respiratory Function	Bowel and Bladder
C1–C4	Tetraplegia Loss of all motor function from neck down	Loss of all sensory functions in the neck and below	Loss of involuntary (phrenic) and voluntary (intercostals) respiratory function Ventilatory support and tracheostomy necessary	No bowel or bladder control
C5	Tetraplegia Loss of all function below upper shoulders Can control head	Loss of sensation below clavicle and in most portions of arms, hands, chest, abdomen, and legs	Phrenic nerve intact but not intercostal muscles	No bowel or bladder control
C6	Tetraplegia Loss of all function below shoulders and upper arms	Loss of everything listed for C5 but greater arm and thumb sensation	Phrenic nerve intact but not intercostal muscles	No bowel or bladder control
C7	Tetraplegia Loss of motor control to portion of arms and hands	Loss of sensation below clavicle and portion of arms and hands	Phrenic nerve intact but not intercostal muscles	No bowel or bladder control
C8	Tetraplegia Loss of motor control to portion of arms and hands	Loss of sensation below chest and in portion of hands	Phrenic nerve intact but not intercostal muscles	No bowel or bladder control
T1–T6	Paraplegia Loss of everything below midchest area	Loss of sensation below midchest area	Phrenic nerve intact Some intercostal muscle impairment	No bowel or bladder control
T6–T12	Paraplegia Loss of motor control below the waist	Loss of sensation below the waist	No interference with respiratory function	No bowel or bladder control
L1–L3	Paraplegia Loss of most control of legs and pelvis	Loss of sensation to the lower abdomen and legs	No interference with respiratory function	No bowel or bladder control
L3–L4	Paraplegia Loss of motor control to portion of lower legs, ankles, and feet	Loss of sensation to portion of lower legs, feet, and ankles	No interference with respiratory function	No bowel or bladder control
L4–S5	Paraplegia Degree varies Segmental motor control of legs, ankles, and feet	Degree varies Loss of sensation to portion of legs, ankles, and feet	No interference with respiratory function	Bowel and bladder control may or may not be impaired

AT THE BEDSIDE
Acute Spinal Cord Injury

A 19-year-old college student was returning home from a party late one night when he struck another vehicle head on. He felt intense pain throughout his neck and body that was soon replaced with a burning sensation in his arms. When the paramedics arrived, he was unable to move his legs and had some gross motor movement of his arms. His heart rate was 42, blood pressure 92/50 (MAP 64), and respirations 28 and shallow. A CT scan and cervical spine x-rays revealed a C5–C6 subluxation with cord compression. His only other injury was a left wrist fracture. He was admitted to the ICU about 4 hours after the accident with methylprednisolone and dopamine infusing. He was placed in halo traction by the neurosurgeon with reduction of his subluxation, with plans for surgical fusion. Intubation was required for increasing respiratory distress and inability to clear secretions about 12 hours after ICU admission.

tients with cervical or thoracic SCI. Abdominal binders can be useful. With time, the intercostal muscles become spastic and the chest wall no longer collapses with inspiration, promoting improved ventilation and facilitating ventilator weaning.

Pulmonary function is closely monitored in patients with cervical and thoracic SCI. Ongoing assessment of maximal inspiratory pressure (MIP) and vital capacity allow early identification of impending respiratory failure. In general, a patient who is unable to generate a MIP of at least -20 cm H_2O or a vital capacity of greater than 10 to 15 mL/kg requires intubation and mechanical ventilation. Noninvasive ventilation may be considered but does not address problems related to inadequate clearance of secretions. Chest physiotherapy and assisted coughing ("quad" coughing) are used in both ventilated and nonventilated patients. In addition, a mechanical cough assist device (in-exsufflator) can be used to clear secretions. This device imitates a physiologic cough by providing a deep breath via positive pressure followed by negative pressure.

Maintaining Spinal Perfusion

Neurogenic shock causes significant hemodynamic alterations. Management focuses on the following:

- Differentiating neurogenic shock from other types of shock. SCI can mask the signs and symptoms of other trauma, including hemorrhage in the abdomen or pelvis.
- Hypotension in neurogenic shock reflects fluid displacement into the vasodilated periphery, not a true lack of fluid volume. Overhydration will not correct hypotension and can lead to pulmonary edema or congestive heart failure. Dopamine and norepinephrine are frequently used to counter the loss of sympathetic tone and to provide inotropic chronotropic support. In the 2002 guidelines for the management of cervical spinal cord injury developed by the American Association of Neurological Surgeons and the Congress of Neurological Surgeons, avoiding hypotension and maintaining a MAP of at least 85 to 90 mm Hg for the first 7 days after injury is recommended as an option with a possible benefit.
- Monitoring for bradycardia. Bradycardia can be profound, even progressing to asystole. Bradycardia occurs more frequently during suctioning; the risk can be lessened by maintaining adequate oxygenation and ventilation. Rapid position changes can cause a decrease in heart rate. Symptomatic bradycardia is treated with atropine, although some patients require a temporary pacemaker.

Administering Methylprednisolone

Although recently its use is the subject of controversy, methylprednisolone is commonly administered after SCI and may improve functional recovery. A loading dose of 30 mg/kg IV is administered over 15 minutes, and followed 45 minutes later by an infusion of 5.4 mg/kg/h. The duration of methylprednisolone therapy varies based on the length of time between injury and initiation of drug therapy. If started within 3 hours of injury, methylprednisolone therapy continues for 23 hours. If started between 3 and 8 hours of injury, the infusion is continued for 48 hours. Because the recommended dose of methylprednisolone is so large, meticulous attention to side effects is essential. All patients on methylprednisolone therapy need prophylaxis against gastrointestinal ulcers and blood glucose monitoring and control.

Fracture Reduction and Decompression of the Spinal Cord

Traction is used in unstable cervical fractures or when subluxation occurred. Traction maintains alignment and prevents movement of unstable bones and bone fragments, and also can be used to reduce fractures and dislocations. Traction devices include Gardner-Wells tongs and a halo device (see manufacturer's literature for more information). Rapid surgical intervention is required if spinal cord compression is unrelieved by traction or if the fracture is unable to be re-

duced. Immediate surgery is also required for hematomas that compromise cord function.

Spine Stabilization

Early surgical intervention to stabilize the spine is dependent on the type of injury and the patient's hemodynamic and pulmonary status. Some spine fractures can be managed without surgery by immobilizing the vertebral column and allowing the bones to heal. Immobilization is achieved with a cervical collar, halo vest, or other orthotic device. Skin care is a primary concern for these patients because skin breakdown can occur at contact points with the brace, especially in patients with decreased sensation.

Bladder and Bowel Management

Areflexia caused by spinal shock leads to urinary retention. An indwelling catheter is placed on admission and maintained until the patient is hemodynamically stable and fluid intake is consistent. Scheduled intermittent catheterizations are then initiated to decrease the incidence of infection associated with indwelling catheters. A bowel program is initiated soon after admission and typically includes daily stool softeners, glycerine or bisacodyl suppositories, and digital stimulation. For patients with injuries at or above T6, an anesthetic jelly is used to decrease the risk of autonomic hyperreflexia.

Managing Pain

Pain following spinal cord injury impacts functional recovery and can be challenging to treat. During the immediate postinjury period, many patients complain of musculoskeletal pain and neuropathic pain (described as a burning sensation, paresthesia, or hypersensitivity). Medications prescribed include opiates and muscle relaxants. Antidepressants and anticonvulsants also are useful in the treatment of neuropathic pain. Some patients benefit from nonpharmacologic methods such as massage, visual imagery, and diversional activities.

Managing Anxiety

Fear, uncertainty, and anxiety are common emotions in the ICU following SCI. The psychological and emotional trauma of SCI can be overwhelming. Sudden paralysis does not allow patients or family to prepare for this major insult. Fear focuses on the injury and life-and-death issues. Anxiety results from the ICU environment, feelings of total dependence, sensory deprivation, powerlessness, and an unknown future.

A trusting relationship must be established between the patient and the ICU staff. For patients on mechanical ventilation, communication strategies are developed based on the individual patient's abilities and needs. Use of eye contact, patience, honesty, and consistency are reassuring to the patient. Encouraging self-care within the patient's abilities decreases feelings of complete dependence. Whenever possible, the patient is allowed choices within the daily care routine. Contracting with the patient may be helpful in setting limits for some patients. The family and significant others are incorporated into the plan of care.

Preventing and Managing Complications

Respiratory complications are the most common cause of morbidity and mortality after SCI. Other complications include:

- *Gastrointestinal problems.* Paralytic ileus is common immediately following injury. An orogastric or nasogastric tube is placed initially for decompression. Nutrition (preferably enteral) is started within the first 3 days after injury. Ulcer prophylaxis is initiated on admission.
- *Skin breakdown.* The patient with SCI is at high risk for skin breakdown due to decreased blood flow to the skin and decreased cutaneous response to focal pressure.
- *Orthostatic hypotension.* Blood pools in the lower extremities due to loss of sympathetic vascular tone. Nursing strategies to decrease orthostatic hypotension include application of graduated compression stockings and elastic wraps to the legs, use of an abdominal binder, hydration, and gradual progression to an upright position.
- *Altered thermoregulation.* Individuals with SCI at or above the T6 level are unable to conserve heat by vasoconstriction or shivering. Heat loss is compromised by the inability to sweat below the level of injury.
- *Deep vein thrombosis.* Preventive strategies include the use of graduated compression stockings, pneumatic compression devices, low-dose subcutaneous unfractionated heparin, low-molecular-weight heparin, and warfarin. In the immediate postinjury period, mechanical devices frequently are used in combination with low-dose subcutaneous unfractionated heparin. Following surgery, low-molecular-weight heparin or warfarin often is started. To prevent pulmonary embolus secondary to DVT, inferior vena cava (IVC) filters can be placed in patients who are at very high risk or who cannot receive pharmacologic prophylaxis. Recently, temporary IVC filters were developed that can later be removed. DVT prophylaxis is recommended for 3 months after injury.
- *Spasticity.* During spinal shock, there is a total loss of motor function below the level of injury. Flaccid paralysis progresses to spastic paralysis as spinal shock resolves. Measures to decrease spasticity in the critical care phase include frequent range-of-motion exercises and medications. Occupational and physical therapy are consulted early in the course of hospitalization.
- *Autonomic hyperreflexia.* Autonomic hyperreflexia is a life-threatening complication that occurs in individuals with SCI at or above T6 due to unopposed sympathetic response below the level of injury. Although it usually appears in the first year following injury, it can occur anytime after spinal shock has resolved. Autonomic hyperreflexia results from a variety of stimuli, including overdistended bladder (most common), full rectum, infection, skin stimulation, pressure sores, pain, and sudden changes in environmental temperature. The stimulus causes massive vasoconstriction that clinically presents with a severe headache, hypertension, nasal congestion, shortness of breath, nausea, blurred vision, flushing and diaphoresis above the level of injury, and pallor and coolness below the level of injury. Treatment includes:
  - Move the patient into a sitting position immediately.
  - Identify and treat the underlying cause (e.g., impaction, bladder distention).
  - Monitor blood pressure and pulse closely. Pharmacologic therapies may be indicated if symptoms continue after removal of the cause. Topical nitroglycerin and hydralazine will dilate blood vessels and help reduce blood pressure. Careful attention to bowel and bladder management aids in the prevention of autonomic hyperreflexia.

BRAIN TUMORS

Etiology, Risk Factors, and Pathophysiology

The epidemiology of brain tumors varies widely based on tumor type. When all brain tumors are grouped together, the incidence is higher in men than women and peaks in the 5th to 7th decades of life. Prognosis varies based on age (younger patients have a better prognosis), tumor type and degree of differentiation, functional status at diagnosis, and anatomic tumor location. The most common brain tumors are gliomas, metastatic lesions, and meningiomas. Intracranial tumors are classified by distinguishing criteria.

Primary Versus Secondary

Primary intracranial tumors originate from the cells and structures in the brain. Secondary or metastatic intracranial tumors originate from structures outside the brain, such as primary tumors of the breast or lung.

Histologic Origins

During the early stage of embryonic development, two types of undifferentiated cells are found—the neuroblasts and the glioblasts. The neuroblasts become neurons. The glioblasts form a variety of cells that support, insulate, and metabolically assist the neurons. The glioblasts are collectively referred to as glial cells and are subdivided into astrocytes, oligodendrocytes, and ependymal cells. This is the basis of a broad category of intracranial tumors called gliomas. Gliomas are subdivided into astrocytomas, oligodendrogliomas, oligoastrocytomas (also called mixed gliomas), and ependymomas. Gliomas are graded based on histologic criteria related to the degree of differentiation from the parent cell. Higher grade tumors are more malignant. Glioblastoma multiforme refers to a tumor in which the cells are so poorly differentiated that the cells of origin cannot be identified. Glioblastoma multiforme is the most aggressive brain tumor and carries the worst prognosis.

A meningioma is a tumor that arises not from the brain itself, but from the meninges that surround the brain. Meningiomas tend to grow slowly and compress rather than invade the brain. Prognosis is excellent if the tumor is in a surgically accessible location. Neuromas (also called schwannomas) are noninvasive, slow-growing tumors that arise from the Schwann cells, which produce myelin. Pituitary adenomas, located in the pituitary gland, can be secretory or nonsecretory. Secretory tumors increase the production of hormones such as prolactin, growth hormone, adrenocorticotrophic hormone, thyrotropin, or gonadotropin. Nonsecretory pituitary tumors cause symptoms through mass effect. Pituitary tumors are treated with pharmacologic agents, surgery, radiation therapy, or a combination of these modalities.

Anatomic Location

This refers to the actual site of the tumor, such as the frontal lobe, temporal lobe, pons, or cerebellum. Knowing the location of the tumor helps in predicting deficits based on the normal functions of that anatomic area. Anatomic location also can refer to the location of the tumor in reference to the tentorium. Supratentorial refers to tumors located above the tentorium (cerebral hemispheres), and infratentorial refers to tumors located below the tentorium (brain stem and cerebellum).

Benign Versus Malignant

The distinction between benign and malignant intracranial tumors is based on histologic examination. Tumors made up of well-differentiated cells are "benign" and the prognosis is generally better than if cells are poorly differentiated. However, a histologically benign tumor can be surgically inaccessible. This "benign" tumor continues to grow and ultimately contributes to a decline in neurologic function and even death. Benign tumors may convert to more histologically malignant types as they develop.

Clinical Presentation

Brain tumors occupy space, causing compression of brain structures, infiltration of tissue that controls functions, and displacement of normal tissue. Brain tumors disrupt the blood–brain barrier and cause cerebral edema. CSF flow may be obstructed by the tumor or edema, leading to hydrocephalus. Tumors are often vascular and may bleed, causing additional neurologic deficits.

The most common initial signs and symptoms of intracranial tumors are related to elevated ICP and include headache, seizures, papilledema, and vomiting. Headache is usually progressive in severity and worse after lying flat, for example, upon awakening from sleep. Clinical presentation may also include decreased level of consciousness, pupillary changes, visual abnormalities, and personality changes. Additional signs and symptoms depend upon the area of the brain that is being compressed or infiltrated (Table 21–4).

Diagnostic Tests

CT and MRI are used to differentiate tumor from abscess and to identify tumor location and characteristics. Functional MRI detects physiologic changes using MRI scanning during physical and cognitive activity and is helpful in mapping language, sensory, and motor function. Magnetic resonance spectroscopy and positive emission tomography scans evaluate cerebral metabolism and are used to provide information about how aggressive a tumor is (a more aggressive tumor will display higher metabolic activity) and to differentiate necrosis or scarring from tumor. Ad-

TABLE 21–4. CLINICAL PRESENTATION OF BRAIN TUMORS RELATED TO LOCATION

Location	Clinical Presentation
Frontal lobe	Inappropriate behavior
	Inattentiveness
	Inability to concentrate
	Emotional lability
	Quiet but flat affect
	Expressive aphasia
	Seizures
	Headache
	Impaired memory
Parietal lobe	Hyperesthesia
	Paresthesia
	Astereognosis (inability to recognize an object by feeling it)
	Autotopagnosia (inability to locate or recognize parts of the body)
	Loss of left–right discrimination
	Agraphia (inability to write)
	Acalculia (difficulty in calculating numbers)
Temporal lobe	Psychomotor seizures
Occipital lobe	Visual loss in half of the visual field
	Seizures
Pituitary and hypothalamus region	Visual deficits
	Headache
	Hormonal dysfunction of the pituitary gland
	Water imbalance and sleep alterations in tumors of the hypothalamus
Ventricles	Symptoms of increased ICP associated with obstruction of CSF flow
Cerebellum	Ataxia
	Incoordination
	Symptoms of increased ICP associated with obstruction of CSF flow

ditional testing includes cerebral angiography, visual field and fundoscopic examination, audiometric studies, and endocrine studies. If the lesion is suspected to be metastatic, additional diagnostic tests are done in an attempt to locate the primary tumor site, if not already known. A biopsy of the lesion determines tumor type and degree of differentiation. Biopsy may be performed via a burr hole using stereotactic guidance or may be done as part of a craniotomy for tumor resection.

Principles of Management of Intracranial Tumors

Treatment modalities are used alone or in any combination. Variables considered in selecting appropriate treatment include the type of tumor, its location and size, related symptoms, and the general condition of the patient.

Corticosteroids

A corticosteroid, typically dexamethasone, is administered to decrease vasogenic cerebral edema. Steroids are started when the tumor is diagnosed and the presence of cerebral edema is noted. Significant improvements in neurologic status can be seen soon after initiation of therapy. Dexamethasone increases gastric acid secretion so prophylactic medication is usually given to prevent gastric ulcer formation (H_2 blocker or proton pump inhibitor). Side effects of steroid therapy include mood swings, fluid retention, hyperglycemia, myopathy, insomnia, and increased risk of infection.

Surgery

The goal of surgery is to resect as much of the tumor as possible with minimal or no harm to normal tissue. In most cases, a craniotomy is done to provide access for resection. Total resection is curative for some tumor types. Some tumors cannot be completely removed because of location or histologic type. A partial resection of the tumor mass temporarily relieves the symptoms of compression, and increased ICP may be relieved. Obstruction of CSF flow is treated by placement of a shunt to reroute CSF from the ventricular system to another part of the body (usually the peritoneal space) where it can be reabsorbed. Transsphenoidal resection uses a special technique to reach pituitary tumors by going through the sphenoid sinus.

Several strategies are available to decrease the morbidity associated with surgery. Intraoperative MRI is available at some centers and is most often used when the lesion is in or near the motor strip, difficult to access, or small and potentially hard to locate. Intraoperative MRI can be used alone or in conjunction with cortical mapping techniques. With cortical mapping, the patient is anesthetized for the initial part of the surgery, then awakened and asked to perform certain tasks, allowing the surgeon to avoid areas that control speech or motor function. Stereotactic techniques allow targeted resection based on previously obtained images, but do not take into account changes, such as edema, that may have occurred since the initial scan was performed.

Most patients undergo elective operations for intracranial tumors and may be admitted to the critical care unit postoperatively. Postoperative management includes monitoring neurologic status, controlling pain, and preventing and managing complications. Potential complications in the immediate postoperative period include:

- *Hematoma formation.* Clinical signs include increasing headache, decreasing level of consciousness, and the development of new focal neurologic signs (e.g., weakness of an arm or leg). If an intracranial bleed is suspected, a CT scan is obtained, and the patient is returned to the OR for surgical removal of the hematoma and management of bleeding points.
- *Cerebral edema.* Postoperative cerebral edema may occur due to the long surgical procedure and/or the retraction of brain tissue to expose the operative area. Cerebral edema is suspected if the patient presents postoperatively with greater neurologic deficits than were present preoperatively. A CT scan is obtained and treatment for increased ICP is initiated. As noted previously, dexamethasone is useful in the management of tumor-related edema.
- *Infection.* Infection can occur following surgery because of contamination in the operating room or a dural tear, which allows communication of the cerebral spinal fluid with the atmosphere. Presence of a dural tear is indicated by clear drainage on the head dressing or from the ear or nose. The drainage on the dressing appears as a "halo sign," with the center bloody or serous and the outer circle clear or yellowish. Drainage from the ear or nose can also be sent to the lab to be tested for tau transferrin, a protein present in CSF. The patient must not be suctioned nasally or allowed to blow the nose. The physician is notified immediately.
- *Thrombophlebitis.* Neurosurgical patients are at increased risk for deep vein thrombosis. Preventive measures to decrease this risk include the use of elastic compression stockings and sequential compression devices, mini-doses of unfractionated heparin or low-molecular-weight heparin, and early progression of activity.
- *Diabetes insipidus* (DI). DI is caused by a disturbance in the posterior lobe of the pituitary gland, which produces antidiuretic hormone (ADH). If ADH is not secreted in sufficient amounts, the patient will produce large volumes of dilute urine with a low specific gravity. Significant fluid and electrolyte imbalances with dehydration can result. Management includes IV therapy that correlates with urine output and administration of aqueous vasopressin or desmopressin acetate (DDAVP). The patient's hydration status, elec-

trolytes (especially sodium), and serum osmolarity are monitored closely. DI is common following surgery for pituitary tumors.

Radiation Therapy

Radiation therapy preferentially destroys tumor cells because they are rapidly dividing, but affects normal cells also. The treatment dose depends on the histologic type, radioresponsiveness, and location of the tumor, and patient tolerance. Increased edema is a common complication of radiation therapy. Patients typically remain on dexamethasone throughout treatment. Brachytherapy refers to the placement of radioactive isotopes into the tumor or resection cavity. Special techniques, such as stereotactic radiosurgery or gamma knife radiation, focus concentrated radiation from many directions on the tumor site and reduce radiation to normal tissue.

Chemotherapy

Chemotherapy is used to slow or stop the proliferation of abnormal cells. Because many chemotherapeutic agents do not cross the blood–brain barrier, alternative delivery methods are being studied. Chemotherapeutic wafers are placed in the tumor bed during surgery or a special port is placed at the tumor site.

Managing Seizures

The incidence of seizures in patients with brain tumors ranges from 20% to 60%. Antiepileptic drugs (usually phenytoin) are often given prophylactically to patients with supratentorial tumors, although this practice recently was questioned. Patients with brain tumors have an increased incidence of side effects (such as severe skin reactions) from antiepileptic drugs. Antiepileptic drugs also interact with many medications commonly prescribed for brain tumor patients, including dexamethasone and chemotherapeutic agents. When seizures do occur, they are managed according to the guidelines described in Chapter 12, Neurologic System. Any seizure in the immediate postoperative period prompts an emergent CT scan to look for hematoma formation.

Advanced Technology: Brain Tissue Oxygen Monitoring

As understanding of the pathophysiology of intracranial processes evolves, the search for improved monitoring techniques intensifies. Simply monitoring intracranial pressure and calculating cerebral perfusion pressure may not be sufficient to guide therapy. A few of the modalities currently in use include jugular venous oxygen monitoring, microdialysis catheters that sample the brain's extracellular fluid, and electrodes that measure the partial pressure of oxygen in the brain tissue. Of these strategies, brain tissue oxygen ($PbtO_2$) monitoring is the most widely used.

The concept of brain tissue oxygenation is based on the understanding of cerebral metabolism and blood flow. As discussed throughout this chapter and Chapter 12, Neuro-

logic System, the brain is dependent on a constant supply of oxygen and glucose. Anything that decreases cerebral perfusion or increases cerebral metabolic demand places brain cells at risk for hypoxia, ischemia, and eventual death. By measuring oxygen in the brain, therapies can be directed at avoiding or promptly treating tissue hypoxia. Tissue hypoxia and ischemia is due to intracranial or extracranial causes. Intracranial causes include elevated intracranial pressure, vasospasm, and seizures. Extracranial causes include anemia, hypotension, and hypoxemia. As discussed, $PaCO_2$ also impacts the diameter of blood vessels and affects oxygen delivery to the tissues.

Brain tissue oxygen monitors are most commonly placed in patients with severe traumatic brain injury or high-grade subarachnoid hemorrhage. The probe is placed into the white matter of the brain via a burr hole. The probe measures regional oxygenation in the area into which it is inserted. In TBI patients, the probe can be placed near the area of injury or on the opposite side. In patients with SAH, the probe is most commonly placed in the vascular distribution, where vasospasm is most likely to occur. Low $PbtO_2$ levels for extended periods are predictive of poor outcome and treatment is aimed at improving cerebral oxygenation. Examples of interventions include:

- Adjusting ventilation to determine the $PaCO_2$ level that achieves the desired $PbtO_2$ level without causing unacceptable increases in ICP
- Administration of blood to correct anemia
- Increasing FiO_2
- Decreasing metabolic demand (measures to avoid fever, sedation/analgesia, neuromuscular blockers, barbiturates)

The goal of therapy is early identification and treatment of conditions that increase secondary injury. While no randomized controlled trials have been published that link improved outcomes directly to $PbtO_2$ monitoring and treatment, several observational study results were reported. These studies demonstrate improved outcomes in patients with TBI following implementation of treatment protocols that include management of cerebral oxygenation. Although additional research is needed, the use of this technology appears promising.

SELECTED BIBLIOGRAPHY

Subarachnoid Hemorrhage

Cavanagh SJ, Gordon VL: Grading scales used in the management of aneurysmal subarachnoid hemorrhage: A critical review. *J Neurosci Nurs* 2002;34:288–295.

Dorsch NWC: Therapeutic approaches to vasospasm in subarachnoid hemorrhage. *Curr Opin Crit Care* 2002;8:128–133.

Hickey JV: *The Clinical Practice of Neurological and Neurosurgical Nursing,* 5th ed. Philadelphia: Lippincott Williams & Wilkins, 2003.

Hinkle JL, et al: Cerebrovascular events of the nervous system. In: Bader MK, Littlejohns LR (eds): *AANN Core Curriculum for Neuroscience Nursing,* 4th ed. St. Louis, MO: Saunders, 2004.

Janjua N, Mayer SA: Cerebral vasospasm after subarachnoid hemorrhage. *Curr Opin Crit Care* 2003;9:113–119.

Kim DH, Joseph M, Ziadi S, Nates J, Dannenbaum M, Malkoff M: Increases in cardiac output can reverse flow deficits from vasospasm independent of blood pressure: A study using xenon computed tomography measurement of cerebral blood flow. *Neurosurgery* 2003;53:1044–1052.

Lindsay KW, Bone I, Callender R: *Neurology and Neurosurgery Illustrated.* Edinburgh: Churchill Livingstone; 1997.

Lysakowski C, Walder B, Costanza MC, Tramèr MR: Transcranial Doppler versus angiography in patients with vasospasm due to a ruptured cerebral aneurysm: A systematic review. *Stroke* 2001;32:2292–2298.

Macdonald RL: Advances in vascular surgery. *Stroke* 2004;35:375–380.

Pfohman M, Criddle LM: Epidemiology of intracranial aneurysm and subarachnoid hemorrhage. *J Neurosci Nurs* 2001;33:39–41.

Solenski NJ, Haley EC, Kassell NF, et al: Medical complications of aneurysmal subarachnoid hemorrhage: A report of the multicenter, cooperative aneurysm study. *Crit Care Med* 1995;23:1007–1017.

Sommargren CE: Electrocardiographic abnormalities in patients with subarachnoid hemorrhage. *Am J Crit Care* 2002;11:48–56.

Teunissen LL, Rinkel GJE, Algra A, van Gijn J: Risk factors for subarachnoid hemorrhage: A systematic review. *Stroke* 1996;27:544–549.

Treggiari MM, Walder B, Suter PM, Romand J: Systematic review of the prevention of delayed ischemic deficits with hypertension, hypervolemia, and hemodilution therapy following subarachnoid hemorrhage. *J Neurosurg* 2003;98:978–984.

Treggiari-Venzi MM, Suter PM, Romand J: Review of medical prevention of vasospasm after aneurysmal subarachnoid hemorrhage: A problem of neurointensive care. *Neurosurgery* 2001;48:246–262.

van Gijn J, Rinkel GJE: Subarachnoid haemorrhage: Diagnosis, causes, and management. *Brain* 2001;124:249–278.

Zaroff JG, Rordorf GA, Newell JB, Ogilvy CS, Levinson JR: Cardiac outcome in patients with subarachnoid hemorrhage and electrocardiographic abnormalities. *Neurosurgery* 1999;44:34–39.

Traumatic Brain Injury

Andrews BT: Head injury management. In: Andrews BT (ed): *Intensive Care in Neurosurgery.* New York: Thieme; 2003.

Bond AE, Draeger CRL, Mandleco B, Donnelly M: Needs of family members of patients with severe traumatic brain injury: Implications for evidence-based practice. *Crit Care Nurse* 2003;23:63–72.

Bulger EM, Nathens AB, Rivara FP, Moore M, MacKenzie EJ, Jurkovich GJ: Management of severe head injury: Institutional variations in care and effect on outcome. *Crit Care Med* 2002;30:1870–1876.

Coles JP, Minhas PS, Fryer TD, et al: Effect of hyperventilation on cerebral blood flow in traumatic head injury: Clinical relevance and monitoring correlates. *Crit Care Med* 2002;30:1950–1959.

Contant CF, Valadka AB, Gopinath SP, Hannay HJ, Robertson CS: Adult respiratory distress syndrome: A complication of induced hypertension after severe head injury. *J Neurosurg* 2001;95:560–568.

Dutton RP, McCunn M: Traumatic brain injury. *Curr Opin Crit Care* 2003;9:503–509.

Elf K, Nilsson P, Enblad P: Outcome after traumatic brain injury improved by an organized secondary insult program and standardized neurointensive care. *Crit Care Med* 2002;30:2129–2134.

Huynh T, Messer M, Sing RF, Miles W, Jacobs DG, Thomason MH: Positive end-expiratory pressure alters intracranial and cerebral perfusion pressure in severe traumatic brain injury. *J Trauma Injury Infect Crit Care* 2002;53:488–493.

Iacono LA: Exploring the guidelines for the management of severe head injury. *J Neurosci Nurs* 2000;21:54–60.

Jeremitsky E, Omert L, Dunham CM, Protetch J, Rodriguez A: Harbingers of poor outcome the day after severe brain injury: Hypothermia, hypoxia, and hypoperfusion. *J Trauma Injury Infect Crit Care* 2003;54:312–319.

Littlejohns LR, Bader MK: Guidelines for the management of severe head injury: Clinical application and changes in practice. *Crit Care Nurse* 2001;21:48–65.

Lovasik D, Kerr ME, Alexander S: Traumatic brain injury research: A review of clinical studies. *Crit Care Nurs Q* 2001;23:24–41.

March K, Wellwood J, Lovasick DA, Madden L, Criddle LM, Hendrickson S: Craniocerebral trauma. In: Bader MK, Littlejohns LR (eds): *AACN Core Curriculum for Neuroscience Nursing,* 4th ed. St. Louis, MO: Saunders, 2004.

McGuire G, Crossley D, Richards J, Wong D: Effects of varying levels of positive end-expiratory pressure on intracranial pressure and cerebral perfusion pressure. *Crit Care Med* 1997;25:1059–1062.

Palmer S, Bader MK, Qureshi A, et al: The impact on outcomes in a community hospital setting of using the AANS traumatic brain injury guidelines. *J Trauma* 2001;50:657–664.

Robertson CS, Valadka AB, Hannay HJ, et al: Prevention of secondary ischemic insults after severe head injury. *Crit Care Med* 1999;27:2086–2095.

Roth P, Farls K: Pathophysiology of traumatic brain injury. *Crit Care Nurs Q* 2000;23:14–25.

Thurman DJ, Alverson C, Dunn KA, Guerrero J, Sniezek JE: Traumatic brain injury in the United States: A public health perspective. *J Head Trauma Rehab* 1999;14:602–615.

Yanko JR, Mitcho K: Acute care management of severe traumatic brain injuries. *Crit Care Nurs Q* 2001;23:1–23.

Zauner A, Daugherty WP, Bullock MR, Warner DS: Brain oxygenation and energy metabolism part I: Biological function and pathophysiology. *Neurosurgery* 2002;51:289–302.

Spinal Cord Injury

Atkinson PP, Atkinson JLD: Spinal shock. *Mayo Clin Proc* 1996;71:384–389.

Ball PA: Critical care of spinal cord injury. *Spine* 2001;26:S27–S30.

Dubendorf P: Spinal cord injury pathophysiology. *Crit Care Nurs Q* 1999;22:31–35.

Hastings RH, Marks JD: Airway management in trauma patients with potential cervical spine injuries. *Anesth Analgesia* 1991; 73:471–482.

Martyn JA, White DA, Gronert GA, Jaffe RS, Ward JM: Up-and-down regulation of skeletal muscle acetylcholine receptors: Effects of neuromuscular blockers. *Anesthesiology* 1992;76: 822–843.

Mcilvoy L, Meyer K, McQuillan KA: Traumatic spine injuries. In: Bader MK, Littlejohns LR (eds): *AANN Core Curriculum for Neuroscience Nursing,* 4th ed. St. Louis, MO: Saunders, 2004.

Prendergast V, Sullivan C: Acute spinal cord injury: nursing considerations for the first 72 hours. *Crit Care Nurs Clin North Am* 2000;12:499–508.

Singhal A, Baker A, Fehlings MG: Spinal cord injury management. In: Andrews BT (ed): *Intensive Care in Neurosurgery.* New York: Thieme; 2003.

Spinal Cord Injury: Facts and Figures at a Glance, from the National SCI Statistical Center. Retrieved March 21, 2004 from www.spinalcord.uab.edu

Stevens RD, Bhardwaj A, Kirsch JR, Mirski MA: Critical care and perioperative management in traumatic spinal cord injury. *J Neurosurg Anesthesiol* 2003;15:215–229.

Brain Tumors

Bohan E: Brain tumors. In: Barker E: *Neuroscience Nursing: A Spectrum of Care,* 2nd ed. St. Louis, MO: Mosby, 2002.

Devroom HL, Smith RK, Mogensen K, Clancey JK: Nervous system tumors. In: Bader MK, Littlejohns LR (eds): *AANN Core Curriculum for Neuroscience Nursing,* 4th ed. St. Louis, MO: Saunders, 2004.

Kanan A, Gasson B: Brain tumor resections guided by magnetic resonance imaging. *AORN J* 2003;77:583–589.

Wen PY, Marks PW: Medical management of patients with brain tumors. *Curr Opin Oncol* 2002;14:299–307.

Central Brain Tumor Registry of the United States: Fact sheet. Retrieved July 22, 2004 from http://www.cbtrus.org/2002/2002report

Advanced Technology: Brain Tissue Oxygen Monitoring

Bader MK, Littlejohns LR, March K: Brain tissue oxygen monitoring in severe brain injury, II: Implications for critical care teams and case study. *Crit Care Nurse* 2003;23:29–44.

Littlejohns LR, Bader MK, March K: Brain tissue oxygen monitoring in severe brain injury, I: Research and usefulness in critical care. *Crit Care Nurse* 2003;23:17–27.

Maloney-Wilensky E, FitzPatrick MK, Sicoutris C, et al: A multidisciplinary team approach to implementation of new clinical technology: Brain tissue oxygenation multi-modality monitoring system. *J Trauma Nurs* 2002;9:96–102.

March K, Wellwood J, Arbour R: Technology. In: Bader MK, Littlejohns LR (eds.): *AANN Core Curriculum for Neuroscience Nursing,* 4th ed. St. Louis, MO: Saunders, 2004.

Evidence-Based Guidelines

Brain Trauma Foundation: *Guidelines for the management of severe traumatic brain injury: Cerebral perfusion pressure.* 2003. Available: www2.braintrauma.org

Brain Trauma Foundation and the American Association of Neurological Surgeons, Joint Section on Neurotrauma and Critical Care: *Management and prognosis of severe traumatic brain injuries, part 1: Guidelines for the management of severe traumatic brain injury.* 2000. Available at www2.braintrauma.org

Chang BS, Lowenstein DH: Practice parameter: Antiepileptic drug prophylaxis in severe traumatic brain injury: Report of the Quality Standards Subcommittee of the American Academy of Neurology. *Neurology* 2003;60:10–16.

Glantz MJ, Cole BF, Forsyth PA, et al: Practice parameter: Anticonvulsant prophylaxis in patients with newly diagnosed brain tumors: Report of the Quality Standards Subcommittee of the American Academy of Neurology. *Neurology* 2000;54:1886–1893.

Guidelines for the Management of Acute Cervical Spine and Spinal Cord Injuries, from the American Association of Neurological Surgeons and the Congress of Neurological Surgeons. *Neurosurgery* 2002;50(Suppl).

Key Reference Information

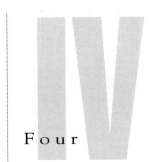

Four

IV

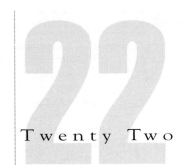

Normal Values Table

Marianne Chulay

Abbreviation	Definition	Normal Value	Formula
BSA	Body surface area	Meters squared (m^2)	Value obtained from a nomogram based on height and weight
MAP	Mean systemic arterial pressure	85–90 mm Hg	Map estimate = diastolic pressure + 1/3 pulse pressure
CVP	Central venous pressure	2–8 mm Hg	
PA	Mean pulmonary artery pressure	10–17 mm Hg	
PCWP	Mean pulmonary capillary wedge pressure	8–12 mm Hg	
CO	Cardiac output	4–6 L/min	
CI	Cardiac index	2.5–3.5 L/min/m^2	$CI\ (L/min/m^2) = \dfrac{\text{cardiac output (L/min)}}{\text{body surface area (}m^2\text{)}}$
SVR	Systemic vascular resistance	900–1200 dynes/sec/cm^5	$SVR\ (TPR)\ (dynes/sec/cm^5) = \dfrac{(MAP\ [mm\ Hg] - CVP\ [mm\ Hg]) \times 79.9}{\text{cardiac output (L/min)}}$
PVR	Pulmonary vascular resistance	120–200 dynes/sec/cm^5	$PVR = dynes/sec/cm^5) = \dfrac{(PA\ [mm\ Hg] - PCWP\ [mm\ Hg]) \times 79.9}{\text{cardiac output (L/min)}}$
HR	Heart rate	60–90 beats/min	
SV	Stroke volume	50–100 mL/beat	$SV\ (mL/beat) = \dfrac{\text{cardiac output (mL)}}{\text{heart rate}}$
SI	Stroke index	35–50 mL/m^2	$SI\ (mL/min/m^2) = \dfrac{\text{stroke volume}}{\text{body surface area}}$
RVSW	Right ventricular stroke work	51–61 g/m/m^2	$RVSW = SI \times MPAP \times 0.0144$
LVSW	Left ventricular stroke work	8–10 g/m/m^2	$LVSW = SI \times MAP \times 0.0144$
EF	Ejection fraction	70%	$\text{Ejection fraction} = \dfrac{SV}{EDV}$
EDV	End-diastolic volume	50–90 mL	
dp/dt	First time derivative of left ventricular pressure	13–14 sec	
Pa_{O_2}	Mean partial pressure of oxygen in alveolus	104 mm Hg	
Pa_{CO_2}	Partial pressure of carbon dioxide in alveolus	40 mm Hg	
Pa_{O_2}	Partial pressure of oxygen in arterial blood	Will vary with patient's age and the Fi_{O_2}. On room air: 80–95 mm Hg. On 100% O_2: 640 mm Hg	
Pa_{CO_2}	Partial pressure of carbon dioxide in arterial blood	35–45 mm Hg	
Pv_{O_2}	Partial pressure of oxygen in mixed venous blood	Will vary with the Fi_{O_2}, cardiac output, and oxygen consumption from 35–40 mm Hg	

continued

Abbreviation	Definition	Normal Value	Formula
Pv_{CO_2}	Partial pressure of carbon dioxide in mixed venous blood	41–51 mm Hg	
$P(A–a)_{O_2}$	Alveolar-arterial oxygen gradient	25–65 mm Hg at $Fio_2 = 1.0$	$P(A–a)_{O_2}$ (mm Hg) = $PA_{O_2} – Pa_{O_2}$
Sa_{O_2}	Percentage of oxyhemoglobin saturation of arterial blood	97% (air)	
Sv_{O_2}	Percentage of oxyhemoglobin saturation of mixed venous blood	75% (air)	
Ca_{O_2}	Arterial oxygen content	Will vary with hemoglobin concentration and Pa_{O_2} on air from 19–20 mL/100 mL	Ca_{O_2} (mL O_2/100 mL blood or vol %) = (Hb $\times$ 1.39) Sa_{O_2} + ($Pa_{O_2} \times 0.0031$)
Cv_{O_2}	Mixed venous oxygen content	Will vary with Ca_{O_2}, cardiac output, and O_2 consumption from 14–15 mL/100 mL	
$C(a–v)_{O_2}$	Arteriovenous oxygen content difference	4–6 mL/100 mL	$C(a–v)_{O_2}$ (mL/100 mL or vol %) = $Ca_{O_2} – Cv_{O_2}$
O_2 avail	Oxygen availability	550–650 mL/min/m^2	O_2 avail (mL/min/m^2 = CI $\times$ $Ca_{O_2} \times$ 10
O_2 ext ratio	Oxygen extraction ratio	0.25	O_2 ext ratio $= \dfrac{C(a–v)_{O_2}}{Ca_{O_2}}$
P_B	Barometric pressure		
V_{O_2}	Oxygen consumption	115–165 mL/min/m^2	O_2 ext ratio $= \dfrac{C(a–v)_{O_2}}{Ca_{O_2}}$
V_{CO_2}	Carbon dioxide production	192 mL/min	
R or RQ	Respiratory quotient	0.8	RQ $= \dfrac{V_{CO_2}}{V_{O_2}}$
FRC	Functional residual capacity	2400 mL	
VC	Vital capacity	65–75 mL/kg	
IF	Inspiratory force	75–100 cm H_2O	
EDC	Effective dynamic compliance	35–45 mL/cm H_2O women 40–50 mL/cm H_2O men	EDC (mL/cm H_2O) $= \dfrac{\text{tidal volume (mL)}}{\text{peak airway pressure (cm } H_2O)}$
V_D	Dead space	150 mL	$V_D/V_T = \dfrac{Pa_{CO_2} – P_{E}co_2}{Pa_{CO_2}}$
V_T	Tidal volume	500 mL	
V_D/V_T	Dead space to tidal volume ratio	0.25–0.40	
Qs/Qt	Right-to-left shunt (percentage of cardiac output flowing past nonventilated alveoli or the equivalent	5–8%	$Qs/Qt(\%) = \dfrac{0.0031 \times P(A–a)_{O_2}}{C(a–v)_{O_2} + (0.0031 \times P[A–a]_{O_2})} \times 100$ Valid only when arterial blood is 100% saturated
CK	Creatinine kinase	<150 mcg/L	
CK-MB	Creatinine kinase MB band	<10 ng/mL or <3% of total	
Troponin I	Troponin J	<0.4 ng/mL	
Troponin T	Troponin I	<0.1 ng/mL	

Adapted from: Hall J, Schmidt G, Wood L: Principles of critical care. New York: McGraw Hill, 1993, cover tables I–IV.

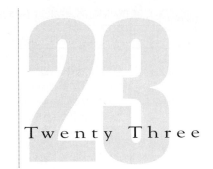

Pharmacology Tables

Twenty Three

Earnest Alexander

TABLE 23–1. INTRAVENOUS MEDICATION ADMINISTRATION GUIDELINES

Drug	Usual IV Dose Range[a]	Standard Dilution	Infusion Times/Comments/Drug Interactions
Abciximab			
Bolus dose	0.25 mg/kg	D_5W in 250 mL	Bolus infused over 10–60 min
Infusion dose	0.125 mcg/kg/min for 12 hours		Maximum infusion rate = 10 mcg/min
Acetazolamide	5 mg/kg/24h or 250 mg qd–qid	Undiluted	Infuse at 500 mg/min
Acyclovir	5 mg/kg q8h	D_5W 100 mL	Infuse over at least 60 min
Adenosine	6 mg initially, then 12 mg ×2 doses	Undiluted	Inject over 1–2 sec Drug interactions: theophylline (1); persantine (2)
Alteplase			
Acute MI	100 mg over 3 hours	100 mg in NS 200 mL	In acute MI infuse 10 mg over 2 min, then 50 mg over
PE	100 mg over 2 hours		1 hour, and then 40 mg over 2 hours.
Amikacin			
Standard dose	7.5 mg/kg q12h	D_5W 50 mL	Infuse over 30 min

Single daily dose	20 mg/kg q24h	D_5W 50 mL	Drug interactions: neuromuscular blocking agents (3)
			Therapeutic levels:
			  Peak: 20–40 mg/L; trough: <8 mg/L
			  Single daily dose: trough level at 24 hours = 0 mg/L; peak
			  levels unnecessary

Aminophylline			
Loading dose	6 mg/kg	D_5W 50 mL	Infuse loading dose over 30 min Maximum loading infusion rate 25 mg/min Aminophylline = 80% theophylline
Infusion dose		500 mg in D_5W 500 mL	Drug interactions: cimetidine, ciprofloxacin, erythromycin, clarithromycin (4)
CHF	0.3 mg/kg/h		Therapeutic levels: 10–20 mg/L
Normal	0.6 mg/kg/h		
Smoker	0.9 mg/kg/h		

Ammonium chloride	mEq Cl = Cl deficit (in mEq/L)
	  × 0.2 × wt (kg)
		100 mEq in NS 500 mL	Maximum infusion rate is 5 mL/min of a 0.2-mEq/mL solution;
			  correct 1/3 to 1/2 of Cl deficit while monitoring pH and Cl;
			  administer remainder as needed

Amphotericin B	0.5–1.5 mg/kg q24h	D_5W 250 mL	Infuse over 2–6 hours Do not mix in electrolyte solutions (e.g., saline, Ringer's lactate)
Ampicillin	0.5–3 g q4–6h	NS 100 mL	Infuse over 15–30 min
Ampicillin/sulbactam	1.5–3 g q6h	NS 100 mL	Infuse over 15–30 min
Anistreplase (APSAC)	30 units IV	SW 5 mL	Infuse over 5 min, give with aspirin 325 mg PO immediately Preparation should be discarded if not used within 6 hours

[a] Usual dose ranges are listed; refer to appropriate disease state for specific dose.

Abbreviations: bid, twice a day; CHF, congestive heart failure; conc, concentration; D_5W, destrose-5%-water; DVT, deep venous thrombosis; HPLC, high-performance liquid chromatography; IM, intramuscular; IV, intravenous; IVP, IV push; IVPB, IV piggy back; MI, myocardial infarction; NS, normal saline; NSAID, nonsteroidal anti-inflammatory drug; PCP, *Pneumocystis carinii* pneumonia; PE, pulmonary embolism; PO, orally; prn, as needed; qd, daily; SW, sterile water.

Drug interactions: (1) antagonizes adenosine effect; (2) potentiates adenosine effect; (3) potentiates effect of neuromuscular blocking agents; (4) inhibits theophylline metabolism; (5) antagonizes effect of neuromuscular blocking agents: (6) metabolism inhibited by cimetidine; (7) metabolism inhibited by ciprofloxacin; (8) increased digoxin concentrations; (9) metabolism inhibited by erythromycin; (10) increased nephrotoxicity; (11) increased heparin requirements.

TABLE 23–1. INTRAVENOUS MEDICATION ADMINISTRATION GUIDELINES (continued)

Drug	Usual IV Dose Range[a]	Standard Dilution	Infusion Times/Comments/Drug Interactions
Argatroban			
Bolus dose	350 mcg/kg	250 mg in NS 250 mL	Titrate to aPTT or ACT
Infusion dose	25 mcg/kg/min		
Atenolol	5 mg IV over 5 min, 5 mg IV 10 min later	Undiluted	Inject 1 mg/min
Atracurium			
Intubating dose	0.4–0.5 mg/kg	Undiluted	Inject over 60 sec to prevent histamine release
Maintenance dose	0.08–0.1 mg/kg	Undiluted	Inject over 60 sec to prevent histamine release
Infusion dose	5–9 mcg/kg/min	1000 mg in D_5W 150 mL	Continuous infusion. Final volume = 250 mL, conc = 4 mg/mL
			Drug interactions: aminoglycosides (3); anticonvulsants (5)
Aztreonam	0.5–2 g q6–12h	D_5W 100 mL	Infuse over 15–30 min
Bivalirudin			
Bolus dose	1 mg/kg	250 mg in D_5W 500 mL	Infuse bolus over 2 min
Infusion dose	2.5 mg/kg/h ×4 hours; if necessary 0.2 mg/kg/h for up to 20 hours		Titrate to aPTT or ACT
Bretylium			
Bolus dose	5–10 mg/kg	Undiluted	Infuse over 5–10 sec
Infusion dose	1–5 mg/min	2 g in D_5W 500 mL	Continuous infusion
Bumetanide			
Bolus dose	0.5–1 mg	Undiluted	Maximum injection rate: 1 mg/min
Infusion dose	0.08–0.3 mg/h	2.4 mg in NS 100 mL	Continuous infusion
Calcium (elemental)	100–200 mg of elemental calcium IV over 15 min followed by 100 mg/h	1000 mg in NS 1000 mL	Ca chloride 1 g = 272 mg (13.6 mEq) of elemental calcium
			Ca gluconate 1 g = 90 mg (4.65 mEq) of elemental calcium
Cefamandole	0.5–2 g q4–8h	D_5W 50 mL	Infuse over 15–30 min
Cefazolin	0.5–1 g q6–8h	D_5W 50 mL	Infuse over 15–30 min
Cefepime	1–2 g q8–12h	1–2 g in D_5W 100 mL	Infuse over 15 min
Cefmetazole	2 g q6–12h	D_5W 50 mL	Infuse over 15–30 min
Cefonicid	1–2 g q24h	D_5W 50 mL	Infuse over 15–30 min
Cefoperazone	1–2 g q12h	D_5W 50 mL	Infuse over 15–30 min
Cefotaxime	1–2 g q4–6h	D_5W 50 mL	Infuse over 15–30 min
Cefotetan	1–2 g q12h	D_5W 50 mL	Infuse over 15–30 min
Cefoxitin	1–2 g q4–6h	D_5W 50 mL	Infuse over 15–30 min
Ceftazidime	0.5–2 g q8–12h	D_5W 50 mL	Infuse over 15–30 min
Ceftizoxime	1–2 g q8–12h	D_5W 50 mL	Infuse over 15–30 min
Ceftriaxone	0.5–2 g q12–24h	D_5W 50 mL	Infuse over 15–30 min
Cefuroxime	0.75–1.5 g q8h	D_5W 50 mL	Infuse over 15–30 min
Chlorothiazide	0.5–1 g qd–bid	SW 18 mL	Inject over 3–5 min
Chlorpromazine	10–50 mg q4–6h	Dilute with NS to a final concentration of 1 mg/mL	Inject at 1 mg/min
Cimetidine			
IVPB	300 mg q6–8h	D_5W 50 mL	Infuse over 15–30 min
			IVP dose may be injected over at least 5 min
Infusion dose	37.5 mg/h	D_5W 250 mL	Continuous infusion
			Drug interactions: theophylline, warfarin, phenytoin, lidocaine, benzodiazepines (6)
Ciprofloxacin	200–400 mg q8–12h	Premix solution 2 mg/mL	Infuse over 60 min
			Drug interactions: theophylline, warfarin (7)
Cisatricurium			
Bolus dose	0.15–0.2 mg/kg	20 mg in D_5W 200 mL	Monitor TOF
Infusion dose	1–3 mcg/kg/min		
Clindamycin	150–900 mg q8h	D_5W 250 mL	Infuse over 30–60 min
Conjugated estrogens	0.6 mg/kg/d ×5 days	NS 50 mL	Infuse over 15–30 min
Cosyntropin	0.25 mg IV	Undiluted	Inject over 60 sec

(continued)

TABLE 23–1. INTRAVENOUS MEDICATION ADMINISTRATION GUIDELINES (continued)

Drug	Usual IV Dose Range[a]	Standard Dilution	Infusion Times/Comments/Drug Interactions
Cyclosporine	5–6 mg/kg q24h	D$_5$W 100 mL	Infuse over 2–6 hours Drug interactions: digoxin (8); erythromycin (9); amphotericin, NSAID (10) IV dose = 1/3 PO dose Therapeutic levels: trough: 50–150 ng/mL (whole blood—HPLC)
Dantrolene			
Bolus dose	1–2 mg/kg	SW 60 mL	Administer as rapidly as possible
Maximum dose	10 mg/kg		Do not dilute in dextrose or electrolyte-containing solutions
Maintenance dose	2.5 mg/kg q4h ×24h	SW 60 mL	Infuse over 60 min
Daptomycin	4–6 mg/kg q24h	250 or 500 mg in NS 50 mL	Infuse over 30 min
Desmopressin	0.3 mg/kg	NS 50 mL	Infuse over 15–30 min
Dexamethasone	0.5–20 mg	NS 50 mL	May give doses ≤10 mg undiluted IVP over 60 sec
Dexmedetomidine			
Bolus dose	1 mcg/kg	200 mcg in NS 50 mL	Infuse bolus over 10 min
Infusion dose	0.2–0.7 mcg/kg/h		
Diazepam	2.5–5 mg q2–4h	Undiluted	Inject 2–5 mg/min Active metabolites contribute to activity
Diazoxide	50–150 mg q5–15 min	Undiluted	Inject over 30 sec Maximum 150 mg/dose
Digoxin			
Digitalizing doco	0.25 mg q4–6h up to 1 mg	Undiluted	Inject over 3–5 min
Maintenance dose	0.125–0.25 mg q24h		Drug interactions: amiodarone, cyclosporine, quinidine, verapamil (8) Therapeutic levels: 0.5–2.0 ng/mL
Diltiazem			
Bolus dose	0.25–0.35 mg/kg	Undiluted	Inject over 2 min
Infusion dose	5–15 mg/h	125 mg in D$_5$W 100 mL	Continuous infusion (final conc = 1 mg/mL)
Diphenhydramine	25–100 mg IV q 2–4h	Undiluted	Inject over 3–5 min Competitive histamine antagonist, doses >1000 mg/24h may be required in some instances
Dobutamine	2.5–20 mcg/kg/min	500 mg in D$_5$W 250 mL	Continuous infusion
Dolasetron	1.8 mg/kg or 100 mg	Undiluted or 100 mg in D$_5$W 50 mL	Infuse undiluted drug over at least 30 sec Infuse piggyback over 15 min Administer 30 min prior to chemo or 1 hour prior to anesthesia
Dopamine			
Renal dose	<5 mcg/kg/min	400 mg in D$_5$W 250 mL	Continuous infusion
Inotrope	5–10 mcg/kg/min	400 mg in D$_5$W 250 mL	Continuous infusion
Pressor	>10 mcg/kg/min	400 mg in D$_5$W 250 mL	Continuous infusion
Doxacurium			
Intubating dose	0.025–0.08 mg/kg	Undiluted	Inject over 5–10 sec
Maintenance dose	0.005–0.01 mg/kg	Undiluted	Inject over 5–10 sec
Infusion dose	0.25 mcg/kg/min	25 mg in D$_5$W 50 mL	Continuous infusion Dose based on lean body weight Drug interactions: aminoglycosides (3); anticonvulsants (5)
Doxycycline	100–200 mg q12–24h	D$_5$W 250 mL	Infuse over 60 min
Drotrecogin alfa	24 mcg/kg/h	100 or 200 mcg/mL dilution in NS	Infuse through dedicated line or lumen (multilumen catheter). Total infusion time is 96 hours
Droperidol	0.625–10 mg q1–4h	Undiluted	Inject over 3–5 min
Enalaprilat	0.625–1.25 mg q6h	Undiluted	Inject over 5 min Initial dose for patients on diuretics is 0.625 mg
Epinephrine	1–4 mcg/min	1 mg in D$_5$W 250 mL	Continuous infusion *(continued)*

[a] Usual dose ranges are listed; refer to appropriate disease state for specific dose.

Abbreviations: bid, twice a day; CHF, congestive heart failure; conc, concentration; D$_5$W, destrose-5%-water; DVT, deep venous thrombosis; HPLC, high-performance liquid chromatography; IM, intramuscular; IV, intravenous; IVP, IV push; IVPB, IV piggy back; MI, myocardial infarction; NS, normal saline; NSAID, nonsteroidal anti-inflammatory drug; PCP, *Pneumocystis carinii* pneumonia; PE, pulmonary embolism; PO, orally; prn, as needed; qd, daily; SW, sterile water.

Drug interactions: (1) antagonizes adenosine effect; (2) potentiates adenosine effect; (3) potentiates effect of neuromuscular blocking agents; (4) inhibits theophylline metabolism; (5) antagonizes effect of neuromuscular blocking agents; (6) metabolism inhibited by cimetidine; (7) metabolism inhibited by ciprofloxacin; (8) increased digoxin concentrations; (9) metabolism inhibited by erythromycin; (10) increased nephrotoxicity; (11) increased heparin requirements.

TABLE 23–1. INTRAVENOUS MEDICATION ADMINISTRATION GUIDELINES (continued)

Drug	Usual IV Dose Range[a]	Standard Dilution	Infusion Times/Comments/Drug Interactions
Eptifibatide			
Bolus dose	180 mcg/kg	Undiluted	Maximum infusion duration of 72 hours
Infusion dose	2 mcg/kg/min until discharge or CABG		
Ertapenem	1 g q24h	1 g in NS 50 mL	Infuse over 30 min
Erythromycin	0.5–1 g q6h	NS 250 mL	Infuse over 60 min
			Drug interactions: theophylline (4); cyclosporine (9)
Erythropoietin	12.5–600 units/kg 1–3 ×per week	Undiluted	Inject over 3–5 min
Esmolol			
Bolus dose	500 mcg/kg	Undiluted	Inject over 60 sec
Infusion dose	50–400 mcg/kg/min	5 g in D_5W 500 mL	Continuous infusion
Ethacrynic acid	50 mg	D_5W 50 mL	Inject over 3–5 min
	May repeat ×1		Maximum single dose 100 mg
Etidronate	7.5 mg/kg qd ×3d	NS or D_5W 500 mL	Infuse over at least 2 hours
Famotidine	20 mg q12h	D_5W 100 mL	Infuse over 15–30 min
Fenoldopam			
Infusion dose	0.1–1.6 mcg/kg/min	20 mg in D_5W 250 mL	Titrate to BP
Fentanyl			
Bolus dose	25–75 mcg q1–2h	Undiluted	Inject over 5–10 sec
Infusion dose	50–100 mcg/h	Undiluted	Continuous infusion
Filgastrim	1–20 mcg/kg ×2–4 weeks	D_5W	Preferred route of administration is subcutaneous
Fluconazole	100–800 mg q24h	Premix solution 2 mg/mL	Maximum infusion rate 200 mg/h (IV rate is 15–30 min)
Flumazenil			
Reversal of conscious sedation	0.2 mg initially, then 0.2 mg q 60 sec to a total of 1 mg	Undiluted	Inject over 15 sec Maximum dose of 3 mg in any 1-hour period
Benzodiazepine overdose	0.2 mg initially, then 0.3 mg ×1 dose, then 0.5 mg q30sec up to a total of 3 mg	Undiluted	Inject over 30 sec Maximum dose of 3 mg in any 1-hour period
Continuous infusion	0.1–0.5 mg/h	5 mg in D_5W 1000 mL	Continuous infusion
Foscarnet			
Induction dose	60 mg/kg q8h	Undiluted	Infuse over 1 hour
Maintenance dose	90–120 mg/kg q24h	Undiluted	Infuse over 2 hours
Fosphenytoin		NS 250 mL	Infuse no faster than 150 mg/min
Status epilepticus			
Loading dose	15–20 mg/kg		
Nonemergency			
Loading dose	10–20 mg/kg		
Maintenance dose	4–6 mg/kg/d		
Furosemide			
Bolus dose	10–100 mg q1–6h	Undiluted	Maximum injection rate 40 mg/min
Infusion dose	1–15 mg/h	100 mg in NS 100 mL	Continuous infusion
Gallium nitrate	100–200 mg/m² qd ×5d	D_5W 1000 mL	Infuse over 24 hours
Ganciclovir	2.5 mg/kg q12h	D_5W 100 mL	Infuse over 1 hour
Gatifloxacin	200–400 mg q24h	200–400 mg in D_5W 200 mL	Infuse over 60 min
Gentamicin			
Loading dose	2–3 mg/kg	D_5W 50 mL	Infuse over 30 min
Maintenance dose	1.5–2.5 mg/kg q8–24h	D_5W 50 mL	Infuse over 30 min
Single daily dose	5–7 mg/kg q24h	D_5W 50 mL	Infuse over 30 min
			Critically ill patients have an increased volume of distribution requiring increased doses
			Drug interactions: neuromuscular blocking agents
			Therapeutic levels:
			Peak: 4–10 mg/L
			Trough: <2 mg/L
			Single daily dose: trough level at 24 hours = 0 mg/L; peak levels unnecessary
Glycopyrrolate	5–15 mcg/kg	Undiluted	Inject over 60 sec

(continued)

TABLE 23–1. INTRAVENOUS MEDICATION ADMINISTRATION GUIDELINES (continued)

Drug	Usual IV Dose Range[a]	Standard Dilution	Infusion Times/Comments/Drug Interactions
Granisetron	10 mcg/kg	D_5W 50 mL	Infuse over 15 min
Haloperidol (lactate)			
Bolus dose	1–10 mg q2–4h	Undiluted	Inject over 3–5 min
Infusion dose	10 mg/h	100 mg in D_5W 100 mL	Continuous infusion
			In urgent situations the dose may be doubled every 20–30 min until an effect is obtained
			Decanoate salt is only for IM administration
Heparin	10–25 units/kg/h	25,000 units in D_5W 500 mL	Drug interactions: nitroglycerin (11)
Hydralazine	10–25 mg q2–4h	Undiluted	
Hydrochloric acid	mEq = $(0.5 \times BW \times (103 - \text{serum Cl}))$	100 mEq in SW 1000 mL	Maximum infusion rate = 0.2 mEq/kg/h
Hydrocortisone	12.5–100 mg q6–12h	Undiluted	Inject over 60 sec
Hydromorphone	1–4 mg q4–6h	Undiluted	Inject over 60 sec
			Dilaudid-HP available as 10 mg/mL
Ibutilide			Infuse over 10 min
Patient >60 kg	1 mg	NS 50 mL	Repeat dose possible 10 min after completion of initial bolus
Patient <60 kg	0.01 mg/kg		
Imamrinone			
Loading dose	0.75–3 mg/kg	Undiluted	Inject over 1–2 min
			Do not mix in dextrose-containing solutions; may be injected into running dextrose infusions through a Y-connector or directly into tubing
Infusion dose	5–20 mcg/kg/min	300 mg in NS 120 mL	
Imipenem	0.5–1 g q6–8h	D_5W 100 mL	Infuse over 30–60 min
Isoproterenol	1–10 mcg/min	2 mg in D_5W 500 mL	Continuous infusion
Ketamine			
Bolus dose	1–4.5 mg/kg	Undiluted	Inject over 60 sec
Infusion dose	5–45 mcg/kg/min	200 mg in D_5W 500 mL	Continuous infusion
Labetalol			
Bolus dose	20 mg, then double q10 min (maximum total dose of 300 mg)	Undiluted	Inject over 2 min
Infusion dose	1–4 mg/min	200 mg in D_5W 160 mL	Continuous infusion
Lepirudin			
Bolus dose	0.4 mg/kg	100 mg in D_5W 50 mL	Titrated to aPTT, 12-hour expiration once compounded
Infusion dose	0.15 mg/kg/h for 2–10 days		
Levofloxacin	250–750 mg q24–48h	D_5W 50 to 150 mL	Infuse over 60 min (250 mg, 500 mg)
			Infuse over 90 min (750 mg)
Levothyroxine	25–200 mg q24h	Undiluted	Inject over 5–10 sec
			IV dose = 75% of PO dose
Lidocaine			
Bolus dose	1 mg/kg	Undiluted	Inject over 60 sec
Infusion dose	1–4 mg/min	2 g in D_5W 500 mL	Continuous infusion
			Drug interactions: cimetidine (6)
			Therapeutic levels: 1.5–5.0 mg/L
Linezolid	600 mg q12h	600 mg in D_5W 300 mL	Infuse over 30–120 min
			Linezolid may exhibit a yellow color that can intensify over time without adversely affecting potency
Lorazepam			
Bolus dose	0.5–2 mg q1–4h	Dilute 1:1 with NS before administration	Inject 2 mg/min
Infusion dose	0.06 mg/kg/h	20 mg in D_5W 250 mL	Monitor for lorazepam precipitate in solution
			Use in-line filter during continuous infusion to avoid infusing precipitate into patient *(continued)*

[a] Usual dose ranges are listed; refer to appropriate disease state for specific dose.

Abbreviations: bid, twice a day; CHF, congestive heart failure; conc, concentration; D_5W, destrose-5%-water; DVT, deep venous thrombosis; HPLC, high-performance liquid chromatography; IM, intramuscular; IV, intravenous; IVP, IV push; IVPB, IV piggy back; MI, myocardial infarction; NS, normal saline; NSAID, nonsteroidal anti-inflammatory drug; PCP, *Pneumocystis carinii* pneumonia; PE, pulmonary embolism; PO, orally; prn, as needed; qd, daily; SW, sterile water.

Drug interactions: (1) antagonizes adenosine effect; (2) potentiates adenosine effect; (3) potentiates effect of neuromuscular blocking agents; (4) inhibits theophylline metabolism; (5) antagonizes effect of neuromuscular blocking agents; (6) metabolism inhibited by cimetidine; (7) metabolism inhibited by ciprofloxacin; (8) increased digoxin concentrations; (9) metabolism inhibited by erythromycin; (10) increased nephrotoxicity; (11) increased heparin requirements.

TABLE 23–1. INTRAVENOUS MEDICATION ADMINISTRATION GUIDELINES (continued)

Drug	Usual IV Dose Range[a]	Standard Dilution	Infusion Times/Comments/Drug Interactions
Magnesium (elemental)			Magnesium 1 g = 8 mEq
Magnesium deficiency	25 mEq over 24 hours followed by 6 mEq over the next 12 hours	25 mEq in D_5W 1000 mL	Continuous infusion
Acute myocardial infarction	15–45 mEq over 24–48 hours followed by 12.5 mEq/d for 3 days	25 mEq in D_5W 1000 mL	Continuous infusion
Ventricular arrythmias	16 mEq over 1 hour followed by 40 mEq over 6 hours	40 mEq in D_5W 1000 mL	16 mEq (2 g) may be diluted in 100 mL D_5W and infused over 1 hour
Mannitol			
Diuretic		Undiluted	Inject over 30–60 min
Bolus dose	0.25–0.5 g/kg		
Maintenance dose	0.25–0.5 g/kg q4h		
Cerebral edema	1.5–2 g/kg over 30–60 min		
Meperidine	25–100 mg q2–4h	Undiluted	Inject over 60 sec Avoid in renal failure
Meropenem	0.5–2 g q8–24h	NS 50 mL or undiluted	Infuse over 15–30 min or bolus dose over 3–5 min
Methadone	5–20 mg qd	Undiluted	Inject over 3–5 min Accumulation with repetitive dosing
Methyldopate	0.25–1 g q6h	D_5W 100 mL	Infuse over 30–60 min
Methylprednisolone	10–500 mg q6h	Undiluted	Inject over 60 sec
Metoclopramide			
Small intestine intubation	10 mg ×1	Undiluted	Inject over 3–5 min
Antiemetic	2 mg/kg before chemo, then 2 mg/kg q2h ×2, then q3h ×3	D_5W 50 mL	Infuse over 15–30 min
Metoprolol	5 mg q2min ×3	Undiluted	Inject over 3–5 min
Metronidazole	500 mg q6h	Premix solution 5 mg/mL	Infuse over 30 min
Mezlocillin	3 g q4h	D_5W 100 mL	Infuse over 15–30 min
Midazolam			
Bolus dose	0.025–0.35 mg/kg q1–2h	Undiluted	Inject 0.5 mg/min
Infusion dose	0.5–5 mcg/kg/min	50 mg in D_5W 100 mL	Continuous infusion Unpredictable clearance in critically ill patients Drug interactions: cimetidine (6)
Milrinone			
Loading dose	50 mcg/kg	1 mg/mL	Infuse over 10 min Available in 5-mL syringe
Maintenance dose	0.375–0.75 mcg/kg/min	50 mg in D_5W 250 mL	Continuous infusion
Mivacurium			
Intubating dose	0.25 mg/kg	Undiluted	Inject over 60 sec
Maintenance dose	0.1 mg/kg	Undiluted	Inject over 60 sec
Infusion dose	9–10 mcg/kg/min	50 mg in D_5W 100 mL	Continuous infusion Drug interactions: aminoglycosides (3); anticonvulsants (5)
Morphine			
Bolus dose	2–10 mg	Undiluted	Inject over 60 sec
Infusion dose	2–5 mg/h	100 mg in D_5W 100 mL	Continuous infusion
Moxifloxacin	400 mg q24h	400 mg in NS 250 mL	Infuse over 60 min
Nafcillin	0.5–2 g q4–6h	D_5W 100 mL	Infuse over 30–60 min
Naloxone			
Postoperative opiate depression			
Loading dose	0.1–0.2 mg q2–3 min	Undiluted	Infuse over 60 min
Infusion dose	3–5 mcg/kg/h	2 mg in D_5W 250 mL	Continuous infusion
Opiate overdose			
Loading dose	0.4–2 mg q2–3 min	Undiluted	Infuse over 60 sec
Infusion dose	2.5–5 mcg/kg/h	2 mg in D_5W 250 mL	Continuous infusion
Neostigmine	25–75 mcg/kg	Undiluted	Inject over 60 sec

(continued)

TABLE 23–1. INTRAVENOUS MEDICATION ADMINISTRATION GUIDELINES (continued)

Drug	Usual IV Dose Range[a]	Standard Dilution	Infusion Times/Comments/Drug Interactions
Nesiritide			
Bolus dose	2 mcg/kg	1.5 mg in preservative-free	Monitor for hypotension
Infusion dose	0.01 mcg/kg/min	D_5W 250 mL	
Nitroglycerin	10–300 mcg/min	50 mg in D_5W 250 mL	Continuous infusion
			Drug interactions: heparin (11)
Nitroprusside	0.5–10 mcg/kg/min	50 mg in D_5W 250 mL	Continuous infusion
			Maintain thiocyanate <10 mg/dL
Norepinephrine	4–10 mcg/min	4 mg in D_5W 250 mL	Continuous infusion
Ofloxacin	200–400 mg q12h	D_5W 100 mL	Infuse over 60 min
Ondansetron			
Chemotherapy-induced nausea and vomiting	32 mg 30 min before chemotherapy	D_5W 50 mL	Infuse over 15–30 min
Postoperative nausea and vomiting	4 mg ×1 dose	Undiluted	Inject over 2–5 min
Oxacillin	0.5–2 g q4–6h	D_5W 100 mL	Infuse over 30 min
Pamidronate	60–90 mg ×1 dose	D_5W 1000 mL	Infuse over 24 hours
Pancuronium			
Intubating dose	0.06–0.1 mg/kg	Undiluted	Inject over 60 sec
Maintenance dose	0.01–0.015 mg/kg	Undiluted	Inject over 60 sec
Infusion dose	1 mcg/kg/min	50 mg in D_5W 250 mL	Continuous infusion
			Metabolite contributes to activity
			Drug interactions: aminoglycosides (3); anticonvulsants (5)
Penicillin G	8–24 MU divided q4h	D_5W 100 mL	Infuse over 15–30 min
Pentamidine	4 mg/kg q24h	D_5W 50 mL	Infuse over 60 min
Pentobarbital			
Bolus dose	5–10 mg/kg	NS 100 mL	Infuse over 2 hours
Infusion dose	0.5–1 mg/kg/h initially, then 0.5–4 mg/kg/h	NS 250 mL 2 g in NS 250 mL	Continuous infusion Therapeutic levels: 20–50 mg/L
Phetobarbital		NS 100 mL	Infuse over 2 hours
Bolus dose	5–10 mg/kg	NS 250 mL	Continuous infusion
Infusion dose	0.5–1 mg/kg/h initially, then 0.5–4 mg/kg/h	2 g in NS 250 mL	Therapeutic levels: 20–50 mg/L
Phentolamine			
Bolus dose	2.5–10 mg prn q 5–15 min	Undiluted	Inject over 3–5 min
Continuous infusion	1–10 mg/min	50 mg in D_5W 100 mL	Continuous infusion
Phenylephrine	20–30 mcg/min	15 mg in D_5W 250 mL	Continuous infusion; 0.5 mg over 20–30 sec
Phenytoin			Maximum infusion rate is 50 mg/min
Status epilepticus		Undiluted	Drug interactions: cimetidine; neuromuscular blocking agents
Bolus dose	15–20 mg/kg		Therapeutic levels: 10–20 mg/L
Infusion dose	5 mg/kg/d (divided into 2 or 3 doses)		
Phosphate (potassium)	0.08–0.64 mmol/kg	Function of K^+ concentration	Infuse over 6–8h 1 mmol of PO_4 = P 31 mg Solution should be made no more concentrated than 0.4 mEq/mL K^+
Piperacillin	2–4 g q4–6h	D_5W 100 mL	Infuse over 15–30 min
Piperacillin/tazobactam	3.375 g IV q6h	D_5W 100 mL	Infuse over 30 min Each 2.25-g vial contains 2 g piperacillin and 0.25 g tazobactam
Plicamycin	15–25 mcg/kg qd ×3–4d	NS 1000 mL	Infuse over 4–6 hours

(continued)

[a] Usual dose ranges are listed; refer to appropriate disease state for specific dose.

Abbreviations: bid, twice a day; CHF, congestive heart failure; conc, concentration; D_5W, destrose-5%-water; DVT, deep venous thrombosis; HPLC, high-performance liquid chromatography; IM, intramuscular; IV, intravenous; IVP, IV push; IVPB, IV piggy back; MI, myocardial infarction; NS, normal saline; NSAID, nonsteroidal anti-inflammatory drug; PCP, *Pneumocystis carinii* pneumonia; PE, pulmonary embolism; PO, orally; prn, as needed; qd, daily; SW, sterile water.

Drug interactions: (1) antagonizes adenosine effect; (2) potentiates adenosine effect; (3) potentiates effect of neuromuscular blocking agents; (4) inhibits theophylline metabolism; (5) antagonizes effect of neuromuscular blocking agents: (6) metabolism inhibited by cimetidine; (7) metabolism inhibited by ciprofloxacin; (8) increased digoxin concentrations; (9) metabolism inhibited by erythromycin; (10) increased nephrotoxicity; (11) increased heparin requirements.

TABLE 23-1. INTRAVENOUS MEDICATION ADMINISTRATION GUIDELINES (continued)

Drug	Usual IV Dose Range[a]	Standard Dilution	Infusion Times/Comments/Drug Interactions
Potassium chloride	5–40 mEq/h	40 mEq in 1000 mL (NS, D_5W, etc)	Cardiac monitoring should be used with infusion rates >20 mEq/h
Prednisolone	4–60 mg q24h	Undiluted	Inject over 60 sec
Procainamide			
Loading dose	15 mg/kg	D_5W 50 mL	Maximum infusion rate 25–50 mg/min
Infusion dose	1–4 mg/min	2 g in D_5W 500 mL	Continuous infusion
			Therapeutic levels:
			Procainamide: 4–10 mg/L
			NAPA: 10–20 mg/L
Propofol			
Bolus dose	0.25–0.5 mg/kg	Undiluted	Infuse over 1–2 min
Infusion dose	5–50 mcg/kg/min	Undiluted	Continuous infusion
Propranolol			
Bolus dose	0.5–1 mg q5–15 min	Undiluted	Infuse over 60 sec
Infusion dose	1–4 mg/h	50 mg in D_5W 500 mL	Continuous infusion
Protamine	<30 min: 1–1.5 units mg/100 units; 30–60 min: 0.5–0.75 mg/100 units; >120 min: 0.25–0.375 mg/100 units	50 mg in SW 5 mL	Inject over 3–5 min; do not exceed 50 mg in 10 min
Pyridostigmine	100–300 mcg/kg	Undiluted	Use to reverse long-acting neuromuscular blocking agents Inject over 60 sec
Quinidine gluconate	600 mg initially, then 400 mg q2h, maintenance 200–300 mg q6h	800 mg in D_5W 50 mL	Infusion rate 1 mg/min; use cardiac monitor Therapeutic levels: 1.5–5 mg/L
Quinupristin/dalfopristin	7.5 mg/kg q8–12h	D_5W 250 mL	Infuse over 60 min Central line preferred Flush with D_5W after peripheral infusion to minimize venous irritation
Ranitidine			
IVPB	50 mg q6–8h	D_5W 50 mL	Infuse over 15–30 min IVP dose should be injected over at least 5 min
Infusion dose	6.25 mg/h	150 mg in D_5W 150 mL	Continuous infusion
Reteplase	10–unit bolus ×2	SW 10 mL	Inject over 2 min, use dedicated IV line, flush heparin-coated catheters with NS D_5W after use
Rocuronium			
Intubating dose	0.45–1.2 mg/kg	Undiluted	Inject over 60 sec
Maintenance dose	0.075–0.15 mg/kg	Undiluted	Inject over 60 sec
Infusion dose	10–14 mcg/kg/min	50 mg in D_5W 100 mL	Continuous infusion
Streptokinase			
Acute MI	1.5 MU	D_5W 45 mL	Infuse over 30 min
DVT, PE	250,000 units over 30 min, then 100,000 units/h over 24–72 hours	D_5W 90 mL	Continuous infusion
Succinylcholine	0.6–2 mg/kg	Undiluted	Inject over 60 sec
Tacrolimus	50–100 mcg/kg/d	5 mg in D_5W 250 mL	
Tenecteplase	30–50 mg	SW 10 mL	Inject over 5 sec
t-PA	100 mg	100 mg in D_5W 100 mL	Infuse 60 mg/h during first hour, then 20 mg/h for 2 hours
Theophylline			Smokers: 0.9 mg/kg/h
Bolus dose	6 mg/kg	800 mg in 500 mL premixed	Nonsmokers: 0.6 mg/kg/h
Infusion dose	0.3–0.9 mg/kg/h		Liver and heart failure: 0.3 mg/kg/h
Thiamine	100 mg qd ×3	D_5W 50 mL	Infuse over 15–30 min
Thiopental	3–4 mg/kg	Undiluted	Inject over 3–5 min
Ticarcillin	3 g q3–6h	D_5W 100 mL	Infuse over 15–30 min
Ticarcillin/clavulanate	3.1 g q4–6h	D_5W 100 mL	Infuse over 15–30 min

(continued)

TABLE 23–1. INTRAVENOUS MEDICATION ADMINISTRATION GUIDELINES (continued)

Drug	Usual IV Dose Range[a]	Standard Dilution	Infusion Times/Comments/Drug Interactions
Tirofiban			
Bolus dose	0.4 mcg/kg/h	25 mg in D_5W 500 mL	Bolus infused over 30 min
Infusion dose	0.1 mcg/kg/min for 12–24 hours after angioplasty or arthrectomy		
Tobramycin			
Loading dose	2–3 mg/kg	D_5W 50 mL	Infuse over 30 min
Maintenance dose	1.5–2.5 mg/kg q8–24h	D_5W 50 mL	Infuse over 30 min
			Critically ill patients have an increased volume of distribution requiring increased doses
			Drug interactions: neuromuscular blocking agents (3)
			Therapeutic levels
			Peak: 4–10 mg/L
			Trough: <2 mg/L
Torsemide	5–20 mg qd	Undiluted	Inject over 60 sec
Trimethaphan	0.5–5 mg/min	500 mg in D_5W 500 mL	Continuous infusion
Trimethaprim-sulfamethoxazole			
Common infections	4–5 mg/kg q12h	TMP 16 mg-SMX 80 mg per D_5W 25 mL	Infuse over 60 min
PCP	5 mg/kg q6h	TMP 16 mg-SMX 80 mg per D_5W 25 mL	Infuse over 60 min
			Therapeutic levels: 100–150 mg/L
Urokinase	4400 units/kg over 10 min,	D_5W 195 mL	Continuous infusion
Pulmonary embolism	then 4400 units/h over 12 hours		
Vancomycin	1 g q12h	D_5W 250 mL	Infuse over at least 1 hour to avoid "red-man" syndrome
			Therapeutic levels
			Peak: 20–40 mg/L
			Trough: <10 mg/L
Vasopressin			
GI hemorrhage	0.2–0.3 units/min	100 units in D_5W 250 mL	Maximum infusion rate 0.9 units/min
Septic shock	0.01–0.04 units/min		
Vecuronium			
Intubating dose	0.1–0.28 mg/kg	Undiluted	Inject over 60 sec
Maintenance dose	0.01–0.015 mg/kg	Undiluted	Inject over 60 sec
Infusion dose	1 mcg/kg/min	20 mg in D_5W 100 mL	Continuous infusion
			Metabolite contributes to activity
			Drug interactions: aminoglycosides (3); anticonvulsants (5)
Verapamil			
Bolus dose	0.075–0.15 mg/kg	Undiluted	Inject over 1–2 min
			Continuous infusion
			Drug interactions: digoxin (8)

[a] Usual dose ranges are listed; refer to appropriate disease state for specific dose.

Abbreviations: bid, twice a day; CHF, congestive heart failure; conc, concentration; D_5W, destrose-5%-water; DVT, deep venous thrombosis; HPLC, high-performance liquid chromatography; IM, intramuscular; IV, intravenous; IVP, IV push; IVPB, IV piggy back; MI, myocardial infarction; NS, normal saline; NSAID, nonsteroidal anti-inflammatory drug; PCP, *Pneumocystis carinii* pneumonia; PE, pulmonary embolism; PO, orally; prn, as needed; qd, daily; SW, sterile water.

Drug interactions: (1) antagonizes adenosine effect; (2) potentiates adenosine effect; (3) potentiates effect of neuromuscular blocking agents; (4) inhibits theophylline metabolism; (5) antagonizes effect of neuromuscular blocking agents: (6) metabolism inhibited by cimetidine; (7) metabolism inhibited by ciprofloxacin; (8) increased digoxin concentrations; (9) metabolism inhibited by erythromycin; (10) increased nephrotoxicity; (11) increased heparin requirements.

TABLE 23–2. NEUROMUSCULAR BLOCKING AGENTS

Agent	Dose	Onset/Duration	Comments
Depolarizing Agents			
Succinylcholine	Intubating dose: 1–2 mg/kg	Onset: 1 min Duration: 10 min	Prolonged paralysis in pseudocholinesterase deficiencies Contraindications: Family history of malignant hyperthermia, neuromuscular disease, hyperkalemia, open eye injury, major tissue injury (burns, trauma, crush), increased intracranial pressure Side effects: bradycardia (especially in children), tachycardia, increased serum potassium concentration
Nondepolarizing Agents ***Short-Acting***			
Mivacurium	Intubating dose: 0.25 mg/kg Maintenance dose: 0.1 mg/kg Continuous infusion: 9.0–10.0 mcg/kg/min	Onset: 5 min Duration: 15–20 min Duration: 15 min	Metabolized by pseudocholinesterase Intubating dose: initial 0.15 mg/kg followed in 30 sec by .01 mg/kg
Intermediate-Acting			
Atracurium	Intubating dose: 0.5 mg/kg Maintenance dose: 0.08–0.10 mg/kg Continuous infusion: 5–9 mcg/kg/min	Onset: 2 min Duration: 30–40 min Duration: 15–25 min	Histamine release with bolus doses >0.6 mg/kg and may precipitate asthma or hypotension Elimination independent of renal hepatic function Metabolized in the plasma by Hoffman elimination and ester hydrolysis Duration not prolonged by renal or liver failure Used when succinylcholine is contraindicated or not preferred
Cisatricurium	Intubating dose: 0.15–0.2 mg/kg Maintenance dose: 0.03 mg/kg Continuous infusion: 1–3 mcg/kg/min	Onset: 2 min Duration: 30–90 min Duration: 15–30 min	Decreased histamine release compared to atracurium Elimination independent of renal or hepatic function Metabolized in the plasma by Hofman elimination and ester hydrolysis Duration not prolonged by renal or liver failure
Rocuronium	Intubating dose: 0.45–1.2 mg/kg Maintenance dose: 0.075–0.15 mg/kg Continuous infusion: 10–14 mcg/kg/min	Onset: 0.7–1.3 min Duration: 22–67 min Duration: 12–17 min	Not associated with histamine release Used when succinylcholine is contraindicated or not preferred Metabolized by liver; duration not significantly prolonged by renal failure, but prolonged in patients with liver disease No adverse cardiovascular effects
Vecuronium	Intubating dose: 0.1–0.15 mg/kg Maintenance dose: 0.01–0.15 mg/kg Continuous infusion: 1 mcg/kg/min	Onset: 2 min Duration: 30–40 min Duration: 15–25 min	Not associated with histamine release Bile is the main route of elimination Metabolized by liver; minimal reliance on renal function, although active metabolite accumulates in real failure Used when succinylcholine is contraindicated or not preferred No adverse cardiovascular effects
Long-Acting			
Doxacurium	Intubating dose: 0.025–0.8 mg/kg Maintenance dose: 0.005–0.01 mg/kg Continuous infusion: 0.25 mcg/kg/min (not generally recommended)	Onset: 4–5 min Duration: 55–160 min Duration: 35–45 min	No adverse cardiovascular effects Predominantly renally eliminated; significant accumulation in renal failure
Pancuronium	Intubating dose: 0.06–0.1 mg/kg 0.1 mg/kg Maintenance dose: 0.01–0.015 mg/kg Continuous infusion: 1 mcg/kg/min (not generally recommended)	Onset: 2–3 min Duration: 60–100 min Duration: 25–60 min	Tachycardia (vagolytic effect) Metabolized by liver; minimal reliance on renal function, although active metabolite accumulates in renal failure

TABLE 23–3. VASOACTIVE AGENTS

Agent and Dose	Receptor Specificity				Pharmacologic Effects					
	α	β_1	β_2	DM	SM	VD	VC	INT	CHT	*Comments*
Inotropes										
Dobutamine										Useful for acute management of low cardiac output
2–10 mcg/kg/min	1+	3+	2+	—	—	1+	1+	3+	1+	states; in chronic CHF intermittent infusions
>10– 20 mcg/kg/min	2+	4+	3+	—	—	2+	1+	4+	2+	palliate symptoms but do not prolong survival
Isoproterenol	—	4+	3+	—	—	3+	—	4+	4+	Used primarily for temporizing treatment of life-
2–10 mcg/kg/min										threatening bradycardia
Inamrinone										Useful for acute management of low cardiac output
Loading dose:										states; can be combined with dobutamine
0.75 mg/kg										Associated with the development of thrombo-
Maintenance dose:										cytopenia
5–15 mcg/kg/min	—	—	—	—	2+	2+	—	3+	3+	
Milrinone										Useful for acute management of low cardiac output
Loading dose:										states; can be combined with dobutamine
50 mcg/kg										
over 10 min										
Maintenance dose:										
0.375–0.75 mcg/kg/min	—	—	—	—	2+	2+	—	3+	3+	
Mixed										
Dopamine										Doses >20–30 mcg/kg/min usually produce no
2–5 mcg/kg/min	—	3+	—	4+	—	—	—	2+	1+	added response; 2 mcg/kg/min may protect
5–10 mcg/kg/min	—	4+	2+	4+	—	—	—	4+	2+	kidneys when giving other vasopressors
10–20 mcg/kg/min	3+	4+	1+	—	—	—	3+	3+	3+	
Epinephrine										Mixed vasoconstrictor/inotrope; stronger inotrope
0.01– 0.05 mcg/kg/min	1+	4+	2+	—	—	1+	1+	4+	2+	than norepinephrine; does not constrict
>0.05 mcg/kg/min	4+	3+	1+	—	—	—	3+	3+	3+	coronary or cerebral vessels; give as needed to
										maintain BP
Vasopressors										
Norepinephrine										Mixed vasoconstrictor/inotrope; useful when
2– 20 mcg/min	4+	2+	—	—	—	—	4+	1+	2+	dopamine inadequate; give as needed to
titrate to effect										maintain BP (usually ≤20 mcg/min)
Phenylephrine										Pure vasoconstrictor without direct cardiac effect;
Start at 30 mcg/min	4+	—	—	—	—	—	4+	—	—	may cause reflex bradycardia; useful when other
IV and titrate										pressors cause tachyarrhythmias; give as much
										as needed to maintain BP
Vasopressin										Pure vasoconstrictor without direct cardiac effect;
0.01–0.04 units/min	—	—	—	—	—	—	4+	—	—	may cause gut ischemia if dose is increased
										>0.04 units/min
Vasodilators										
Nitroglycerin										Tachyphylaxis, headache
20–100 mcg/min	—	—	—	—	4+	4+ A<V	—	—	1+	
Nitroprusside										Monitor thiocyanate levels if infusion duration
0.5–10 mcg/kg/min	—	—	—	—	4+	4+ A=V	—	—	1+	>48 hours; maintain thiocyanate level <10 mg/dL

Abbreviations: α_1: α_1-adrenergic; β_1: β_1-adrenergic; β_2: β_2-adrenergic; DM: dopaminergic; SM: smooth muscle; VD: vasodilator; VC: vasoconstrictor; INT: inotropic; CHT: chronotropic. Vasoconstrictors usually are given by central vein and should be used only in conjunction with adequate volume repletion. All can precipitate myocardial ischemia. All except phenylephrine can cause tachyarrhythmias.

Modified from: Gonzalez ER, Meyers DG: Assessment and management of cardiogenic shock. In Oronato JC (ed): Clinics in Emergency Medicine: Cardiovascular Emergencies, *p. 125. New York: Churchill Livingstone; 1986, with permission.*

TABLE 23–4. ANTIARRHYTHMIC AGENTS

Agents	Indications	Dosage	Comments
Class IA			
Procainamide	Ventricular ectopy; conversion of atrial fibrillation and atrial flutter; WPW	Loading dose: (IV) 15 mg/kg at 25–50 mg/min, (PO) 1 g Maintenance dose: (IV) 2–5 mg/min; (PO): 500 mg q3h or SR 500–1500 mg q6h	N-acetyl procainamide is active metabolite; lupus-like syndrome; rash; agranulocytosis; QT prolongation Therapeutic range: PA 4–10 mg/L, NAPA 10–20 mg/L
Quinidine	Ventricular ectopy; conversion of atrial fibrillation and atrial flutter; WPW	Quinidine sulfate: 200–300 mg PO q6h Quinidine sulfate: 324–648 mg PO q8h	Diarrhea, nausea, headache dizziness; hypersensitivity reactions including thrombocytopenia; hemolysis; fever hepatitis; rash QT prolongation; increased digoxin level Dosage adjustment should be made when switching from one salt to another: Quinidine sulfate (83% quinidine), gluconate (62% quinidine), polygalacturonate (60% quinidine) Therapeutic range: 2.5–5 mg/L
Disopyramide	Ventricular ectopy; conversion of atrial fibrillation and atrial flutter; WPW	100–300 mg PO q6h; SR: 100–300 mg PO q12h	Anticholinergic effects; negative inotropy; QT prolongation Therapeutic range: 2–4 mg/L
Class IB			
Lidocaine	Malignant ventricular ectopy; WPW	1.5 mg/kg IV over 2 min, then 1–4 mg/min	No benefit in atrial arrhythmias Seizures; paresthesias; delirium; levels increased by cimetidine; minimal hemodynamic effects Therapeutic range: 1.5–5 mg/L
Mexiletine	Malignant ventricular ectopy	150–300 mg PO q6–8h with food	No benefit in atrial arrhythmias Less effective than IA and IC agents Nausea; tremor; dizziness; delirium; levels increased by cimetidine Therapeutic range: 0.5–2 mg/L
Tocainide	Malignant ventricular ectopy	200–600 mg PO q8h with food	No benefit in atrial arrhythmias Less effective than IA and IC agents Nausea; tremor; dizziness; delirium; agranulocytosis; pneumonitis; minimal hemodynamic effects Therapeutic range: 4–10 mg/L
Class IC			
Flecainide	Life-threatening ventricular arrhythmias refractory to other agents Prevention of symptomatic, disabling, paroxysmal supraventricular arrhythmias, including atrial fibrillation or flutter and WPW in patients without structural heart disease	100–200 mg PO q12h	Proarrhythmic effects; moderate negative inotropy; dizziness; conduction abnormalities Therapeutic range: 0.2–1 mg/L
Propafenone	Life-threatening ventricular arrythmias refractory to other agents SVT, WPW, and paroxysmal atrial fibrillation or flutter in patients without structural heart disease	150–300 mg PO q8h	Proarrhythmic effects; negative inotropy; dizziness; nausea; conduction abnormalities
Class IB/IC (hybrid electrophysiologic effects)			
Moricizine	Life-threatening ventricular arrythmias refractory to other agents	100–300 mg PO q8h	Proarrhythmic effects; dizziness; nausea; headache

(continued)

TABLE 23–4. ANTIARRHYTMIC AGENTS (continued)

Agents	Indications	Dosage	Comments
Class II (beta-blocking agents)			
Propranolol	Slowing ventricular rate in atrial fibrillation, atrial flutter, and SVT; suppression of PVCs	Up to 0.5–1 mg IV, then 1–4 mg/hour (or 10–100 mg PO q6h)	Not cardioselective; hypotension; bronchospasm; negative inotropy
Esmolol	Slowing ventricular rate in atrial fibrillation, atrial flutter, SVT, and MAT	Loading dose: 500 mcg/over 1 min Maintenance dose: 50 mcg/kg/min; rebolus and increase q5min by 50 mcg/kg/min to maximum of 400	Cardioselective at low doses; hypotension; negative inotropy; very short half-life
Metoprolol	Slowing ventricular rate in atrial fibrillation, atrial flutter, SVT, and MAT	Initial IV dose: 5 mg q5min up to 15 mg, then 25–100 mg PO q8–12h	Cardioselective at low doses; hypotension; negative inotropy
Class III			
Amiodarone	Life-threatening ventricular arrhythmias, supraventricular arrhythmias, including WPW refractory to other agents	800–1600 mg PO qd for 1–3 weeks, then 600–800 mg PO qd for 4 weeks, then 100–400 mg PO qd	Half-life >50 days; pulmonary fibrosis; corneal microdeposits; hypo/hyperthyroidism; bluish skin; hepatitis; photosensitivity; conduction abnormalities; mild negative inotropy; increased effect of coumadin; increased digoxin level Therapeutic range: 1–2.5 mg/L
Bretylium	Refractory ventricular tachycardia and ventricular fibrillation	5–10 mg/kg IV boluses q10min up to 30 mg/kg, then 0.5–2 mg/min	Initial hypertension, then postural hypotension; nausea and vomiting; parotitis; catecholamine sensitivity
Sotalol	Life-threatening ventricular arrythmias	80–160 mg PO q12h; may increase up to 160 mg PO q8h	Beta-blocker with class III properties; proarrhythmic effects; QT prolongation
Dofetilide	Conversion of atrial fibrillation	250–500 mcg orally twice a day	Dose adjusted based on QTc interval and creatinine clearance
Class IV (calcium channel antagonists)			
Verapamil	Conversion of SVT; slowing ventricular rate in atrial fibrillation, atrial flutter, and MAT	IV bolus: 5–10 mg over 2–3 min (repeat in 30 min prn), continuous infusion: 2.5–5 mcg/kg/min PO: 40–160 mg PO q8h	Hypotension; negative inotropy; conduction disturbances; increased digoxin level; generally contraindicated in WPW
Diltiazem	Conversion of SVT; slowing ventricular rate in atrial fibrillation, atrial flutter, and MAT	IV bolus: 0.25 mg/kg over 2 min (repeat in 15 min prn with 0.35 mg/kg IV); Maintenance infusion: 5–15 mg/h PO: 30–90 mg PO q6h	Hypotension; less negative inotropy than verapamil; conduction disturbances; rare hepatic injury; generally contraindicated in WPW
Miscellaneous agents			
Adenosine	Conversion of SVT, including WPW	6-mg rapid IV bolus; if ineffective, 12-mg rapid IV bolus 2 min later; follow bolus with fast flush; use smaller doses if giving through central venous line	Flushing; dyspnea; nodal blocking effect increased by dipyridamole and decreased by theophylline and caffeine; very short half-life ($\approx$10 sec)
Atropine	Initial therapy for symptomatic bradycardia	0.5-mg IV bolus; repeat q5 min prn to total of 2 mg IV	May induce tachycardia and ischemia
Digitalis	Slowing AV conduction in atrial fibrillation and atrial flutter	Loading dose: 0.5 mg IV, then 0.25 mg IV q4–6h up to 1 mg; Maintenance dose: 0.125–0.375 mg PO/IV qd	Heart block; arrhythmias; nausea; yellow vision; numerous drug interactions, generally contraindicated in WPW Therapeutic range: 0.5–2.0 mg/mL

Abbreviations: AV, atrioventricular; MAT, multifocal atrial tachycardia; SR: sustained release; SVT, supraventricular tachycardia; WPW, Wolff-Parkinson-White.

TABLE 23–5. THERAPEUTIC DRUG MONITORING

Drug	Usual Therapeutic Range	Usual Sampling Time
Antibiotics		
Amikacin	Peak: 20–40 mg/L Trough: <10 mg/L Single daily dose: 0 mg/L at 24 h	Peak: 30–60 min after a 30-min infusion Trough: just before next dose Single daily dose: trough level just before next dose
Chloramphenicol	Peak: 10–25 mg/L Trough: 5–10 mg/L	Peak: 30–90 min after a 30-min infusion Trough: just before the next dose
Flucytosine	Peak: 50–100 mg/L Trough: <25 mg/L	Peak: 1–2 hours after an oral dose Trough: just before the next dose
Gentamicin	Peak: 4–10 mg/L Trough: <2 mg/L Single daily dose: 0 mg/L at 24 h	Peak: 30–60 min after a 30-min infusion Trough: just before the next dose Single daily dose: trough level just before next dose
Tobramycin	Peak: 4–10 mg/L Trough: <2 mg/L	Peak: 30–60 min after a 30-min infusion Trough: just before the next dose
Netilmicin	Peak: 4–10 mg/L Trough: <2 mg/L Single daily dose: 0 mg/L at 24 h	Peak: 30–60 min after a 30-min infusion Trough: just before the next dose Single daily dose: trough level just before next dose
Vancomycin	Peak: 20–40 mg/L Trough: <10 mg/L	Peak: 1 hour after end of a 1-hour infusion Trough: just before the next dose
Sulfonamides (sulfamethoxazole, sulfadiazine, cotrimoxazole)	Peak: 100–150 mg/L	Peak: 2 hours after 1-hour infusion Trough: not applicable
Antiarrhythmics		
Amiodarone	0.5–2 mg/L	Trough: just before next dose
Digoxin	0.5–2 mcg/L	Peak: 8–12 hours after administered dose Trough: just before next dose
Disopyramide	2–4 mg/L	Trough: just before next dose
Flecainide	0.2–1.0 mg/L	Trough: just before next dose
Lidocaine	1.5–5 mg/L	Anytime during a continuous infusion
Mexiletine	0.5–2 mg/L	Trough: just before next dose
Procainamide/NAPA	Procainamide: 4–10 mg/L NAPA: 10–20 mg/L	IV: immediately after IV loading dose: anytime during continuous infusion PO: trough: just before next dose
Quinidine	2.5–5 mg/L	Trough: just before next dose
Tocainide	4–10 mg/L	Trough: just before next dose
Anticonvulsants		
Carbamazepine	4–12 mg/L	Trough: just before next dose
Pentobarbital	20–50 mcg/L	IV: immediately after IV loading dose: anytime during continuous infusion
Phenobarbital	15–40 mg/L	Trough: just before next dose
Phenytoin	10–20 mg/L	IV: 2–4 hours after dose Trough: PO/IV: just before next dose Free phenytoin level: 1–2 mg/L
Valproic acid	50–100 mg/L	Trough: just before next dose
Bronchodilators		
Theophylline	10–20 mg/L	IV: prior to IV bolus dose, 30 min after end of bolus dose, anytime during continuous infusion PO: peak: 2 hours after rapid-release product, 4 hours after sustained-release product Trough: just before next dose
Miscellaneous		
Cyclosporine	50–150 ng/mL (whole blood, HPLC)	Trough: IV, PO: just before next dose

Advanced Cardiac Life Support Algorithms

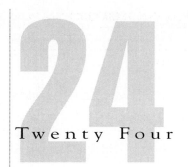

Twenty Four

Marianne Chulay

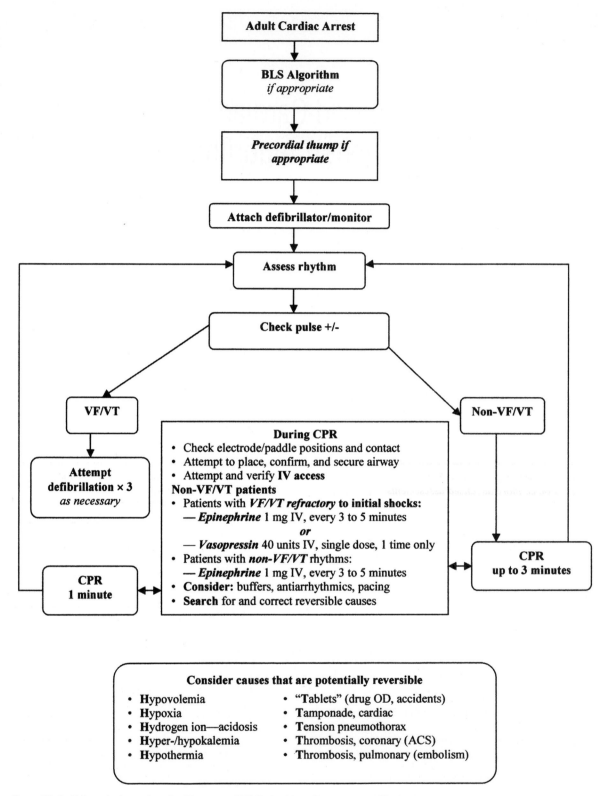

Figure 24–1. Universal advanced cardiac life support (ACLS) algorithm. *Abbreviations:* ACS, acute coronary syndrome; BLS, basic life support, CPR, cardiopulmonary resuscitation; OD, overdose; VF, ventricular fibrillation; VT, ventricular tachycardia. (*Reproduced with permission from the* Handbook of Emergency Care for Healthcare Providers, ©2004, American Heart Association, page 6.)

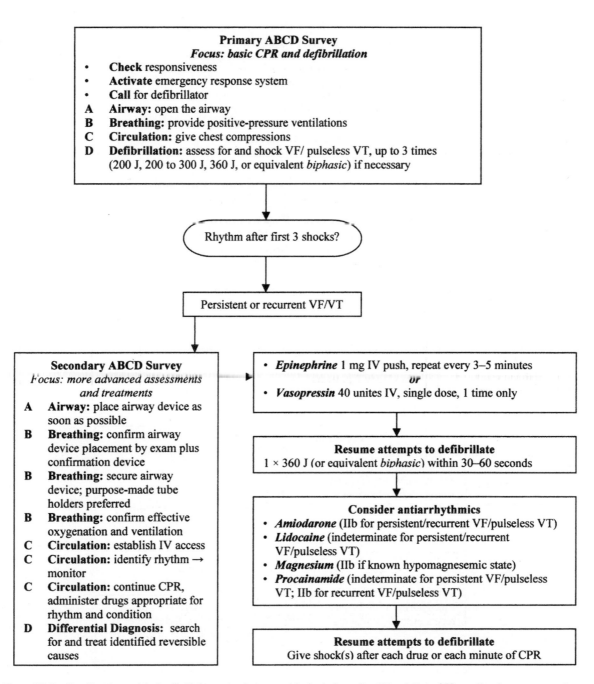

Figure 24–2. Algorithm for ventricular fibrillation and pulseless ventricular tachycardia. *Abbreviations:* CPR, cardiopulmonary resuscitation; VF, ventricular fibrillation; VT, ventricular tachycardia. (*Reproduced with permission from the* Handbook of Emergency Care for Healthcare Providers, *©2004, American Heart Association, page 8.*)

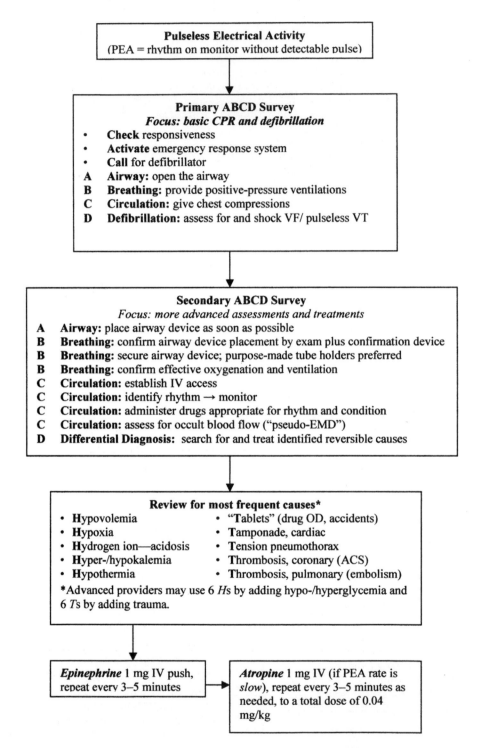

Figure 24–3. Algorithm for pulseless electrical activity (PEA) (electromechanical dissociation [EMD]). *Abbreviations:* ACS, acute coronary syndrome; CPR, cardiopulmonary resuscitation; OD, overdose; VF, ventricular fibrillation; VT, ventricular tachycardia. (*Reproduced with permission from the* Handbook of Emergency Care for Healthcare Providers, ©2004, American Heart Association, page 10.)

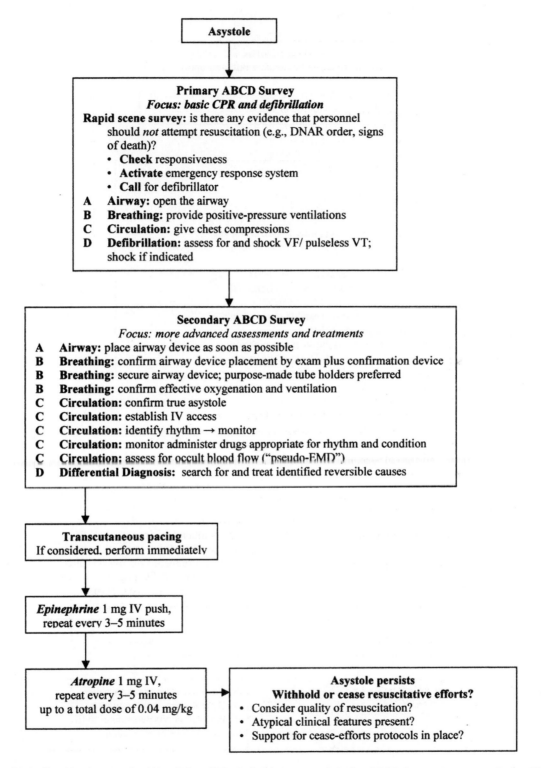

Figure 24–4. Algorithm for asystole. *Abbreviations:* CPR, cardiopulmonary resuscitation; DNAR, do not attempt resuscitation; EMD, electromechanical dissociation; VF, ventricular fibrillation; VT, ventricular tachycardia. (*Reproduced with permission from the* Handbook of Emergency Care for Healthcare Providers, ©*2004, American Heart Association, page 11.*)

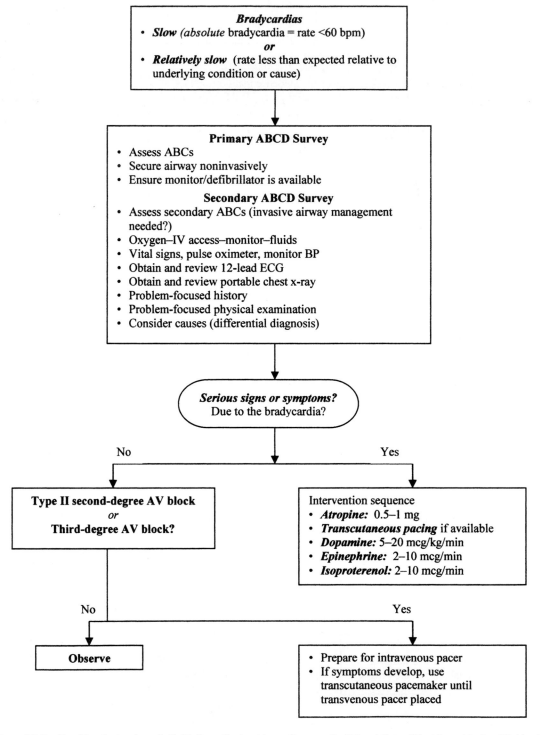

Figure 24–5. Algorithm for bradycardia (with the patient not in cardiac arrest). *Abbreviations:* AV, atrioventricular; BP, blood pressure. (*Reproduced with permission from the* Handbook of Emergency Care for Healthcare Providers, ©*2004, American Heart Association, page 12.*)

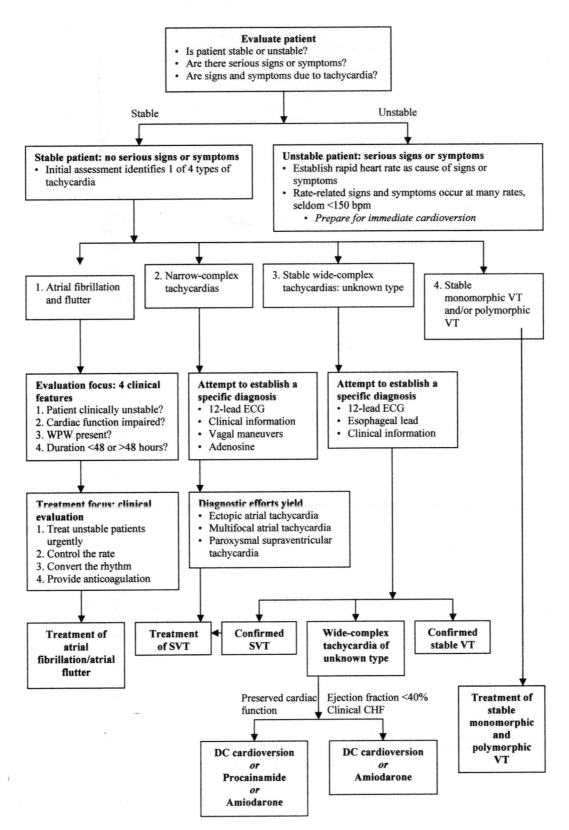

Figure 24–6. Algorithm for tachycardia—overview. *Abbreviations:* CHF, congestive heart failure; PSVT, paroxysmal supraventricular tachycardia; SVT, supraventricular tachycardia; VF, ventricular fibrillation; VT, ventricular tachycardia; WPW, Wolff-Parkinson-White syndrome. (*Reproduced with permission from the* Handbook of Emergency Care for Healthcare Providers, ©*2004, American Heart Association, page 13.*)

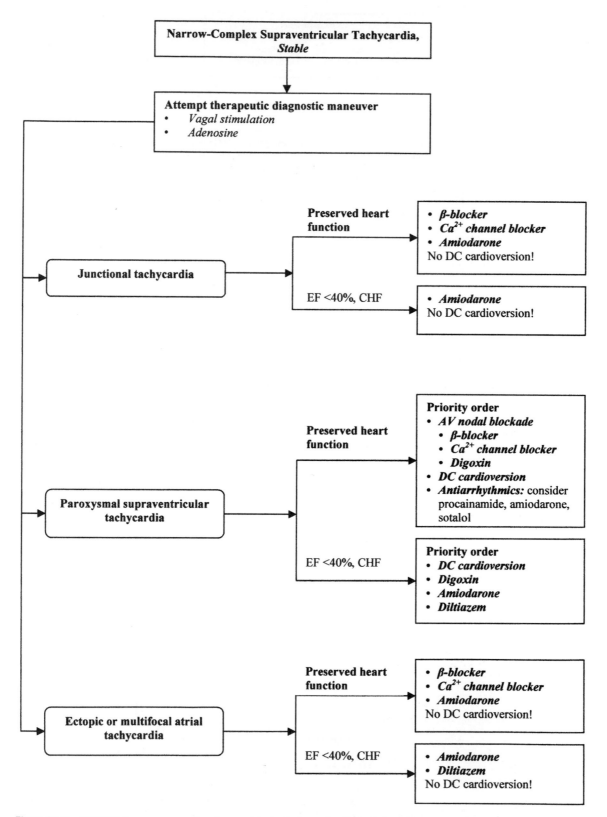

Figure 24–7. Algorithm for narrow-complex supraventricular tachycardia. *Abbreviations:* AV, atrioventricular; CHF, congestive heart failure; EF, ejection fraction. (*Reproduced with permission from the* Handbook of Emergency Care for Healthcare Providers, ©*2004, American Heart Association, page 16.*)

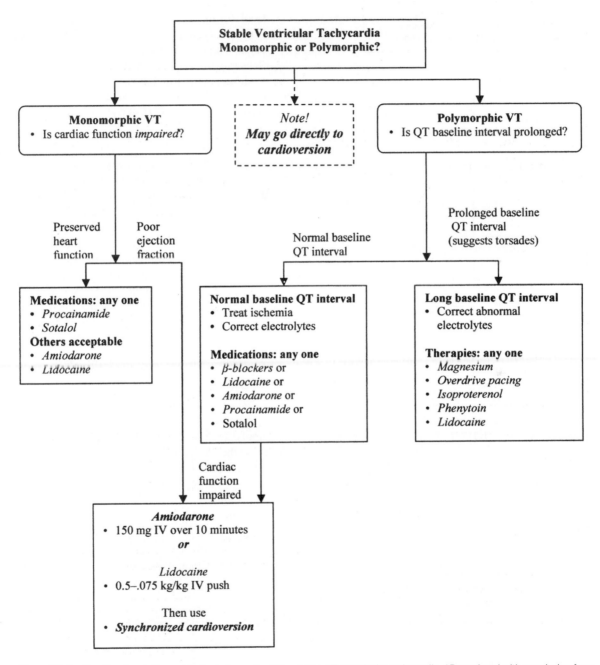

Figure 24–8. Algorithm for stable ventricular tachycardia. *Abbreviation:* VT, ventricular tachycardia. (*Reproduced with permission from the* Handbook of Emergency Care for Healthcare Providers, *©2004, American Heart Association, page 17.*)

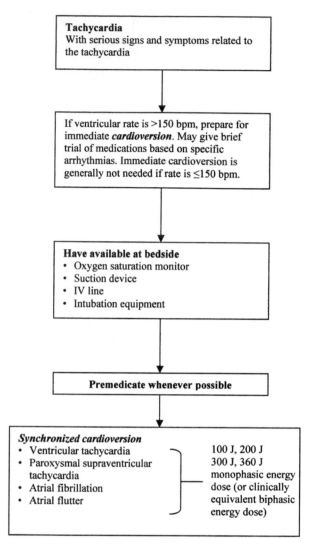

Tachycardia
With serious signs and symptoms related to the tachycardia

If ventricular rate is >150 bpm, prepare for immediate *cardioversion*. May give brief trial of medications based on specific arrhythmias. Immediate cardioversion is generally not needed if rate is ≤150 bpm.

Have available at bedside
• Oxygen saturation monitor
• Suction device
• IV line
• Intubation equipment

Premedicate whenever possible

Synchronized cardioversion
• Ventricular tachycardia
• Paroxysmal supraventricular tachycardia
• Atrial fibrillation
• Atrial flutter

100 J, 200 J 300 J, 360 J monophasic energy dose (or clinically equivalent biphasic energy dose)

Figure 24–9. Algorithm for Synchronized Electrical Cardioversion (with the Patient Not in Cardiac Arrest). [a]Effective regimens have included a sedative (e.g., diazepam, midazolam, barbiturate, etomidate, ketamine, methohexital) with or without an analgesic agent (e.g., fentanyl, morphine, meperidine). Many experts recommend anesthesia if service is readily available. [b]Both monophasic and biphasic waveforms are acceptable if documented as clinically equivalent to reports of monophasic shock success. [c]Paroxysmal supraventricular tachycardia and atrial flutter often respond to lower energy levels (start with 50 J). (*Reproduced with permission from the* Handbook of Emergency Care for Healthcare Providers, ©*2004, American Heart Association, page 20.*)

Steps for Synchronized Cardioversion

1. Consider sedation.
2. Turn on defibrillator (monophasic or biphasic).
3. Attach monitor leads to the patient ("white to right, red to ribs, what's left over to the left shoulder") and ensure proper display of the patient's rhythm.
4. Engage the synchronization mode by pressing the "sync" control button.
5. Look for markers on R waves indicating sync mode.
6. If necessary, adjust monitor gain until sync markers occur with each R wave.
7. Select appropriate energy level.
8. Position conductor pads on patient (or apply gel to paddles).
9. Position paddle on patient (sternum-apex).
10. Announce to team members:
    "Charging defibrillator—stand clear!"
11. Press "charge" button on apex paddle (right hand).
12. When the defibrillator is charged, begin the final clearing chant. State firmly in a forceful voice the following chant before each shock:
    • *"I am going to shock on three. One, I'm clear."* (Check to make sure you are clear of contact with the patient, the stretcher, and the equipment.)
    • *"Two, you are clear."* (Make a visual check to ensure that no one continues to touch the patient or stretcher. In particular, check the person providing ventilations. That person's hands should not be touching the ventilatory adjuncts, including the tracheal tube! Be sure oxygen is not flowing across the patient's chest. Turn oxygen off or direct flow away from the patient's chest.)
    • *"Three, everybody's clear."* (Check yourself one more time before pressing the "shock" buttons.)
13. Apply 25 lb pressure on both paddles.
14. Press the "discharge" buttons simultaneously.
15. Check the monitor. If tachycardia persists, increase the joules according to the electrical cardioversion algorithm.
16. Reset the sync mode after each synchronized cardioversion because most defibrillators default back to unsynchronized mode. This default allows an immediate shock if the cardioversion produces VF.

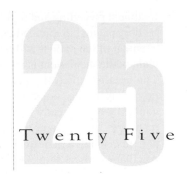

Guidelines for the Transfer of Critically Ill Patients[a]

Twenty Five

Marianne Chulay

TRANSFERS WITHIN THE HOSPITAL

Transport Personnel

- A minimum of two people should accompany the patient
- One of the accompanying personnel should be the critical care nurse assigned to the patient or a specifically trained critical care transfer nurse. This critical care nurse should have completed a competency-based orientation and meet the described standards for critical care nurses.
- Additional personnel may include a respiratory therapist, registered nurse, critical care technician, or physician. A respiratory therapist should accompany all patients requiring mechanical ventilation.

Transport Equipment Requirements

The following minimal equipment should be available:

- Cardiac monitor/defibrillator.
- Airway management equipment and resuscitation bag of proper size and fit for the patient.
- Oxygen source of ample volume to support the patient's needs for the projected time out of the ICU, with an additional 30-minute reserve.
- Standard resuscitation drugs: epinephrine, lidocaine, atropine.
- Blood pressure cuff (sphygmomanometer) and stethoscope.
- Ample supply of the IV fluids and continuous drip medications (regulated by battery-operated infusion pumps) being administered to the patient.
- Additional medications to provide the patient's scheduled intermittent medication doses and to meet anticipated needs (e.g., sedation) with appropriate

orders to allow their administration if a physician is not present.

- For patients receiving mechanical support of ventilation, a device capable of delivering the same volume, pressure, and PEEP and an FiO_2 equal to or greater than what the patient is receiving in the ICU. For practical reasons, in adults an FiO_2 of 1.0 is most feasible during transfer because this eliminates the need for an air tank and air–oxygen blender. During neonatal transfer, FiO_2 should be precisely controlled.
- Resuscitation cart and suction equipment need not accompany each patient being transferred, but such equipment should be stationed in areas used by critically ill patients and be readily available (within 4 minutes) by a predetermined mechanism for emergencies that may occur en route.

Monitoring During Transfer

- If technologically possible, patients being transported should receive the same physiologic monitoring during transfer that they were receiving in the ICU.
- Minimally, all critically ill patients being transferred must have continuous monitoring of ECG and pulse oximetry and intermittent measurement and documentation of blood pressure, respiratory rate, and pulse rate.
- In addition, selected patients, based on clinical status, may benefit from monitoring by capnography; continuous measurement of blood pressure, PAP, and ICP; and intermittent measurement of CVP, PaO_2, and CO.
- Intubated patients receiving mechanical support of ventilation should have airway pressure monitored. If a transfer ventilator is used, it should have alarms to indicate disconnects or excessively high airway pressures.

Pretransfer Coordination and Communication

- Physician-to-physician and/or nurse-to-nurse communication regarding the patient's condition and

---

[a]From: American Association of Critical Care Nurses: *Guidelines for the Transfer of Critically Ill Patients.* Aliso Viejo, CA: AACN; 1998.

treatment preceding and following the transfer should be documented in the medical record when the management of the patient will be assumed by a different team while the patient is away from the ICU.

- The area to which the patient is being transferred (x-ray, operating room, nuclear medicine, etc.) must confirm that it is ready to receive the patient and immediately begin the procedure or test for which the patient is being transferred.
- Ancillary services (e.g., security, respiratory therapy, escort) must be notified as to the timing of the transfer and the equipment and support needed.
- The responsible physician must be notified either to accompany the patient or to be aware that the patient is out of the ICU at this time and may have an acute event requiring the physician's response to provide emergency care in another area of the hospital.
- Documentation in the medical record must include the indication for transfer, the patient's status during transfer, and whether the patient is expected to return to the ICU.

TRANSFERS BETWEEN HOSPITALS

Transport Personnel

- A minimum of two people, in addition to the vehicle operator, should accompany the patient.
- One of the accompanying personnel should be a registered nurse, physician, or advanced EMT capable of providing advanced airway management, including endotracheal intubation, IV therapy, arrhythmia interpretation and treatment, and basic and advanced cardiac and trauma life support.
- When a physician does not accompany the patient, there should be a mechanism available to communicate with a physician regarding the patient's condition. Standing orders should be authorized if direct communication is not possible.

Transport Medication Requirements

Transfer medications include drugs for advanced cardiac resuscitation, the management of acute physiologic derangements, and the specific needs of that patient (e.g., sedatives, analgesics, antibiotics). The following is a complete list of transfer medications:

(1) Dextrose 50%/50 mL
(1) calcium chloride 1 g/10 mL
(2) atropine sulfate 1 mg/10 mL
(2) lidocaine 100 mg/10 mL
(1) lidocaine 2 g/10 mL
(4) sodium bicarbonate 50 mEq/50 mL

(4) epinephrine 1:10,000/10 mL
(1) local anesthetic spray
(10) blood glucose monitoring strips
(1) potassium chloride 20 mEq/10 mL
(2) verapamil hydrochloride 5 mg/2 mL (Calan, Isoptin)
(1) nitroglycerin tablets 0.4 mg/tablet
(1) nitroprusside 50 mg/vial (Nipride)
(1) heparin sodium 1000 units/mL
(2) dexamethasone 20 mg/mL, 5 mL vial (Decadron)
(1) diphenhydramine hydrochloride 50 mg/mL (Benadryl)
(1) digoxin 0.25 mg/mL (Lanoxin)
(2) metroprolol 5 mg/5 mL (Lopressor)
(2) naloxone hydrochloride 2.0 mg/2 mL vial (Narcan)
(1) procainamide 100 mg/mL—10 mL total (Pronestyl)
(3) epinephrine 1:1000 ampules
(2) bretylium tosylate 500 mg/10 mL (Bretylol)
(2) fosphenytoin 500 mg/10 mL (Cerebyx)
(2) phenytoin sodium 250 mg/5 mL—20 mL total (Dilantin)
(1) furosemide 100 mg/10 mL (Lasix)
(1) mannitol 12.5 g/50 mL, 50–100 g/50 mL
(1) nitroglycerin vial 5 mg/mL
(1) aminophylline 500 mg/20 mL
(2) dopamine 200 mg/5 mL (Intropin)
(1) isoproterenol 1 mg/5 mL (Isuprel)
(1) normal saline 30 mL
(1) sterile water 10 mL
(2) adenosine 6 mg/2 mL (Adenocard)
(2) labetalol 200 mg/40 mL, 40 mg/8 mL (Normodyne)

Narcotics, sedatives, neuromuscular paralyzing agents added, based on anticipated patient need.

Transfer Equipment

The following minimal equipment should be available:

- Cardiac monitor/defibrillator.
- Airway management equipment and resuscitation bag of proper size and fit for the patient.
- Oxygen source of ample volume to support the patient's needs for the projected time out of the ICU, with an additional 30-minute reserve.
- Standard resuscitation drugs: epinephrine, lidocaine, atropine.
- Blood pressure cuff (sphygmomanometer) and stethoscope.
- Materials for IV therapy including cannulas, solutions, tubing needles and syringes, and devices for regulation of continuous IV infusions.
- Spinal immobilization devices.
- Communication equipment to allow contact between the transporting vehicle and the referring and receiving hospital.

A complete listing of equipment is contained in Table 25–1.

TABLE 25–1. TRANSFER EQUIPMENT

Airway Management—Adult and Pediatric
(1) adult bag—valve system with oxygen reservoir
(1) end-tidal CO_2 monitor
(1) PEEP valve
(1) small pediatric mask
(1) medium pediatric mask
(1) large pediatric mask
(1) small adult mask
(1) medium adult mask
(1) large adult mask
(2) O_2 tubing
(1) 50-mL flex tube with patient adapter
(1) pediatric bag—valve system with
  oxygen reservoir
(1) pressure gauge with airway
  adapter tubing and test lung
(1) tonsil suction
(2) #T-63 5/6 French suction catheters
(2) #5 suction catheters
(2) #8 suction catheters
(2) #10 suction catheters
(2) #14 suction catheters
(1) nasal cannula

Arterial Line Tubing and Monitoring Equipment
(3) three-way pressure stopcocks
(1) 6-ft pressure tubing
(1) 1-ft pressure tubing
(1) flush system
(1) adaptor tubing
(1) mercury manometer
(1) roll 1/2″ adhesive tape
(1) roll 2″ adhesive tape
(1) roll 2″ Elastoplast tape

Syringes
(6) 1 oo TB
(3) 3 cc with 20-gauge needle
(3) 3 cc with 22-gauge needle
(3) 5 cc
(3) 10 cc
(2) 60 cc

Alcohol Wipes

IV Catheters
(2) #14
(2) #16
(2) #18
(2) #20
(2) #22
(2) #24
(2) #22 (1 inch)
(2) #24 (1.6 cm)

Butterfly Needles
(2) #23
(2) #25

Intubation Kit
(1) #1 Macintosh blade
(1) #2 Macintosh blade
(1) #3 Macintosh blade
(1) #4 Macintosh blade
(1) #0 Miller blade
(1) #1 Miller blade
(1) #2 Miller blade
(1) pediatric laryngoscope handle
(1) pediatric ET stylet
(1) adult ET stylet
(1) roll 1″ adhesive tape
(1) wrist restraints
(1) Heimlich valve
(1) pediatric Magil forceps
(1) adult Magil forceps
(2) 10-cc syringes
(1) booted hemostat
(1) #2.5 uncuffed ET tube
(1) #3.0 uncuffed ET tube
(1) #3.5 uncuffed ET tube
(1) #4.0 uncuffed ET tube
(1) #4.5 uncuffed ET tube
(1) #5.0 uncuffed ET tube
(1) pair disposable scissors
(4) water-soluble lubricant
(1) #26 nasopharyngeal airway
(1) #30 nasopharyngeal airway
(1) #0 oral airway
(1) #1 oral airway
(1) #2 oral airway
(1) #3 oral airway
(1) #4 oral airway
(1) #5.0 cuffed ET tube
(1) #5.5 cuffed ET tube
(1) #6.0 cuffed ET tube
(1) #6.5 cuffed ET tube
(1) #7.0 cuffed ET tube
(1) #7.5 cuffed ET tube
(1) #8.0 cuffed ET tube
(1) scalpel with blade for cricothyroidotomy
(1) infant medium concentration mask with tubing
(1) pediatric rebreather mask
(1) adult rebreather mask
(1) adult Venturi mask

Dressing Sponges
(4) surgical combines
(8) 2 × 2 sponges
(8) 4 × 4 sponges
(1) 3″ Kling
(1) Kerlix

IV Administration Sets
(3) regular (macro) drip administration sets

(3) mini (pediatric) drip administration sets
(2) Y-blood tubing drip sets
(5) three-way stopcocks with extensions

IV Solutions
(2) 1000 mL normal saline
(2) 1000 mL Ringer's lactate
(2) 500 mL normal saline
(4) 250 mL D_5W
(4) 360 mL D_5 1/2NS
(4) 250 mL D_5 1/4NS

Arm Boards
(1) short arm board
(1) pediatric arm board

Nasogastric Tubes
(1) #10 NG Tube
(1) #14 NG Tube
(1) #18 NG Tube
(1) catheter tip (60-cc) irrigating syringe
(4) blood pump bags
(1) 250-mL bottle normal saline for irrigation
(1) set pediatric electrodes
(1) set adult electrodes
(1) tube electrode jelly
(1) neonatal BP cuff
(1) infant BP cuff
(1) child BP cuff
(1) adult BP cuff
(1) stethoscope
(1) pair trauma scissors
(1) rubber tourniquets
(1) tube Betadine ointment
(1) roll 1″ adhesive tape
(1) Kelly clamp

Needles
(6) 19-gauge needles
(6) 20-gauge needles
(6) 22-gauge needles
(6) 25-gauge needles
(1) bone marrow needle

Equipment
external pacemaker
monitor/defibrillator
transport ventilator
suction apparatus
MAST—adult and pediatric spinal immobilization
  device
pulse oximeter
infusion pumps
neonatal isolette (if appropriate for mission)

Monitoring During Transfer

- All critically ill patients being transferred should have continuous ECG monitoring as a minimal level of monitoring.

- Intermittent measurement of blood pressure, respiratory rate, and pulse rate should be done and documented.
- Continuous monitoring of pulse oximetry is strongly recommended.

- Selected patients, based on clinical status, may benefit from monitoring by capnography; continuous measurement of blood pressure, measurement of CVP, PAP, or ICP; and/or end-tidal CO_2.

- Intubated patients receiving mechanical support of ventilation should have airway pressure monitored. If a transfer ventilator is used, it should have alarms to indicate disconnects or excessively high airway pressures.

Transfer Algorithm

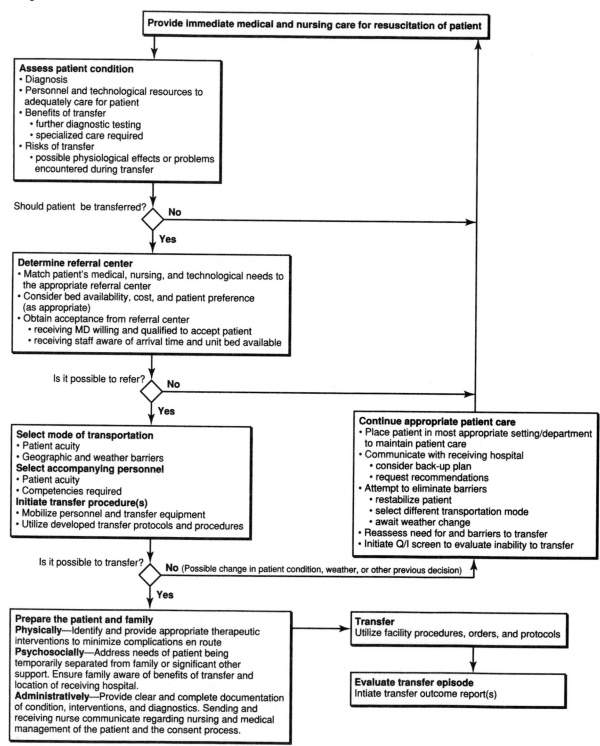

Figure 25–1. *From: American Association of Critical Care Nurses:* AACN's Guidelines for the Transfer of Critically Ill Patients. *Aliso Viejo, CA: AACN; 1998.*

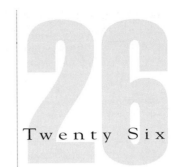

Hemodynamic Troubleshooting Guide

Leanna R. Miller

TABLE 26–1. PROBLEMS ENCOUNTERED WITH ARTERIAL CATHETERS

Problem	Cause	Prevention	Treatment
Hematoma after withdrawal of needle	Bleeding or oozing at puncture site	Maintain firm pressure on site during withdrawal of catheter and for 5–15 min (as necessary) after withdrawal. Apply elastic tape (Elastoplast) firmly over puncture site.	Continue to hold pressure to puncture site until oozing stops.
		For femoral arterial puncture sites, leave a sandbag on site for 1–2 hours to prevent oozing. If patient is receiving heparin, discontinue 2 hours before catheter removal.	Apply sandbag to femoral puncture site for 1–2 hours after removal of catheter.
Decreased or absent pulse distal to puncture site	Spasm of artery	Introduce arterial needle cleanly, nontraumatically.	Inject lidocaine locally at insertion site and 10 mg into arterial catheter.
	Thrombosis of artery	Use 1 unit of heparin/1 mL IV fluid.	Arteriotomy and Fogarty catheterization both distally and proximally from the puncture site result in return of pulse in >90% of cases if brachial or femoral artery is used.
Bleedback into tubing or transducer	Insufficient pressure on IV bag Loose connections	Maintain 300 mm Hg pressure on IV bag. Use Luer-Lok stopcocks; tighten periodically.	Replace transducer. "Fast flush" through system. Tighten all connections.
Hemorrhage	Loose connections	Keep all connecting sites visible. Observe connecting sites frequently. Use built-in alarm system. Use Luer-Lok stopcocks.	Tighten all connections.
Emboli	Clot from catheter tip into bloodstream	Always aspirate and discard before flushing. Use continuous flush device. Gently flush <2–4 mL.	Remove catheter.
Local infection	Forward movement of contaminated catheter	Carefully suture catheter at insertion site.	Remove catheter.
	Break in sterile technique Prolonged catheter use	Always use aseptic technique. Remove catheter after 72–96 hours. Leave dressing in place until catheter is removed, changed, or dressing becomes damp, loosened, or soiled.	Prescribe antibiotic.
Sepsis	Break in sterile technique Prolonged catheter use	Use percutaneous insertion. Always use aseptic technique. Remove catheter after 72–96 hours.	Remove catheter. Prescribe antibiotic.
	Bacterial growth in IV fluid	Change IV fluid bag, stopcocks, dome, and tubing no more frequently than at 72-hour intervals. Do not use IV fluid containing glucose. Use sterile dead-end caps on all ports of stopcocks. Carefully flush remaining blood from stopcocks after blood sampling.	

From: Daily E, Schroeder J: Techniques in Bedside Hemodynamic Monitoring, *5th ed, pp. 165–166. St. Louis, MO: CV Mosby; 1994.*

TABLE 26–2. INACCURATE ARTERIAL PRESSURE MEASUREMENTS

Problem	Cause	Prevention	Treatment
Damped pressure tracing	Catheter tip against vessel wall	Usually cannot be avoided.	Pull back, rotate, or reposition catheter while observing pressure waveform.
	Partial occlusion of catheter tip by clot	Use continuous infusion under pressure. Briefly "fast flush" after blood withdrawal (2–4 mL).	Aspirate clot with syringe and flush with saline (<2–4 mL). Consider line removal.
	Clot in stopcock or transducer	Carefully flush catheter after blood withdrawal and reestablish IV drip. Use continuous flush device.	Flush stopcock and transducer; if no improvement, change stopcock and transducer.
	Air bubbles in transducer or connector tubing	Carefully flush transducer and tubing when setting up system and attaching to catheter.	Check system; flush rapidly; disconnect transducer and flush out air bubbles.
	Compliant tubing	Use stiff, short tubing.	Shorten tubing or replace softer tubing with stiffer tubing.
Abnormally high or low readings	Change in transducer air-reference level	Maintain air-reference port of transducer at midchest and/or catheter tip level for serial pressure measurements.	Recheck patient and transducer positions.
No pressure available	Transducer not open to catheter	Follow routine, systematic steps for setting up system and turning stopcocks.	Check system—stopcocks, monitor, and amplifier setup.
	Settings on monitor amplifiers incorrect—still on zero, cal, or off		
	Incorrect scale selection	Select scale appropriate to expected range of physiologic signal.	Select appropriate scale.

From: Daily E, Schroeder J: Techniques in Bedside Hemodynamic Monitoring, 5th ed, p. 161. St. Louis, MO: CV Mosby; 1994.

TABLE 26–3.   PROBLEMS ENCOUNTERED WITH PULMONARY ARTERY (PA) CATHETERS[a]

Problem	Cause	Prevention	Treatment
Phlebitis or local infection at insertion site	Mechanical irritation or contamination	Prepare skin properly before insertion. Use sterile technique during insertion and dressing change. Insert smoothly and rapidly. Use Teflon-coated introducer. Change dressings, stopcocks, and connecting tubing every 72 hours. Remove catheter or change insertion site.	Remove catheter. Apply warm compresses. Give pain medication as necessary.
Ventricular irritability	Looping of excess catheter in right ventricle	Suture catheter at insertion site; check chest film.	Reposition catheter; remove loop.
	Migration of catheter from PA to RV	Position catheter tip in main right or left PA.	Inflate balloon to encourage catheter flotation out to PA. Advance rapidly out to PA.
	Irritation of the endocardium during catheter passage	Keep balloon inflated during advancement; advance gently.	
Apparent wedging of catheter with balloon deflated	Forward migration of catheter tip caused by blood flow, excessive loop in RV, or inadequate suturing of catheter at insertion site	Check catheter tip by radiograph or fluoroscopy; position in main right or left PA. Suture catheter in place at insertion site.	Aspirate blood from catheter; if catheter is wedged, sample will be arterialized and obtained with difficulty. If not wedged, slowly pull back catheter until PA waveform appears. If not wedged, gently aspirate and flush catheter with saline; catheter tip can partially clot, causing damping that resembles damped PAW waveform.
Pulmonary hemorrhage or infarction, or both	Distal migration of catheter tip	Check chest film immediately after insertion and 12–24 hours later; remove any catheter loop in RA or RV. Leave balloon deflated.	Deflate balloon (passively). Place patient on side (catheter tip down). Stop anticoagulation. Consider "wedge" angiogram.
	Continuous or prolonged wedging of catheter	Suture catheter to prevent inadvertent advancement. Position catheter in main right or left PA. Pull catheter back to pulmonary artery if it spontaneously wedges. Do not flush catheter when in wedge position.	
	Overinflation of balloon while catheter is wedged	Inflate balloon slowly with only enough air to obtain a PAW waveform.	
	Failure of balloon to deflate	Do not inflate 7-Fr catheter with more than 1.25–1.5 mL air.	

(continued)

TABLE 26–3. PROBLEMS ENCOUNTERED WITH PULMONARY ARTERY (PA) CATHETERS[a] (Continued)

Problem	Cause	Prevention	Treatment
"Overwedging" or damped PAW	Overinflation of balloon	Do not inflate if resistance is met. Watch waveform during inflation; inject only enough air to obtain PAW pressure. Do not inflate 7-Fr catheter with more than 1.25–1.5 mL air.	Deflate balloon; reinflate slowly with only enough air to obtain PAW pressure.
	Eccentric inflation of balloon	Check inflated balloon shape before insertion.	Deflate balloon; reposition and slowly reinflate.
PA balloon rupture	Overinflation of balloon Frequent inflations of balloon Syringe deflation damaging wall of balloon	Inflate slowly with only enough air to obtain a PAW pressure. Monitor PAD pressure as reflection of PAW and LVEDP. Allow passive deflation of balloon. Remove syringe after inflation.	Remove syringe to prevent further air injection. Monitor PAD pressure.
Infection	Nonsterile insertion techniques	Use sterile techniques. Use sterile catheter sleeve.	Remove catheter. Use antibiotics.
	Contamination via skin	Prepare skin with effective antiseptic (chlorhexidine). Leave dressing in place until catheter is removed, changed, or the dressing becomes damp, loosened, or soiled. Reassess need for catheter after 3 days. Avoid internal jugular approach.	
	Contamination through stopcock ports or catheter hub	Use sterile dead-end caps on all stopcock ports. Change tubing, continuous flush device and flush solution every 72 hours. Do not use IV flush solution that contains glucose.	
	Fluid contamination from transducer through cracked membrane	Check transducer for cracks. Change transducers every 96 hours. Do not use IV flush solution that contains glucose.	
	Prolonged catheter placement	Change catheter and/or insertion site with any local signs of infection and for infections without an obvious source (should obtain cultures). Remove catheter as soon as clinically feasible.	
Heart block during insertion of catheter	Mechanical irritation of His bundle in patients with preexisting left bundle branch block	Insert catheter expeditiously with balloon inflated. Insert transvenous pacing catheter before PA catheter insertion.	Use temporary pacemaker or flotation catheter with pacing wire.

[a]PAW, pulmonary artery wedge; RV, right ventricle; PA, pulmonary artery.

From Daily E, Schroeder J: Techniques in Bedside Hemodynamic Monitoring, 5th ed, pp. 134–136. St. Louis, MO: CV Mosby; 1994.

TABLE 26–4. INACCURATE PULMONARY ARTERY (PA) PRESSURE MEASUREMENTS[a]

Problem	Cause	Prevention	Treatment
Damped waveforms and inaccurate pressures	Partial clotting at catheter tip	Maintain adequate flush bag pressures. Hand flush occasionally. Flush with large volume after blood sampling.	Aspirate, then flush catheter with fluid (not in PAW position).
	Tip moving against wall; Kinking of catheter	Obtain more stable catheter position. Restrict catheter movement at insertion site.	Reposition catheter. Reposition to straighten catheter. Replace catheter.
Abnormally low or negative pressures	Incorrect air-reference level (above midchest level)	Maintain transducer air-reference port at midchest level; rezero after patient position changes.	Remeasure level of transducer air-reference and reposition at midchest level; rezero.
	Incorrect zeroing and calibration of monitor; Loose connection	Zero and calibrate monitor properly. Use Luer-Lok stopcocks. Use Luer-Lok stopcocks.	Recheck zero and calibration of monitor. Check all connections.
Abnormally high pressure reading	Pressure trapped by improper sequence of stopcock operation	Turn stopcocks in proper sequence when two pressures are measured on one transducer.	Thoroughly flush transducers with IV solution; rezero and turn stopcocks in proper sequence.
	Incorrect air-reference level (below midchest level)	Maintain transducer air-reference port at midchest level; recheck and rezero after patient position changes.	Check air-reference level; reset at midchest and rezero.
Inappropriate pressure waveform	Migration of catheter tip (e.g., in RV or PAW instead of in PA)	Establish optimal position carefully when introducing catheter initially. Suture catheter at insertion site and tape catheter to patient's skin.	Review waveform; if RV, inflate balloon; if PAW, deflate balloon and withdraw catheter slightly. Check position under x-ray and/or fluoroscopy after reposition.
No pressure available	Transducer not open to catheter; Amplifiers still on cal, zero, or off	Follow routine, systematic steps for pressure measurement.	Check system, stopcocks.
Noise or fling in pressure waveform	Excessive catheter movement, particularly in PA	Avoid excessive catheter length in ventricle.	Try different catheter tip position.
	Excessive tubing length; Excessive stopcocks	Use shortest tubing possible (<3–4 ft). Minimize number of stopcocks.	Eliminate excess tubing. Eliminate excess stopcocks.

[a]PAW, pulmonary artery wedge; RV, right ventricle; PA, pulmonary artery.
From: Daily E, Schroeder J: Techniques in Bedside Hemodynamic Monitoring, 5th ed, p. 137. St. Louis, MO: CV Mosby; 1994.

TABLE 26–5. TROUBLESHOOTING PROBLEMS WITH THERMODILUTION CARDIAC OUTPUT MEASUREMENTS

Problem	Cause	Action
Cardiac output values lower than expected	Injectate volume greater than designated amount	Inject exact volume to correspond to computation constant used.
		Discontinue rapid infusion through proximal or distal port.
	Catheter tip in RV or RA	Verify PA waveform from distal lumen. Reposition catheter.
	Incorrect variables entered into monitor	Recheck and correct variables (height, weight).
	Left-to-right shunt (VSD)	Check RA and PA oxygen saturations.
		Use alternative CO measurement technique.
	Catheter kinked or thermistor partially obstructed with clot	Check for kinks at insertion site; straighten catheter; aspirate and flush catheter. Replace catheter.
	Faulty catheter (communication between proximal and distal lumens)	
Cardiac output values higher than expected	Injectate volume less than designated amount	Inject exact volume to correspond to computation constant.
		Carefully remove all air bubbles from syringe.
	Catheter too distal (PAW)	Verify PA waveform from distal lumen.
		Pull catheter back.
	RA port lies within sheath	Advance catheter.
	Thermistor against wall of PA	Reposition patient.
		Rotate catheter to turn thermistor away from wall.
		Reposition catheter.
	Fibrin covering thermistor	Check a-vDo$_2$; change catheter.
	Incorrect variables	Recheck and correct variables (height, weight).
	Right-to-left shunt (VSD)	Use alternative CO measurement technique.
	Severe tricuspid regurgitation	
	Incorrect injectate temperature	Use closed injectate system with in-line temperature probe.
		Handle syringe minimally.
		Do not turn stopcock to reestablish IV infusion through proximal port between injections; reduce or discontinue IV flow through VIP port.
		Try to determine cause of interference.
Irregular upslope of CO curve	Magnetic interference producing numerous spikes in CO curve	
	Long lag time between injection and upstroke of curve	Press start button after injection completed to delay computer sampling time.
	Uneven injection technique	Inject smoothly and quickly (10 mL in ≤4 sec).
	RA port partially occluded with clot	Always check catheter patency by withdrawing, then flushing proximal port before CO determinations.
	Catheter partially kinked	Check for kinks, particularly at insertion site; straighten catheter; reposition patient.
Irregular downslope of CO curve	Cardiac dysrhythmias (PVC, AF, etc.)	Note ECG during CO determinations.
		Try to inject during a stable period.
		Increase the number of CO determinations.
	Marked movement of catheter tip	Obtain x-ray film to determine position of tip.
		Advance catheter tip away from pulmonic value.
	Marked variation in PA baseline temperature	Use iced temperature injectate to increase signal/noise ratio.
		Increase the number of CO determinations.
		Inject at various times during respiratory cycle.
	Curve prematurely terminated	Press start button after injection completed to delay computer sampling time.
	Right-to-left shunt	Use alternative CO measurement technique.

Abbreviations: AV, atrioventricular; CO, cardiac output; CPR, cardiopulmonary resuscitation; ECG, electrocardiogram; IV, intravenous; NSR, normal sinus rhythm; MAT, multifocal atrial tachycardia; PAC, premature atrial contraction; PJC, premature junctional complex; PVC, premature ventricular complexes; VT, ventricular tachycardia.

From: Daily E, Schroeder J: Techniques in Bedside Hemodynamic Monitoring, *5th ed, pp. 183–184. St. Louis, MO; CV Mosby; 1994. Cardiac output waveforms from: Gardner P: Cardiac output: Theory, technique and troubleshooting. In Underhill SL, Woods S, Froelicher E, et al:* Cardiac Nursing, *2nd ed, p. 465. Philadelphia: JB Lippincott; 1989.*

Ventilatory Troubleshooting Guide

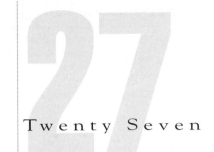

Twenty Seven

Robert E. St. John and Suzanne M. Burns

Problem	Causes	Management
Low Exhaled Tidal Volume (V$_t$)		Ventilate patient as necessary with manual resuscitation bag if exhibiting signs and symptoms of respiratory insufficiency and problem cannot be immediately corrected. Obtain appropriate assistance.
	Patient Related Cuff leak caused by • Insufficient air added to cuff or malfunctioning cuff • Higher airway pressures, which create the need for higher cuff pressure to seal the trachea • Leak in air inflation port • Displaced endotracheal tube	Evaluate for cause of leak. Inflate cuff properly to minimally occlude trachea and provide effective ventilation. • If leak is in cuff, call for assistance in reintubation. Attempt to maintain ventilation in the interim by increasing V$_t$ to compensate for gas escaping or bag the patient until help arrives. Inform and reassure patient. Observe for potential gastric distension caused by leakage of air into stomach. Maintain gastric suction. • If leak is in air inflation port, seal port by placing three-way stopcock or leaving syringe on port. Tape syringe hub to prevent cuff deflation. Do not use a clamp; it may further damage inflation tubing. • If endotracheal tube is displaced, reposition or obtain assistance as necessary.
	Factors that increase airway resistance and/or decrease compliance (see increased Airway Pressure) will increase inspiratory pressures and trigger high airway pressure alarm, causing the volume which is not delivered to be vented to the atmosphere (Volume-cycled ventilators deliver the prescribed volume unless the pressure limit is exceeded.)	• Assess and correct causes of increased airway pressure (see Increased Airway Pressure). Increase airway pressure upper limit as necessary to allow for ventilation (last step after other assessments and management).
	Bronchopleural air leak, which results in passage of air from airways to pleural space causing a pneumothorax.	• Refer to respiratory acidosis section for management.
	If a pressure mode of ventilation is being used such as pressure support ventilation (PSV) or pressure control (PC), increased resistance or decreased compliance will result in decreased VA and often an increase in RR. Airway pressure will not increase.	• Explore etiology of decreased VA described above. May also need to increase PSV level to assure adequate VA.
	Ventilator Related Loose, cracked, ill-fitted connectors to humidifier.	• Check for loose, cracked, or ill-fitted humidification system; replace if necessary.
	Loose tubing, connections.	• Check for and tighten loose tubing connections.

(continued)

Abbreviations: ARDS, acute respiratory distress syndrome; CNS, central nervous system; CO, cardiac output; COPD, chronic obstructive pulmonary disease; CPAP, continuous positive airway pressure; CVP, central venous pressure; Fio$_2$, percentage of inspired oxygen; IMV, intermittent mandatory ventilation; PAOP, pulmonary artery occlusion pressure; PEEP, positive end-expiratory pressure; V$_t$, tidal volume.

Problem	Causes	Management
	Tears in tubing. Flow rate may become too high because of a combination of high ventilator V_t rate, or flow rate settings. High flow rates may result in an inability to deliver the total prescribed volume.	• Change tubing as necessary. • Be aware of potential volume loss resulting from combinations of high ventilator V_t respiratory rate, or peak flow settings, which exceed capabilities of the ventilator. (The effect of higher flow rates on volume delivery should be evaluated.) Correct problem by lowering the flow rate (decrease peak flow or lengthen inspiratory time; lower dialed-in respiratory rate or volume settings). • Support patient with manual resuscitation bag if unable to correct problem rapidly. Call for assistance to change ventilators.
No Exhaled V_t	**Patient Related** Patient disconnected from ventilator. Large cuff leak; endotracheal tube displaced so that cuff is above the vocal cords (may lead to inability to seal the pharyngeal area despite addition of large volume of air to cuff).	• Check patient to ensure the ventilator circuit adaptor is securely attached to tracheostomy or endotracheal tube. • Evaluate and correct cuff leaks, endotracheal tube displacement.
	Ventilator Related Tubing disconnections, large tears in tubing, loss of wall electrical or compressed air source.	• Evaluate for disconnected tubing, holes in tubing, loss of power of air/oxygen source.
Increased Airway Pressure (generally refers only to volume-targeted ventilation modes)	**Patient Related** Higher airway pressures are required to deliver the prescribed volume because of various factors that increase airway resistance, including secretions, mucous plugs, endotracheal tube factors (becomes kinked or narrowed, biting on orally placed tube), bronchospasm, or decreased lung compliance, including pneumothorax, atelectasis, pulmonary edema. The upper airway pressure alarm sounds when the peak inspiratory pressure reaches the preset alarm limit. Endotracheal tube in right mainstem bronchus. Inspiratory pressures can become higher because of resistance of the chest wall to expansion, increased abdominal pressure, chest-wall injury, external restrictions, abdominal contractions during coughing or breathing efforts. Coughing because of tracheal irritation caused by jarring of the endotracheal or tracheostomy tube; air leak around cuff, which causes air and secretion movement; head movement; tip of tube touching carina. Need for communication of concerns and problems; may not be sufficiently informed or comprehending explanations regarding inability to verbally communicate; alternative methods of communication are not used or are inappropriate or ineffective.	• Suction as necessary. • Assess for difficulty passing suction catheter through tube or observable kinking. Notify physician and respiratory care if necessary. • If patient bites on tube, explain purpose of tube, reason for not biting. May need bite block. • Anchor tube using tape or commercially designed tube holder if necessary. • Auscultate chest regularly to detect changes in breath sounds that may coincide with increased inspiratory pressures. • Notify physician of decreased breath sounds. Obtain chest x-ray film to evaluate for proper endotracheal tube placement. After readjustment, mark tube depth and anchor tube securely. • Reposition patient for optimal ventilation. Increase upper pressure limit setting 10–15 cm H_2O higher than the pressure required for ventilation when certain positions that create higher pressures are necessary for patient management. • Evaluate for causes of coughing (minimal or no volume delivery may occur if the high airway pressure alarm sounds because, when the set pressure limit is reached, inspiration is discontinued and expiration begins). • Avoid jarring or moving tube during turning. • Evaluate for optimum cuff inflation. Add air to cuff as necessary to obtain minimum leak. • Chest x-ray studies to evaluate for proper tube placement. • Evaluate with intradisciplinary team whether patient is a candidate for weaning/extubation, which may resolve the problem. • Explain reason for inability to communicate verbally and implement alternative method(s) to meet needs. Anticipate needs, ask "yes or no" questions. • Convey calm, confident, reassuring approach; explain procedures.

(continued)

Problem	Causes	Management
	Increased respiratory rate from anxiety, fear, pain, inadequate oxygenation, inadequate ventilation (hypercarbia), acidemia, or CNS malfunction. The higher the breathing rate, the faster the flow rates. If the ventilator peak flow rate is set too low or inspiratory time is too long, the patient will be attempting to exhale during the ventilator inspiratory phase. Forceful contraction of the thoracoabdominal musculature during the inspiratory phase causes the ventilator pressure limit to be exceeded, thus terminating air delivery prematurely.	• Evaluate for causes of increased ventilatory requirements, patient–ventilator dyssynchrony. Implement measures to correct problem(s). Provide calm, confident, reassuring approach. Explain interventions and use touch to relieve anxiety and fear. Provide analgesics as appropriate. Evaluate for increased work of breathing caused by inadequate oxygenation or ventilation caused by air leaks in the ventilator system. • Evaluate whether inspiratory flow rate setting is set optimally to match patient's breathing pattern. Observe chest/abdomen during inspiratory phase and evaluate whether patient appears to exhale (as evidenced by chest/abdominal contraction) during ventilator inspiratory cycle. Readjust peak flow setting, shorten inspiratory time, and/or increase respiratory rate setting (higher setting results in increased flow rate) as necessary to match patient's rapid inspiratory phase. • Observe trends in airway pressures which may signal changes in compliance or resistance.
	Ventilator related Airway upper pressure limit alarm is set too low. Unusually high V_t for the patient. Compliance may be decreased when PEEP is applied, possibly as a result of overdistension of alveoli.	• Set upper pressure limit 10–15 cm H_2O higher than the patient's maximum inspiratory pressure. • Evaluate whether the patient is receiving too large a V_t (normal: 6–12 mL/kg normal body weight). • Increase upper pressure limit. • Monitor for adverse effects of PEEP (see Decreased CO). • Review reasons for decreased compliance and treat as appropriate. • Monitor for adverse effects of PEEP (see Decreased CO).
Decreased V_t with Pressure-Targeted Modes of Ventilation	**Patient Related** With pressure modes, V_t will decrease with increases in resistance and decreases in compliance. Airway pressure will remain the same. **Ventilator Related** PSV level set too low.	• As per section on Increased Airway Pressure. • Remember that with decreases in V_t, respiratory rate increases to compensate. Adjust pressure level to obtain appropriate V_t.
Respiratory Alkalosis	**Patient Related** Factors that may increase respiratory rate or minute ventilation, include anxiety, restlessness, discomfort, pain; hypoxemia; CNS malfunction; metabolic acidosis; sensation of dyspnea caused by underlying lung pathology. Mechanical hyperventilation ($Paco_2$ <30 mm Hg) may be used rarely as therapy to decrease intracranial pressure.	• Assist in decreasing feelings of anxiety and fear through calm, confident, reassuring approach, providing explanations and other measures to decrease stress. • Evaluate ventilator for proper functioning (receiving prescribed V_t flow rate adjusted to match breathing pattern). • Check Pao_2, provide adequate oxygenation. • Evaluate and treat metabolic disturbance when warranted. • Consider different ventilation mode. • Hyperventilation may not be corrected by various interventions if CNS dysfunction is present. • Mechanically hyperventilate as prescribed for purpose of decreasing intracranial pressure (generally no longer than 24 hours).

Abbreviations: ARDS, acute respiratory distress syndrome; CNS, central nervous system; CO, cardiac output; COPD, chronic obstructive pulmonary disease; CPAP, continuous positive airway pressure; CVP, central venous pressure; Fio_2, percentage of inspired oxygen; IMV, intermittent mandatory ventilation; PAOP, pulmonary artery occlusion pressure; PEEP, positive end-expiratory pressure, V_t, tidal volume.

Problem	Causes	Management
	Ventilator Related High tidal or minute volume settings on ventilator which cause overventilation, decreased Pa_{CO_2}, increased pH.	• Set initial V_t at 6–12 mL/kg and set rate at 10–15 breaths/min. If patient has COPD, select lower V_ts to reduce the risk of barotrauma and hypoventilation. Check arterial blood gases to ensure acid–base goal (generally allow 20 min for equilibration). • Decrease V_t or respiratory rate if hypocarbia persists. (*Note:* Decreasing respiratory rate setting while in assist/control mode will not correct the problem if the patient is triggering the ventilator. Decreasing V_t may not correct the problem in patients who can maintain their desired Pa_{CO_2} level by increasing their respiratory rate.) • If a pressure mode is in use it may be that the pressure level is set too high. Reevaluate and adjust as necessary.
	Ventilator trigger sensitivity dial is set too positively causing machine to automatically cycle without patient effort, resulting in unintentional hyperventilation (Pa_{CO_2} below normal).	• Maintain sensitivity setting so that it takes between -1 or -2 cm H_2O spontaneous effort to trigger a respiration. • Most ventilators automatically adjust sensitivity to the PEEP level. However, in the presence of auto-PEEP, patient triggering will be more difficult because the auto-PEEP is not sensed by the ventilator. In this example, the patient must generate negative pressure equal to the selected sensitivity level plus the auto-PEEP. The work of breathing is greatly increased. • When patient is receiving PEEP, avoid air leaks in cuff or ventilator system (air leaks may cause loss of PEEP and machine self-cycling may occur).
Respiratory Acidosis	**Patient Related** Inadequate V_t to provide adequate gas exchange. Insufficient respiratory rate. Some COPD patients have chronically elevated Pa_{CO_2} levels.	• Increase V_t. • Maintain Pa_{CO_2} at the patient's normal baseline level. Do not attempt to ventilate to a normal Pa_{CO_2} level if the patient has COPD with chronic carbon dioxide retention. Instead, the goal should be normalization of pH. • Make changes gradually to patient's baseline Pa_{CO_2} and pH. (Rapid changes may cause respiratory alkalosis with risk of cardiac arrhythmias, tetany, seizures.)
	Increased carbon dioxide production results from the provision of excess calories. Increased ventilation is observed as a result of increased carbon dioxide production. In mechanically ventilated patients unable to increase their minute ventilation (e.g., patients with chronic lung disease, those with normal lungs who develop compromised lung function because of acute lung disorder), the increase in carbon dioxide production is paralleled by an increase in Pa_{CO_2}.	• Monitor effects of nutrition therapy on ventilatory status including measurements of minute ventilation, respiratory rate, oxygen consumption, carbon dioxide production, arterial blood gases. • With pressure modes, adjust the pressure level to attain the desired V_t. In pressure control modes, selection of a rate is also necessary.
	Bronchopleural air leak results in passage of air from airways to pleural space secondary to factors that increase intrathoracic pressure. Examples include high peak flow rate, high airway resistance, increased mean intrathoracic pressure throughout the respiratory cycle, inflation hold, and PEEP, and CPAP. Higher negative suction pressure will augment leak independent of factors as outlined.	• Implement measures that minimize the bronchopleural pressure gradient and maintain adequate pH, oxygenation, and ventilation. Suggested conservative management includes: – Deliver lowest number of mechanical breaths compatible with adequate ventilation (spontaneous ventilation if possible). – Reduce exhaled V_t to 6. – Avoid inflation hold. – Minimize PEEP/CPAP levels. – Use lowest effective level of chest tube suction. – Consider sedating with or without paralysis if spontaneous movements accentuate leak and clinical condition is unstable. – Treat underlying cause for respiratory failure while maintaining nutritional and respiratory care support.

(continued)

Problem	Causes	Management
	Ventilator Related Patient not receiving prescribed V_t because of air leaks. Reduction of volume delivered to the patient because of tubing system compliance and gas compression. This correction is generally in the range of 3 mL/cm H_2O of peak inspiratory pressure for adult ventilator circuits; however, may be negligible on some ventilator circuits.	• Evaluate and correct air leaks (refer to Low/No exhaled V_t sections). • Be aware of reduced delivered volume, which may be significant if high inflation pressures are required. • Increase V_t as necessary to provide adequate ventilation.
Thick Secretions	**Patient Related** Dehydration. Infection.	• Maintain accurate intake, output, weight, CVP, LAP, PAOP recordings. Notify physician of abnormalities. • Maximize systemic hydration. • Monitor sputum for changes in color, amount, consistency. Obtain culture and sensitivity if indicated. If signs of infection, check with physician regarding antibiotics. Monitor for improvements after treatment initiated. • Suction as necessary if secretions present.
	Ventilator Related Heating unit set too low or not functioning properly. Insufficient water in humidifier system.	• Check sensor that monitors temperature of inspired humidified gas (should be located close to patient airway). Maintain temperature at 98°F or 37°C (most are set between 35° and 37° but can be adjusted as needed). • Notify respiratory therapist that heating unit not functioning properly. • Add water to refill system as necessary. • Drain water from tubing every 2 hours and as needed.
Tracheostomy/Endotracheal Tube Discomfort	**Patient Related** Insufficient attention to observing patient's airway, guiding tubing, and providing extra tubing during turning or other movement. Tube movement with turning. Tube not secured adequately.	• Obtain necessary assistance so that one person can pay attention to guiding tubing and prevent pulling or jarring during patient activities. • Disconnect the patient from the ventilator, turn and reconnect. Do not leave off ventilator longer than 10–15 sec. (Disconnection may be undesirable for unstable patients requiring high oxygen concentrations, PEEP, or if they are paralyzed or sedated.) • Stabilize tracheostomy or endotracheal tube with one hand when reconnecting the ventilator adapter. • Anchor tube securely with ties, tape, or other tube securing device. • Position ventilator tubing on support system to minimize pulling.
High Pao_2/Sao_2	**Ventilator Related** Improvement in gas exchange because of improvement in disorder that caused increased oxygen requirement. Oxygen concentration setting on ventilator is too high.	• Decrease inspired oxygen concentration. • Monitor Sao_2 and/or reevaluate arterial blood gases in 15–20 min. • If on PEEP therapy, consider decreasing PEEP if $Fio_2 < 0.5$. • Decrease PEEP in increments of 3–5 cm H_2O and evaluate Sao_2 and/or arterial blood gases within 20 min. • Refer to Decreased CO section for other management procedures related to PEEP.

Abbreviations: ARDS, acute respiratory distress syndrome; CNS, central nervous system; CO, cardiac output; COPD, chronic obstructive pulmonary disease; CPAP, continuous positive airway pressure; CVP, central venous pressure; Fio_2, percentage of inspired oxygen; IMV, intermittent mandatory ventilation; PAOP, pulmonary artery occlusion pressure; PEEP, positive end-expiratory pressure, V_t, tidal volume.

Problem	Causes	Management
Low PaO_2/SaO_2	**Patient Related** Various abnormalities causing ventilation–perfusion disturbances and shunting, such as secretions, bronchospasm, pulmonary edema, pulmonary embolism.	• Correct pathophysiologic state causing the abnormal oxygenation. • Manually ventilate with self-inflating bag and 100% O_2 if unable to quickly fix problem or for drop in PaO_2/SaO_2 expecially if <90%. • Hyperoxygenate before and after suctioning as necessary (refer to Arrhythmias during suctioning section). Preoxygenation is important even when using closed-suction catheter systems.
	Arterial blood gas drawn immediately after suctioning.	• Wait at least 15–20 min after suctioning before obtaining blood gas measurement.
	Changes in position causing alveolar hypoventilation, ventilation-perfusion disturbances.	• Assess whether certain positions cause decreased PaO_2. Refrain from placing in positions which precipitate respiratory discomfort, PaO_2 or SaO_2 deterioration. Obtain order to increase FiO_2, V_t, rate or pressure level to maintain adequate oxygenation, ventilation.
	Right mainstem bronchus intubation, pneumothorax causing decreased ventilation (airway pressure will increase).	• Evaluate for, and correct, tube malposition, pneumothorax. • Obtain chest x-ray film.
	Ventilator Related Oxygen concentration setting on ventilator is too low.	• Increase FiO_2, PEEP as necessary to avoid unsafe high oxygen concentrations.
	Air leak around tracheostomy or endotracheal tube cuff, or in ventilator system, or both, leading to inadequate oxygenation, ventilation, loss of PEEP therapy.	• Evaluate for air leaks, and correct (see Low/No exhaled V_t).
	Inaccurate oxygen percentage from oxygen source failure or oxygen analyzer error.	• Notify respiratory therapist to determine accuracy of oxygen analyzer or whether oxygen concentration is being delivered. • Provide oxygen as necessary to maintain acceptable PaO_2, saturation (SaO_2), and/or manually ventilate patient on 100% O_2 until problem identified and corrected.
Decreased CO with Hypotension	**Patient Related** Significant stimulation (hypoxemia, hypercarbia, acidemia) of the autonomic system in a patient requiring ventilator support. Physiologic stress is frequently compounded by a state of anxiety and fear. These factors lead to arterial and venous constriction, as well as myocardial stimulation. Support of ventilation usually relieves work of breathing, and reverses hypercarbia, acidemia, and hypoxemia. It also produces relaxation and sleep. The combination of relief of the work of breathing and improved oxygenation and ventilation often leads to a profound and sudden decrease in sympathetic stimulation to the cardiovascular system. Arteriolar and venous relaxation result in hypotension.	• Be aware of potential hypotension following institution of positive pressure ventilation. Monitor blood pressure, pulse, rhythm. • Stabilize cardiovascular system by correcting relative hypovolemia with appropriate intravenous fluid administration. • Elevate lower extremities 20–30° from horizontal position if hypotension is severe. • During this period, augment spontaneous ventilation initially by manual ventilation (using technique which maintains synchrony with the patient's varying inspiratory efforts.
	Sudden "relative hypovolemia" may occur because the patient cannot mobilize extravascular fluid rapidly. Positive ventilator pressure increases intrathoracic pressure and accentuates interference with venous return.	• Make sure the manual ventilation bag is capable of providing adequate FiO_2 delivery to meet the patient's requirements. • Place patient on ventilator when relaxed. Shorten inspiratory time or increase peak flow setting as necessary to simulate normal breathing pattern. • Monitor vital signs, hemodynamic parameters, if pulmonary artery catheter in place, including: (1) arterial-venous oxygen content difference and CO measurements (aids assessment of perfusion and oxygen extraction); (2) intrapulmonary shunt calculations (aids assessment of pulmonary effects of

(continued)

Problem	Causes	Management
		PEEP); and (3) pulmonary artery occlusion pressures (aids in the assessment of intravascular fluid administration). Notify physician of abnormalities.
	Patients with airflow obstruction may trap air so that alveolar pressure remains positive at end-expiration, even when PEEP is not applied intentionally. This "autoPEEP" effect can cause increased intrathoracic pressure and severely depress CO. It is a result of inadequate expiratory time.	• Evaluate auto-PEEP in patients with airflow obstruction (performed by pressing end-expiration hold button on some ventilators). If auto-PEEP is present the baseline pressure (0 or existing set PEEP level) will elevate reflecting the amount of auto-PEEP. No spontaneous respiratory efforts should be present nor any gas flow from a supplemental source, such as that used with medication nebulization.
		• Treat hemodynamic effects of auto-PEEP by measures that lower mean intrathoracic pressure.
		– Adjust inspiratory time or peak flow setting to allow maximal time for exhalation between cycles (shorten inspiratory time or increase peak flow) and to avoid progressive increases in end-expiratory lung volume.
		– Reduce minute ventilation to minimal amount consistent with acceptable pH.
		– Manage fever, agitation, metabolic acidosis, to diminish ventilatory requirements.
		– Continue medical therapy for treatment of airflow obstruction.
		• Administer fluids to correct hypovolemia.
		• Administer inotropic agents as necessary.
	Level of PEEP is high yet still required to assure adequate oxygenation with Fio_2 levels >0.5.	• Use the lowest of PEEP necessary to correct severe hypoxemia while allowing a reduction of the Fio_2.
		• Provide PEEP if an Fio_2 of >0.5 is required for more than 24 hours to achieve a Pao_2 >50–60 mm Hg.
		• "Lung recruitment" in ARDs requires that PEEP levels that "open" and "keep-open" the lung be maintained. Different methods of applying PEEP may be used to accomplish this goal (see Chapter 20).
	Ventilator Related Positive pressure ventilation and PEEP may decrease CO by impeding venous return, which decreases right and subsequently left ventricular stroke volume. Other factors proposed may include release of humoral substances during lung expansion, which depress left ventricular function and CO reduction secondary to endocardial blood supply impairment. Factors that may increase positive intrathoracic pressure and mean airway pressure include high V_t PEEP, continuous mechanical ventilation, and increased respiratory rate (more positive pressure).	• May need to decrease V_t to avoid high peak inspiratory pressures.
		• If pressure mode, may need to decrease pressure level to decrease V_t.
		• Use V_t and PEEP that maintain "optimal compliance."
		• May try shortening inspiratory time or increasing peak flow to shorten the amount of time that positive pressure remains in the thorax.
		• Use lowest PEEP level necessary to meet therapeutic goal.
		• Increase Fio_2 and remove PEEP as necessary until the patient is hemodynamically stable or fluids and vasopressors may be used.
	A higher intrapleural pressure and lower CO may be produced when PEEP is used with control modes of ventilation.	• Modes that allow spontaneous breathing may enhance venous return and CO.

Abbreviations: ARDS, acute respiratory distress syndrome; CNS, central nervous system; CO, cardiac output; COPD, chronic obstructive pulmonary disease; CPAP, continuous positive airway pressure; CVP, central venous pressure; Fio_2, percentage of inspired oxygen; IMV, intermittent mandatory ventilation; PAOP, pulmonary artery occlusion pressure; PEEP, positive end-expiratory pressure, V_t, tidal volume.

Problem	Causes	Management
Anxiety and Fear	**Patient Related** Decreased ability to communicate because of tracheostomy/endotracheal tube. Fear of unknown, unfamiliar environment and people.	• Assess most effective method(s) of communication: paper and pencil, lip reading, gestures, alphabet board, cards indicating major needs, and electric larynx. Communicate method on care plan. • Ask "yes and no" questions. • Keep call light in reach at all times. • Obtain assistance if unable to interpret communications. Use touch to ease frustrations. • Evaluate and manage psychosocial factors that may be creating anxiety and fear. • Convey calm, confident, reassuring approach. • Explain all procedures; allow patient participation in decisions to the extent possible. • Maintain familiarity in environment (family visits, significant personal belongings, radio, television, clock, consistency in personnel caring for patient).
	Effects of surgery or various other interventions, which create discomfort, pain. Decreased arterial oxygenation related to suctioning.	• Identify factors creating discomfort, pain, shortness of breath, and implement measures to modify or resolve problem. • See Low Pa_{O_2} and Arrhythmias during suctioning.
	Ventilator Related Ventilator settings not optimally adjusted to meet patient's needs. Air leaks causing patient to receive inadequate ventilation, oxygenation; incorrect settings.	• Assess whether ventilator is optimally adjusted to meet patient's needs. Readjust flow rate setting higher or inspiratory time shorter as necessary to match faster breathing pattern. • Evaluate whether prescribed V_t is being delivered and whether settings are correct. Manually ventilate as necessary. • Efficiently identify and correct problem using a calm, confident approach.

Arrhythmias During or After Suctioning	**Patient Related**
	Suctioning induces arterial desaturation. Other adverse effects include bronchoconstriction, vasovagal reactions, cardiac arrhythmias, unexplained cardiovascular collapse, and sudden death.
	
	There are considerable differences in the rate of fall in oxygen tension. Variables affecting the degree of hypoxemia include: (1) the ratio of suction catheter size to endotracheal tube size, (2) the duration of suctioning, (3) whether or not hyperoxygenation was performed before or after suctioning, (4) the patient's initial Pa_{O_2}, (5) the magnitude of pulmonary shunt, (6) suction induced alveolar collapse, and (7) the ability to breathe spontaneously.
		• Implement measures to minimize or prevent suction related hypoxemia and vagal reactions:
		  – Assess need for suctioning. Suction only as necessary, not on a "routine" basis.
		  – Use catheter no greater than half the internal diameter of the tube through which it is passed.
		  – Inform patient that you will be suctioning.
		  – Insert catheter without applying suction.
		  – Spend <15 sec total time off ventilator. Limit applied suction time to 10 sec.
		  – Administer hyperoxygenation (100% O_2) with a manual resuscitation bag or the ventilator for 3–5 breaths before and after each suctioning pass.
		  – Use ventilator for hyperoxygenation when PEEP >10 cm H_2O or when removal from ventilator results in distress or hypoxemia.
		  – Monitor blood pressure, heart rate, rhythm during suctioning procedures. If arrhythmias or significant changes in heart rate occur, discontinue suctioning and ventilate patient immediately using 100% O_2 for several breaths. Be certain that vital signs have recovered to baseline values before repeating suction process.
		  – Modify procedure for pre- and post-hyperoxygenation to fit the individual patient's physiologic requirements.
		• Assess whether an increase in Fi_{O_2} or mechanical hyperinflation with oxygen is needed to raise the Pa_{O_2} to a sufficient level. If mechanical hyperinflation is needed, avoid large changes in pH (respiratory alkalosis) which may produce hazards related to myocardial and central nervous system excitability.

(continued)

Problem	Causes	Management
	Large lung volumes have been reported to cause bradycardia and hypotension.	• Stop hyperinflation if serious hypotension or bradycardia is observed. • Be knowledgeable about oxygen delivery performance of resuscitation bag or device used (oxygen delivery varies with different types). If the FiO_2 is increased on the ventilator, keep in mind that a variable lag time will elapse before the patient receives the increased oxygen concentration because of the "washout" time of the ventilator. • Keep patient on the ventilator during hemodynamic pressure measurements. • Consider use of closed suction catheter systems that allow the patient to remain on the ventilator during suctioning. *Note:* May produce smaller decreases in PaO_2 than does suctioning when the ventilator is removed.
	Receptors for the vagus nerve are found throughout the tracheobronchial tree, to the level of the carina. Stimulation of this nerve produces slowing of the heart rate. Positive pressure ventilation increases intrathoracic pressures and sometimes stimulates a Valsalva maneuver. Increased intrathoracic pressure that occurs during Valsalva's maneuver (coughing, vomiting, defecating) causes rapid changes in preload and afterload. Venous return to the heart is decreased and systolic and pulse pressures decrease. Paroxysms of coughing without taking a deep breath are Valsalva strains at high expiratory pressures.	• Monitor blood pressure and heart rate during suctioning procedure. Discontinue suctioning if significant decrease in blood pressure and heart rate occurs and ventilate patient. • Be alert to potential complications related to coughing, etc. Monitor for slowing of heart rate, decreased blood pressure. • Withdraw the catheter from the trachea as quickly as possible following a suctioning procedure.
Incorrect PEEP Setting	**Patient Related** Air leak in patient (cuff site) or ventilator system causing inability to maintain end-expiratory pressure.	• Evaluate and correct air leaks (see Low/No Exhaled Volume). • Recheck PEEP value after leak is corrected, readjust PEEP as necessary.
	Ventilator Related PEEP incorrectly set on machine.	• Assess whether PEEP is correctly set. Reset as necessary.
Pneumothorax/Tension Pneumothorax	**Patient Related** Underlying lung pathology (COPD, emphysematous blebs, lung surgery), which makes some persons more susceptible to the effects of positive pressure.	

	Ventilator Related
	Positive pressure created by ventilator, which causes pulmonary barotrauma. High-volume or high-pressure settings, PEEP.
		• Judicious use of PEEP.
		• Maintain minimal PEEP levels necessary for adequate oxygenation.
		• Use low volume, low rate ventilation in those at risk of barotrauma.
		• Monitor for signs, symptoms of pneumothorax, tension pneumothorax. Notify physician of abnormalities.
		• If symptoms are mild, obtain chest x-ray film and notify physician immediately.
		• If tension pneumothorax occurs:
		  – disconnect patient from ventilator and ventilate with manual resuscitation bag
		  – increase FiO_2 to 1.0

Abbreviations: ARDS, acute respiratory distress syndrome; CNS, central nervous system; CO, cardiac output; COPD, chronic obstructive pulmonary disease; CPAP, continuous positive airway pressure; CVP, central venous pressure; FiO_2, percentage of inspired oxygen; IMV, intermittent mandatory ventilation; PAOP, pulmonary artery occlusion pressure; PEEP, positive end-expiratory pressure, V_t, tidal volume.

Problem	Causes	Management
		– have someone else notify physician immediately, prepare chest tube insertion equipment for immediate use and set up chest drainage unit
		– have a large-bore needle ready for insertion as a life-saving maneuver for tension pneumothorax. *Note:* A medium- or large-bore needle is inserted into the affected hemithorax anteriorly through the second or third interspace in the midclavicular line. The needle should pass through the middle of the interspace to avoid intercostal blood vessels.
		• Increase fluids to maintain blood pressure.
		• Reassure and remain with the patient.
		• Obtain chest x-ray film.
		• Monitor oxygenation and saturation hourly until stable.
Inability to Tolerate Mode of Ventilation	**Patient Related** Increased work of breathing from various physiologic factors that increase airway resistance, decrease lung compliance, decrease respiratory muscle strength, endurance or alter mechanics of breathing, includes: Secretions, respiratory muscle fatigue, infections, pleural effusions, inappropriate ventilator settings.	• Support on ventilator mode that provides patient comfort. • Suction airway as necessary. Provide call light so that capable patient can inform of need. • Rest the respiratory muscles for 12–24 hours (see Chapter 20). • Provide medications as ordered for management of respiratory infection.
	• Narrowed airway because of endotracheal tube. Airway resistance increases threefold and the work of breathing almost twofold with decreasing tube diameter.	• Consider endotracheal tube diameter as one of the factors that may increase airway resistance and work of breathing during spontaneous breathing. • Change to different mode of ventilation or add pressure support if it provides breathing comfort. • Weaning trials of spontaneous breathing (i.e., CPAP or T-piece) should not be excessively long. Generally 30 minutes to 2 hours is adequate.
	• Brochospasm. • Certain positions, which provide less than optimal ventilation–perfusion matching. • Acute or chronic lung disorder, or both.	• Evaluate, treat bronchospasm. • Place in positions that maximize ventilation and breathing comfort (usually with head of bed elevated). • Evaluate whether the patient is physiologically stable enough to be weaned.
	• Excessive sedative or narcotic use. • Decreased respiratory muscle strength and endurance from effects of malnutrition.	• Provide necessary ventilator support for goals of breathing comfort, ability to rest and sleep, and maintain normal ventilation, oxygenation. Changing the mode of ventilation may help. • Obtain nutrition consult (see Chapter 9).
	Increased carbon dioxide production from excessive caloric intake (see Respiratory Acidosis).	• Support patient on the ventilatory mode, which provides respiratory comfort, usually assist/control mode. • Thoroughly assess and correct any physiologic and equipment factors interfering with success. • Protocols are effective tools for weaning trials. Adhere to signs of tolerance/intolerance and duration of trial (see Chapter 20).
	Ventilator Related Various equipment factors can significantly increase resistance and work of breathing, which result in signs and symptoms of respiratory distress.	• Evaluate patient comfort and synchrony with the ventilator. If unable to determine etiology of respiratory distress, bag the patient and work with respiratory therapist to determine and correct cause.
	Deleterious effects on hemodynamic status may occur when patients with poor ventricular function are changed from controlled mechanical ventilation to spontaneous breathing modes (e.g., CPAP). Oxygen consumption can increase significantly.	• Monitor for deleterious effects of partial ventilator support on hemodynamic status, particularly in some patients, such as those with cardiac problems.

(*continued*)

Problem	Causes	Management
	Myocardial ischemia has been shown to occur more often on CPAP versus full ventilator support. Mechanical ventilator support may be beneficial to the failing heart in several ways: optimizes left ventricular end-diastolic volume (increases intrapleural pressure, which decreases right heart preload; increased airway pressure may restrict left ventricular filling); in clinical states of compromised oxygen delivery (cardiogenic shock), full ventilatory support may decrease inspiratory oxygen demands and release oxygen for use by other systems; patients can be safely sedated and sympathetic outflow is decreased, which prevents hypertension and tachycardia thereby decreasing left ventricular strain.	• In the presence of cardiogenic shock, provide optimum ventilator support to decrease inspiratory oxygen demands.
	Kinked tubing, obstruction of tubing with water.	• Drape tubing to avoid kinks and optimum drainage of water into water traps. Empty water from tubing every 2 hours or more frequently as indicated by assessment.
	Setting incorrectly calculated, set on machine.	• Evaluate whether IMV settings are correctly set on ventilator. Correct errors or notify respiratory therapist.
	Inappropriate inspiratory time or flow rate setting.	• Evaluate for appropriate inspiratory time or peak flow setting by observing chest expansion on positive pressure breaths. (Rapid rise of the chest and airway pressure manometer may be indicators that the inspiratory time is too short or peak flow too fast.) Notify respiratory therapist or make appropriate inspiratory time or peak flow adjustments.
	Not receiving prescribed V_t because of air leaks in ventilator system or cuff.	• Correct leaks (described earlier). • Switch to assist/control mode as necessary. If ready for weaning, use PSV or other spontaneous method (CPAP or T-piece).

Cardiac Rhythms, ECG Characteristics, and Treatment Guide

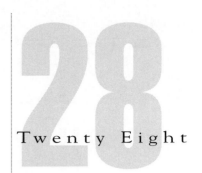

Twenty Eight

Carol Jacobson

Rhythm	ECG Characteristics	ECG Sample	Treatment
Normal sinus rhythm (NSR)	• Rate: 60–100 beats/min • Rhythm: Regular • P waves: Precede every QRS; consistent shape • PR Interval: 0.12–0.20 sec • QRS complex: 0.04–0.10 sec		• None
Sinus bradycardia	• Rate: <60 beats/min • Rhythm: Regular • P waves: Precede every QRS; consistent shape • PR interval: Usually normal (0.12–0.20 sec) • QRS complex: Usually normal (0.04–0.10 sec) • Conduction: Normal through atria, AV node, bundle branches, and ventricles		• Treat only if symptomatic. • Atropine 0.5–1 mg IV.
Sinus tachycardia	• Rate: >100 beats/min • Rhythm: Regular • P waves: Precede every QRS; consistent shape • PR interval: Usually normal (0.12–0.20 sec); may be difficult to measure if P waves are buried in T waves • QRS complex: Usually normal (0.04–0.10 sec) • Conduction: Normal through atria, AV node, bundle branches, and ventricles		• Treat underlying cause.
Sinus arrhythmia	• Rate: 60–100 beats/min • Rhythm: Irregular; phasic increase and decrease in rate, which may or may not be related to respiration • P waves: Precede every QRS; consistent shape • PR interval: Usually normal • QRS complex: Usually normal • Conduction: Normal through atria, AV node, bundle branches, and ventricles		• Treatment usually not required. • Hold digoxin if due to digitalis toxicity.
Sinus arrest	• Rate: Usually within normal range, but may be in the bradycardia range • Rhythm: Irregular due to absence of sinus node discharge • P waves: Present when sinus node is firing and absent during periods of sinus arrest. When present, they precede every QRS complex and are consistent in shape. • PR interval: Usually normal when P waves are present • QRS complex: Usually normal when sinus node is functioning and absent during periods of sinus arrest, unless escape beats occur. • Conduction: Normal through atria, AV node, bundle branches, and ventricles when sinus node is firing. When the sinus node fails to form impulses, there is no conduction through the atria.		• Treat underlying cause. • Discontinue drugs that may be causative. • Minimize vagal stimulation. • For frequent sinus arrest causing hemodynamic compromise, atropine 0.5–1 mg IV may increase heart rate. • Pacemaker may be necessary for refractory cases.

(continued)

(continued)

Premature atrial contraction

- Rate: Usually within normal range
- Rhythm: Usually regular except when PACs occur, resulting in early beats. PACs usually have a noncompensatory pause.
- P waves: Precede every QRS. The configuration of the premature P wave differs from that of the sinus P waves.
- PR interval: May be normal or long depending on the prematurity of the beat. Very early PACs may find the AV junction still partially refractory and unable to conduct at a normal rate, resulting in a prolonged PR interval.
- QRS complex: May be normal, aberrant (wide), or absent, depending on the prematurity of the beat.
- Conduction: PACs travel through the atria differently from sinus impulses because they originate from a different spot. Conduction through the AV node, bundle branches, and ventricles is usually normal unless the PAC is very early.

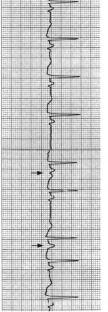

PACs conducted normally in the ventricle.

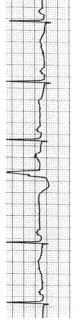

PAC conducted abnormally in the ventricle.

Treatment:
- Treatment usually not necessary.
- Treat underlying cause.
- Drugs (e.g., beta-blockers, calcium channel blockers, procainamide) can be used if necessary.

Wandering atrial pacemaker

- Rate: 60–100 beats/min. If the rate is faster than 100 beats/minute, it is called *multifocal atrial tachycardia* (MAT).
- Rhythm: May be slightly irregular.
- P waves: Varying shapes (upright, flat, inverted, notched) as impulses originate in different parts of the atria or junction. At least three different P-wave shapes should be seen.
- PR interval: May vary depending on proximity of the pacemaker to the AV node.
- QRS complex: Usually normal
- Conduction: Conduction through the atria varies as they are depolarized from different spots. Conduction through the bundle branches and ventricles is usually normal.

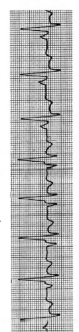

Treatment:
- Treatment usually not necessary.
- Treat underlying cause.
- For symptoms from slow rate can use atropine.
- Anti-arrhythmic therapy often ineffective, but beta-blockers, verapamil, flecainide, amiodarone, or magnesium may be successful.

Atrial tachycardia

- Rate: Atrial rate is 150–250 beats/min.
- Rhythm: Regular unless there is variable block at the AV node.
- P waves: Differ in shape from sinus P waves because they are ectopic. Precede each QRS complex but may be hidden in preceding T wave. When block is present, more than one P wave appears before each QRS complex.
- PR interval: May be shorter than normal but often difficult to measure because of hidden P waves.
- QRS complex: Usually normal but may be wide if aberrant conduction is present.
- Conduction: Usually normal through the AV node and into the ventricles. In atrial tachycardia with block some atrial impulses do not conduct into the ventricles. Aberrant ventricular conduction may occur if atrial impulses are conducted into the

Treatment:
- Eliminate underlying cause and decrease ventricular rate.
- Sedation.
- Vagal stimulation.
- Digitalis (unless it is the cause of atrial tachycardia with block).
- Propranolol, verapamil, or diltiazem.
- Cardioversion for significant symptoms.
- Procainamide, flecainide, amiodarone may be effective to prevent recurrences.
- Radiofrequency ablation often successful.

Rhythm	ECG Characteristics	ECG Sample	Treatment
Atrial flutter	ventricles while the ventricles are still partially refractory. • Rate: Atrial rate varies between 250 and 350 beats/min, most commonly 300. Ventricular rate varies depending on the amount of block at the AV node, most commonly 150 beats/min and rarely 300 beats/min. • Rhythm: Atrial rhythm is regular. Ventricular rhythm may be regular or irregular due to varying AV block. • P waves: F waves (flutter waves) are seen, characterized by a very regular, "sawtooth" pattern. One F wave is usually hidden in the QRS complex, and when 2:1 conduction occurs, F waves may not be readily apparent. • FR interval (flutter wave to the beginning of the QRS complex): May be consistent or may vary. • QRS complex: Usually normal; aberration can occur. • Conduction: Usually normal through the AV node and ventricles.	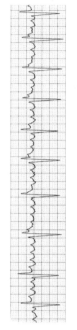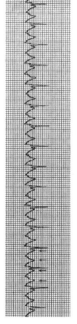	• Treatment depends on hemodynamic consequences of arrhythmia. • Cardioversion for markedly reduced cardiac output. • Beta-blockers, calcium channel blockers to slow ventricular rate. • Procainamide, flecainide, amiodarone, ibutilide, dofetilide, sotalol may convert to sinus. • Use drugs that slow atrial rate (procainamide, flecainide, propafenone) *only* after prior treatment to ensure AV block (e.g., beta-blockers, calcium channel blockers). • Radiofrequency ablation usually successful.
Atrial fibrillation	• Rate: Atrial rate is 400–600 beats/min or faster. Ventricular rate varies depending on the amount of block at the AV node. In new atrial fibrillation, the ventricular response is usually quite rapid, 160–200 beats/min; in treated atrial fibrillation, the ventricular rate is controlled in the normal range of 60–100 beats/min. • Rhythm: Irregular. One of the distinguishing features of atrial fibrillation is the marked irregularity of the ventricular response. • P waves: Not present. Atrial activity is chaotic with no formed atrial impulses visible. Irregular f waves are often seen and vary in size from coarse to very fine. • PR interval: Not measurable; there are no P waves. • QRS complex: Usually normal; aberration is common. • Conduction: Conduction within the atria is disorganized and follows a very irregular pattern. Most of the atrial impulses are blocked within the AV junction. Those impulses that are conducted through the AV junction are usually conducted normally through the ventricles. If an atrial impulse reaches the bundle branch system during its refractory period, aberrant intraventricular conduction can occur.	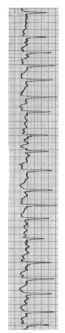	• Cardiovert if hemodynamically unstable. • Calcium channel blockers and beta-blockers to slow ventricular rate. Procainamide, flecainide, propafenone, amiodarone, sotalol, ibutilide, dofetilide to convert to sinus. • Radiofrequency ablation may be successful.

(continued)

Premature junctional complexes

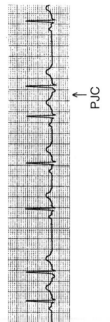

↑
PJC

- Rate: 60–100 beats/min or whatever the rate of the basic rhythm.
- Rhythm: Regular except for occurrence of premature beats.
- P waves: May occur before, during, or after the QRS complex of the premature beat and are usually inverted.
- PR interval: Short, usually 0.10 sec or less, when P waves precede the QRS.
- QRS complex: Usually normal but may be aberrant if the PJC occurs very early and conducts into the ventricles during the refractory period of a bundle branch.
- Conduction: Retrograde through the atria; usually normal through the ventricles.

- Treatment usually not necessary.

Junctional rhythm

- Rate: Junctional rhythm, 40–60 beats/min; accelerated junctional rhythm, 60–100 beats/min; junctional tachycardia, 100–250 beats/min.
- Rhythm: Regular.
- P waves: May precede or follow QRS.
- PR interval: Short, 0.11 sec or less if P waves precede QRS.
- QRS complex: Usually normal.
- Conduction: Retrograde through the atria; normal through the ventricles.

- Treatment rarely needed unless rate too slow or too fast to maintain adequate CO.
- Atropine used to increase rate.
- Verapamil, propranolol, or digitalis used to decrease rate.
- Cardioversion for rapid rate with severely reduced CO.
- Withhold digitalis if digitalis toxicity suspected.

Premature ventricular complexes

- Rate: 60–100 beats/min or the rate of the basic rhythm.
- Rhythm: Irregular because of the early beats.
- P waves: Not related to the PVCs. Sinus rhythm is usually not interrupted by the premature beats, so sinus P waves can often be seen occurring regularly throughout the rhythm.
- PR interval: Not present before most PVCs. If a P wave happens, by coincidence, to precede a PVC, the PR interval is short.
- QRS complex: Wide and bizarre; greater than 0.10 sec in duration. May vary in morphology (size, shape) if they originate from more than one focus in the ventricles.
- Conduction: Wide QRS complexes. Some PVCs may conduct retrograde into the atria, resulting in inverted P waves following the PVC.

- Eliminate underlying cause.
- Drug therapy not usually used, but if desired, lidocaine, amiodarone, procainamide, beta-blockers may be effective.

(continued)

Rhythm	ECG Characteristics	ECG Sample	Treatment
Ventricular rhythm	• Rate: <50 beats/min for ventricular rhythm and 50–100 beats/min for accelerated ventricular rhythm. • Rhythm: Usually regular. • P waves: May be seen but at a slower rate than the ventricular focus, with dissociation from the QRS. • PR interval: Not measured. • QRS complex: Wide and bizarre. • Conduction: If sinus rhythm is the basic rhythm, atrial conduction is normal. Impulses originating in the ventricles conduct via muscle cell-to-cell conduction, resulting in the wide QRS complex.		• For ventricular escape rhythms, atropine to increase sinus rate and overdrive ventricular rhythm. • Ventricular pacing to increase ventricular rate if escape rhythm is too slow.
Ventricular tachycardia	• Rate: Ventricular rate is faster than 100 beats/min. • Rhythm: Usually regular but may be slightly irregular. • P waves: P waves may be seen but will not be related to QRS complexes (dissociated from QRS complexes). If sinus rhythm is the underlying basic rhythm, regular P waves are often buried within QRS complexes. • PR interval: Not measurable because of dissociation of P waves from QRS complexes. • QRS complex: Wide and bizarre; >0.10 sec in duration. • Conduction: Impulse originates in one ventricle and spreads via muscle cell-to-cell conduction through both ventricles. There may be retrograde conduction through the atria, but more often the sinus node continues to fire regularly and depolarize the atria normally.		• Treatment depends on how rhythm is tolerated. • Lidocaine, amiodarone, procainamide, or magnesium if patient is stable. • Cardioversion for hemodynamic instability. • Defibrillation if VT is pulseless.
Ventricular fibrillation	• Rate: Rapid, uncoordinated, ineffective. • Rhythm: Chaotic, irregular. • P waves: None seen. • PR interval: None. • QRS complex: No formed QRS complexes seen; rapid, irregular undulations without any specific pattern. • Conduction: Multiple ectopic foci firing simultaneously in ventricles and depolarizing them irregularly and without any organized pattern. Ventricles are not contracting.	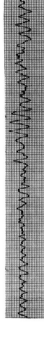	• Immediate defibrillation. • CPR required until defibrillator available. • Lidocaine, amiodarone, procainamide, magnesium commonly used. • After conversion, use IV anti-arrhythmic that facilitated conversion to prevent recurrence.

(continued)

Ventricular asystole

- Rate: None.
- Rhythm: None.
- P waves: May be present if the sinus node is functioning.
- PR interval: None.
- QRS complex: None.
- Conduction: Atrial conduction may be normal if the sinus node is functioning. There is no conduction into the ventricles.

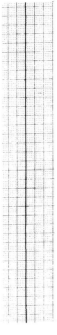

- Immediate CPR.
- IV epinephrine.
- Atropine.
- Pacemaker.

First-degree AV block

- Rate: Can occur at any sinus rate, usually 60–100 beats/min.
- Rhythm: Regular.
- P waves: Normal; precede every QRS.
- PR interval: Prolonged above 0.20 sec.
- QRS complex: Usually normal.
- Conduction: Normal through the atria, usually delayed through the AV node. Ventricular conduction is normal.

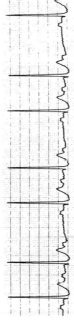

- Treatment usually not necessary.

Second-degree AV block type I (Wenckebach; Mobitz I)

- Rate: Can occur at any sinus or atrial rate.
- Rhythm: Irregular. Overall appearance of the rhythm demonstrates "group beating."
- P waves: Normal. Some P waves are not conducted to the ventricles, but only one at a time fails to conduct to the ventricle.
- PR interval: Gradually lengthens in consecutive beats. The PR interval preceding the pause is longer than that following the pause.
- QRS complex: Usually normal unless there is associated bundle branch block.
- Conduction: Normal through the atria, progressively delayed through the AV node until an impulse fails. Conduction ratios can vary, with ratios as low as 2:1 (every other P wave is blocked), up to high ratios such as 15:14 (every fifteenth P wave blocked).

- Treatment depends on conduction ratio, ventricular rate, and symptoms.
- Atropine used for slow ventricular rate.
- No treatment with normal ventricular rate.
- Discontinue digitalis, beta-blockers, and calcium channel blockers.
- Temporary pacemaker may be needed for slow ventricular rate.

(continued)

557

Rhythm	ECG Characteristics	ECG Sample	Treatment
Second-degree AV block type II (Mobitz II)	• Rate: Can occur at any basic rate. • Rhythm: Irregular due to blocked beats. • P waves: Usually regular and precede each QRS. Periodically a P wave is not followed by a QRS complex. • PR interval: Constant before conducted beats. The PR interval preceding the pause is the same as that following the pause. • QRS complex: Usually wide due to associated bundle branch block. • Conduction: Normal through the atria and through the AV node but intermittently blocked in the bundle branch system and fails to reach the ventricles. Conduction through the ventricles is abnormally slow due to associated bundle branch block. Conduction ratios can vary from 2:1 to only occasional blocked beats.		• Pacemaker often needed. • CPR for slow rate and severely decreased cardiac output. • Atropine usually not effective.
High AV block	• Rate: Atrial rate less than 135 beats/min. • Rhythm: Regular or irregular, depending on conduction pattern. • P waves: Normal; present before every conducted QRS, but two or more consecutive P waves may not be followed by QRS complexes. • PR interval: Constant before conducted beats; may be normal or prolonged. • QRS complex: Usually normal in type I and wide in type II advanced blocks. • Conduction: Normal through the atria. Two or more consecutive atrial impulses fail to conduct to the ventricles. Ventricular conduction is normal in type I and abnormally slow in type II advanced blocks.		• Treatment necessary if patient is symptomatic. • Atropine may increase ventricular rate. • Pacemaker often required.
Third-degree AV block	• Rate: Atrial rate is usually normal; ventricular rate is <45 beats/min. • Rhythm: Regular. • P waves: Normal but dissociated from QRS complexes. • PR interval: No consistent PR intervals because there is no relationship between P waves and QRS complexes. • QRS complex: Normal if ventricles controlled by a junctional rhythm; wide if controlled by a ventricular rhythm. • Conduction: Normal through the atria. All impulses are blocked at the AV node or in the bundle branches, so there is no conduction to the ventricles. Conduction through the ventricles is normal if a junctional escape rhythm occurs, and abnormally slow if a ventricular escape rhythm occurs.		• Pacemaker. • Atropine usually not effective. • With severely decreased cardiac output, perform CPR until pacemaker available.

(continued)

Ventricular paced rhythm with capture

- Rate: Depends on type of pacemaker.
- Rhythm: Regular.
- P waves: Absent, or present but dissociated from QRS complexes.
- PR interval: None.
- QRS complex: Pacemaker spike followed immediately by wide, bizarre QRS complex.

- None.

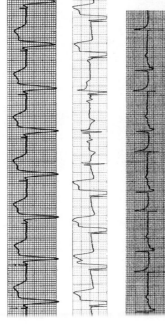

Ventricular paced rhythm without capture

- Conduction: Abnormal.
- ECG characteristics depend on nature of intrinsic rhythm.
- Pacemaker spike has no fixed relationship to QRS complexes.

- If hemodynamically stable, elective correction/replacement of pacemaker.
- If hemodynamically unstable, treatment as for third-degree AV block.

Index

AACN (American Association of Critical-Care Nurses), 199–200
ABCDE acronym, 4–6, 4t
Abciximab
administration guidelines, 505t
Abdominal trauma
etiology and pathophysiology, 380–381
management, 381
Absence seizures, 300
Accelerated hypertension, 243
Accelerated junctional rhythm, 50, 50f
Accelerated ventricular rhythm, 51–52, 52f
Acetazolamide
administration guidelines, 505t
Acidemia, 113–115
ACLS (universal advanced cardiac life support), algorithm for, 520f
Activated coagulation time, 307
Activated partial thromboplastin time (APTT), 307
Activated protein C (drotrecogin alfa), 185
Acute coronary syndromes (ACS), 218, 221
Acute hypoglycemia
clinical presentation, 364–365
etiology, risk factors, and pathophysiology, 364, 364t
following traumatic brain injury, 484
management, 365, 365t
overview, 364
Acute ischemic heart disease
alleviating pain, 228
clinical presentation, 221–222, 226t–227t
diagnostic tests
myocardial infarction, 222–223
unstable angina, 222, 228f
etiology and pathophysiology, 218–221, 223f–224f, 224t
management
medical, 224, 230f, 230t–231t
principles, 223–224, 228t, 229f
surgical, 224–225, 231f
overview, 218
preventing complications associated with coronary obstruction, 225, 228
reducing anxiety, 228–229
Acute ischemic stroke
clinical presentation

cerebellar or brainstem stroke, 297
stroke in a cerebral hemisphere, 297
diagnostic tests, 297
etiology, risk factors, and pathophysiology
embolism, 297
overview, 296
thrombosis, 296
management, 297–299, 298t–299t
Acute pancreatitis
clinical presentation, 329
diagnostic tests, 329
etiologies, risk factors, and pathophysiology, 329, 329t
imaging studies, 329
management
fluid resuscitation, 330
pain management, 330
rest the pancreas, 330
treat local complications in the pancreas, 330
treat multisystem failure, 330–331
overview, 329
Acute renal failure (ARF)
clinical presentation, 344
diagnostic tests, 344
etiology, risk factors, and pathophysiology, 341–343, 342t
management
correction of fluid imbalance, 344–345, 344t
improving nutritional status, 345–346
overview, 344
preventing additional kidney damage, 345
preventing and treating infection, 345
preventing and treating life-threatening electrolyte imbalances, 345
treating acidosis, 345
overview, 341
Acute respiratory distress syndrome (ARDS), 384–385
clinical presentation, 257
etiology, risk factors, and pathophysiology, 256–257, 257t
management, 257–258
overview, 256
recent studies on, 463–464

Acute respiratory failure
clinical presentation, 255
etiology, risk factors, and pathophysiology, 253–255, 254t
airway obstruction, 254, 254f
impaired gas exchange, 253–254, 254f
impaired ventilation, 253
ventilation–perfusion abnormalities, 254–255, 255f
management, 255–256
overview, 252–253
in patients with COPD
clinical presentation, 258
etiology, risk factors, and pathophysiology, 258, 258t
management, 259–260, 259t
overview, 258
Acute upper GI bleeding
clinical presentation, 319–320
diagnostic tests, 320
etiology, risk factors, and pathophysiology, 317–319, 318t–319t, 319f–320f
management
hemodynamic stabilization, 320–321, 321t
identify bleeding site, 321
institute therapies to control or stop bleeding, 321–323, 322f, 323t
newer therapies to control bleeding, 324
overview, 320
reducing anxiety, 324–325
surgical therapies to stop bleeding, 323–324, 323f–324f
overview, 317
Acyclovir
administration guidelines, 505t
Adenosine, 182
administration guidelines, 505t, 517t
Admission
comprehensive assessment. See Comprehensive admission assessment
quick check assessment
airway and breathing, 6
chief complaint, 6
circulation and cerebral perfusion, 6
drugs and diagnostic tests, 6–7, 7t
equipment, 7, 7t
overview, 5–6

Advanced concepts in caring for critically ill patient
  advanced cardiovascular concepts. *See* Cardiovascular concepts, advanced
  advanced ECG concepts. *See* ECG concepts, advanced
  advanced neurologic concepts. *See* Neurologic concepts, advanced
  advanced respiratory concepts. *See* Respiratory concepts, advanced
Afterload, 70–72, 104–105, 105*t*
Air emboli, 263
Airway and ventilatory management
  airway management
    artificial airways
      cuff inflation, 122–123
      cuff pressure measurement, 123–124, 123*f*
      endotracheal suctioning, 124–125, 124*t*
      extubation, 125
      insertion, 121–122, 121*f*–122*f*
      overview, 120
      types, 120–121, 120*f*
    nasopharyngeal airway
      combitube, 120
      laryngeal mask airway (LMA), 120
      overview, 120
    oropharyngeal airway, 118–119, 119*f*
    overview, 118
  basic ventilatory management
    communication
      alphabet board/picture board, 140
      common problems, 139
      gesturing, 140
      nonvocal treatments, 139
      overview, 139
      teaching communication methods, 141
      vocal treatments, 140–141, 140*f*–141*f*
      writing, 139–140
    complications
      barotrauma, 135
      hemodynamic compromise, 135
      overview, 135
      positive fluid balance and hyponatremia, 135–136
      upper GI hemorrhage, 136
      ventilator-associated pneumonia, 135, 136*f*
      ventilator malfunction, 136
      volutrauma, 135
    general principles
      overview, 129–130, 130*f*
      patient-ventilator system, 130, 131*f*
      ventilator control panel, 131–132, 132*f*–133*f*
      ventilator tubing circuit, 130–131
    indications, 129, 129*t*
    modes
      assist-control ventilation, 133–134
      control ventilation, 132–133
      overview, 132
      PEEP/CPAP, 134
      pressure support, 134
      spontaneous breathing, 134
      synchronized intermittent mandatory ventilation (SIMV), 134

    principles of management
      maximizing communication, 142
      maximizing oxygenation and ventilation, 141–142
      preventing complications, 42
      reducing anxiety and providing psychosocial support, 142–143
    troubleshooting ventilators, 138–139, 138*f*
    weaning from short-term mechanical ventilation
      methods, 137–138
      overview, 136
      readiness assessment, 136–137, 137*t*
      weaning trials, 137
  oxygen therapy
    complications
      absorption atelectasis, 127
      alveolar hypoventilation, 125, 127
      overview, 125
      oxygen toxicity, 127
    overview, 125, 125*t*
    oxygen delivery
      invasive devices
        manual resuscitation bags, 127
        mechanical ventilators, 127
        T-piece, 128–129
        tracheal gas insufflation (TGI), 128
        transtracheal oxygen therapy, 128–129
      noninvasive devices, 126*f*, 127
  respiratory assessment techniques, diagnostic tests, and monitoring systems
    arterial blood gas (ABG) monitoring
      analysis
        acid–base analysis, 113–115, 114*t*
        overview, 112–113
        oxygenation, 115–116, 115*f*
      overview, 111, 112*t*
      techniques
        arterial puncture, 112
        indwelling arterial catheters, 111–112, 113*f*
    pulmonary function assessment
      end-tidal carbon dioxide monitoring, 118, 118*f*–119*f*
      overview, 118
    pulse oximetry, 116–117, 117*f*
    venous blood gas monitoring, 116
  ventilatory troubleshooting guide
    anxiety and fear, 546*t*
    arrhythmias during or after suctioning, 546*t*–547*t*
    decreased CO with hypotension, 544*t*–545*t*
    decreased tidal volume with pressure-targeted modes of ventilation, 541*t*
    high PaO$_2$/SaO$_2$, 543*t*
    inability to tolerate mode of ventilation, 548*t*–549*t*
    incorrect PEEP setting, 547*t*
    increased airway pressure, 540*t*–541*t*
    low exhaled tidal volume, 539*t*–540*t*
    low PaO$_2$/SaO$_2$, 544*t*
    no exhaled tidal volume, 540*t*
    pneumothorax/tension pneumothorax, 547*t*–548*t*
    respiratory acidosis, 542*t*–543*t*
    respiratory alkalosis, 541*t*–542*t*

    thick secretions, 543*t*
    tracheostomy/endotracheal tube discomfort, 543*t*
Airway pressure release ventilation (APRV), 467, 468*t*
Albuterol, 187
Alcohol overdose
  clinical presentation, 274
  diagnostic tests, 274–275
  etiology, risk factors, and pathophysiology, 274
  management, 276–277
  overview, 274
Alkalemia, 113–114
Allen test, 80, 84*f*
Alpha-adrenergic blocking agent (phentolamine), 178
Alpha- and beta-adrenergic blocking agent (labetalol), 178
Alteplase, 183
  administration guidelines, 505*t*
American Association of Critical-Care Nurses (AACN), 199–200
American Nurses Association (ANA), 199–200, 205, 209
Amikacin
  administration guidelines, 505*t*
  therapeutic monitoring, 518*t*
Aminoglycosides, 185–186
Aminophylline
  administration guidelines, 505*t*
Amiodarone, 182
  administration guidelines, 517*t*
  therapeutic monitoring, 518*t*
Ammonium chloride
  administration guidelines, 505*t*
Amphotericin B
  administration guidelines, 505*t*
Ampicillin
  administration guidelines, 505*t*
Ampicillin/sulbactam
  administration guidelines, 505*t*
ANA (American Nurses Association), 199–200, 205, 209
Anemia, 484
  clinical signs and symptoms, 309
  etiology, risk factors, and pathophysiology, 308–309
  management, 309–310
Angioplasty, 216–217
Anistreplase
  administration guidelines, 505*t*
Antacids, 188
Antiarrhythmics, 516*t*–517*t*
  adenosine, 182
  amiodarone, 182
  atropine, 182
  class I agents, 180
  class Ia agents, 180
  class Ib agents, 180
  class Ib/Ic agents, 180
  class Ic agents, 180
  class II agents, 180–181
  class III agents, 181
  class IV agents, 181
  class V agents, 181
  digoxin, 182

dofetilide, 182
ibutilide, 181–182
therapeutic monitoring, 518*t*
Antibiotics
therapeutic monitoring, 518*t*
Anticoagulants
heparin, 191
low-molecular-weight heparin, 192
warfarin, 192–193
Anticonvulsants
therapeutic monitoring, 518*t*
Antidotes, 277
Anti-infective pharmacology
aminoglycosides, 185–186
linezolid, 186–187
vancomycin, 186
Aortic aneurysm
clinical presentation, 444–445
diagnostic tests, 445
etiology and pathophysiology, 443–444
management, 445–446
overview, 443
Aortic dissection, 445
Aortic insufficiency, 437, 439*f*
Aortic rupture, 445
Aortic stenosis, 437, 439*f*
Aphasia, 281
APRV (airway pressure release ventilation),
467, 468*t*
APTT (activated partial thromboplastin time),
307
ARDS (acute respiratory distress syndrome).
See Acute respiratory distress syndrome
(ARDS)
ARF (acute renal failure). *See* Acute renal
failure (ARF)
Argatroban, 193
administration guidelines, 506*t*
Arrhythmias, advanced interpretation of atrial
fibrillation in Wolff-Parkinson-White
syndrome, 414–415, 415*f*
atrioventricular nodal reentry tachycardia,
412, 413*f*–414*f*
circus movement tachycardia, 413–414, 415*f*
differentiating wide QRS beats and rhythms
electrocardiographic clues
concordance, 419, 420*f*, 420*t*
P waves, 416–417, 416*f*–417*f*
QRS morphology, 417–418, 418*f*–419*f*
mechanisms of aberration, 416, 416*f*
overview, 415–416
overview, 411
supraventricular tachycardia (SVT), 412
Arrhythmias, basics of
arrhythmias originating in the atrioventricular
junction
accelerated junctional rhythm, 50, 50*f*
junctional rhythm, 50, 50*f*
junctional tachycardia, 50
overview, 49, 49*f*
premature junctional complexes, 50, 50*f*
arrhythmias originating in the ventricles
accelerated ventricular rhythm, 51–52, 52*f*
overview, 50*f*, 51
premature ventricular complexes, 51, 51*f*
ventricular asystole, 53–54, 53*f*

ventricular fibrillation, 53, 53*f*
ventricular rhythm, 51–52, 52*f*
ventricular tachycardia, 52–53, 52*f*
overview, 43
rhythms originating in the atria
atrial fibrillation, 48–49, 48*f*–49*f*
atrial flutter, 47–48, 47*f*–48*f*
atrial tachycardia, 47, 47*f*
overview, 45*f*
premature atrial complex (PAC), 46, 46*f*
wandering atrial pacemaker, 46–47, 46*f*
rhythms originating in the sinus node
normal sinus rhythm, 44, 44*f*
overview, 43*f*
sinus arrest, 45, 45*f*
sinus arrhythmia, 45, 45*f*
sinus bradycardia, 44, 44*f*
sinus tachycardia, 44–45, 44*f*
Arterial catheters
catheter insertion and removal
complications, 80, 84, 85*t*
insertion, 80, 84*f*
overview, 80
removal, 80
problems encountered with, 533*t*
Artificial airways
cuff inflation, 122–123
cuff pressure measurement, 123–124, 123*f*
endotracheal suctioning, 124–125, 124*t*
extubation, 125
insertion, 121–122, 121*f*–122*f*
overview, 120
types, 120–121, 120*f*
Aspiration, reducing risk of, 335–336, 336*t*
Assessment of critically ill patients and families
admission quick check assessment
airway and breathing, 6
chief complaint, 6
circulation and cerebral perfusion, 6
drugs and diagnostic tests, 6–7, 7*t*
equipment, 7, 7*t*
overview, 5–6
assessment framework, 3–4
admission quick check, 4, 4*t*
comprehensive admission assessment, 4
ongoing assessment, 4
prearrival assessment, 4
comprehensive admission assessment
overview, 7, 8*t*
past medical history, 8, 8*t*
physical assessment by body system
cardiovascular system, 10–11, 10*t*–11*t*
endocrine system, 12
gastrointestinal system, 12
hematologic system, 12
immune system, 12
integumentary system, 12
nervous system, 9–10
overview, 9, 9*t*
renal system, 11
respiratory system, 11
psychosocial assessment
anxiety and stress, 13
coping styles, 13
family needs, 13
general communication, 12–13

overview, 12
referrals, 14, 14*t*
unit orientation, 14
social history, 8–9
ongoing assessment, 14–15, 14*t*
overview, 3
prearrival assessment, 4–5, 4*t*–5*t*
Asystole, algorithm for, 523*f*
Atenolol, 179
administration guidelines, 506*t*
Atonic seizures, 301
Atracurium
administration guidelines, 506*t*, 514*t*
Atrial fibrillation, 48–49, 48*f*–49*f*
algorithm for, 554*t*
Atrial fibrillation in Wolff-Parkinson-White
syndrome, 414–415, 415*f*
Atrial flutter, 47–48, 47*f*–48*f*
algorithm for, 554*t*
Atrial tachycardia, 47, 47*f*
algorithm for, 553*t*–554*t*
Atrioventricular blocks
first-degree, 54, 54*f*
high-grade, 56, 56*f*
overview, 54
second degree, 54–56
type I, 54–55, 54*f*–55*f*
type II, 55–56, 56*f*
third-degree (complete block), 56–57, 56*f*–57*f*
Atrioventricular nodal reentry tachycardia, 412,
413*f*–414*f*
Atropine, 182
administration guidelines, 517*t*
Autoregulatory mechanisms, loss of, 484
Aztreonam
administration guidelines, 506*t*

Backward failure, 239
Bacteremia, 268*t*
Balloon angioplasty, 216–217
Barbiturates
overview, 169
pentobarbital, 169
Beneficence, 201
Benign hypertension, 243
Benzodiazepines, 176
diazepam, 168
lorazepam, 167–168
midazolam, 167
monitoring parameters, 167
overview, 167
Best interest standard, 206–207
Beta-adrenergic blocking agents, 178
Bi-level positive airway pressure (BIPAP),
465–466, 466*t*
Billroth I and II procedures, 323, 324*f*
Bi-phasic ventilation, 467, 468*t*
Bivalirudin, 193
administration guidelines, 506*t*
Blood glucose monitoring
equipment-related discrepancies, 357
overview, 357, 358*f*
patient-related discrepancies, 357–358, 358*t*
patient teaching, 358
Blunt cardiac injury, 379

Bowel infarction/obstruction
  clinical presentation, 331
  etiology, risk factors, and pathophysiology, 331
  management, 331–332
Bowel sounds, 336, 336*t*
Bradycardia, algorithm for, 524*f*
Brain injury. *See* Traumatic brain injury (TBI)
Brain tumors
  advanced technology: brain tissue oxygen
    monitoring, 497
  clinical presentation, 495, 495*t*
  diagnostic tests, 495–496
  etiology, risk factors, and pathophysiology,
    494–495
  management
    chemotherapy, 497
    corticosteroids, 496
    postoperative complications, 496–497
    radiation therapy, 497
    seizures, 497
    surgery, 496
Breathing techniques, 26
Bretylium
  administration guidelines, 506*t*, 517*t*
Bumetanide, 190
  administration guidelines, 506*t*
Bundle branch block, 399–401
  left bundle branch block, 400–401, 403*f*
  right bundle branch block, 399–400, 402*f*

CABG (coronary artery bypass grafting),
    223–225
Calcium
  administration guidelines, 506*t*
Calcium imbalance
  hypercalcemia, 347–348, 350
  hypocalcemia, 348, 350
CAM-ICU (Confusion Assessment Method for
    the Intensive Care Unit), 281, 282*f*
Capacity, 205
Carbamazepine, therapeutic monitoring of, 518*t*
Carbon dioxide rebreathing, 100
Cardiac life support algorithms, advanced
  asystole, 523*f*
  bradycardia, 524*f*
  electromechanical dissociation (EMD), 522*f*
  pulseless electrical activity (PEA), 522*f*
  pulseless ventricular tachycardia, 521*f*
  synchronized electrical cardioversion, 528*f*
  tachycardia, narrow-complex
    supraventricular, 526*f*
  tachycardia, overview, 525*f*
  tachycardia, stable ventricular, 527*f*
  universal advanced cardiac life support
    (ACLS), 520*f*
  ventricular fibrillation, 521*f*
Cardiac pacemakers
  DDD pacemaker evaluation
    atrial capture, 428
    atrial sensing, 428
    overview, 427–428
    ventricular capture, 428
    ventricular sensing, 429, 429*f*
  evaluating pacemaker function, 423
  overview, 422–423, 423*t*

VVI pacemaker evaluation
    capture, 424–425, 425*f*–426*f*
    overview, 423–424, 424*f*
    sensing, 425–426, 426*f*–427*f*
    stimulation threshold testing, 427
    stimulus release, 424, 425*f*
Cardiac rhythms, ECG characteristics, and
    treatment guide
  atrial fibrillation, 554*t*
  atrial flutter, 554*t*
  atrial tachycardia, 553*t*–554*t*
  first-degree AV block, 557*t*
  high AV block, 558*t*
  junctional rhythm, 555*t*
  normal sinus rhythm (NSR), 552*t*
  premature atrial contraction, 553*t*
  premature junctional complexes, 555*t*
  premature ventricular complexes, 555*t*
  second-degree AV block type I (Mobitz II),
    558*t*
  second-degree AV block type I
    (Wenckebach; Mobitz I), 557*t*
  sinus arrest, 552*t*
  sinus arrhythmia, 552*t*
  sinus bradycardia, 552*t*
  sinus tachycardia, 552*t*
  third-degree AV block, 558*t*
  ventricular asystole, 557*t*
  ventricular fibrillation, 556*t*
  ventricular paced rhythm with capture, 559*t*
  ventricular rhythm, 556*t*
  ventricular tachycardia, 556*t*
  wandering atrial pacemaker, 553*t*
Cardiac rhythms, interpretation and
    management of
  atrioventricular blocks
    first-degree, 54, 54*f*
    high-grade, 56, 56*f*
    overview, 54
    second degree, 54–56
      type I, 54–55, 54*f*–55*f*
      type II, 55–56, 56*f*
    third-degree (complete block), 56–57,
      56*f*–57*f*
  basic electrophysiology, 37–38, 38*f*
  cardiac monitoring, 39–40, 40*t*–41*t*, 41*f*, 42
  cardiac rhythm determination, 42
  cardioversion, 62, 62*f*
  common arrhythmias
    arrhythmias originating in the
      atrioventricular junction
      accelerated junctional rhythm, 50, 50*f*
      junctional rhythm, 50, 50*f*
      junctional tachycardia, 50
      overview, 49, 49*f*
      premature junctional complexes, 50, 50*f*
    arrhythmias originating in the ventricles
      accelerated ventricular rhythm, 51–52,
        52*f*
      overview, 50*f*, 51
      premature ventricular complexes, 51, 51*f*
      ventricular asystole, 53–54, 53*f*
      ventricular fibrillation, 53, 53*f*
      ventricular rhythm, 51–52, 52*f*
      ventricular tachycardia, 52–53, 52*f*
    overview, 43

rhythms originating in the atria
      atrial fibrillation, 48–49, 48*f*–49*f*
      atrial flutter, 47–48, 47*f*–48*f*
      atrial tachycardia, 47, 47*f*
      overview, 45*f*
      premature atrial complex (PAC), 46, 46*f*
      wandering atrial pacemaker, 46–47, 46*f*
    rhythms originating in the sinus node
      normal sinus rhythm, 44, 44*f*
      overview, 43*f*
      sinus arrest, 45, 45*f*
      sinus arrhythmia, 45, 45*f*
      sinus bradycardia, 44, 44*f*
      sinus tachycardia, 44–45, 44*f*
  defibrillation
    automatic external defibrillator (AED),
      61–62
    overview, 60–61, 61*f*–62*f*
  ECG waveforms, complexes, and intervals
    overview, 38, 39*f*
    PR interval, 38
    P wave, 38
    QRS complex, 38, 39*f*–40*f*
    QT interval, 39
    ST segment, 38
    T and U waves, 348
  heart rate determination, 42, 42*f*–43*f*, 43*t*
  overview, 37
  temporary pacing
    basics of pacemaker operation
      asynchronous (fixed-rate) pacing mode,
        59
      capture and sensing, 58–59, 59*f*
      demand mode, 59
      overview, 58
    components of a pacing system, 57–58, 58*f*
    ECG characteristics of paced rhythms, 60,
      60*f*
    epicardial pacing, 57, 58*f*
    external (transcutaneous) pacemakers, 60,
      61*f*
    indications, 57
    initiating epicardial pacing, 60
    initiating transvenous ventricular pacing, 60
    transvenous pacing, 57, 58*f*
Cardiac tamponade, 379
Cardiac transplantation
  candidate selection, 447, 447*t*
  management
    monitoring altered immune response and
      graft protection, 449–451, 451*f*, 451*t*
    overview, 448
    providing posttransplant psychological
      adjustment, 451–452
    stabilizing cardiovascular function, 448–
      449
  overview, 446–447
  pretransplant process, 447–448
  transplant surgical techniques, 448, 448*f*–449*f*
Cardiogenic shock, 238–239, 242–243
Cardiomyopathy
  clinical presentation
    dilated cardiomyopathy, 433
    hypertrophic cardiomyopathy, 433–434
    overview, 433
    restrictive cardiomyopathy, 434

diagnostic tests
  dilated cardiomyopathy, 434
  hypertrophic cardiomyopathy, 434
  restrictive cardiomyopathy, 434
etiology and pathophysiology
  dilated cardiomyopathy, 431–432
  hypertrophic cardiomyopathy, 432–433
  overview, 431, 433t
  restrictive cardiomyopathy, 433
management
  dilated cardiomyopathy, 435
  facilitating coping, 435–436
  hypertrophic cardiomyopathy, 435
  preventing and managing complications,
    436
  restrictive cardiomyopathy, 435
overview, 431, 432f
Cardiovascular concepts, advanced
  pathologic conditions
    aortic aneurysm
      clinical presentation, 444–445
      diagnostic tests, 445
      etiology and pathophysiology, 443–444
      management, 445–446
      overview, 443
    cardiac transplantation
      candidate selection, 447, 447t
      management
        monitoring altered immune response
          and graft protection, 449–451, 451f,
          451t
        overview, 448
        providing posttransplant
          psychological adjustment, 451–452
        stabilizing cardiovascular function,
          448–449
      overview, 446–447
      pretransplant process, 447–448
      transplant surgical techniques, 448,
        448f–449f
    cardiomyopathy
      clinical presentation
        dilated cardiomyopathy, 433
        hypertrophic cardiomyopathy, 433–434
        overview, 433
        restrictive cardiomyopathy, 434
      diagnostic tests
        dilated cardiomyopathy, 434
        hypertrophic cardiomyopathy, 434
        restrictive cardiomyopathy, 434
      etiology and pathophysiology
        dilated cardiomyopathy, 431–432
        hypertrophic cardiomyopathy,
          432–433
        overview, 431, 433t
        restrictive cardiomyopathy, 433
      management
        dilated cardiomyopathy, 435
        facilitating coping, 435–436
        hypertrophic cardiomyopathy, 435
        preventing and managing
          complications, 436
        restrictive cardiomyopathy, 435
      overview, 431, 432f
    intra-aortic balloon pump therapy
      indications and contraindications, 452

management, 453–455
overview, 452, 452f
timing, 452–453, 453f–454f
weaning, 453
pericarditis
  clinical presentation, 442
  diagnostic tests, 442
  etiology and pathophysiology, 442, 442f
  management, 442–443
  overview, 441–442
valvular disease
  clinical presentation
    mitral and aortic disease, 438–440
    tricuspid and pulmonary valve
      disease, 440
  etiology and pathophysiology
    aortic insufficiency, 437, 439f
    aortic stenosis, 437, 439f
    mitral insufficiency, 437, 438f
    mitral stenosis, 436, 438f
    overview, 436, 437t
    pulmonic insufficiency, 438
    pulmonic stenosis, 438
    tricuspid insufficiency, 437
    tricuspid stenosis, 437
  management, 440–441
  overview, 436
ventricular assist devices
  indications, 455
  management, 457–458, 458t
  overview, 455
  principles, 455–457, 456f
  weaning and recovery, 457
Cardiovascular system
  pathologic conditions
    acute ischemic heart disease
      alleviating pain, 228
      clinical presentation, 221–222, 226t–227t
      diagnostic tests
        myocardial infarction, 222–223
        unstable angina, 222, 228f
      etiology and pathophysiology, 218–221,
        223f–224f, 224t
      management
        medical, 224, 230f, 230t–231t
        principles, 223–224, 228t, 229f
        surgical, 224–225, 231f
      overview, 218
      preventing complications associated
        with coronary obstruction, 225, 228
      reducing anxiety, 228–229
    congestive heart failure
      clinical presentation, 234–235, 235t–236t
      diagnostic tests, 235–236
      etiology, risk factors, and
        pathophysiology, 230–232,
        233f–235f, 234
      management, 236–238
      overview, 230
    hypertension
      clinical presentation, 244
      diagnostic tests, 244
      etiology, risk factors, and
        pathophysiology, 243–244
      follow-up, 245
      management, 244–245, 244t

overview, 243
patient education on lifestyle
  modification, 245
shock
  clinical presentation, 242
  diagnostic tests, 242
  etiology, risk factors, and
    pathophysiology, 238–239, 239f, 239t
  management, 242–243
  overview, 238
  stages of shock, 239–240, 240f–241f, 242
special assessment techniques, diagnostic
  tests, and monitoring systems
  chest pain assessment, 215, 216t
  coronary angiography
    complications, 216, 220t
    interpretation of results, 216, 218f
    overview, 215, 216t
    procedure, 215–216, 217f
  percutaneous coronary interventions
    (PCIs), 216–218, 221f
    complications, 217, 221t
Cardiovascular system pharmacology
  activated protein C (drotrecogin alfa), 185
  inotropic agents
    catecholamines
      dobutamine, 184
      dopamine, 184
      epinephrine, 184–185
      isoproterenol, 184
    phosphodiesterase inhibitors
      inamrinone, 185
      milrinone, 185
  miscellaneous agents
    fenoldopam, 177
    nesiritide, 176–177
  parenteral vasodilators
    alpha-adrenergic blocking agent
      (phentolamine), 178
    alpha- and beta-adrenergic blocking agent
      (labetalol), 178
    angiotensin-converting enzyme (ACE)
      inhibitor (enalapril), 179
    antiarrhythmics
      adenosine, 182
      amiodarone, 182
      atropine, 182
      class I agents, 180
      class Ia agents, 180
      class Ib agents, 180
      class Ib/Ic agents, 180
      class Ic agents, 180
      class II agents, 180–181
      class III agents, 181
      class IV agents, 181
      class V agents, 181
      digoxin, 182
      dofetilide, 182
      ibutilide, 181–182
    arterial vasodilating agents
      hydralazine, 177–178
      beta-adrenergic blocking agents, 178
      calcium channel blocking agent
        (nicardipine), 179
      central sympatholytic agent (clonidine), 180
      diazoxide, 178

parenteral vasodilators, *continued*
  ganglionic blocking agent (trimethaphan), 178
  nitrates
    nitroglycerin, 177
    sodium nitroprusside, 177
  thrombolytic agents
    alteplase, 183
    overview, 182–183
    reteplase, 183
    streptokinase, 183
    tenecteplase, 183
  vasoconstricting agents, 183–184
Cardioversion, 62, 62*f*
CBC (complete blood cell) count, 305
Cefamandole
  administration guidelines, 506*t*
Cefazolin
  administration guidelines, 506*t*
Cefepime
  administration guidelines, 506*t*
Cefmetazole
  administration guidelines, 506*t*
Cefonicid
  administration guidelines, 506*t*
Cefoperazone
  administration guidelines, 506*t*
Cefotaxime
  administration guidelines, 506*t*
Cefotetan
  administration guidelines, 506*t*
Cefoxitin
  administration guidelines, 506*t*
Ceftazidime
  administration guidelines, 506*t*
Ceftizoxime
  administration guidelines, 506*t*
Ceftriaxone
  administration guidelines, 506*t*
Cefuroxime
  administration guidelines, 506*t*
Central nervous system (CNS) infections
  encephalitis, 302
  intracranial abscess, 302–303
  meningitis, 302
Central nervous system (CNS) pharmacology
  analgesics
    narcotics
      fentanyl, 170
      morphine, 170
      overview, 170
    NSAID (ketorolac), 171
    opioid antagonist (naloxone), 170–171
  anticonvulsants
    barbiturates
      pentobarbital, 175–176
      phenobarbital, 176
    benzodiazepines, 176
    hydantoins
      fosphenytoin, 174–175
      phenytoin, 173–174
  neuromuscular blocking agents (NMBAs)
    depolarizing agent (succinylcholine), 171–172
    nondepolarizing agents, 172–173
    overview, 171

sedatives
  barbiturates
    overview, 169
    pentobarbital, 169
  benzodiazepine antagonist (flumazenil), 168
  benzodiazepines
    diazepam, 168
    lorazepam, 167–168
    midazolam, 167
    monitoring parameters, 167
    overview, 167
  miscellaneous agents
    dexmedetomidine, 169–170
    ketamine, 169
    propofol, 169
  neuroleptic (haloperidol), 168
  overview, 167
Central venous pressure (CVP), 85–88, 86*f*–87*f*, 503
Cerebral angiography, 289
Cerebral contusion, 483
Cerebral edema, 291
Cerebral laceration, 483
Chest pain assessment, 216*t*
Chest tubes, 252, 252*f*–253*f*, 252*t*
Chest x-rays
  basic views of the chest, 247–248
  helpful hints, 251
  invasive lines, 250–251, 251*f*
  normal variants and common abnormalities, 248–250, 250*t*
  overview, 247, 248*t*
  systematic approach to interpretation, 248, 248*t*, 249*f*
Chloramphenicol, therapeutic monitoring of, 518*t*
Chlorothiazide, 190
  administration guidelines, 506*t*
Chlorpromazine
  administration guidelines, 506*t*
Cimetidine
  administration guidelines, 506*t*
Ciprofloxacin
  administration guidelines, 506*t*
Circus movement tachycardia, 413–414, 415*f*
Cisatricurium
  administration guidelines, 506*t*, 514*t*
Clindamycin
  administration guidelines, 506*t*
Clonic seizures, 301
Clonidine, 180
Clostridium difficile, 337
CNS (central nervous system). *See* entries for Central nervous system (CNS)
Coagulation studies
  activated coagulation time, 307
  activated partial thromboplastin time (APTT), 307
  D-dimer, 308
  fibrin degradation products (FDP), 308
  fibrinogen, 307
  fibrin split products (FSP), 308
  international normalizing ratio, 307
  miscellaneous tests, 308
  partial thromboplastin time (PTT), 307
  prothrombin time (PT), 307

Coagulopathies
  clinical signs and symptoms, 314
  etiology, risk factors, and pathophysiology, 312–314, 313*f*, 313*t*–314*t*
  management, 315
Code for Nurses, 199–200, 205, 209
Combitube, 120
Competence, 205
Complete blood cell (CBC) count, 305
Complex partial seizures, 300
Comprehensive admission assessment
  overview, 7, 8*t*
  past medical history, 8, 8*t*
  physical assessment by body system
    cardiovascular system, 10–11, 10*t*–11*t*
    endocrine system, 12
    gastrointestinal system, 12
    hematologic system, 12
    immune system, 12
    integumentary system, 12
    nervous system, 9–10
    overview, 9, 9*t*
    renal system, 11
    respiratory system, 11
  psychosocial assessment
    anxiety and stress, 13
    coping styles, 13
    family needs, 13
    general communication, 12–13
    overview, 12
    referrals, 14, 14*t*
    unit orientation, 14
  social history, 8–9
Confidentiality and privacy, 202–203
Confusion Assessment Method for the Intensive Care Unit (CAM-ICU), 281, 282*f*
Congestive heart failure
  clinical presentation, 234–235, 235*t*–236*t*
  diagnostic tests, 235–236
  etiology, risk factors, and pathophysiology, 230–232, 233*f*–235*f*, 234
  management, 236–238
  overview, 230
Conjugated estrogens
  administration guidelines, 506*t*
Continuous mixed venous oxygen monitoring (SVO$_2$), 97–99, 99*t*
Continuous positive airway pressure (CPAP), 138, 257
Continuous renal replacement therapy, 195
Continuous venovenous hemodialysis (CVVHD), 355
Continuous venovenous hemofiltration (CVVH), 354–355
Contractility, 72, 103
Coronary angiography
  complications, 216, 220*t*
  interpretation of results, 216, 218*f*
  overview, 215, 216*t*
  procedure, 215–216, 217*f*
Coronary artery bypass grafting (CABG), 223–225
Cosyntropin
  administration guidelines, 506*t*
Cotrimoxazole, therapeutic monitoring of, 518*t*

CPAP (continuous positive airway pressure), 138, 257
Cranial nerve assessment and assessment of brainstem function
corneal reflex, 285
extraocular eye movements, 285–286, 286f
gag and cough reflexes, 285
overview, 285, 285t
pupil size and reaction to light, 285
Cushing's response, 287
Cutaneous stimulation, 155, 156f
CVP (central venous pressure), 85–88, 86f–87f, 503
CVVH (continuous venovenous hemofiltration), 354–355
CVVHD (continuous venovenous hemodialysis), 355
Cyclosporine, 193–194
administration guidelines, 507t
therapeutic monitoring, 518t

Dantrolene
administration guidelines, 507t
Daptomycin
administration guidelines, 507t
D-dimer, 308
DDD pacemaker evaluation
atrial capture, 428
atrial sensing, 428
overview, 427–428
ventricular capture, 428
ventricular sensing, 429, 429f
Death by neurologic criteria, 287
Deep venous thrombosis (DVT), prevention of, 18, 23, 264–265, 382, 384t
Defibrillation
automatic external defibrillator (AED), 61–62
overview, 60–61, 61f–62f
Delirium, 281
Dementia, 281
Dermatomes, 284, 284f
Desmopressin
administration guidelines, 507t
Dexamethasone
administration guidelines, 507t
Dexmedetomidine, 158, 169–170
administration guidelines, 507t
Diabetes insipidus
clinical presentation, 367–368
diagnostic tests, 368
etiology, risk factors, and pathophysiology, 367, 367f, 368t
management, 368–369, 368t
Diabetes mellitus (DM), 359
Diabetic ketoacidosis, 359–361, 360t–361t, 361f
Diazepam, 159, 168
administration guidelines, 507t
Diazoxide, 178
administration guidelines, 507t
DIC (disseminated intravascular coagulation), 307–308, 313–314
Digitalis
administration guidelines, 517t

Digoxin, 182
administration guidelines, 507t
therapeutic monitoring, 518t
Dilated cardiomyopathy
clinical presentation, 433
diagnostic tests, 434
etiology and pathophysiology, 431–432
management, 435
Diltiazem
administration guidelines, 507t, 517t
Diphenhydramine
administration guidelines, 507t
Direct thrombin inhibitors
argatroban, 193
bivalirudin, 193
lepirudin, 193
Disopyramide
administration guidelines, 516t
therapeutic monitoring, 518t
Disseminated intravascular coagulation (DIC), 307–308, 313–314
Distraction techniques, 26, 155
Distributive shock, 239, 242–243
Diuretics
loop diuretics, 190
osmotic diuretic (mannitol), 190–191
overview, 190
thiazide diuretics, 190
DM (diabetes mellitus), 359
Dobutamine, 69t, 184
actions and effects, 515t
administration guidelines, 507t
Dofetilide, 182
administration guidelines, 517t
Dolasetron
administration guidelines, 507t
Do not resuscitate (DNR) orders, 209
Dopamine, 69t, 183–184
actions and effects, 515t
administration guidelines, 507t
Doxacurium
administration guidelines, 507t, 514t
Doxycycline
administration guidelines, 507t
Droperidol
administration guidelines, 507t
Drotrecogin alfa
administration guidelines, 507t
Drug overdose
clinical presentation, 275t, 276
diagnostic tests, 276
etiology, risk factors, and pathophysiology, 275
management, 276–277
overview, 274
DVT (deep venous thrombosis), prevention of, 18, 23, 264–265, 382, 384t
Dysarthria, 281

ECG concepts, advanced
advanced arrhythmia interpretation
atrial fibrillation in Wolff-Parkinson-White syndrome, 414–415, 415f
atrioventricular nodal reentry tachycardia, 412, 413f–414f

circus movement tachycardia, 413–414, 415f
differentiating wide QRS beats and rhythms
electrocardiographic clues
concordance, 419, 420f, 420t
P waves, 416–417, 416f–417f
QRS morphology, 417–418, 418f–419f
mechanisms of aberration, 416, 416f
overview, 415–416
overview, 411
supraventricular tachycardia (SVT), 412
cardiac pacemakers
DDD pacemaker evaluation
atrial capture, 428
atrial sensing, 428
overview, 427–428
ventricular capture, 428
ventricular sensing, 429, 429f
evaluating pacemaker function, 423
overview, 422–423, 423t
VVI pacemaker evaluation
capture, 424–425, 425f–426f
overview, 423–424, 424f
sensing, 425–426, 426f–427f
stimulation threshold testing, 427
stimulus release, 424, 425f
12-lead electrocardiogram
axis determination, 396–399, 397f–400f, 397t
bundle branch block, 399–401
left bundle branch block, 400–401, 403f
right bundle branch block, 399–400, 402f
description, 391–394, 392f–396f, 396
myocardial ischemia, injury, and infarction
description, 401, 404, 404f–406f
locating infarction from ECG, 404–405, 404f, 406f–409f, 407, 407t
preexcitation syndromes
overview, 407
Wolff-Parkinson-White syndrome, 407, 409–411, 409f–411f
ST-segment monitoring, 419–422, 422t
ECG concepts, basic
overview, 38, 39f
PR interval, 38
P wave, 38
QRS complex, 38, 39f–40f
QT interval, 39
ST segment, 38
T and U waves, 348
Edema rating scale, 10t
EDH (epidural hematoma), 483, 483f
EEG (electroencephalography), 290
Elderly patients
pain, sedation, and neuromuscular blockade management
assessment, 157
interventions, 157
overview, 156–157
physiologic effects of aging, 9t
special dosing considerations, 195
Electrocardiograph (ECG). See ECG concepts, advanced; ECG concepts, basic

Electroencephalography (EEG), 290
Electrolyte imbalances, life-threatening
  calcium imbalance
    hypercalcemia, 347–348, 350
    hypocalcemia, 348, 350
  magnesium imbalance
    hypermagnesemia, 348, 350
    hypomagnesemia, 348, 350
  overview, 346
  phosphate imbalance
    hyperphosphatemia, 348–350
    hypophosphatemia, 349–350
  potassium imbalance
    hyperkalemia, 347, 349
    hypokalemia, 347, 350
  sodium imbalance
    hyperosmolar disorders, 346, 349
    hypoosmolar disorders, 346–347, 349
Electromechanical dissociation (EMD),
    algorithm for, 522f
Electromyography (EMG), 290
Enalapril and enalaprilat, 179
  administration guidelines, 507t
Encephalitis, 302
Endocrine system
  pathologic conditions
    acute hypoglycemia
      clinical presentation, 364–365
      etiology, risk factors, and
        pathophysiology, 364, 364t
      management, 365, 365t
      overview, 364
    diabetes insipidus
      clinical presentation, 367–368
      diagnostic tests, 368
      etiology, risk factors, and
        pathophysiology, 367, 367f, 368t
      management, 368–369, 368t
    hyperglycemic emergencies
      clinical presentation, 362
      diabetic ketoacidosis, 359–361,
        360t–361t, 361f
      etiology, risk factors, and
        pathophysiology, 359
      hyperosmolar hyperglycemic states,
        361–362
      management, 362–364, 362t, 364t
      overview, 359
    syndrome of inappropriate antidiuretic
      hormone secretion (SIADH)
      clinical presentation, 366
      etiology, risk factors, and
        pathophysiology, 365–366, 366t
      management, 366–367
      overview, 365
  special assessment techniques, diagnostic
    tests, and monitoring systems
    blood glucose monitoring
      equipment-related discrepancies, 357
      overview, 357, 358f
      patient-related discrepancies, 357–358,
        358t
      patient teaching, 358
End-of-life issues
  decisions to forego life sustaining treatments,
    207–208

nutrition and hydration, 208
pain management, 208–209
resuscitation decisions, 209
  do not resuscitate (DNR) orders, 209
  partial codes, 209
  slow codes, 209
Endotracheal suctioning, 124–125, 124t
Enteral nutrition, 333, 333t–334t
Epidural analgesia
  local anesthetics, 154
  opioids, 153–154, 154f
  overview, 153
  titrating, 154–155
Epidural hematoma (EDH), 483, 483f
Epinephrine, 69t, 184–185
  actions and effects, 515t
  administration guidelines, 507t
Eptifibatide
  administration guidelines, 508t
Ertapenem
  administration guidelines, 508t
Erythrocyte sedimentation rate (ESR), 307
Erythromycin
  administration guidelines, 508t
Erythropoietin
  administration guidelines, 508t
Esmolol, 179
  administration guidelines, 508t, 517t
Esophageal Doppler cardiac output, 100, 101f
Ethacrynic acid
  administration guidelines, 508t
Ethical and legal considerations
  building an ethical environment
    engage in collaborative decision making,
      210
    provide information and clarify issues,
      209–210
    recognize moral distress, 210
    values clarification, 209
  contemporary ethical issues
    advance directives, 206–207
      best interests, 206–207
      substituted judgment, 206
    determining capacity, 205–206
    end-of-life issues
      decisions to forego life-sustaining
        treatments, 207–208
      nutrition and hydration, 208
      pain management, 208–209
      resuscitation decisions, 209
        do not resuscitate (DNR) orders, 209
        partial codes, 209
        slow codes, 209
    informed consent, 205
  foundation for ethical decision making
    care, 203–204
    institutional policies, 200
    legal standards, 200–201
    patient advocacy, 204
    position statements and guidelines, 200
    principles of ethics
      beneficence, 201
      fidelity, 203
      justice, 202
      nonmaleficence, 201
      overview, 201

privacy and confidentiality, 202–203
respect for persons (autonomy), 202
utility, 202
veracity, 203
professional codes and standards,
  199–200
overview, 199
process of ethical analysis
  assessment, 204
  evaluation, 205
  implementation, 204
  overview, 204
  plan, 204
Etidronate
  administration guidelines, 508t
Extraocular eye movements, 285–286, 286f

Family-focused care, 28–29, 28t
Famotidine
  administration guidelines, 508t
Fat emboli, 263
Fenoldopam, 177
  administration guidelines, 508t
Fentanyl, 170
  administration guidelines, 508t
Fibrin degradation products (FDP), 308
Fibrinogen, 307
Fibrin split products (FSP), 308
Fidelity, 203
Filgastrim
  administration guidelines, 508t
First-degree atrioventricular block, 54, 54f
  algorithm for, 557t
Flail chest, 378–379
Flecainide
  administration guidelines, 516t
  therapeutic monitoring, 518t
Fluconazole
  administration guidelines, 508t
Flucytosine, therapeutic monitoring of, 518t
Flumazenil, 168
  administration guidelines, 508t
Focal motor or sensory seizures, 300
Forward failure, 239
Foscarnet
  administration guidelines, 508t
Fosphenytoin, 174–175
  administration guidelines, 508t
Fractured ribs, 378
Frank-Starling response, 231, 234f
FSP (fibrin split products), 308
Furosemide, 190
  administration guidelines, 508t

Gallium nitrate
  administration guidelines, 508t
Galvanometer, 37
Ganciclovir
  administration guidelines, 508t
Gastric tonometry (pH), 100–101, 102f
Gastrointestinal system
  nutritional support for critically ill patients.
    See Nutritional support for critically ill
    patients

pathologic conditions
  acute pancreatitis
    clinical presentation, 329
    diagnostic tests, 329
    etiologies, risk factors, and
      pathophysiology, 329, 329t
    imaging studies, 329
    management
      fluid resuscitation, 330
      pain management, 330
      rest the pancreas, 330
      treat local complications in the
        pancreas, 330
      treat multisystem failure, 330–331
    overview, 329
  acute upper GI bleeding
    clinical presentation, 319–320
    diagnostic tests, 320
    etiology, risk factors, and
      pathophysiology, 317–319,
      318t–319t, 319f–320f
    management
      hemodynamic stabilization, 320–321,
      321t
      identify bleeding site, 321
      institute therapies to control or stop
      bleeding, 321–323, 322f, 323t
      newer therapies to control bleeding,
      324
      overview, 320
      reducing anxiety, 324–325
      surgical therapies to stop bleeding,
      323–324, 323f–324f
    overview, 317
  bowel infarction/obstruction
    clinical presentation, 331
    etiology, risk factors, and
      pathophysiology, 331
    management, 331–332
  liver failure
    clinical presentation, 327–328
    diagnostic tests, 328
    etiology, risk factors, and pathogenesis
      acid–base disturbance, 326
      acute gastrointestinal bleeding, 326
      acute respiratory distress syndrome,
      326
      ascites, 326
      electrolyte imbalance, 326
      hepatic encephalopathy, 326
      hepatorenal syndrome, 326
      jaundice, 326
      malnutrition, 327
      overview, 325, 325t–326t
    management, 328–329
    overview, 325, 325t
  stress ulcer prophylaxis
    antacids, 188
    H_2 antagonists, 188
    overview, 188
    sucralfate, 188–189
Gatifloxacin
  administration guidelines, 508t
GCS (Glasgow Coma Scale), 9, 280–281, 280t,
  281f
Generalized seizures, 300–301

Gentamicin
  administration guidelines, 508t
  therapeutic monitoring, 518t
Glasgow Coma Scale (GCS), 9, 280–281, 280t,
  281f, 481
Glycoprotein IIb/IIIa inhibitors, 193
Granisetron
  administration guidelines, 509t
Guillain-Barré syndrome, 303
Gunshot wounds, 482

Haloperidol, 168
  administration guidelines, 509t
H_2 antagonists, 188
Helicobacter pylori, 317
Hematocrit, 306
Hematology and immunology systems
  pathologic conditions
    anemia
      clinical signs and symptoms, 309
      etiology, risk factors, and
      pathophysiology, 308–309
      management, 309–310
    coagulopathies
      clinical signs and symptoms, 314
      etiology, risk factors, and
      pathophysiology, 312–314, 313f, 313t–
      314t
      management, 315
    immunocompromise
      clinical signs and symptoms, 311
      etiology, risk factors, and
      pathophysiology, 310–311
      management, 311–312
      system-specific evidence, 311
  pharmacology
    anticoagulants
      heparin, 191
      low-molecular-weight heparin, 192
      warfarin, 192–193
    direct thrombin inhibitors
      argatroban, 193
      bivalirudin, 193
      lepirudin, 193
    glycoprotein IIb/IIIa inhibitors, 193
  special assessment techniques, diagnostic
    tests, and monitoring systems
    coagulation studies
      activated coagulation time, 307
      activated partial thromboplastin time
      (APTT), 307
      D-dimer, 308
      fibrin degradation products (FDP), 308
      fibrinogen, 307
      fibrin split products (FSP), 308
      international normalizing ratio, 307
      miscellaneous tests, 308
      partial thromboplastin time (PTT), 307
      prothrombin time (PT), 307
    complete blood cell (CBC) count, 305
    erythrocyte sedimentation rate (ESR), 307
    hematocrit, 306
    hemoglobin, 306
    overview, 305, 306t
    platelet count, 307

    red blood cell (RBC) count, 305–306
    red blood cell indices, 306
    total white blood cell (WBC) count, 306
    white blood cell differential, 306–307
Hemodynamic monitoring
  application of hemodynamic parameters
    high cardiac output states, 106–107, 106t
    low cardiac output states
      hypovolemia, 105–106
      left ventricular dysfunction, 103–105,
      104t
      overview, 102–103
  basic components of hemodynamic
    monitoring systems
    alarms, 74
    arterial catheter, 72, 74f
    overview, 72
    pressure amplifier, 74, 74f
    pressure bag and flush device, 74, 75f
    pressure transducer, 73–74, 74f
    pressure tubing, 72–73, 74f
    pulmonary artery (PA) catheter, 72, 73f,
    73t
  catheter insertion and removal
    arterial catheters
      complications, 80, 84, 85t
      insertion, 80, 84f
      overview, 80
      removal, 80
    pulmonary artery (PA) catheters
      complications, 79–80, 82t–83t
      insertion, 79, 79f, 81t
      removal, 79
  continuous mixed venous oxygen monitoring
    (SVO_2)
    clinical application examples
      SVO_2 and blood loss, 99, 99t
      SVO_2 and high output states, 99
      SVO_2 and low cardiac output, 98
      troubleshooting SVO_2 catheter, 99
    principles, 97–98
  hemodynamic parameters
    cardiac output
      components of cardiac output/cardiac
      index
        ejection fraction (EF), 68
        heart rate and rhythm, 67–68
        stroke volume and stroke volume
        index. *See* Stroke volume and stroke
        volume index
      high cardiac output/cardiac index, 67
      low cardiac output/cardiac index, 67
      overview, 65–67, 66f, 66t
  minimally invasive hemodynamic
    monitoring
    carbon dioxide rebreathing, 100
    esophageal Doppler cardiac output, 100,
    101f
    gastric tonometery (pH), 100–101, 102f
    sublingual capnometry, 101
    thoracic bioimpedance, 100, 101f
  obtaining accurate hemodynamic values
    calibration of transducer/amplifier system,
    77
    ensuring accurate waveform transmission,
    77, 78f, 78t–79t

obtaining accurate hemodynamic values,
continued
leveling transducer to catheter tip, 75–76,
75*f*–76*f*, 75*t*
zeroing the transducer, 74–75
obtaining and interpreting hemodynamic
waveforms
arterial and ventricular waveforms, 88–89,
90*f*
artifacts, 91–92, 92*f*–95*f*
cardiac output
interpreting cardiac output and cardiac
index, 95, 97, 97*t*
measurement, 92–93, 95, 96*f*–97*f*
overview, 92
interpretation
atrial and venous waveforms, 84–88,
86*f*–89*f*
overview, 84
overview, 84, 85*f*
patient positioning, 84, 86*f*
PA waveforms, 89–91, 91*f*
systemic arterial pressures, 91
overview, 65, 66*t*
right ventricular ejection fraction catheters
monitoring principles, 99, 100*t*
troubleshooting, 99–100
Hemodynamic troubleshooting guide
arterial catheters, problems encountered
with, 533*t*
inaccurate arterial pressure measurements,
534*t*
inaccurate pulmonary artery pressure
measurements, 537*t*
pulmonary catheters, problems encountered
with, 535*t*–536*t*
thermodilution cardiac output measurements,
troubleshooting problems with, 538*t*
Hemoglobin, 306
Hemorrhagic gastritis, 318
Hemorrhagic stroke
clinical presentation, 300
diagnostic tests, 300
etiology, risk factors, and pathophysiology,
299–300
management, 300
Hemothorax, 378
Heparin, 191
administration guidelines, 509*t*
Hepatitis, 325*t*
Hexaxial reference system, 396
High AV block, algorithm for, 558*t*
High-frequency oscillation (HFO), 468–469,
469*t*
High-frequency ventilation (HFV), 468–469,
469*t*
High-grade atrioventricular blocks, 56, 56*f*
Hospital-acquired infections
overview, 23
prevention, 23–24, 23*t*
Hydralazine, 177–178
administration guidelines, 509*t*
Hydrocortisone
administration guidelines, 509*t*
Hydromorphone
administration guidelines, 509*t*

Hypercalcemia, 347–348, 350
Hypercapnia, 485
Hyperglycemic emergencies
clinical presentation, 362
diabetic ketoacidosis, 359–361, 360*t*–361*t*,
361*f*
etiology, risk factors, and pathophysiology,
359
following traumatic brain injury, 484*f*
hyperosmolar hyperglycemic states,
361–362
management, 362–364, 362*t*, 364*t*
overview, 359
Hyperkalemia, 347, 349
Hypermagnesemia, 348, 350
Hyperosmolar disorders, 346, 349
Hyperosmolar hyperglycemic states, 361–362
Hyperphosphatemia, 348–350
Hypertension
clinical presentation, 244
diagnostic tests, 244
etiology, risk factors, and pathophysiology,
243–244
follow-up, 245
management, 244–245, 244*t*
overview, 243
patient education on lifestyle modification, 245
Hypertensive crisis, 243
Hypertrophic cardiomyopathy
clinical presentation, 433–434
diagnostic tests, 434
etiology and pathophysiology, 432–433
management, 435
Hypocalcemia, 348, 350
Hypocapnia, 485
Hypoglycemia, acute. *See* Acute hypoglycemia
Hypokalemia, 347, 350
Hypomagnesemia, 348, 350
Hypoosmolar disorders, 346–347, 349
Hypophosphatemia, 349–350
Hypotension, 268*t*, 484
Hypovolemic shock, 239, 239*t*, 242–243
Hypoxemia, 484

Ibutilide, 181–182
administration guidelines, 509*t*
IM (intramuscular) administration, 165
Imagery, 26, 155
Imamrinone
administration guidelines, 509*t*
Imipenem
administration guidelines, 509*t*
Immunocompromise
clinical signs and symptoms, 311
etiology, risk factors, and pathophysiology,
310–311
management, 311–312
system-specific evidence, 311
Immunology system. *See* Hematology and
immunology systems
Immunosuppression, 449–450
Immunosuppressive agents
cyclosporine, 193–194, 450–451
sirolimus, 194–195
tacrolimus (FK506), 194

Inamrinone, 185
actions and effects, 515*t*
Informed consent, 205
Insulin-dependent (type I) diabetes mellitus, 359
International normalizing ratio, 307
Intra-aortic balloon pump (IABP) therapy
indications and contraindications, 452
management, 453–455
overview, 452, 452*f*
timing, 452–453, 453*f*–454*f*
weaning, 453
Intracerebral hematoma, 483
Intracoronary stents, 217–218, 222*f*
Intracranial abscess, 302–303
Intracranial pressure, 484–485
causes of increased intracranial pressure,
291–292, 292*f*
cerebral blood flow, 291
management, 294–296
monitoring, 292–294, 293*f*–294*f*
overview, 290–291, 290*f*
Intramuscular (IM) administration, 165
Intranasal administration, 166
Intravenous (IV) medication administration, 165
guidelines, 505*t*–513*t*
Ischemia, 218
Ischemic heart disease, acute. *See* Acute
ischemic heart disease
Ischemic stroke, acute. *See* Acute ischemic stroke
Isolation, 23, 23*t*
Isoproterenol, 69*t*, 184
actions and effects, 515*t*
administration guidelines, 509*t*
IV (intravenous) medication administration, 165
guidelines, 505*t*–513*t*

Junctional rhythm, 50, 50*f*
algorithm for, 555*t*
Junctional tachycardia, 50
Justice, 202

Ketamine, 158, 169
administration guidelines, 509*t*
Ketorolac, 171
Key reference information. *See* Reference
information
Killip Classification, 234, 236*t*

Labetalol, 178
administration guidelines, 509*t*
Laryngeal mask airway (LMA), 120
Left bundle branch block, 400–401, 403*f*
Left-sided heart failure, 235*t*
Legal considerations. *See* Ethical and legal
considerations
Lepirudin, 193
administration guidelines, 509*t*
Levalbuterol, 188
Level of consciousness (LOC), 9–10, 279–280,
280*t*
terms used to describe, 280*t*
Levofloxacin
administration guidelines, 509*t*

Levothyroxine
   administration guidelines, 509*t*
Lidocaine
   administration guidelines, 509*t*, 516*t*
   therapeutic monitoring, 518*t*
Linezolid, 186–187
   administration guidelines, 509*t*
Liver failure
   clinical presentation, 327–328
   diagnostic tests, 328
   etiology, risk factors, and pathogenesis
      acid–base disturbance, 326
      acute gastrointestinal bleeding, 326
      acute respiratory distress syndrome, 326
      ascites, 326
      electrolyte imbalance, 326
      hepatic encephalopathy, 326
      hepatorenal syndrome, 326
      jaundice, 326
      malnutrition, 327
      overview, 325, 325*t*–326*t*
   management, 328–329
   overview, 325, 325*t*
LMA (laryngeal mask airway), 120
LOC (level of consciousness). *See* Level of
   consciousness (LOC)
Loop diuretics, 190
Lorazepam, 158–159, 167–168
   administration guidelines, 509*t*
Low-molecular-weight heparin, 192
Lumbar puncture, 287–288

Magnesium
   administration guidelines, 510*t*
   imbalance
      hypermagnesemia, 348, 350
      hypomagnesemia, 348, 350
Malignant hypertension, 243
Mallory-Weiss syndrome, 317–318
Mannitol, 190–191
   administration guidelines, 510*t*
Manual resuscitation bags, 127
Mechanical ventilation, 127
   alternative modes of
      alternative ventilator options
         flow-by, 469
         minimum minute volume, 469
      new concepts in, 463–464
         acute lung injury and acute respiratory
            distress syndrome, 463–464
      volume versus pressure ventilation
         airway pressure release ventilation
            (APRV), 467, 468*t*
         bi-level positive airway pressure (BIPAP),
            465–466, 466*t*
         bi-phasic ventilation, 467, 468*t*
         high-frequency oscillation (HFO),
            468–469, 469*t*
         high-frequency ventilation (HFV),
            468–469, 469*t*
         overview, 464–465, 464*f*
         pressure control and pressure
            controlled/inverse ratio ventilation, 466,
            466*t*

         pressure support ventilation, 465
         volume-guaranteed pressure modes of
            ventilation, 466–467, 467*f*–468*f*, 468*t*
         weaning patients from. *See* Weaning, from
            long-term mechanical ventilation
Meningitis, 302
Mental status, 281, 282*f*, 283
Meperidine
   administration guidelines, 510*t*
Meropenem
   administration guidelines, 510*t*
Metabolic acidemia, 114
Metabolic alkalemia, 114
Methadone
   administration guidelines, 510*t*
Methyldopate
   administration guidelines, 510*t*
Methylprednisolone, 493
   administration guidelines, 510*t*
Metoclopramide
   administration guidelines, 510*t*
Metolazone, 190
Metoprolol, 179
   administration guidelines, 510*t*, 517*t*
Metronidazole
   administration guidelines, 510*t*
Mexiletine
   administration guidelines, 516*t*
   therapeutic monitoring, 518*t*
Mezlocillin
   administration guidelines, 510*t*
Midazolam, 158, 167
   administration guidelines, 510*t*
Milrinone, 69*t*, 185
   actions and effects, 515*t*
   administration guidelines, 510*t*
Minimally invasive hemodynamic monitoring
   carbon dioxide rebreathing, 100
   esophageal Doppler cardiac output, 100,
      101*f*
   gastric tonometery (pH), 100–101, 102*f*
   sublingual capnometry, 101
   thoracic bioimpedance, 100, 101*f*
Mitral and aortic disease
   clinical presentation, 438–440
Mitral insufficiency, 437, 438*f*
Mitral stenosis, 436, 437*t*, 438*f*
Mivacurium
   administration guidelines, 510*t*, 514*t*
MODS (multiple organ dysfunction), 268*t*, 270,
   272–273
Moral distress, 210
Moricizine
   administration guidelines, 516*t*
Morphine, 170
   administration guidelines, 510*t*
Motor assessment, 283, 283*f*, 283*t*
Moxifloxacin
   administration guidelines, 510*t*
Multiple organ dysfunction (MODS), 268*t*, 270,
   272–273
Multisystem problems
   overdoses
      alcohol overdose
         clinical presentation, 274
         diagnostic tests, 274–275

         etiology, risk factors, and
           pathophysiology, 274
      drug overdose
         clinical presentation, 275*t*, 276
         diagnostic tests, 276
         etiology, risk factors, and
           pathophysiology, 275
         management, 276–277
         overview, 274
   pathologic conditions
      sepsis and multiple organ dysfunction
         syndrome
         clinical presentation, 270, 272
         diagnostic tests, 272
         etiology, risk factors, and
           pathophysiology
            MODS (multiple organ dysfunction),
               270
            sepsis, 269–270, 270*t*–271*t*–272*t*
            systemic inflammatory response
              syndrome (SIRS), 267–269, 269*f*
         management, 272–274, 273*t*
         overview, 267, 268*t*, 269*f*
Muscle relaxation, 26
Musculoskeletal trauma
   etiology and pathophysiology, 381–382,
      382*f*
   management, 382, 383*t*–384*t*
Myasthenia gravis, 303
Myocardial infarction
   clinical presentation, 226*t*–227*t*
   diagnostic tests, 222–223
Myocardial ischemia, 218, 226*t*–227*t*
Myoclonic seizures, 301

Nafcillin
   administration guidelines, 510*t*
Naloxone, 170–171
   administration guidelines, 510*t*
Nasopharyngeal airway
   combitube, 120
   laryngeal mask airway (LMA), 120
   overview, 120
Neostigmine
   administration guidelines, 510*t*
Nesiritide, 176–177
   administration guidelines, 511*t*
Netilmicin
   therapeutic monitoring, 518*t*
Neurologic concepts, advanced. *See also*
   Neurologic system
   brain tumors
      advanced technology: brain tissue oxygen
         monitoring, 497
      clinical presentation, 495, 495*t*
      diagnostic tests, 495–496
      etiology, risk factors, and pathophysiology,
         494–495
      management
         chemotherapy, 497
         corticosteroids, 496
         postoperative complications, 496–497
         radiation therapy, 497
         seizures, 497
         surgery, 496

Neurologic concepts, *continued*
subarachnoid hemorrhage
clinical presentation, 477
diagnostic tests
cerebral angiography, 479
CT scan, 479
lumbar puncture (LP), 479
MRA, 479
MRI, 479
etiology, risk factors, and pathophysiology,
477, 478*f,* 479*t*
management
complication prevention, 481
hydrocephalus, 480
miscellaneous strategies, 481
overview, 479
rebleeding, 479–480, 480*f*
vasospasm, 480–481
traumatic brain injury
clinical presentation, 485
diagnostic tests, 485
etiology, risk factors, and pathophysiology,
481–482
mechanism of injury, 482
primary brain injury
cerebral contusion, 483
cerebral laceration, 483
diffuse injury, 484
epidural hematoma (EDH), 483, 483*f*
intracerebral hematoma, 483
overview, 482–483
subdural hematoma (SDH), 483, 483*f*
traumatic subarachnoid hemorrhage,
483–484
secondary brain injury
anemia, 484
biochemical changes, 485
hypercapnia, 485
hyperglycemia, 484
hypocapnia, 485
hypoglycemia, 484
hypotension, 484
hypoxemia, 484
increased intracranial pressure,
484–485
increased metabolic demands, 484
loss of autoregulatory mechanisms, 484
overview, 484
skull fractures, 482
management
airway, 485–486
cerebral perfusion, 486
family education and support, 487
fluid and volume management, 486
high-dose barbiturates, 487
increased intracranial pressure, 486
overview, 485
oxygenation, 486
preventing increased cerebral oxygen
demand, 486–487
preventing secondary complications, 487
ventilation, 486
traumatic spinal cord injury
clinical presentation, 489–490, 490*t,* 491*f,*
492*t*
diagnostic tests, 490

etiology, risk factors, and pathophysiology
overview, 487–488, 488*f*–489*f*
future treatment, 490
management
airway, 490
anxiety, 493–494
bladder and bowel, 493
complications, 494
fracture reduction and decompression of
spinal cord, 493
immobilization and prevention of further
injury, 490
maintaining spinal perfusion, 493
methylprednisolone, 493
oxygenation and ventilation, 490, 492
pain, 493
spine stabilization, 493
Neurologic system. *See also* Neurologic
concepts, advanced
acute ischemic stroke
clinical presentation
cerebellar or brainstem stroke, 297
stroke in a cerebral hemisphere, 297
diagnostic tests, 297
etiology, risk factors, and pathophysiology
embolism, 297
overview, 296
thrombosis, 296
management, 297–299, 298*t*–299*t*
CNS infections
encephalitis, 302
intracranial abscess, 302–303
meningitis, 302
diagnostic testing
cerebral angiography, 289
computed tomography (CT), 288
electroencephalography (EEG), 290
electromyography (EMG), 290
lumbar puncture, 287–288
magnetic resonance imaging (MRI),
288–289
transcranial Doppler ultrasound, 290
hemorrhagic stroke
clinical presentation, 300
diagnostic tests, 300
etiology, risk factors, and pathophysiology,
299–300
management, 300
intracranial pressure concepts and monitoring
causes of increased intracranial pressure,
291–292, 292*f*
cerebral blood flow, 291
management, 294–296
monitoring, 292–294, 293*f*–294*f*
overview, 290–291, 290*f*
neuromuscular diseases
Guillain-Barré syndrome, 303
myasthenia gravis, 303
seizures
clinical presentation
generalized seizures, 300–301
partial seizures, 300
status epilepticus, 301
diagnostic testing, 301
etiology, risk factors, and pathophysiology,
300

management
maintaining patient safety and airway
management, 301–302
medication administration for status
epilepticus, 302
principles, 301
treatment options, 302
special assessment techniques, diagnostic
tests, and monitoring systems
cranial nerve assessment and assessment of
brainstem function
corneal reflex, 285
extraocular eye movements, 285–286,
286*f*
gag and cough reflexes, 285
overview, 285, 285*t*
pupil size and reaction to light, 285
death by neurologic criteria, 287
Glasgow Coma Scale, 280–281, 280*t,* 281*f*
level of consciousness, 279–280, 280*t*
mental status, 281, 282*f,* 283
motor assessment, 283, 283*f,* 283*t*
overview, 279
sensation, 283–284, 284*f*
vital sign alterations in neurologic
dysfunction, 286–287
Neuromuscular blockade (NMB), 159
agents for, 160–161, 171–173, 514*t*
management, 161, 163
monitoring
airway pressure monitoring, 161, 163*f*
overview, 161
peripheral nerve stimulator (PNS), 161,
162*f*
New York Heart Association Functional
Classification System, 234, 236*t*
Nicardipine, 179
Nitroglycerin, 69*t,* 177
actions and effects, 515*t*
Nitroglycerin
administration guidelines, 511*t*
Nitroprusside
actions and effects, 515*t*
administration guidelines, 511*t*
NMB (neuromuscular blockade). *See*
Neuromuscular blockade (NMB)
Nociceptors, 145, 146*f*–147*f*
Non–insulin-dependent (type II) diabetes
mellitus, 359
Nonmaleficence, 201
Norepinephrine
actions and effects, 515*t*
administration guidelines, 511*t*
Normal sinus rhythm (NSR)
algorithm for, 552*t*
Normal values table, 503*t*–504*t*
NSAIDs (nonsteroidal anti-inflammatory drugs),
149–150
Nutritional support for critically ill patients
aspiration
detection, 335
overview, 335
reducing aspiration risk
body position, 335
feeding rate, 336
overview, 336*t*

pharmacologic interventions, 336
tube size and placement, 335
bowel sounds, 336, 336*t*
diarrhea, 337, 337*t*
enteral nutrition, 333, 333*t*–334*t*
flow rates and hours of infusion, 337–338, 338*t*
formula selection, 338
nausea and vomiting, 336–337, 336*t*
nutrition needs, 332–333, 333*t*
osmolality or hypertonicity of formula, 337, 337*t*
overview, 332
residual volume, 334, 334*t*–335*t*
total parenteral nutrition, 333, 333*t*

Octreotide, 189
Ofloxacin
administration guidelines, 511*t*
Ondansetron
administration guidelines, 511*t*
Open pneumothorax, 378
Opioids
intravenous, 151
overview, 150, 150*t*
patient-controlled analgesia (PCA), 151–152
side effects, 150–151, 151*t*
switching from IV to oral, 152–153
Oral (PO) administration, 166
Oropharyngeal airway, 118–119, 119*f*
Overdamping, 77, 78*f*
Overdoses
alcohol overdose
clinical presentation, 274
diagnostic tests, 274–275
etiology, risk factors, and pathophysiology, 274
drug overdose
clinical presentation, 275*t*, 276
diagnostic tests, 276
etiology, risk factors, and pathophysiology, 275
management, 276–277
overview, 274
Oxacillin
administration guidelines, 511*t*
Oxygen therapy
complications
absorption atelectasis, 127
alveolar hypoventilation, 125, 127
overview, 125
oxygen toxicity, 127
overview, 125, 125*t*
oxygen delivery
invasive devices
manual resuscitation bags, 127
mechanical ventilators, 127
T-piece, 128–129
tracheal gas insufflation (TGI), 128
transtracheal oxygen therapy, 128–129
noninvasive devices, 126*f*, 127

PAC (premature atrial complex), 46, 46*f*
PA (pulmonary artery) catheters. *See* Pulmonary artery (PA) catheters

Pain, sedation, and neuromuscular blockade
cutaneous stimulation, 155, 156*f*
distraction, 155
elderly patients
assessment, 157
interventions, 157
overview, 156–157
end-of-life pain, 208–209
epidural analgesia
local anesthetics, 154
opioids, 153–154, 154*f*
overview, 153
titrating, 154–155
imagery, 155
neuromuscular blockade (NMB), 159
management, 161, 163
monitoring
airway pressure monitoring, 161, 163*f*
overview, 161
peripheral nerve stimulator (PNS), 161, 162*f*
neuromuscular blocking agents, 160–161
NSAIDS, 149–150
opioids
intravenous, 151
overview, 150, 150*t*
patient-controlled analgesia (PCA), 151–152
side effects, 150–151, 151*t*
switching from IV to oral, 152–153
overview, 145
pain assessment, 148, 148*t*
pain management, multilevel approach to, 148–149, 149*f*, 149*t*
physiologic mechanisms of pain, 146*f*
central processing, 147
peripheral mechanisms, 143, 146*f*–147*f*, 147
spinal cord integration, 147
relaxation and sedation techniques
deep breathing and progressive relaxation, 156
overview, 155
presence, 156
responses to pain, 147–148, 148*t*
sedation
drugs for delirium, 159
drugs for sedation, 158–159
goals of, 159
management, 159, 162*f*
monitoring, 159, 160*t*–161*t*
overview, 157
reasons for, 157–158
traumatic spinal cord injury, 493
Pamidronate
administration guidelines, 511*t*
Pancreatitis, acute. *See* Acute pancreatitis
Pancuronium
administration guidelines, 511*t*, 514*t*
Pantoprazole, 189
Partial codes, 209
Partial seizures, 300
Partial thromboplastin time (PTT), 307, 457
Pathologic conditions
cardiovascular system. *See* Cardiovascular system
endocrine system. *See* Endocrine system

gastrointestinal system. *See* Gastrointestinal system
hematology and immunology systems. *See* Hematology and immunology systems
multisystem problems. *See* Multisystem problems
neurologic system. *See* Neurologic system
renal system. *See* Renal system
respiratory system. *See* Respiratory system
trauma. *See* Trauma
Patient advocacy, 204
Patient-controlled analgesia (PCA), 151–152
Patient Self-Determination Act (PSDA), 201, 206
PCIs (percutaneous coronary interventions), 216–218, 221*f*, 221*t*
PEA (pulseless electrical activity), algorithm for, 522*f*
PEEP (positive end-expiratory pressure), 463–464
PEEP/CPAP (positive end expiratory pressure/continuous positive airway pressure), 134, 256–257
Penicillin G
administration guidelines, 511*t*
Pentamidine
administration guidelines, 511*t*
Pentobarbital, 175–176
administration guidelines, 511*t*
therapeutic monitoring, 518*t*
Percutaneous coronary interventions (PCIs), 216–218, 221*f*, 221*t*
Percutaneous transluminal coronary angioplasty (PTCA), 216–217, 221*f*
Pericarditis
clinical presentation, 442
diagnostic tests, 442
etiology and pathophysiology, 442, 442*f*
management, 442–443
overview, 441–442
Peripheral nerve stimulator (PNS), 161, 162*f*
Peripheral pulse rating scale, 11*t*
Pharmacology
acute peptic ulcer bleeding
proton pump inhibitor (pantoprazole), 189
anti-infective pharmacology
aminoglycosides, 185–186
linezolid, 186–187
vancomycin, 186
cardiovascular system pharmacology
activated protein C (drotrecogin alfa), 185
antiarrhythmics, 180–182, 516*t*–517*t*
arterial vasodilating agents
hydralazine, 177–178
beta-adrenergic blocking agents, 178
calcium channel blocking agent (nicardipine), 179
central sympatholytic agent (clonidine), 180
diazoxide, 178
ganglionic blocking agent (trimethaphan), 178
inotropic agents
catecholamines
dobutamine, 184
dopamine, 184

catecholamines, *continued*
  epinephrine, 184–185
  isoproterenol, 184
  phosphodiesterase inhibitors
    inamrinone, 185
    milrinone, 185
  miscellaneous agents
    fenoldopam, 177
    nesiritide, 176–177
  nitrates
    nitroglycerin, 177
    sodium nitroprusside, 177
  parenteral vasodilators
    alpha-adrenergic blocking agent
      (phentolamine), 178
    alpha- and beta-adrenergic blocking
      agent (labetalol), 178
    angiotensin-converting enzyme (ACE)
      inhibitor (enalapril), 179
  thrombolytic agents
    alteplase, 183
    overview, 182–183
    reteplase, 183
    streptokinase, 183
    tenecteplase, 183
  vasoconstricting agents, 183–184
central nervous system pharmacology
  analgesics
    narcotics
      fentanyl, 170
      morphine, 170
      overview, 170
    NSAID (ketorolac), 171
    opioid antagonist (naloxone), 170–171
  anticonvulsants
    barbiturates
      pentobarbital, 175–176
      phenobarbital, 176
    benzodiazepines, 176
    hydantoins
      fosphenytoin, 174–175
      phenytoin, 173–174
  neuromuscular blocking agents
    (NMBAs)
    depolarizing agent (succinylcholine),
      171–172
    nondepolarizing agents, 172–173
    overview, 171
  sedatives
    barbiturates
      overview, 169
      pentobarbital, 169
    benzodiazepine antagonist (flumazenil),
      168
    benzodiazepines
      diazepam, 168
      lorazepam, 167–168
      midazolam, 167
      monitoring parameters, 167
      overview, 167
    miscellaneous agents
      dexmedetomidine, 169–170
      ketamine, 169
      propofol, 169
    neuroleptic (haloperidol), 168
    overview, 167

gastrointestinal pharmacology
  stress ulcer prophylaxis
    antacids, 188
    H$_2$ antagonists, 188
    overview, 188
    sucralfate, 188–189
hematologic pharmacology
  anticoagulants
    heparin, 191
    low-molecular-weight heparin, 192
    warfarin, 192–193
  direct thrombin inhibitors
    argatroban, 193
    bivalirudin, 193
    lepirudin, 193
  glycoprotein IIb/IIIa inhibitors, 193
immunosuppressive agents
  cyclosporine, 193–194
  sirolimus, 194–195
  tacrolimus (FK506), 194
intravenous medication administration
  guidelines, 505t–513t
medication administration methods
  intramuscular (IM), 165
  intranasal, 166
  intravenous (IV), 165
  oral (PO), 166
  subcutaneous (SC), 165
  sublingual, 166
  transdermal, 166–167
neuromuscular blocking agents, 514t
overview, 165
pulmonary pharmacology
  albuterol, 187
  levalbuterol, 188
  theophylline, 187
renal pharmacology
  diuretics
    loop diuretics, 190
    osmotic diuretic (mannitol), 190–191
    overview, 190
    thiazide diuretics, 190
special dosing considerations
  continuous renal replacement therapy, 195
  elderly patients, 195
  therapeutic drug monitoring, 195–197
tables
  antiarrhythmic agents, 516t–517t
  intravenous medication administration
    guidelines, 505t–513t
  neuromuscular blocking agents, 514t
  therapeutic drug monitoring, 518t
  vasoactive agents, 515t
therapeutic drug monitoring, 518t
variceal hemorrhage
  octreotide, 189
  propranolol, 189
  vasopressin, 189
vasoactive agents, 515t
Phenobarbital, 176
  administration guidelines, 511t
  therapeutic monitoring, 518t
Phentolamine, 178
  administration guidelines, 511t
Phenylephrine
  actions and effects, 515t

administration guidelines, 511t
Phenytoin, 173–174
  administration guidelines, 511t
  therapeutic monitoring, 518t
Phosphate
  administration guidelines, 511t
  imbalance
    hyperphosphatemia, 348–350
    hypophosphatemia, 349–350
Piperacillin
  administration guidelines, 511t
Piperacillin/tazobactam
  administration guidelines, 511t
Planning care for critically ill patients and
    families
  multidisciplinary plan of care and critical
    pathways, 17–18, 19f–22f
  overview, 17
  prevention of common complications
    deep venous thrombosis (DVT), 18, 23
    family-focused care, 28–29, 28t
    hospital-acquired infections
      overview, 23
      prevention, 23–24, 23t
    overview, 18
    patient and family education
      assessment of learning readiness, 26, 27t
      outcome measurement, 27, 27t
      overview, 26
      strategies to address patient and family
        education, 27, 27t
    physiologic instability, 18
    psychosocial impact
      anxiety, 26
      basic tenets, 25
      delirium, 25
      depression, 25–26
    skin breakdown, 24
    sleep pattern disturbance, 24–25, 24t–25t
  transporting the critically ill patient. *See*
    Transporting the critically ill patient
  supporting patients and families during the
    dying process, 33
  transitioning to the next stage of care, 32–33
Platelet count, 307
Plicamycin
  administration guidelines, 511t
Pneumonia
  clinical presentation, 261–262
  etiology, risk factors, and pathophysiology,
    260–261, 260f, 261t
  management, 262–263, 262t
  overview, 260
PNS (peripheral nerve stimulator), 161, 162f
PO (oral) administration, 166
Positive end-expiratory pressure (PEEP),
    463–464
Positive end expiratory pressure/continuous
    positive airway pressure (PEEP/CEEP),
    134, 256–257
Potassium chloride
  administration guidelines, 512t
Potassium imbalance
  hyperkalemia, 347, 349
  hypokalemia, 347, 350
PQRST nomogram, 215, 216t

Prednisolone
  administration guidelines, 512*t*
Preexcitation syndromes
  overview, 407
  Wolff-Parkinson-White syndrome, 407,
    409–411, 409*f*–411*f*
Preload, 68–70, 69*f*–71*f*, 103–104
Premature atrial complex (PAC), 46, 46*f*
Premature atrial contraction, algorithm for, 553*t*
Premature junctional complexes, 50, 50*f*
  algorithm for, 555*t*
Premature ventricular complexes, 51, 51*f*
  algorithm for, 555*t*
Presence, 156
Pressure control and pressure controlled/inverse
    ratio ventilation, 466, 466*t*
Pressure support ventilation (PSV), 465
Primary brain injury
  cerebral contusion, 483
  cerebral laceration, 483
  diffuse injury, 484
  epidural hematoma (EDH), 483, 483*f*
  intracerebral hematoma, 483
  overview, 482–483
  subdural hematoma (SDH), 483, 483*f*
  traumatic subarachnoid hemorrhage, 483–484
Privacy and confidentiality, 202–203
Procainamide
  administration guidelines, 512*t*, 516*t*
Procainamide/NAPA, therapeutic monitoring of,
    518*t*
Professional codes and standards, 199–200
Pronator drift assessment, 283*f*
Propafenone
  administration guidelines, 516*t*
Propofol, 158, 169
  administration guidelines, 512*t*
Propranolol, 179, 189
  administration guidelines, 512*t*, 517*t*
Protamine
  administration guidelines, 512*t*
Prothrombin time (PT), 307
PSDA (Patient Self-Determination Act), 201,
    206
PSV (pressure support ventilation), 465
PTCA (percutaneous transluminal coronary
    angioplasty), 216–217, 221*f*
PTT (partial thromboplastin time), 307, 457
Pulmonary angiograms, 252
Pulmonary artery (PA) catheters
  catheter insertion and removal
    complications, 79–80, 82*t*–83*t*
    insertion, 79, 79*f*, 81*t*
    removal, 79
  problems encountered with, 535*t*–536*t*
Pulmonary contusion, 378
Pulmonary embolism, 362, 384*t*
  clinical presentation, 263–264
  etiology, risk factors, and pathophysiology,
    263, 263*t*
  management, 264–265, 264*t*, 265*f*
Pulmonary pharmacology
  albuterol, 187
  levalbuterol, 188
  theophylline, 187
Pulmonic insufficiency, 438

Pulmonic stenosis, 438
Pulseless electrical activity (PEA), algorithm
    for, 522*f*
Pulseless ventricular tachycardia, algorithm for,
    521*f*
P wave, 38
Pyridostigmine
  administration guidelines, 512*t*

QRS complex, 38, 39*f*–40*f*
QT interval, 39
Quinidine
  administration guidelines, 516*t*
  therapeutic monitoring, 518*t*
Quinidine gluconate
  administration guidelines, 512*t*
Quinupristin/dalfopristin
  administration guidelines, 512*t*

Ranitidine
  administration guidelines, 512*t*
Red blood cell (RBC) count, 305–306
Red blood cell indices, 306
Reference information
  advanced cardiac life support algorithms
    asystole, 523*f*
    bradycardia, 524*f*
    electromechanical dissociation (EMD),
      522*f*
    pulseless electrical activity (PEA), 522*f*
    pulseless ventricular tachycardia, 521*f*
    synchronized electrical cardioversion, 528*f*
    tachycardia, narrow-complex
      supraventricular, 526*f*
    tachycardia, overview, 525*f*
    tachycardia, stable ventricular, 527*f*
    universal advanced cardiac life support
      (ACLS), 520*f*
    ventricular fibrillation, 521*f*
  cardiac rhythms, ECG characteristics, and
      treatment guide
    atrial fibrillation, 554*t*
    atrial flutter, 554*t*
    atrial tachycardia, 553*t*–554*t*
    first-degree AV block, 557*t*
    high AV block, 558*t*
    junctional rhythm, 555*t*
    normal sinus rhythm (NSR), 552*t*
    premature atrial contraction, 553*t*
    premature junctional complexes, 555*t*
    premature ventricular complexes, 555*t*
    second-degree AV block type I (Mobitz II),
      558*t*
    second-degree AV block type I
      (Wenckebach; Mobitz I), 557*t*
    sinus arrest, 552*t*
    sinus arrhythmia, 552*t*
    sinus bradycardia, 552*t*
    sinus tachycardia, 552*t*
    third-degree AV block, 558*t*
    ventricular asystole, 557*t*
    ventricular fibrillation, 556*t*
    ventricular paced rhythm with capture,
      559*t*

    ventricular rhythm, 556*t*
    ventricular tachycardia, 556*t*
    wandering atrial pacemaker, 553*t*
  guidelines for transfer of critical ill patients.
      See Transporting the critically ill patient,
      guidelines
  hemodynamic troubleshooting guide
    arterial catheters, problems encountered
      with, 533*t*
    inaccurate arterial pressure measurements,
      534*t*
    inaccurate pulmonary artery pressure
      measurements, 537*t*
    pulmonary catheters, problems encountered
      with, 535*t*–536*t*
    thermodilution cardiac output
      measurements, troubleshooting problems
      with, 538*t*
  normal values table, 503*t*–504*t*
  pharmacology tables
    antiarrhythmic agents, 516*t*–517*t*
    intravenous medication administration
      guidelines, 505*t*–513*t*
    neuromuscular blocking agents, 514*t*
    therapeutic drug monitoring, 518*t*
    vasoactive agents, 515*t*
  ventilatory troubleshooting guide
    anxiety and fear, 546*t*
    arrhythmias during or after suctioning,
      546*t*–547*t*
    decreased CO with hypotension, 544*t*–545*t*
    decreased tidal volume with pressure-
      targeted modes of ventilation, 541*t*
    high PaO_2/SaO_2, 543*t*
    inability to tolerate mode of ventilation,
      548*t*–549*t*
    incorrect PEEP setting, 547*t*
    increased airway pressure, 540*t*–541*t*
    low exhaled tidal volume, 539*t*–540*t*
    low PaO_2/SaO_2, 544*t*
    no exhaled tidal volume, 540*t*
    pneumothorax/tension pneumothorax,
      547*t*–548*t*
    respiratory acidosis, 542*t*–543*t*
    respiratory alkalosis, 541*t*–542*t*
    thick secretions, 543*t*
    tracheostomy/endotracheal tube
      discomfort, 543*t*
Relaxation and sedation techniques
  deep breathing and progressive relaxation,
    156
  overview, 155
  presence, 156
Renal failure, acute. *See* Acute renal failure
    (ARF)
Renal replacement therapy
  access, 351–352
  dialysate, 352
  dialyzer, 352
  hemofilters, 352
  overview, 350–351, 351*t*, 355
  procedures
    continuous renal replacement therapy, 352,
      354–355
    hemodialysis, 352, 353*f*
    peritoneal dialysis, 352, 354

Renal system
  pathologic conditions
    acute renal failure (ARF)
      clinical presentation, 344
      diagnostic tests, 344
      etiology, risk factors, and
        pathophysiology, 341–343, 342t
      management
        correction of fluid imbalance,
          344–345, 344t
        improving nutritional status, 345–346
        overview, 344
        preventing additional kidney damage,
          345
        preventing and treating infection, 345
        preventing and treating life-
          threatening electrolyte imbalances,
          345
        treating acidosis, 345
      overview, 341
    life-threatening electrolyte imbalances
      calcium imbalance
        hypercalcemia, 347–348, 350
        hypocalcemia, 348, 350
      magnesium imbalance
        hypermagnesemia, 348, 350
        hypomagnesemia, 348, 350
      overview, 346
      phosphate imbalance
        hyperphosphatemia, 348–350
        hypophosphatemia, 349–350
      potassium imbalance
        hyperkalemia, 347, 349
        hypokalemia, 347, 350
      sodium imbalance
        hyperosmolar disorders, 346, 349
        hypoosmolar disorders, 346–347,
          349
    renal replacement therapy
      access, 351–352
      dialysate, 352
      dialyzer, 352
      hemofilters, 352
      overview, 350–351, 351t, 355
      procedures
        continuous renal replacement therapy,
          352, 354–355
        hemodialysis, 352, 353f
        peritoneal dialysis, 352, 354
    pharmacology
      loop diuretics, 190
      osmotic diuretic (mannitol), 190–191
      overview, 190
      thiazide diuretics, 190
    special assessment techniques, diagnostic
      tests, and monitoring systems, 341,
      342t
Respect for persons (autonomy), 202
Respiratory acidemia, 115
Respiratory alkalemia, 114–115
Respiratory concepts, advanced. See also
    Respiratory system
  advanced modes of mechanical ventilation
    alternative ventilator options
      flow-by, 469
      minimum minute volume, 469

new concepts in mechanical ventilation,
      463–464
    acute lung injury and acute respiratory
      distress syndrome, 463–464
  volume versus pressure ventilation
    airway pressure release ventilation
      (APRV), 467, 468t
    bi-level positive airway pressure
      (BIPAP), 465–466, 466t
    bi-phasic ventilation, 467, 468t
    high-frequency oscillation (HFO),
      468–469, 469t
    high-frequency ventilation (HFV),
      468–469, 469t
    overview, 464–465, 464f
    pressure control and pressure
      controlled/inverse ratio ventilation, 466,
      466t
    pressure support ventilation, 465
    volume-guaranteed pressure modes of
      ventilation, 466–467, 467f–468f, 468t
  weaning patients from long-term mechanical
    ventilation
    overview, 470
    wean assessment, 470–471, 471t
    weaning trials, modes, and methods, 471
      critical pathways, 473
      protocol-directed glucose control, 473
      protocol-directed sedation management,
        473
      respiratory fatigue, rest, and
        conditioning, 471–472
      systematic institutional management
        initiatives, 473
      wean trial protocols, 472–473, 472t–473t
    wean planning, 471
Respiratory distress syndrome, acute. See
    Acute respiratory distress syndrome
    (ARDS)
Respiratory failure, acute. See Acute respiratory
    failure
Respiratory system. See also Respiratory
    concepts, advanced
  pathologic conditions
    acute respiratory distress syndrome
      (ARDS)
      clinical presentation, 257
      etiology, risk factors, and
        pathophysiology, 256–257, 257t
      management, 257–258
      overview, 256
    acute respiratory failure
      clinical presentation, 255
      etiology, risk factors, and
        pathophysiology, 253–255, 254t
        airway obstruction, 254, 254f
        impaired gas exchange, 253–254,
          254f
        impaired ventilation, 253
        ventilation–perfusion abnormalities,
          254–255, 255f
      management, 255–256
      overview, 252–253
    acute respiratory failure in patient with
      COPD
      clinical presentation, 258

etiology, risk factors, and
        pathophysiology, 258, 258t
      management, 259–260, 259t
      overview, 258
    pneumonia
      clinical presentation, 261–262
      etiology, risk factors, and
        pathophysiology, 260–261, 260f, 261t
      management, 262–263, 262t
      overview, 260
    pulmonary embolism
      clinical presentation, 263–264
      etiology, risk factors, and
        pathophysiology, 263, 263t
      management, 264–265, 264t, 265f
  special assessment techniques, diagnostic
    tests, and monitoring systems
    chest tubes, 252, 252f–253f, 252t
    chest x-rays
      basic views of the chest, 247–248
      helpful hints, 251
      invasive lines, 250–251, 251f
      normal variants and common
        abnormalities, 248–250, 250t
      overview, 247, 248t
      systematic approach to interpretation,
        248, 248t, 249f
    computed tomography (CT), 251
    magnetic resonance imaging (MRI), 251
    pulmonary angiograms, 252
Restrictive cardiomyopathy, 431, 432f
  clinical presentation, 434
  diagnostic tests, 434
  etiology and pathophysiology, 433
  management, 435
Resuscitation decisions, 209
  do not resuscitate (DNR) orders, 209
  partial codes, 209
  slow codes, 209
Reteplase, 183
  administration guidelines, 512t
Right bundle branch block, 399–400, 402f
Right-sided heart failure, 235t
Rocuronium
  administration guidelines, 512t, 514t

SAH (subarachnoid hemorrhage). See
    Subarachnoid hemorrhage (SAH)
SC (subcutaneous) administration, 165
SCD (sequential compression device), 264, 265f
SCUF (slow continuous ultrafiltration), 354
SDH (subdural hematoma), 483, 483f
Secondary brain injury
  anemia, 484
  biochemical changes, 485
  hypercapnia, 485
  hyperglycemia, 484
  hypocapnia, 485
  hypoglycemia, 484
  hypotension, 484
  hypoxemia, 484
  increased intracranial pressure, 484–485
  increased metabolic demands, 484
  loss of autoregulatory mechanisms, 484
  overview, 484

Second degree atrioventricular blocks, 54–56
    type I, 54–55, 54*f*–55*f*, 557*t*
    type II, 55–56, 56*f*, 558*t*
Sedation
    drugs for
        barbiturates, 169
            pentobarbital, 169
        benzodiazepine antagonist (flumazenil), 168
        benzodiazepines
            diazepam, 159, 168
            lorazepam, 158–159, 167–168
            midazolam, 158, 167
            monitoring parameters, 167
            overview, 167
        miscellaneous agents
            dexmedetomidine, 158, 169–170
            ketamine, 158, 169
            propofol, 158, 169
        neuroleptic (haloperidol), 168
        overview, 158–159, 167
    goals of, 159
    management, 159, 162*f*
    monitoring, 159, 160*t*–161*t*
    overview, 157
    reasons for, 157–158
    scales, 159, 160*t*
Seizures
    clinical presentation
        generalized seizures, 300–301
        partial seizures, 300
        status epilepticus, 301
    diagnostic testing, 301
    etiology, risk factors, and pathophysiology, 300
    management
        maintaining patient safety and airway management, 301–302
        medication administration for status epilepticus, 302
        principles, 301
        treatment options, 302
Sensation, 283–284, 284*f*
Sepsis and multiple organ dysfunction syndrome (MODS)
    clinical presentation, 270, 272
    diagnostic tests, 272
    etiology, risk factors, and pathophysiology
        MODS, 270
        sepsis, 269–270, 270*t*–271*t*–272*t*
        systemic inflammatory response syndrome (SIRS), 267–269, 269*f*
    management, 272–274, 273*t*
    overview, 267, 268*t*, 269*f*
Septic shock, 268*t*
Sequential compression device (SCD), 264, 265*f*
Severe sepsis, 268*t*, 270, 271*t*, 272, 273*t*
Shock
    clinical presentation, 242
    diagnostic tests, 242
    etiology, risk factors, and pathophysiology, 238–239, 239*f*, 239*t*
    management, 242–243
    overview, 238
    stages of shock, 239–240, 240*f*–241*f*, 242

SIADH (syndrome of inappropriate antidiuretic hormone secretion). *See* Syndrome of inappropriate antidiuretic hormone secretion (SIADH)
Simple partial seizures, 300
SIMV (synchronized intermittent mandatory ventilation), 134
Sinus arrest, 45, 45*f*
    algorithm for, 552*t*
Sinus arrhythmia, 45, 45*f*
    algorithm for, 552*t*
Sinus bradycardia, 44, 44*f*
    algorithm for, 552*t*
Sinus tachycardia, 44–45, 44*f*
    algorithm for, 552*t*
Sirolimus, 194–195
SIRS (systemic inflammatory response syndrome), 267–270, 268*t*, 269*f*, 385
Skull fractures, 482
Slow codes, 209
Slow continuous ultrafiltration (SCUF), 354
Sodium imbalance
    hyperosmolar disorders, 346, 349
    hypoosmolar disorders, 346–347, 349
Sodium nitroprusside, 177
Sotalol
    administration guidelines, 517*t*
Spinal cord injury
    clinical presentation, 489–490, 490*t*, 491*f*, 492*t*
    diagnostic tests, 490
    etiology, risk factors, and pathophysiology
        overview, 487–488, 488*f*–489*f*
    future treatment, 490
    management
        airway, 490
        anxiety, 493–494
        bladder and bowel, 493
        complications, 494
        fracture reduction and decompression of spinal cord, 493
        immobilization and prevention of further injury, 490
        maintaining spinal perfusion, 493
        methylprednisolone, 493
        oxygenation and ventilation, 490, 492
        pain, 493
        spine stabilization, 493
Square wave test, 77
Standards of nursing practice, 199
Status epilepticus, 301
Streptokinase, 183
    administration guidelines, 512*t*
Stress ulcer prophylaxis
    antacids, 188
    H₂ antagonists, 188
    overview, 188
    sucralfate, 188–189
Stroke volume and stroke volume index
    factors affecting
        afterload, 70–72
            clinical indicators, 71
            pulmonary vascular resistance, 72
            systemic vascular resistance, 71–72
        contractility, 72
        preload

clinical indicators, 69–70
    left ventricular preload (PAOP or LAP), 70, 70*f*–71*f*
    right ventricular preload (VCP or RAP), 69–70
    determinants, 69, 69*t*
    overview, 68–69, 69*f*
    overview, 68, 503*t*
ST segment, 38, 419–422, 422*t*
Subarachnoid hemorrhage (SAH)
    clinical presentation, 477
    diagnostic tests
        cerebral angiography, 479
        CT scan, 479
        lumbar puncture (LP), 479
        MRA, 479
        MRI, 479
    etiology, risk factors, and pathophysiology, 477, 478*f*, 479*t*
    management
        complication prevention, 481
        hydrocephalus, 480
        miscellaneous strategies, 481
        overview, 479
        rebleeding, 479–480, 480*f*
        vasospasm, 480–481
Subcutaneous (SC) administration, 165
Subdural hematoma (SDH), 483, 483*f*
Sublingual administration, 166
Sublingual capnometry, 101
Substantia gelatinosa, 147
Substituted judgment, 206
Succinylcholine, 171–172
    administration guidelines, 512*t*, 514*t*
Sucralfate, 188–189
Sulfadiazine, therapeutic monitoring of, 518*t*
Sulfamethoxazole, therapeutic monitoring of, 518*t*
Supraventricular tachycardia (SVT), 412
Synchronized electrical cardioversion, algorithm for, 528*f*
Synchronized intermittent mandatory ventilation (SIMV), 134
Syndrome of inappropriate antidiuretic hormone secretion (SIADH)
    clinical presentation, 366
    etiology, risk factors, and pathophysiology, 365–366, 366*t*
    management, 366–367
    overview, 365
Systemic inflammatory response syndrome (SIRS), 267–270, 268*t*, 269*f*, 385

Tachycardia, algorithms for
    narrow-complex supraventricular, 526*f*
    overview, 525*f*
    stable ventricular, 527*f*
Tacrolimus, 194
    administration guidelines, 512*t*
TBI. *See* Traumatic brain injury
Temporal lobe seizures, 300
Temporary pacing
    basics of pacemaker operation
        asynchronous (fixed-rate) pacing mode, 59

basics of pacemaker operation, *continued*
 capture and sensing, 58–59, 59*f*
 demand mode, 59
 overview, 58
 components of a pacing system, 57–58, 58*f*
 ECG characteristics of paced rhythms, 60,
  60*f*
 epicardial pacing, 57, 58*f*
 external (transcutaneous) pacemakers, 60, 61*f*
 indications, 57
 initiating epicardial pacing, 60
 initiating transvenous ventricular pacing, 60
 transvenous pacing, 57, 58*f*
Tenecteplase, 183
 administration guidelines, 512*t*
Theophylline, 187
 administration guidelines, 512*t*
 therapeutic monitoring, 518*t*
Therapeutic drug monitoring, 195–197, 518*t*
Thermodilution cardiac output measurements,
  troubleshooting problems with, 538*t*
Thiamine
 administration guidelines, 512*t*
Thiazide diuretics, 190
Thiopental
 administration guidelines, 512*t*
Third-degree (complete block) atrioventricular
  blocks, 56–57, 56*f*–57*f*, 558*t*
Thoracic bioimpedance, 100, 101*f*
Thoracic trauma
 etiology and pathophysiology, 378–379, 379*f*
 management, 379–380
Thrombocytes, 307
Thromboemboli, 263
Thrombolytic agents
 alteplase, 183
 overview, 182–183
 reteplase, 183
 streptokinase, 183
 tenecteplase, 183
Thrombolytic therapy, 230*t*, 297
Ticarcillin
 administration guidelines, 512*t*
Ticarcillin/clavulanate
 administration guidelines, 512*t*
Tirofiban
 administration guidelines, 513*t*
Tobramycin
 administration guidelines, 513*t*
 therapeutic monitoring, 518*t*
Tocainide
 administration guidelines, 516*t*
 therapeutic monitoring, 518*t*
Tonic-clonic seizures, 301
Tonic seizures, 301
Torsemide, 190
 administration guidelines, 513*t*
Total parenteral nutrition, 333, 333*t*
Total white blood cell (WBC) count, 306
t-PA
 administration guidelines, 512*t*
T-piece, 128–129
Transcranial Doppler ultrasound, 290
Transdermal administration, 166–167
Transjugular intrahepatic portosystemic shunt
  (TIPS), 324

Transporting the critically ill patient
 assessment of risk for complications
  cardiovascular complications, 30
  gastrointestinal complications, 30
  neurologic complications, 30
  overview, 29, 29*t*
  pain, 30
  respiratory complications, 29–30
 guidelines, 529–532
  algorithm, 532
  monitoring during transfer, 529
  pretransfer coordination and
   communication, 529–530
  transfers between hospitals
   monitoring during transfer, 531–532
   transfer equipment, 530
   transport medication requirements, 530
   transport personnel, 530
  transport equipment requirements, 529
  transport personnel, 529
 interfacility transfers, 32
 level of care required during transport, 30,
  31*t*
 overview, 29
 preparation, 31, 31*t*
 transport, 31–32
Transtracheal oxygen therapy, 128–129
Trauma
 brain. *See* Traumatic brain injury (TBI)
 common injuries in the critically ill trauma
  patient
  abdominal trauma
   etiology and pathophysiology, 380–381
   management, 381
  musculoskeletal trauma
   etiology and pathophysiology, 381–382,
    382*f*
   management, 382, 383*t*–384*t*
  thoracic trauma
   etiology and pathophysiology, 378–379,
    379*f*
   management, 379–380
 complications of traumatic injury in severe
  multisystem trauma
  acute respiratory distress syndrome
   (ARDS), 384–385
  infection/sepsis, 385
  overview, 382, 384
  systemic inflammatory response syndrome
   (SIRS), 385
 major complications in, 372*t*–373*t*
 psychological consequences, 385–386, 386*t*
 specialized assessment techniques, diagnostic
  tests, and monitoring systems
  diagnostic studies
   cervical spine radiograph, 376
   computed axial tomography (CAT), 374,
    376, 376*t*
   diagnostic peritoneal lavage (DPL), 374,
    376, 376*t*
   ultrasound, 374, 376, 376*t*
  mechanism of injury, 376–377,
   377*f*–378*f*
  overview, 371, 372*t*–373*t*, 383*t*
  physiologic consequences of trauma,
   377–378

  primary and secondary trauma survey
   assessment, 371, 374, 374*t*–375*t*
  spinal cord. *See* Spinal cord injury
Traumatic aortic disruption, 379
Traumatic brain injury (TBI)
 clinical presentation, 485
 diagnostic tests, 485
 etiology, risk factors, and pathophysiology,
  481–482
  mechanism of injury, 482
  primary brain injury
   cerebral contusion, 483
   cerebral laceration, 483
   diffuse injury, 484
   epidural hematoma (EDH), 483, 483*f*
   intracerebral hematoma, 483
   overview, 482–483
   subdural hematoma (SDH), 483, 483*f*
   traumatic subarachnoid hemorrhage,
    483–484
  secondary brain injury
   anemia, 484
   biochemical changes, 485
   hypercapnia, 485
   hyperglycemia, 484
   hypocapnia, 485
   hypoglycemia, 484
   hypotension, 484
   hypoxemia, 484
   increased intracranial pressure,
    484–485
   increased metabolic demands, 484
   loss of autoregulatory mechanisms, 484
   overview, 484
  skull fractures, 482
 management
  airway, 485–486
  cerebral perfusion, 486
  family education and support, 487
  fluid and volume management, 486
  high-dose barbiturates, 487
  increased intracranial pressure, 486
  overview, 485
  oxygenation, 486
  preventing increased cerebral oxygen
   demand, 486–487
  preventing secondary complications, 487
  ventilation, 486
Traumatic spinal cord injury. *See* Spinal cord
  injury
Traumatic subarachnoid hemorrhage, 483–484
Tricuspid and pulmonary valve disease, 440
Tricuspid insufficiency, 437
Tricuspid stenosis, 437
Trimethaphan, 178
 administration guidelines, 513*t*
Trimethaprim-sulfamethoxazole
 administration guidelines, 513*t*
T waves, 348
Type I diabetes mellitus, 359, 364
Type II diabetes mellitus, 359

Underdamping, 77, 78*f*
Universal advanced cardiac life support
  (ACLS), algorithm for, 520*f*

Unstable angina, 218–219
  diagnostic tests, 222, 228*f*
Upper GI bleeding, acute. *See* Acute upper GI
  bleeding
Urokinase
  administration guidelines, 513*t*
Utility, 202
U waves, 348

VADs (ventricular assist devices). *See*
  Ventricular assist devices (VADs)
Valproic acid, therapeutic monitoring of, 518*t*
Valvular disease
  clinical presentation
    mitral and aortic disease, 438–440
    tricuspid and pulmonary valve disease, 440
  etiology and pathophysiology
    aortic insufficiency, 437, 439*f*
    aortic stenosis, 437, 439*f*
    mitral insufficiency, 437, 438*f*
    mitral stenosis, 436, 438*f*
    overview, 436, 437*t*
    pulmonic insufficiency, 438
    pulmonic stenosis, 438
    tricuspid insufficiency, 437
    tricuspid stenosis, 437
  management, 440–441
  overview, 436
Vancomycin, 186
  administration guidelines, 513*t*
  therapeutic monitoring, 518*t*
Variances, 18
Variceal hemorrhage
  octreotide, 189
  propranolol, 189
  vasopressin, 189
Vasoactive agents, 515*t*
Vasoconstricting agents, 183–184
Vasopressin, 189
  actions and effects, 515*t*
  administration guidelines, 513*t*

Vecuronium
  administration guidelines, 513*t*–514*t*
Ventilatory management. *See* Airway and
  ventilatory management
Ventricular assist devices (VADs)
  indications, 455
  management, 457–458, 458*t*
  overview, 455
  principles, 455–457, 456*f*
  weaning and recovery, 457
Ventricular asystole, 53–54, 53*f*
  algorithm for, 557*t*
Ventricular failure, 68, 69*f*
Ventricular fibrillation, 53, 53*f*
  algorithm for, 521*f*, 556*t*
Ventricular paced rhythm with capture,
  algorithm for, 559*t*
Ventricular rhythm, 51–52, 52*f*
  algorithm for, 556*t*
Ventricular tachycardia, 52–53, 52*f*
  algorithm for, 556*t*
Veracity, 203
Verapamil
  administration guidelines, 513*t*, 517*t*
Viral hepatitis, 325*t*
Volume-guaranteed pressure modes of
  ventilation, 466–467, 467*f*–468*f*, 468*t*
Volume versus pressure ventilation
  airway pressure release ventilation (APRV),
    467, 468*t*
  bi-level positive airway pressure (BIPAP),
    465–466, 466*t*
  bi-phasic ventilation, 467, 468*t*
  high-frequency oscillation (HFO), 468–469,
    469*t*
  high-frequency ventilation (HFV), 468–469,
    469*t*
  overview, 464–465, 464*f*
  pressure control and pressure
    controlled/inverse ratio ventilation, 466,
    466*t*
  pressure support ventilation, 465

volume-guaranteed pressure modes of
  ventilation, 466–467, 467*f*–468*f*,
  468*t*
VVI pacemaker evaluation
  capture, 424–425, 425*f*–426*f*
  overview, 423–424, 424*f*
  sensing, 425–426, 426*f*–427*f*
  stimulation threshold testing, 427
  stimulus release, 424, 425*f*

Wandering atrial pacemaker, 46–47, 46*f*
  algorithm for, 553*t*
Warfarin, 192–193
Weaning
  from long-term mechanical ventilation
    overview, 470
    wean assessment, 470–471, 471*t*
    weaning trials, modes, and methods, 471
      critical pathways, 473
      protocol-directed glucose control, 473
      protocol-directed sedation management,
        473
      respiratory fatigue, rest, and
        conditioning, 471–472
      systematic institutional management
        initiatives, 473
      wean trial protocols, 472–473,
        472*t*–473*t*
    wean planning, 471
  from short-term mechanical ventilation
    methods, 137–138
    overview, 136
    readiness assessment, 136–137, 137*t*
    weaning trials, 137
Wenckebach block, 54
White blood cell differential, 306–307
Willis, circle of, 477, 478*f*
Wolff-Parkinson-White syndrome, 407,
  409–411, 409*f*–411*f*
  atrial fibrillation in, 414–415, 415*f*
Wound care, 381